Principles and Practice of Primary Care Sports Medicine

Principles and Practice of Primary Care Sports Medicine

Editors

WILLIAM E. GARRETT, JR., MD, PhD
Frank C. Wilson Professor and Chairman
Department of Orthopaedics
University of North Carolina School of Medicine
Chapel Hill, North Carolina

DONALD T. KIRKENDALL, PhD
Clinical Assistant Professor
Department of Orthopaedics
University of North Carolina School of Medicine
Chapel Hill, North Carolina

DEBORAH L. SQUIRE, MD
Assistant Professor
Departments of Pediatrics and
Community and Family Medicine
Duke University Medical Center
Durham, North Carolina

Medical Illustrations by
Marsha Dohrmann Kitkowski

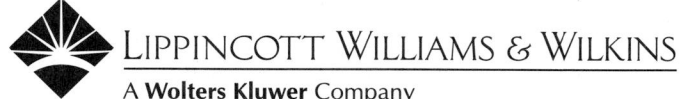

A **Wolters Kluwer** Company
Philadelphia • Baltimore • New York • London
Buenos Aires • Hong Kong • Sydney • Tokyo

Acquisitions Editor: James Merritt
Developmental Editors: Sonya L. Seigafuse, Tanya Lazar
Production Editor: P. M. Gordon, P. M. Gordon Associates
Manufacturing Manager: Tim Reynolds
Cover Designer: Catherine Lau Hunt
Compositor: Bi-Comp/PRD Group
Printer: Maple Press

© 2001 by LIPPINCOTT WILLIAMS & WILKINS
530 Walnut Street
Philadelphia, PA 19106
LWW.com

All rights reserved. This book is protected by copyright. No part of this book may be reproduced in any form or by any means, including photocopying, or utilized by any information storage and retrieval system without written permission from the copyright owner, except for brief quotations embodied in critical articles and reviews. Materials appearing in this book prepared by individuals as part of their official duties as U.S. government employees are not covered by the above-mentioned copyright.

Printed in the USA

Library of Congress Cataloging-in-Publication Data

Principles and practice of primary care sports medicine/editors, William E. Garrett, Jr., Donald T. Kirkendall, Deborah L. Squire; medical illustrations by Marsha Dohrmann Kitkowski.
    p.; cm.
  Includes bibliographical references and index.
  ISBN 0-7817-2956-4
  1. Sports medicine. 2. Primary care (Medicine) I. Garrett, William E. II. Kirkendall, Donald T. III. Squire, Deborah L.
    [DNLM: 1. Athletic Injuries—therapy. 2. Sports—psychology. 3. Sports Medicine. QT 261 P957 2001]
RC1210 .P735 2001
617.1′027—dc21
                                                                                          00-032257

Care has been taken to confirm the accuracy of the information presented and to describe generally accepted practices. However, the authors, editors, and publisher are not responsible for errors or omissions or for any consequences from application of the information in this book and make no warranty, expressed or implied, with respect to the currency, completeness, or accuracy of the contents of the publication. Application of this information in a particular situation remains the professional responsibility of the practitioner.

    The authors, editors, and publisher have exerted every effort to ensure that drug selection and dosage set forth in this text are in accordance with current recommendations and practice at the time of publication. However, in view of ongoing research, changes in government regulations, and the constant flow of information relating to drug therapy and drug reactions, the reader is urged to check the package insert for each drug for any change in indications and dosage and for added warnings and precautions. This is particularly important when the recommended agent is a new or infrequently employed drug.

    Some drugs and medical devices presented in this publication have Food and Drug Administration (FDA) clearance for limited use in restricted research settings. It is the responsibility of the health care provider to ascertain the FDA status of each drug or device planned for use in their clinical practice.

10 9 8 7 6 5 4 3 2 1

To my family: Both the family at home who make work meaningful
and the extended family at the office, laboratory, clinic,
and operating theater who make work productive and fun.

WEG, Jr.

To Mac and Louise for every opportunity
Fritz for the direction,
Sara, Trevor, and Katy for the reason.

DTK

This book is dedicated to Samuel L. Katz, MD, teacher and mentor, who
first encouraged me to explore the developing field of primary care
sports medicine, and to Frank H. Bassett III, MD, mentor and colleague,
who first taught me the science and craft of caring for athletes.
Thank you all for your support.

DLS

Contents

Contributing Authors xi
Preface xvii

Part One: General Considerations

1. The Team Physician 3
   John McKenzie Henderson
2. Preparticipation Physical Examination 11
   Paul R. Stricker
3. On-the-Field Emergencies 23
   David G. Carfagno and A. J. Cianflocco
4. Medical Coverage of Endurance Events 33
   Warren A. Scott and William O. Roberts
5. The Law and Sports Medicine 47
   Matthew J. Mitten
6. Sports Medicine Imaging 57
   Nancy M. Major

Part Two: Special Populations

7. The Young Athlete 87
   David T. Bernhardt
8. The Female Athlete 93
   Aurelia Nattiv, Elizabeth A. Arendt, and Suzanne S. Hecht
9. The Disabled Athlete 115
   Brian C. Halpern, Rosemarie Boehm, and Dennis A. Cardone

Part Three: Psychosocial Issues

10. Drug Abuse in Athletes 133
    Gary Alan Green and Bassil Aish
11. Drug Testing in Sports 151
    Richard T. Ferro and Douglas B. McKeag
12. Eating Disorders 185
    J. Sundgot-Borgen
13. Psychological Impact of Injury and Rehabilitation 191
    John Heil and Edmund A. O'Connor

14. Pain and Injury in Sport 205
    Stephan R. Walk

15. Gender: Its Relevance to Sports Medicine 215
    Cynthia A. Hasbrook

16. Disability and Sport: A Sociological Analysis 221
    Sharon R. Guthrie and Shirley Castelnuovo

Part Four: General Medical Problems

17. Sports Dermatology 231
    Thomas N. Helm and Wilma F. Bergfeld

18. Infectious Mononucleosis in Athletes 239
    Warren B. Howe

19. Blood-Borne Pathogens in Sports 247
    Christopher McGrew

20. The Athletic Heart Syndrome 251
    Bryan W. Smith and Mario F. Ciocca

21. Exercise-Induced Anaphylaxis and Urticaria 261
    Gregory L. Landry

22. The Athlete with Epilepsy 265
    Tom W. Bartsokas

23. The Athlete with Asthma or Other Pulmonary Disease 273
    David M. Orenstein

24. Headache and the Athlete 281
    William Primos and Robert Nahouraii

25. The Athlete with Type 1 Diabetes 287
    Kris Berg

26. Hematological Problems in Athletes 293
    E. Randy Eichner

27. Renal Problems in the Athlete 299
    Thomas H. Trojian and Douglas B. McKeag

28. Cold-Related Injury in Athletes and Active People 311
    William O. Roberts

Part Five: Overuse and Trauma

29. Catastrophic Injuries in High School and College Sports 321
    Frederick O. Mueller

30. Head Injuries 331
    Margot Putukian

31. Abdominal Injuries 353
    Cindy J. Chang, Howard C. Lin, and Julie A. Pryde

32. Genital Injuries in Sports 373
    Andrew W. Nichols

33.	Physeal Injuries	381
	Manuel Leyes and Jack T. Andrish	
34.	Traction Apophysitis	397
	Douglas F. Hoffman and Robert J. Johnson	
35.	Avulsion Injuries	413
	Keith L. Stanley	
36.	Stress Fractures	429
	Thomas P. Knapp and William E. Garrett, Jr.	

Part Six: Sports Epidemiology

37.	The Applied Physiology of Baseball	441
	Kevin E. Wilk	
38.	Cycling	453
	Arnie Baker	
39.	Dance	471
	William T. Hardaker, Jr.	
40.	Football	477
	John A. Bergfeld and Jonathan J. Paul	
41.	Golf	493
	Thomas J. Noonan and William J. Mallon	
42.	Ice Hockey	499
	Robert J. Johnson	
43.	Lacrosse and Field Hockey	513
	Leslie S. Matthews and Jeffrey B. Yurkofsky	
44.	Martial Arts	525
	Leonard A. Wilkerson	
45.	Oar Sports	531
	Jo A. Hannafin and Timothy M. Hosea	
46.	Running	541
	Karl B. Fields and Steven G. Reece	
47.	Skiing	553
	Antero Natri and Robert J. Johnson	
48.	Soccer	563
	Lawrence L. Golusinski, Jr.	
49.	Swimming	571
	James C. Puffer	
50.	Tennis	577
	W. Ben Kibler and T. Jeff Chandler	
51.	Volleyball	591
	Lee Rice and Allen Richburg	
52.	Water-Skiing	603
	Peter I. Sallay	

53.	Weightlifting (Strength-Power Activities)	609
	Richard T. Herrick	
54.	Wrestling	637
	William M. Heinz	

Part Seven: Management of Injuries

55.	Principle-Centered Rehabilitation	645
	P. Gunnar Brolinson and Gary Gray	
56.	Athletic Taping	653
	Brent S. E. Rich and Brent C. Mangus	
57.	PRICE: Management of Injuries	665
	Brent S. E. Rich	
Index	....	669

Contributing Authors

Bassil Aish, MD
Clinical Instructor and Sports Medicine Fellow
UCLA Department of Family Medicine/Sports
  Medicine
10833 Le Conte Avenue
Los Angeles, California 90095–1683

Jack T. Andrish, MD
Section of Sports Medicine
Section of Pediatric Orthopaedics
Department of Orthopaedics
Cleveland Clinic Foundation
9500 Euclid Avenue, Desk A-41
Cleveland, Ohio 44195

Elizabeth A. Arendt, MD
Associate Professor
Department of Orthopaedic Surgery
University of Minnesota Hospital
420 Delaware St. SE, No. 492
Minneapolis, Minnesota 55455

Arnie Baker, MD
1820 Washington Place
San Diego, California 92103

Tom W. Bartsokas, MD
Bone and Joint Clinic
206 Bedford Way
Franklin, Tennessee 37064

Kris Berg, MD
School of Health, Physical Education, and
  Recreation
University of Nebraska–Omaha
Omaha, Nebraska 68182–0216

John A. Bergfeld, MD
Executive Director
Cleveland Clinic Sports Health
Cleveland Clinic Foundation
9500 Euclid Avenue, Desk A-41
Cleveland, Ohio 44195

Wilma F. Bergfeld, MD, FACP
Head, Section of Dermatologic Research
Cleveland Clinic Foundation
9500 Euclid Avenue
Cleveland, Ohio 44195

David T. Bernhardt, MD
Assistant Professor
Department of Pediatrics
Section of Sports Medicine
University of Wisconsin Medical School
600 Highland Avenue, H6/440
Madison, Wisconsin 53792–4116

Rosemarie Boehm, MD
Department of Orthopedic Surgery
Columbia Presbyterian Medical Center
New York, New York 10032

P. Gunnar Brolinson, DO, FAOASM
Sports Care
Wildwood Health Pavilion
Toledo, Ohio 43615

Dennis A. Cardone, DO
Department of Orthopedic Surgery
Columbia Presbyterian Medical Center
New York, New York 10032

David G. Carfagno, DO
Southwest Sports Medicine and Surgery
9700 N. 91st Street, Suite B115
Scottsdale, Arizona 85258

Shirley Castelnuovo, PhD
Departments of Political Science and Women's
  Studies
Saddleback College
28000 Marguerite Parkway
Mission Viejo, California 92692–3635

T. Jeff Chandler, EdD
Associate Professor
Division of Exercise Science, Sport, and
  Recreation
Marshall University
Huntington, West Virginia 25755

Cindy J. Chang, MD, FACSM
Head Team Physician
Intercollegiate Athletics and University Health
 Services
University of California–Berkeley
Berkeley, California 94720;
Assistant Clinical Professor
Departments of Family and Community
 Medicine
University of California–San Francisco and
 University of California–Davis
San Francisco, California 94110 and
 Sacramento, California 95817

Alfred J. Cianflocco, MD
Department of Orthopedic Surgery
Cleveland Clinic Foundation
9500 Euclid Avenue, Desk A-51
Cleveland, Ohio 44195

Mario F. Ciocca, Jr., MD
University of North Carolina
Student Health Service at Chapel Hill
Chapel Hill, North Carolina 27599–7470

E. Randy Eichner, MD, FACSM
Professor of Medicine
University of Oklahoma Health Sciences
 Center
5505 N. Stonewall Drive
Oklahoma City, Oklahoma 73190

Richard T. Ferro, MD
Assistant Professor
Department of Community and Family
 Medicine
Division of Orthopaedic Surgery;
Director, Primary Care Sports Medicine
 Fellowship
Duke University Medical Center
Durham, North Carolina 27710

Karl B. Fields, MD
Family Practice Center
1125 North Church Street
Greensboro, North Carolina 27401

Lawrence L. Golusinski, Jr., MD
Emory University School of Medicine
478 Peachtree Street, Suite 818A
Atlanta, Georgia 30306

Gary Gray, PT
Gary Gray and Associates
770 Riverside
Professional Building 10
Adrian, Michigan 49221

Gary Alan Green, MD, FACP, FACSM
Clinical Associate Professor
UCLA Division of Sports Medicine
10833 Le Conte Avenue
Los Angeles, California 90095–1683

Sharon R. Guthrie, PhD
Department of Kinesiology and Physical
 Education
California State University, Long Beach
Long Beach, California 90840

Brian C. Halpern, MD
The Hospital for Special Surgery
535 East 70th Street
New York, New York 10021

Jo A. Hannafin, MD, PhD
Orthopaedic Surgery and Sports Medicine
Hospital for Special Surgery
535 E. 70th Street
New York, New York 10021

William T. Hardaker, Jr., MD
Division of Orthopaedic Surgery
Duke University Medical Center
Durham, North Carolina 27710

Cynthia A. Hasbrook, PhD
Professor and Chair
Department of Human Kinetics
University of Wisconsin–Milwaukee
2400 E. Hartford Avenue
Milwaukee, Wisconsin 53201

Suzanne S. Hecht, MD
Assistant Professor
Departments of Family Medicine and
 Orthopaedic Surgery
UCLA School of Medicine
924 Westwood Boulevard, Suite 650
Los Angeles, California 90095–0794

John Heil, DA
Lewis-Gale Clinic
Valley View Medical Center
4910 Valley View Boulevard, NW
Roanoke, West Virginia 24012

William M. Heinz, MD
Orthopaedic Associates of Portland
33 Sewall Street
Portland, Maine 04102

Thomas N. Helm, MD
Assistant Clinical Professor of Dermatology
State University of New York at Buffalo
6255 Sheridan Drive, Building B
Williamsville, New York 14221

John McKenzie Henderson, DO, FAAFP
Hughston Sports Medicine Center
2300 Manchester Expressway, Building G
Columbus, Georgia 31904

Richard T. Herrick, MD
Herrick Orthopaedic Clinic;
Adjunct Associate Professor
Department of Industrial Engineering
Auburn University
Opelika, Alabama 36802

Douglas F. Hoffman, MD
Department of Orthopedics and Sports
 Medicine
St. Mary's Duluth Clinic
400 East Third Street
Duluth, Minnesota 55805

Timothy M. Hosea, MD
Orthopaedic Surgery and Sports Medicine
Hospital for Special Surgery
535 E. 70th Street
New York, New York 10021

Warren B. Howe, MD, FACSM
Team Physician
Western Washington University
4222 Northridge Way
Bellingham, Washington 98226

Robert J. Johnson, MD
Director, Division of Primary Care Sports
 Medicine
Department of Family Practice
Hennepin County Medical Center
Five West Lake Street
Minneapolis, Minnesota 55408

Robert J. Johnson, MD
Head, Division of Sports Medicine
Department of Orthopedics and Rehabilitation
The University of Vermont, College of
 Medicine
Stafford Hall
Burlington, Vermont 05405-0084

W. Ben Kibler, MD
Department of Orthopaedics
Lexington Sports Medicine Center
Lexington Clinic
1221 South Broadway
Lexington, Kentucky 40507

Thomas P. Knapp, MD
Santa Monica Orthopaedic and Sports
 Medicine Group
1301 Twentieth Street, Suite 150
Santa Monica, California 90404

Gregory L. Landry, MD
Professor of Pediatrics
University of Wisconsin–Madison
600 Highland Avenue
Madison, Wisconsin 53792-4116

Manuel Leyes, MD, PhD
Fellow, Section of Sports Medicine
Department of Orthopaedics
Cleveland Clinic Foundation
9500 Euclid Avenue
Cleveland Ohio 44195

Howard C. Lin, MD
Team Physician
Intercollegiate Athletics and University Health
 Services
University of California at Berkeley
222 Bancroft Way
Berkeley, California 94720;
Staff Physician
Departments of Internal Medicine and Sports
 Medicine
Kaiser Permanente Medical Center
Santa Clara, California 95051

Nancy M. Major, MD
Assistant Professor, Department of Radiology
Musculoskeletal Division
Duke University Medical Center
Box 3808, Erwin Rd.
Durham, North Carolina 27710

William J. Mallon, MD
Associate Consulting Professor
Duke University Medical Center;
Assistant Consulting Professor
University of North Carolina Medical School;
Triangle Orthopedic Associates
2609 North Duke Street, Suite 905
Durham, North Carolina 27710

Brent C. Mangus, EdD, ATC
Arizona Orthopedic and Sports Medicine
 Specialists
7777 S. Point Parkway Sports Club
Phoenix, Arizona 85044

Leslie S. Matthews, MD
Department of Orthopaedic Surgery
The Union Memorial Hospital
The Johnston Professional Building #400
333 N. Calvert Street
Baltimore, Maryland 21218

Christopher McGrew, MD
*Department of Orthopaedics and
  Rehabilitation
University of New Mexico
2211 Lomas NE
Albuquerque, New Mexico 87131–5296*

Douglas B. McKeag, MD, FACSM
*Department of Family Medicine
Family Practice Center
Indiana University School of Medicine
University Hospital and Outpatient Center
  2007
550 North University Boulevard
Indianapolis, Indiana 46202–5102*

Matthew J. Mitten, JD
*Professor of Law
Director, National Sports Law Institute
Marquette University Law School
Milwaukee, Wisconsin 53233*

Frederick O. Mueller, MD
*Chairman, Department of Exercise and Sport
  Science
University of North Carolina at Chapel Hill
Chapel Hill, North Carolina 27599–8605*

Robert Nahouraii, MD
*Sport Science Center
335 Billingsley Road
Charlotte, North Carolina 28211*

Antero Natri, MD, PhD
*The University of Vermont, College of
  Medicine
Department of Orthopedics and Rehabilitation
Sports Medicine Division
McClure Musculoskeletal Research Center
Burlington, Vermont 05405;
Section of Orthopaedics
Department of Surgery
Tampere University Hospital
University of Tampere;
Tampere Research Centre of Sports Medicine
Tampere, Finland*

Aurelia Nattiv, MD
*Associate Professor
Departments of Family Medicine and
  Orthopaedic Surgery
UCLA School of Medicine
924 Westwood Boulevard, Suite 650
Los Angeles, California 90095–7087*

Andrew W. Nichols, MD
*Associate Professor and Director of Sports
  Medicine
John A. Burns School of Medicine
University of Hawaii at Manoa
1960 East-West Road, Room T-101
Honolulu, Hawaii 96822*

Thomas J. Noonan, MD
*Charlotte Orthopaedic Specialists
1915 Randolph Road
Charlotte, North Carolina 28207*

Edmund A. O'Connor, Jr., PhD
*Pain and Headache Rehabilitation Programs
Rehabilitation Professionals, LLC
350 Lafayette, SE
Grand Rapids, Michigan 49503*

David M. Orenstein, MD
*Professor of Pediatrics
School of Medicine;
Professor of Health, Physical and Recreation
  Education
School of Education
University of Pittsburgh;
Director, Cystic Fibrosis Center
Children's Hospital of Pittsburgh
3705 Fifth Avenue
Pittsburgh, Pennsylvania 15213*

Jonathan J. Paul, MD
*Orthopaedic Group of Concord
354 Copperfield Boulevard
Concord, North Carolina 28025*

William Primos, MD
*Director, Primary Care Sports Medicine
Metrolina Orthopedics and Sports Medicine
335 Billingsley Road
Charlotte, North Carolina 28211*

Julie A. Pryde, MS, PT
*Adjunct Assistant Professor
Department of Physical Therapy
Samuel Merritt College
Oakland, California 94609*

James C. Puffer, MD
*Professor and Chief
Division of Sports Medicine
UCLA School of Medicine
924 Westwood Boulevard, Suite 650
Los Angeles, California 90095–7087*

Margot Putukian, MD, FACSM
Director, Primary Care Sports Medicine
Penn State University;
Associate Professor
Department of Orthopedics and Rehabilitation
Hershey Medical Center
Penn State Center for Sports Medicine
1850 East Park Avenue, Suite 112
University Park, Pennsylvania 16803

Steven G. Reece
Family Practice Specialists
1471 Johnston Willis Drive
Richmond, Virginia 23235-4730

Lee Rice, MD
San Diego Sports Medicine
6719 Alvarado Road S., Suite 200
San Diego, California 92120

Brent S. E. Rich, MD
Arizona Orthopaedic and Sports Medicine
  Specialists
7777 S. Point Parkway Sports Club
Phoenix, Arizona 85044

Allen Richburg, MD
San Diego Sports Medicine
6719 Alvarado Road S., Suite 200
San Diego, California 92120

William O. Roberts, MD, FACSM
MinnHealth Family Physicians
4786 Banning Avenue
White Bear Lake, Minnesota 55115;
Department of Family Practice and
  Community Health
University of Minnesota Medical School
Minneapolis, Minnesota 55454

Peter I. Sallay, MD
Methodist Sports Medicine Center
1815 North Capital Avenue
Indianapolis, Indiana 46202

Warren A. Scott, MD, FACSM
Medical Director, Monterey Sports Center
Executive Director, Monterey Bay Triathlon
Soquel, California 95073;
Founder of the Sports Medicine Fellowship
Kaiser Permanente Medical Center
Santa Clara, California 95051

Bryan W. Smith, MD, PhD
University of North Carolina at Chapel Hill
Student Health Service
Chapel Hill, North Carolina 27599-7470

Keith L. Stanley, MD
Eastern Oklahoma Orthopaedic
6585 South Yale
Tulsa, Oklahoma 74136

Paul R. Stricker, MD
Sports Medicine Physician
Department of Orthopedics
Scripps Clinic
10666 N. Torrey Pines Road
La Jolla, California 92037

J. Sundgot-Borgen, MD
Department of Sports Medicine
The Norwegian University of Sport and
  Physical Education
Oslo, Norway

Thomas H. Trojian, MD
Assistant Professor
Asylum Hill Family Practice Center
Saint Francis Hospital and Medical Center
University of Connecticut Health Center
99 Woodland Street
Hartford, Connecticut 06105

Stephan R. Walk, PhD
Division of Kinesiology and Health
  Promotion
California State University, Fullerton
800 North State College Boulevard
Fullerton, California 92834-6870

Kevin E. Wilk, PT
Director, Rehabilitative Research
American Sports Medicine Institute;
Health South Rehabilitation Corporation
1201 11th Avenue South, Suite 100
Birmingham, Alabama 35205

Leonard A. Wilkerson, DO, MBA, MPH
Medical Director of Medical Management
CIGNA HealthCare of Tennessee
6555 Quince Road
Memphis, Tennessee 38119

Jeffrey B. Yurkofsky, MD
Department of Orthopaedic Surgery
The Union Memorial Hospital
The Johnston Professional Building, #400
333 N. Calvert Street
Baltimore, Maryland 21218

Preface

Principles and Practice of Primary Care Sports Medicine is the primary care component of a three-volume series on sports medicine. Although the subject matter is complex and the audience is diverse, including exercise physiologists, biomechanists, and sports medicine physicians, we hope that the text will serve as the definitive reference for all serious students of sports medicine.

Perhaps the simplest component of sports medicine is the study of "performance" as applied to exercise of athletic participation. All of the basic science of sports medicine builds from that component. For exercise physiologists, the study of sports medicine has led to investigations of the responses to exercise and the adaptations to training of those individuals with acute or chronic disease, normal or untrained persons, and competitive athletes. Biomechanists have defined the mechanics of both the specific skills required in each sport and the injuries that can occur in that sport, and they have also described cellular and tissue biomechanics.

Primary care sports medicine is a challenging discipline that requires a knowledge base in many varied fields. The content of this volume reflects this variety, presenting those topics not covered in the sport science and musculoskeletal volumes of this series. The prepreparticipation physical examination is reviewed, and special populations and their challenges to exercise are presented. Sociological and psychological issues facing the athlete are highlighted. The epidemiology of sport injuries is discussed on a sport-specific basis, with recommendations for treatment and prevention of these injuries provided where appropriate. More generalized discussions cover a spectrum of chronic and overuse injuries in the growing and skeletally mature athletes. The role of imaging in diagnosing athletic injuries is reviewed, and the variety of therapies and modalities available to treat athletic injuries is considered. Diagnosis and treatment of acute head injury is discussed in detail. The management of various chronic medical conditions in the exercising individual is presented. The authors are recognized experts in the subjects of their chapters and have ongoing research or clinical experience in the various subject areas. Their writing reflects the most current standard of care and, where appropriate, indicates areas in which ongoing research may lead to modifications in clinical practice. Our hope is that this volume will be useful to primary care physicians who treat exercising individuals, whether on an individual or team basis.

We hope that this volume will be useful not only to the basic scientists involved in the study of sports medicine but to all other experts in the discipline, because the understanding of these topics will form the basis of future developments in sports medicine. In other volumes we cover exercise and sport science and primary care aspects of sports medicine.

All of us involved in this project are indebted to the staff at Lippincott Williams & Wilkins: Darlene Cook and Fran Klass, who helped us get this project underway, and Danette Knopp, Tanya Lazar, and Sonya Seigafuse, whose continued patience throughout this project must be commended. The guidance of Lottie Applewhite, author's editor, and the efforts of Marsha Dohrmann Kitkowski, medical illustrator, cannot be overstated. Without the help of these people, we would still be way over our heads and still struggling to complete our work.

William E. Garrett, Jr., MD, PhD
Donald T. Kirkendall, PhD
Deborah L. Squire, MD

Principles and Practice of Primary Care Sports Medicine

PART I
General Considerations

CHAPTER 1

The Team Physician

John McKenzie Henderson

INTRODUCTION

Among the pressing issues in sports medicine is the role of the modern team physician. Witness the fact that every athletic team of any size or sophistication has some sort of medical support, yet the operational, technical, administrative, and medico-legal backgrounds for these relationships are poorly understood.

This chapter traces the evolution of the wide range of roles seen in the practice of sports medicine and discusses some of the dilemmas facing today's team doctors.

BACKGROUND

This chapter is not intended to trace the development of sports medicine per se, but rather to focus on the physician as a team doctor. Like any focus of medical practice, sports medicine is an integral part of medicine in general. The application of exercise as a treatment modality, the traumatology of sports, athletic conditioning and rehabilitation, and nutrition as a means of performance enhancement can be traced to ancient times.

The practice of medicine in the past, both distant and recent, has set the stage for all modern team physicians. For convenience this discussion is divided into the distant past, the military model, and the recent past. Throughout all of this, however, recurring themes are found.

TEAM PHYSICIANS IN THE DISTANT PAST (6000 B.C.–1935)

Ancient history includes many instances in which physicians laid the basis for modern sports medicine practice. Almost six thousand years ago physicians were trying to keep active people active by treating them with functional methods. In the 19th century Edwin Smith found a surgical papyrus describing injury treatment by Imhotep, chief physician (and team doctor) to King Djoser, who designed the earliest pyramids at Saqqarah three millennia B.C. The earliest recorded use of exercise as treatment belongs to the Hindus in the Atharua-Veda and to the Chinese in the book of Kung Fu around 1000 B.C.

The Olympiad, held every four years in honor of Zeus at Mount Olympus, began in 776 B.C. Before competing in the Olympics, the athletes were required to train for ten months under the supervision of physicians. Professional jealousies grew between the athletic trainers and the sports physicians, so ultimately, the physicians did not participate in the care and training of the athlete except to treat their acute injuries. This dichotomy continued for centuries, but in the early 1950s, several sports medicine physicians were prominent in assisting the founding members of the National Athletic Trainers Association to establish that association successfully. Herodicus may have been the first sports medicine professional in 500 B.C. He insisted that athletic training be systematized, include a balance in exercise and diet, and have a medical component. Herodicus' student Hippocrates helped to make physical education a necessary part of a Greek youth's overall training.

In A.D. 200 Claudius Galen of Pergamum and Rome was "team physician" to the gladiators. He was appointed by Pontifex Maximus in Pergamum. Galen used his experiences in treating gladiators' injuries as the substance of his published findings. He also advocated weight training and resistance exercises to promote health. He was called to Rome by Marcus Aurelius to be his personal physician. When Commodus succeeded Marcus, Galen was his physician also, particularly attending to this emperor's own wounds sustained as a gladiator in the arena. With the fall of the Roman Empire, sports medicine in western Europe, like all medical science, was stifled. During the Dark Ages Galen's

---

J. M. Henderson: Hughston Sports Medicine Center, Columbus, Georgia 31904.

works, whether accurate or not, were preserved and promulgated by the medieval Church. Team doctors have traditionally gained their appointment through two main pathways: whom they know, i.e., through their association with the team's key management, or what they know, i.e., through their own progression in medical training and skill acquisition.

Advances in sports medicine continued elsewhere, though. In A.D. 1000 a Middle Eastern physician, Hakimibn-e-Sina (better known now as Avicenna), recommended the use of medical gymnastics, massage, and warm baths to promote rehabilitation from injuries (*The Canon of Medicine*). During the Second Crusades in 1270, physicians to King Richard II noted how combatants wearing armor were more susceptible to heat injuries than their peasant servants were. Since the Crusades no group has ever engaged in battle without medical support. Medical intelligence is a key part of preparation for any campaign, sportive or military.

Bergerius (1370–1440), a professor of logic and "team physician" at the University of Padua, advocated the inclusion of regular physical exercise for all children in school. The educational curriculum in 15th century Italy saw the reemergence of physical education and exercise due to the efforts of Vittorino de Feltre. In 1569 Geronimo Mercuriali published the first book on sports medicine, *Artis gymnasticae apud antiquos celeberrimae nostris temporibus ignoratae.* This text described the relationship between medicine, sports, and the role of exercise in gaining and preserving health. In the mid-1950s the first President's Council on Physical Fitness recommended curriculum changes in response to the poor fitness status of U.S. youth.

In 16th-century France Laurent Joubert of Montpelier introduced therapeutic exercise into the medical school curriculum. In the 1980s the American Academy of Family Physicians (AAFP) made suggestions about the inclusion of team physician function into the curriculum of family practice residents.

In 18th-century France a physician collected the known practice of musculoskeletal medicine into one text. Nicolas Andry's book *Orthopaedia* validated this body of knowledge as a distinct entity. Bernardino Ramazzini's classic work of 1700, *De Morbis Artificum* ("Diseases of Workers"), detailed industrial injuries and included diseases that affected runners and athletes. He recognized exercise-induced asthma and hematuria. Team physicians today still chronicle the different presentations of medical conditions in athletes.

In 1854 Edward Hitchcock, M.D., was appointed Amherst College's first instructor of physical education and hygiene. Hitchcock is credited with the advent of collegiate sports medicine in the United States. He integrated traditional European training in gymnastics and running with American sports that would later become baseball and basketball. As the school's physician he instituted anthropometric studies of the students, recorded the incidence of sports injuries at the school, and published 161 topics on athletics and medicine. In 1899 E.A. Darling of Harvard College published *The Effects of Training,* a study of the fitness of Harvard crews. In the 1970s the team physicians of the National Collegiate Athletic Association (NCAA) were instrumental in developing the Committee on the Medical Aspects of Sports.

From the death of a Portuguese runner due to heat stroke in the 1912 Stockholm Olympic marathon came the requirement for physical examinations for all marathoners, the first such requirement since the modern Olympic Games were reestablished in 1896. Nonetheless, the United States did not send athletic trainers with its teams until the 1920 Antwerp Olympic Games, and team physicians were not included until the Paris games of 1924. Medical contingents were initially viewed as potential troublemakers, not as an integral part of the team. In the Rome Olympics of 1960 a tragedy similar to the one in 1912 sparked more advances.

At the second Winter Games of 1928 in Saint Moritz, Switzerland, the first international sports medicine organization was formed. Beginning with 33 team physicians from 11 nations, the International Association of Sports Medicine (Association Internationale Medico-Sportive, or AIMS) was established. This group met formally at the First International AIMS Congress at the Amsterdam Olympics in 1928. Membership growth was encouraging, with 280 team physicians from 20 countries participating. At a subsequent meeting in Chamonix, France, in 1934 the organization changed its name to the International Federation of Sports Medicine (Federation Internationale de Medecine Sportive, or FIMS). These team physicians were a blend of generalists, academics, surgical specialists, and physiologists.

TEAM PHYSICIANS IN THE RECENT PAST (1935–1995)

The 60 years from 1935 to 1995 started with the empowerment of Nazism in Europe. Never before had a state controlled its people's activities to include its sports community and its medical community. Even medical education and medical practice were affected. The burgeoning military-industrial complex included sports medicine trials executed by deluded team physicians who believed that their efforts were justified by the end results. Applications of amphetamines and anabolic androgenic steroids exceeded then-known boundaries. Chronicling the natural course of exposure to cold environments and the extremes of enforced catabolism passed the borders of barbarism, but such investigations were conducted "in the name of science." These methodologies would, fortunately, never be repeated.

The middle third of the 20th century was tumultuous with political change but rich in terms of the team physician's evolution. Mal Stevens, a team physician for the New York Yankees professional baseball team, got his start at Yale University, where he was head coach of the football team while he attended medical school there. With Winthrop Phelps he coauthored *The Control of Football Injuries* in 1935. He recommended the use of pneumatic padding in football helmets. In 1938 Angus Thorndike published *Athletic Injuries: Prevention, Diagnosis, and Treatment*. This remains one of the models of sports medicine texts. Thomas "Bart" Quigley began serving his 30-year tenure as Harvard's team physician in the 1940s. His "Athletes' Bill of Rights" set forth in concrete terms solid athletic medical care, always with the rights of the athlete taking precedence over any other consideration.

World War II created the demand for getting more performance out of the soldier-athlete. Whether ethical or not, human use studies challenged the morals and mores of the third and fourth decades. Sports medicine advanced through all of these macabre and morbid developments because physicians learned more about the biologic limits of the human body and psyche.

After World War II sports and medicine tried to return to peacetime, and sports medicine started to earn a scientific base. Thomas DeLorme and A. L. Watkins published *Progressive Resistance Exercise* in 1951. Hettinger and Muller published *Isometric Training* just two years later. Also in 1951 the National Athletic Trainer's Association (NATA) was formed. The NATA was formed to adopt standards and enhance the professional stature of professional trainers. Many team physicians were instrumental in establishing this organization for members of their "sports medicine team."

Political ideology flavored the Olympics starting with the 1952 Helsinki Games. Team physicians from the Warsaw Pact countries were an integral part of the Eastern Bloc sports machine, which applied sports medicine for cheating in the areas of ergogenic aids and gender falsification.

In 1954 the American College of Sports Medicine was founded as the U.S. counterpart of FIMS. The American College of Sports Medicine developed as the national organization representing the interests of sports scientists such as exercise physiologists, anatomists, kinesiologists, biomechanists, fitness counselors, and rehabilitation therapists. Team physicians were, and still are, in the distinct minority in the ACSM. In 1958 the American College Health Association created its Athletic Medicine Section, formed primarily of team physicians from its member colleges and universities. In 1960 the American Medical Association formed its Committee on the Medical Aspects of Sports, but this group was driven more by the medical politics of the AMA and its university-tertiary care base than by the concerns of the team physicians.

Orthopedists took on the task of developing U.S. sports medicine from the sideline to the operating room and laboratory and back to the sports venue. Jack C. Hughston of Columbus, Georgia, served as the first chairman of the American Academy of Orthopaedic Surgery's Committee on Sports Medicine in 1964. As team physician for Auburn University he found that he could make the most accurate diagnosis by being on the sidelines and witnessing the mechanism of injury and then examining the injured athlete immediately after the injury was sustained. His *Classification of Knee Ligament Instabilities* was based on his intimate understanding of the functional anatomy of the knee and a self-critical assessment of his patients' surgical outcomes. It is still a standard today.

Don O'Donoghue of Oklahoma City, Oklahoma, became the first president of the American Orthopaedic Society for Sports Medicine (AOSSM). Among his many contributions as team physician for the University of Oklahoma were his focus on the exact diagnosis to arrive at accurate decision-making and a surgical approach to orthopedic injuries. His *Treatment of Injuries to Athletes* was first published in 1962 and has gone through many updated editions.

The International Olympic Committee (IOC) formed its Medical Commission in 1966 in response to blood-doping scandals at the Rome (1960) and Tokyo (1964) Olympic Games. Wider television coverage spurred the IOC to finally respond to longstanding medical problems.

During the Munich (1972) Games, Palestinian terrorists posed as team medical personnel to gain entrance to the Israeli team headquarters, beginning one of the darkest acts in Olympic history. Since then the team physician's credentials have been highly scrutinized and exquisitely controlled.

The American Orthopaedic Society for Sports Medicine was formed in 1972 by a group of orthopedic surgeons and team physicians who wanted to pursue their interests more intently than they were previously able. Three members, Ben Goode, Bill Stinton, and Jack Hughston, established the *American Journal of Sports Medicine* during a period when it was difficult for sports medicine papers to be published in the then-current medical and orthopedic journals.

Title IX of the Education Amendments of 1972 brought gender equity to the forefront. Together with greater awareness of women socially through the women's movement, this legislation made it necessary for the team physician to understand the particular needs of the female athlete. These changes broadened the general acumen of the team physician.

Japanese investigators Tagaki, Watanabe, Takeda, and Ikeuchi refined the application of fiber optics so that arthroscopy could be used as a diagnostic and therapeutic tool. In 1976 the first U.S. text on arthroscopy was published by team physicians, R. W. Jackson and

D. J. Dandy. *Arthroscopy of the Knee* ignited a procedural-based deluge away from the patient and diverted attention toward structures that are accessible through "the 'scope." Team physicians needed to reassess their function within the team. Biomechanical and clinical studies supported the use of the arthroscope to diagnose and manage intra-articular pathology. The trap of making "sports medicine" into "sports surgery," that is, avoiding the evolution of the sports medicine specialist into a sports arthroscopist, was a challenge the team physician had to meet.

Just as the 1950s through the 1970s brought several orthopedists to the forefront of sports medicine through their involvement as team physicians, the 1970s through the 1990s was a time for primary care physicians to become more deeply involved. Major universities, orthopedic surgery referral centers, and the U.S. Olympic Committee (USOC) realized the usefulness of primary care specialists as team physicians. The leaders in orthopedic sports medicine began to attract primary care sports medicine physicians as highly valued allies and partners. In 1984 the Hughston Orthopaedic Clinic in Columbus, Georgia, established the first formal fellowship program for primary care physicians. Today there are 58 such fellowships training about 75 physicians a year. The combination of an orthopedic surgeon and a primary care specialist as a sports medicine duo became a formidable standard at higher levels of competition. Every level of the NCAA, National Junior College Athletic Association (NJCAA), and National Association of Intercollegiate Athletics (NAIA) boasted teams that were served by team physicians.

In 1985 there were no widely accepted curricula for sports medicine in the primary care residency training programs, even though many teaching centers were beginning to offer elective experiences such as clinical clerkships for physicians. The orthopedic surgery residencies, however, saw sports medicine as a distinct entity, albeit not a full-fledged, "board-able" subspecialty (like hand or spine). The mid-1980s saw the establishment and proliferation of fellowship training for primary care specialists. These fellowships stressed the need for an organized approach as a team physician with close coordinated efforts among the physician, the school, the team, and the athletes with their families. By the late 1980s many primary care residencies boasted access to their own sports medicine resource, whether organic to their faculty as a full-time physician educator or affiliated as a part-time position. Essentials for the residency curricula were suggested by groups that were intent on providing structure to heretofore informal efforts.

The Olympic Games, both Winter and Summer, were studded with primary care team doctors who had leadership roles. The USOC discovered that primary care sports medicine physicians possessed sophisticated organizational skills, a broad medical acumen, and the ability to coordinate the efforts of a mix of sports medicine professionals while keeping the administrative requisites satisfied. Bob Voy, M.D., in the Seoul (1988) Games, Jim Puffer, M.D., in the Los Angeles (1984) Games, and John Lombardo, M.D., in the Calgary (1988) Games are just three of the many dozen physicians who made this country's teams so successful.

The Americans with Disabilities Act of 1990 was designed to prevent mistreatment of people who have physical or mental impairments. In sports medicine this meant that the team doctor has had to be fluent in interpreting this legislation in regards to sports activity participation.

The American Medical Society for Sports Medicine (AMSSM) was established in 1990 to provide a forum and foster a collegial relationship among the primary care sports medicine providers, including family physicians, internists, pediatricians, emergency physicians, and physiatrists. The members of the AMSSM were all team physicians at various levels, from youth recreation leagues to professional leagues. In cooperation with the AOSSM, the AMSSM has presented clinical symposia and published monographs on pertinent team physician topics (Preparticipation Screening monograph and the Blood-borne Diseases in Athletes monograph).

The early 1990s were ripe for formalizing the recognition and validation of physicians who practice sports medicine. In 1993 family physicians, internists, pediatricians, and emergency medicine specialists were able to earn the first Certificate of Added Qualifications through their respective boards acting as one coordinated examiner. By the mid-1990s the growth of the field continued with formalizing the accreditation process for the sports medicine fellowship programs through the ACGME.

TEAM PHYSICIANS DURING THE LAST HALF OF THE 1990s

During the last half of the 1990s, three main issues became the subjects of focus for the team physician: litigation, managed care, and the Centennial Olympic Games.

There has continued to be a proliferation of litigation involving team physicians based on what patient-plaintiffs expect from their team physician and what the sports medicine community is really able to provide. As with general medical jurisprudence, the majority of cases involve allegations of failure to diagnose, failure to provide protection, loss of potential earnings, and lack of availability. The different components of the cases against the team physician show some of the shortcomings faced in the most recent past. "Negligence" is defined as doing something that an ordinary prudent person would not have done under similar circumstances or failure to meet the "standard of care." This has been difficult when the "standard" may be in the literature but not scientifically substantiated or even practiced. "Causation" is an act performed in a breach of duties resulting in physical harm, death, or economic or property damage. Causation is difficult to prove in sports because of the doctrines of assumption of risk and contributory negligence. Assumption of risk involves the athlete's consent to expose himself or herself to a known risk. Contributory negligence involves the athlete's own attention to safety during sports participation. Perceptions and realities are often discordant. The question is not usually malice but rather a departure from "the usual and customary diligence and practice of medicine." The team physician has often been found in situations that are not covered by the Good Samaritan principle and in a medico-legal quagmire regardless of his or her intended efforts.

Health maintenance organizations (HMOs) have grown from metropolitan pockets of southern California and the Boston-Washington corridor to cover the entire country, including even beneficiaries of federally funded health programs. Having a team physician who is outside the athlete's provider network or referral of an athlete by a primary care team physician to an out-of-network specialist has become a common predicament. The need to balance student health services, team physician services, and HMO guidelines presents a significant dilemma to the team physician who wants to provide his or her athletes with high-quality sports medicine care. Similarly, HMOs are adopting clinical pathways and chronic disease surveillance algorithms that do not allow for the individualization practiced by team physicians. Financial credentialing and resource utilization review also are potential stumbling blocks that are confronted more and more in sports medicine. The training room as a cost center and clinical outcome center is growing into a reality. Cost-shifting, cost-sharing, and HEDIS guidelines all challenge the team doctor's resourcefulness.

The Summer Games of the XXVI Olympiad took place in and around Atlanta, Georgia, in the summer of 1996. These Games were the centennial celebration of the modern Olympics and were duly focused on two prime topics that team physicians dread: using medical science to cheat and applying medical science to avoid environmental injuries. Regarding the former, gender verification and doping control were the main IOC programs involving team doctors as intermediaries. Environmental monitoring using wet-bulb globe thermometers was an interface of high-tech and low-tech for the benefit of the competitors and spectators alike. Owing to a preventive medicine focus of the team physicians' preparations in the years leading up to these Games and because the medical specialty mix at each venue underwent exquisite scrutiny, the medical support of these Games was commendable even by IOC standards.

At a considerable distance from Atlanta, a few competition venues, such as soccer (in Athens), sailing (in Savannah), softball (in Columbus), and kayaking (in Ocoee), involved extremes in the logistics of sports medicine. The team physicians who volunteered at these sites combined orthopedic and primary care skills to provide high-quality care.

ISSUES CONFRONTING THE MODERN TEAM PHYSICIAN

Being a team physician is a coveted honor and an immense responsibility. "It can be rewarding and at times demanding, inconvenient but entertaining, even obligatory but soul satisfying." The modern team physician must have an immensely broad knowledge base that, in some areas, must also be deep. This can be obtained only by combining formal didactics (pedagogy) with practical experiences gained over time. The following areas represent the current issues confounding the modern team doctor's practice.

Primary Care Sports Medicine

The actual content of sports medicine has been the subject of debate. The care of any active individual, or anyone who wants to be active, is the accepted description of "sports medicine," but as medical practices adjust to societal changes, this may also change. The content of modern sports medicine is, in part, reflected in the content of the sports medicine CAQ (Certificate of Added Qualification) examination. This includes knowledge of exercise physiology, biomechanics, management of acute and chronic musculoskeletal injuries, management of chronic medical illnesses, management of acute medical conditions caused by or affecting physical activity, sports psychology, medico-legal issues, and preparation for and management of emergent conditions on the athletic field. The respective certifying boards must stay vigilant to make certain this test actually does reflect current knowledge and practice.

Even though the types of medical specialties have been effectively frozen at their present number, the function of many primary care specialists includes sports medicine to some extent. To excel as a team physician, a primary care specialist cannot strive to become as accomplished with an arthroscope as his or her orthopedic colleague but should try to excel in his or her own primary care specialty. The team doctor should take advantage of the myriad opportunities to stay skillful and current that are available today.

Approach to Problem Solving

Today's problems are sometimes not as straightforward as the textbook would lead the modern team doctor to believe. Complex situations call for more sophisticated decision making. At times traditional paradigms just do not fit the situation. When the data are lacking or vague or when established guidelines fly in the face of common sense, the modern team physician should have the composure and tact to work toward an acceptable, albeit imperfect, solution. Only practice will allow the physician to develop this ability. At times different approaches of Western medicine—allopathic, osteopathic, homeopathic, and others—may need consideration. Eastern medical philosophy can also give structure to problem solving. The modern team physician needs to stay alert to methods used by colleagues worldwide to accomplish common goals.

Among the most frustrating developments in the practice of the team physician is the repeat visit of the athlete who should have resolved a seemingly trivial problem or repeat visits by an athlete who has a succession of complaints. The modern team physician will be most successful by applying the biopsychosocial model of disease and health to the interface between biology and behavior.

Ethics in Medical Practice: Divided Loyalties

The team physician's loyalty is to the patient-athlete. In the extreme case the team physician who is also a part-owner of the athlete's team franchise cannot make a truly objective decision about that athlete's playing status. In more common scenarios team physicians who may have divided allegiances may also have more difficulties in making these decisions. Pressures from the coaching staff, athletic directors, alumni, sponsors, media, and countless others can cloud the team physician's objectivity.

The two main oaths taken by medical graduates in this country, the Oath of Hippocrates (taken by allopathic physicians earning the M.D. degree) and the Osteopathic Oath (taken by osteopathic physicians earning the D.O. degree), require the physician to hold the well-being of the patient uppermost in all thoughts and actions. When the team physician identifies a situation in which he or she feels that objectivity may be jeopardized, the physician must exercise enough self-discipline to request assistance.

Specific Problem Situations

Almost every organized group of sports medicine professionals, physicians or not, develops an official stance on a provocative topic. These official statements, called position statements, are circulated widely among the membership and the media. The modern team physician must be well grounded in these controversial topics. This will involve a reasonable familiarity based on a broad, balanced approach to the current literature and sound medical practice. All this may fly in the face of the position statement. In those instances, the team physician must be a strong individual who will be accountable for his or her actions. Case in point: In the mid-1980s the AAFP disseminated a position against its member physicians' serving as ringside physician in wrestling because such service seemed to condone violence. After appropriate discussion this position was repealed.

A subtle problem lies in the mechanics of the position paper process. These papers may take 12 to 18 months to develop. If the position paper is a consensual statement from several organizations, the time needed for approval by all groups involved may take two years or more.

From time to time, new topics may merit the attention of the modern team physician. Topics such as return to play criteria after blunt, closed head injuries; injury prevention in the skeletally immature athlete; and long-term care of uninsured athletes are all current subjects under discussion.

Associated Clinical Knowledge Bases

The primary care knowledge bases are, by their nature, very broad. These specialties are called the cognitive specialties because decision making is the hallmark activity of its practitioners. The modern team physician needs maximal latitude to offer his or her patients a wide array of management alternatives. To this end, a variety of eye-hand procedural skills should be included in the armamentarium of the team doctor. Intra-articular injections, osteopathic manipulative therapy, fracture management, use of prostheses and orthoses, cardiac stress testing, and minor surgical skills are among the most commonly sought procedural skills.

Other cognitive knowledge bases that are useful for the primary care trained team physician include parts of the following disciplines: physical medicine and rehabilitation, wilderness medicine, orthopedics, preventive medicine, cardiovascular medicine, and psychology.

The team physician should have an open mind about other approaches to solving similar problems. As in treating common warts, there are many methods to deal with any one problem. The physician should be aware of multiple methods, sometimes involving different expenses, toxicity, invasiveness, and other factors, to approach common problems. Similarly, Western medical philosophy might not satisfy all the needs of the team physician's patients. Other philosophies of medicine hold promise in many cases. Pain management, headache, dysmenorrhea, reflex sympathetic dystrophy, exercised-induced syndromes, sciatica, and muscle spasm represent only a few of the many thousands of entities that respond favorably to traditional Hindu, Chinese, and Arab medicine.

Associated Nonclinical Knowledge Bases

The technological advances of the current age demand that the modern team physician be well versed in topics such as practice management, medical economics, information management, and even estate planning that actually do affect patient care. Practice management can influence the conduct of the training room clinic to involve record keeping and patient tracking. Medical economics influence resource utilization in a time of downsizing and shrinking budgets. Information management includes the use of computer science in daily medical practice and record archiving to include imaging modalities. Estate planning allows the modern team physician the latitude to provide noncompensable services to his or her teams without becoming a pauper.

Needs of the Team Physician

The modern team physician has several professional needs that should be met by all the people who affect the milieu in which the team physician functions. These needs include the following:

1. The team physician should have professional autonomy over all medical decisions. Medical decision making is not negotiable and cannot be compromised by peripheral influences.

2. The team physician should be protected against any coercive pressures. Repudiation and retaliation are strictly out of the question.

3. The team physician needs to establish an explicit formal relationship between the physician and the school, league, or team. This should take place before the season begins and should include definitions of the relationship that are integral to daily functioning. This should include the job description, a statement of expectations from both parties, any fiscal arrangements, chain of command/accountability, scope of services at home and away, remuneration/reimbursements, other benefits, and any other expectations of the institution or the physician. This document should be in writing and mutually agreed upon by the team physician and a spokesperson for the team.

4. The team physician is a member of the sports medicine team needing lateral and vertical integration into the team. If the team has an athletic trainer, that person is the pivotal medical resource around which the team physician functions. The sports medicine team is made up of the athletic trainer and the team physician who have daily or weekly contact with the team and other health care professionals whose services are directed by the doctor and the trainer. These might include, for instance, the dentist, psychologist, nutritionist, orthotist, and medical and surgical subspecialists who may be called on from time to time to provide care in the area of their expertise. The sports medicine team interacts with the equipment managers, NGB/NCAA compliance specialists, coaching staff, including the strength training coaches, administrative and legal personnel, and even the sports information/media personnel.

THE ROLES OF THE TEAM PHYSICIAN

For the team physician to be professionally gratified through his or her activities as a team physician, there needs to be more than just the clinical role. Additional roles include, but are not limited to, the following:

1. **Medico-legal role:** The team physician should stay aware of trends in medical jurisprudence and maintain a prudent practice. The team physician should know where he or she stands in terms of liability in all his or her activities.

2. **Educational role:** Because of the team concept of our athletic medicine delivery system, the team physician is an educator as well as a student. The physician has many opportunities to share his or her knowledge base with the other health care professionals of the sports medicine team (athlete trainees, physical therapists, occupational therapists, exercise physiologists, psychologists, orthodontists, etc.). The doctor can also learn from these other team members. Additionally, the team physician has the privilege of those singular moments when lessons on perseverance, courage, self-discipline, and self-control can be presented to the athlete.

3. **Research role:** It is critical that clinically relevant research be conducted by team physicians at all levels. Clinicians cannot relegate research activities to applied and basic scientists and expect the results to be readily applicable to their sports medicine practice. Additionally, the longstanding traditional practice patterns, unfounded by medical science, cannot be improved upon without solidly designed and meticulously executed sports medicine research.

4. **Political role:** The team physician should be an active participant in the continued refinement of the practice of sports medicine. Active membership in representative organizations leads to avenues for change and control of the change process in sports medicine. Despite all the recent changes in the delivery of health care in the United States, the physician, including the team physician, will be looked to for leadership through these organizations.

5. **Clinical role:** Although listed last, this role is the bedrock on which the preceding roles all have their foundation. The team physician must practice the most current brand of medicine possible. This would be based on being broadly educated and widely experienced in general medicine with a knowledge base that should include BCLS (basic cardiac life support), ACLS (advanced cardiac life support), ATLS (advanced

trauma life support), and on-the-field sports medicine. Preventive efforts, for both athletic injuries and medical conditions, should be the main focus. Proper conditioning in preparation for play and proper safeguards during play should be in the team physician's vernacular. The team physician should be certified (and recertified) in his or her primary care specialty (family practice, pediatrics, emergency medicine, or internal medicine) or orthopedic surgery. Team physicians should successfully pass the CAQ in sports medicine if it is available to them, as well as staying current with CME (continuing medical education).

BIBLIOGRAPHY

Adams J. The development of sports medicine. *NC Med J* 1994; 55(10):488–492.

Albright J, Noyes F. Role of the team physician in sports injury studies. *Am J Sports Med* 1988;16[Suppl]:S1–S4.

Appelboom J, Rouffin C, Fierens E. Sports and medicine in ancient Greece. *Am J Sports Med* 1988;16(6):594–596.

Buchanan W. Bernardino Ramazzini (1633-1714): physician of tradesmen and possibly one of the fathers of sports medicine. *Clin Rheumatol* 1991;10(2):136–137.

Committee on Sports Medicine: The team physician. *Bulletin of the American Academy of Orthopaedic Surgeons* 1972;20(3):22.

Howe W. The team physician. *Prim Care* 1991;18(4):763–776.

Howe W. The team physician: a part-timer's perspective. *Phys Sportsmed* 1988;16(1):103–114.

Hughston J. The role of the team physician. In Baker C, ed. *The Hughston Clinic sports medicine book.* Baltimore, MD: Williams & Wilkins, 1995:3–4.

Jackson D. The history of sports medicine: part 2. *Am J Sports Med* 1984;12(4):255–257.

LaCava G. Sports medicine in modern times: a short historical survey. *J Sports Med Phys Fitness* 1973;13(3):155–158.

Lombardo J. Sports medicine: a team effort. *Phys Sportsmed* 1985;13(4):72–81.

Maron B, Mitchell J. Revised eligibility recommendations for competitive athletes with cardiovascular abnormalities. *MSSE* 1994: 26(Suppl 10):S223–S226.

McKeag D, Hugh D. *Primary care sports medicine.* Dubuque, IA: Brown & Benchmark, 1993.

Mellion M, Walsh M. Medical supervision of the athlete. In Mellion M, Walsh M, eds. *The team physician's handbook.* Philadelphia: Hanley & Belfus, 1997:1–8.

Miller T. American Medical Society for Sports Medicine. *Journal of the Georgia American Academy of Family Physicians* 1993;15(3):24.

Mitten M, Maron M. Legal considerations that affect medical eligibility for competitive athletes. *MSSE* 1994;26(Suppl 10):S238–S241.

Peltier L. The classic Geronimo Mercuriali (1530–1606) and the first illustrated book on sports medicine. *Clin Orth Rel Res* 1985;198: 21–24.

Peltier L. The lineage of sports medicine. *Clin Orthop* 1987;216: 4–12.

Puffer J. Sports medicine delivery systems for the athlete: a multi-sport model. *Advances in Sports Medicine and Fitness* 1989;2:287–294.

Rich B. All physicians are not created equal: understanding the educational background of the sports medicine physician. *Journal of Athletic Training* 1993;28(2):177–179.

Ryan AJ. Sports medicine in the world today. In Ryan AJ, Allman FL, Jr, eds. *Sports medicine.* San Diego: Academic Press, 1989:3–21.

Ryan A. Sportsmedicine history. *Phys Sportsmed* 1978;6(10):77–82.

Samples P. The team physician: no official job description. *Phys Sportsmed* 1988;16(1);169–175.

Smith RD, Levandowski R. The history of sports medicine: a full circle. In Birrer RB, ed. *Sports medicine for the primary care physician,* 2nd ed. Boca Raton, FL: CRC Press, 1994.

Snook G. The history of sports medicine: part 1. *Am J Sports Med* 1984;12(4):252–254.

Snook G. The father of sports medicine. *Am J Sports Med* 1978; 6(3):128–131.

Souryal T. Liability and risk management in sports medicine. in Baker C, ed. *The Hughston Clinic sports medicine book.* Baltimore, MD: Williams & Wilkins, 1995:14–18.

Tittel K, Knuttgen G. The development, objectives and activities of FIMS. In Dirix A, Knuttgen H, Tittel K, eds. *The Olympic book of sports medicine,* vol 1. *The encyclopaedia of sports medicine.* Boston: Blackwell Scientific, 1988:7–12.

Walsh M, Mellion M. The team physician. In DeLee J, Drez D, eds. *Orthopaedic sports medicine: principles and practice.* Philadelphia: WB Saunders, 1994:346–355.

CHAPTER 2

Preparticipation Physical Examination

Paul R. Stricker

Millions of young people, including grade school, middle school, high school, and college students, are involved in sporting activities, whether competing on organized teams or participating in school activities or unstructured play. It is well known that exercise and sports participation can enhance general fitness, improve cholesterol, increase self-esteem, and provide social development (1).

Most physicians agree on the importance of exercise and encourage young and old alike to take part in some degree of regular physical activity. To help support the idea of safe participation, a preparticipation physical examination (PPE) is usually required. Although the American Academy of Pediatrics recommends that health maintenance exams be performed every two years, most schools require annual sports participation examinations. Physicals are performed for university and high school athletes across the country, and this practice is supported by investigative work that shows that college and high school athletes are more likely to have significant findings on PPE than junior high athletes (33.9% versus 15.4% versus 3.4%, respectively) (2). Unfortunately, the large majority of the PPEs are used as a substitute for their regular health maintenance exam, and this quick screening will be the individual's only interaction with a physician for over 78% of athletes (3–4). Although no easy solution exists to this problem, physicians and health care professionals should be proactive in stressing the critical importance of yearly exams in addition to sports physicals. This allows for more continuity of care, the ability to adequately address issues that are not timely or appropriate for the PPE, and time to investigate findings without conflicting with practice or coaching schedules.

Contrary to many young athletes' perceptions, the PPE is not performed to disqualify certain athletes from participation in sports, but rather to screen individuals for conditions that may result in significant morbidity and mortality. It may also be an opportunity to provide educational input to encourage athletes to modify unhealthy behavior. The drive and intensity that help athletes to succeed in sports can also result in their taking risks in other activities. It has been shown that maladaptive lifestyles are more prevalent in athletes, especially males who are involved in contact sports (5). Some of the high-risk behaviors in which athletes participate more frequently than nonathlete controls are lack of use of seatbelts and helmets, alcohol and drug use, sexual promiscuity, and fighting. The PPE is an important tool to detect abnormalities that might place an individual at risk for injury or death or that may worsen with continued participation. Despite the countless numbers of PPEs that are performed, only 0.3–1.3% of athletes are actually denied clearance, while 3.2–13.5% need further evaluation before clearance can be provided (3,6–9).

Objectives have been emphasized in the most recent monograph regarding the PPE (10). The first edition of the monograph was published in 1992, and the second edition was published in 1997 as a joint effort of the American Academy of Family Practice (AAFP), American Academy of Pediatrics (AAP), American Medical Society for Sports Medicine (AMSSM), American Orthopaedic Society for Sports Medicine (AOSSM), and American Osteopathic Association for Sports Medicine (AOASM). Primary objectives of the PPE include detecting conditions that may predispose the person to injury, detecting conditions that may be life-threatening or disabling, and meeting legal and insurance requirements. Secondary objectives are to determine general health, counsel the person about health-related issues, and assess the person's fitness level for specific sports.

Physicians conducting the PPE usually examine the athletes either as individual patients in the doctor's office or as large groups of athletes in a setting that can accommodate a station-based exam. A doctor who is

---

P. R. Stricker: Scripps Clinic, San Diego, California 92037.

familiar with the athlete from previous years of contact with the athlete and family may be best suited to examine that athlete (11) because of continuity of care, rapport with the athlete, and knowledge of certain conditions (e.g., murmur, previous surgery) that will not require further investigation or delay of clearance. Some physicians with busy schedules find it extremely difficult to fit in a number of physicals and may need to block out time or have alternative schedules to perform the examinations. Besides the fact that a number of athletes do not have a personal physician, other disadvantages of the individual office exam include cost, the examining physician's potential lack of specific sports medicine expertise, and the potential for problems in communication from the private physician and athlete to the school, athletic trainer, coach, and team physician.

To compensate for some of these difficulties, the station-based mass screening approach is often used to conduct large numbers of PPEs efficiently and in a more cost-effective manner. It has been reported that the station-based exam can identify abnormalities better than private office exams (12,13). Multiple health care personnel can be used for the different aspects of the exam to aid in maximizing the flow of participating athletes. This provides access to health care professionals with specialized expertise and may provide more organized communication, since coaches and/or athletic trainers are also often present. Adequate numbers of examiners must be present for the station approach to be effective, since exam flow is only as fast as the slowest station. Having the athletes arrive in appropriate clothing and using private rooms helps with efficiency and confidentiality. Keeping a record of individuals who are not cleared or who need further workup is critical to ensure close follow-up of these individuals with either their personal physician or a specialist. Necessary stations include weight and height, vision, vital signs, and the actual exam areas. Additional stations such as dental and nutrition may be used optionally if time, space, and personnel are available.

It is commonly agreed that the PPE should be carried out at least six weeks before practices are to begin (10,14). This is very important to allow time for further workup of certain conditions, adequate rehabilitation of a deficit or injury, and conditioning for athletes who are out of shape or beginning a new sport. Even though this timing is most logical, it is often very difficult to carry out, and unfortunately, many physicals are done the week practice begins. Physicians should build on good relationships with coaches and stress the importance of appropriate and optimal timing of the PPE.

There are differing opinions about the frequency of exams (15,16). At this time there is still no unanimous consensus on the best frequency. Lack of unanimity stems from needing to individualize specific sports and the need to meet institutional or liability requirements. Important points for examination frequency include school or state requirements, the sport's level of risk, and availability of people to perform the exams.

Although controversial, additional screening studies are not recommended, since their predictive value as well as their ability to reduce morbidity and mortality has not been established. No consistent support exists in the literature for using urinalysis, CBC, chemistries, lipid profile, ferritin, or sickle trait (17–19). Urinalyses are often confounded by increased protein in the urine due to vigorous exercise, increased muscle mass, or benign orthostatic proteinuria and are not recommended in healthy asymptomatic individuals (20,21). CBC and ferritin may be useful in special athletic populations such as wrestlers and gymnasts or athletes with positive signs and symptoms, but these laboratory studies are usually unrewarding and are not cost-effective for large groups of athletes. Even though laboratory tests should be individualized, a value that should be obtained on everyone is blood pressure. Pulse and blood pressure may be elevated because of anxiety or inappropriate cuff size (22) and should be repeated if elevated initially. Measurements that remain elevated require repeat testing at a later time, and clearance should be prohibited until the values either are normal or have been investigated further and the athlete started on treatment. Classifications of hypertension by age categories may be found in the PPE monograph (10). In addition, a recent update by the National Heart Lung and Blood Institute Task Force regarding high blood pressure in children provides blood pressure percentiles by height (23).

Every physician would like to have a screening test to automatically determine which athletes are at risk for sudden death. However, no one definitive test exists. Unfortunately, some congenital anomalies do not manifest any signs or symptoms until the sudden death occurs. Mass screening with extensive cardiac testing has not been shown to be cost effective (24–26) and often fails to identify significant abnormalities (27), since the prevalence of potentially lethal conditions is very low. Recent work in which almost 3000 echocardiograms were performed found no disqualifying conditions and had poor correlation of echocardiogram results with the history and physical examination (27).

Sudden death events have tremendous impact, yet it is difficult for physicians to a automatically predict these events despite the many methods that are used to attempt identification of such lethal entities. However, abnormalities that can be detected from a thorough screening event may allow interventions that ultimately prevent a sudden death episode. To provide guidance with respect to cardiovascular screening, the American Heart Association (AHA) consensus panel recently provided a statement addressing recommendations and guidelines for practical and effective screening procedures (28). These AHA guidelines suggest that the screening should be performed by someone who has the training, skills, and background to adequately take a detailed history, perform a thorough examination, and recognize cardiovascular disease. Questions should be included in the history to determine previous episodes of chest pain, syncope or near-syncope with exercise, unexplained dyspnea with exercise, previous findings of a heart murmur or hypertension, family history of early death or significant cardiovascular disease in a close relative younger than 50 years of age, and knowledge of specific cardiac conditions. Physical examination should at least include auscultation of the precordium in both the supine and standing positions, palpation of femoral artery pulses, examination for signs of Marfan syndrome, and sitting blood pressure measurement (28).

The primary aim of the PPE is to identify individuals who are at risk for morbidity and mortality. However, just because an athlete has undergone a PPE does not guarantee that injury or sudden death will not occur. The screening questionnaire and physical examination are frequently being updated and refined to provide the best possible opportunity for physicians to detect potential catastrophic problems. However, these recommendations from major medical organizations cannot be effective unless they are adequately used. Recent investigations paint a disappointing picture of the current practices of medical evaluations of athletes in high school and college (29–30). Surveys of Division I, II, and III colleges and universities revealed that only 26% of schools used at least nine of the 1996 American Heart Association (AHA) consensus panel recommendations for cardiovascular screening and that many forms did not include relevant and important items (30). Similar work investigating the programs used in high schools in all 50 states and the District of Columbia found that athletic screening for cardiovascular disease is dependent on state-approved questionnaires, which are often incomplete or inadequate (29). Eight states had no approved history and physical forms, and only 17 states had forms that were adequate and included at least nine of the AHA recommendations. Both of these studies underscore the reality that preparticipation screening processes in U.S. colleges and high schools are frequently inadequate to detect potentially lethal cardiovascular abnormalities (31). It is hoped that more uniformity of the screening process would optimize the detection of such lethal congenital problems.

In addition to cardiac screening, studies have revealed that simple screening tests such as resting spirometry do not consistently identify athletes with exercise-induced bronchospasm (32–34). Exercise challenge tests and field tests are more useful (32–34) yet are not convenient for available time and location.

Laboratory tests including urinalysis, lipid profile, hepatitis B, and HIV should be performed only if signs and symptoms, history, physical examination, and risk factors warrant. Factors necessitating laboratory studies or other diagnostic tests will usually become apparent in reviewing the medical history and discussing the findings with the athlete and/or parents.

The history form is a critical part of the PPE. Certainly, there are athletes who fill out the form themselves and purposefully omit important details for fear of being disqualified. It is best if the athlete and parents fill out the form together. However, in general, accurate histories can be obtained. This is important because about 75% or more of problems will be identified via the history (3), and most disqualifying conditions show up on the form (3,35). Using accepted forms aids in providing consistency between examiners and in including questions that are thought to be crucial from the PPE Task Force. The history questionnaire and physical exam from the second edition PPE monograph are shown in Figure 2–1. Unfortunately, only 17 states use all or part of this form, and at least 13 states have no state form (personal communication, J. B. Robinson, presented at Advanced Team Physicians course, December 4, 1997).

The history form attempts to cover many areas concisely and efficiently and to provide information to the physician that will help in determining which areas need further questioning. The basic areas covered in the history include medical illnesses and medications, allergies, cardiovascular, skin, head/neurologic, heat illness, respiratory, special needs, eyes/vision, orthopedic/injury, eating habits, psychosocial, immunizations, and menses. A history of prior head injuries must be addressed to determine the total number of concussions and the most recent events. Any symptoms that are still present require further evaluation before clearance. Athletes who are symptomatic from a concussion may sustain a minor head injury, which may result in the development of the fatal second impact syndrome (36). Previous surgeries or significant injuries need to be ascertained to perform a more directed examination and address rehabilitative issues, since reinjury of a previously injured joint is a common occurrence (1). Recent illnesses such as mononucleosis have definite implications on clearance to play. In addition to decreased fitness level, other risks of mononucleosis include splenic rupture, hepatitis, and encephalitis (37). Febrile illness requires limitations of activity due to risks of dehydration and viral myocarditis (38). Positive responses to questions in the history about syncope or dizziness with exercise of family history of sudden death requires thorough cardiac evaluation. Menstrual history is important in female athletes and may provide an opportunity to educate the athlete about issues of body fat, nutrition, and bone health.

Detailed descriptions of the physical examination already exist in other publications as well as in the PPE monograph (10). Certain aspects will be highlighted here because of their importance. Documentation of symmetry or asymmetry between pupils provides a base-

Preparticipation Physical Evaluation

HISTORY

DATE OF EXAM _____

Name _____ Sex _____ Age _____ Date of birth _____

Grade ____ School _____ Sport(s) _____

Address _____ Phone _____

Personal physician _____

In case of emergency, contact

Name _____ Relationship _____ Phone (H) _____ (W) _____

Explain "Yes" answers below. Circle questions you don't know the answers to.

	Yes	No
1. Have you had a medical illness or injury since your last check up or sports physical?	☐	☐
Do you have an ongoing or chronic illness?	☐	☐
2. Have you ever been hospitalized overnight?	☐	☐
Have you ever had surgery?	☐	☐
3. Are you currently taking any prescription or nonprescription (over-the-counter) medications or pills or using an inhaler?	☐	☐
Have you ever taken any supplements or vitamins to help you gain or lose weight or improve your performance?	☐	☐
4. Do you have any allergies (for example, to pollen, medicine, food, or stinging insects)?	☐	☐
Have you ever had a rash or hives develop during or after exercise?	☐	☐
5. Have you ever passed out during or after exercise?	☐	☐
Have you ever been dizzy during or after exercise?	☐	☐
Have you ever had chest pain during or after exercise?	☐	☐
Do you get tired more quickly than your friends do during exercise?	☐	☐
Have you ever had racing of your heart or skipped heartbeats?	☐	☐
Have you had high blood pressure or high cholesterol?	☐	☐
Have you ever been told you have a heart murmur?	☐	☐
Has any family member or relative died of heart problems or of sudden death before age 50?	☐	☐
Have you had a severe viral infection (for example, myocarditis or mononucleosis) within the last month?	☐	☐
Has a physician ever denied or restricted your participation in sports for any heart problems?	☐	☐
6. Do you have any current skin problems (for example, itching, rashes, acne, warts, fungus, or blisters)?	☐	☐
7. Have you ever had a head injury or concussion?	☐	☐
Have you ever been knocked out, become unconscious, or lost your memory?	☐	☐
Have you ever had a seizure?	☐	☐
Do you have frequent or severe headaches?	☐	☐
Have you ever had numbness or tingling in your arms, hands, legs, or feet?	☐	☐
Have you ever had a stinger, burner, or pinched nerve?	☐	☐
8. Have you ever become ill from exercising in the heat?	☐	☐
9. Do you cough, wheeze, or have trouble breathing during or after activity?	☐	☐
Do you have asthma?	☐	☐
Do you have seasonal allergies that require medical treatment?	☐	☐

	Yes	No
10. Do you use any special protective or corrective equipment or devices that aren't usually used for your sport or position (for example, knee brace, special neck roll, foot orthotics, retainer on your teeth, hearing aid)?	☐	☐
11. Have you had any problems with your eyes or vision?	☐	☐
Do you wear glasses, contacts, or protective eyewear?	☐	☐
12. Have you ever had a sprain, strain, or swelling after injury?	☐	☐
Have you broken or fractured any bones or dislocated any joints?	☐	☐
Have you had any other problems with pain or swelling in muscles, tendons, bones, or joints?	☐	☐

If yes, check appropriate box and explain below.

☐ Head	☐ Elbow	☐ Hip
☐ Neck	☐ Forearm	☐ Thigh
☐ Back	☐ Wrist	☐ Knee
☐ Chest	☐ Hand	☐ Shin/calf
☐ Shoulder	☐ Finger	☐ Ankle
☐ Upper arm		☐ Foot

	Yes	No
13. Do you want to weigh more or less than you do now?	☐	☐
Do you lose weight regularly to meet weight requirements for your sport?	☐	☐
14. Do you feel stressed out?	☐	☐

15. Record the dates of your most recent immunizations (shots) for:

Tetanus _____ Measles _____
Hepatitis B _____ Chickenpox _____

FEMALES ONLY

16. When was your first menstrual period? _____
When was your most recent menstrual period? _____
How much time do you usually have from the start of one period to the start of another? _____
How many periods have you had in the last year? _____
What was the longest time between periods in the last year? _____

Explain "Yes" answers here: _____
_____
_____
_____
_____
_____

I hereby state that, to the best of my knowledge, my answers to the above questions are complete and correct.

Signature of athlete _____ Signature of parent/guardian _____ Date _____

FIG. 2–1. PPE monograph history questionnaire and physical exam forms. (© 1997 American Academy of Family Physicians, American Academy of Pediatrics, American Medical Society for Sports Medicine, American Orthopaedic Society for Sports Medicine, and American Osteopathic Academy of Sports Medicine.)

Preparticipation Physical Evaluation

PHYSICAL EXAMINATION

Name _____ Date of birth _____

Height _____ Weight _____ % Body fat (optional) _____ Pulse _____ BP ___/____ (___/___, ___/___)

Vision R 20/ _____ L 20/ _____ Corrected: Y N   Pupils: Equal _____ Unequal _____

	NORMAL	ABNORMAL FINDINGS	INITIALS*
MEDICAL			
Appearance			
Eyes/Ears/Nose/Throat			
Lymph Nodes			
Heart			
Pulses			
Lungs			
Abdomen			
Genitalia (males only)			
Skin			
MUSCULOSKELETAL			
Neck			
Back			
Shoulder/arm			
Elbow/forearm			
Wrist/hand			
Hip/thigh			
Knee			
Leg/ankle			
Foot			

* Station-based examination only

CLEARANCE

❑ Cleared

❑ Cleared after completing evaluation/rehabilitation for: _____

_____

_____

❑ Not cleared for: _____ Reason: _____

Recommendations: _____

_____

_____

Name of physician (print/type) _____ Date _____

Address _____ Phone _____

Signature of physician _____, MD or DO

FIG. 2–1. *Continued.*

Preparticipation Physical Evaluation
CLEARANCE FORM

☐ **Cleared**

☐ **Cleared after completing evaluation/rehabilitation for:** _____

_____

_____

_____

☐ **Not cleared for:** _____ **Reason:** _____

Recommendations: _____

_____

_____

_____

Name of physician (print/type) _____ **Date** _____

Address _____ **Phone** _____

Signature of physician _____, MD or DO

FIG. 2–1. *Continued.*

---

line for comparison if an athlete has a head injury at a later date. Neck range of motion must be unrestricted. If motion is not normal, investigation with radiographs and treatment with physical therapy will be necessary. Individuals with Down syndrome who want to participate in collision or contact sports require cervical spine radiographs because of a 10–20% incidence of atlantoaxial instability (1). Cardiac examination should be performed in the supine and standing positions, since the murmur of hypertrophic cardiomyopathy tends to be louder when standing than when sitting (10). Auscultation should be carried out at rest and with the valsalva/squatting maneuvers. Athletes commonly have functional murmurs due to increased stroke volume. However, these benign murmurs should diminish with change in position (supine to standing) or with decreased venous return as occurs with the valsalva maneuver. Murmurs due to pathologic ventricular septum thickness and outlet obstruction such as aortic stenosis increase when heart blood volume is decreased as with the valsalva maneuver. Unfortunately, hypertrophic cardiomyopathy can exist without a murmur (31). Abdominal organomegaly, especially splenomegaly, warrants further investigation. If there has been a recent

---

FIG. 2–2. The general musculoskeletal screening examination consists of the following: (1) Inspection, athlete standing, facing toward examiner (symmetry of trunk upper extremities); (2) forward flexion, extension, rotation, lateral flexion of neck (range of motion, cervical spine); (3) resisted shoulder shrug (strength, trapezius); (4) resisted shoulder abduction (strength, deltoid); (5) internal and external rotation of shoulder (range of motion, glenohumeral joint); (6) extension and flexion of elbow (range of motion, elbow); (7) pronation and supination of elbow (range of motion, elbow and wrist); (8) clench fist, then spread fingers (range of motion, hand and fingers); (9) inspection, athlete facing away from examiner (symmetry of trunk, upper extremities); (10) back extension, knees straight (spondylolysis/spondylokisthesis); (11) back flexion with knees straight, facing toward and away from examiner (range of motion, thoracic and lumbosacral spine; spine curvature; hamstring flexibility); (12) inspection of lower extremities, contraction of quadriceps muscles (alignment symmetry); (13) "duck walk" four steps (motion of hip, knee, and ankle; strength; balance); (14) standing on toes, then on heels (symmetry, calf; strength; balance). (Drawings 1–9, 11–14: © 1997, Rebekah Dodson; drawing 10: Terry Boles.)

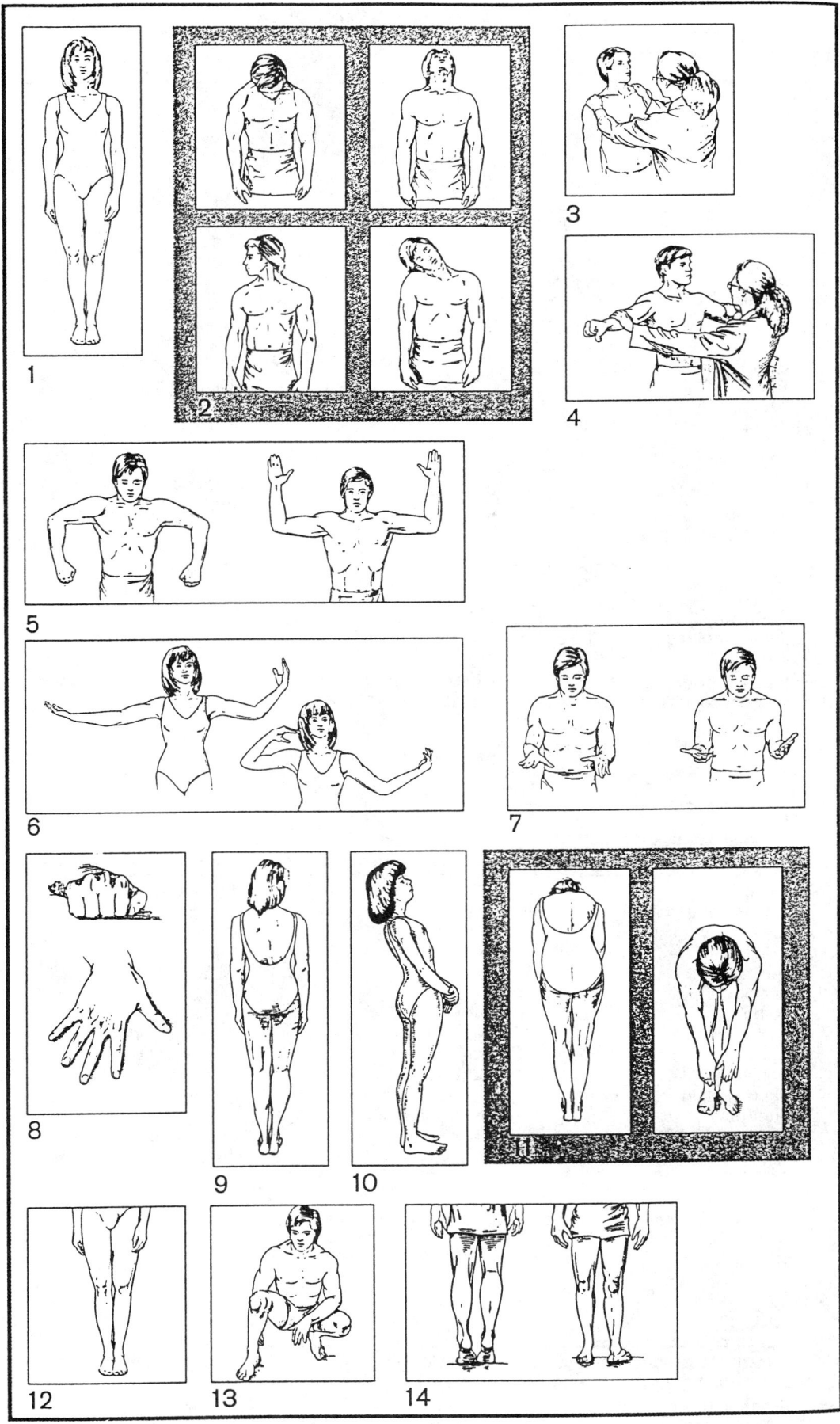

TABLE 2-1. *Classification of sports by contact*

Contact/collision	Limited contact	Noncontact
Basketball	Baseball	Archery
Boxing*	Bicycling	Badminton
Diving	Cheerleading	Body building
Field hockey	Canoeing/Kayaking (white water)	Canoeing/Kayaking (flat water)
Football	Fencing	Crew/Rowing
Flag	Field	Curling
Tackle	High jump	Dancing
Ice hockey	Pole vault	Field
Lacrosse	Floor hockey	Discus
Martial arts	Gymnastics	Javelin
Rodeo	Handball	Shot put
Rugby	Horseback riding	Golf
Ski jumping	Racquetball	Orienteering
Soccer	Skating	Power lifting
Team handball	Ice	Race walking
Water polo	In-line	Riflery
Wrestling	Roller	Rope jumping
	Skiing	Running
	Cross-country	Sailing
	Downhill	Scuba diving
	Water	Strength training
	Softball	Swimming
	Squash	Table tennis
	Ultimate Frisbee	Tennis
	Volleyball	Track
	Windsurfing/Surfing	Weight lifting

* Participation not recommended by the AAP. The AAFP, AMSSM, AOASM, and AOSSM have no stand against boxing.

Reprinted with permission from American Academy of Pediatrics Committee on Sports Medicine and Fitness: Medical conditions affecting sports participation. *Pediatrics* 1994;94(5):757–760

TABLE 2-2. *Classification of sports by strenuousness*

High-to-moderate intensity		
High-to-moderate dynamic and static demands	High-to-moderate dynamic and low static demands	High-to-moderate static and low dynamic demands
Boxing*	Badminton	Archery
Crew/Rowing	Baseball	Auto racing
Cross-country skiing	Basketball	Diving
Cycling	Field hockey	Equestrian
Downhill skiing	Lacrosse	Field events (jumping)
Fencing	Orienteering	Field events (throwing)
Football	Ping-Pong	Gymnastics
Ice Hockey	Race walking	Karate or judo
Rugby	Racquetball	Motorcycling
Running (sprint)	Soccer	Rodeoing
Speed skating	Squash	Sailing
Water polo	Swimming	Ski jumping
Wrestling	Tennis	Water skiing
	Volleyball	Weight lifting

Low intensity
Low dynamic and low static demands
Bowling
Cricket
Curling
Golf
Riflery

* Participation not recommended by the AAP. The AAFP, AMSSM, AOASM, and AOSSM have no stand against boxing.

Reprinted with permission from American Academy of Pediatrics Committee on Sports Medicine and Fitness: Medical conditions affecting sports participation. *Pediatrics* 1994;94(5):757–760

TABLE 2-3. *Medical conditions and sports participation*

This table is designed to be understood by medical and nonmedical personnel. In the "Explanation" section below, "needs evaluation" means that a physician with appropriate knowledge and experience should assess the safety of a given sport for an athlete with the listed medical condition. Unless otherwise noted, this is because of the variability of the severity of the disease or of the risk of injury among the specific sports, or both.

Condition	May participate
Atlantoaxial instability* (instability of the joint between cervical vertebrae 1 and 2)	Qualified yes
Explanation: Athlete needs evaluation to assess risk of spinal cord injury during sports participation.	
Bleeding disorder*	Qualified yes
Explanation: Athlete needs evaluation.	
Cardiovascular diseases	
Carditis (inflammation of the heart)	No
Explanation: Carditis may result in sudden death with exertion.	
Hypertension (high blood pressure)	Qualified yes
Explanation: Those with significant essential (unexplained) hypertension should avoid weight and power lifting, body building, and strength training. Those with secondary hypertension (hypertension caused by a previously identified disease), or severe essential hypertension, need evaluation.	
Congenital heart disease (structural heart defects present at birth)	Qualified yes
Explanation: Those with mild forms may participate fully; those with moderate or severe forms, or who have undergone surgery, need evaluation.†	
Dysrhythmia (irregular heart rhythm)	Qualified yes
Explanation: Athlete needs evaluation because some types require therapy or make certain sports dangerous, or both.	
Mitral valve prolapse (abnormal heart valve)	Qualified yes
Explanation: Those with symptoms (chest pain, symptoms of possible dysrhythmia) or evidence of mitral regurgitation (leaking) on physical examination need evaluation. All others may participate fully.	
Heart murmur	Qualified yes
Explanation: If the murmur is innocent (does not indicate heart disease), full participation is permitted. Otherwise, the athlete needs evaluation (see "Congenital heart disease" and "Mitral valve prolapse" above).	
Cerebral palsy*	Qualified yes
Explanation: Athlete needs evaluation.	
Diabetes mellitus*‡	Yes
Explanation: All sports can be played with proper attention to diet, hydration, and insulin therapy. Particular attention is needed for activities that last 30 minutes or more.	
Diarrhea§	Qualified no
Explanation: Unless disease is mild, no participation is permitted, because diarrhea may increase the risk of dehydration and heat illness. See "Fever" below.	
Eating disorders	Qualified yes
Anorexia nervosa, Bulimia nervosa	
Explanation: These patients need both medical and psychiatric assessment before participation.	
Eyes	
Functionally one-eyed athlete, loss of an eye, detached retina, previous eye surgery or serious eye injury	Qualified yes
Explanation: A functionally one-eyed athlete has a best corrected visual acuity of <20/40 in the worse eye. These athletes would suffer significant disability if the better eye was seriously injured as would those with loss of an eye. Some athletes who have previously undergone eye surgery or had a serious eye injury may have an increased risk of injury because of weakened eye tissue. Availability of eye guards approved by the American Society for Testing Materials (ASTM) and other protective equipment may allow participation in most sports, but this must be judged on an individual basis.	
Fever‡	No
Explanation: Fever can increase cardiopulmonary effort, reduce maximum exercise capacity, make heat illness more likely, and increase orthostatic hypotension during exercise. Fever may rarely accompany myocarditis or other infections that may make exercise dangerous.	
Heat illness, history of	Qualified Yes
Explanation: Because of the increased likelihood of recurrence, the athlete needs individual assessment to determine the presence of predisposing conditions and to arrange a prevention strategy.	
HIV infection§	Yes
Explanation: Because of the apparent minimal risk to others, all sports may be played that the state of health allows. In all athletes, skin lesions should be properly covered, and athletic personnel should use universal precautions when handling blood or body fluids with visible blood.	
Kidney: absence of one	Qualified yes
Explanation: Athlete needs individual assessment for contact/collision and limited contact sports.	

continued

TABLE 2-3. Continued

Condition	May participate
Liver, enlarged	Qualified yes
Explanation: If the liver is acutely enlarged, participation should be avoided because of risk of rupture. If the liver is chronically enlarged, individual assessment is needed before contact/collision or limited contact sports are played.	
Malignancy*	Qualified yes
Explanation: Athlete needs individual assessment.	
Musculoskeletal disorders	Qualified yes
Explanation: Athlete needs individual assessment.	
Neurologic	
History of serious head or spine trauma, severe or repeated concussions, or craniotomy	Qualified yes
Explanation: Athlete needs individual assessment for contact/collision or limited contact sports, and also for noncontact sports if there are deficits in judgment or cognition. Recent research supports a conservative approach to management of concussion.	
Convulsive disorder, well controlled	Yes
Explanation: Risk of convulsion during participation is minimal.	
Convulsive disorder, poorly controlled	Qualified yes
Explanation: Athlete needs individual assessment for contact/collision or limited contact sports. Avoid the following noncontact sports: archery, riflery, swimming, weight or power lifting, strength training, or sports involving heights. In these sports, occurrence of a convulsion may be a risk to self or others.	
Obesity	Qualified yes
Explanation: Because of the risk of heat illness, obese persons need careful acclimatization and hydration.	
Organ transplant recipient*	Qualified yes
Explanation: Athlete needs individual assessment.	
Ovary: absence of one	Yes
Explanation: Risk of severe injury to the remaining ovary is minimal.	
Respiratory	
Pulmonary compromise including cystic fibrosis*	Qualified yes
Explanation: Athlete needs individual assessment, but generally all sports may be played if oxygenation remains satisfactory during a graded exercise test. Patients with cystic fibrosis need acclimatization and good hydration to reduce the risk of heat illness.	
Asthma	Yes
Explanation: With proper medication and education, only athletes with the most severe asthma will have to modify their participation.	
Acute upper respiratory infection	Qualified yes
Explanation: Upper respiratory obstruction may affect pulmonary function. Athlete needs individual assessment for all but mild disease. See "Fever" above.	
Sickle cell disease	Qualified yes
Explanation: Athlete needs individual assessment. In general, if status of the illness permits, all but high-exertion, contact/collision sports may be played. Overheating, dehydration, and chilling must be avoided.	
Sickle cell trait	Yes
Explanation: It is unlikely that individuals with sickle cell trait (AS) have an increased risk of sudden death or other medical problems during athletic participation except under the most extreme conditions of heat, humidity, and possibly increased altitude. These individuals, like all athletes, should be carefully conditioned, acclimatized, and hydrated to reduce any possible risk.	
Skin: boils, herpes simplex, impetigo, scabies, molluscum contagiosum	Qualified yes
Explanation: While the patient is contagious, participation in gymnastics with mats, martial arts, wrestling, or other contact/collision or limited contact sports is not allowed. Herpes simplex virus probably is not transmitted via mats.	
Spleen, enlarged	Qualified yes
Explanation: Patients with acutely enlarged spleens should avoid all sports because of risk of rupture. Those with chronically enlarged spleens need individual assessment before playing contact/collision or limited contact sports.	
Testicle: absent or undescended	Yes
Explanation: Certain sports may require a protective cup.	

* Not discussed in text of the monograph.

† Mild, moderate, and severe congenital heart disease are defined in 26th Bethesda Conference: Recommendations for determining eligibility for competition in athletes with cardiovascular abnormalities. January 6–7, 1994. *Med Sci Sports Exerc* 1994;26(10 suppl):S246–253

‡ Well controlled

§ AAP recommendation as indicated; see text for qualifications by other commentators.

Reprinted with permission from: American Academy of Pediatrics Committee on Sports Medicine and Fitness: Medical conditions affecting sports participation. *Pediatrics* 1994;94(5):757–760 history of mononucleosis, then ultrasonography may be necessary to determine splenomegaly. It has been shown that physical examination will not always definitively reveal abnormal increases in splenic size (37,39). Documentation of a single testicle is important for appropriate protective recommendations for contact sport participation.

The musculoskeletal examination can be effectively and efficiently carried out in approximately 90–120 seconds (40); it includes contour, range of motion, stability, and symmetry of neck, back, shoulder, elbow, wrist, hand, hip, knee, ankle, and foot (Fig. 2–2). The brief orthopedic screening has been evaluated in a prospective single blind study (41). The overall sensitivity was moderate at 50.8% with a specificity of 97.5%. Interestingly, 92% of significant findings were discovered by the orthopedic history alone; therefore the screening exam should be used in conjunction with the history. Previously injured areas, including areas of fractures or significant sprains, areas requiring arthroscopy or surgery, or areas injured in the interim since the last PPE will require more detailed examination.

After review and discussion of the history and conduct of the physical examination, the physician then makes a determination of clearance. There are various means of clearance for the athlete: complete clearance without restriction, clearance pending further tests, evaluation or therapy, limited clearance for certain sports, or no clearance. It is valuable from a physiologic and psychologic standpoint to determine whether an athlete can be redirected to another activity if he or she is not cleared in a certain sport (10). Guidelines established by the AAP Committee on Sports Medicine and Fitness (42) and the 26th Bethesda Conference for Cardiovascular Abnormalities (43) can help in clearance determination. These guidelines categorize activities by contact and by strenuousness (Tables 2–1 and 2–2). Guidelines for participation with certain medical conditions established by the AAP appear in the monograph (Table 2–3) and should guide individualized clearance of these athletes. If an athlete desires to participate, then complete documentation of explanations of risk must occur. Exculpatory waivers signed by the athlete and parents are written agreements stating that the physician will not be sued. However, the reality of that type of protection is suspect (44). Certainly each case requires adequate legal advice.

Too often, the preparticipation physical examination is viewed as the evil stepchild of sports medicine. Athletes often see physicals as a hassle and a ritual that they must undergo every year just so that they can proceed with their sport. Physicians usually dread them as a time-eating behemoth involving hundreds of man-hours every fall and spring. However, the PPE truly has a purpose of quickly assessing an athlete's risk for morbidity and mortality. It is clear that the PPE is not a panacea, yet many organizations involved in the care of athletes have put tremendous effort into devising a history and physical form to provide the best risk assessment of athletes. If such information is used more consistently across the United States, then it is hoped that a more productive experience and accurate screening will be provided for athletes and the physicians who provide care for them.

REFERENCES

1. Hulse E, Strong WB. Preparticipation evaluation for athletics. *Pediatr Rev* 1987;9:1–10.
2. Briner WW Jr, Farr C. Athlete age and sports physical examination findings. *J Fam Pract* 1995;40:370–375.
3. Goldberg B, Saraniti A, Witman P, et al. Pre-participation sports assessment: an objective evaluation. *Pediatrics* 1980;66:736–t745.
4. Risser WL, Hoffman HM, Bellah GG Jr. Frequency of preparticipation sports examinations in secondary school athletes: are the University Interscholastic League guidelines appropriate? *Tex Med* 1985;81:35–39.
5. Nattiv A, Puffer JC, Green GA. Lifestyles and health risks of collegiate athletes: a multicenter study. *Clin J Sport Med* 1997;7:262–272.
6. Linder CW, DuRant RH, Seklecki RM, et al. Preparticipation health screening of young athletes: results of 1268 examinations. *Am J Sports Med* 1981;9:187–193.
7. Thompson TR, Andrish JT, Bergfeld JA. A prospective study of preparticipation sports examinations of 2670 young athletes: method and results. *Cleve Clin Q* 1982;49:225–233.
8. Tennant FS Jr, Sorenson K, Day CM. Benefits of preparticipation sports examinations. *J Fam Pract* 1981;13:287–288.
9. Magnes SA, Henderson JM, Hunter SC. What conditions limit sports participation? Experience with 10,540 athletes. *Phys Sportsmed* 1992;20:143–160.
10. American Academy of Family Physicians, American Academy of Pediatrics, American Medical Society for Sports Medicine, American Orthopaedic Society for Sports Medicine, American Osteopathic Association for Sports Medicine. *Preparticipation Physical Evaluation Monograph,* 2nd ed., 1997:1–49.
11. Puffer JC. Sports medicine and the adolescent. *Seminars in Family Medicine* 1981;1:201.
12. Garrick JG. Sports medicine. *Pediatr Clin North Am* 1977;24:737.
13. DuRant RH, Seymore C, Linder CW, et al. The participation examination of athletes. *Am J Dis Child* 1985;139:657–661.
14. Lombardo JA. Pre-participation physical evaluation. *Prim Care* 1984;11:3–21.
15. Johnson MD, Kibler WB, Smith D, et al. Keys to successful preparticipation exams. *Phys Sportsmed* 1993;21:108–123.
16. Committee on Sports Medicine. *Sports medicine: health care for young athletes.* Evanston, IL: American Academy of Pediatrics, 1983.
17. Peggs JF, Reinhardt RW, O'Brien JM. Proteinuria in adolescent sports physical examinations. *J Fam Pract* 1986;22:80–81.
18. Taylor WC III, Lombardo JA. Preparticipation screening of college athletes: value of the complete blood count. *Phys Sportsmed* 1990;18:106–118.
19. Vehaskari VM, Rapola J. Isolated proteinuria: analysis of a school-age population. *Pediatrics* 1982;101:661–668.
20. Woolhandler S, Pels RJ, Bor DH, et al. Dipstick urinalysis screening of a symptomatic adults for urinary tract disorders. *JAMA* 1989;262:1214–1219.
21. Ryan AJ, West CD, Shapiro FL, et al. Proteinuria in the athlete. *Phys Sportsmed* 1978;45–55.
22. Strong WB. Hypertension in sports. *Pediatrics* 1979;64:693.
23. National Heart Lung and Blood Institute Task Force on High Blood Pressure in Children. *Blood pressure percentiles for children age 1 to 17 years by height* (update), Bethesda, MD, 1996.
24. Epstein SE, Maron BJ. Sudden death and the competitive athlete:

perspectives on preparticipation screening studies. *J Am Coll Cardiol* 1986;7:220–230.
25. Feinstein RA, Colvin E, Oh MK. Echocardiographic screening as part of a preparticipation examination. *Clin J Sport Med* 1993;3:149–152.
26. Maron BJ, Bodison SA, Wesley YE, et al. Results of screening a large group of intercollegiate competitive athletes for cardiovascular disease. *J Am Coll Cardiol* 1987;10:1214–1221.
27. Weidenbener EJ, Krauss MD, Waller BF, et al. Incorporation of screening echo cardiography in the preparticipation exam. *Clin J Sport Med* 1995;5:86–89.
28. Maron BJ, Thompson PD, Puffer JC, et al. American Heart Association statement: cardiovascular preparticipation screening of competitive athletes. *Circulation* 1996;94:850–856.
29. Glover DW, Maron BJ. Profile of preparticipation cardiovascular screening for high school athletes. *JAMA* 1998;279:1817–1819.
30. Maron BJ, Lange SK, Puffer JC. Profile of the preparticipation screening process for competitive athletes in U.S. colleges and universities (abstract). Paper presented at the AHA Annual Scientific Session; New Orleans, LA, 1996.
31. Maron BJ, Shirani J, Poliac LC, et al. Sudden death in young competitive athletes. *JAMA* 1996;276:199–204.
32. Rupp NT, Brudno DS, Guill MF. The value of screening for risk of exercise-induced asthma in high school athletes. *Ann Allergy* 1993;70:339–342.
33. Rupp NT, Guill MF, Brudno DS. Unrecognized exercise-induced bronchospasm in adolescent athletes. *Am J Dis Child* 1992;146:941–944.
34. Feinstein RA, LaRussa J, Wang-Dohlman A, et al. Screening adolescent athletes for exercise-induced asthma. *Clin J Sport Med* 1996;6:119–123.
35. Hara JH, Puffer JC. The preparticipation physical examination. In: Mellion, MB, ed. *Office management of sports injuries & athletic problems*. Philadelphia: Hanley & Belfus, 1988.
36. Cantu RC, Voy R. Second impact syndrome a risk in any contact sport. *Phys Sportsmed* 1995;23:27.
37. Doolittle R. Pharyngitis and mononucleosis. In: Fields KB, Fricker PA, eds. *Medical problems in athletes*. Malden, MA: Blackwell Science, 1997.
38. Kramer JS. Pericarditis and myocarditis. In: Fields KB, Fricker PA, eds. *Medical problems in athletes*. Malden, MA: Blackwell Science, 1997.
39. Eichner ER. Infectious mononucleosis: recognition and management in athletes. *Phys Sportsmed* 1987;15:61–72.
40. Garrick JG. Sports medicine. *Pediatr Clin North Am* 1977;24:737–747.
41. Gomez JE, Landry GL, Bernhardt DT. Critical evaluation of the 2-minute orthopedic screening examination. *Am J Dis Child* 1993;147:1109–1113.
42. American Academy of Pediatrics Committee on Sports Medicine and Fitness. Medical conditions affecting sports participation. *Pediatrics* 1994;94:757–760.
43. 26th Bethesda Conference: Recommendations for determining eligibility for competition in athletes with cardiovascular abnormalities. *Med Sci Sports Exerc* 1994;26:5223–5283.
44. Herbert DL. Prospective releases: will their use protect sports medicine physicians from suit? *Sports Med Stand Malpract Rep* 1994;6:33–36.

CHAPTER 3

On-the-Field Emergencies

David G. Carfagno and A. J. Cianflocco

INTRODUCTION

Medical coverage of present-day athletics has evolved vastly since the early days of humankind. The concept of sport arose as an offshoot from the basic skills needed for survival and to wage war (1). As the popularity of sport increased from the beginnings of the Olympic movement around 776 B.C., so did the frequency of injuries. Sporting events in ancient times such as boxing, wrestling, and track and field had their share of injuries. As a result, the need for sports physicians developed.

The first sports physician-trainers, called *gymnastes,* were involved in all aspects of an athlete's training and care. The first recorded "team physician" was Claudius Galen in A.D.160. He was the chief physician to the gladiators (2). He provided surgical services and exercise for the treatment of many forms of disease or injury.

Medical coverage of sporting events has come a long way in 2000 years, yet preparation remains the key to successful coverage. It is important to first know your ancillary medical and nonmedical personnel. The nonmedical personnel involved are the coaches and officials. These individuals play an integral role in emergency situations. It is important to become familiar with them and to introduce yourself before the game and identify yourself as the team physician. The coaches should be aware that you are the team physician. You may be the team physician for both teams; therefore the opposing athletic trainer and coach need to be aware of your presence.

The medical personnel involved are the athletic trainers and emergency medical technicians. Knowledge of the local hospital/trauma center and local on-call medical and surgical specialists is also important.

The team physician's medical bag must include medications and equipment required for any injury from minor to serious (Table 3–1). Limited space is available in the bag; therefore only essential and frequently used items should be included. This will vary depending on the extent of the equipment provided by the school or facility, but knowledge of this in advance of the event is important.

HEAD INJURIES

Head injuries are most frequent in sports such as boxing, football, ice hockey, rugby, skiing, and gymnastics. The incidence of minor head injuries per year, including concussions in the high school football athlete, is approximately 20% (3); five to ten football players per year die from head injuries (4).

The initial approach to the athlete with a suspected head injury should be one of precaution. An athlete who doesn't awaken readily after a blow to the head must be assumed to have a severe head injury. The differential diagnosis includes concussion, intracranial hemorrhage, epidural hematoma, subdural hematoma, and intracerebral hematoma. The aforementioned medical and nonmedical personnel need to be aware of the necessary precautions. Frequently, players and referees will wave the athletic trainer or team physician onto the field. The team physician or trainer should assess the athlete immediately, following basic life support protocol and determining level of consciousness. The conscious athlete who is breathing spontaneously but complains of focal neck pain, paralysis, or paresis of bilateral extremities should be managed as a cervical spine trauma. A brief but thorough neurologic exam must be performed, including assessment of mental status, motor and sensory function, and reflexes. If the athlete is unconscious, suspect a cervical spine injury. If the player is face down, he or she must be

---

D. G. Carfagno: Southwest Sports Medicine and Orthopaedic Surgery, Scottsdale, Arizona 85258.
A. J. Cianflocco: Department of Orthopaedic Surgery, Cleveland Clinic Foundation, Cleveland, Ohio 44195.

TABLE 3-1. *Medical bag: head trauma, basic CPR/advanced cardiac life support**

Spine board	Stethoscope
Stretcher	Automated external defibrillator
Rigid cervical collar	Communication device (cellular phone)
Sand bags	
Orthopedic Trauma	Pocket Equipment
Cotton cast padding	Airway
Crutches	Knife for cutting a football facemask
Knee immobilizer	Penlight
Splint material	Reflex hammer
Plaster, 4 & 6 inch	Scissors, bandage
Sling	Gloves
Bolt cutter	Power screw driver
Gloves, sterile	Cardiac meds (atropine, epinephrine, lidocaine)
Surgical Equipment	
Oral and nasal airway	Defibrillator (if available)

Miscellaneous: alcohol swabs, antibiotics, anti-inflammatories, antihistamines, betadine swabs, asthma meds, analgesics

*Ambulance usually supplies oxygen, suction, intravenous lines and fluids, cardiac monitor and defibrillator, blood pressure cuff, crash cart, and endotracheal kit.

brought face up by a logroll technique (Figs. 3-1 and 3-2) (5-7).

Once the player is in a supine position, airway, breathing, and circulation can be assessed. If spontaneous breathing is not present, establish an airway. The helmet should not be removed. The face mask can be either snapped off or removed with a screwdriver or bolt cutter (Fig. 3-3). The jaw-thrust, head-tilt, or chin-lift technique can be used to open the airway. The jaw-thrust technique (Fig. 3-4) is the safest approach, since the neck does not extend. Clear the airway of any foreign body with a finger sweep, checking for dental trauma and any mouth guard. An oral airway should be used to maintain air exchange, but with caution because it may cause vomiting, resulting in aspiration.

With the airway secured, rescue breathing can be initiated with mouth-to-mouth, mouth-to-mask, or mouth-to-nose ventilation. Supplemental oxygen should be used when available. Rescue breathing as above (ventilation using exhaled air) provides 16-17% oxygen to patient, producing an alveolar oxygen tension of 80 mm Hg. Hypoxemia can develop, resulting in metabolic acidosis, which can blunt the beneficial effects of subsequent chemical and electric therapy. Therefore 100% inspired oxygen is recommended when available.

If needed, nasotracheal intubation is preferred over endotracheal intubation in suspected cervical spine injuries to avoid causing further cervical spine trauma. If ventilation cannot be established because of massive facial trauma, laryngeal edema, or laryngeal fracture, consider a needle cricothyroidotomy (Fig. 3-5). After palpating the cricothyroid membrane, insert a no. 14 catheter over needle angulated at 45'. Aspirate for air to confirm the catheter's position in the tracheal lumen. Ventilation can be continued through the catheter. Once ventilation is established, inspect and auscultate the

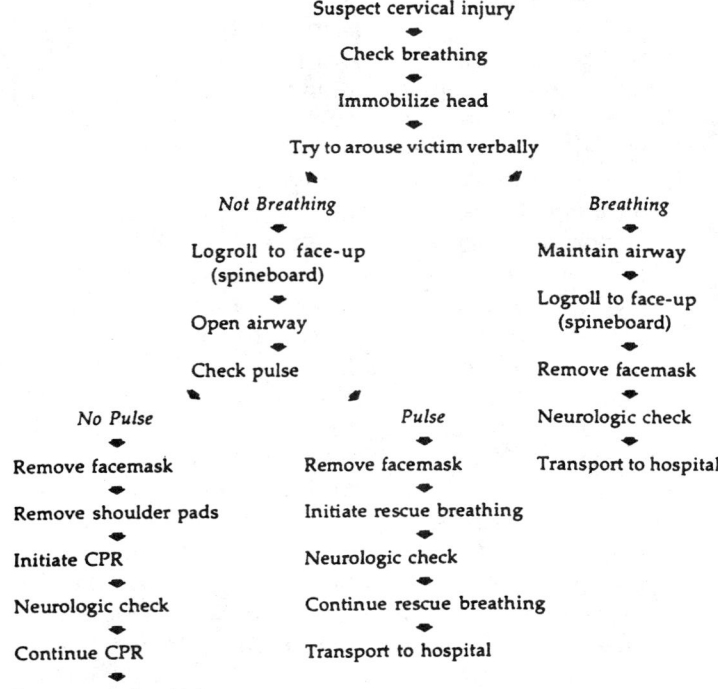

FIG. 3-1. Field decision making. (Reprinted with permission from Veggo JJ, Lehman R. Field evaluation and management of head and neck injuries. *Clin Sports Med.* 1987;1-15.)

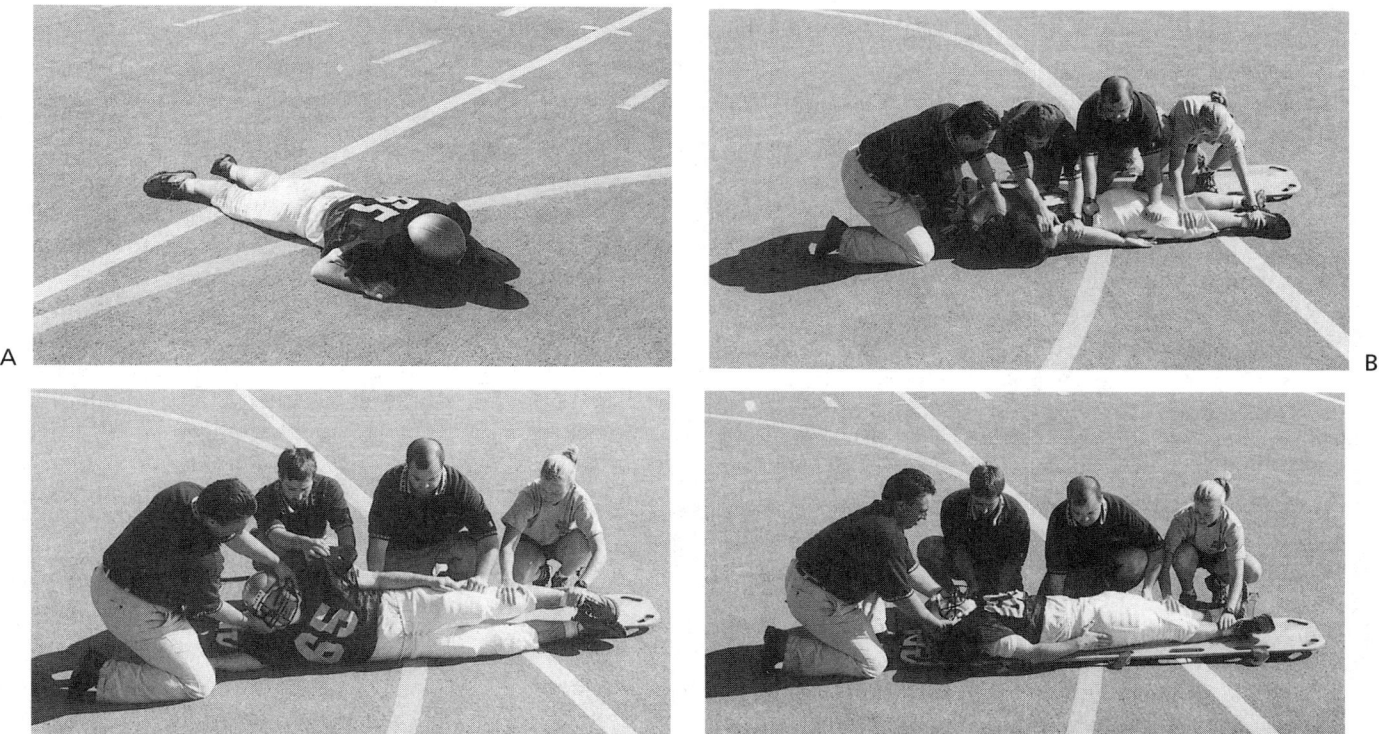

FIG. 3-2. Logroll technique.

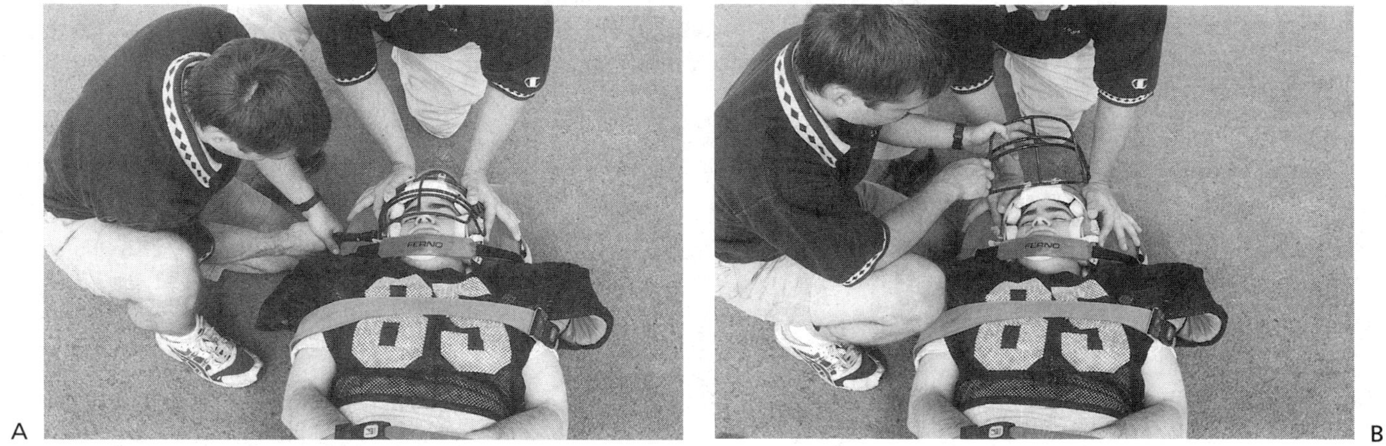

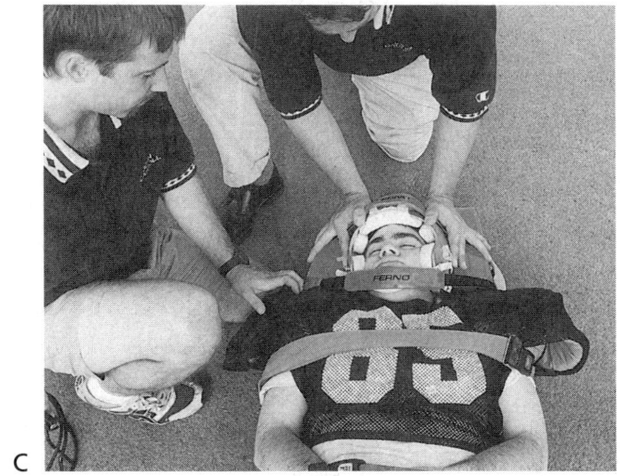

FIG. 3-3. Removal of face mask with a bolt cutter.

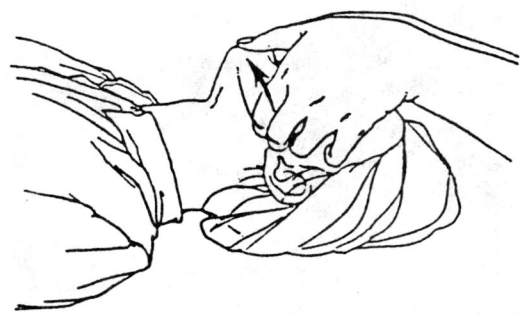

FIG. 3–4. Jaw-thrust technique for opening the airway in a player with suspected cervical spine injury. (Reprinted with permission from American Heart Association, 1992, JAMA.)

chest for symmetrical movement and air entry to confirm good placement.

Once on a spine board and properly immobilized (Fig. 3–6), the athlete should be transferred to a nearby emergency facility, preferably a trauma center. The team physician should communicate with the emergency room and/or the neurosurgeon. A more thorough neurologic exam can be performed during transport to the hospital. Observe abnormal posturing, lateralized weakness, pupillary asymmetry, vomiting, prolonged unconsciousness, bradycardia, and elevated blood pressure, which are signs of increasing intracranial pressure and imminent cerebral herniation. The most life-threatening intracranial injury is the epidural hematoma, which can be associated with a skull fracture. If the injury is not recognized and treated promptly, deterioration follows an early "lucid interval" indicative of brainstem compression, which can progress to death. Subdural hematomas can compress underlying parenchyma, causing cerebral ischemia, shift, and herniation. Treatment en route to the emergency facility can include hyperventilation through artificial ventilation and intravenous (IV) mannitol (50–100 g) to reduce intracerebral edema (8).

If the conscious athlete is breathing spontaneously and has a normal screening neurologic exam and no cervical tenderness, the athlete can perform active range of motion of the neck. If no pain or limitation of neck motion is present, the player may walk, with assistance, off the field. Postconcussive symptoms include headache, confusion, blurred vision, amnesia, and unsteadiness. Athletes with a mild concussion may return to the game once symptoms subside and do not recur with activity. Athletes must be carefully reexamined before reentry to prevent second-impact syndrome (9).

CARDIOVASCULAR EMERGENCIES

The incidence of fatal collapse is approximately 1 in every 300,000 high school and college athletes but is more frequent with marathons (1 in 50,000). Sudden death in athletes over 35 years old results from coronary artery disease. Congenital heart disease such as hypertrophic cardiomyopathy, anomalous coronary artery, and Marfan syndrome is the primary cause with individuals under 35 (10). Other causes of collapse include exercise-associated collapse, insulin reaction, asthma exacerbation, or shock secondary to hypovolemia from dehydration.

The collapsed player must be treated as a cardiac emergency once head and cervical spine injury is excluded and a thorough exam has been completed. If the player is unconscious, a sternal rub to the midsternum may awaken the athlete. Do not use ammonia or vigorously shake the athlete, since there may be spinal cord injury. If the athlete remains unconscious, then emergency medical services and BCLS (basic cardiac life support) protocol should be activated.

Cardiac monitoring is the next priority. The most common cause of sudden cardiac arrest is ventricular fibrillation (11,12). Studies have proven the benefit of early defibrillation, in particular with an automated external defibrillator, which can be kept on the sideline (12).

Exercise-associated collapse typically occurs during endurance events such as marathons and triathlons. Signs and symptoms include exhaustion, nausea, cramps, abnormally high or low core body temperature, muscle spasms, and an inability to walk unassisted. Treatment is aimed at replacing fluid and electrolyte losses, correcting body temperature, and alleviating leg cramps. Recommended fluid replacement is with oral

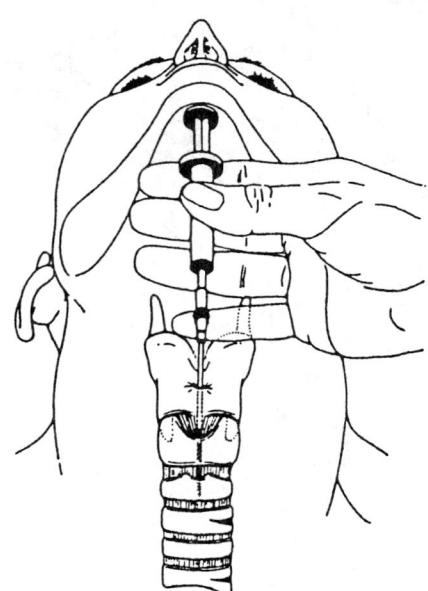

FIG. 3–5. Needle cricothyroidectomy. (Reprinted with permission from American Heart Association, 1992, JAMA.)

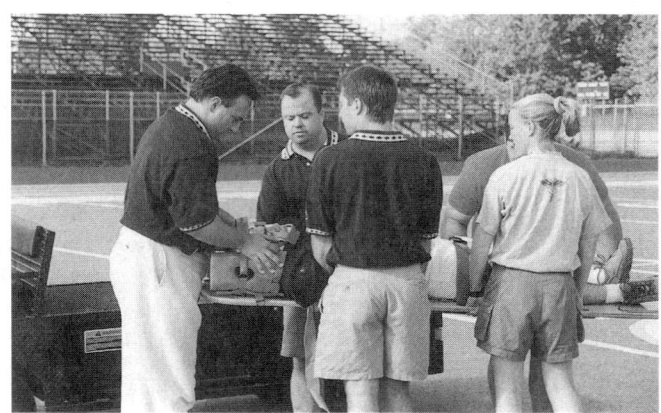 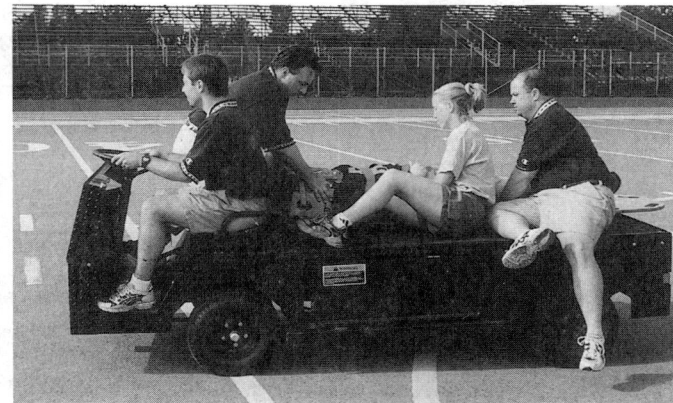

FIG. 3–6. Immobilized patient ready for transport.

fluids such as 6–7% carbohydrate solution if tolerated; if not, intravenous fluid (e.g., 500–1000 mL of 5% dextrose in 0.5 normal saline) can be used. The hyperthermic athlete can be cooled by applying ice bags to areas of major heat loss (face, neck, axilla, and groin) and fanning with cool mist. The hypothermic athlete can be warmed by removing any wet clothing, drying the skin, insulating with warm blankets, and using a portable heater. If not alleviated with initial oral or IV fluids, leg cramps can be treated with D50W. If cramps persist beyond one hour, intravenous diazepam, up to 5 mg slowly injected, can be used.

PULMONARY EMERGENCIES

The most common pulmonary emergency encountered on the field is exercise-induced bronchospasm (EIB). Athletes typically present with hyperpnea and dyspnea, repeatedly depending on their inhaler. Bronchoconstriction results from airway sensitization by cool air triggering an obstructive-bronchospasm pattern (13–15). Others have implicated elevated histamine and neutrophil chemotactic factor of anaphylaxis levels in individuals with exercise-induced asthma (14,16). McFadden theorized that obstruction is due to hyperreactive airways; with exercise-associated hyperpnea, bronchial vasoconstriction occurs (17).

Treatment focuses on the use of mast cell membrane stabilizers, such as cromolyn sodium, given 30–45 minutes before exercise. A synergistic effect occurs with beta-2 agonists (18). Albuterol, a beta-2 agonist, does play a role in the acute asthmatic attack, and the bronchdilatatory effects can last up to 4–6 hours. Glucocorticoids have no role in the acute exacerbation but have some effect in late phase bronchoconstriction approximately 4–6 hours after exercise.

Encountered less frequently is exercise-induced anaphylaxis. The athlete typically presents with warmth, pruritus, urticaria, and, less commonly, stridor. These individuals usually have a food-borne allergy, for example to nuts, certain fruits such as strawberries, and monosodium glutamate (food additive). The mechanism is similar to EIB with elevated levels of histamine and degranulation of mast cells. With EIA, there is a temporal relationship between the ingestion of a particular food and the onset of symptoms after the initiation of exercise (19).

Management of these athletes on the field includes epinephrine 1:10,000 SQ (Epi-Pen), oxygen, bronchodilator (e.g., albuterol), and antihistamines. For severe cases, such as impending respiratory failure, securing the airway by intubation is necessary. If shock develops, IV fluids and stress-dose steroids (hydrocortisone, 100 mg IV) need to be given.

Pneumothorax is typically seen in contact sports such as hockey, football, and lacrosse. The typical presentation is an athlete complaining of acute dyspnea with decreased breath sounds over the traumatic area. If the pneumothorax is small, dyspnea may not be severe; however, checking a pulse oximetry is warranted. A larger pneumothorax will require oxygenation and placing a sterile gauze or cloth over the open wound, if present. Secure the bandage on three sides, leaving the fourth side open; if all four sides are taped, a tension pneumothorax can develop. The athlete should be transported immediately for placement of a chest tube.

A tension pneumothorax presents with tachypnea, dyspnea, tracheal deviation, hypotension, unilateral absence of breath sounds, distended neck veins, and possibly cyanosis. Oxygenate first; then insert a large-bore needle (14 gauge) into the second intercostal space in the midclavicular line of the involved side. Transport immediately for placement of a chest tube.

Flail chest typically presents with asymmetry of the chest wall usually secondary to multiple rib fractures. Initial management consists of applying direct pressure manually or with a sandbag over the flail segment, which improves the efficiency of ventilation. Intubation may be necessary. Transport immediately.

GASTROINTESTINAL EMERGENCIES

The majority of abdominal injuries that occur in sports arise from contact sports, such as football, rugby, skiing, soccer, and wrestling. The injuries are classified as either penetrating or blunt trauma. Penetrating injury is relatively uncommon and can result from impalement or spearing. Blunt trauma is more common and typically involves the liver, spleen, or kidneys; initially, the severity may be difficult to assess.

The initial management of the acute abdominal injury involves determination of the mechanism of the injury. Blunt trauma can present with immediate or insidious onset of pain. Typically, the location of the pain can define the extent of an injury. Focal tenderness at the site of impact is usually a contusion. Extensive tenderness or pain that radiates to the shoulder, to the back, or throughout the abdomen, in association with rigidity and/or loss of bowel sounds, is indicative of more extensive intraabdominal trauma. The athlete should be removed from play. Once he or she is on the sideline, evaluation includes assessment of pulse and blood pressure, skin for color/pallor, heart sounds, breath sounds, pulses in the upper and lower extremities, and palpation of the ribs for any fractures. Oral fluid intake or analgesics may obscure physical findings that would prompt surgical intervention.

MUSCLE INJURIES

The most common injury of abdominal musculature is a rectus abdominus muscle contusion from a direct blow, occasionally with hemorrhage into the muscle. Abdominal wall muscle strain can occur at the tendinous insertion on the pelvis, which can be confused with a hernia. Management includes ice and direct pressure to prevent swelling and hematoma formation.

SPLENIC INJURIES

The spleen is the most common organ injured. An enlarged spleen, due to viral infection such as infectious mononucleosis, is at greater risk of injury. The likelihood of this occurring is 1%, with a mortality rate of approximately 50%. A blow to the left upper quadrant, and/or lower ribs, causing fractures, typically of the tenth to the twelfth ribs, places the spleen at risk for rupture. If shock (tachycardia and hypotension) develops with abdominal symptoms and signs such as nausea, vomiting, rebound tenderness, rigid abdomen, or diminished bowel sounds, splenic rupture should be considered, and IV fluid resuscitation should begin immediately, maintaining systolic blood pressure above 90 mm Hg. If shock does not respond to IV fluids, intravenous dopamine at 1 to 5 $\mu g/kg/min$ may be given en route to the emergency facility. The role of pneumatic antishock garments in abdominal trauma remains controversial. Diagnosis can be confirmed with either an ultrasound or a scan; if it is inconclusive, then arteriography can be done. Any of the following causes of splenomegaly should restrict an athlete from contact sports: a recent history of mononucleosis, a blood dyscrasia, or reactive lymphoid hyperplasia such as may occur with a viral infection.

LIVER INJURIES

The liver is the second most common frequently injured organ with blunt abdominal trauma. The typical mechanism is a blow to the midabdomen/right lower chest. The athlete may complain of pain not only in the right upper quadrant but also in the right shoulder. Management is similar to that of splenic injury. Diagnosis can be confirmed by ultrasound or computed tomography (CT) scan.

KIDNEY INJURIES

Contusions can result in flank pain and ecchymoses. Microscopic or gross hematuria may develop. More than 25% of boxers, college basketball players, college football players, and long-distance runners can develop occult hematuria without radiographic evidence of injury after competition, practice, or training (20,21). Athletes with gross hematuria secondary to trauma should be evaluated at an emergency facility. Continuous monitoring of the pulse and blood pressure and administration of IV fluids is recommended. An IVP or CT scan with contrast can be done to evaluate for hematoma or laceration (Fig. 3–7). Transport these athletes immediately with notification of a urologist.

Athletes who present with hematuria postexercise, called march hematuria, will present with blood in their urine after exercise. A repeat urinalysis at rest will demonstrate no hematuria. Treatment is reassurance.

PANCREATIC INJURIES

Injuries to the pancreas occur infrequently but can be life threatening. The typical injury is a direct blow to the midabdomen, occurring most commonly in football, motorcycle and auto racing, and cycling (from handlebars or steering wheel). The athlete complains of severe midabdominal pain progressing to diffuse pain suggestive of peritonitis. Rapid recognition, supportive care, and transportation are key to successful management.

Management includes routine blood test with a com-

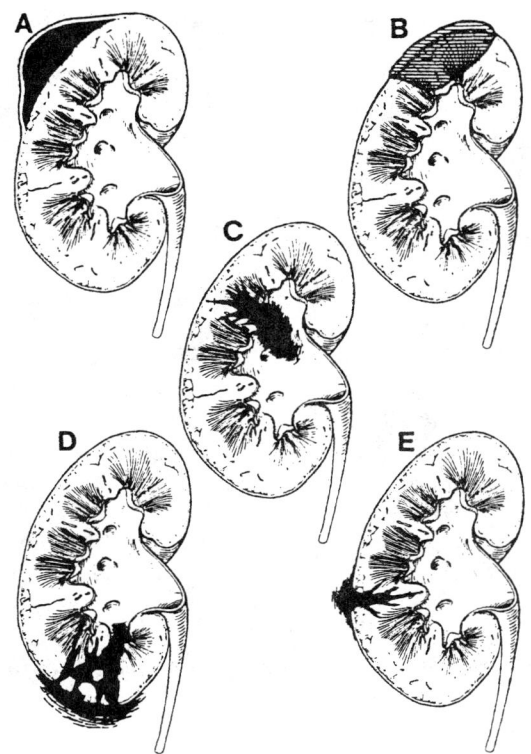

FIG. 3–7. Kidney injuries. (Reprinted with permission from Diamond DL. Sports-related abdominal trauma. *Clin Sports Med* 1989;8:91–99.)

plete blood cell count, chemistry profile, amylase, and lipase. Serum amylase measurement is often recommended as a screening measure in cases of suspected pancreas trauma (22,23). A CT scan of the abdomen can visualize any pancreatic abnormalities from trauma.

GENITOURINARY EMERGENCIES

Testicular trauma occurs commonly in sports such as soccer, football, and karate. Scrotal pain and swelling with inability to void are typical presenting complaints. The most common injury of the testicles is a contusion. Palpate the testicle for congruity. Transillumination can reveal either a hematocele, which poorly transilluminates, or a hydrocele, revealing a shadow. An ultrasound of the testes is the study of choice to rule out acute scrotal pathology. Management includes analgesics and bed rest with the athlete lying supine with the scrotum supported with towels.

The most serious consequence of testicular trauma is rupture, a surgical emergency. The tunica albuginea, the soft tissue covering the vascular and tubular structure of the testes, can rupture with impact. Bleeding can subsequently occur, causing swelling, constriction, and necrosis. Immediate urologic consultation is mandatory. An ultrasound of the testis should be done initially. A Doppler of the testis may follow the ultrasound if rupture is suspected.

MUSCULOSKELETAL EMERGENCIES

Dislocations of the knee are infrequent but are associated with a high risk of vascular injury and morbidity if not recognized and treated (24). The popliteal artery is commonly involved. The athlete presents with knee pain but may have no deformity; suspect a dislocation if recurvatum greater than 30°, positive Lachman maneuver with excursion greater than 10 mm indicating both anterior and posterior cruciate ligament disruption, and rapid hemarthrosis are noted (25).

Immediate management is directed at the assessment of the neurovascular status of the extremity on the field. Assess sensory or motor function as well as pulses distally. Reduction of both anterior and posterior dislocation is accomplished with longitudinal traction. After reduction, immobilize the knee in 5–10° of flexion. The athlete should be transported to a nearby emergency facility that has a vascular surgeon available.

More common are shoulder dislocations, which occur in football, hockey, and lacrosse. Most are either anterior or posterior. A fall on an outstretched upper extremity with abduction and external rotation of the shoulder is the typical mechanism in anterior dislocations. Posterior dislocations occur with a fall on a forwardly flexed and adducted arm.

Suspected shoulder dislocations should be evaluated on the sideline but preferably in the training room. A history of prior dislocation, subluxation, or instability is important from the standpoint of treatment. Examine the neck and cervical spine initially. Examine *both* shoulders and neurovascular status of the extremities. Provocative maneuvers such as the apprehension test, relocation test, fulcrum test, and sulcus sign should be performed.

Reduction of an anterior dislocation can be accomplished closed with a variety of techniques. The preferred technique is to have the athlete lying prone with the affected shoulder hanging off the side of the treatment table. While applying downward traction from the forearm or with a weight tied to the athlete's wrist, internally rotate the scapula until the shoulder is reduced. Other techniques such as the Stimson maneuver are discouraged because of increased risk of proximal humeral fractures and the Hippocratic method because of patient-required cooperation. Reevaluate neurovascular status after reduction. Once the dislocation is reduced, sling the shoulder and transport the athlete to the nearest emergency facility for postreduction X-rays. Reasons not to reduce any dislocations in the training room include suspicion of a fracture, compromised neurovascular status, or inexperience of the physician in doing reductions. When a fracture is suspected, the first priority is to assess the neurovascular status of the extremity.

Compound fractures should be covered with a sterile dressing that has been soaked in sterile saline or betadine. The joints above and below the fracture should be immobilized with splinting. Most fractures can be splinted with an inflatable air splint or plaster. A compressive ice pack can be applied to the affected area. En route to the hospital, observe the athlete for any signs of neurovascular compromise or shock. Estimates of blood loss from individual fractures vary. Blood loss from elbow, knee, or ankle fractures can range from 1 to 2 L, whereas pelvic and hip fractures can cause the loss of as much as 5 L.

EYE, EAR, NOSE, AND THROAT EMERGENCIES

The most common eye injuries encountered are corneal abrasions. The mechanism of injury is usually a finger in the eye. The typical symptoms are pain, photophobia, foreign body sensation, and tearing. Diagnosis can be confirmed by identifying an epithelial staining defect with fluorescein. The treatment includes antibiotic eye drops or ointment and a patch for 24 hours then recheck.

Hyphema is a more serious problem indicating significant trauma. Hyphema is a collection of blood in the anterior chamber, which can lead to visual deficits and a permanent loss of vision. A complete ocular exam should be performed. The treatment of hyphema is bed rest with the head of the bed elevated, eye shield, atropine 1% drops three to four times daily, and analgesics. The athlete should take no aspirin products.

Worrisome signs and symptoms associated with ocular injuries include loss of visual acuity, lack of movement of one eye, abnormal pupil size, laceration or penetration of the eyelid or globe, blood in between the cornea and iris, and abnormal pupil size or shape. Immediately tape a sterile eye pad over the eye, and cover this with a hard shield. A shield may be sufficient in some injuries in which the patch may cause excessive pressure on the globe. The athlete should then be transported to the nearest emergency facility for evaluation by an ophthalmologist.

Auricular hematoma, known as cauliflower ear, is most commonly seen in wrestling, football, and hockey. Typical presentation is a throbbing, painful, and swollen ear. Management is aspiration of the hematoma. Under sterile technique, a small-gauge needle (25δ) is inserted into the hematoma. After aspiration is complete, apply a compressive dressing to the ear using a colloidion pack or Paris cast. The player must keep this on for 24 hours or longer. It is suggested that antibiotics be administered if there is any signs of infection present (i.e., fever, pus, erythema).

The most common nasal injury is epistaxis resulting from a blow to the nose as in football, soccer, or hockey. In the absence of gross deformity, the epistaxis can be treated with ice and compression. If deformity is present or blood is noted in the posterior pharynx, then a fracture of the nasal bone or a posterior source of the bleeding is likely. Reduction on the sideline can be performed. More extensive fractures involving orbital bones may present with ecchymoses, or periorbital pain, which requires immediate evaluation by a maxillofacial surgeon or otolaryngologist. Posterior epistaxis will also require an ear-nose-throat consult.

Dental injuries include fracture or avulsion of a tooth, usually with contact sports such as football, hockey, wrestling, and lacrosse. Once the athlete is on the sideline, perform a thorough exam. Check for missing or loose teeth and for any hemorrhage or swelling around the teeth and gums by palpating the gum lines and each tooth. Examine the mandible for tenderness and range of motion. Initial management of any suspected fracture involving the teeth or mandible includes having the athlete breathe through his or her nose, applying a compression packing in the mouth with sterile gauze, and referral to a dental specialist. Immediate referrals include fracture through the enamel, dentin, and pulp and displacement or avulsion of a tooth.

An avulsion will be more obvious than the fracture. Take the avulsed tooth and place it in Hank's solution, saliva, or milk as a preservative. The tooth can be replaced intraorally within 30 minutes. If this is not possible, keep it in the preservative solution and refer the athlete to a dentist.

CONCLUSION

In summary, on-the-field emergencies will exist as long as sports are played. Management has improved because of communication and technology, as well as emphasis on prevention.

Many of the emergencies that are encountered on the field—such as sudden death, head injuries, or fractures—are not preventable. But more careful preparticipation physical examination to screen athletes; educating coaches, parents and athletes; and improvements in protective equipment will help decrease the incidence of serious athletic injuries.

REFERENCES

1. Garnder EN. *Athletics of the ancient world.* Oxford: Clarendon, 1930.
2. Clendening L. *Source book of medical history.* New York: Dover, 1960.
3. Gerberich SG, Priest JD, Boen JR, et al. Concussion incidences

and severity in secondary school varsity football players. *Am J Public Health* 1983;73:1370–1375.
4. Wilberger JE, Maroon JC. Head Injuries in Athletes. *Clin Sports Med* 1989;8:1–9.
5. American National Red Cross. *Cardiopulmonary resuscitation.* Washington, DC: American National Red Cross, 1981:25.
6. Emergency Cardiac Care Committee and Subcommittee, American Heart Association. Guidelines for the cardiopulmonary resuscitation and emergency cardiac care: adult basic life support. *JAMA* 1992;268:2184–2198.
7. Emergency Cardiac Care Committee and Subcommittee, American Heart Association. Guidelines for the cardiopulmonary resuscitation and emergency cardiac care: adult advanced cardiac life support. *JAMA* 1992;268:2199–2241.
8. Lehman LB, Ravich SJ. Closed head injuries in athletes. *Clin Sports Med* 1990;9:247–260.
9. Saunders RL, Harbaugh RE. The second impact in catastrophic contact-sports head trauma. *JAMA* 1984;252:538–539.
10. Maron BJ, Epstein SE, Roberts WC. Causes of sudden death in competitive athletes. *J Amer Coll Cardiol* 1986;7:204–214.
11. Bayes de Luna A, Coumel P, Leclercq JF. Ambulatory sudden cardiac death: mechanisms of production of fatal arrhythmia on the basis of data from 157 cases. *Am Heart J* 1989;117:151–159.
12. Weaver WD, Hill D, Fahrenbruch CE, et al. Use of the automatic external defibrillator in the management of out-of-hospital cardiac arrest. *N Engl J Med* 1988;319:661–666.
13. McFadden ER Jr, Denison DM, Waller JF, et al. Direct recordings of the temperatures in the tracheobronchial tree in normal man. *J Clin Invest* 1982;69:700–705.
14. Morgan DJ, Moodley I, Phillips MJ, et al. Plasma histamine in asthmatic and control subjects following exercise: Influence of circulating basophils and different assay techniques. *Thorax* 1983;38:771–777.
15. Strauss RH, McFadden ER, Ingram RH, et al. Enhancement of exercise-induced asthma by cold air. *N Engl J Med* 1977;297: 743–747.
16. Lee TH, Brown MJ, Nagy L, et al. Exercise-induced release of histamine and neutrophil chemotactic factor in atopic asthmatics. *J Allergy Clin Immunol* 1982;70:73–81.
17. McFadden ER Jr. Exercise-induced asthma: assessment of current etiologic concepts. *Chest* 1987;91:151S–157S.
18. Katz RM, Pierson WE. Exercise-induced asthma: current perspective. *Adv Sports Med Fitness* 1988;1:83–95.
19. Kidd JM, Cohen SH, Sosman AJ, et al. Food-dependent exercise-induced anaphylaxis. *J Allergy Clin Immunol* 1983;71:407–411.
20. Boone AW, Haltiwanger E, Chambers RL, et al. Football hematuria. *JAMA* 1955;158:1516–1517.
21. Kleiman AH. Renal trauma in sports. *West J Surg Obstet Gynecol* 1961;69:331–340.
22. Buechter KJ, Arnold M, Steele B, et al. The use of serum amylase and lipase in evaluating and managing blunt abdominal trauma. *Adv Sports Med Fitness* 1990;56(4):204–208.
23. Mure AJ, Josloff R, Rothberg J, et al. Serum amylase determination in blunt abdominal trauma. *Am Surg* 1991;57(4):210–213.
24. Green NE, Allen BL: Vascular injuries associated with dislocation of the knee. *J Bone Joint Surg Am* 1977;59A:236–239.
25. Varnell RN, et al. Arterial injury complicating knee disruption. *Am Surg* 1989;55:699.

CHAPTER 4

Medical Coverage of Endurance Events

Warren A. Scott and William O. Roberts

INTRODUCTION

The sphere of medical care at endurance sporting events will vary according to the activity, the intensity of the race, and the condition of the participants. Athletic activity can stress the body in a variety of ways and can unmask occult disease, including coronary artery disease (1). Imagine providing medical care for the Ironman Triathlon on the Big Island of Hawaii with a course 140 miles long in extremely hot, humid, and windy conditions (2), or managing the medical logistics for the New York City Marathon with nearly 30,000 entrants and the potential for millions of spectators, or the Birkebiner Nordic Ski Race with 8000 skiers in potentially frigid conditions through 55 kilometers of rural hilly terrain that has motor vehicle access at only four points along the course. Remote area event rescue attempts are very difficult and, when casualties occur, become an issue of survival. Issues of safety, injury prevention, and disaster management for the racers and spectators are in the domain of medical operations for mass participation events. Proactive involvement of the medical team will maximize safety and minimize morbidity. Much of the information presented in this chapter is taken from the medical operations and databases of the Twin Cities Marathon, the Falmouth Road Race, the Boston Marathon, the Hawaiian Ironman Triathlon, and numerous events around the world. These recommendations encompass the best of many plans and should provide the background to develop a well-managed medical care team for any race or event. With this information a medical director should be able to develop a working plan based on a model of a particular race setting. The model for race preparation is based on the areas outlined in Table 4–1. Event type, distance, participants, and anticipated environment will require race planners to adapt the model to each specific race.

PRERACE OPERATIONS

There are very few indexed publications on the approach to fieldside medical care at endurance sporting events. Although the how-to of individual race operations is sometimes outlined, comprehensive reporting of injury rates and patterns is often missing. Some references are given for medical care at athletic venues such as swimming meets, Olympic and pre-Olympic competitions (multiple sports), road races, and triathlons (3–16). It is important to note that every race has unique dimensions, including the course profile, weather conditions, and participant mix. Therefore it is necessary to individually design the best medical plan for each race site and condition according to both the shared and individual parameters of the activity.

There are many variables to address in developing medical operations for an event. Studying medical care experiences at a variety of endurance events will provide a framework for developing a medical team and event care plan. A local ten-kilometer race can easily attract several thousand runners. The medical care for this race can usually be accomplished with two or three health professionals and minimal first aid supplies. Some important aspects to consider that may increase the need for medical personnel include the expected age range of participants, the number of children, the number of seniors, and the number of walkers. Each group has the potential to alter the medical needs of the event. During hot, humid weather at this race distance, athletes who run at a fast pace can

---

W. A. Scott: Monterey Sports Center, Soquel, California 95073; and Kaiser Permanente Medical Center, Santa Clara, California 95051.

W. O. Roberts: MinnHealth Family Physicians, White Bear Lake, Minnesota 55110; and Department of Family Practice and Community Health, University of Minnesota Medical School, Minneapolis, Minnesota 55454.

TABLE 4–1. Race preparation areas

Competitor safety	Preparticipation screening	Supply type and distribution
Competitor education	Course setup	Staffing type and distribution
Race scheduling	Transportation	Medical and race records
Race start time	Communications	Medical care protocols
Emergency medical services notification	Fluids type and distribution	Medical volunteer safety precautions
Hazardous conditions	Equipment type and distribution	Adverse event protocol
Impaired competitor policy		

easily develop heatstroke, especially unacclimatized runners (17). Hot, humid conditions would require a larger medical staff and ice water tubs for onsite cooling protocols (18–20).

Even at shorter distances, a very large participant field will require a larger medical staff and more detailed plan. Very large runs, such as the Bloomsday Road Race with 50,000 entrants and the Bay to Breakers with 75,000 entrants, have the potential to tax the medical delivery system because of their sheer size. The potential for chance medical events rises with the large numbers as the statistics of background disease begin to play a role in the medical problems presenting to the medical team (21). These large races yield many individuals participating in physical exercise in various states of health, who complicate the risk equation. Preparticipation medical screening is usually not done for these citizen running races. Although the athletes sign a waiver attesting that they are familiar with the strenuous nature of running and that they are well prepared, the waiver will not ensure runner safety or event immunity from liability exposure. It is also possible that competitors will engage in "heroic exercise" and collapse from myocardial infarction, exertional heatstroke, or rhabdomyolysis (22). These very large events, when conducted in hot conditions, can yield numerous collapsed runners, some suffering with life threatening heatstroke. The medical team must have a broad capability for medical care in such a venue.

A small marathon may draw 500–1000 runners; however, the medical requirements will significantly increase as the injury rate increases with the marathon distance. Average conditioned athletes may push too hard and suffer from the problems common to the marathon race finish line, such as exercise-associated collapse, dehydration, exercise-associated muscle cramping, hypothermia, exertional hyperthermia, exercise exhaustion, and a variety of lower extremity musculoskeletal and skin injuries.

Very large numbers of participants in urban locations, as in the New York City Marathon or the London Marathon, with 25,000 to 30,000 runners, combine the increased injury rate of the marathon race with large participant numbers. The result can be large numbers of casualties, and the entire city must be ready for what in reality is a metropolitan disaster drill because of the mass of people who are at risk for injury. In addition to the runners, these highly populated urban center races often attract substantial numbers of spectators, who can become trapped inside the race and, should they become ill, may seek first aid from the race medical crew. Near the start of a local triathlon, a spectator collapsed in cardiac arrest. The medical team and on-site ambulance responded immediately, initiated resuscitation, and transported the downed spectator to a nearby hospital, where he made an excellent recovery. All large gatherings of athletes and spectators (25,000–50,000) present the possibility of spontaneous medical problems developing during the event with the medical team responding for first aid and transition to the emergency medical delivery system. Be prepared for chest pain, abdominal pain, allergic reactions, acute asthma, and other common medical problems. The race must not hamper the normal medical system access of the general populace. Most race medical facilities do not treat spectators except in a first response capacity, and a security team must be available to limit access to the medical tent and divert the spectators to local medical care facilities.

Bicycle events produce more trauma causalities owing to high speeds approaching 60 miles per hour with little protective equipment to guard the rider in a crash or fall. The problem is greatly compounded when prize money is involved and the racers take chances descending hills and cornering at high speed. In 1996 the Italian rider Casterili was killed in the Tour de France when he hit a wall at high speed. He was not wearing a helmet. High speeds yield major trauma, most of which should be immediately directed to the closest trauma center via an advanced life support (ALS) ambulance. The transfer and treatment protocols for resuscitation of major trauma victims should be defined in advance to ensure rapid transport to an emergency facility for definitive care. The local emergency facilities should be informed of the race and the potential for casualties. Always inform the medical officer at the receiving hospital of the incoming trauma victim if transport of an athlete from the race site is required. The medical team must decide in advance what trauma care will be offered on site, when to transfer the athletes for more extended care, and what special supplies will be required for on-site care.

A triathlon venue includes open water swimming in addition to biking and running. There are two transition stations (swim-bike and bike-run) that will require a medical station. The courses can be loops or point to point, both of which spread the athletes over a large area with increased needs for communication systems to allow the medical team to respond within reasonable time parameters. The lifeguards join the medical team, and all must be prepared for treating hypothermia and near drowning. The Chicago Triathlon is the largest in the United States, and many novice competitors participate. A participant in the Chicago Triathlon died from a myocardial infarction during the swim portion of the race, and his body was not discovered until several hours after his death. As the number of racers increases, there is a critical mass beyond which adequate surveillance of the participants to ensure safety and timely rescue becomes impossible.

Ultramarathon runs, usually defined as any distance greater than 42 kilometers, can be conducted on a standard track, in 1- to 3-mile loops on trails, or on point-to-point courses such as bike pathways and roads. The shorter loops keep the athletes in close observation, and the medical team can be centralized. The point-to-point races require mobile medical teams or very frequent stationary teams. Other ultradistance events involving bikes, canoes, horses, or skis may course through many miles of wilderness area, making surveillance and medical care very difficult. Wilderness route races (skiing, snowshoeing, ultramarathons, triathlon, and adventure racing) pose additional hazards for the athletes and new challenges for the medical team. Multiday endurance events expand the problems of the one-day ultra events. Multiday events may require several transition and check-in stations and a portable medical tent and team. Individual responsibility is very high in multiday events, and each athlete should have a support crew to assist in routine care. During the event emphasis is placed on helping the athletes to recover from their ailments or patching their injuries to allow safe completion of the race. Weather conditions may change unexpectedly, producing dangerous conditions for the athletes during the competition. The athletes participating in these races often require medical attention for skin problems (chafing, blisters, sunburn, abrasions); gastrointestinal problems (indigestion, nausea, cramps, vomiting, diarrhea); muscle cramping; and exhaustion. An experienced medical team providing care at ultra races uses an extensive array of products and medical tricks during the race to allow the athletes to continue in a more comfortable manner. The medical team must develop race-specific experience to appropriately advise the participants who seek medical attention. Fortunately, most of the athletes are well prepared for this type of event.

A majority of ultraendurance and multiday races conducted in off-road or wilderness settings require medical clearance before final acceptance into the event. The medical director should review all records and make note of at-risk individuals. Some athletes will have unusual and or unreasonable requests to participate in an event that has serious consequences. Each case should be reviewed well in advance of the race with the safety of the individual, the other participants, and the medical team taken into consideration before any exceptions to the race participation criteria are allowed. High-velocity sports (e.g., bicycling, skiing, canoeing, kayaking) have the potential for major trauma. Helicopters, four-wheel all-terrain vehicles, and snowmobiles will be required to replace ambulance transport in mountainous and wilderness settings. The medical team must be prepared to stabilize victims of shock, closed head injuries, or spinal cord injuries in remote areas.

Visually impaired, hearing impaired, and physically challenged athletes require special handlers, special routes, special equipment, and equipment transport vehicles on race day. Unique problems affecting these athletes include nerve compression injuries, injuries to insensate areas, and disruption of skin integrity in insensate areas and under a prosthesis. Spinal-cord-injured athletes have unique problems with thermoregulation and may develop autonomic dysreflexia in response to an occult injury.

The medical team must decide whether or not to be responsible for spectator medical care. The race administration will have to address spectator control during the race. Crowds can impede race flow, traffic flow, and ambulance pathways. Carefully review anticipated spectator flow before, during, and after the race so that the security team can effectively control spectators and their access to the medical areas.

RISK ASSESSMENT AND RISK REDUCTION

Before the event, it is essential to assess the risks specific to each race with respect to safety and medical issues. The race medical team must be aware of the event location, the course route and length, the participant profile, and the expected race weather conditions to structure the race health and safety plan with a goal of eliminating potential problems. The medical and safety plan should be established well in advance of race. Race site visits at different times of the day can reveal potential problems and are best conducted as a group project by the race board of directors and medical representatives. Given an expected range of weather conditions, the race management team must also prepare for unseasonably cold, hot, humid, windy, or rainy weather or other adverse conditions. The race distance is also important as faster-paced races in hot, humid conditions have a higher risk of exertional heatstroke than slower-paced races in the same conditions.

Longer races in milder temperatures will yield an increase in exercise-associated collapse. Predicting casualty numbers, peak injury locations, and peak injury volume is a guessing game until the race has historical data to more accurately predict injuries and injury types. High-speed events such as bicycle racing, especially on wet or icy surfaces, will dramatically increase the potential for crashes, resulting in major trauma and shock. It is very difficult to get athletes to slow down, even in adverse conditions. Event cancellation or modification may be the only safe alternative in situations with extremes of environment or unexpected and unsafe conditions.

What is really practical when it comes to risk reduction? Some situations are clearly beyond the control of the race administration and medical team. The responsibility of the race is to schedule and modify the event within the safest known parameters. An event can develop a life of its own, and as the spirit of the event gains momentum, all those participating cheer for the race to carry on, regardless of the potential consequences. Race organizers, sponsors, and athletes can lose sight of potential risks and vote for the race to proceed despite obvious safety hazards. Severe environmental hazards such as high surf, lightning, tornadoes, and hurricanes place all athletes and volunteers at risk for accidental death or injury, and the event may have to be rescheduled or modified immediately before the start or during the event. At a recent California triathlon, a first-year race director was forced to deal with unexpected high surf on race morning. The waves were six feet high and pounding the beach with great force. The first group of swimmers paddled through the waves, and two dozen athletes were washed back with the incoming surf. The race was postponed, and the swimmers were eventually sent off between the sets of surf. Of note in this race, the beach site was specifically selected for the swim because of its typically small surf. The higher than usual winter rains had caused the rivers to dump sand on the beach, which changed the sandbars and resulted in giant surf on race day. The lifeguards on duty at the beach were concerned about the safety of the participants and the responsibility they had as officials on the beach. This raises the question of authority to cancel an event. The safety of a race can change dramatically with the environment and may have to be canceled or part of the race venue may have to be altered. Who has the authority in this situation to change or cancel the event. Does the lifeguard have authority over the race director? Could the lifeguards have canceled the swim portion of the race? These are important situations that need to be fully analyzed by the race board of directors in advance of race day, and the participants should be informed of known potential event changes in the race literature. The safety of the participants should take precedent over the perception that the event must be completed in its original form.

High altitude, extreme cold, or high heat and humidity, although inherently dangerous, pose a more subtle threat, and not all athletes will be harmed in a similar fashion (23–26). Many in the athletic arena do not consider these conditions, especially high heat and humidity, to carry significant risk to the athlete, and it is difficult to cancel a large event because of heat and humidity. The International Federation for Skiing does impose a lower limit of $-20°C$ on the coldest point of the course as a cancellation or postponement benchmark for Nordic ski races.

The American College of Sports Medicine recommends canceling long-distance endurance events above a wet bulb globe temperature of 28°C (82°F), and the U.S. military suspends training above a wet bulb globe temperature of 90°F. Organizers of major races have been hesitant to commit to these recommendations. Hazardous conditions and the event response plan should be determined in advance of the race and be publicized for the participants so that there are no surprises on race day.

Extreme environment conditions, such as intense solar radiation, high wind, high altitude, extremes of the temperature range, high humidity, lightning, high surf, rain, hail, and snow, will profoundly affect the safety and medical outcome of many races. When these hazardous conditions are present, consideration must be given to canceling the event for the protection of the participants and the volunteers. In July 1992, a half Ironman triathlon race (swim one mile, bike 56 miles, and run 10 miles) was held in Evergreen, Colorado, at an elevation of 7000 feet above sea level. The temperature at the 6:30 A.M. start on race morning was 70°F. The bike route took the competitors up to 11,500 feet elevation. In the midmorning it began to snow and hail at the higher elevations. This weather change caught many of the participants on the bike portion of the race dressed in bathing suits and tank tops. The bike segment of the race included a long descent, causing the bikers to be wet, cold, and shaking uncontrollably while traveling over 45 miles per hour on the bike. There were a dozen crashes on the bicycle section of the race due to the weather changes and poor traction. The number of major trauma casualties overwhelmed the medical team. Postrace interviews revealed that the crash victims had tried to maintain race pace despite the slick road conditions, compared to those who did not crash, who had proceeded at a cautious pace to a lower elevation with clear roads and warmer weather. Unexpected situations arise during races, and it is unlikely that all the athletes will make the safest choices, which places them, their fellow competitors, and the race volunteers in jeopardy. Was anyone negligent in this situation? Can the race director make an improvement here? Should the race administration reserve the right to cancel when unexpected hazards arise on the course during the race or immediately before the start?

In 1990 Hurricane Bob hit Cape Cod with a vengeance. This storm made land one day after the Falmouth Road Race. Had the storm come in one day earlier, the area could have been packed with racers. Plans for potential disasters from weather-related activities should be considered in advance.

The swimming leg of a recent midsummer triathlon was held in a reservoir that served the nearby town. The race directors and the participants assumed that the water was safe, since the reservoir was the source of the drinking water for the town's residents. Over 100 triathlon participants contracted a very severe flu-like illness. One of the infected athletes was a medical doctor, and he eventually made the diagnosis of leptospirosis, which was confirmed as the pathogen in over 40 of the cases that resulted from the single exposure of swimming in the reservoir. Should the water be tested before mass participation swimming events? Is there testing that can be performed just before the event to detect any possible pathogens or toxins in the water?

What motivates risk taking? Athletes may sacrifice safety for speed. Reckless behavior is difficult to control during the event. Elite racers sometimes act as though they are above the law by proceeding in a fashion that maximizes performance but increases risk. Professional athletes can create additional risk for the event. Race officials should meet with the elite athletes before the race to explain any safety-related competitive rules and specifically state what behaviors will dictate time penalties or disqualification. Penalties for unsafe conduct help to control athletes who take excessive risks. As an example, an athlete who was trying to gain advantage tried to pass quickly through an uncontrolled intersection during the bike portion of a triathlon. He collided with a truck and was rendered quadriplegic. The bike course was not completely closed to traffic during the race. The prerace contestant information should outline the bike course and the potential traffic hazards. Athletes must be proactive when racing on courses that are not completely closed to traffic and continuously monitor their own safety. Safety dictates that competitors must obey all traffic rules in bike races and triathlons on noncontrolled roadways. Competitive athletes sometimes run stop signs to gain advantage if left to their own accord. Renegade behavior will increase the risk of trauma secondary to high-velocity accidents. Should there be a penalty for demonstrated reckless riding in these races? The more effective safety intervention is monitored traffic control and a course that is closed to traffic. This adds another dimension to race administration as police support to control race flow increases operating costs. Even with traffic control, motorists may drive through the barricades, putting competitors at undue risk. At the Twin Cities Marathon in 1997 an angry motorist who was delayed by the race drove around the barricades and across the course despite the presence of marathon safety personnel. In a separate episode in the late 1980s a driver inadvertently entered the race course when the traffic barriers were placed one block off the race course. An older gentleman left his home through the alley one-half block off the course. He took his usual route to church and ended up on the race course, where he struck a runner. The runner heard the car approaching and was able to tuck and roll after the impact. Fortunately, the runner was not injured. The barricades are now placed at the course intersection to prevent the access from the alleys and driveways that are within a block of the course.

Are there risks that have been inadvertently or intentionally ignored by the race administration? Promoters may overlook safety concerns to save time and money or to satisfy sponsors. Ignoring a potential problem does not reduce the liability exposure of the medical team, and it is the obligation of the medical team to protect the athletes from these abuses. The legal system requires race promoters to produce a safe event and to identify and disclose all of the known risks to the athletes. Participants should sign a waiver acknowledging those risks and assume personal responsibility for their participation. The waiver should serve as an educational tool for the athletes and help every participant to achieve a successful outing on race day. Some issues and situations during or after the race are beyond the control of the organizers and medical personnel. Document these incidents, and explain in detail the race medical team response and future modifications to prevent repeat episodes.

Medical Disqualification of Athletes

The medical staff should reserve the option to evaluate competitors who appear to be in distress during the event. Athletes should be informed before the race of the potential for a medical disqualification and that they may receive an evaluation and first aid from medical volunteers without disqualification during the event. The medical team should develop the criteria for a competitor to continue participating before race day and disseminate the impaired competitor policy to the medical team, administration, race volunteers, and athletes. The race executive committee should approve and support the criteria for the event. The ability to assess the athlete and return him or her to competition is critical for the safety of the athletes. If the ability to assess and return to competition is not allowed, athletes will take unnecessary risks in hot and cold conditions. The usual criteria to proceed in an event include being oriented to person, place, and time; knowing details of the event;

making straight-line progress toward the finish; maintaining a good competitive posture; and appearing clinically fit. The medical risk to an individual athlete in good health competing in an endurance race is low, and the likelihood of a life- or limb-threatening accident is small. If injury or illness occurs during the event, the medical staff should assess the athlete, provide initial first aid treatment, and determine whether the athlete can return to the event. When a true medical emergency occurs, the chance for successful completion of the event has ended, and the emphasis is on minimizing the risk of morbidity or mortality to the athlete. The decision to return an athlete to the event is based on the provider's knowledge and experience and may in some circumstances seem subjective. The return to activity decision should be conservative and temporary until the athlete can obtain definitive assessment and treatment from his or her physician of choice. When it is determined that it is unsafe for the athlete to return to the event, the race managers must be notified that the athlete is medically disqualified. Disqualification is often required when interventions such as intravenous fluids are instituted. The medical spotters (nonmedical volunteers) should be provided with some specific instructions to help identify potentially impaired athletes and direct them toward evaluation and definitive care.

PRERACE CONTESTANT INFORMATION

Education of athletes is an important first step in preventing medical problems that may develop during the race. Competitor education is an active primary prevention strategy that requires the cooperation of the athlete and is not as effective as the passive strategies that are out of the athlete's control. The medical team should identify and disclose all safety and hazard issues the athletes may encounter. Recommendations regarding nutrition, fluids, heat and altitude acclimatization, and equipment selection will help athletes to reduce their risk. More extensive individual preparation is required for longer and more challenging events, and the educational effort should reflect the complex issues that will confront the participants. The contestant education information should be included in the waiver, the registration materials, the acceptance notification, the medical preparticipation questionnaire, and the prerace packet. The education materials should inform athletes of the race volunteer services and how to access the race medical volunteers during the race. If there are specific situations in which the medical team cannot provide assistance during the race, describe when and where the athletes must assume personal responsibility for their health and safety. In situations in which athletes will not have full medical coverage during an event, inform the athletes in a mandatory prerace meeting immediately before the start to provide last-minute directions and corrections that may influence injury patterns.

PREPARTICIPATION MEDICAL QUESTIONNAIRE AND EXAMINATION

More arduous races lasting longer than eight hours often require thorough screening and medical documentation of fit state of health by a physician before participation is allowed. These events usually have a manageable number of entrants, and the medical director should review each medical record before the race. Participants in all races should be instructed to record special problems and medications on the back of the race number, but it is difficult to ensure compliance. This medical information is especially helpful in longer races in remote wilderness areas. The preparticipation exchange of information provides an opportunity for the athlete to relay any special needs to the race director and medical team.

MEDICAL OPERATIONS

Administrative Responsibilities

The medical director should serve on the executive board of the race committee. A presence on the board allows the medical director to establish the chain of authority regarding critical race decisions involving the health and safety of the participants. The medical director is an advocate for the participants and in the best position to protect the race and the racers from unsafe practices. It is important to review all medical policies with the board before the event. Safety and medical issues should be clarified, and the chain of command for race day should be established. It is important for medical directors to know who is ultimately responsible for health and safety decisions on race day and to be aware of potential conflicts of interest in the person who is designated to make the decisions. Ideally, this responsibility should rest with the medical director or jointly with the medical director and the president or chairman of the race executive board. Many races have millions of sponsor dollars invested in the event, and a conflict can easily arise if safety considerations point toward cancellation of the event. Sponsors may lobby for the race to carry on, with seeming disregard for the safety of the participants. A preventable adverse event, when engaging in risky practices in the public sector, may be considered negligent, putting both the medical team and the event at risk if the actual or anticipated conditions warranted modification or cancellation of the event. The medico-legal recommendation for the medical director is to act in a responsible manner, attempting to provide the standard of medical care and advice to protect the participants despite external pressures to the contrary.

The Race Medical Director's Objectives and Goals

A race medical director should provide an effective plan for the care of athletes in medical emergencies. The medical director should be able to identify the types of medical emergencies that are likely to occur during the event, determine the personnel and equipment needed to deliver emergency medical care at the event, and describe an appropriate plan of care for injured athletes. A race medical emergency is an acute illness or injury that poses an immediate threat to an athlete's life or carries the risk of prolonged disability. The medical director's duties include designing treatment protocols, dispensing written guidelines for the medical team, and estimating the volume and cost of medical supplies and services for all the medical problems that are likely to be encountered during the event. The medical volunteer expectations should be written to ensure uniform and consistent throughout the event. Medical volunteers should be instructed not to exceed the limits of their training and licensure and should understand what to do if they encounter a distressed athlete. It is important for all event volunteers to know how to access the medical care system.

Medical team planning should begin at least one year in advance to ensure a successful outcome. A first-time event will require more organization and may require more than a year of planning for large events. A working timeline is helpful to appreciate the dynamic nature of providing medical care at sporting events. Charting the preparation steps on the calendar will decrease the risk of omissions in prerace preparation. List all the steps and equipment that are required to assemble and outfit the medical team. A separate timeline for race day, specifically addressing medical access to the course and participants and the expected staffing and duration of service at specific stations during the race, should be included in the medical planning. The medical team requires unlimited access to all parts of the race course and finish area. Maps can assist with the overall perspective of the event. It is helpful to construct a series of maps to focus on different areas of the event, including the race course, the finish area, the medical tent layout, the communications network, the course well-athlete pickup vehicle flow, the course emergency vehicle flow, the on-course vehicle traffic flow, the off-course vehicle traffic flow, the athlete flow, and the spectator flow. The flow patterns will be time specific, and the need for medical care will change as the flow of runners peaks and wanes along the race course. For example, a 19-mile marathon medical aid station will not need staffing at the start of the race but will need to be staffed with the medical providers at 85 minutes for the runners and at 75 minutes if wheelchair racers are participating. The peak staffing for the 19-mile aid station at the Twin Cities Marathon would be at 150 minutes into the race, which would correspond to the peak flow of runners on the course.

Medical Protocols

The medical team must decide in advance of the race what problems will be treated on site and how long an athlete with a medical problem will be cared for on site during the race and after the race is concluded. In advance of the event, it is important to determine which medical and trauma problems will require immediate triage to an emergency facility in a hospital setting. A simple classification system of injury and illness is listed in Figure 4–1. Race course and finish line triage can be classified in several categories, including medical, musculoskeletal, psychologic, dermatologic, and traumatic. Panic attacks can ensue in open water swims and extreme environment situations. Head and neck trauma can occur in high-speed activities and requires the ability to stabilize the injured athlete's neck before transport to an emergency facility. Major trauma requires immediate access to emergency medical services transport, and an on-site ambulance dedicated to the race is essential in high-risk situations. Minor trauma can be handled on site if the equipment and materials necessary to provide this treatment are available. Medical protocols for fluid and electrolyte, cardiac, asthma, anaphylaxis, insulin shock, and thermal injury should be available for the medical team (27–35).

Common problems in the marathon include exercise associated muscle cramping, hypothermia, hyperthermia, exercise associated collapse, dehydration, and exhaustion. Evaluation and treatment of exhaustion and dehydration during the race and at the finish area should be standardized so that seriously ill athletes are identified quickly (36–45). Mild muscle cramps can be treated with stretching, massage, accupressure, oral electrolyte-carbohydrate solutions, and rest. More severe cramping may require pharmacologic intervention with intravenous fluids and diazepam or magnesium sulfate. Exertional hyponatremia is an emerging problem in endurance activities, especially in events lasting longer than 4–5 hours. The working hypothesis for the onset of exertional hyponatremia is overhydration with resultant water intoxication presenting with cerebral and pulmonary edema. Several fatal and severe nonfatal cases have been reported in the past 2–3 years. Medical personnel should be cautioned not to assume all collapse is from dehydration, and the use of on-site diagnostic laboratory devices for $Na+$, $K+$, O_2 saturation, glucose, and hematocrit may be useful in distinguishing the etiology of collapse in the finish area medical tent. Slow marathoner runners and other long-endurance participants should be warned and taught to match fluid intake to fluid losses rather than following the current replacement schedules for water and fluids that run the risk of overhy-

```
MARATHON MEDICAL RECORD - CONFIDENTIAL©                          19_____
Race # _____  Location: Finish / Aid Station Mile _____   Arrival Time: _____
Name _____          Discharge time: _____
Age: _____  Gender: M / F   Finish Time: _____
Previous marathons: # Entered: _____ ; # Finished: _____  Best previous time: _____
Weekly Mileage: _____        Pre-race injury/illness: Y / N
                                 Describe _____
```

Skin, Bones, & Joints

Complaint:	Pain	Blister	Abrasion	Bleeding	Cramps	Swelling
	Other _____					
Tissue:	Skin	Muscle	Tendon	Ligament	Bone	
	Other _____					

Location: Toe   R / L   Knee   R / L
           Foot R / L   Thigh R / L
           Ankle R / L   Hip   R / L
           Calf R / L   Back   R / L
           Other _____

Diagnosis: Blister   Tendinitis
           Sprain   Abrasion
           Strain   Cramps
           Bursitis   Stress Fx (suspected)
           Fasciitis
           Other _____

Notes:

(side 2)
Medical Problems   Arrival Time _____
Race # _____   Discharge time _____
Symptoms & Signs
Exhaustion   Lightheaded   Stomach cramps
Fatigue   Confused   Leg cramps
Hot or Fever   Headache   Rapid heart rate
Vomiting   Nausea   Palpitations'
Unconscious   CNS changes   Muscle spasms
Other _____

Mental Status: Alert   or   Responds to: Voice / Touch / Pain
Orientation: Person / Place / Time
Walking Status: Alone / With assistance / Unable
Other _____

Time	Temp (rectal)	BP	Pulse	IV fluids	Meds/Rx

Notes:

Diagnosis
EAC   Other _____   IV fluid   Y / N
Hyperthermic: mild / mod / severe   _____ $D_{50}W$ Y / N
Normothermic: mild / mod / severe   _____   ER transfer   Y / N
Hypothermic: mild / mod / severe   _____   Discharge home   Y / N
☺☺

FIG. 4–1. Example of a medical data collection card.

dration if the sweat rate is surpassed (46). Ultradistance races frequently rely on medical checkpoints and weigh stations to help ensure individual racer safety. Abrasions and blisters are common in all endurance events, and the medical team should be instructed in a uniform skin care protocol. The protocols should address the issues of chance medical events and have a simple method to activate emergency medical service (EMS) providers and transportation. An ALS ambulance should be on site at the finish area and other high-risk areas on the course. Experienced volunteers and racers will have favorite methods for treating race-induced ailments that can be incorporated into the medical protocols. On the course and in the finish area, crowds can hamper access to injured runners. Response plans should account for crowding along the course, and the finish area should be secured to improve access to the competitors.

The medical staff should be well versed in modified universal precautions, and the medical care areas should be restricted to casualties and providers. Nonmedical volunteers should be instructed in the blood-borne pathogen policy and risk. All volunteers in the medical area should be immunized for hepatitis B, and minors should have their parents' permission before being placed in pathogen-risk sections of the medical area. Red bag waste and sharps containers should be conveniently placed throughout the medical area. Large basins should be available for emesis, and a wheelchair-accessible portable toilet should be located near the medical tent for competitors who develop diarrhea during and after the competition.

Staffing an Event Medical Team

The medical team will require both medical and nonmedical personnel. Nonmedical personnel are necessary for medical communications, medical transportation, medical security, stocking medical supply tables, fetching dry clothing, communication with family members waiting outside the medical area, cleanup, and record keeping. Nurses and physicians can be recruited from hospitals, clinics, and residency programs. Other medically trained personnel can be obtained from local EMS groups, local hospitals, state athletic training Associations, American Red Cross chapters, military units, National Ski Patrol, National Bicycle Patrol, Explorer Scout troops, and medical schools.

Medical Record Keeping

Medical records are essential to record treatment rendered by the medical team and for epidemiologic data on your race to assess future needs for medical supplies and staffing. Accurate records allow the medical director to begin to predict the potential for injury when the injury rates are correlated to the weather conditions. Tracking the meteorologic conditions for race day should become a part of the race record system along with entrants, starters, finishers, and medical casualties. The medical record can be designed to be processed in many different ways on a computer database. Table 4–2 and Figure 4–1 are examples of various medical records. Comprehensive forms, tailored to the common medical problems at a specific event seem to work well. It may be best to review examples from other races. Forms printed on heavyweight paper or cardboard will withstand the rigors of the medical tents better than standard weight paper. Over time the event medical record will evolve to improve data collection and provide useful data for developing race strategies that increase participant safety and reduce morbidity.

Hospital and Emergency Medical Services Notification

The local hospitals and emergency medical services should be notified in advance of the event, especially if the hospitals will be receiving event casualties. The letter of notification should describe the event type, location, and course route; the number of participants; event medical staffing; ambulance transport support, anticipated casualities and usual medical problems; and the medical team's goals for on-site and hospital-based care. It is also helpful to send information about your capacity as medical director to local police, fire, ambulance, and hospital personnel.

Medical Volunteer Education

A review of medical operations and medical services should be presented at team meeting before the event, either in didactic presentation or, at a minimum, as a written handout. A second meeting should occur on race day, conducted by the lead physician at each aid station. The education sessions should emphasize the medical protocols and the need for all encounters to be recorded.

Race Day Transportation

Transportation should be arranged for well dropouts and ill or injured participants. This can be as simple as shuttle vans or golf carts picking up the runners who are unable to continue. In remote areas, snowmobiles and all-terrain vehicles may be required for motorized access to participants. Transportation and shelter for well dropouts is critical in cool or cold conditions to prevent the onset of hypothermia in competitors who are wet with sweat and can lose body heat rapidly.

Ill or injured participants will require more sophisticated transportation with the ability to deliver medical

TABLE 4–2. *Medical services data summary*

Date:	Venue:	Location:	
Number of Doctors: Nurses:		Phys Therapy:	Students
Water temperature:			
Start air temperature:			
Minimum ambient air temperature:			
Maximum ambient air temperature:			
Relative humidity at start:			
Dewpoint at start:			
Dewpoint at 1- to 4-hour intervals:			
Black globe temperature at start:			
Black globe temperature at 1- to 4-hour intervals:			
Entrants:	Starters:	Finishers:	% Finishers:
Number Treated:	Athletes:	Spectators:	Staff/Volunteers:
Minor injuries:		Treated and returned to race:	
Minor sprains and strains:			
Minor contusions and abrasions:			
Major injuries (requiring more than an ice bag or Band-Aid):			
Major sprains and strains:			
Major contusions and abrasions:			
Treatment and disposition:			
Treated and released:			
Treated and not able to return to race:			
IV starts, number and percent:			
ALS transport:			
BLS transport:			
Self-transport (recommended follow-up at emergency department or urgent care site):			
Patients who were transported:			
Patient's Name: Athlete No.: Reason for Transport: Mode: Receiving Facility:			

care. Ambulance services should be enlisted to provide on course response to downed runners and to transport casualties from the finish area medical tent. In remote race sites, helicopter, snow cat, or toboggan transport may be required for rapid evacuation of injured competitors.

Race Day Communications and Surveillance

Communication systems are essential for rapid response to injury or illness during an event. The communication system should connect the medical providers and connect the medical team with the event administration. In large events, communications systems may need to link lifeguards, rescue boats, paddlers, first aid tents, mobile medical units, medical headquarters, a hospital emergency department, an EMS ambulance, police units, security teams, race command, and medical personnel. A person who is skilled in communications networking should be recruited to coordinate a comprehensive communication system for the event. Cellular phones, short-wave radio, and hardwired phones are all useful, but a well-designed ham radio network will give widespread, coordinated communications along the course. The central communications unit is ideally located in the medical area to keep the medical director and tent personnel informed of problems on a race course. A race course is often spread out over many miles, and communications between the finish area medical personnel and the course aid stations is essential. A radio-equipped vehicle should follow the last participant on the race course to provide radio contact with the director for course closure and withdrawal of medical support teams.

Drug Testing and Doping Control

A race that offers prize money or of international significance may be required to provide doping control testing for a national or international governing body. Individuals participating in the event may be selected for testing on the basis of finish order or random draw at the discretion of the governing body. The drug-testing personnel are often provided by the organization requesting the testing, but the event will be expected to provide the facility and ancillary personnel. It is best to separate the medical team from the drug-testing team so that there is no perceived conflict of interest. The drug-testing team should get the full cooperation of the race administration and medical team. Cooperation with the drug-testing team is critical when an athlete is temporarily detained in the medical tent for evaluation and treatment. The medical team can be proactive on several fronts by stocking only USOC-approved medications and fluids and by educating volunteers in the doping control process.

TABLE 4-3. *Medical supplies (in alphabetical order)*

Acetaminophen	Diazepam: injectable, tablets	Oto-ophthalmoscope
ACLS supplies, medications	Diphenhydramine: tablet, injectable	Penlights
Adrenaline	Duct tape	Pens
Albuterol inhaler	EKG monitor	Petroleum jelly
Alcohol wipes	Elastic wraps	Pocket airways
Ambu bag	Endotracheal tubes	Podiatric supplies
Aminophylline	Epinephrine	Polysporin ointment
Amoxicillin	Epi-Pen	Povidone-iodine: ointment, solution, soap, scrub-brush
Anaphylaxis kit	Erythromycin: tablet, topical; skin, eye	
Anesthetics: oral, topical, injectable, eye	Eye pads	Prewrap
Antacid tablets	Eye wash	Q-Tips
Antibiotic ointment: skin, eye	Flashlights	Scissors: bandage, iris, suture, heavy duty
Antibiotics: tablet, injectable	Garbage can	Scrub brushes
Antifungal: topical, tablets	Gauze: pads, rolls	Sharps container
Antihistamines: tablet, injectable	Gloves: exam	Sheets
Antinausea: tablet, injectable, topical patch	Gloves: sterile	Signs
Asthma kit	Glucose monitor	Slings, arm
Atropine	Goggles (or eye protection)	Soap
Band-Aids	Gooseneck lamp	Spine board
Basins	Hand wipes	Splints: arm, leg, ankle, wrist, finger
BCLS supplies	Hydrogen peroxide	Steri strips
Beds	Ibuprofen	Stethoscope
Bee sting kit	Ice	Sunscreen
Biohazard spill kit	Intubation kit	Suture packs
Blankets	IV dressings	Syringes various sizes
Blood pressure cuffs	IV fluids setups	Tables
Cardiac medications	IV fluids	Tape: cloth, elastic, paper
Cervical collars	Kling gauze	Tegaderm
Chairs	Knee immobilizer	Telfa pads (any nonstick)
Clipboards	Lidocaine: oral, topical, injectable	Tent
Clothesline	Magnesium sulfate: injectable	Thermometer sheaths
Coban	Marcaine 0.5%	Thermometers: rectal (high- and low-temperature ranges)
Cooler	Medical reporting forms	
Corticosteroids: tablets, injectable, topical, inhaled	Medical staff shirts, ID badges	Tongue blades
	Naloxone	Tourniquets
Cots	Narcotic analgesics	Towels
Crash cart supplies	Needles: angiocath 16g, 21g,	Tube gauze
Crutches	Needles: standard 16g, 21g, 25g, 27g	Xeroform gauze
Defibrillator	Normal saline irrigation	Ziplock bags
Defibrillator pads	Ophthalmologic kit	
Dextrose: 50 gr in water	Oral airways	

Medical First Aid and Treatment Stations

The location and level of care provided at medical aid stations will vary according to the type and frequency of injury seen most frequently along the course. Aid stations can be classified as stationary or mobile and as minor care or major care. The level of care offered at each aid station will determine staffing and supply needs (see Table 4-3). Major aid stations usually provide full medical care, including intravenous fluids, and minor aid stations usually offer comfort cares with first aid, shelter, and injury stabilization. Minor aid stations depend on the emergency transport system to move casualties to the nearest emergency facility or major aid station. The athletes should be informed of the location of aid stations and what level of care will be provided at each station. In some circumstances athletes will be expected to provide for themselves, especially in backcountry locations and events. Stationary medical aid stations are often located near the fluid stations. Stationary locations should be located in areas that are easily visible to the competitors and easily accessible by the emergency medical services responsible for transport of casualties.

The finish area should have a major medical station. Large events with high injury rates may require more than one tent to accommodate all the casualties. The tent or buildings should provide shelter as well as privacy. Medical area entry triage can speed the care process by moving casualties to the proper evaluation and treatment section. It is prudent to designate a team to respond to cardiac arrest and competitors who present to the medical area in an unconscious state. The finish line medical area should be equipped to evaluate and stabilize cardiac arrest and other forms of syncope while awaiting transfer to a medical facility. The chest pain protocol at the Twin Cities Marathon calls for runners with chest pain to be evaluated in the ALS ambulance and be either transferred to the emergency room or released to the medical tent if the problem does not have a cardiac origin.

SPECIAL RACES AND SITUATIONS

Triathlon Races

The obvious difference in the triathlon competition is the water hazard in the open water swim portion of the race. The large geographic area involved in an Ironman length triathlon (2.4 km swim, 180 km bike, and 42 km run) usually dictates the need for a main medical tent and several satellite or mobile clinics for adequate medical coverage. The bike portion of the race will increase the risk of major trauma.

Swim Races

Open water swimming involves a new set of risks and hazards that requires the inclusion of lifeguards and water-based personnel on the medical team. Lifeguards are necessary for near drowning and open water rescues. In most open water races, hypothermia is a risk owing to immersion in cool water. In water that is less than 65°F, a wet suit is often required for added insulation and heat retention to decrease the risk of hypothermia. Digital, facial, and eye trauma are common at the start and during the race when swimmers bunch up and collide with one another. Skin trauma may require a temporary closure until it can be definitively fixed after the race. It is not unusual for swimmers to develop psychological problems such as panic attack during the start and race portions of an open water swim. Storms, fog, and high surf will increase the risk to all competitors and make surveillance of the athletes a risk for the volunteers in and on the water. Postponement or cancellation may be necessary. Toxic chemicals and biological infectious agents can be unseen risks in open water swims.

Bike Races

Bicycles or other wheeled vehicles (roller skis, in-line skates, and wheelchairs) increase the forward velocity of the athlete and increase the risk of major trauma (47). An athlete with major trauma is best transported to an emergency medical center, but the medical team will need to be prepared to initiate the evaluation and first aid on site while waiting for the transport team. A course that is designed for safety will decrease the risk in these high-speed events.

Nordic Skiing Races

Cold temperatures and the dangers of high-speed events complicate the medical care of Nordic ski races, especially if conducted at higher altitudes (48,49). By their nature, most long-distance races are held in fairly remote areas on trails that are not easily accessible by the usual urban rescue and transport vehicles. Volunteers who are inadequately prepared for cold weather duty can be at risk for cold-induced problems. Many competitors assume that the cold protects them from fluid loss and do not adequately hydrate along the course. Downhill starts and turns at the bottoms of hills are particularly dangerous in mass participation ski races. Wave starts and attention to course design can dramatically reduce injury risk. Frostbite is a risk from both actual and relative windchill. Cold weather modification and cancellation parameters should be determined and published in advance. Eye protection should be recommended to help prevent frostbite of the cornea.

Ultraendurance Events

Ultraendurance events (bicycle, run, equestrian, ski, snowshoe, canoe/kayak, and dogsled racing) require serious and intensive prerace preparation by the athlete. The medical team places less emphasis on rescue and more emphasis on athlete monitoring and maintenance during the event. The 5- to 30-hour events (50–100 miles of running, 100–200 miles of cycling) are becoming more common. Many of these events cross vast expanses of poorly accessible wilderness area. A massage team, course monitors, and a roving medical team can help athletes to complete the event more safely. Blister treatment is very important. A large variety of skin and foot care products should be available to the medical team and the athletes. Many ultraendurance athletes will be skillful in applying their own favorite bandage during the race if a problem develops. Treatment of indigestion takes on a new meaning during ultraracing. It is essential to process fluids and calories over many hours. A variety of over-the-counter medications are the safest approach to controlling acid reflux symptoms during ultraendurance events. Sometimes it is necessary for an athlete to lie down to overcome the feeling of malaise associated with ultraendurance activities. Slowing down for an hour or two may also prove helpful for many competitors.

Multiple-Day Races

In multiple-day races there is a need for more stringent prerace screening and more assumption of risk by athletes. The athletes must be well prepared for these challenging endurance events. As in ultraraces, skin and foot care are of paramount importance. Rehydration requirements and physical performance standards are common for these events and provide a yardstick for measuring safety and injury risk. The emphasis of the medical team is to monitor the athlete and minimize the need for heroic rescues.

Wilderness routes, such as the Western States 100-mile endurance run, carry the runners over mountainous trails to high elevations. These routes are nearly inaccessible except for emergency helicopter rescues. The racers are rigorously tested before the race and are given extensive instructions on the possibility of injuries and medical problems they are likely to encounter during the race. Mandatory weigh-in stations are located along the race course. To ensure proper maintenance of hydration, the athletes cannot proceed past the checkpoints if their weight is 10% or more below the starting weight. The medical team must be prepared for frostbite, hypothermia, acute mountain sickness, high-altitude cerebral edema, and high-altitude pulmonary edema.

Physically Challenged Athletes

The special needs of physically challenged athletes present a unique set of problems for the medical team. Wheelchair athletes develop unusual problems under the strain of athletic competition, especially in the hot, humid conditions that can precipitate dehydration. A thorough prerace screening should be conducted to ensure the safety of the physically challenged competitor (and the surrounding athletes). A preparticipation medical history submitted to the race medical team before the race should be mandatory in high-risk activities. A physician of the athlete's choice must sign a physical readiness medical form before acceptance into the event. Special transition areas and access routes may need to be included. Other problems include thermoregulatory concerns, indwelling urinary catheters, high-speed safety issues, special support crew to transport the athlete's equipment, special access areas, skin care protocols, occult skin and musculoskeletal trauma, and autonomic dysreflexia. The medical director should be informed of any special equipment, medications, or extra personnel required for the physically challenged athletes participating in the event.

POSTRACE OPERATIONS

After the race it is important to assess the effectiveness of the prevention strategies in place for the event and the performance of the medical team during the event. Look at the effective strategies, the ineffective strategies, the workload of the volunteers, the injury types, supplies used for the race, what strategies need improvement, and what can be added or dropped to improve the effectiveness of the medical team. Modify the data collection survey to capture the information that is most helpful to the event medical operation, and assess the usefulness of the medical record for the medical care providers. Consider altering the race to improve the safety profile. Continue to record medical encounters and analyze the race records, as event-specific past experience is the best predictor of future needs of the race and of what is required to minimize casualties during an event.

REFERENCES

1. Elchner ER, Scott WA. Exercise as disease detector. *Phys Sportsmed* 1998;26:41–52.
2. Laird RH. Medical care at ultra endurance triathlons. *Med Sci Sports Exerc* 1989;21(5 Supp):S222–S225.
3. Elias S, Roberts WO, and Thorson DC. Team sports in hot weather: guidelines for modifying youth soccer. *Phys Sportsmed* 1991;19:67–80.
4. Baker WM, Simone BM, Neimann JT. Special event medical care at the 1984 LA Summer Olympics experience. *Ann Emerg Med* 1986;51:185–190.
5. Hannay DR, English BK, Usherwood TP. The provision and use of medical services during the 1991 World Student University Games. *J Public Health Med* 1993;15:229–234.
6. Laskowski ER, Najarian MM, Smith AM. Medical coverage for multiple sports competition: a comprehensive analysis of the injuries in the 1994 Star of the North Summer Games. *Mayo Clin Proc* 1995;70:549–555.
7. Martin RK, Yesalis CE, Foster D. Sports injuries at the 1985 Junior Olympics: an epidemiologic analysis. *Am J Sports Med* 1987;15:603–608.
8. Gonzalez D. Medical coverage of endurance events. *Prim Care* 1991;18:867–887.
9. Sanders AB, Criss E, Steckl P. An analysis of medical care at mass gatherings. *Ann Emerg Med* 1986;15:515–519.
10. Franaszek J. Medical care at mass gatherings. *Ann Emerg Med* 1986;15:600–601.
11. Hadden W, Kelly S, Pumford N. Medical care for the golf championship. *Br J Sport Med* 1992;26:125–127.
12. Crouse B, K Beattie. Marathon medical services: strategies to reduce runner morbidity. *Med Sci Sports Exerc* 1996;28:1093–1096.
13. Jones BH, Roberts WO. Medical management of endurance events. In Cantu RC, Micheli LJ, eds. *ACSM: guidelines for the team physician.* Philadelphia: Lea & Febiger, 1991.
14. Laird RH, ed. *Medical coverage of endurance events.* Ross Symposium, Columbus, OH: Ross Laboratories, 1988.
15. Noble HB, Bachman D. Medical aspects of distance race planning. *Phys Sportsmed.* 1979;7:78–84.
16. Richards D, Richards R, Schofield PJ, et al. Management of heat exhaustion in Sydney's The Sun City-to-Surf Fun Run. *Med J Aust* 1979:2:457–461.
17. Booth J, Marino F, Ward JJ. Improved running performance in hot humid conditions following whole body precooling. *Med Sci Sports Exerc* 1997;29:943–949.
18. American College of Sports Medicine. Position statement on heat and cold illnesses during distance running. *Med Sci Sports Exerc* 1996;28:i–vii.
19. Armstrong LE, Maresh CM. The induction and decay of heat acclimatisation in trained athletes. *Sports Med* 1991;12:302–312.
20. Barthel HJ. Exertion-induced heat stroke in a military setting. *Military Med* 1990;155:116–119.
21. Maron B, Poliac LC, Roberts WO. Risk for sudden death associated with marathon running. *J Am Coll Cardiol* 1996;28:428–431.
22. Eichner ER. Editorial: Sacred cows and straw men. *Phys Sportsmed* 1991;19:24.
23. Bracher MD. Environment and thermal injury. *Clin Sports Med* 1992;11:419–436.
24. Heggers JP, MC Robson, et al. Experimental and clinical observations on frostbite. *Ann Emerg Med* 1987;16:1056–1062.
25. Mills WJ. Field care of the hypothermic patient. *Int J Sports Med* 1992;13(Supp 1):199–202.
26. Roberts WO. Environmental concerns. In Kibler WB, ed. *ACSM's handbook for the team physician.* Baltimore: Williams & Wilkins, 1996.
27. Roberts WO. Exercise associated collapse in endurance events: a classification system. *Phys Sportsmed* 1989;17:49–55.

28. England AC. Preventing severe heat injury in runners. *Ann Inter Med* 1982;92:196–201.
29. Gardner JW, Kark JA, Karnei K, et al. Risk factors predicting exertional heat illness in Marine Corps recruits. *Med Sci Sports Exerc* 1996;28:939–944.
30. Holtzhausen LM, Noakes TD, Kroning B, et al. Clinical and biochemical characteristics of collapsed ultramarathon runners. *Med Sci Sports Exerc* 1994;26:1095–1101.
31. Whipkey RR. Paris PM, Stewart RD. Marathon medicine. *Emer Med* 1985;Sept:64–90.
32. Noakes TD. Dehydration during exercise: what are the real dangers? *Clin J Sport Med* 1995;5:123–128.
33. Noakes TD, Berlinski N, Solomon E, et al. Collapsed runners: blood biochemical changes after IV fluid therapy. *Phys Sportsmed* 1991;19:70–82.
34. Noakes TD, Myburgh KH, du Pliessis J, et al. Metabolic rate, not percent dehydration, predicts rectal temperature in marathon runners. *Med Sci Sports Exerc* 1991;23:443–449.
35. O'Toole ML, Douglas PS, Laird RH, et al. Fluid and electrolyte status in athletes receiving medical care at an ultradistance triathlon. *Clin J Sport Med* 1995;5:116–122.
36. Roberts WO. Assessing core temperature in collapsed athletes. *Phys Sportsmed* 1994;22:49–55.
37. Roberts WO. Managing heatstroke: on-site cooling. *Phys Sportsmed* 1992;20:17–28.
38. Armstrong LE, Crago AE, Adams R, et al. Whole-body cooling of hyperthermic runners: comparison of two field therapies. *Am J Emerg Med* 1996;14:355–358.
39. Armstrong LE, Maresh CM, Crago AE, et al. Interpretation of aural temperatures during exercise, hyperthermia, and cooling therapy. *Med Exerc Nut Health* 1994;3:9–16.
40. Brodeur VB, Dennett SR, Griffin LS. Exertional hyperthermia, ice baths, and emergency care at The Falmouth Road Race. *Journal of Emergency Nursing* 1989;15:304–312.
41. Costrini AM. Emergency treatment of exertional heat stroke and comparison of whole body cooling techniques. *Med Sci Sports Exerc* 1990;22:15–18.
42. Deschamps A, Levy RD, Cosio MG, et al. Tympanic temperature should not be used to assess exercise induced hyperthermia. *Clin J Sports Med* 1992;2:27–32.
43. McCann DJ, Adams WC. Wet bulb globe temperature index and performance in competitive distance runners. *Med Sci Sports Exerc* 1997;29:955–961.
44. Sawka MN, Young AJ, Latzka WA, et al. Human tolerance to heat strain during exercise: influence of hydration. *J Appl Physiol* 1992;73:368–375.
45. Shearer S. Dehydration and serum electrolyte changes in South African gold miners with heat disorders. *Am J Ind Med* 1990;17:225–239.
46. Ayrus JC, Varon J, Areiff AI. Hyponatremia, cerebral edema, and noncardiogenic pulmonary edema in marathon runners. *Ann Int Med* 2000;132(9):711–714.
47. Mclennan JG, Mclennan JC, Ungersma J. Accident prevention in competitive cycling. *Am J Sports Med* 1988;16:266–268.
48. Gannon DM, Derse AR, Bronkema PJ. Emergency care network of a ski marathon. *Am J Sports Med* 1985;13:318–320.
49. Murphy P. Treating the wounded and the weary at a large ski marathon. *Phys Sport Med* 1987;15:170–183.

CHAPTER 5

The Law and Sports Medicine

Matthew J. Mitten

INTRODUCTION

This chapter identifies important legal issues that arise in connection with the provision of sports medicine care to athletes. Currently there exists little judicial precedent and few statutes establishing the legal duties of a physician in providing sports medicine care and treatment to athletes. Although recently several lawsuits have alleged physician malpractice in connection with medical treatment rendered to athletes, virtually all of them have been settled by the involved parties before judicial resolution of their merits and establishment of precedent for resolving future similar disputes. This chapter discusses the developing law concerning the provision of sports medicine care to athletes (1).

THE NATURE OF THE PHYSICIAN-ATHLETE RELATIONSHIP

The nature of the physician-athlete relationship is unique in many respects and differs from the ordinary physician-patient relationship. Athletes generally are highly motivated to participate in their chosen sports and are reluctant to spend time on the sideline because of an injury or illness. Both a typical patient and an athlete want a cure or treatment for a specific physical malady, but an athlete usually also seeks the quickest possible return to competition. Competitive athletes often feel invincible, have a strong desire to play a sport for psychological or economic reasons, and may be willing to sacrifice their bodies to accomplish an athletic objective. For these reasons, athletes may not readily accept a physician's medical recommendations that delay a return to play or advise against further participation in a sport.

Sports medicine physicians may encounter the sometimes conflicting objectives of protecting the athlete's health while minimizing the time spent away from athletic competition. Sports medicine is evolving and often lacks definitive scientific data on which a physician can rely in providing care and treatment to athletes. In addition to facing medical uncertainty, a physician may be subjected to extreme pressure from an athlete and/or team officials to provide medical clearance or treatment necessary for the athlete to play. Moreover, the playing season and team's need for a player's services continue while the athlete's medical condition is being evaluated and treated, thereby creating an environment that is not optimal for making well-considered and medically sound judgments that protect the athlete's health.

A physician has special knowledge, training, and skill in diagnosing and treating diseases and injuries that a patient such as an athlete lacks, which is the primary reason that patients seek medical services from physicians. Because an athlete entrusts his or her physical well-being to his physician and relies on the physician to protect the athlete's health in providing sports medicine care and treatment, the physician-athlete relationship is characterized as fiduciary in nature. This means that a physician has a legal obligation to act primarily for the athlete's benefit in connection with medical matters.

Even if a physician is selected and/or paid by an institution, the physician must provide medical care, treatment, and advice that are consistent with an individual athlete's best health interests because there is a physician-patient relationship with the athlete. It is important for a physician to be aware of this potential conflict of interest and not to place his or her own economic interests or the team's needs before an athlete's medical best interests. Although one of a sports medicine physician's objectives is to avoid the unnecessary restriction of athletic activity, the physician's paramount responsibility is to protect the athlete's health, and the physician's judgment should be governed only

---

M. J. Mitten: National Sports Law Institute, Marquette University Law School, Milwaukee, Wisconsin 53233.

by medical considerations rather than economic or psychological factors.

THE PHYSICIAN'S GENERAL LEGAL DUTY OF CARE

While providing medical care to a patient, a physician has a legal obligation to have and use the knowledge, skill, and care ordinarily possessed and used by members of his or her specialty in good standing, considering the state of medical science at the time such care is rendered. The law generally permits the medical profession to establish the parameters of appropriate medical care as well as to designate any specific medical practices or treatment that a physician should follow within those boundaries. Thus, the medical standard of care, which must be established by physician expert testimony, becomes the legal standard of care for malpractice purposes. Malpractice liability for harm caused to an athlete may arise if a physician deviates from reasonable or accepted practices within his or her area of specialty in providing medical care, but the physician will not be liable for failing to use the highest degree of medical care, skill, and judgment exercised within his or her specialty.

Team physicians often are either family practitioners or orthopedic surgeons. Other specialists such as internists, cardiologists, pediatricians, dermatologists, and gynecologists also practice sports medicine. Currently, the American Board of Medical Specialties does not recognize a specialized practice area for sports medicine, but the American Osteopathic Association now has a certification board for sports medicine.

Sports medicine physicians have a legal duty to conform to the standard of care corresponding to their actual specialty training; for example, an orthopedic surgeon will be held to the standard of an orthopedist providing sports medicine care. In the past, courts have not recognized sports medicine as a separate medical specialty, presumably because no national medical specialty board certification or standardized training previously existed. However, this judicial view may change as sports medicine becomes more standardized as an area of specialization within the medical profession.

In medical malpractice litigation the trend of the law is to apply a national standard of care because national specialty certification boards, standardized training, and certification procedures exist. A national standard of care for team physicians is preferable because appropriate sports medicine care and treatment should not vary with the geographic location in which these services are provided. As sports medicine continues to develop as a medical specialty, it is likely that courts will hold that a national standard of care applies to team physicians, which will facilitate the provision of high-quality sports medicine care to athletes.

There have been few reported appellate cases discussing the appropriate standard of care in a malpractice suit involving a sports medicine physician. The general legal standard of physician conduct is "good medical practice" within the physician's type of practice. In other words, what is commonly done by physicians in the same specialty generally serves as the standard by which a physician's conduct is measured. Courts traditionally have equated "good medical practice" with what is customarily and usually done by physicians under the circumstances.

More recently, some courts have adopted an "accepted practice" standard of care (2). Under this standard, acceptable medical practices establish a physician's legal duty of care in treating athletes. In other words, what should have been done under the circumstances, not what is commonly done, controls. Physicians have a legal obligation to keep abreast of new developments and advances in sports medicine and may be liable for using outdated treatment methods that no longer have a sound medical basis or do not currently constitute appropriate care. In many situations customary practices reflect accepted medical practices, so a determination of malpractice liability may be the same under either standard. Like custom, proof of accepted practice for litigation purposes will require expert medical testimony.

The most likely potential areas of malpractice liability for sports medicine physicians are failing to conduct appropriate preparticipation screening or diagnostic tests, misinterpreting test results or misdiagnosing injuries, providing improper treatment of an identified medical condition, improperly prescribing or monitoring the use of prescription drugs, improperly clearing an athlete to play with a known physical abnormality, and/or incomplete disclosure of the medical risks of playing with an injury, illness, or abnormal medical condition. These specific topics are discussed in detail in the following sections of this chapter.

PREPARTICIPATION PHYSICALS AND SCREENING EXAMINATIONS

The law requires that a medical examination of an athlete to determine his or her fitness to play a sport be reasonable under the circumstances; the law relies on the collective judgment of the medical profession to establish the appropriate nature and scope of a screening examination or preparticipation evaluation to discover physical abnormalities and potentially life-threatening conditions in athletes. This necessarily involves the development of reliable diagnostic procedures considering cost-benefit and feasibility factors as well as the current state of medical science. The medical and legal acceptability or reasonableness of the comprehensiveness of a physical fitness evaluation appears to depend on the individual athlete's level of competition, the physical demands of the particular sport and level of competition, and the economic ability of the team, athletic sponsoring organization, or athlete to pay for an extensive examination.

A consortium of five medical organizations whose members practice sports medicine has developed a monograph that includes guidelines for the recommended scope of a preparticipation physical evaluation for youth athletes (3). These guidelines are evidence of the medically appropriate scope of a physical examination for youth athletes but do not conclusively establish a physician's legal duty of care.

A physician is not necessarily legally liable for failing to discover a latent medical condition during screening or evaluation of an athlete. Potential liability arises only if the examining physician deviates from customary, accepted, or reasonable medical practice, the use of which would have led to detection of the subject condition in the athlete.

In *Rosensweig* v. *State* (4), the court ruled that a physician was not liable for failing to discover a boxer's preexisting brain injury from a previous fight. The court found that the physician had conducted a standard examination (without discussing its nature and scope) that did not reveal a prior brain injury. The court also observed that the boxer's medical history indicated no symptoms of concussions or brain injury and that the physician had relied on the opinions of other physicians who had examined the boxer after his prior fight without finding any indications of a brain injury. Similarly, in *Classen* v. *State* (5), the court found that a physician had conducted an extensive physical and neurological examination of a boxer in accordance with accepted medical practice and was not liable for malpractice in medically clearing the boxer to fight. It is important to recognize that a "standard examination" must conform to the medical state of the art and may not alone be sufficient for all individual athletes.

An athlete's malpractice claim arising out of alleged negligence in connection with preparticipation screening or evaluation must be encompassed within the scope of the physician's agreed duty to provide medical care or advice to the athlete. In *Murphy* v. *Blum* (6), the court held that a physician who had been hired by the National Basketball Association (NBA) solely to advise it whether a referee would be physically capable of performing his duties did not have a physician-patient relationship with the referee that could form the basis of a malpractice claim. The NBA physician had informed an NBA league official of the abnormal results of the referee's stress test, and the official forwarded these results to the referee's personal physician. The NBA physician did not directly advise the referee of the abnormal test results and did not recommend or provide any treatment for his heart condition. After suffering a heart attack that prevented his continuing to referee, the referee sued the NBA physician for malpractice in a suit that the court dismissed because of the lack of a physician-patient relationship between the parties.

The *Murphy* case suggests that a physician who conducts preparticipation examinations solely for the benefit of an athletic team is not legally required to directly inform an athlete of discovered medical abnormalities. Nevertheless, to minimize potential legal liability, an examining physician should directly inform both the athlete and the athlete's personal physician of any discovered abnormalities in writing. Even if a physician who merely provides routine mass screening for certain medical conditions has no legal duty to provide follow-up medical care, it is strongly recommended that the physician inform athletes of the limited nature of the medical services the physician is providing in conducting preparticipation examinations and either promptly treat or refer symptomatic athletes to other physicians for treatment.

DIAGNOSIS AND TREATMENT OF ATHLETE'S MEDICAL CONDITION AND INJURIES

A sports medicine physician must adhere to customary or accepted sports medicine practice in diagnosing or treating an athlete's injuries. In some instances it may be necessary to consult with specialists to provide proper sports medicine care, and the team physician may be negligent for failing to do so. Protecting the athlete's health should always be the team physician's paramount objective in providing medical care.

A physician may be liable for not using recognized and appropriate tests or examinations to gather information necessary to determine the proper treatment of an athlete's injury or illness. In *Speed* v. *State* (7) the Iowa Supreme court upheld a finding that a team physician negligently failed to order testing to diagnose a basketball player's condition. The player complained of persistent headache and body aches and had other symptoms of an infection. A cranial infection that caused a blockage in the flow of blood to his eyes ultimately resulted in the player's blindness. The court relied on expert testimony that the team physician should have given the player a more thorough physical examination and various tests in light of his symptoms.

A physician generally does not warrant the correctness of a diagnosis, and a doctor is not liable for honest mistakes of judgment if the appropriate diagnosis is in reasonable doubt. However, a physician may be liable for malpractice if he or she does not use the requisite degree of care and skill ordinarily possessed by those within the physician's specialty in interpreting test results and determining a patient's need for treatment.

In *Gardner* v. *Holifield* (8), a basketball player's surviving mother alleged that a cardiologist misinterpreted two echocardiograms that had been ordered to confirm an initial diagnosis during a routine physical examination that the player had Marfan's syndrome. As a result, proper follow-up care, including the probable need for cardiovascular surgery, was not provided, and the athlete died six months after being initially evaluated by the cardiologist. Medical experts testified that a proper confirming diagnosis and treatment would have prevented the athlete's death and given him a normal life expectancy. This testimony created a factual issue regarding the physician's alleged malpractice for resolution by the jury.

A physician has a legal duty to either provide appropriate sports medicine care or ensure that an athlete with a known injury, illness, or medical condition receives necessary treatment in a timely manner. In *Dailey* v. *Winston* (9), expert testimony that a surgeon negligently failed to immediately hospitalize a basketball player for an arteriogram after discovering an arterial blockage and not informing the athlete of the seriousness of his condition created an issue of malpractice liability for resolution by a jury.

A team physician may be liable for failing to provide proper emergency medical care to an injured athlete. In *Welch* v. *Dunsmuir Joint Union High School District* (10), a physician was found negligent for failing to promptly attend to an injured football player and supervise his removal from the playing field. Moving the plaintiff without a stretcher was found to be an improper medical practice in view of his symptoms and caused his permanent paralysis.

In prescribing rehabilitation therapy for an injured athlete, the team physician also must adhere to good medical practice consistent with an athlete's best health interests. If there are various recognized and accepted methods of treatment, a physician may select the one he or she deems best and is not liable for malpractice because some physicians use other procedures. The athlete's unique physiology and physical condition, as well as the level of athletic competition, are factors in determining the appropriate treatment. Professional and college players may be able to recover from injuries more rapidly because of their superior conditioning, physical development, and team-provided rehabilitation. Because of their still-developing bodies, different rehabilitation procedures and longer periods of inactivity may be appropriate for high school athletes.

PRESCRIPTION OF DRUGS

Team physicians may be liable for negligently prescribing anesthetics and painkillers to athletes to facilitate athletic participation. Medication to relieve pain masks the seriousness of an injury and may cause aggravation or reinjury of a preexisting condition. In prescribing drugs to athletes, team physicians should follow accepted medical practices regarding the appropriate type and dosage of pharmaceutical treatment. They should prescribe drugs to enable athletic participation only if doing so is consistent with an athlete's best health interests. A physician may be subject to liability for injury to an athlete caused by improperly delegating his or her authority to dispense prescription drugs to an athletic trainer or failing to monitor or keep accurate records on drugs taken by athletes (11).

In 1990 Hank Gathers collapsed and died of a heart attack while playing in a basketball game for Loyola Marymount University. Gathers had previously been diagnosed as having a potentially life-threatening heart rhythm disorder. After his death Gathers's heirs sued his treating physicians, claiming, among other things, that he was given a nontherapeutic dosage of heart medication to enable him to continue playing basketball at an elite level. Although this lawsuit ultimately was settled, this claim, if proven, would constitute actionable negligence.

In an unreported case, *Mendenhall* v. *Oakland Raiders*, an NFL player was awarded a $35,000 verdict against a team physician who improperly prescribed amphetamines, thereby precluding the player from fully appreciating his potential for injury by playing and contributing to the reinjury of his knee during a game. Dick Butkus, a former Chicago Bears linebacker, settled a negligence suit for $600,000 against physicians for the alleged negligent administration of drugs causing his permanent knee injury.

INFORMED CONSENT REQUIREMENTS AND MEDICAL CLEARANCE RECOMMENDATIONS

A physician must have an athlete's informed consent before providing medical treatment. The informed consent doctrine is based on the principle of individual autonomy, namely, that a competent adult has the legal right to determine what to do with his or her body. This autonomy includes the right to accept or refuse medical treatment. A competent adult athlete has the legal capacity to consent to medical care, but consent for treatment of athletes who are minors generally must be obtained from the athlete's parents or legal guardian.

For an athlete's consent to be legally valid, it must be the product of an informed decision regarding the proposed medical treatment. The average person has little understanding of medicine and relies on a physician to provide the information necessary to make a responsible decision regarding treatment. The extent of a physician's duty to disclose to a patient traditionally has been determined by prevailing practices in the medical profession. Physician custom or what a reasonable physician would disclose under the circumstances has been the controlling legal standard. The recent judicial trend, however, is to focus on the patient and require physicians to disclose all material information to enable the patient to make an informed decision. A risk is material "when a reasonable person, in what the physician knows or should know to be the patient's position, would be likely to attach significance to the risk or cluster of risks in deciding whether or not to forego the proposed therapy" (12). Therefore, a physician should ask himself or herself what information about the athlete's medical condition and treatment the athlete would want and need to know and then disclose this medical information to the athlete in a timely manner.

A physician should fully disclose to an athlete the material medical risks of playing with the subject injury, illness, or abnormality and the potential health consequences of using or forgoing a given medication or treatment. The availability and pros and cons of accepted alternative methods of treatment also need to be considered and discussed with the athlete. All material short- and long-term medical risks of continued athletic participation and treatment, including any potentially life-threatening or permanently disabling health consequences, must be disclosed.

Treating physicians have a duty to disclose material medical risks to an athlete in plain and simple language. Information about the athlete's medical condition, proposed treatment and alternatives, probability of future injury and severity of harm from continued athletic participation, and potential long-term health effects should preferably be in writing and tape-recorded when given verbally. It also is advisable to discuss any conflicting second opinions about medical care of the athlete and not to downplay other physicians' conclusions about the athlete's medical condition and potential consequences of playing. A physician would be prudent to take affirmative steps to ensure that an athlete understands the available treatment options, their side effects, and the potential consequences of engaging in athletics with a cardiovascular condition; these steps might include questioning the athlete or asking the athlete to write down his or her understanding of what he or she has been told.

A failure to provide an athlete with full disclosure of material information about playing with the athlete's medical condition or the potential consequences of proposed treatment may create physician liability for negligence or fraud. In *Krueger* v. *San Francisco Forty Niners* (13), the court held that the conscious failure to inform a player that he risked a permanent knee injury by continuing to play was fraudulent concealment of a material fact regarding his medical treatment. The court found that physicians had not informed Charley Krueger of the true nature and extent of his knee injuries, the consequences of steroid injection treatment, or the long-term dangers associated with playing professional football with his medical condition. The court also found that the purpose of this nondisclosure was to induce Krueger to continue playing football despite his injuries. The jury accepted Krueger's testimony that he would have rejected the proposed treatment and discontinued playing football, thereby preventing his subsequent permanent harm from occurring. The jury awarded Krueger $2.366 million in damages.

The *Krueger* case illustrates that a physician may incur legal liability for not fully disclosing material information about an athlete's medical condition that is necessary to enable the athlete to determine whether to accept proposed medical treatment or to continue playing a sport. To prevail in litigation against a physician for negligent or fraudulent nondisclosure of medical information, an athlete must prove that he or she would not have played or undergone the treatment that caused the harm if he or she had been properly informed of the material risks of doing so. Physicians providing sports medicine care to athletes can minimize potential legal liability by communicating openly and honestly with their patients.

Physicians should provide all material information about an athlete's medical condition directly to the athlete and obtain permission, preferably in writing, before communicating any medical information about the athlete to team officials. Ethically, a physician is prohibited from disclosing a patient's medical condition to others without patient consent or legal requirement. Unauthorized disclosure of information about an athlete's medical condition to third parties may create legal liability. In *Chuy* v. *Philadelphia Eagles Football Club* (14), a federal appellate court affirmed a jury finding that the Philadelphia Eagles' team physician intentionally inflicted emotional distress on a professional football player by falsely informing the press that the player suffered from a fatal blood disease. The physician's statement was found to be intolerable professional conduct because he knew that the player did not have the reported condition. Moreover, a physician's unauthorized disclosure of even accurate information about an athlete's medical condition, such as HIV positive status, creates potential legal liability for invasion of the athlete's privacy.

Even if an athlete's illness or condition has been properly diagnosed and the athlete has been warned of the potential health consequences of continued play, in extreme cases a physician may be liable for making a negligent medical clearance recommendation. In *Mikkelson* v. *Haslam* (15), a patient alleged that her physician had negligently provided medical clearance to snow ski after her hip replacement surgery. The jury found the physician negligent on the basis of undisputed testimony that advising a total hip replacement patient that skiing is permissible "is a departure from orthopedic medical profession standards."

In *Gathers* v. *Loyola-Marymount University* (16), the

Gathers heirs asserted, along with claims of other negligent medical treatment, that Hank Gathers was not fully informed of the seriousness of having ventricular tachycardia and should not have been medically cleared to play college basketball with this condition. This 1990 lawsuit asserted that physicians providing such clearance acted negligently because the 16th Bethesda Conference guidelines (17), which were in effect at that time, recommended that individuals with ventricular tachycardia should not participate in any competitive sports. The Gathers heirs contended that Gathers was "sacrificed on the altar of college basketball" in Loyola Marymount University's quest for basketball success, notoriety and economic gain.

In *Lillard* v. *State of Oregon* (18), Earnest Killum's mother alleged that her son's physicians did not inform him of the material medical risks of continuing to play college basketball with an impaired vascular condition caused by two prior strokes. She also claimed that these physicians negligently cleared her son to resume playing basketball, although doing so subjected him to an increased risk of death or serious injury. She further contended that the physicians breached their duty to refuse to provide medical clearance to avoid allowing an athlete to expose himself to an enhanced risk of death or serious harm and not compromise an athlete's medical care to advance a university's economic interests.

Both the *Gathers* and *Lillard* lawsuits were settled before their judicial resolution established legal precedent regarding physician liability for negligent medical clearance recommendations. However, these cases illustrate the need for physicians to consider carefully the parameters of the acceptable medical risks of athletic participation with an injury, illness, or physical abnormality and always to adhere to their paramount obligation to protect an athlete's health. It is a serious violation of a physician's ethical and legal duties to an athlete to allow nonmedical factors to impair the exercise of his or her medical best judgment in making clearance recommendations and/or not to fully inform an athlete of the health risks of athletic participation with the athlete's condition. A physician should refuse to clear an athlete to participate if the physician believes that there is a significant medical risk of harm from sports participation, irrespective of the team's need for the player or the player's strong psychologic or economic motivation to play and willingness to risk his or her health.

In formulating a participation recommendation a physician should consider only the athlete's medical best interest. The following factors may be appropriately considered: the athlete's unique physiology; the intensity and physical demands of the subject sport; whether the athlete has previously participated in the sport with his or her physical condition; available clinical evidence; medical organization and society guidelines; the probability and severity of harm from athletic participation with the athlete's condition; and whether medication or monitoring or protective devices will minimize potential health risks and enable safe athletic participation. In cases in which there is an uncertain potential for life-threatening or permanently disabling harm to an athlete, it is advisable to err on the side of caution and recommend against athletic participation.

There has been at least one case in which an athlete brought a malpractice action against a physician for refusing to medically clear him to play a sport. In *Penny* v. *Sands* (19), Anthony Penny filed a malpractice suit against a cardiologist who had diagnosed him as having cardiomyopathy and recommended against his continued participation in intercollegiate basketball. Two other cardiologists had concurred with this opinion, and Central Connecticut State University refused to allow Penny to participate in its basketball program for two years. Penny ultimately obtained medical clearance to play competitive sports from two other cardiologists. He alleged that Dr. Sands' negligence caused economic harm to his anticipated professional basketball career because of his involuntary two-year exclusion from college basketball. Penny voluntarily dismissed his malpractice suit before he collapsed and died while playing in a 1990 professional basketball game in England.

Although Penny's allegations were not judicially resolved, it is unlikely that a court would permit an athlete to recover any economic damages for loss of a speculative professional career because team officials accept a physician's medical recommendation against permitting the athlete to participate in a sport. Legal recognition of such claims would unduly impair a physician's medical judgment and may cause the physician to place greater weight on legal rather than medical considerations. This also would create the paradoxical and undesirable situation of imposing legal liability on a physician for complying with his primary obligation to protect an athlete's health.

THE ATHLETE'S RESPONSIBILITY TO PROTECT HIS OR HER OWN HEALTH

An athlete has a legal duty to reasonably protect his or her own health. One court has defined a patient's duties regarding the receipt of medical care as follows:

> A patient is required to cooperate in a reasonable manner with his treatment. This means that a patient has a duty to listen to his doctor, truthfully provide information to his doctor upon request, follow reasonable advice given by his doctor, and cooperate in a reasonable manner with his treatment. A patient also has a duty to disclose material and significant information about his condition or habits when requested to do so by his physician (20).

An athlete must satisfy these obligations to comply with his duty to reasonably protect his or her health. Otherwise, the athlete may be found to be contributorily negligent for exposing himself or herself to an unreasonable risk of harm.

Physicians and patients have corresponding legal obligations to facilitate the provision of quality medical care. A physician has a duty to obtain a complete and accurate medical history from an athlete. In turn, an athlete must exercise due care for his or her own safety by truthfully relating his or her medical history to the physician. Although an athlete has no general duty to diagnose his or her own condition or to volunteer information, the athlete should disclose known information about his or her physical condition that may expose the athlete to a risk of future harm if he or she knows that the physician has failed to ascertain these facts while taking the athlete's medical history.

An athlete generally may rely on the recommendations of the treating physicians without seeking a second medical opinion. It ordinarily is reasonable for athletes to rely on their physicians' recommendations about the athletes' medical care and treatment because of the physicians' superior knowledge and expertise. In *Mikkelson* v. *Haslam* (15), the court found that the patient was not contributorily negligent for following her physician's advice that she could snow ski after total hip replacement surgery without seeking a second opinion from other physicians. She did not assume the risk of her permanently disabling injury, which occurred while skiing, because her physician had not informed her of this potential risk and it was not an obvious risk to a layperson.

Courts have held that an athlete's failure to use reasonable care to protect his or her health may totally bar or reduce the athlete's recoverable damages in a malpractice suit against his or her treating physicians. In *Gillespie* v. *Southern Utah State College* (21), a college basketball player was found to be solely responsible for aggravating an ankle injury by not following physician instructions. He iced his ankle for longer than the physician's prescribed period of time, causing thrombophlebitis and frostbite, requiring amputation of his toe and other foot tissue.

If an athlete fails to take prescribed medication in the required dosage or deliberately takes steps to reduce its therapeutic effectiveness, such conduct would be an unreasonable disregard for his or her own safety. Similarly, disobeying a physician's restrictions on athletic activity would constitute contributory negligence.

LEGAL ENFORCEABILITY OF LIABILITY WAIVERS

Under certain circumstances the law permits an adult to agree to waive his or her right to recover damages in litigation for harm caused by another's breach of his legal duty. A waiver of legal rights signed by a minor usually is not enforceable even if it also is signed by the minor's parents or legal guardian or is entered into with their approval because minors have only a limited legal capacity to enter into binding contracts. In general, an adult may prospectively agree to knowingly and voluntarily waive his or her legal right to recover for future harm attributable to another's wrongful conduct unless such an agreement violates public policy. Some courts may uphold waivers of liability from future negligence, but courts generally hold that waivers of liability for more culpable conduct such as intentional, reckless, or grossly negligent torts are unenforceable because they violate public policy.

As was discussed more fully in an earlier section, a physician providing sports medicine care to an athlete has a legal duty to comply with reasonable, customary, or accepted medical practice and may be liable for malpractice for breach of this obligation. Courts generally will not enforce waivers that purport to release physicians from liability for negligent medical care of their patients. Such waivers have been held to violate public policy because medical services are essential public services; the patient places himself or herself under the physician's control but remains subject to the risks of the physician's negligence; and the physician may have superior bargaining power, thereby enabling him or her to require a release from negligence liability as a condition of providing medical treatment.

Although a court might not enforce a waiver signed by an athlete in which the athlete agrees not to hold a physician liable for providing negligent sports medicine care that causes injury, a physician will incur malpractice liability only if he or she deviates from the appropriate medical standard of care or fails to comply with the requirements of the informed consent doctrine. It is important to recognize that merely informing an athlete about the risks of participation with the athlete's condition does not discharge a physician's legal duty of care in providing medical care and medical clearance recommendations. For example, advising an athlete not to play a sport with his or her injury, illness, or physical abnormality but then medically clearing the athlete to play in exchange for a waiver of liability probably will not protect a physician from malpractice liability if the physician acted negligently. Conforming to current accepted standards of sports medicine practice and fully apprising the athlete of all material information about his or her condition are the best means by which a physician can avoid legal liability.

IMMUNITY FROM MALPRACTICE LIABILITY

In some instances, sports medicine physicians may be immune from legal liability for malpractice claims brought by athletes. Several states have enacted so-called Good Samaritan statutes protecting licensed physicians from negligence liability for emergency medical care rendered to athletes in good faith and without compensation. Immunity generally is not provided for emergency medical treatment that is found to be grossly negligent, reckless, or willful or wanton. Preparticipation physical exams, general nonemergency medical care rendered to athletes, and physician medical clearance recommendations are not normally subject to tort immunity.

In some jurisdictions, state law immunizes physicians employed by public educational institutions from malpractice liability in suits brought by athletes. In *Gardner* v. *Holifield* (8), the court ruled that alleged negligent medical care provided to a college basketball player by a physician is encompassed within the scope of tort immunity under Florida law if the physician was acting in his capacity as director of a public university's student health center when such treatment was rendered. Florida state employees, including physicians, are immune from liability for negligence committed within the scope and course of their employment.

Similarly, in *Sorey* v. *Kellett* (22), a federal court held that a public university's team physician was immune from a negligence suit brought by the mother of a deceased football player. The player collapsed during a football practice, was given allegedly negligent medical treatment by the team physician, and died while being transported to the hospital. The court ruled that public employees have a qualified immunity from tort claims based on their discretionary acts. Finding that the physician was performing a discretionary function in administering emergency medical care to the decedent, the court dismissed the lawsuit.

In some states a professional athlete's claim against a physician for negligent medical care may be barred by a state workmen's compensation statute prohibiting actions against coemployees for injuries caused to fellow employees when acting within the scope of their employment. If so, the athlete's legal remedy is limited to receipt of the statutorily determined workmen's compensation benefits under state law. In *Hendy* v. *Losse* (23), the court dismissed a professional football player's suit against a team physician for negligently diagnosing and treating his knee injury and medically clearing him to continue playing football. The court held that California's workmen's compensation law bars tort suits between coemployees for injuries caused within the scope of employment. The player's malpractice claim was dismissed because both he and the physician were employed by the San Diego Chargers team and the physician acted within the scope of his employment in treating the player. However, the court stated that a physician who is an employee of a professional team is subject to malpractice liability for improper medical services provided to athletes that are outside of the scope of the services the physician agrees to provide to players pursuant to his employment agreement with the team.

JUDICIAL RESOLUTION OF ATHLETIC PARTICIPATION DISPUTES

Ideally, whether an athlete will participate in a sport with a physical impairment should be the product of mutual agreement between the team physician and consulting specialists, team or school officials, and the athlete and his or her family. However, it is not uncommon for physicians to disagree in their medical clearance recommendations or for highly motivated athletes at all levels of competition to be reluctant to accept a medical recommendation not to continue playing a sport. Disagreements about medical eligibility to participate in a sport will be judicially resolved on a case-by-case basis under federal or state laws prohibiting discrimination against individuals with physical impairments.

Both the Americans With Disabilities Act of 1990 (ADA) (24) and the Rehabilitation Act of 1973 (25) prohibit unjustified discrimination against athletes who have physical impairments within the meaning of these statutes. These federal laws apply to virtually all professional teams and intercollegiate or interscholastic sports programs but do not hold a physician personally liable for determining that an athlete is medically ineligible to participate in a sport. State education, human rights, and/or employment laws also may prohibit medically unwarranted discrimination by educational institutions or professional teams against athletes with physical impairments.

Federal law entitles an athlete with the physical capabilities and skills necessary to play a sport despite a physical impairment to have his or her condition individually evaluated in light of current medical evidence. Exclusion from an athletic team or event must be based on reasonable medical judgments by physicians, given the current state of medical knowledge. The ADA and the Rehabilitation Act require a careful balancing of an impaired athlete's right to participate in athletic activities within his or her physical abilities, physician evaluation of the medical risks of athletic participation, and the team's interest in conducting a safe athletics program (26).

Exclusion of an athlete because his or her physical impairment increases the risk of personal injury to others or to the athlete himself or herself while engaging in athletic activity must be based on "reasonable medical judgments given the state of medical knowledge" (27) Relevant medical factors include the nature, duration, probability, and severity of harm from athletic participation as well as whether the risk of injury can be effectively reduced by medication, monitoring or protective devices, or other reasonable accommodations to enable athletic participation. An athlete may be legally excluded from an athletic event or competition if his or her participation exposes others to significant health and safety risks. In *School Board of Nassau County, Florida* v. *Arline* (27), the Supreme Court held that excluding an individual from a particular program or activity because of a risk of harm to others must be based on "reasonable medical judgments given the state of medical knowledge." The nature, duration, probability, and severity of harm likely to result from a physically impaired athlete's participation in an activity and whether reasonable accommodations will eliminate the risk of injury to others are factors to be considered. In *Montalvo* v. *Radcliffe, II* (28), a federal appellate court upheld the exclusion of a 12-year-old boy with AIDS from full contact group karate classes because his participation posed a direct threat to the health and safety of other students.

Even if such participation does not expose others to significant harm, developing judicial precedent holds that a physically impaired college or high school athlete may be excluded from a sport to prevent exposing himself or herself to a significant risk of injury. To date, there have been no reported cases in which professional athletes have asserted a legal right to play a sport with a physical impairment. Although the medical issues may be the same, courts may develop a different legal framework for resolving participation disputes involving professional athletes because sports is their livelihood rather than an extracurricular activity that is merely a component of a high school or college education (29).

In recent years courts have expanded the legal rights of athletes with a missing or nonfunctioning paired organ, such as an eye or a kidney, to participate in interscholastic and intercollegiate contact sports (30). In these cases the athlete was able to convince a court that his exclusion was illegal based on the opinion of medical specialists that his physical condition did not increase the probability of personal injury and evidence that available protective equipment would adequately protect his functioning organ.

If a physically impaired athlete's medical condition may create an enhanced risk of death or serious injury during athletic competition, courts are reluctant to require an educational institution to allow the athlete to participate in sports. In *Knapp* v. *Northwestern University* (31), a federal appellate court held that Northwestern University did not violate the Rehabilitation Act in following its team physician's recommendation that an athlete with idiopathic ventricular fibrillation not play intercollegiate basketball. As a high school senior, Nicholas Knapp suffered sudden cardiac arrest while playing recreational basketball, which required cardiopulmonary resuscitation and defibrillation to restart his heart. Thereafter, he had an internal cardioverter-defibrillator implanted in his abdomen. He subsequently played competitive recreational basketball without any incidents of cardiac arrest and received medical clearance to play college basketball from three cardiologists who examined him.

Northwestern agreed to honor its commitment to provide Knapp with an athletic scholarship, although it adhered to its team physician's medical disqualification from intercollegiate basketball. This recommendation was based on Knapp's medical records and history, the 26th Bethesda Conference guidelines for athletic participation with cardiovascular abnormalities, and opinions of two consulting cardiologists who concluded that Knapp would expose himself to a significant risk of ventricular fibrillation or cardiac arrest during competitive athletics.

All medical experts agreed that: Knapp had suffered sudden cardiac death due to ventricular fibrillation; even with the internal defibrillator, playing college basketball places Knapp at a higher risk of suffering another event of sudden cardiac death compared to other male college basketball players; the internal defibrillator has never been tested under the conditions of intercollegiate basketball; and no person currently plays or has ever played college or professional basketball after suffering sudden cardiac death and having a defibrillator implanted.

The court held that a university legally may establish legitimate physical qualifications that an individual must satisfy to participate in its athletic program. An athlete may be medically disqualified from athletics if necessary to avoid a significant risk of personal physical injury to himself or herself that cannot be eliminated through the use of reasonable medical accommodations. The court explained that Knapp's exclusion from Northwestern's basketball team was legally justified:

> We disagree with the district court's legal determination that such decisions are to be made by the courts and believe instead that medical determinations of this sort are best left to team doctors and universities as long as they are made with reason and rationality and with full regard to possible and reasonable accommodations. In cases such as ours, where Northwestern has examined both Knapp and his medical records, has considered his medical history and the relation between his prior sudden cardiac death and the possibility of future occurrences, has considered the severity of the potential injury, and has rationally and reasonably reviewed consensus medical opinions or recommendations in the pertinent field—regardless whether conflicting medical opinions exist—the university has the right to determine that an individual is not otherwise medically qualified to play without violating the Rehabilitation Act. The place of the court in such cases is to make sure that the decision-maker has reasonably considered and relied upon sufficient evidence specific to the individual and the potential injury, not to determine on its own which evidence it believes is more persuasive.

Similarly, in *Pahulu* v. *University of Kansas* (32), a federal court upheld the team physician's "conservative" medical disqualification of a college football player with an abnormally narrow cervical canal after an episode of transient quadriplegia during a scrimmage. After consulting with a neurosurgeon, the team physician concluded that the athlete was at extremely high risk of sustaining permanent, severe neurologic injury, including permanent quadriplegia, if he resumed playing football. The athlete wanted to resume playing because three other medical specialists concluded that he was at no greater risk of permanent paralysis than any other player. The university agreed to honor the athlete's scholarship, although he was not allowed to play football.

CONCLUSION

Like sports medicine itself, the law of sports medicine is evolving. As a general rule, the law requires sports medicine physicians to act reasonably when caring for athletes. The best means of avoiding legal liability is for a physician to adhere to his or her primary responsibility of protecting an athlete's health and safety by providing high-quality sports medicine care and treatment.

REFERENCES

1. See Mitten MJ. Team physicians and competitive athletes; allocating legal responsibility for athletic injuries. *University of Pittsburgh Law Review* 1993;55(1):129–169.
2. *Classen* v. *Izquierdo,* 520 N.Y.S. 2d 999, 1002 (NY Sup Ct 1987); *Classen* v. *State,* 500 N.Y.S. 2d 460, 466 (Ct. Cl. 1985).
3. American Academy of Family Physicians, American Academy of Pediatrics, American Medical Society for Sports Medicine, American Orthopedic Society for Sports Medicine, American Osteopathic Academy of Sports Medicine. Preparticipation Physical Evaluation 2d, 1997 at 34-35. Guidelines also have been developed for cardiovascular screening. Maron BJ, Thompson PD, Puffer PC, et al. Cardiovascular preparticipation screening of competitive athletes. *Circulation* 1996;94:850–856.
4. *Rosensweig* v. *State,* 171 N.Y.S. 2d 912 (NY App 3d Dept. 1958), aff'd, 185 N.Y.S. 2d 521 (NY 1958).
5. *Classen* v. *State,* 500 N.Y.S. 2d 460 (NY App 2d Dept. 1990).
6. *Murphy* v. *Blum,* 554 N.Y.S. 2d 640 (NY App 2d Dept. 1990).
7. *Speed* v. *State,* 240 N.W. 2d 901 (Iowa 1976).
8. *Gardner* v. *Holifield,* 639 So. 2d 656 (Fla. App. 1994).
9. *Dailey* v. *Winston,* 1986 WL 12063 (Tenn. App. 1986) (slip opinion available on WESTLAW).
10. *Welch* v. *Dunsmuir Joint Union High School District,* 326 P2d 633 (Cal. Ct. App. 1958).
11. *Wallace* v. *Broyles,* 961 S.W. 2d 712 (Ark. 1998).
12. *Canterbury* v. *Spence,* 464 F.2d 772, 787 (D.C. 1972), cert denied, 409 U.S. 1064 (1972).
13. *Krueger* v. *San Francisco Forty Niners,* 234 Cal. Rptr. 579 (Cal. Ct. App. 1987).
14. *Chuy* v. *Philadelphia Eagles Football Club,* 595 F.2d 1265 (3d Cir. 1979).
15. *Mikkelson* v. *Haslam,* 764 P.2d 1384 (Utah Ct. App. 1988).
16. *Gathers* v. *Loyola-Marymount University,* No. C 795027 (Los Angeles, CA Super. Ct., filed April 20, 1990).
17. Mitchell JH, Maron BJ, Epstein SJ. 16th Bethesda Conference: cardiovascular abnormalities in the athlete: recommendations regarding eligibility for competition. *J Am Coll Cardiol* 1985;6:1185–1232. These guidelines were updated in 1994. Maron BJ, Mitchell JH. 26th Bethesda Conference: recommendations for determining eligibility for competition in athletes with cardiovascular abnormalities. *J Am Coll Cardiol* 1994;2 (4):845–899.
18. *Lillard* v. *State of Oregon,* No. BC 2941 (Los Angeles, CA Super. Ct. Filed Jan. 19, 1993).
19. *Penny* v. *Sands,* No. H89280 (D. Conn., filed May 3, 1989).
20. *Benedict* v. *St. Luke's Hospital,* 365 N.W. 2d 499, 505 (N.D. 1985).
21. *Gillespie* v. *Southern Utah State College,* 669 P. 2d 861 (Utah 1983).
22. *Sorey* v. *Kellett,* 849 F.2d 960 (5th Cir. 1988).
23. *Hendy* v. *Losse,* 819 P.2d 1 (Cal. 1991). See also *Daniels* v. *Seattle Seahawks,* 968 P.2d 883 (Wash. Ct. App. 1998).
24. Americans With Disabilities Act of 1990, 42 USCA §§12101–12213 (West 1995 and 1997 Supp.).
25. Rehabilitation Act of 1973, 29 USCA §§701–796 (West 1999 and 1999 Supp.).
26. Mitten MJ. Amateur athletes with handicaps or physical abnormalities: who makes the participation decision? *Nebraska Law Review* 1992;71:987–1032.
27. *School Board of Nassau County, Florida* v. *Arline,* 480 U.S. 273 (1987).
28. 167 F.3d 873 (4th Cir. 1999), cert. denied, 120 S. Ct. 145 (1999).
29. Mitten MJ. Enhanced risk of harm to one's self as a justification for exclusion of athletics. *Marq Sports L. J.* 1998;8:189–223.
30. *Grube* v. *Bethlehem Area School Dist.,* 550 F. Supp 418 (ED Pa 1982); *Wright* v. *Columbia Univ.,* 520 F. Supp. 789 (ED Pa 1981); *Poole* v. *South Plainfield Bd of Education,* 490 F. Supp. 948 (D.N.J. 1980).
31. *Knapp* v. *Northwestern University,* 101 F.3d 473 (7th Cir. 1996), cert. Denied, 117 U.S. 2454 (1997).
32. *Pahulu* v. *University of Kansas,* 897 F. Supp. 1387 (D. Kan. 1995).

CHAPTER 6

Sports Medicine Imaging

Nancy M. Major

IMAGING OF SPORTS INJURIES

Diagnostic radiology remains a vital part of diagnosis of sports-related injuries, especially because the technology continues to improve and the number of examinations requested continues to increase. The goals of this chapter are to review the basic principles of the major diagnostic imaging methods and to discuss the advantages and disadvantages of each technique as it relates to imaging the various tissue types in the body that may become injured during the course of sports participation.

Plain Film Radiography

Plain film examination remains fundamental to the practice of radiology. X-rays use radiant energy, which has a very short wavelength that is able to penetrate many substances within the human body. As X-rays pass through the body, they are attenuated by interaction with body tissues, resulting in an image that is recognizable as human anatomy.

An X-ray view is named by the way the beam passes through the patient. An anteroposterior (AP) view is obtained when the X-ray beam passes from the front of the patient to the back. Other views are named by the position of the patient in relation to the beam. For instance, an axillary view is obtained when the patient's arm is abducted and the film cassette is placed behind the shoulder. The X-ray beam is directed at the axilla. A notch view of the knee angles the beam of the X-ray machine to image into the notch and eliminates the bone overlap of the patella and condyles.

Air attenuates very little of an X-ray beam, allowing the film to blacken. Bone and metal attenuate a large proportion of the beam, allowing very little radiation through to blacken the film. Thus bone and metal appear white on radiographs. Anatomic structures are seen on radiographs when they are outlined in whole or in part by tissues of different X-ray density. The high density of bones allows their details to be visualized through overlying soft tissues.

Conventional Tomography

Conventional tomography provides radiographic slices of a patient. Both the X-ray tube and the film are simultaneously moved about a pivot point centered in the patient in the plane of the structure to be imaged. Structures above and below the focal plane are blurred by the motion, and objects in the focal plane are visualized with improved detail because of the blurring of the other structures. Tomography is a useful adjunct to conventional radiographs whenever improved detail is needed for diagnosis. For instance, a nonunion of a fracture can be more readily evaluated by tomography because the overlying structures have essentially been removed from obscuring the fracture line because of the superimposition of blurred structures.

Computed Tomography

Computed tomography (CT) uses a computer to mathematically reconstruct a cross-sectional image of the body from measurements of X-ray transmission through thin slices of patient tissue. Unlike conventional tomography, CT displays the imaged slice without the superimposition of blurred structures. Most CT units allow slice thickness between 1 and 10 mm. Data are acquired in 1–2 seconds. Advantages of CT include rapid scan time, exquisite bone detail, and demonstration of calcifications. CT is generally limited to the axial plane. In some instances direct coronal images can be obtained in the

---

N. M. Major: Department of Radiology, Musculoskeletal Division, Duke University Medical Center, Durham, North Carolina 27710.

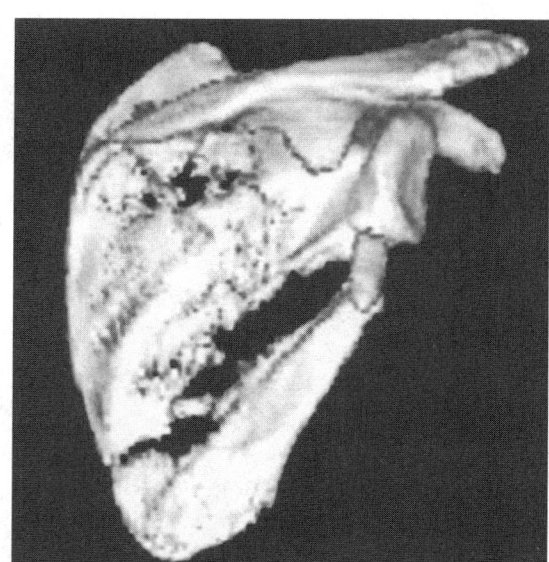 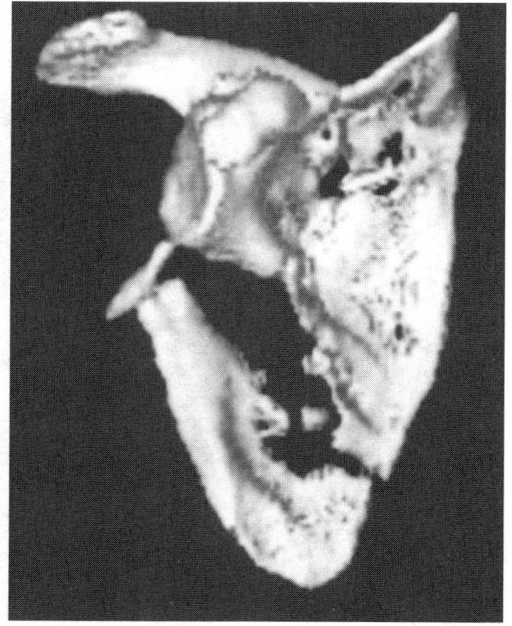

FIG. 6–1. This 52-year-old male was playing touch football and sustained a comminuted fracture of his scapula. The initial CT exam was performed with 1-mm contiguous axial images to obtain three-dimensional reconstruction, which shows the degree of the fracture.

foot and ankle, and direct sagittal, coronal, and axial images can be obtained in the wrist. If the slice is thin enough (1 mm), reformations can be obtained in any plane depending on the software capability of the computer. Additionally, three-dimensional reconstruction can be performed to assess for the complex fractures around a joint (Fig. 6–1). Again a slice thickness of 1 mm is recommended to get satisfactory reconstruction. Optimal bone detail is viewed by using bone windows.

CT has been performed with the assistance of intraarticular contrast agents to identify subtle abnormalities within a joint. This technique is especially useful in evaluating the glenoid labrum. The patient initially undergoes fluoroscopic guidance of a contrast injection using a small amount of contrast (usually 1 cc) with about 12 cc of air. This is immediately followed by CT examination in both internal and external rotation to evaluate the integrity of the labrum.

Some imaging artifacts occur with CT. These include volume averaging, beam hardening, motion artifact, and streak artifacts. Volume averaging is a result of a three-dimensional volume of tissue displayed in a two-dimensional image. Beam hardening is a result of greater attenuation of a low-energy X-ray beam than a high-energy X-ray beam as it passes through tissue. The mean energy of the X-ray beam is increased. This results in streaks of low density extending from structures of high attenuation such as the shoulders and the hips. Motion artifact occurs as objects move to different positions during image acquisition. The result is a blurred or duplicated image. Streak artifacts emanate from high-density sharp-edged objects such as metal. Reconstruction algorithms are not possible when significant artifacts exist because of problems with misregistration as detected by the computer.

Ultrasound

Ultrasound uses sound waves to evaluate tissues. The ultrasound transducer converts electrical energy to a brief pulse of high-frequency sound energy that is transmitted into the patients' tissues. The transducer then becomes a receiver, detecting the echoes reflected from the tissues. The transducer is applied directly to the patient's skin using a water-soluble gel as a coupling agent to ensure good contact and conduction. By adjusting the angle of the transducer and the position of the patient, images may be produced in any anatomic plane. The quality of all ultrasound examinations depends heavily on the skill and diligence of the sonographer. Ultrasound examinations provide the most diagnostic information when they are directed at answering a particular clinical question. Visualization of anatomic structures by ultrasound is severely limited by bone and by gas-containing structures such as the bowel and lung. Acoustic shadowing from the bone limits visualization of structures deep to the bone surface and precludes imaging of the bones.

Bone Scinitigraphy

A bone scan is a map of osteoblastic activity that occurs in response to a variety of conditions. It is an excellent complement to other radiographic studies of the skeletal system. Blood flow is required to deliver the radiopharmaceutical to functioning osteoblasts. Skeletal scinitigraphy has a resolution of about 5 mm in the best conditions. Adult intravenous doses of 20 mCi or more of Tc-99m diphosphonates are adequate for static imaging 3–4 hours after injection. Conditions stimulating skeletal blood flow, pathologic and nonpathologic, as well as vigorous osteoblastic activity such as that seen in the juvenile skeleton or healing fractures increase bone labeling. Spot view, whole-body, and single-photon emission computed tomography imaging technology may be used.

Magnetic Resonance Imaging

Magnetic resonance imaging (MRI) is a technique that produces tomographic images by means of magnetic fields and radio waves. While CT evaluates only a single tissue parameter, that is, X-ray attenuation, MRI analyzes multiple tissue characteristics, including hydrogen or proton density, T1 and T2 relaxation times of tissue, and blood flow within tissue. The soft tissue contrast provided by MRI is substantially better than that of any other imaging modality. Differences in the density of protons available to contribute to the MRI signal discriminate one tissue from another.

The physics of MRI is beyond the scope of this chapter. However, put simply, MRI is based on the ability of a small number of protons within the body to absorb and emit radio wave energy when the body is placed within a strong magnetic field. The two major components of MRI machine settings are TR and TE. The time between the administered radio frequency pulses, or the time allowed for protons to align with the main magnetic field, is TR. The time allowed for absorbed radio wave energy to be released and detected is TE. T1 weighted (T1WI) images are obtained by selecting short TR (<500 ms) and short TE (<20 ms) settings. T1WI usually provide the best anatomic detail and are good for identifying fat and subacute hemorrhage. A T2 weighted image (T2WI) is selected by using a long TR (>2000 ms) and long TE (>80 ms) values. T2WI usually provides the most sensitive detection of pathologic lesions.

The MRI signal is weak; therefore prolonged imaging time is often required for optimal images. An entire series of images covering a specified body area is obtained during the imaging time as compared with CT, which produces images one slice at a time. Gradient-echo and fast spin-echo techniques have significantly decreased imaging times.

The advantages of MRI are its outstanding soft-tissue contrast resolution, ability to provide images in any anatomic plane, and absence of ionizing radiation. It is limited by the inability to demonstrate exquisite bone detail or small calcifications. It suffers from long imaging times, limited spatial resolution compared with CT, limited availability in many areas, and expense. The patient is physically confined in the magnet, and claustrophobia can be a problem. This can often be alleviated by sedation, but occasionally a patient simply cannot tolerate the procedure.

MRI is contraindicated for patients who have electrical, magnetic, or mechanical implants such as pacemakers, pumps, cochlear implants, and stimulators (bone or neuro), to name a few. Ferromagnetic implants such as aneurysm clips, vascular clips, and skin staples are at risk of dislodging or causing burns. Bullets or metallic fragments may move, dislodge, or become projectiles in the magnetic field. Metal workers and patients with a history of penetrating eye injuries should be screened with plain radiographs of the orbits to detect intraocular metallic foreign bodies that may dislodge and cause blindness. A number of implants have been confirmed to be safe for MRI, including nonferromagnetic vascular clips and orthopedic devices.

A number of artifacts can occur with MRI. These include ferromagnetic, motion, chemical shift, truncation, and aliasing. Ferromagnetic artifacts result from focal distortion in the main magnetic field due to the presence of objects such as orthopedic devices, surgical clips and wires, and metallic foreign bodies in the patient. A signal void is seen at the location of the metal device, and the image is distorted in the vicinity (Fig. 6–2). Motion artifact is common because of prolonged image acquisition time. The image will appear blurred or double-exposed. Chemical shift occurs at an interface between fat and water. The artifact appears as a line of high signal intensity on one side of the fat-water interface and a line of signal void at the opposite side of the fat-water interface. Truncation occurs adjacent to sharp boundaries between tissues of markedly different tissue contrast. This appears as regular intervals of alternating parallel bands of bright and dark signal. Aliasing is image wraparound and occurs when anatomy outside the designated field of view but still within the image plane is mismapped onto the opposite side of the image.

Basic principles are necessary for MRI interpretation. Water is generally low in signal on T1WI and gets bright on T2WI. This holds true for extracellular water and edema. Proteinaceous fluids are bright on both T1 and T2WI. Muscles have intermediate signal intensity on both T1 and T2WI, owing to the predominance of intracellular water. Hyaline cartilage has a predominance of extracellular water, but the water is extensively bound to a mucopolysaccharide matrix. Therefore its signal

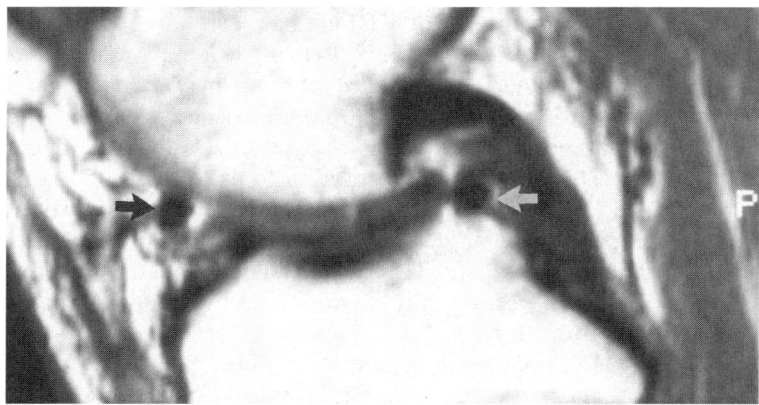 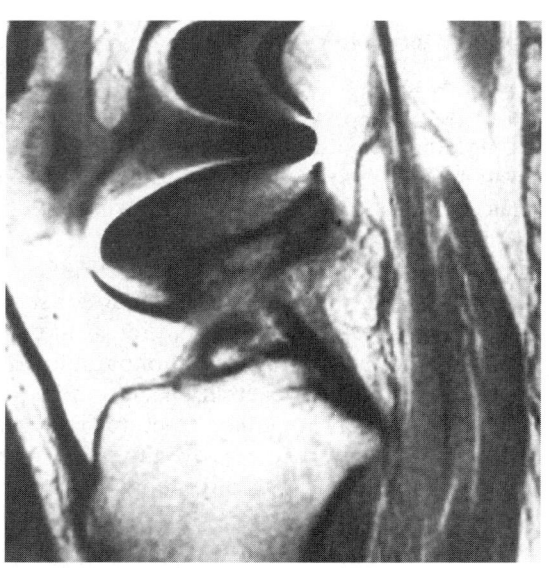

FIG. 6–2. **A:** A metallic artifact is noted mimicking a loose body (*arrows*). Note the low signal with high-signal rim. This represents a metallic artifact from previous arthroscopy. **B:** Metallic artifact from intramedullary rod obscures femur. A torn anterior cruciate ligament is noted.

characteristics resemble cellular soft tissues and is intermediate in strength on most imaging sequences. Fat is bright on T1WI and is lower in signal intensity relative to water on a T2WI. Using fat saturation techniques, pathologic processes are more visible because these areas remain abnormally bright on T2WI. Hemorrhage may have many different signal characteristics depending on its intracellular, extracellular methemaglobin state or on whether it has already matured to hemosiderin. The latter is dark on all sequences. The appearance of blood may be bright on T1WI and bright on the T2WI, low in signal on T1WI and bright on T2WI or bright on T1WI and low in signal on T2WI (see Fig. 6–3).

MRI arthrography has been employed to evaluate small structures within a joint as well as loose bodies. A contrast agent that has been developed for MRI, gadolinium, has been used to evaluate intra-articular

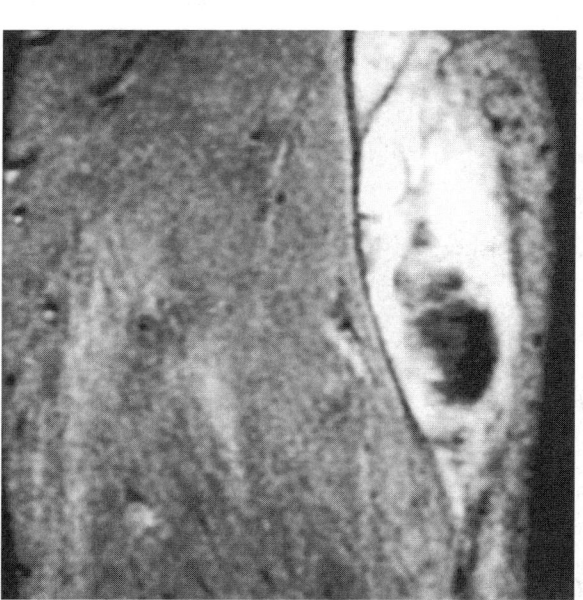 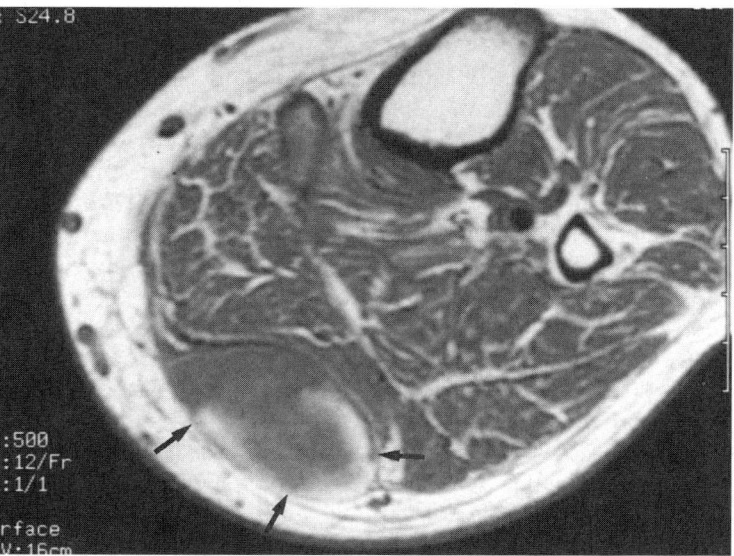

FIG. 6–3. Hemorrhage in a Baker's cyst. **A:** Coronal GRE (716/15 *15) shows low-signal globular structures in a Baker's cyst. **B:** The axial T1WI (400/12) reveals a mixture of high and low signals within the Baker's cyst (*arrows*) which has dissected down into the lower leg. Hemorrhage can be high in signal on a T1WI.

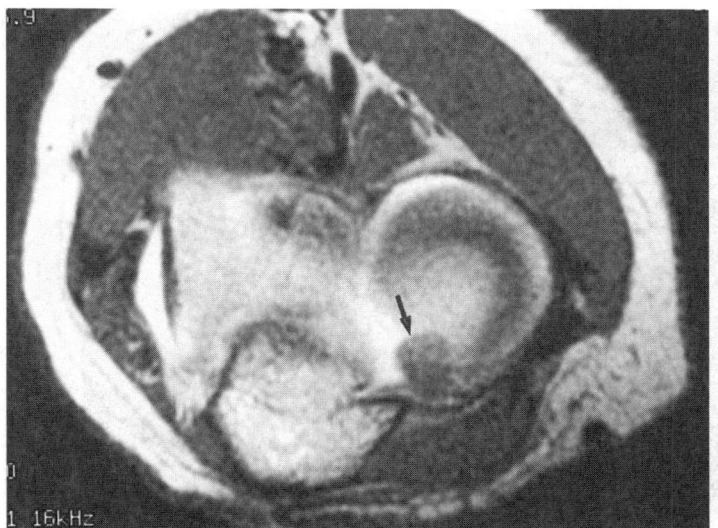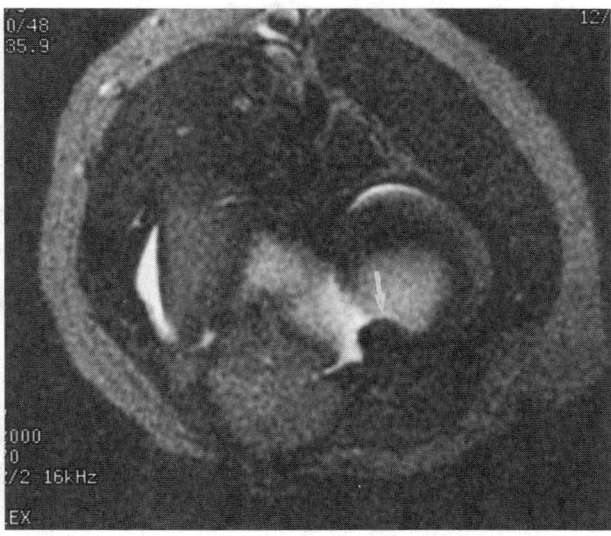

FIG. 6–4. This 13-year-old female fell off a horse and was unable to fully extend the elbow joint. **A:** Axial T1 (600/20) with intraarticular gadolinium and an axial T2WI. **B:** The loose body (*arrow*) adjacent to the radial head.

pathology, in much the same way as CT arthrography. A dilute injection using 1:200 gadolinium to saline is injected into a joint to evaluate subtle structures such as labral abnormalities in the hip or shoulder, to assess the integrity of a rotator cuff repair, and to evaluate for loose bodies (see Fig. 6–4). The procedure is performed as it is for CT in a fluoroscopy suite, followed by MRI. Fat saturation techniques are used, resulting in increased conspicuity of the gadolinium.

Using this brief review of the imaging modalities, the different tissue types will be discussed with the best imaging technique for that injured tissue type.

BONE

In deciding what modality to order in imaging a patient, the suspected injured tissue should be considered. Generally, the initial screening examination to evaluate an injury is a plain radiograph. At least two views at orthogonal planes are obtained and, when possible, three views. Plain films are useful for evaluating fractures and dislocations. At least two views are necessary to characterize the fracture and to assess for distraction and displacement. To satisfactorily reduce the fracture, knowledge of the direction of displacement is necessary (Fig. 6–5).

In setting a dislocation, it is imperative to know whether it is anteriorly or posteriorly positioned. Although this assessment can often be made clinically, the reduction can be made more difficult when an associated fracture is present. It is recommended that if an X-ray was not taken before reduction, such as in the acute shoulder dislocation, a series of postreduction films be obtained to exclude the not infrequently associated greater tuberosity fracture. Similarly, finding a volar plate fracture after reducing an interphalangeal dislocation is important to identify, as it may require additional treatment. Additional imaging can be performed with CT to evaluate the possibility of tiny intra-articular bone fragments after a dislocation (Fig. 6–6). The ability to have high resolution and thin slice thickness is a significant advantage of CT over conventional tomography. However, conventional tomography can be useful if hardware is present that would result in streak artifacts on CT and a suboptimal examination. Additional imaging with bone scan is not useful. In setting an associated fracture, the bone scan will show increased uptake at the fracture site. Ultrasound, because of its inherent inability to image the bones, is not useful for evaluating bone injury. Since dislocations are best managed with timely reduction, an MRI would delay the time to reduction. MRI becomes useful after a reduction in the clinical setting of persistent pain or failed reduction. The joint can be assessed for additional abnormalities such as soft tissue injuries, occult bone fractures, contusions, or entrapped soft tissues. These findings are not going to be visualized on the plain films.

Periosteal reactions such as that seen with stress fractures are also well demonstrated on a plain film examination. The plain film X-ray shows marked benign cortical thickening in the area of the stress fracture. Identifying this abnormality is imperative to appropriately rest the athlete. The consequences of untimely detection of a stress fracture can lead to unfortunate

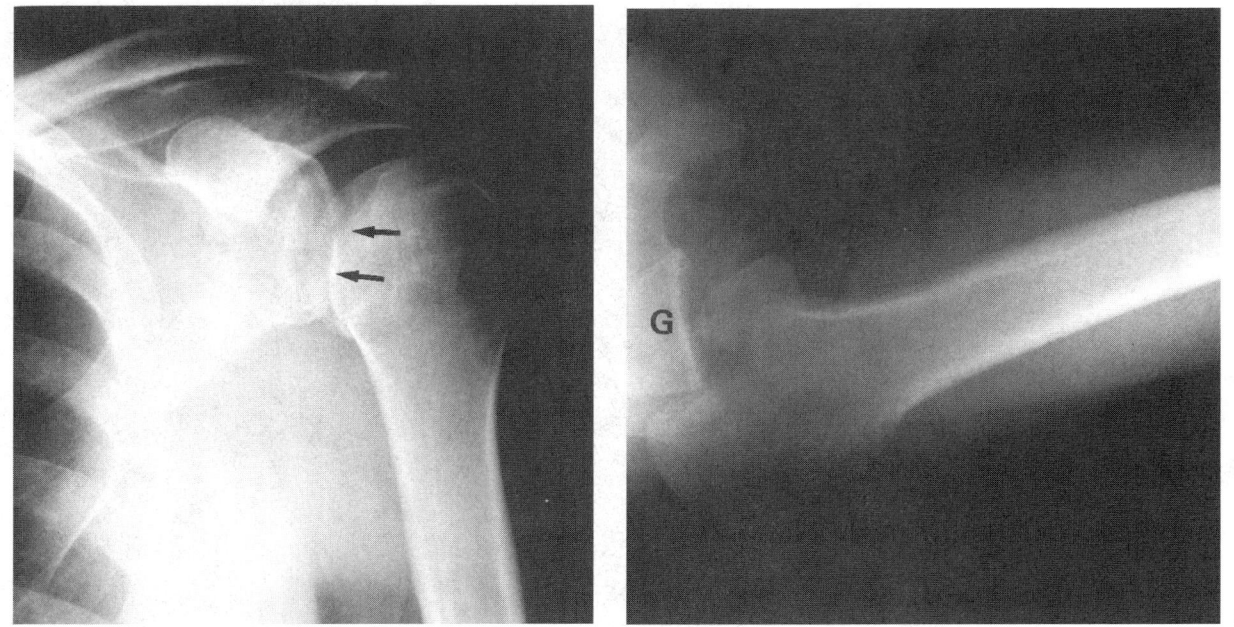

FIG. 6–5. This 50-year-old male suffered a posterior dislocation. **A:** AP view shows trough from impaction fracture (*arrows*), but a "normal" appearing joint space. **B:** Axillary view reveals posterior dislocation, fracture, and impaction. (G, glenoid.)

complications such as completing the fracture (Fig. 6–7). With a stress fracture in the hip, this complication could be devastating. However, the plain film is not always abnormal. With a high clinical suspicion for a stress fracture and a negative plain film, additional imaging is necessary. Conventional tomography was used for years to identify the subtle lucency associated with a stress fracture. Today there are more sophisticated techniques that use far less radiation and take far less time. A bone scan is often a useful imaging modality. The stress fracture will demonstrate characteristic focal linear uptake along the fracture site. The additional benefit of a bone scan is to precisely localize the area of the fracture.

Occasionally, the patient cannot precisely localize the pain on exam, resulting in numerous plain films. When a bone scan shows the precise location, additional imaging of the fracture can then be performed. It is often not necessary to perform additional imaging once the diagnosis on bone scan has been made. However, many clinicians prefer to visualize the fracture site. This can be done with CT. The subtle change in the periosteum can often be appreciated on the CT when the long bones are involved. For instance, a subtle lucency in the navicular is nicely demonstrated on CT owing to its intrinsic exquisite bone detail. The ability to use small slice thickness and the multiple planes of imaging make CT in

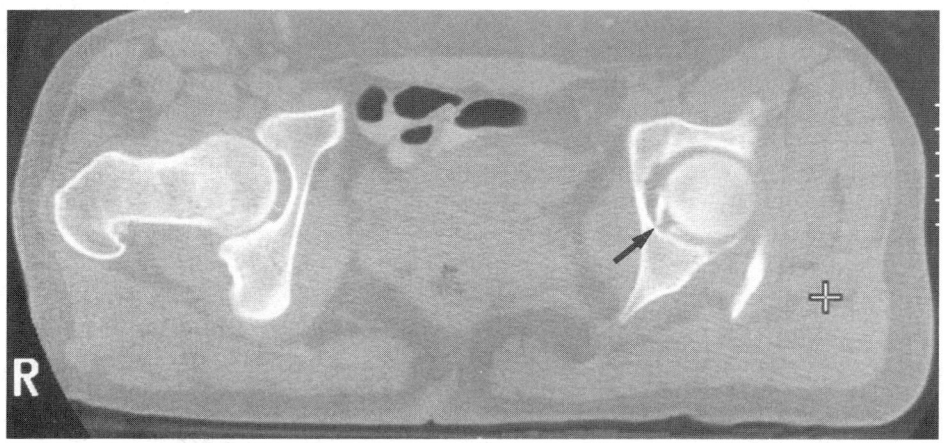

FIG. 6–6. This 21-year-old female sustained a hip dislocation. Axial CT, 1-mm thickness with bone algorithm demonstrating intraarticular bone fragments (*arrow*) from hip dislocation. Bone fragment represents a piece from an acetabular fracture not shown here.

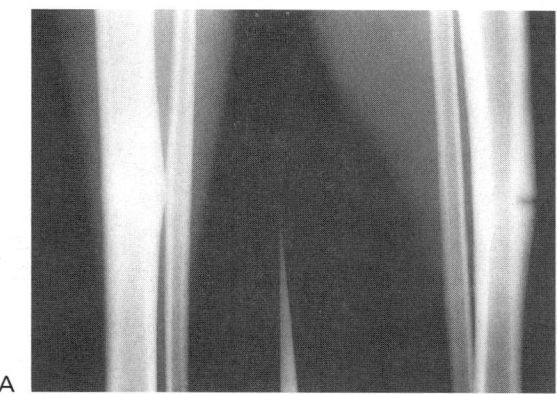
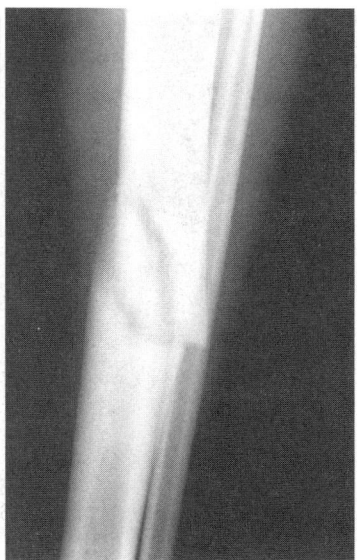

FIG. 6–7. A: This 19-year-old male continued to play basketball with the diagnosis of a stress fracture of the tibia. Note the cortical thickening and the lucency through the cortex. B: Follow-up X-ray reveals the completed fracture.

this situation a very useful diagnostic tool (Fig. 6–8). MRI is also extremely sensitive in evaluating for a stress fracture. It is important to have a more precise location of injury, as the sensitivity for the exam drops as the field of view becomes larger to incorporate an entire extremity, for instance. Once the area has been localized, either clinically or by bone scan imaging, an MRI can show the amount of periosteal reaction and associated bone marrow edema. This is demonstrated as low signal of the thickened periosteum on both T1 and T2WI. The associated marrow edema will be high in signal on the T2WI and should be focal in the area of the fracture site. The T1WI will demonstrate a linear low-signal band in the marrow representing the stress fracture (Fig. 6–9). The ability to evaluate the fracture in multiple planes and lack of ionizing radiation makes MR an attractive diagnostic study. Ultrasound provides no useful information for evaluation of this type of injury.

Avulsion injuries such as a Segond fracture or gamekeeper's injury are well visualized on plain film radiographs, but the associated soft tissue abnormalities such as the anterior cruciate ligament (ACL) tear or Stener lesion, respectively, will not be seen. When the lateral capsule of the knee avulses a piece of the posterior tibial plateau, a Segond fracture, there is a 99% correlation

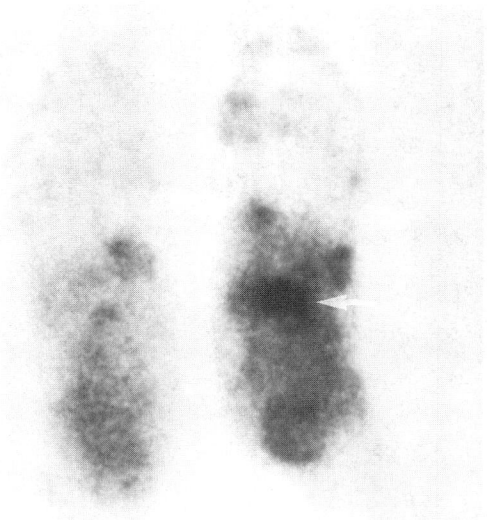
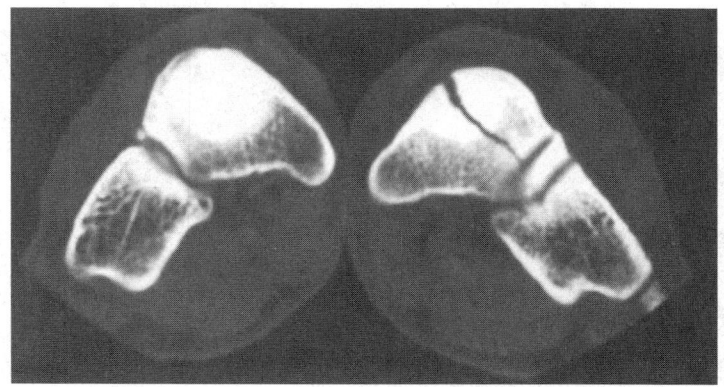

FIG. 6–8. A 28-year-old professional basketball player complained of foot pain. Plain films were negative. A: Bone scan showed increased uptake in the left navicular (*arrow*) and to a lesser degree in the tarsometatarsal joints. B: CT through the foot shows a nondisplaced fracture through the navicular.

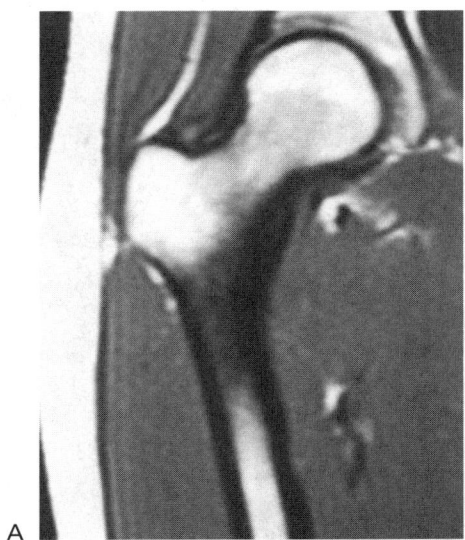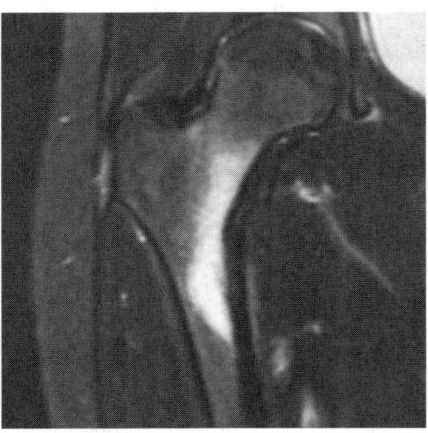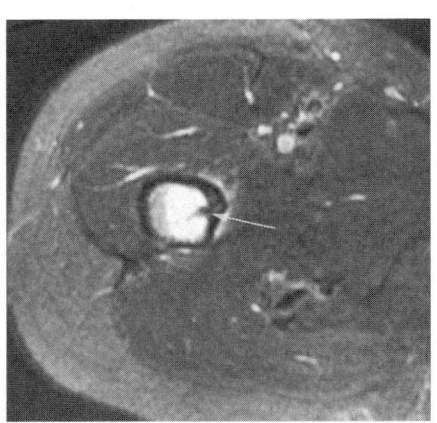

FIG. 6–9. This 40-year-old female was training for a marathon and developed groin pain. Plain films were negative. **A:** The T1WI coronal image (600/20) reveals low signal along the medial neck of femur. **B:** The corresponding FSE with fat saturation (3500/75Ef) shows the edema as high signal. **C:** FSE with fat saturation (3500/75Ef) reveals, in addition to the edema, a linear fracture line (*arrow*).

with a tear of the ACL (Fig. 6–10). The actual tear of the ACL is not visualized on plain radiographs, but the associated joint effusion should be easily seen. Similarly, the avulsion caused by the ulnar collateral ligament (UCL) in the thumb identifies the gamekeeper's injury. However, plain X-ray will not identify whether the adductor aponeurosis is trapped beneath the UCL preventing healing (a Stener lesion) (Fig. 6–11). Additional imaging with MRI eases the diagnostic dilemma. Because of MRI's exquisite tissue contrast, both bone and soft tissue abnormalities are readily appreciated. A T1WI will show diffuse low signal in the marrow at the site of the avulsion injury and even within the avulsed fragment. High signal will be seen in the T2WI as a

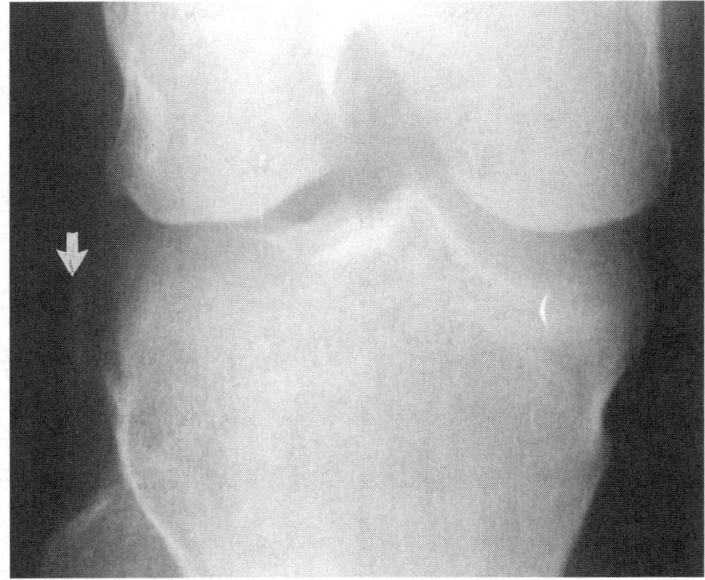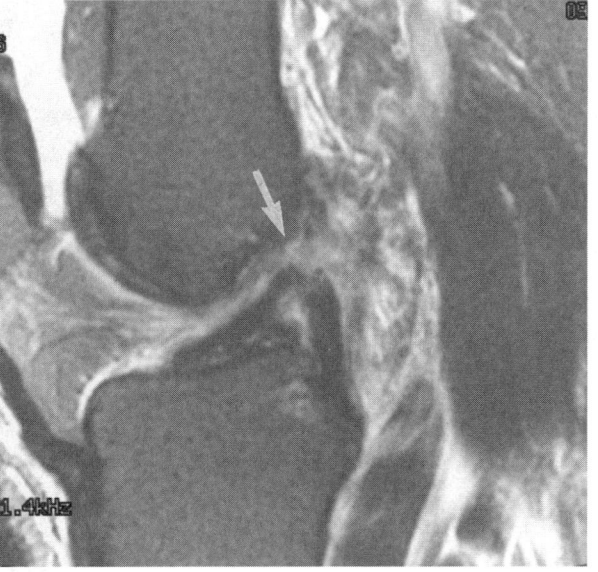

FIG. 6–10. This 22-year-old male fell while skiing and heard a "pop." **A:** Plain AP (*notch*) reveals a flake fracture from the posterolateral tibial plateau (*arrow*), a Segond fracture. **B:** The sagittal FSE with fat saturation (3500/75Ef) shows avulsion of ACL from femoral origin (*arrow*). A large joint effusion is also quite apparent.

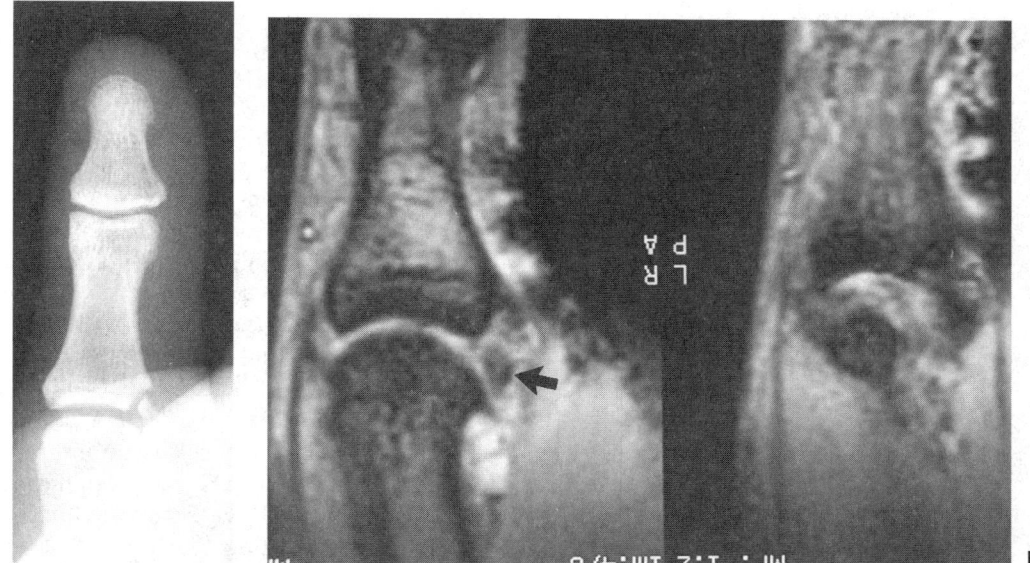

FIG. 6–11. This 16-year-old male fell while skiing and injured his thumb. **A:** Plain film X-ray shows an avulsion of ulnar aspect at first MCP joint (*arrow*), diagnostic of a gamekeeper's thumb. **B:** MR coronal GRE (400/20 *30) shows avulsion of the ulnar collateral ligament with adductor aponeurosis (*arrow*) trapped beneath the UCL.

result of the edema and hemorrhage at the avulsion site. When a nonhealing avulsion injury is identified, MRI can determine whether there is tissue present within the fracture site. CT is not as tissue contrast sensitive as MR is and therefore is unable to satisfactorily assess for the associated and important soft tissue injuries (Fig. 6–12). Similarly, bone scan imaging will show abnormal uptake in the bone associated with the avulsion injury at the donor site but will give no indication of the soft tissue abnormality. Conventional tomography has limitations similar to those of CT in that it can identify an avulsion but not any of the soft tissue abnormalities. The role for ultrasound in this type of injury is limited. In the hand, while the bone detail is not appreciated by ultrasound, the tissue planes can be imaged. Interpretation of ultrasound images for tendon avulsions is opera-

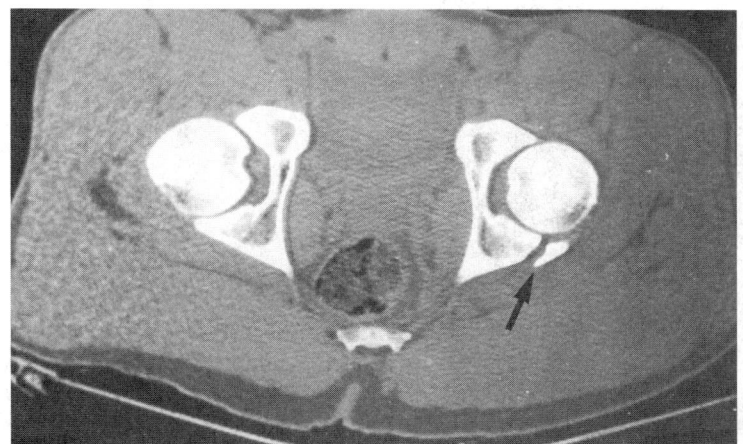
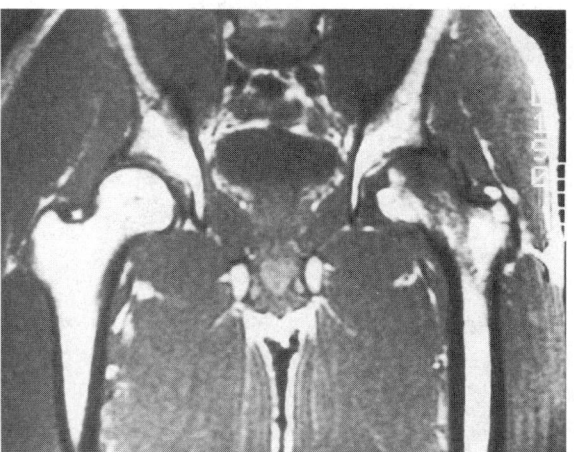

FIG. 6–12. CT axial image using bone algorithm in a 28-year-old male professional football player who was thought to have suffered a "hip pointer." **A:** CT shows avulsed fragment from posterior column of acetabulum (*arrow*). **B:** The MR T1 coronal image (600/20) shows, in addition to the acetabular abnormality, abnormal marrow signal in the left femoral head compatible with a contusion. This progressed to a focal area of avascular necrosis. The CT and MRI were very useful, as the injury was diagnosed to be much more serious than originally anticipated.

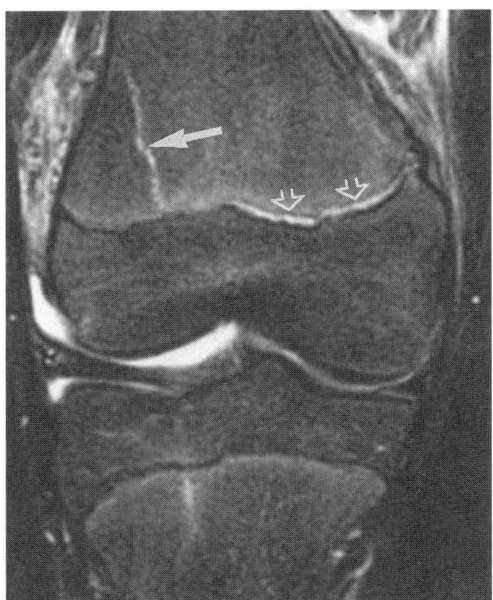

FIG. 6–13. A 13-year-old male was playing football and complained of knee pain. Plain films were normal. MRI was obtained because pain persisted. Coronal FSE T2 with fat saturation (3500/85Ef) shows a linear fracture (*arrow*) compatible with an occult Salter-Harris II fracture. Note the increased signal along the growth plate (*arrows*).

tor dependent and therefore does not have universal application.

In the setting of an occult fracture, the standard AP and lateral views may not show a fracture. Most reported data of utilization of MRI in evaluating occult bone injuries are around the knee and hip. However, a similar role exists for wrist, hand, and foot fractures. Fractures of the radial head and scaphoid fractures are two examples of injuries that can be detected with MRI. The T1WI will show linear low signal representing the fracture line. The T2WI will show the fracture (sometimes less conspicuously) but will show the associated edema and hemorrhage as high signal. In the setting of a normal plain film and clinical suspicion for a fracture, an MR can be performed to exclude the possibility of an occult fracture (Figs. 6–13 and 6–14). If there is no abnormal signal on the MRI, the examination is negative, and no fracture is present. Bone scan, however, still represents an effective, sensitive method for the diagnosis of an occult bone injury. The bone scan will show linear uptake of radiopharmaceutical along the fracture site. Bone scan is helpful, additionally, in specifically localizing the area of abnormality, which may be difficult on clinical exam. However, in an osteoporotic patient the bone scan could take up to 48 hours to become positive. CT examination and conventional tomography can identify subtle bone abnormalities, making them both sensitive and specific, but conventional tomography uses more radiation and is more time consuming. The advantages of CT are that it is fast, uses thin slice thickness, and can be performed in different imaging planes (not as many as MRI). A disadvantage is that it uses ionizing radiation. There is no role for ultrasound in the evaluation of occult fractures.

Bone contusions are not identified on plain X-ray or CT but are easily diagnosed on MRI and bone scan. With a normal plain film and clinical suspicion for an

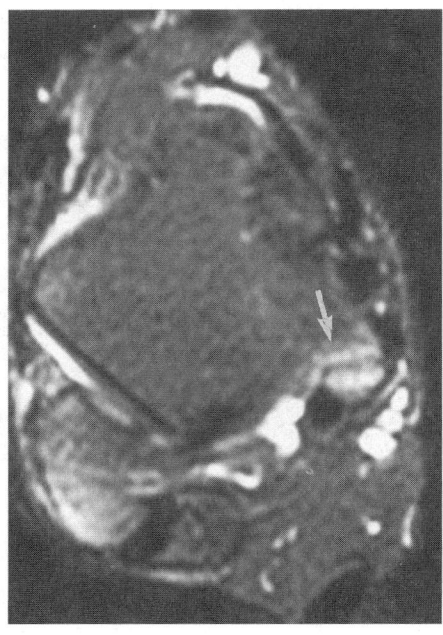 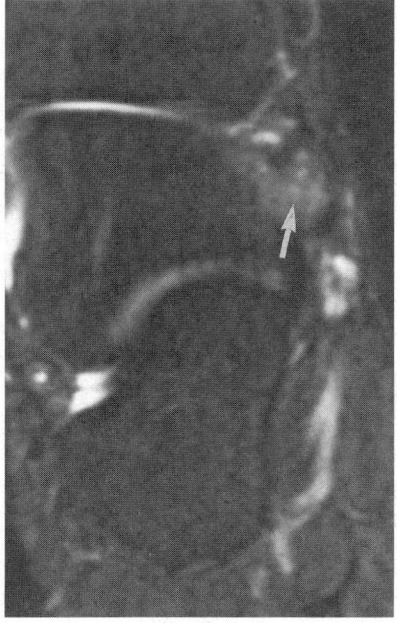

FIG. 6–14. This 20-year-old male football player had complaints referable to the posteromedial joint line of the ankle. Plain X-rays were normal. Axial (**A**) and coronal (**B**) fast spin echo with fat saturation (3850/65Ef) show increased signal in the medial tubercle of the talus (*arrows*). This is a contusion or possible occult fracture.

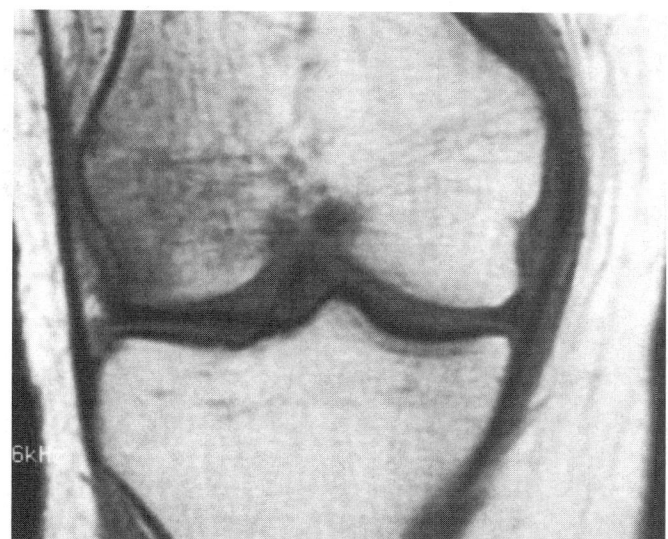 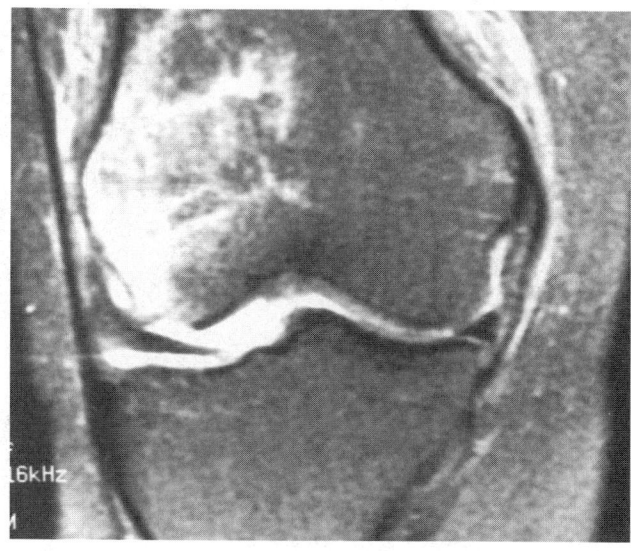

FIG. 6-15. This 22-year-old female dislocated her patella during a soccer match. The T1WI coronal image (**A**) (600/13) shows low signal in the anterior lateral femoral condyle, which on the FSE with fat saturation image (**B**) (3000/54Ef) is high in signal. This is a characteristic location of contusion as a result of a patella dislocation.

abnormality, additional imaging is recommended with MRI. The examination shows abnormal marrow signal in a geographic distribution that is low in signal on T1WI and becomes high in signal on T2WI (Fig. 6–15). Occasionally, the contusion is the only abnormality noted on the MRI and is the source of the patient's pain. When these contusions are large and are left unprotected, they can go on to osteochondritis dissecans. MRI is extremely useful in the setting of a normal plain X-ray and a high clinical suspicion of an injury. Proper treatment can be instituted more quickly and effectively, potentially preventing an unfortunate outcome. Bone scan is sensitive but not specific for the evaluation of contusions. Increased uptake can be seen with a geographic distribution, but a similar pattern can be seen with tumors and avascular necrosis. Therefore, MRI is the examination of choice.

In summary, when an injury to bone is suspected or needs to be evaluated, plain X-rays are the first radiologic examination obtained. The soft tissue structures around bones and joints are not effectively evaluated, although a joint effusion may be appreciated on plain films because of the tissue contrast between joint fluid and the fat pads that surround the joint. MRI demonstrates exquisite tissue contrast, and if the plain radiographs are negative for an abnormality and the clinical suspicion remains high for pathology, this is the study of choice. It has remarkable abilities to evaluate the bone marrow to assess for stress fracture, occult fractures, and associated soft tissue injuries. CT is sensitive and specific for evaluating bone abnormalities. A disadvantage is that it uses ionizing radiation, but the examinations can be performed quickly. Soft tissue abnormalities are not nearly as well depicted as they are on MRI. Conventional tomography is useful when a patient has a lot of hardware that could impede the interpretation of the MRI or CT examination. It is quite adequate for evaluating nonunion and subtle fractures but is limited by its inability to evaluate soft tissue structures. Bone scan is very sensitive for identifying fractures, stress, or occult. Often, further imaging is required, either CT or MRI, to visualize the fracture site. Additionally, the geographic increased uptake seen in a contusion, while sensitive for an abnormality, is not specific. There is essentially no role for ultrasound in evaluating bone detail.

CARTILAGE

Different cartilaginous structures exist in and around a joint. These include the hyaline articular cartilage lining the joint surfaces and the fibrocartilaginous structures, labrum in the shoulder and hip (limbus), and the menisci in the knee. In assessing cartilaginous structures, MRI is the modality of choice. Recently, the literature has touted a number of imaging techniques to better assess the cartilage. The most easily identified articular cartilage is in the knee. Evaluation of the articular cartilage in the shoulder, hip, and ankle is much more difficult, and techniques have not been perfected to adequately assess for abnormalities in these locations. It has been shown that standard imaging of the knee using fat-saturated fast spin echo T2WI is more than adequate for assessing articular cartilage abnormalities. The normal

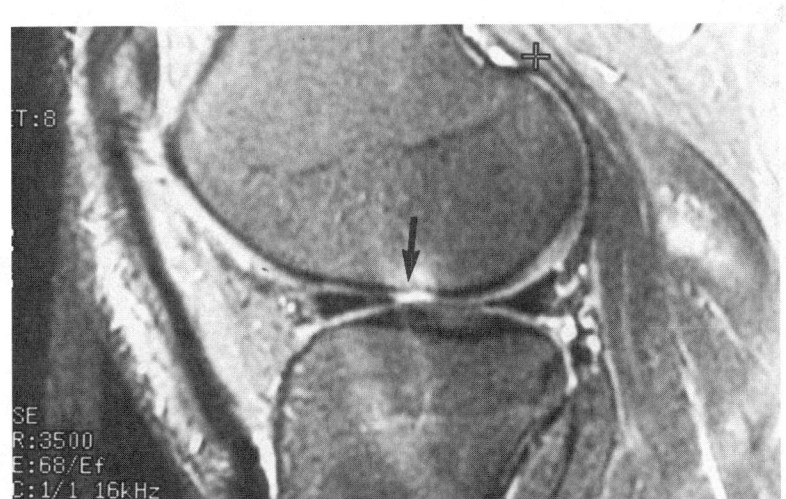
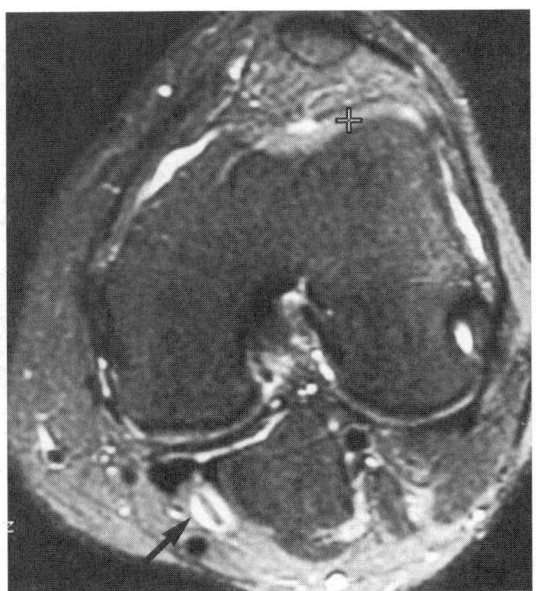

FIG. 6–16. **A:** A 19-year-old basketball player with knee pain. Focal cartilage defect (*arrow*) is noted adjacent to normal appearing cartilage on sagittal FSE with fat saturation (3500/65Ef). **B:** The loose cartilage (*arrow*) is identified in a small Baker's cyst.

cartilage lining the bone should be intermediate (gray) in signal. An abnormality is diagnosed if there is focal signal abnormality. That is, if a focus of high signal is identified within the cartilage, an abnormality is present (Fig. 6–16). Unfortunately, it is not possible to determine with certainty whether the cartilage abnormality represents a delaminating injury, a focus of a partial thickness abnormality, or an area of severe chondromalacia. Generally, completely denuded cartilage can readily be detected (Fig. 6–17). This information is extremely useful to the surgeon. If the cartilage abnormality can be localized, that area can be probed at the time of arthroscopy, and an otherwise unappreciated cartilage defect can be exposed. Therefore, the imaging guides the surgeon to the location of the abnormality, but MRI cannot always reliably determine the degree of cartilage injury.

In the shoulder and hip, the cartilage is more difficult to evaluate. The hip articular cartilage can occasionally be imaged by using a surface coil and a very small field of view with a very thin slice thickness. It is important that enough signal to noise be maintained to adequately visualize this small structure. If cartilage abnormalities are suspected, a smaller field of view can be obtained with small slice thickness, keeping in mind the important signal-to-noise ratio necessary for MRI to be so sensitive. The signal abnormalities in the shoulder, hip, and ankle articular cartilage are interpreted in the same way as those in the knee. The area is localized and described for the surgeon, but no attempt is made to suggest the

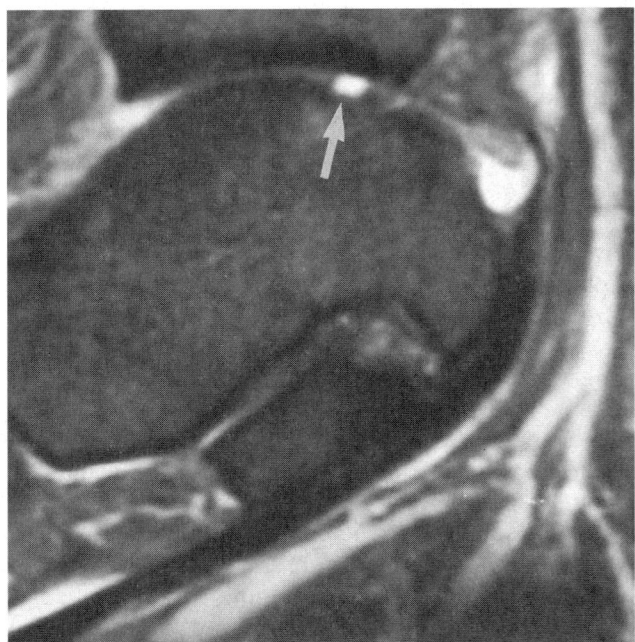

FIG. 6–17. This 20-year-old college basketball player suffered an inversion injury. Sagittal fast spin echo with fat saturation (3333/75Ef) shows a focal cartilage abnormality along the talar dome (*arrow*). Joint fluid is noted where the defect in the cartilage exists. (Anterior is to the left.)

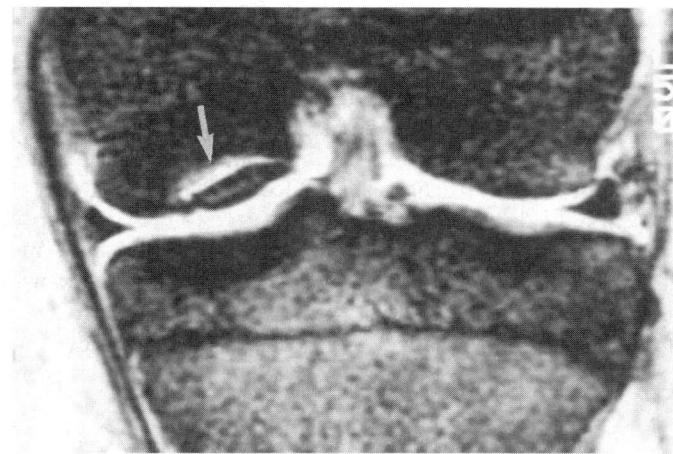 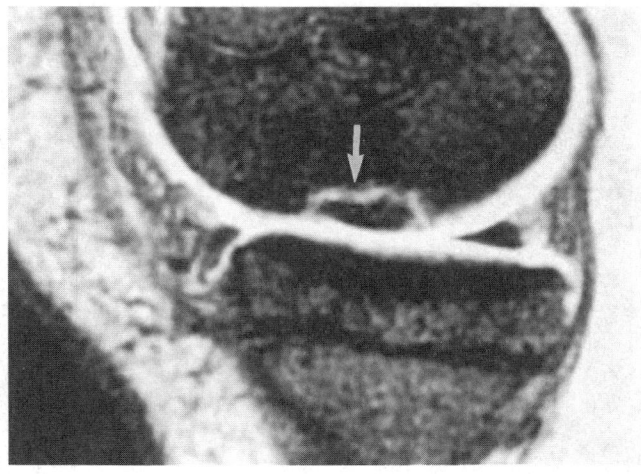

FIG. 6–18. This 13-year-old female has an osteochondritis dissecans of the medial femoral condyle. (A) Note the high signal around the fragment (*arrow*) on the coronal and (B) sagittal GRE (600/20 *30) images. This would be compatible with an unstable fragment.

severity except in the situation of an osteochondral injury.

Osteochondritis dissecans (OCD) or an osteochondral injury from trauma is important to identify. MRI is superb at determining whether the fragment is stable or unstable. OCD is identified as a focal area of low signal on T1W1 in a subchondral location. Three different appearances exist on MRI if the fragment is unstable: high signal around the fragment on the T2WI, high signal on T2WI in the bed where the expected osteochondral fragment would be, and, additionally, the osteochondral fragment itself can demonstrate high signal on T2WI (Fig. 6–18). MRI is extremely useful because even when not apparent on plain films, the focus of osteochondritis dissecans can be identified and its stability assessed. Bone scan can identify the area of osteochondritis dissecans as focal increased uptake but is nonspecific and cannot determine whether the fragment is stable or unstable. CT can demonstrate the fragment and with thin slice thickness can also demonstrate the donor site (Fig. 6–19). Plain films may identify the OCD but cannot assess stability of the fragment (Fig. 6–20).

In evaluating the meniscus of the knee, the MRI sequence of choice is a sagittal image using an imaging sequence with a short TE. This includes a T1WI, a proton density image, and a gradient echo image. The normal meniscus is identified as uniformly low in signal on these sequences with several body segments and several anterior and posterior horn images (Fig. 6–21). A simple oblique tear is diagnosed when the articular surface (either superior or inferior) is disrupted by linear

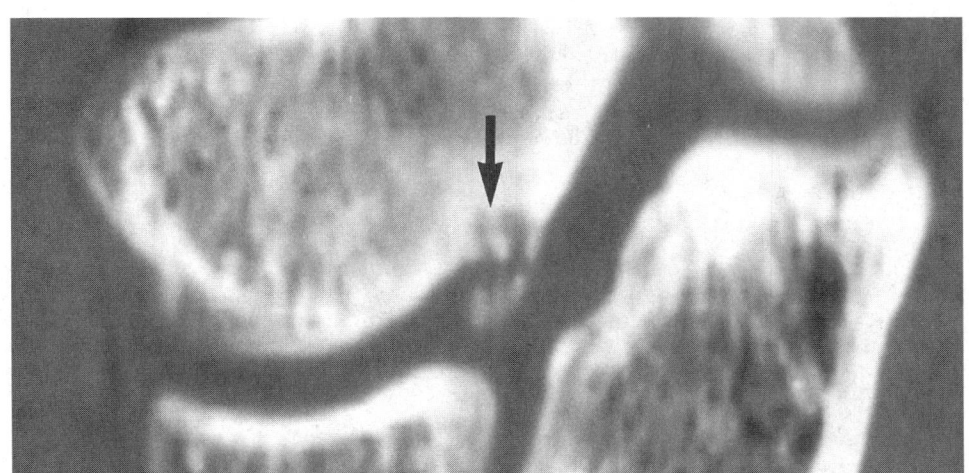

FIG. 6–19. An 18-year-old male basketball player had a complaint of inability to completely extend the elbow. CT at 1-mm acquisition with coronal reformations was obtained. Osteochondritis dissecans with a loose body (*arrow*) is noted in the capitellum.

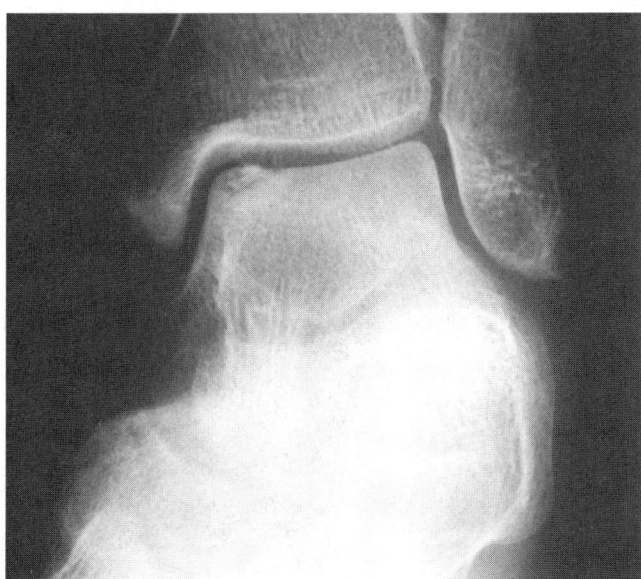

FIG. 6–20. This 28-year-old male sustained an inversion injury of the ankle and complained of persistent pain. Evaluation of the superior medial dome of the talus reveals osteochondritis dissecans. The stability of the fragment cannot be assessed on the plain film.

diagnosed when there is abnormal rounded high signal within the meniscus that seems to cause bowing of the surface of the meniscus (Fig. 6–25). A tear is not always identified on MRI when a meniscal cyst is identified. Horizontal linear high signal through the meniscus suggests a horizontal cleavage tear, and a thorough search for a parameniscal cyst is necessary (Fig. 6–26). It is thought that the horizontal cleavage tear is a collapsed meniscal cyst that has expressed its fluid out through the meniscus into a well-contained parameniscal component. This is seen as a well-defined high-signal focus on the T2WI that can be seen arising from the meniscus.

Evaluation of the labrum in the shoulder is best done with MRI arthrography. Conventional MRI is not as adequate to assess for labral detachments as MRI arthrography unless there is native joint fluid present. A dilution of gadolinium with saline instilled in the

high signal (Fig. 6–22). It has been established that a long TE (T2WI) can mask signal that would ordinarily diagnose a meniscal tear and is therefore not recommended as a sequence for evaluating the meniscus. Additional tears of the meniscus are diagnosed by a change in the morphology. A parrot beak tear or radial tear is identified as a truncation of meniscal tissue (Fig. 6–23). Rather than demonstrating a triangular morphology, the edge of the meniscus is squared. This is a tear that occurs on the free edge of the meniscus. A commonly overlooked meniscal tear is the bucket handle tear. It is not possible always to rely on the signal characteristics of the abnormal meniscus to diagnose this type of tear. Careful evaluation of the morphology of the meniscus is required. The normal meniscus averages about 9–12 mm in width. When sagittal images of 4-mm slices are used, the mensicus should resemble a slab of tissue that is uniformly low in signal on at least two to three images. If fewer than that number are identified, the possibility of a bucket handle tear is raised. Occasionally, the torn meniscus will be displaced into the notch and mimic a second posterior cruciate ligament (PCL). This appearance has been termed the "double PCL sign" (Fig. 6–24). In the case of discoid meniscus the meniscal tissue will be bigger than expected, and therefore more than three slabs of meniscal tissue will be identified. Discoid menisci are more common laterally and are reported to occur in 3–6% of the population. They are prone to meniscal tears and meniscal cysts. Meniscal cysts are

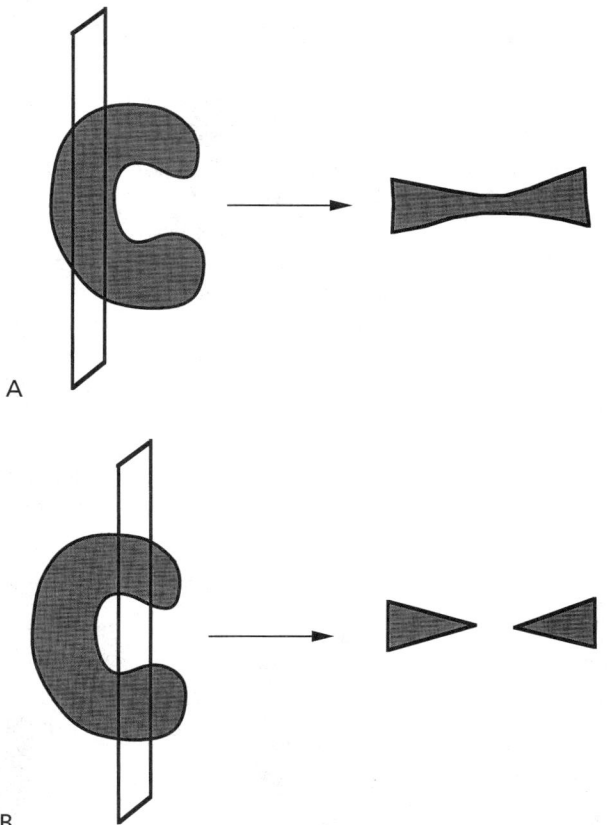

FIG. 6–21. A: Shape and size of the meniscus. When sagittal images are obtained through the body, a full "slab" of meniscus should be present. **B:** When a sagittal image is obtained through the anterior and posterior horns, two triangles are present. If the meniscus is narrow (such as a bucket handle tear), then fewer body segments are noted, and many more anterior and posterior horns are present instead. In contrast, a discoid meniscus will have an increase in the number of body segments and a smaller number of anterior and posterior horns.

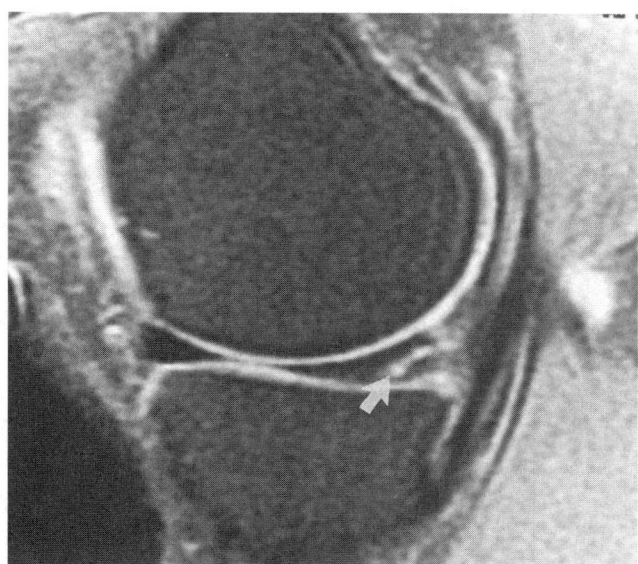

FIG. 6–22. This 47-year-old male demonstrates high signal in an oblique orientation in the posterior horn and body of the medial meniscus on the proton density with fat saturation image (2000/20). At arthroscopy a large tear was identified in the body and posterior horn.

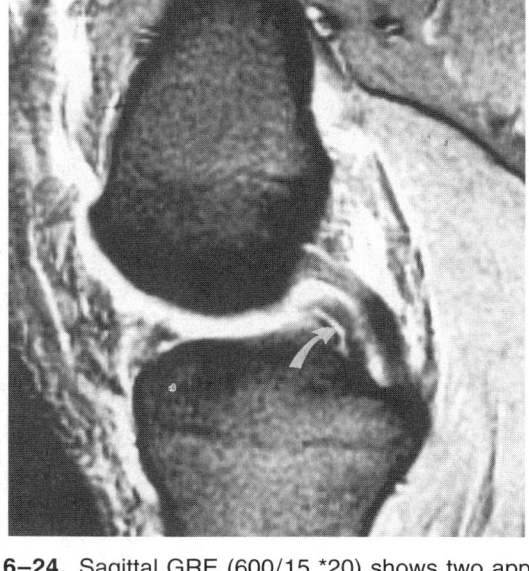

FIG. 6–24. Sagittal GRE (600/15 *20) shows two apparent posterior cruciate ligaments. The more inferiorly located low-signal curvilinear structure (*arrow*) is the torn bucket handle of the medial meniscus. This is what is referred to as "a double PCL sign."

shoulder to the point of joint distention allows for better visualization of labral tears. Tears are identified as fluid extending through the substance of the labrum or identifying the labrum as detached from the glenoid (Fig. 6–27). An exception to this definition is in the superior-anterior labrum above the equator of the glenoid. The sublabral foramen is located in this area, and an isolated tear in this portion of the labrum is difficult to diagnose (Fig. 6–28). The lack of fluid in the joint can make assessment of labral pathology difficult. However, labral tears can still be diagnosed (Figs. 6–29 and 6–30).

Before MRI became readily available, CT was used in combination with arthrography to evaluate instability and assess the labrum. This is done by introducing a mixture of iodinated contrast with air into the joint to distend the joint capsule and imaging the patient immediately with axial CT scans and thin slice thickness. This technique allows for superior imaging of the la-

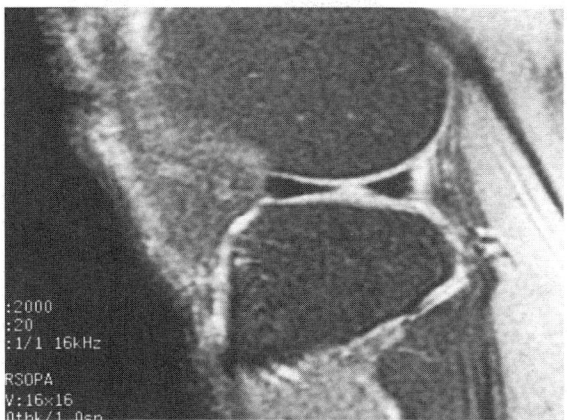

FIG. 6–23. Lateral meniscus of the same patient in Figure 6–22. Note the slightly blunted appearance to the anterior and posterior horn on this sagittal proton density image with fat saturation (2000/20). High signal is noted in the gap where meniscal tissue should be demonstrating a parrot beak or radial tear.

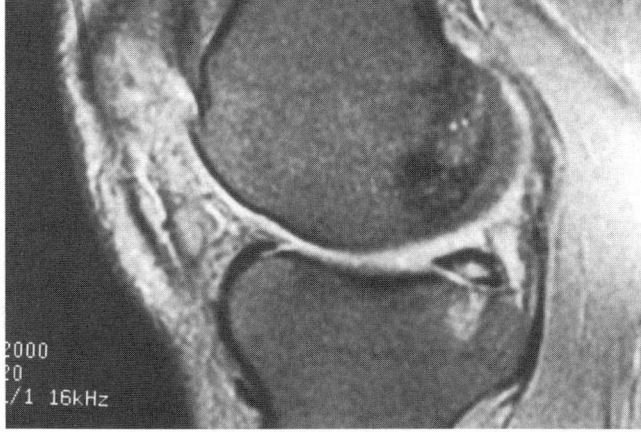

FIG. 6–25. Thirty-nine-year-old male with medial joint pain. Sagittal proton density image with fat saturation (2000/20) shows globular marked high signal within the posterior horn of the medial meniscus. This is the appearance of an intrameniscal cyst.

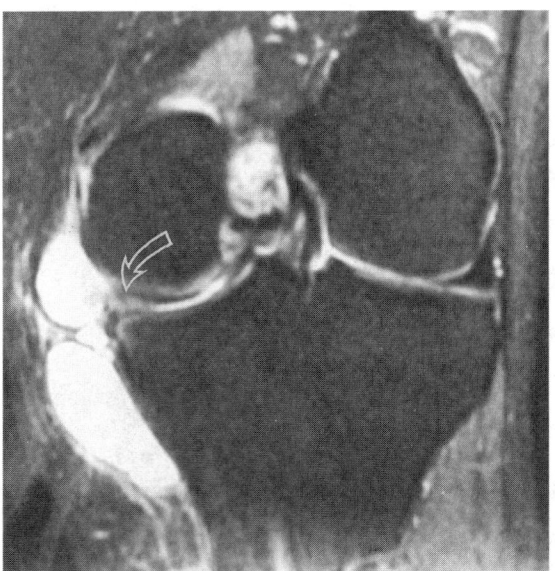

FIG. 6-26. Coronal FSE with fat saturation (3500/85Ef) shows well-contained high-signal collection with a neck (*arrow*) arising from the medial meniscus. The appearance is compatible with a parameniscal cyst.

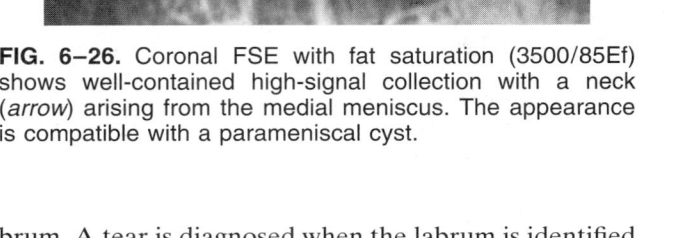

FIG. 6-28. Axial FSE with fat saturation (3500/54Ef) demonstrates native joint fluid with some debris (low signal in the joint fluid). A sublabral foramen is noted (*curved arrow*). Incidentally seen is a thickened middle glenohumeral ligament (*arrow*).

brum. A tear is diagnosed when the labrum is identified as detached from the glenoid or when contrast is identified extending through the labrum (Fig. 6-31). CT arthrography is still used, especially in a patient who is not MRI compatible—that is, a patient with a pacemaker device or internal metallic device (e.g., pump, cochlear implant, aneurysmal clips) that may torque and result in injury or a patient whose body habitus precludes fitting in the bore of the magnet.

In evaluating the labrum in the hip, MRI is the best way to assess for an abnormality in these patients. By using a small field of view, surface coil, and thin slices,

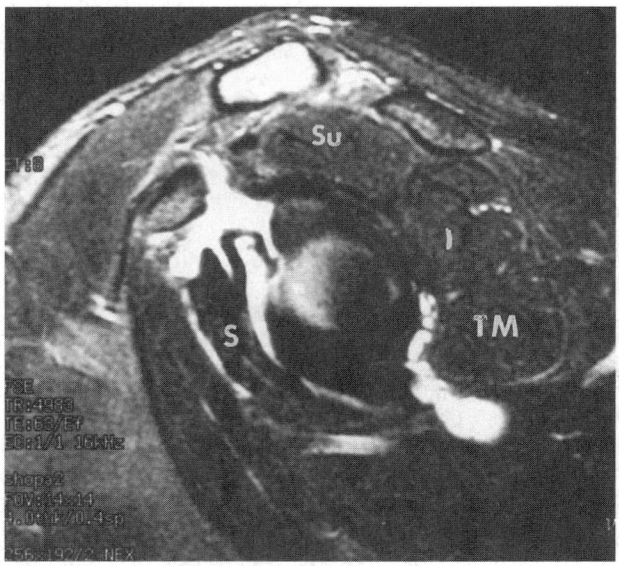
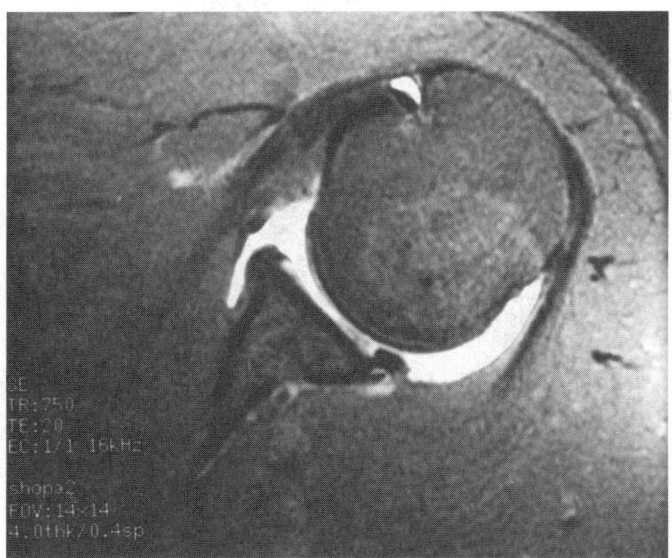

FIG. 6-27. Thirty-year-old recreational basketball player. **A:** Sagittal (anterior is to the left). FSE with fat saturation (4983/68Ef) and intraarticular gadolinium show gadolinium posteriorly in a large labral cyst. (Su, supraspinatus, I, infraspinatus, TM, teres minor, and S, subscapularis.) There is a 100% correlation of a labral tear when a labral cyst is identified. **B:** The axial T1WI (750/20) with fat saturation shows a blunted anterior labrum and torn posterior labrum. (Anterior is to the top.)

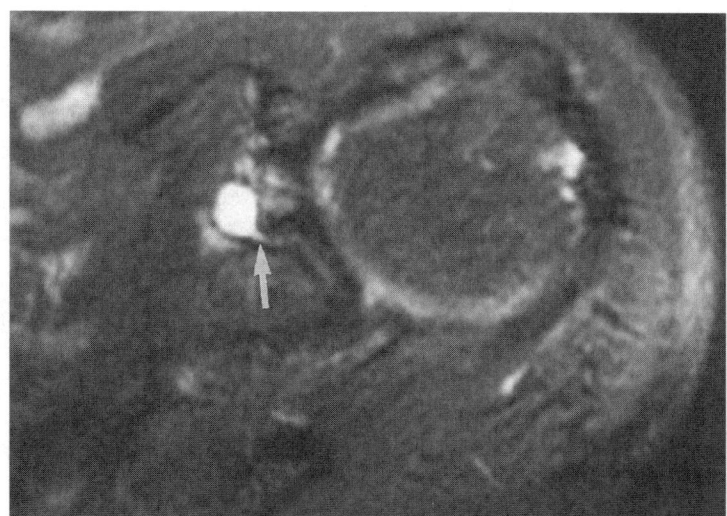 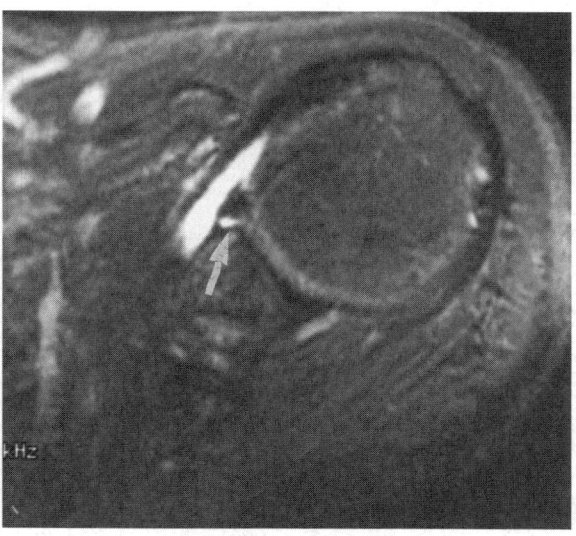

FIG. 6–29. These are adjacent axial images. (Anterior is to the top.) **A:** Fast spin echo with fat saturation (3580/65Ef) without intraarticular gadolinium reveals a small anterior ganglion (*arrow*). **B:** The next axial image demonstrates joint fluid beneath the anterior labrum (*arrow*). This is a labral tear.

the labrum can be evaluated in both the axial and coronal plane. Ideally, if joint fluid is present, a tear is more conspicuously identified. As in the shoulder, instilling dilute gadolinium into the joint is a helpful way of diagnosing a tear. A tear is diagnosed when fluid is noted through the labrum or the labrum is completely detached from the acetabulum (Figs. 6–32 and 6–33). Variable appearances to the limbus are seen normally. It can be round, blunted, and partly attached. The labrum is always uniform in low signal on all imaging sequences unless it has been injured. CT arthrography can be performed for a patient who, for one reason or another, cannot tolerate an MRI. An arthrographic procedure is performed initially, followed by thin-section CT. A tear is diagnosed when contrast is identified through the

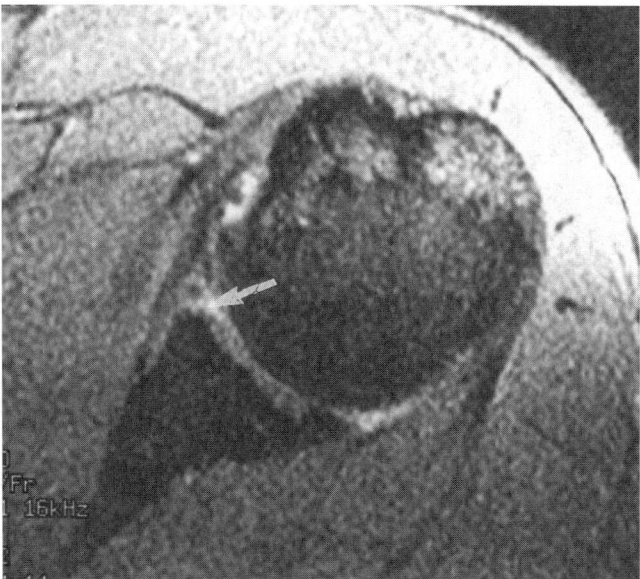

FIG. 6–30. A 27-year-old weight lifter complained of anterior shoulder pain. Noncontrast MR axial GRE image (500/15 *20) shows a torn anterior labrum (*arrow*) in this very muscular patient.

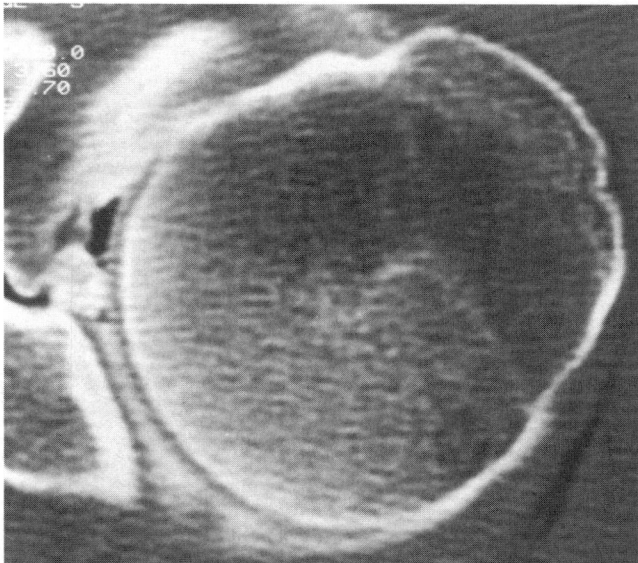

FIG. 6–31. This 39-year-old male with anterior shoulder instability shows on CT arthrography an abnormal anterior labrum that is irregular in appearance with globular configuration. The CT arthrogram should show the labrum as a "filling defect," as is demonstrated in the posterior labrum.

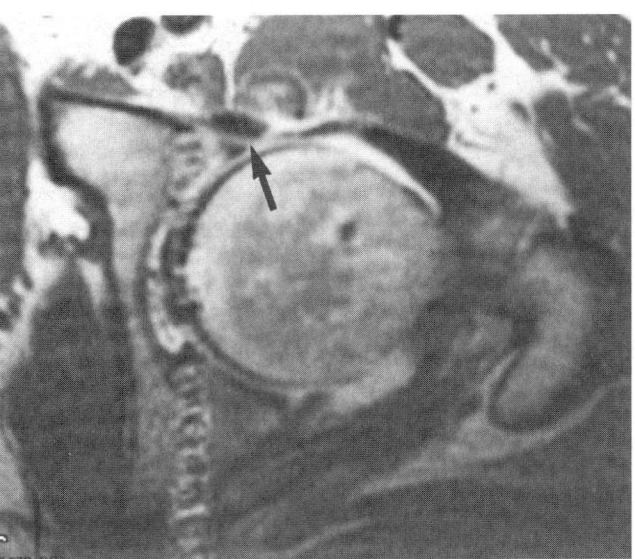

FIG. 6-32. This 34-year-old female jogger had a one-year history of clicking in the right hip. MRI arthrogram T1WI axial image (500/12) reveals linear high signal in the anterior labrum (*arrow*). This is a labral tear.

labrum or the labrum is noted to be detached. CT is not able to determine whether the labrum has been injured in any way other than being torn, whereas MRI can show intrinsic signal abnormalities suggesting contusion, as demonstrated by abnormal high signal throughout the labrum with preservation of morphology.

Cartilaginous structures are not well evaluated by plain X-ray. As was mentioned previously, an osteochondral defect may be appreciated on plain film, but this is due to the associated bony fragment. A bone scan will show increased uptake at the site of the osteochondral injury. Conventional tomography may identify an osteochondral injury, but this is time consuming and requires more radiation than CT. CT will show the bone defect but does not show cartilage detail. Conventional arthrography has been done to force fluid around the osteochondral defect to demonstrate whether this is an unstable fragment. When a forcible injection of contrast material is used, fluid should theoretically get around an unstable fragment. This can be painful for the patient, and the advent of MRI has precluded conventional arthrography and tomography as necessary for evaluating an unstable fragment. The labrum in the shoulder and hip and menisci in the knee are not assessed with plain film. There is no role for bone scan or ultrasound in assessing abnormalities of these structures.

In summary, the best way to evaluate cartilaginous structures is with MRI. Carefully designed protocols can adequately visualize the meniscus and labrum. Alternative imaging with CT arthrography is useful for labral imaging but will not give the additional imaging information that MRI will, such as the surrounding soft tissue structural integrity and potential associated injuries to the cuff, bone, or biceps. Conventional tomography and ultrasound provide no useful information. Bone scan is helpful in the specific situation of an osteochondral defect or injury, but the bone scan, while sensitive, is not specific.

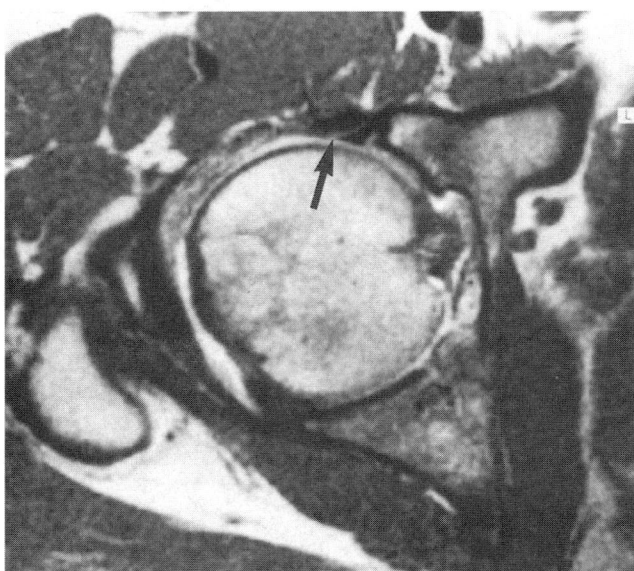

FIG. 6-33. Thirty-five-year-old male. MR arthrogram shows abnormal high signal in the anterior labrum (*arrow*) on the axial T1WI (400/12). The high signal at the labral bone interface represents cartilage. This is a labral tear.

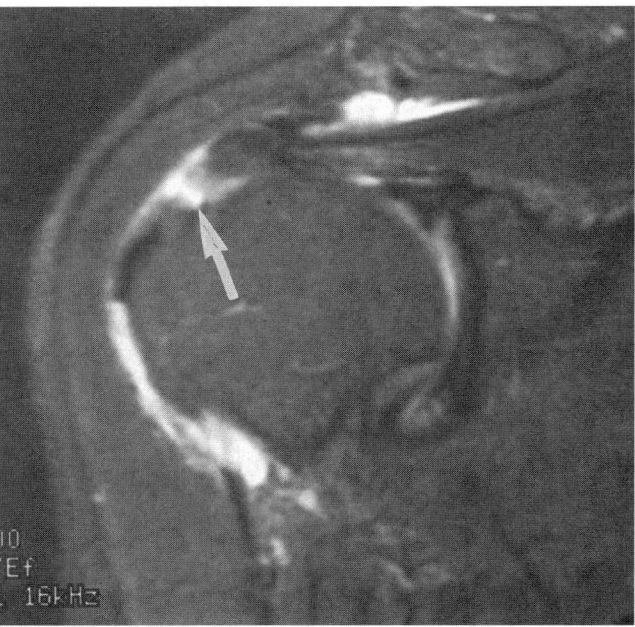

FIG. 6-34. Sixty-seven-year-old female recreational golfer. Oblique coronal FSE with fat saturation (4000/63Ef) shows high signal and a small gap (*arrow*) in the tendon of the rotator cuff. This is a full-thickness tear. Note the joint fluid and the fluid in the subacromial/subdeltoid bursa.

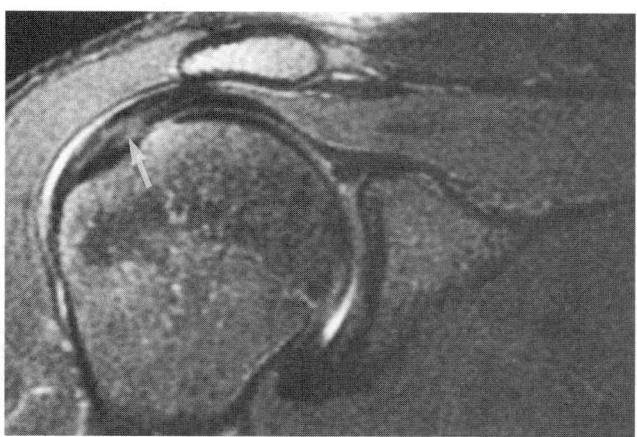

FIG. 6–35. This 22-year-old weight lifter complained of rotator cuff symptoms. Oblique coronal FSE with fat saturation (5000/65Ef) shows high signal in the tendon of the rotator cuff (*arrow*). No gap is identified in the tendon to suggest a full-thickness tear. Note that fibers of the tendon are seen to be contiguous. This high signal can be seen with a partial tear or tendinitis. It is termed tendinopathy.

LIGAMENTS AND TENDONS

The only imaging modality that can accurately assess tendon and ligament abnormalities is MRI. Limited application of ultrasound exists, and this will be discussed briefly. The other imaging modalities will not be discussed to any length. The most commonly injured structures will be discussed in this section.

Both ligaments and tendons are uniformly low in signal on T1 and T2WI on MRI when the structures are normal. Abnormalities in these structures are diagnosed when abnormal high signal is identified in the tendon or ligament on the T2WI. The abnormalities consist of strain (tendons) or sprain (ligaments), a partial tear, tendinopathy, or full-thickness tear. A full-thickness tear of a tendon or ligament is identified when the fibers of these structures are no longer visualized as a continuous low-signal band (Fig. 6–34). Partial tear or strain of a tendon has the same signal characteristics as tendinopathy. That is, some high signal will be identified within the tendon, but some visible low-signal fibers will be seen to still be intact. It is not possible by signal criteria to distinguish the difference between partial tear, a strain, or "tendonitis." The abnormality is collectively referred to as tendinopathy (Figs. 6–35 and 6–36). Occasionally, high signal can be seen in a tendon on the T1WI. This finding is not very significant, as there are numerous causes for this appearance. They include partial volume averaging with some adjacent fat, focus of calcification within the tendon, magic angle phenomenon (an artifact of imaging that occurs when anisotropic fibers in a structure run at an angle 55° to the bore of the magnet), and hemorrhage from a partial tear. When high signal is identified on the T2WI, then pathology is diagnosed. The type of pathology is based on whether intact fibers can be identified.

Within the foot and ankle, specific pathologic processes are worth mentioning. The tendons around the foot and ankle are easy to recognize and identify. All of the tendons demonstrate homogeneous low signal on all sequences when normal. As was described previously, if high signal is identified in the substance of

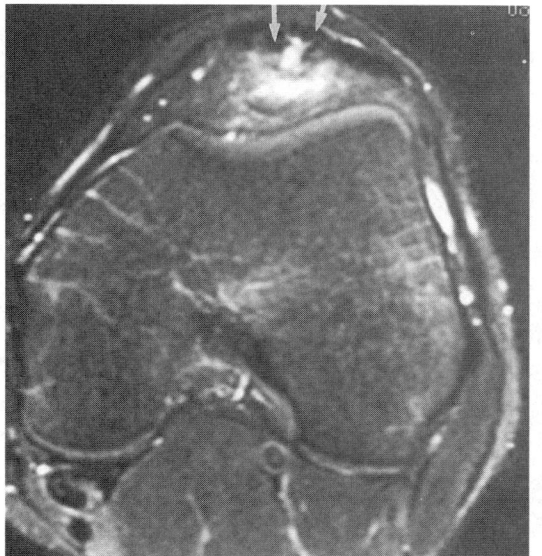
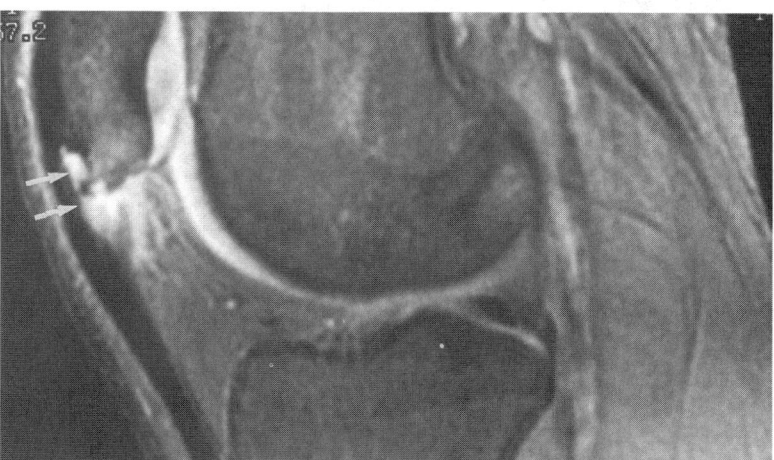

FIG. 6–36. Nineteen-year-old basketball player with complaints relating to jumper's knee. (**A**) Axial and (**B**) sagittal fast spin echo with fat saturation (3050/68Ef) reveal high signal in the inferior pole of the patella and patella tendon with attenuation of the patella tendon (*arrows*). MRI is a a helpful way to monitor the prognosis of jumper's knee, especially in an elite athlete.

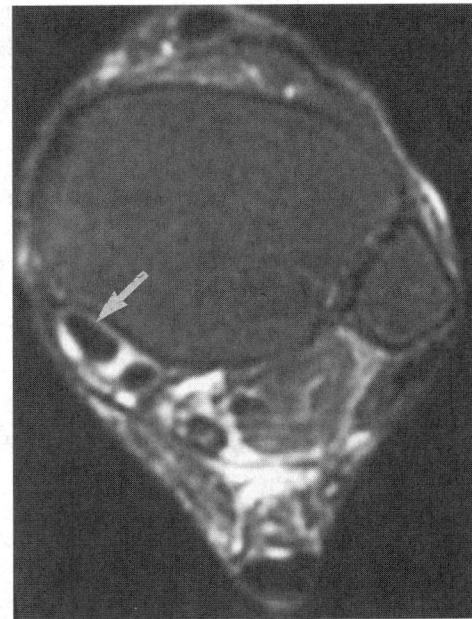 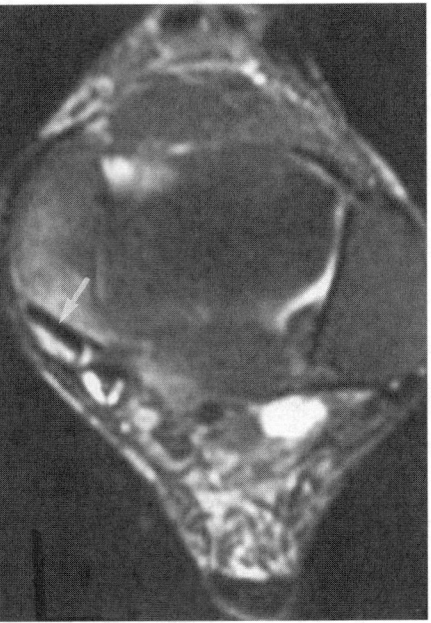

FIG. 6–37. The posterior tibial tendon is partially torn in this patient, who is an avid user of the stairstepper. **A:** The axial fast spin echo with fat saturation (4300/90Ef) shows a normal-size tendon (*arrow*) with abnormal signal around it. **B:** A more distal axial image shows marked attenuation of the posterior tibial tendon (*arrow*). This is the appearance of a partial tear or severe tendinopathy.

the tendon on T2WI, tendinopathy is diagnosed (Fig. 6–37). A full-thickness tear is noted when the tendon is discontinuous. The peroneal tendons are unique in that they are bounded by a retinaculum and are intimately associated with the fibula. When an ankle has sustained a forced inversion injury, the peroneus longus, which is located slightly more dorsal than the peroneus brevis, can wedge the brevis into the fibula, causing a longitudinal split tear in the peroneus brevis. The peroneus longus then gets trapped in the split tear, preventing the brevis from healing (Fig. 6–38). MRI is the only nonoperative way of making this diagnosis.

Increased fluid can often be seen in an ankle joint of a normal individual. This is usually due to prolonged standing and is seen at imaging at the end of the day. Fluid can normally be seen in the flexor halluces tendon sheath (analogous to fluid in the biceps tendon sheath) when there is fluid in the ankle joint. A normal communication exists between these structures in about 20% of patients. However, fluid is not normally seen around the tendon sheaths of the other tendons of the foot and ankle. If fluid is seen in these tendon sheaths or is noted around the flexor hallucis longus (FHL) out of proportion to the joint fluid, then a diagnosis of tenosynovitis should be entertained.

Ultrasound, in some radiologists' hands, can be diagnostic for full-thickness rotator cuff tears and to assess Achilles tendon abnormalities. This technique is extremely operator dependent. That is, a less experienced ultrasonographer may yield unreliable results. Ultrasound is inexpensive and is performed without the use of radiation. However, it does not provide any additional tissue information, such as labral integrity, biceps appearance, or any bone changes that may provide an explanation for the patient's symptomatology. Often, a coexisting injury is present. Ultrasound is not widely practiced as a definitive diagnostic tool for evaluating tendon structures.

In assessing a ligament, similar criteria exist as described for the tendons. However, specific ligaments require slightly more discussion. These ligaments are located in the knee, ankle, and elbow. In the knee several ligaments have the potential to be injured. These include both the anterior and posterior cruciate ligaments, the medial and lateral collateral ligament complex, and the posterior oblique and arcuate ligaments; the latter are not technically ligaments, but rather thickenings of the joint capsule.

The collateral ligaments are best evaluated with coronal imaging using T2WI. It is necessary to identify the fluid within and around these structures to be able to determine their integrity. Coronal T1WI will not be able to distinguish fluid (which will be low in signal) from the ligament (which will also be low in signal). Therefore, all imaging of the collateral ligaments should be performed with T2WI. Pathology in the medial collateral ligament (MCL) is normally graded by its signal appearance. That is, a grade 1 sprain is diagnosed if fluid is seen external to the intact normal-appearing low signal MCL (Fig. 6–39). Grade 2 sprain is diagnosed when fluid is identified within the fibers of the MCL but at least some of the ligament's low-signal fibers are seen to be intact. Grade 3 sprain is equivalent to a full-thickness tear. Fluid is seen around the MCL, and the ligament is seen

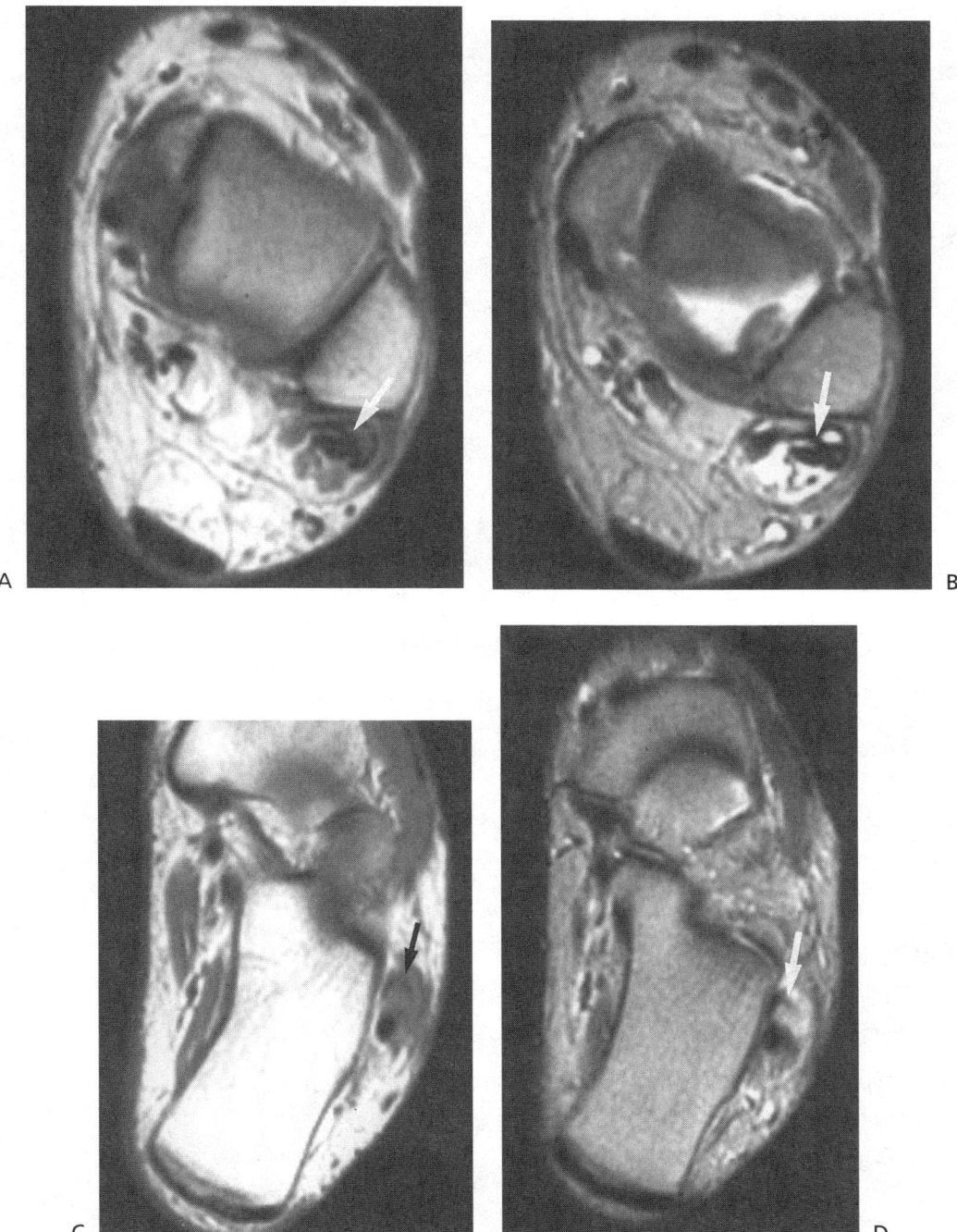

FIG. 6–38. This 37-year-old female sustained an ankle inversion injury and complains of chronic lateral ankle pain. Axial proton density (**A**) and SE T2 (2000/20 and 80) (**B**) reveal abnormal shape and signal of the peroneus brevis with invagination of the longus (*arrow*) between the portions of the brevis. The brevis has a chevron shape. Slightly more distal proton density (**C**) and SE T2 image (**D**) reveal a markedly attenuated brevis (*arrow*). This is the appearance of a longitudinal split tear of the peroneus brevis.

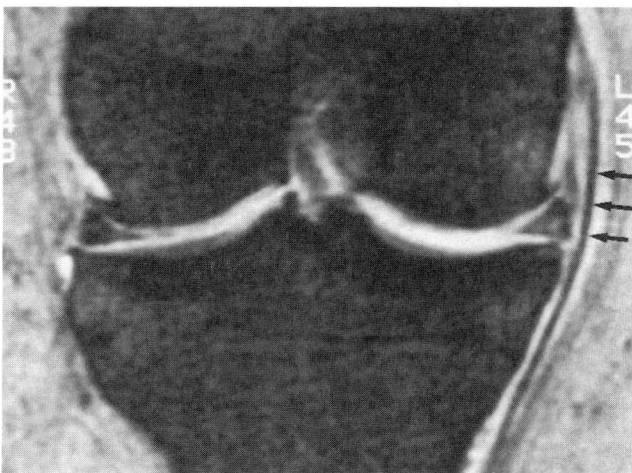

FIG. 6–39. This 46-year-old female injured her knee while skiing. Coronal GRE (600/13 *30) shows intact fibers of the medial collateral ligament (*arrows*) with high signal superficial to the fibers. This is the appearance of a grade 1 MCL sprain.

to be completely torn at the origin, insertion, or midsubstance (Fig. 6–40).

The cruciate ligaments are best evaluated in the sagittal plane. A normal ACL is a uniform low-signal linear structure on all sequences that parallels the roof of the intercondylar notch. The optimal sequence for identifying a tear of the ACL is a T2WI, which will show the fluid that has replaced the location of the ACL. A tear is diagnosed by MRI criteria when fluid replaces the normally seen low-signal structure on the T2WI. Also, if the fibers of the ACL do not parallel the intercondylar notch and appear to be lax and not straight or are more flat in its orientation, a tear is diagnosed (see Fig 6–2B). The tear may be intrasubstance, at its origin or insertion (see Fig. 6–10). Many secondary signs have been reported to identify an ACL tear if the sagittal images are equivocal. These include a hooked appearance of the PCL due to the redundancy from joint laxity, uncovering of the posterior horn of the lateral meniscus, a drawer sign that is identified by the tibia anteriorly translocating in relationship to the femur, and bone contusions that are identified in the midportion of the lateral femoral condyle and posterior lateral tibial plateau.

A PCL tear does not have the same appearance as an ACL tear. That is, the structure is not replaced by fluid. In fact, identifying a PCL tear is more difficult because often the only perceptible alteration is a change in the morphology. The PCL is normally low in signal on all sequences and has a gentle curve. When it tears, it can become swollen and may have some hemorrhage within its substance. These findings are best identified on sequences that have a short echo time, that is, a short TE such as a proton density image, T1WI, or GRE with a short TE (T2*). These are the same sequences that are recommended for evaluating the meniscus. A tear is identified when the short TE images reveal a swollen ligament or a ligament that has intrinsic high signal. The T2WI might not confirm the high signal in all cases, and a false conclusion of a normal PCL mighty be drawn. The tears may be within the substance, at the origin or the insertion of the ligament (Figs. 6–41 and 6–42). Unlike the ACL, no additional secondary signs exist to aid in this diagnosis. Occasionally, an associated anterior tibial plateau contusion may be present.

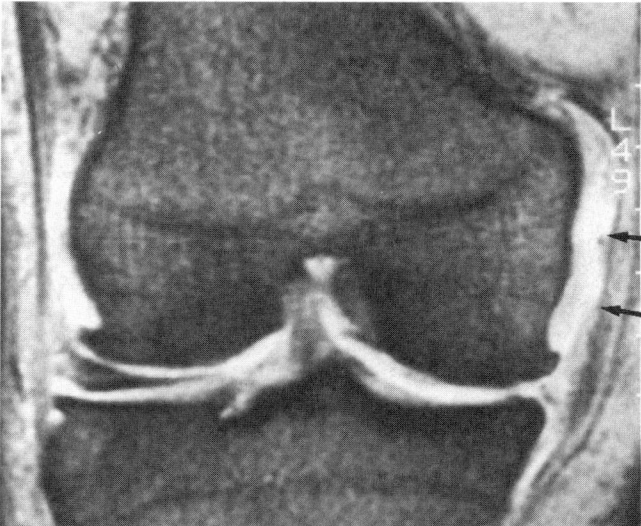

FIG. 6–40. The coronal gradient (600/20 *30) reveals complete disruption of the MCL fibers (*arrows*). The MCL normally is closely adherent to the medial femoral condyle. This is a tear of the MCL or grade 3 sprain. A T2WI must be performed to appreciate the high signal of the fluid in order to visualize the fibers separate from the fluid.

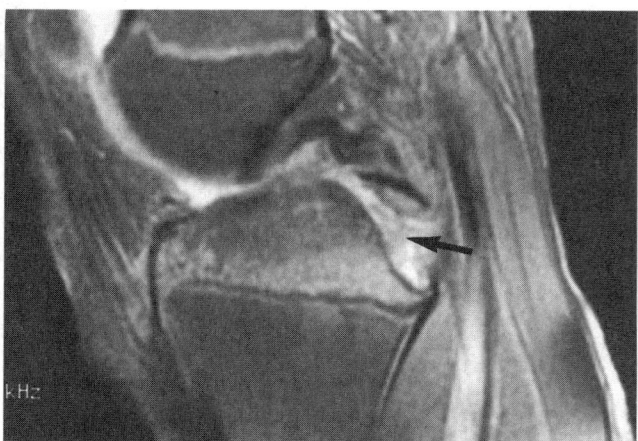

FIG. 6–41. This 14-year-old male was in an all-terrain vehicle race. Sagittal proton density with fat saturation (2000/20) shows the posterior cruciate ligament avulsed from the tibia (*arrow*).

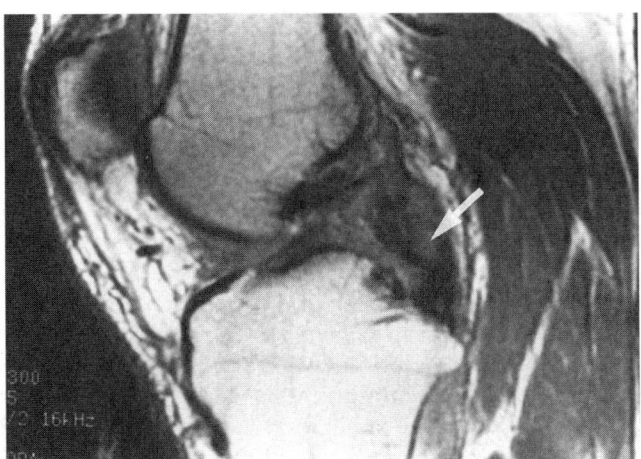

FIG. 6–42. This 40-year-old male caught his foot in a hole during a softball game. Sagittal proton density (2300/15) image reveals abnormal signal in the posterior cruciate ligament (*arrow*) compatible with a tear.

In the foot and ankle there are numerous ligamentous structures that are responsible for the support of the ankle joint. These include laterally the anterior tibiofibular, posterior tibiofibular, anterior talofibular, and posterior talofibular as well as calcaneofibular ligaments. The anterior and posterior tibiofibular ligaments are identified above the ankle joint. The remaining three ligaments are identified below the ankle joint at the level where the fibula has its malleolar fossa. The order in which the latter three ligaments tear with an ankle inversion injury is the anterior talofibular followed by the calcaneofibular ligament. The posterior talofibular ligament is said to tear infrequently. These small ligamentous structures are uniformly low in signal on all sequences when normal. When torn, the end of the ligament is noted to be surrounded by fluid and not attached at its insertion. A particular entity associated with injury to the lateral ligament complex results in fibrous tissue which collects in the lateral recess (lateral gutter). This finding has been termed anterolateral impingement syndrome. It consists of a torn anterior tibiofibular ligament with intermediate signal identified on both the T1 and T2WI images. The intermediate signal on the T2WI is significant because this cannot represent fluid. This scarring or fibrous tissue often has to be addressed surgically (Fig. 6–43). No additional imaging is necessary, and the MRI is diagnostic for this entity. Medially located is the thick ligament known as the deltoid ligament. When it is considered sprained, high signal is identified within the substance of the deltoid ligament.

The ulnar collateral ligament (medial collateral ligament) in the elbow deserves special mention. Magnetic resonance arthrography is useful in evaluating the integrity of the ulnar collateral ligament (UCL) in the

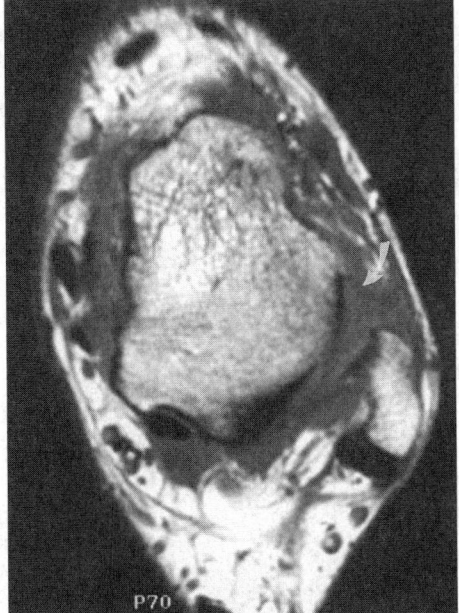
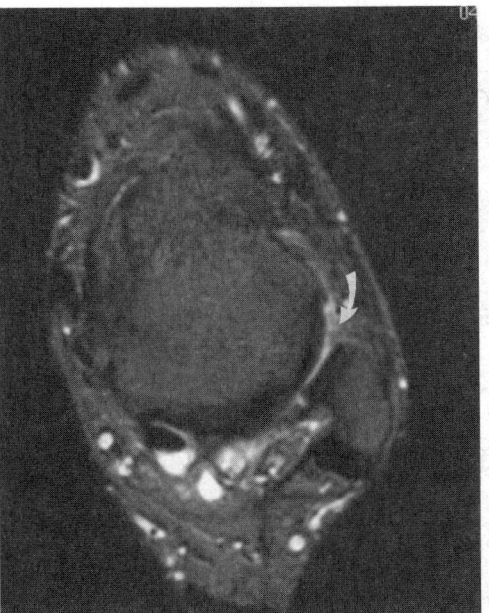

FIG. 6–43. This patient is a 22-year-old male who complained of chronic anterolateral ankle pain 6 months after an inversion injury. **A:** The axial T1 (500/15) shows low signal in the anterolateral gutter (*arrow*). **B:** Axial SE T2 (3000/80) shows persistent low signal in the anterolateral gutter compatible with fibrosis (*arrow*). At arthroscopy this was found to be meniscoidlike tissue representing scar and fibrosis seen in anterolateral impingement syndrome.

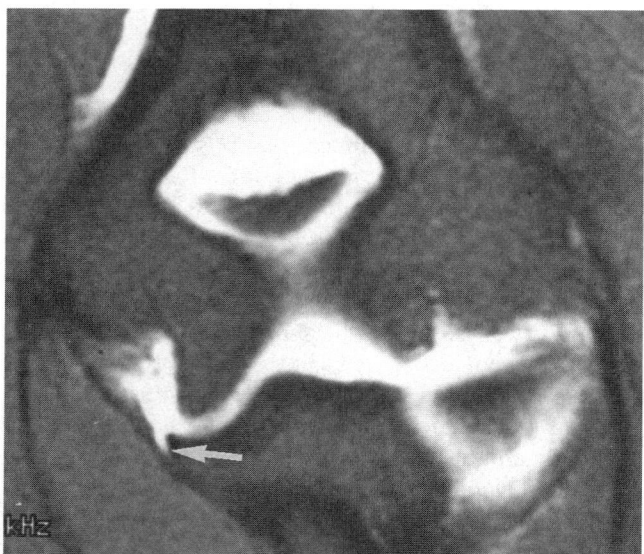

FIG. 6–44. Twenty-one-year-old female field hockey player with complaints of medial elbow joint pain. Clinical concern for an ulnar collateral ligament tear existed. An MRI arthrogram was performed, and disruption of the deep fibers (*arrow*) of the UCL can be seen on the coronal T1 (500/14) with fat saturation as demonstrated by the "T" sign. Intraarticular gadolinium makes this diagnosis much easier to identify.

elbow. A partial tear that occurs to the deep fibers of the UCL is extremely difficult to detect without fluid in the joint. At surgery, when an external approach to the joint is used, the tear is not identified. A characteristic "T" sign is noted when the deep fibers are torn (Fig. 6–44).

Plain X-rays have limited use in evaluating tendons and ligaments. Occasionally, mineralization can be identified within the location of a tendon, and calcific tendinopathy can be diagnosed. MRI can readily identify this calcium structure as either a low- or high-signal focus within the tendon. The signal characteristics of the calcification depend on the amount of hydration around the calcium molecules. There is no role for tomography in evaluating tendons and ligaments. Computed tomography may show the gross integrity of a tendon, generally only on axial imaging, but will not show the intrinsic abnormality such as tendinopathy. The ankle ligaments are not well appreciated on CT exam, nor are the cruciate or collateral ligaments.

MUSCLES

Muscles can undergo a variety of changes, from injury or contusion to atrophy and edema. Muscle injury is not possible to diagnose by any imaging modality other than MRI. The exception to this statement is the diagnosis of myositis ossificans in which peripheral ossification is noted within the injured muscle. This ossification occurs over time and represents maturing of a hematoma and muscle injury (Fig. 6–45). It is important to recognize the characteristics of myositis on a plain X-ray in order not to confuse the diagnosis with something more sinister. If a biopsy were to be done on myositis, the increased number of mitotic figures present would suggest to the pathologist that an aggressive lesion, such as an osteosarcoma, is present. Therefore identifying the mineralization as peripheral in nature is important and diagnostic for myositis. If the pattern of mineralization is difficult to appreciate on a plain X-ray, a CT examination can determine where the mineralization is located within the injured muscle (Fig. 6–46). Before ossification the CT examination is not very useful. CT will show a muscle abnormality as an area of mixed density and mixed enhancement pattern following contrast administration, but this is a nonspecific finding. History can sometimes be helpful; however, many patients do not remember being injured or think of the trauma as incidental. Ultrasound is not very useful in evaluating muscles. If an injury has occurred to a muscle, the ultrasound findings may demonstrate the injured muscle to be of mixed echogenicity. This is a nonspecific finding and can be seen with infection and even tumors. Therefore for muscle evaluation, ultrasound is not recommended except in evaluating whether a cystic component is present such as a seroma or organizing hematoma (fluid collections). Bone scan may show increased uptake in the region of mineralization because of the bone

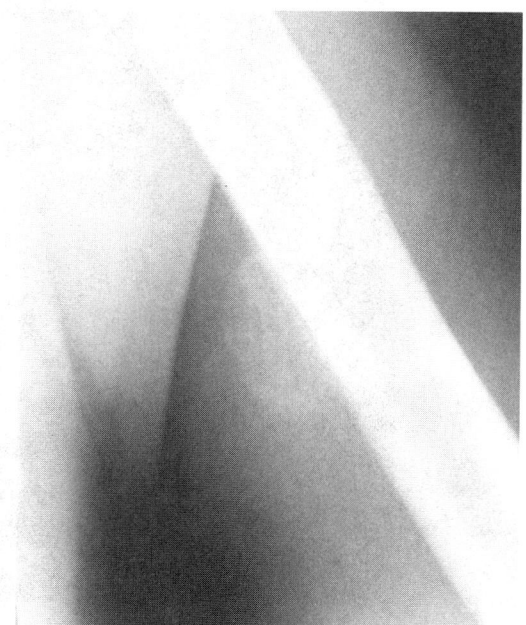

FIG. 6–45. The plain film in this 21-year-old male shows peripheral calcification adjacent to the proximal left humerus. The patient reported being hit by a racquet during a game of racquetball 4 weeks earlier.

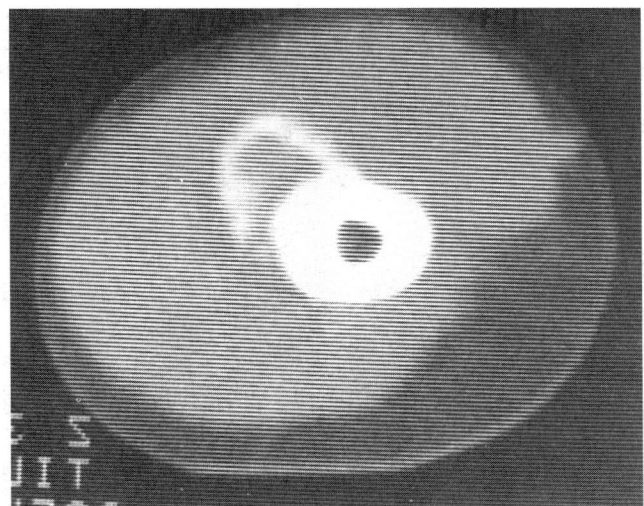

FIG. 6–46. This is the same patient as in Figure 6–44. Axial CT image demonstrates the peripheral nature of the calcification.

turnover in this area. Conventional tomography may show the peripheral mineralization but not to the degree that will be demonstrated by CT.

Muscles appear as intermediate to low signal on all MR sequences. Muscles are not as low in signal as tendons and ligaments but are not as high in signal as fluid or fat. When muscle is injured, it changes signal characteristics on the basis of the hemorrhage and edema (increased water) in the muscle. Therefore the signal becomes brighter on a T2WI. Fluid that is low in signal on a T1WI will be isointense to the muscle signal and can easily be overlooked. Therefore, appropriate evaluation with MR requires a T2WI (Figs. 6–47 and 6–48). Hemorrhage can demonstrate a variety of signal characteristics, which include occasionally being high in signal on the T1WI. When this is identified, it is very useful, as not many substances can be high in signal on the T1WI. Hemorrhage can be definitively diagnosed if the area of high signal on the T1WI remains high in signal on the T2WI (Fig. 6–49). The other possibilities for the high signal on T1WI includes fat, which would become lower in signal on a T2WI, and gadolinium. Administration of gadolinium should be known, and a pregadolinium image would be necessary to determine whether enhancement has occurred. Another possibility for high signal on a T1WI is calcification. Calcification is most often low in signal on T1WI; however, the signal characteristics are entirely dependent on the amount of hydration around the calcium molecules (number of protons available).

It is known that after exercising, the muscles used during the exercise can change in signal. Similarly, the weekend warrior who attempts to perform activities beyond his or her muscle capabilities can develop delayed onset muscle soreness. Over a 2-week period the muscle continues to demonstrate increased signal on the T2WI. The signal characteristics for muscle injury on MRI are not specific for trauma. However, the muscle planes and fascia are preserved. A soft tissue mass such as a tumor would have similar signal characteristics, but generally, muscle distortion can be appreciated. This is not a hard-and-fast rule because in the setting of blunt trauma, the muscle or muscle groups may swell in addition to the changing signal. This can make distinguishing

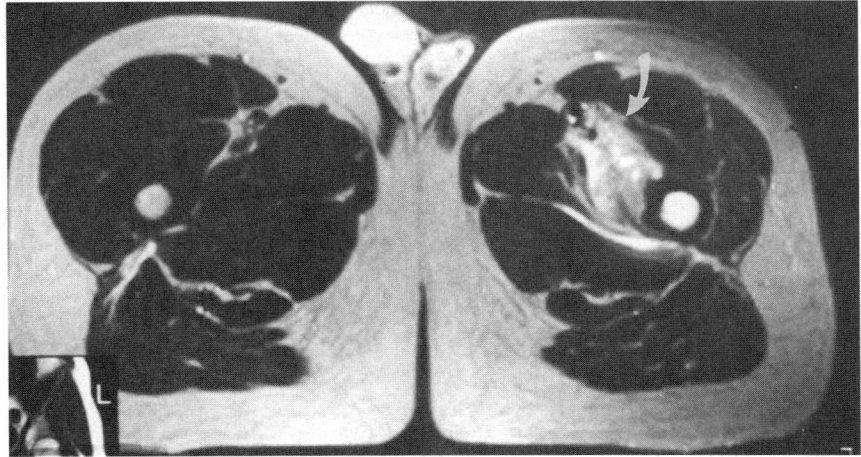
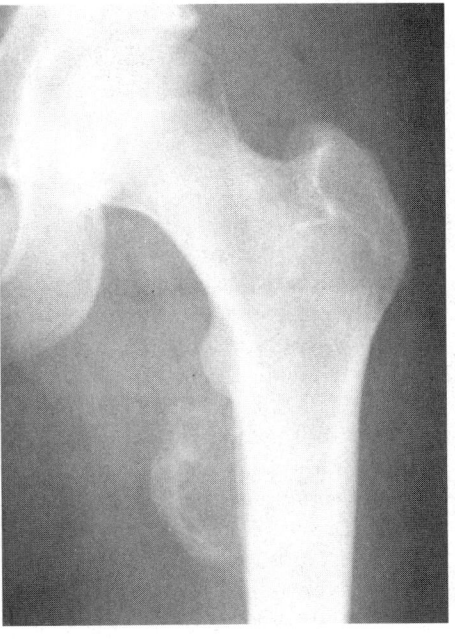

FIG. 6–47. A 17-year-old male presented with complaint of proximal left thigh mass. Axial T2WI (4950/105) (**A**) reveals mixed high and intermediate signal in a mass located in the medial proximal thigh (*arrow*). A history of trauma was elicited after the MRI, and a plain film was obtained (**B**), which shows peripheral calcification around the soft tissue mass compatible with myositis ossificans.

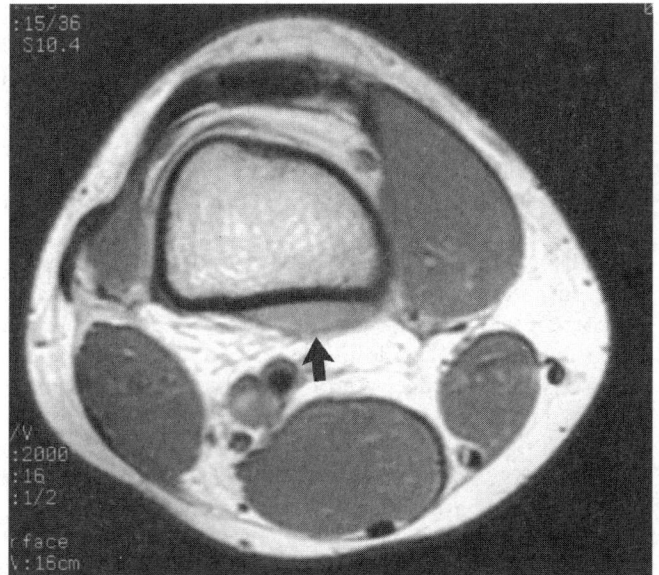
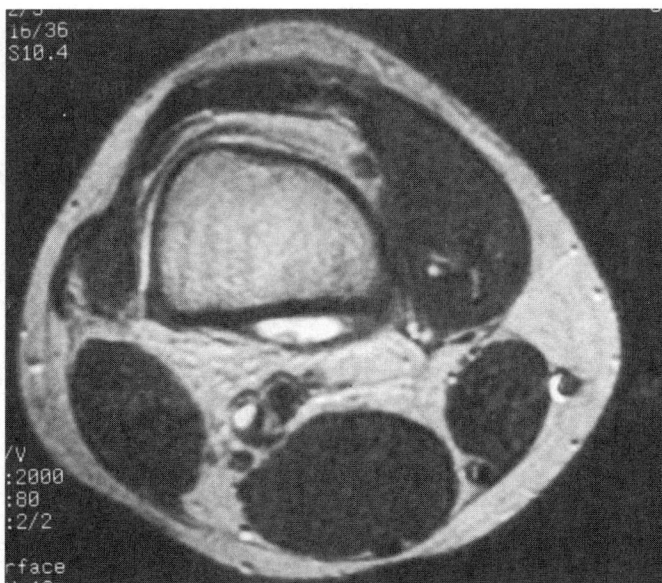
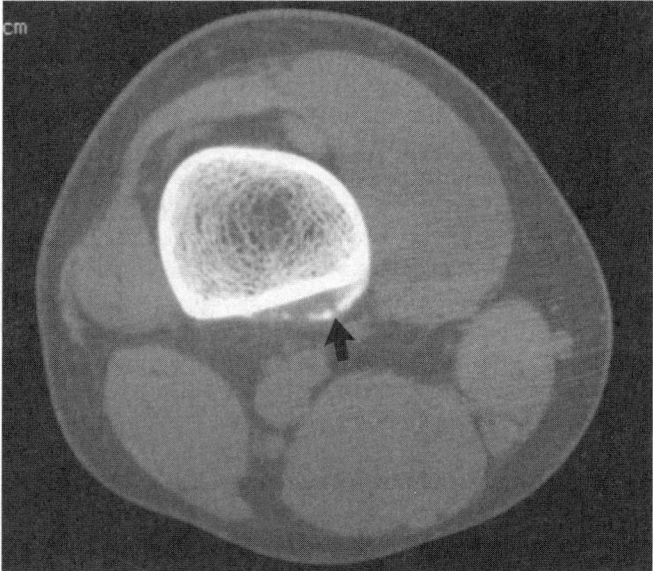

FIG. 6–48. This 15-year-old male was hit with a baseball. **A:** The axial proton density (2000/20) image shows increased signal intensity adjacent to the periosteum (*arrow*). **B:** Axial T2 (2000/80) shows increased signal compatible with fluid or hemorrhage. Low signal is noted peripherally, likely representing calcification or hemosiderin. No abnormal marrow signal is noted. **C:** An axial CT 1 month later reveals peripheral calcification around the periosteum (*arrow*).

trauma from a mass more difficult. The presence of blood or blood products can be very useful in diagnosing a traumatic muscle injury, although there are masses that can hemorrhage. The clinical history will be very helpful in distinguishing these entities.

Other changes in muscle can be diagnosed only with MRI. For instance, muscle changes due to nerve injury are not appreciated on other modalities. Neurogenic edema in a muscle can be diagnosed when the muscle size is normal, but the signal on the T2WI is diffusely high throughout the entire muscle. This entity is seen most often in the muscles of the rotator cuff but can be seen anywhere in the body (Fig. 6–50). Occasionally, a remote injury to the brachial plexus will result in high signal within the muscle belly innervated by the injured nerve roots. The MRI cannot reliably visualize the nerve, but the resultant changes in the muscle belly of the nerve distribution are diagnostic. Masses that have pressure on a nerve can cause resultant abnormalities in the muscle innervated by the affected nerve. For example, in the shoulder, if a mass is identified in the spinoglenoid notch, atrophy or abnormal signal may be identified in the infraspinatus muscle. The muscle is innervated by the suprascapular nerve, which is located within the spinoglenoid notch. A mass in this location will affect the nerve and result in the changes in the infraspinatus. The most commonly encountered mass to cause these findings is a ganglion that occurs as a result of a torn posterior labrum. Atrophy is identified as a small muscle belly with more high signal within it on the T1WI as a result of fat infiltrating the muscle belly. Quadrilateral space syndrome is diagnosed when the teres minor is noted to be atrophic or demonstrates abnormal signal in its muscle belly. The teres minor is innervated by the axillary nerve, which gets entrapped between the teres minor and major, long head of triceps, and humeral head. The resultant signal change or development of atrophy helps in determining the cause of the patient's pain. These patients generally present with rotator cuff symptomatology.

The best imaging modality for a suspected muscle injury or abnormality is MRI. It is particularly useful when it reveals an unsuspected cause of pain such as neurogenic edema or atrophy of a muscle, which may identify a nerve injury as the problem. CT and ultrasound are less sensitive and specific. Tomography has essentially no role, and the use of bone scan is limited to the known case of myositis ossificans as identified on a plain X-ray. The plain X-ray is not at all sensitive for muscle injury except in the specific setting of myositis ossificans.

In this chapter a great deal of material was covered. The imaging techniques and their advantages and disadvantages were reviewed with respect to imaging of specific tissue types. Although all sports-related injuries could not adequately be discussed in this chapter, gen-

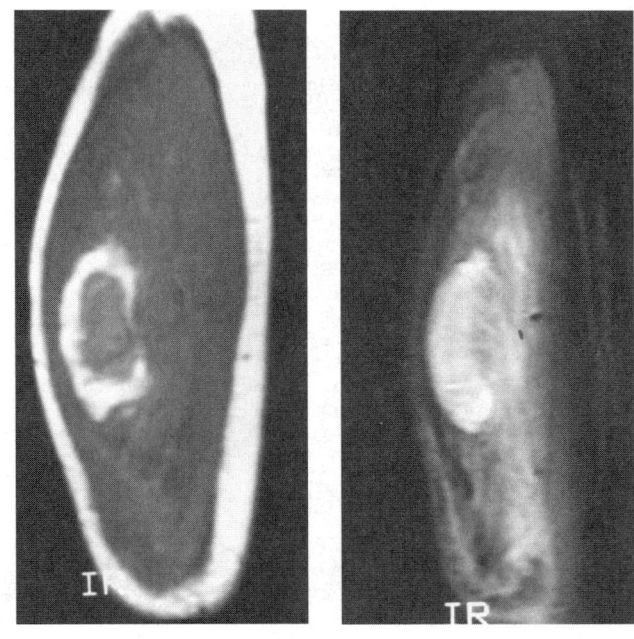

FIG. 6–49. This 18-year-old male had direct trauma to the thigh. (**A**) T1 coronal (600/20) shows some high signal in the vastus medialis, which on the FSE T2WI (3500/65Ef) (**B**) shows mixed high and low signal compatible with a hematoma.

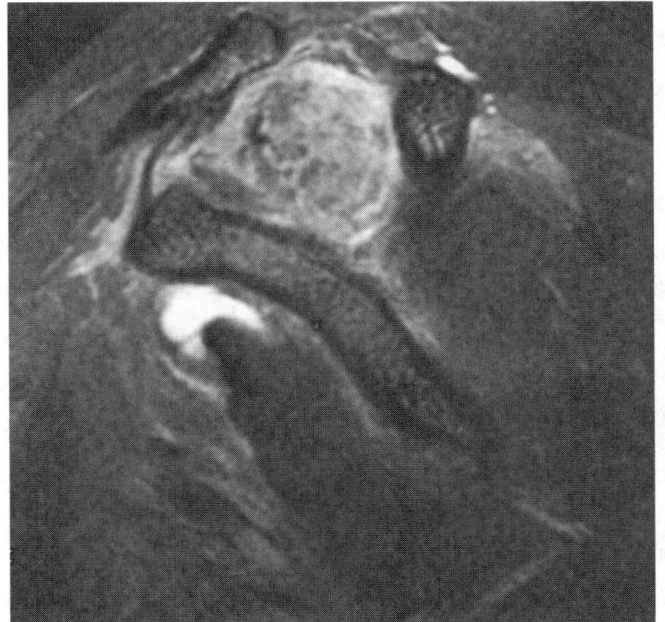
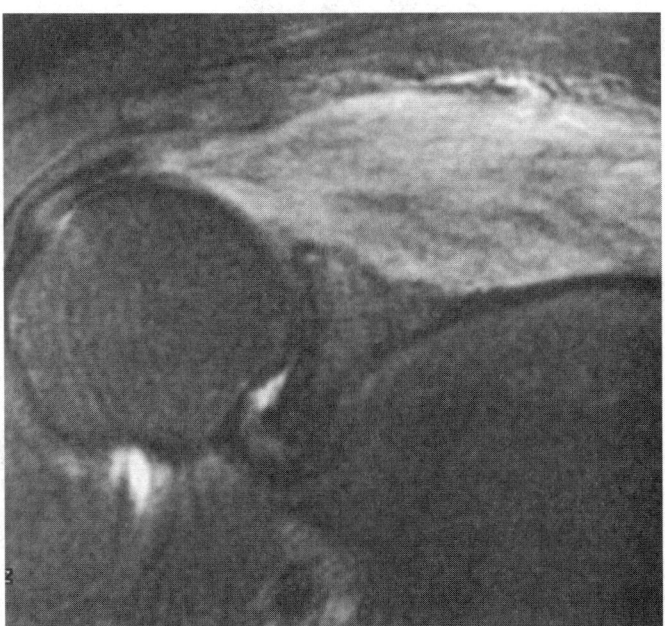

FIG. 6–50. An oblique (**A**) sagittal (anterior to the left) and (**B**) oblique coronal FSE with fat saturation (3000/78Ef) show high signal in the supraspinatus muscle and a small amount of high signal in the infraspinatus muscle relative to the adjacent muscles. This is a pattern compatible with neurogenic edema.

eral concepts were reviewed to help provide the clinician with a knowledge base to help guide the selection of studies to best address the clinical question.

BIBLIOGRAPHY

Ahovuo J, Paavolainen P, Slatis P. Diagnostic value of sonography in lesions of the biceps tendon. *Clin Orthop* 1986;282:184–188.

Beltran J, Munchow A, Khabiri H, et al. Ligaments of the lateral aspect of the ankle and sinus tarsi: an MR imaging study. *Radiology* 1990;177:455–458.

Brant WE, Helms CA. *Fundamentals of diagnostic radiology.* Baltimore, MD: Williams & Wilkins, 1994:Chapters 1, 34–43.

Breitenseher MJ, Metz VM, Gilula LA, et al. Radiographically occult scaphoid fractures: value of MR imaging in detection. *Radiology* 1997;203(1):245–50.

Czerny C, Hofmann S, Neuhold A, et al. Lesions of the acetabular labrum: accuracy of MR imaging and MR arthrography in detection and staging. *Radiology* 1996;200(1):225–230.

Desmet AA, Ilahi OA, Graf BK. Reassessment of the MR criteria for stability of osteochondritis dissecans in the knee and ankle. *Skeletal Radiol* 1996;25(2):159–163.

Fleckenstein JL, Watumull D, Conner KE, et al. Denervated human skeletal muscle: MR imaging evaluation. *Radiology* 1993;187(1):213–218.

Fritz RC, Helms CA, Steinbach LS, Genant HK. Suprascapular nerve entrapment: evaluation with MR imaging. *Radiology* 1992;182(2):437–444.

Helgason JW, Chandnani VP, Yu JS. MR arthrography: a review of current technique and applications [Review]. *Am J Roentgenol* 1997;168(6):1473–1480.

Heyman P, Gelberman R, Duncan K, Hipp J. Injuries of the ulnar collateral ligament of the thumb metacarpophalangeal joint. *Clinical Orthop* 1993;292:165–171.

Higgins CB, Hricak H, Helms CA. *Magnetic resonance imaging of the body.* 3rd ed. Philadelphia: Lippincott-Raven, 1996:Chapter 11.

Hodler J, Resnick D. Current status of imaging of articular cartilage [Review]. *Skeletal Radiol* 1996;25(8):703–709.

Hunter J, Blatz D, Escobedo E. SLAP lesions of the glenoid labrum: CT arthrographic and arthroscopic correlation. *Radiology* 1992;184:513–518.

Kingston S. Magnetic resonance imaging of the ankle and foot. *Clin Sports Med* 1988;7(1):15–28.

Lecouvet FE, Vandeberg BC, Malghem J, et al. MR imaging of the acetabular labrum: variations in 200 asymptomatic hips. *Am J Roentgenol* 1996;167(4):1025–1028.

Middleton WD, Reinus WR, Totty WG, et al. Ultrasonographic evaluation of the rotator cuff and biceps tendon. *J Bone Joint Surg Am* 1986;68(3):440–450.

Monu J, Pope T, Chabon S, Vanarthos W. MR diagnosis of superior labral anterior posterior (SLAP) injuries of the glenoid labrum: value of routine imaging without intraarticular injection of contrast material. *Am J Roentgenol* 1994;163:1425–1429.

Munk PL, Helms CA. *MRI of the knee.* 2nd ed. Philadelphia: Lippincott-Raven, 1996.

Patten RM. Overuse syndromes and injuries involving the elbow: MR imaging findings. *Am J Roentgenol* 1995;164(5):1205–1211.

Rafii M, Firooznia H, Sherman O, et al. Rotator cuff lesions: signal patterns at MR imaging. *Radiology* 1990;177(3):817–823.

Rizzo P, Gould E, Lyden J, Asnis S. Diagnosis of occult fractures about the hip: MRI compared with bone-scanning. *J Bone Joint Surg Am* 1993;75-A:395–401.

Schneck C, Mesgarzadeh M, Bonakdarpour A, Ross G. MR imaging of the most commonly injured ankle ligaments. Part 1: Ankle anatomy. *Radiology* 1992;184:499–506.

Schwartz ML, al-Zahrani S, Morwessel RM, Andrews JR. Ulnar collateral ligament injury in the throwing athlete: evaluation with saline-enhanced MR arthrography. *Radiology* 1995;197(1):297–299.

Snearly WN, Kaplan PA, Dussault RG. Lateral-compartment bone contusions in adolescents with intact anterior cruciate ligaments. *Radiology* 1996;198(1):205–208.

Spaeth HJ, Abrams RA, Bock GW, et al. Gamekeeper thumb: differentiation of nondisplaced and displaced tears of the ulnar collateral ligament with MR imaging. Work in progress. *Radiology* 1993;188(2):553–556.

Tirman PF, Feller JF, Janzen DL, Peterfy CG, Bergman AG. Association of glenoid labral cysts with labral tears and glenohumeral instability: radiologic findings and clinical significance. *Radiology* 1994;190(3):653–658.

Tirman P, Feller JF, Palmer WE, et al. The Buford complex:a variation of normal shoulder anatomy: MR arthrographic imaging features. *Amer J Roentgenol* 1996;166(4):869–873.

Tuckman G. Abnormalities of the long head of the biceps tendon of the shoulder: MR imaging findings. *Amer J Roentgenol* 1994;163:1183–1188.

West GA, Haynor DR, Goodkin R, et al. Magnetic resonance imaging signal changes in denervated muscles after peripheral nerve injury. *Neurosurgery* 1994;35(6):1077–1085.

PART II

Special Populations

CHAPTER 7

The Young Athlete

David T. Bernhardt

The future health and well-being of youth across our country is determined largely by their level of physical activity. A sedentary lifestyle will have serious implications for their physical health and their psychological well-being. Physical activity plays a significant role in disease prevention and health promotion at all ages. One of the three major goals of *Healthy People 2000* is to "increase the span of healthy life for Americans" by promoting physical activity and nutrition (1). Positive attributes of sport such as discipline, time management, respect for others, structured recreation, and teamwork apply beyond the scope of the sport. Health care professionals should strive to identify obstacles to exercise and provide exercise and nutrition counseling to their young patients in an attempt to promote daily physical activity and a life long healthy lifestyle.

The number of younger children who are involved in competitive sports may have both important physical and psychological implications. Increased pressure, either self-imposed or from overbearing parents and coaches, to develop future champions can subject a young athlete to physical and psychological risks. These risks include growth plate injuries, stress fractures, eating disorders, depression, burnout, and renouncing sport and physical activity. The adoption of an unhealthy lifestyle and other high-risk behavior may result. The primary care provider must be familiar with the many complicated aspects of exercise that are unique to the young athlete to promote safe participation in daily physical activity and prevent injury.

Promoting daily physical activity is also critical to children and adolescents with physical disabilities and chronic illness. Exercise can have significant impact on the youngster with disabilities and chronic disease such as Down syndrome, cystic fibrosis, or rheumatoid arthritis or the young wheelchair athlete.

Many of the topics to be highlighted in this chapter are discussed in detail in other chapters in this text. The purpose of this chapter is to introduce aspects of sport and exercise that are particular to the child and adolescent. Any provider who cares for healthy and physically challenged youngsters should be proficient in promoting the physical and psychological benefits of exercise. In addition, the provider should have an understanding of the inherent risks of unhealthy pressure, training, and competition.

ADVANTAGES OF EXERCISE

The prevalence of obesity has increased in both children and adults (2). The chance of becoming obese in adulthood when the patient is obese as a child ranges from 8 percent, for 1- to 2-year-olds without obese parents, to 79 percent for 10- to 14-year-olds with at least one obese parent (3).

In adults, regular physical exercise is associated with fewer coronary heart disease (CHD) risk factors (4,5), including less obesity (6), hypertension (7), and an improved lipoprotein/cholesterol profile (8). In childhood and adolescence the link between physical activity and reduction in coronary risk profile is less well established. Although college athletic participation has been shown to lower the subsequent risk of CHD (9), college athletes are not a representative sample of general active adolescents. Substantial evidence supports the role of physical activity in preventing osteoporosis (10). Psychologically, participation in exercise programs is associated with improved self-esteem (11) and reduced anxiety and depression (12).

One of the best reasons to support increased activity among children is the increased chance of their remaining physically active as adults. Dennison and col-

---

D. T. Bernhardt: Department of Pediatrics, Section of Sports Medicine, University of Wisconsin Medical School, Madison, Wisconsin 53792–4116.

leagues showed that physically active adults had better standardized fitness scores as children. In addition, physically active adults participated in more organized sports per year after high school and reported greater parental encouragement of exercise as children (13). Adult lifestyle habits are often established during the formative childhood and adolescence years. Although a healthy lifestyle does not always track to adult life, increased physical activity as a child has the potential to continue as an integral part of an adult's healthy lifestyle. Therefore, it is imperative that parents, physical education teachers, athletic trainers, and primary care providers take advantage of certain windows of opportunity to set an example and promote physical activity for today's youth. The increasing evidence of childhood obesity tracking to adulthood supports the role of promoting physical activity in the young in hopes of lowering coronary risk factors for a lifetime.

When studies are looked at critically, however, there is little scientific evidence that documents the effect of adolescent activity levels on CHD profiles, chronic disease prevention, tracking of activity levels into adult life, risk-taking behaviors, or injury prevention (14). Further research must be completed in an attempt to solidify the blind promotion of physical activity for youth.

EPIDEMIOLOGY OF INJURIES

A commonly asked question in the physician's office is "Are sports safe for my son or daughter?" Minor injuries that do not require medical attention or are treated by a team's athletic trainer are frequent in youth sports. Sports medicine physicians and athletic organizations are emphasizing time lost from practice or competition

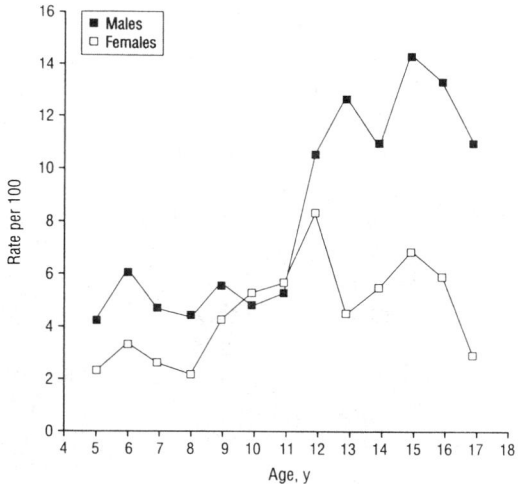

FIG. 7–1. Rates of sports and recreational injuries by age and gender. (From Bijur PE, Trumble A, Harel Y, et al. Sports and recreation injuries in U.S. children and adolescents. *Arch Pediatr Adolesc Med* 1995;149:1009–1016.)

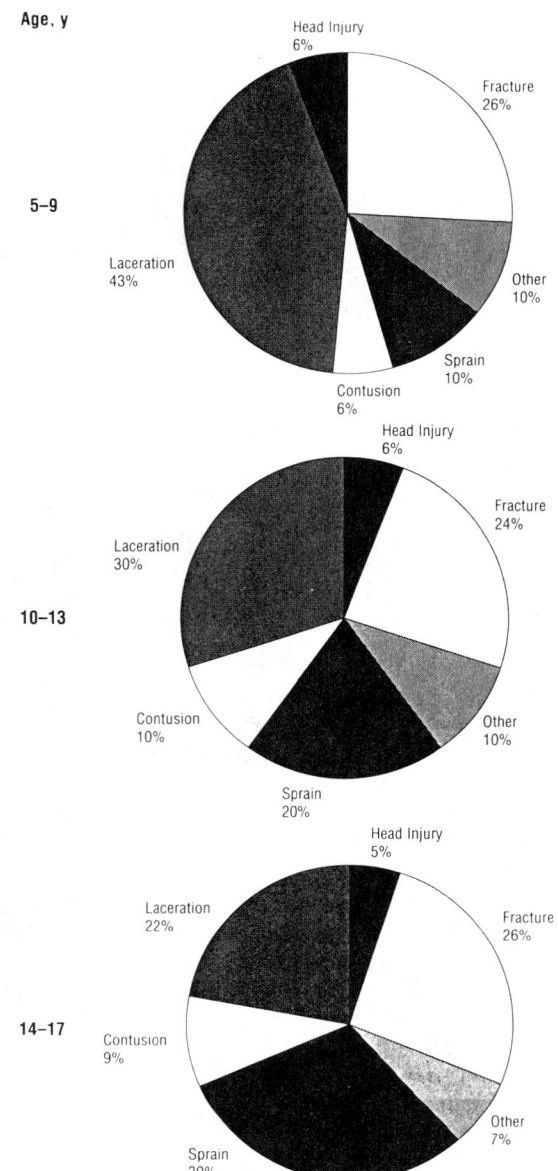

FIG. 7–2. Distribution of nature of sports and recreational injuries by age. (From Bijur PE, Trumble A, Harel Y, et al. Sports and recreation injuries in U.S. children and adolescents. *Arch Pediatr Adolesc Med* 1995;149:1009–1016.)

as a measure of injury severity. Significant injury causes loss of at least one practice or game.

To help answer the safety question, a survey of over 11,840 children and adolescents aged 5 to 17 years, conducted by the National Center for Health Statistics, showed that sports and recreation accounted for 35.8% of all injuries (15). Almost 3 million sports and recreational injuries occur annually in 5- to 17-year-olds in the United States. Approximately 978,000 serious sports and recreational injuries occur annually, resulting in an estimated 80,750 hospitalizations. Serious injuries were defined as injury-producing events that resulted in half a day or more in bed or missed from school, one or more nights in the hospital, or surgical treatment. The highest-risk age group for injury was the adolescents 14 to 17 years of age (Fig. 7–1). The most common reported injury was sprain followed by fracture and dislocation and laceration (Fig. 7–2). Cause of injury was most commonly overexertion and strenuous movements, followed by bicycles and being struck by a person or object (Fig. 7–3).

Three million injuries per year would seem to be an astonishing number. However, one must recognize that an estimated 35 million boys and girls currently participate in organized sports annually in the United States (16). Youth sports are relatively safe and have low injury rates. A study involving over 14,000 junior high and high school athletes cited an injury rate of 0.78 injuries per athlete during the 8 years of the study. When football and wrestling data were removed from the injury totals, there was no substantial difference between the injury rate for boys (0.58 injuries per athlete) and girls (0.64 injuries per athlete). The majority of the injuries (94%) were minor (no time lost from sport) or mild (one to seven days lost) (17).

A contact/collision sport such as ice hockey has very low injury rates at the youth level (18,19). As athletes reach puberty and muscle mass increases, the physical forces that cause serious injury are generated (Table 7–1). The incidence of injury in high school hockey (34.4 per 1000 player game hours) is less than that in Junior A (96.1 per 1000 player game hours) (20).

At the high school level the sports of football, gymnastics, and wrestling have the highest rates of injury. For high school football an injury rate of 0.506 per athlete per year and 0.031 serious injuries per athlete per year (requiring surgery or hospitalization) was shown in a study of 100 high schools in Texas during the 1989 football season (21).

Because of varied methodologies, it is very difficult to compare studies and make firm recommendations to parents about safety. Nevertheless, there is no risk-free sport, and children tend to select the sports they wish to participate in on the basis of their own desire, peer pressure, and their own talent, regardless of injury rates (22).

TABLE 7–1. *Number of players injured and rate of injuries during practice sessions and games for youth hockey players, stratified by level of participation*

Division	Ages (years)	Total injuries per 1000 hours
Squirt	9–10	1.0
Peewee	11–12	1.8
Bantam	13–14	4.3
High School	14–18	34.4
Junior A	17–19	96.1

Adapted from Stuart MJ, Smith AM, Nieva JJ, Rock MG. Injuries in youth hockey: a pilot surveillance strategy. *Mayo Clin Proc* 1995;70:350–356; and Smith AM, Stuart MJ, Wiese-Bjornstal DM, et al. Predictors of injury in ice hockey players: a multivariate, multidisciplinary approach. *Am J Sports Med* 1997;25(4):500–507.

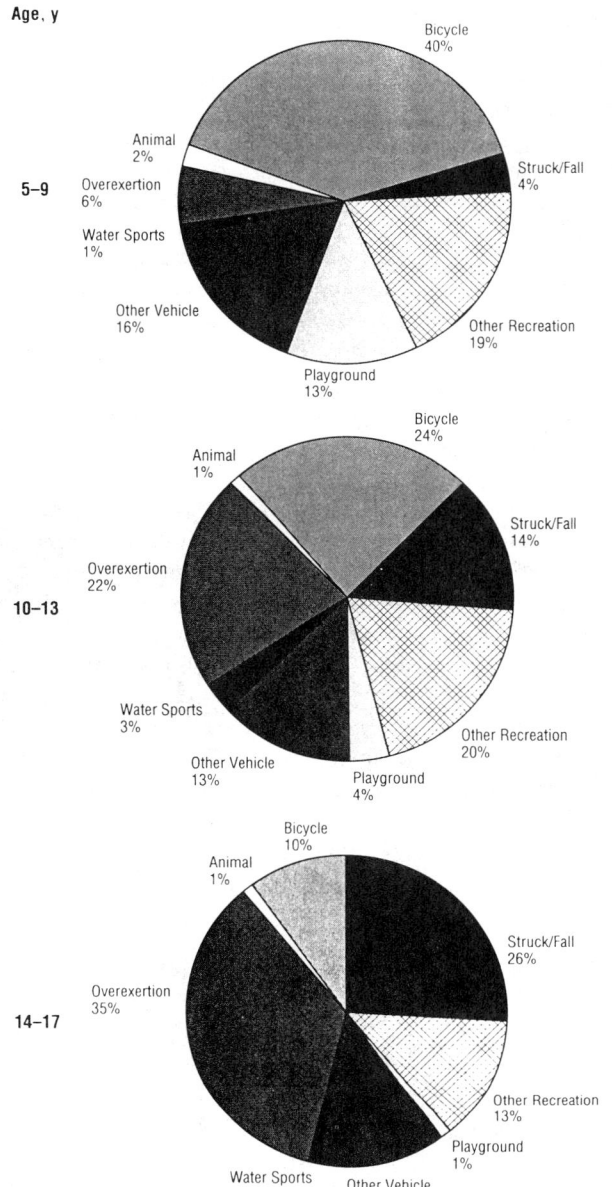

FIG. 7–3. Distribution of cause of sports and recreational injuries by age. (From Bijur PE, Trumble A, Harel Y, et al. Sports and recreation injuries in U.S. children and adolescents. *Arch Pediatr Adolesc Med* 1995;149:1009–1016.)

INJURIES UNIQUE TO THE YOUNG ATHLETE

Growth phases in the young athlete place stresses on tissues that are unique to the child or adolescent. The growing bones of youngsters 4 to 10 years of age are different from the bones of older children. Growing bones are weak at the physis (growth plate), making them susceptible to injury in this area. A relatively strong ligament attached to a physeal area may be able to withstand a rapidly applied force with resultant growth plate injury.

Repetitive micro traumatic injury to the immature physis can result in serious injury to a developing skeleton. Stress injuries to the physis may be difficult to detect with plain radiographs. MRI may be used as an adjunct when there is suspicion of physeal injury (23). The sports medicine practitioner must be keenly aware of the vulnerability of this primary growth center in diagnosing and treating the young athlete.

In the younger age group, the muscles are relatively weak. Muscle strain injury is relatively uncommon, owing to the insufficient force generation by these immature muscles.

In children skeletal growth occurs in advance of soft tissue growth (particularly in the axial plane), resulting in periods of disproportionate growth. The muscle–tendon unit extending across the bones and joints becomes sequentially tighter with growth (24). Inflexibility of the soft tissue develops more rapidly during high growth times. This inflexibility can then place undue stress on secondary growth centers (apophyses), resulting in acute avulsion fractures or chronic overuse apophysitis. Although this has not been proven, soft tissue stretching to maintain flexibility during phases of rapid growth has been thought to reduce the chance of injury and is recommended as an essential part of a warm-up routine for children of any age (25).

The articular, epiphyseal cartilage is also at risk for injury during childhood. Osteochondritic lesions involving the immature joint surface may occur at any bone and are most commonly seen at the knee. The etiology of this condition is unknown, and treatment depends on location, the joint involved, and the stability of the lesion.

HEAD INJURIES

Concussion, or mild traumatic brain injury, is defined by a minimum of an alteration in an athlete's mental function. Concussions are frequently encountered in the contact/collision sports of football, soccer, hockey, wrestling, and basketball. Controversy exists regarding determination of concussion severity and when to allow an athlete who has sustained a head injury to return to practice and competition. At this time there is no scientific basis for any grading scheme or return to play guidelines. Sports medicine physicians attempting to evaluate children and high school athletes with mild traumatic brain injury need to know the athlete's baseline mental status. Among uninjured high school athletes, only 51% are able to successfully complete serial sevens, whereas 78% can perform serial threes and 89% can complete the month of the year in reverse (26). A sensitive and specific test must be developed to aid in the assessment and treatment of mild head injury among athletes of all ages.

STRENGTH TRAINING

Strength training is the use of several methods of exercise (free weights, weight machines, plyometrics) to increase strength, endurance, and power. Although the general belief is that resistance training would be ineffective in increasing strength before adolescence because of inadequate hormonal stimulation, the majority of studies now support the notion that resistance training can result in significant increases in strength in preadolescence (27).

Preadolescents make similar relative percentage gains but smaller absolute gains in strength compared to their adolescent and adult counterparts. Despite the increased strength, there is a paucity of information about the potential performance benefits of strength training among this population. There is even less information showing the positive effects on injury rate or recovery from injury. The increased strength in the young athlete may be secondary to neural activation and improved motor coordination in contrast to adolescents and adults, who rely more on muscle hypertrophy to improve strength.

The risks of resistance training are also an area with little in the way of epidemiologic studies to provide any practical information. A cohort study of junior and senior high school football players showed an incidence of 7.6% (27/354) for weight-training injuries requiring more than 7 missed days of participation. The incidence among freshman/junior varsity athletes was 9.4% compared to 5.2% among high school athletes. It was noted in the study that the varsity athletes had more supervision and teaching about proper technique compared to the younger counterparts as one possible explanation for the reduced injury rate. (28) The back is the most frequent site of injury associated with resistance training in children, adolescents, and adults.

In designing a strength program for the youngster, the athlete and his or her family should be advised to lift only with the adequate supervision of a properly trained educator or coach (one with a National Strength and Conditioning Association Certification). Free weights should be recommended for the younger age groups because resistance machines are designed for adults with inconsistent adjustment settings for children. Most experts recommend avoiding maximum lifts because of a higher associated injury rate and increased stress on the physis. As with adults, weight training should be only a part of an overall conditioning program and should be performed on alternate days in an attempt to avoid overuse injury.

INTENSE PARTICIPATION

The amount of exercise that is necessary to produce adverse effects in young athletes is unknown. Despite concern, there is no scientific evidence to demonstrate significant direct effects of exercise on growth, age at peak height velocity, or skeletal maturity in most sports. An exception to this may be ballet, gymnastics, and wrestling in which dietary restriction combined with intense training at the elite level may result in growth impairment and delayed puberty. A recent prospective study demonstrated that heavy training in gymnastics (more than 18 hours per week), starting before puberty and maintained through puberty, can diminish growth velocity to such an extent that final adult height is less than would be expected (29).

Psychologically, intense sports participation can have a damaging effect, depending on the qualifications and training of the coach. Because of time and budget constraints, many high school athletes are now being coached by coaches who have had very little education in coaching children and adolescents (30). Overtraining, burnout, eating disorders, and increasing risky behavior are seen regularly among elite athletes as a direct result of excessive pressure, whether self-imposed or a result of an overzealous parent or coach.

SUMMARY

As with adults, promoting physical activity among children and adolescents is a challenge for any medical provider. In the adult population studies of supervised exercise programs demonstrate that poor compliance with an exercise program is related to failure to attain goals, lack of program accessibility, schedule conflicts, and lack of spousal support (31). In the pediatric population fun is thought to be the key to maintaining a successful exercise program. As with adults, social influences that sway compliance with physical activity need further study. Social support from friends and family is thought to affect compliance and therefore exercise promotion in the pediatric setting needs to be a family matter.

REFERENCES

1. U.S. Department of Health and Human Services. *Healthy people 2000: national health promotion and disease prevention objectives.* DHHS Publication No. (PHS) 91-50212. Washington, DC: U.S. Government Printing Office, 1991.
2. Troiano RP, Flegal KM, Kuczarski RJ, et al. Overweight prevalence and trends for children and adolescents: the National Health and Nutrition Examination Surveys, 1963 to 1991. *Arch Pediatr Adolesc Med* 1995;149:1085–1091.
3. Whitaker RC, Wright JA, Pepe MS, et al. Predicting obesity in young adulthood from childhood and parental obesity. *N Engl J Med* 1997;337:869–873.
4. Poole W. Exercise, coronary heart disease, and risk factors: a brief report. *Sports Med* 1984;1:341–349.
5. Gibbon LW, Blair SN, Cooper KH, et al. Association between coronary heart disease risk factors and physical fitness in healthy adult women. *Circulation* 1983;67:977–983.
6. Corbin CB, Pletcher P. Diet and physical activity patterns of obese and non obese elementary school children. *Res Q Am Assoc Health Phys Educ* 1968;39:922–924.
7. Fraser GE, Phillips RL, Harris R. Physical fitness and blood pressure in school children. *Circulation* 1983;67:405–412.
8. Heath GW, Ehsani AA, Hagberg JM, et al. Exercise training improves lipoprotein lipid profiles in patients with coronary artery disease. *Am Heart J* 1983;105:889–895.
9. Paffenbarger RS, Hyde RT, Wing AL, Steinmetz CH. A natural history of athleticism and cardiovascular health. *JAMA* 1984;252:491–495.
10. Morris FL, Naughton GA, Gibbs JL, et al. Prospective ten-month exercise intervention in premenarcheal girls: positive effects on bone and lean mass. *J Bone Miner Res* 1997;12(9):1453–1462.
11. Sonstroem RJ. Exercise and self-esteem. In: Terjung, RL, ed. *Exercise and sports science reviews,* Vol 12. Lexington, MA: The Collamore Press, 1984:123–155.
12. Taylor CB, Sallis JF, Needle R. The relation of physical activity and exercise to mental health. *Public Health Rep* 1985;100:195–201.
13. Dennison BA, Straus JH, Mellits D, Charney E. Childhood physical fitness tests: predictor of adult physical activity levels? *Pediatrics* 1988;82:324–330.
14. Aaron DJ, LaPorte RE. Physical activity, adolescence and health: an epidemiologic perspective. *Exercise and Sport Science Reviews* 1997;25:391–405.
15. Bijur PE, Trumble A, Harel Y, et al. Sports and recreation injuries in US children and adolescents. *Arch Pediatr Adolesc Med* 1995;149:1009–1016.
16. Seefeldt V, Ewing M, Walk S. *An overview of youth sports programs in the United States.* New York: Carnegie Council on Adolescent Development, Carnegie Corporation of New York, 1991.
17. Beachy G, Akau CK, Martinson M, et al. High school sports injuries: a longitudinal study at Punahou School: 1988–1996. *Am J Sports Med* 1997;25(5):675–681.
18. Brust JD, Leonard BJ, Pheley A, Roberts WO. Children's ice hockey injuries. *Am J Dis Child* 1992;146:741–747.
19. Stuart MJ, Smith AM, Nieva JJ, Rock MG. Injuries in youth ice hockey: a pilot surveillance strategy. *Mayo Clin Proc* 1995;70:350–356.
20. Smith AM, Stuart MJ, Wiese-Bjornstal DM, et al. Predictors of injury in ice hockey players: a multivariate, multidisciplinary approach. *Am J Sports Med* 1997;25(4):500–507.
21. DeLee JC, Farney WC. Incidence of injury in Texas high school football. *Am J Sport Med* 1992;20:575–580.
22. Landry GL. Sports injuries in childhood. *Pediatr Ann* 1992;21:165–168.
23. DiFiori JP, Mandelbaum BR. Wrist pain in a young gymnast: unusual radiographic findings and MRI evidence of growth plate injury. *Med Sci Sports Exerc* 1996;28(12):1453–1458.
24. Malina RN. Adolescent changes in size, build, composition and performance. *Hum Biol* 1974;46:117.
25. American Academy of Pediatrics Committee on Sports Medicine and Fitness. Assessing physical activity and fitness in the office setting. *Pediatrics* 1994;93:686–689.
26. Young CC, Jacobs BA, Clavette K, et al. Serial sevens: not the most effective test of mental status in high school athletes. *Clin J Sports Med* 1997;7(3):196–198.
27. Blimpkie C. Resistance training during preadolescence: issues and controversies. *Sports Med* 1993;15(6):389–407.
28. Risser WL, Risser JMH, Preston D. Weight-training injuries in adolescents. *Am J Dis Child* 1990;144:1015–1017.
29. Theintz GE, Howald H, Weiss U, et al. Evidence for a reduction of growth potential in adolescent female gymnasts. *J Pediatr* 1993;122:306–313.
30. Brown BR, Butterfield SA. Coaches: a missing link in the health care system. *Am J Dis Child* 1992;146:211–217.
31. Andrew GM, Oldridge NB, Parker JO, et al. Reasons for dropout from exercise programs in post coronary patients. *Med Science Sports Exerc* 1981;13:164–168.

CHAPTER 8

The Female Athlete

Aurelia Nattiv, Elizabeth A. Arendt, and Suzanne S. Hecht

HISTORY

"Women's sports are against the laws of nature and the most unaesthetic sight human eyes could contemplate."
    Baron Pierre de Coubertin, 1902,
    Father of the Modern Olympics (1)

What would Pierre de Coubertin think today if he knew that 34% of the athletes who competed in the 1996 Atlanta Summer Olympic Games were women? Would he have been able to watch the gold medal–winning performances of women athletes in basketball, swimming, gymnastics, soccer, and softball? What about the gold medal–winning victory of the U.S. women's hockey team in the 1998 Winter Olympics? The role of women and exercise has changed dramatically since the beginnings of the modern Olympics in 1896 and even more since the ancient Greek Olympics. Today, women are participating in sports at all levels in record numbers. This role change has significantly improved both the athletic opportunities and the competitive environments for today's young female athletes.

The origins of the modern Olympic games began in Greece as a tribute to the Greek god Zeus. The ancient Greek Olympics were strictly for men. Women were not allowed to compete in or even watch the ancient Olympics. In fact, the Olympic champions were often awarded "a beautiful and good woman for life" (2).

The Victorian era had significant impact on women's health and exercise. For upper-class urban women of the 19th century, the ideal woman was one who was frail, passive, and weak. If a woman's husband was successful, then she was able to stay indoors and let the servants perform the chores. A pale, weak wife was a status symbol. Accepted sports for upper-class women during this era were archery, croquet, bowling, tennis, and golf. Of course, exertion levels were kept to a minimum, and any type of competition was frowned upon (3).

The health of a 19th century woman was thought to revolve around her reproductive ability. The medical community commonly linked any physical and psychiatric ailments to the uterus. It was believed that hysteria would result if a woman overexerted herself. Only mild exercise was allowed for women because sweating, in addition to being socially unacceptable, was believed to be unhealthy. Strict bed rest was mandated by physicians during the "monthly sexual storms" (menses) and also during and after pregnancy (3).

The period from 1920 to 1970 was one of substantial progress for women and athletics, despite resistance to competition from physical educators. The 1920s brought forth two athletic female stars who gained worldwide attention. Helen Wills reigned as the women's tennis champion during this time, and Gertrude Ederle swam the English Channel two hours faster than anyone ever had, including men (3). In spite of great athletic accomplishments by some women, the Association of Directors of Physical Education for Women believed that all women should participate in athletics but firmly resisted the idea of intercollegiate or professional competition for women. Instead, they developed "playdays" or "sportsdays," when teams from other schools would get together to participate in sports but not to compete. The Committee of Women's Athletics and the Women's Division of the Amateur Athletic Union actually opposed sending women to the 1928 and 1932 Olympics. The U.S. Olympic Committee, however, sent women's teams despite the opposition of these committees (4).

Public recreation took on a prominent role of promoting exercise and sports during the 1930s. Offering organized sports to the general public made exercise available to more people, regardless of their income.

A. Nattiv and S. Hecht: Departments of Family Medicine and Orthopaedic Surgery, UCLA School of Medicine, Los Angeles, California 90095-1683.

E. A. Arendt: Department of Orthopaedic Surgery, University of Minnesota Hospital, Minneapolis, Minnesota 55455.

Industry-sponsored city leagues developed from the recognition that employees were healthier if they exercised. Babe Didrikson, a 1932 Olympic champion, developed her athletic abilities through sports sponsored by industry (3). With the start of World War II, women found themselves in traditionally male jobs that required strength and endurance. Rosie the Riveter, an image that represented the strong, independent American woman, was popularized. The All-American Girls' Baseball League was formed to fill the void created in men's professional sports because of the war (4,5).

The late 1960s was the first time that physical educators began to accept and sponsor activities for the high-level female athlete. Intercollegiate athletic competition for women, including national championships, began to develop in 1967. It was during this time that the U.S. Olympic Development Committee took an interest in developing programs for female athletes with Olympic potential. These programs were initiated in conjunction with the Division of Girls and Women's Sports, formally known as the Association of Directors of Physical Education for Women from the 1920s. This Division was replaced with the Association for Intercollegiate Athletics for Women (AIAW) in 1971, which agreed to athletic scholarships for women in 1973 and by 1975 sponsored championships in 19 sports (5).

Although tremendous strides in women's athletics were made between 1920 and 1970, the explosion of women's athletics occurred in the early 1970s. The spark for this explosion came from the passage of Title IX of the 1972 Education Amendments Act by the U.S. Congress. Title IX stated that "No person in the United States shall on the basis of sex be excluded from participation in, be denied the benefits of, or be subjected to discrimination under any education program or activity receiving Federal financial assistance." The guidelines of Title IX were passed into federal law in 1975, and one of them stated that institutions receiving federal aid must provide equal opportunity for women's and men's sport. By 1986–1987 there were 82,979 women participating in intercollegiate sports compared to only 31,852 in 1971–1972. The number of athletic scholarships for women rose from 60 in 1974 to 500 in 1981. Marked increases were also seen in high school athletic participation, with 35% of all high school girls competing in interscholastic sports in 1981 compared to only 7% in 1971 (5).

Today, women's participation in sports is at record highs. Over the last decade the number of women competing in intercollegiate athletics has increased by almost 50% (6), and the number of athletic scholarships has grown to over 25,000 (7). Now women can have successful professional careers as athletes, newscasters, sports writers, coaches, and officials. Female athletes have the opportunity to compete at the professional level in sports including basketball, soccer, softball, bodybuilding, volleyball, and skiing, in addition to the more traditional women's professional sports of tennis, figure skating, and golf. Athletic companies such as Adidas, Nike, and Reebok are offering prominent female athletes lucrative contracts to endorse their products. The role of women in sports has been revolutionized over the last 25 years. Like her predecessors, the female athlete of the future will continue to break new ground, forever changing the role of women in sports.

WOMEN IN SPORTS: PHYSIOLOGIC CONSIDERATIONS AND GENDER DIFFERENCES

Understanding the anatomic and physiologic similarities and differences between male and female athletes is valuable for enhancing athletic performance and well-being (Table 8–1). It is extremely important to remember that there is great variability among individuals, regardless of their gender or athletic abilities. As the scientific body of knowledge about female athletes continues to grow, female athletes will be able to reach new heights and face a variety of challenges in all athletic arenas.

The Adult Female Athlete

Body Composition

Women generally have 8–10% more body fat than men (8–9). Body fat can be divided into two components: essential and storage. A portion of essential fat consists of gender-specific fat such as that in the breasts, buttocks, and thighs. Storage fat is approximately 15% in both sexes (10). Essential fat contributes 9–12% of body weight in women compared to 3% in men (9,11).

The average percent body fat for female college students is approximately 25%, while male college students average about 15% body fat. This difference is main-

TABLE 8–1. *Physiologic parameters important to exercise: adult females compared to adult males*

Physiologic parameter	Females as compared to males
Percent body fat	More
Strength	Less
Muscle fiber size	Smaller
Proportion of muscle fiber types	Similar
Aerobic capacity	Less
Stroke volume	Smaller
Lung volumes	Smaller
Left ventricular mass	Smaller
Hemoglobin/hematocrit	Less
Mitochondrial density	Less
Anaerobic capacity	Less
Thermoregulation	Similar

tained or decreased in female athletes as compared to male athletes in the same sport (10,12). For example, the average body fat percent in female track athletes is 10–15% compared to less than 7% for male track athletes (13). Body fat percent in many female athletes is less than the body fat percent in sedentary men and women of comparable age (9) This is especially true for female athletes who compete in sports such as cross-country running and gymnastics (9). Female athletes in sports such as basketball, volleyball, swimming, and tennis average 18–24% body fat (14), while body fat estimates of elite female soccer players range from 19.7 to 22.0% (15). A women's higher body fat is thought to hinder performance in most endurance sports, although evidence supporting this theory is lacking. A higher body fat actually provides an advantage in swimming. Buoyancy is increased with higher body fat, which, in turn, decreases drag and reduces energy expenditure by about 20% (9,16).

Strength

Overall, a woman's strength is approximately 67% of that of her male counterpart. Absolute strength in women is approximately 50% less in the upper body and 25% less in the lower body compared to men. These differences diminish when absolute strength is expressed as relative strength by taking body mass into account. Relative leg strength in women is similar to that of men when expressed in this manner, but relative upper body strength is still less (14,17–20). Total muscle mass in women is approximately 23% of their total body weight, compared to 40% in men (14). This difference in muscle mass is due to muscle fibers that are 15–40% smaller in females than in males (9,14). However, the proportions of fast- and slow-twitch muscle fiber types are similar between the sexes (9,11,12). Men and women demonstrate similar gains in relative strength with weight-training programs (9,17,21).

Skeletal Differences

Maturation is reached earlier in females. Skeletal maturation in females is generally complete by 18–19 years of age in contrast to males, who reach skeletal maturity at 21–22 years old (22). On average men attain greater height and weight than women (23). Average American men are about 18 kg heavier and 13 cm taller than average American women (24). Generally, women have smaller bones and thus less articular surface area (13). Compared to males, females tend to have narrower shoulders, wider pelvic structure, and increased knee valgus and hip varus angles (9,13). These increased angles are often blamed for some of the overuse injuries seen in female athletes (see the section entitled "Common Musculoskeletal Problems in the Female Athlete"). Finally, it is important to remember that there is great variation in skeletal structure between individuals of the same and opposite sex.

Aerobic Performance

Energy for prolonged exercise is supplied predominantly by metabolic pathways that require oxygen. The ability of the heart, lungs, and skeletal muscle cells to utilize oxygen during sustained exercise is referred to as aerobic capacity or power. Maximal aerobic capacity is measured as Vo_2max. Vo_2max is generally accepted as the best measure of an individual's cardiovascular fitness. Maximal aerobic capacity is reached when oxygen uptake is maximized despite continued increases in work and energy requirements (12). A high Vo_2max reflects a large aerobic capacity. A large aerobic capacity does not necessarily predict successful sports performances, particularly in comparing athletes of similar competitive levels (8). Vo_2max depends on physiologic, genetic, and psychological factors. There is great variation in Vo_2max between individuals. Although all three factors are important, the following discussion will be limited to the physiologic components. Physiologic factors can be divided into three areas: body composition, oxygen transportation, and oxidative capacity (25).

As we discussed earlier, men and women have different body compositions. Women have more body fat, while men have more muscle mass. On average, a larger body with less body fat will be able to generate a higher Vo_2max. It requires extra energy to carry body fat; therefore less energy is available for exercise. Absolute Vo_2max (mL/min) is 40–60% higher in males than in females. To remove the body mass advantage of males, since males are generally larger than females, relative Vo_2max can be calculated. Relative Vo_2max (mL/kg/min) is calculated by dividing the absolute Vo_2max by body weight. Relative Vo_2max is 20–30% greater in males even after accounting for body weight. If it is calculated with fat-free mass instead of total body weight, the difference between genders declines to 10–15% (9,10).

To study the effect of extra body fat on Vo_2max, Cureton and Sparling (26) had males exercise with external weights added. This was done in an attempt to replicate the extra body fat load with which women must exercise. They found that the differences in relative Vo_2max were reduced to insignificant levels when males exercised with extra weight. Although the Vo_2max was equalized, men still had approximately 20–30% better performances in terms of distance, time, and efficiency of running (26). Gender differences in aerobic capacity narrow when athletes in the same sport are compared, but elite male athletes still have higher Vo_2max than elite female athletes (14). Helgerud and colleagues compared performance-matched male and female marathon runners and found a similar $\text{V}_{\text{O}_2}\text{max}$ (approximately 60 mL/kg/min) for each group (27). The largest aerobic capacities are seen in male and female long-distance runners and cross-country skiers (12). Males and females demonstrate similar increases in $\text{V}_{\text{O}_2}\text{max}$ with endurance training (11,28). Women athletes who participate in endurance exercise have higher relative $\text{V}_{\text{O}_2}\text{max}$ compared to most men (29,30).

Although body composition appears to account for a significant proportion of the gender differences in aerobic capacity, oxygen transportation also plays a role. Systemic oxygen transportation is a function of respiratory function, cardiac output, and the oxygen-carrying capacity of red blood cells. Women have smaller lung volumes than men owing to a smaller thoracic cavity. Average total lung capacity in females is 4200 mL compared to 6000 mL in males (9). Although this difference exists, respiratory volumes are not thought to limit maximal aerobic capacity at low altitudes (25).

Heart volumes are approximately 10–15% less in women, resulting in a smaller stroke volume and maximal cardiac output (11). Females have a smaller left ventricular mass even when calculated relative to lean body mass. If men and women exercise at the same intensity, women demonstrate higher heart rates (approximately 5–8 beats per minute) and lower stroke volumes (9,11). Women have been shown to increase their left ventricular end diastolic volumes with endurance training, resulting in increased stroke volume and cardiac output (11).

In addition to a smaller heart, women also have lower hemoglobin levels and plasma volumes than men. Adult males have 6% more red blood cells and 10–15% greater hemoglobin concentrations than females. Since 1 g of hemoglobin can combine maximally with 134 mL of oxygen, it is not surprising that this difference may effect $\text{V}_{\text{O}_2}\text{max}$. Thus, for the same amount of exercise, females must transport more oxygen to the tissues or extract more oxygen from the red blood cells than males (9,25). Endurance training has been shown to decrease hemoglobin and plasma volume differences between males and females (11).

Oxidative capacity of skeletal muscle also contributes to aerobic capacity. The density of mitochondria in skeletal muscle is thought to reflect the muscle's oxidative ability. Endurance training increases the mass of mitochondria up to two times the original mass. This increase in mitochondrial density is seen in both slow- and fast-twitch muscle fibers. Slow-twitch muscle fibers can extract three to five times more oxygen than fast-twitch fibers, owing to a higher mitochondrial density. It is postulated that increased mitochondrial density improves endurance by improving the ability of muscle to metabolize fats, thereby conserving muscle glycogen stores. Another benefit of increased mitochondrial density may be increased clearance of lactic acid by oxidation. Since females have less muscle mass than males, their mitochondrial density is lower, thus contributing to lower maximal aerobic capacity (30).

Since women first started competing in marathons in the early 1970s, their winning times have dramatically improved. Although women have not been able to equal the winning times of male marathoners, there is research to suggest that women may outperform men in ultraendurance events. A study of performance-matched male and female athletes found that women performed significantly better than men in a 90-km race. This superior performance by the female athletes was not related to greater maximal aerobic capacity, running economy, training level, or fatty acid metabolism (31). Another study compared the performances of male and female athletes matched for 56-km race times, age, and training over racing distances of 5–90 km. Men had better performances in race distances from 5 to 42.2 km but not at 90 km. The authors of this study suggest that women ultramarathon runners have greater fatigue resistance than male athletes, who have better performances in marathon distances (32).

Anaerobic Performance

Unlike aerobic exercise, anaerobic performance is required for activities that consist of quick bursts of energy usually lasting less than 3 minutes total duration. This type of exercise predominantly utilizes metabolic pathways that are oxygen independent to provide energy, even though anaerobic metabolism is less efficient. If exercise intensity is strenuous, aerobic metabolism will not be able to generate energy fast enough to meet the energy demands of the exercising muscle (8). In this situation anaerobic metabolism will be used to a greater extent. Fast-twitch muscle fibers are predominantly recruited for anaerobic activities because of their reliance on oxygen independent metabolism. Anaerobic metabolism of glucose and/or glycogen generates lactic acid. Removal of lactic acid from the bloodstream requires oxidation. Thus, the lactic acid concentration in the bloodstream reflects the degree of anaerobic metabolism. The exercise level that generates a lactic acid concentration greater than 4 mM is termed the lactate threshold (LT) or anaerobic threshold (25). Prolonged exercise is difficult once the LT has been reached, owing to inefficient energy production by anaerobic metabolism. Although research on gender differences in anaerobic capacity is limited, it is known that females (athletes and nonathletes) generally have a lower maximal LT than males. This may be due to less muscle mass and/or training differences (12). LT is often expressed as a percent of $\text{V}_{\text{O}_2}\text{max}$. When LT is expressed in this way, there are no differences between genders, although females reach the LT at a lower absolute exercise intensity (25,27). This suggests that in females a larger amount of the total energy required for strenuous exercise is derived from anaerobic metabolism.

Thermoregulation

The ability to regulate core body temperature appears to be more closely related to fitness level and acclimatization than to gender (25,33–34). For many years it was believed that women were less tolerant of exercise in hot temperatures than men. The early studies that led to this erroneous conclusion were flawed by lack of comparable fitness levels between the male and female subjects (35–36). These previously reported differences in heat tolerance disappeared when women and men with matched fitness levels were studied (13,37,38). Now it is also known that sweating and vasodilation occur sooner in people who are acclimatized to the heat and are more physically fit, regardless of their gender (14,37). Women acclimate to hot weather conditions as well as men do (39,40).

When exercising in hot, humid temperatures, women may have an advantage over men because of their larger body surface area (BSA), which enhances heat loss (25). A study by Shapiro and colleagues found no differences in rectal temperatures and heart rates for men and women exercising in hot, humid conditions who were matched for BSA (41). When exercising in a cold environment, women lose body heat more readily than men, because of their larger BSA. Some of this heat loss is compensated for by the greater body fat content of females, which provides an insulating effect (25).

Effect of Menstrual Cycle on Performance

One of the most obvious physiologic differences between men and women is the menstrual cycle. Approximately once a month, women experience a complex interaction of hormonal shifts. Athletes, coaches, and researchers alike have wondered whether the menstrual cycle has any influence on athletic performance. Many Olympic and world record performances have been set by women athletes during all phases of the menstrual cycle (23), although individual athletes may complain of altered performance during certain phases of the menstrual cycle. Multiple studies have looked at physical and psychologic performance characteristics such as speed, endurance, strength, cognition, and perceived exertion at various phases of the menstrual cycle. The conclusions of these studies generally suggest that there is no significant relationship between the phase of the menstrual cycle (follicular or luteal) and performance, though some subtle differences may exist (11,13,23,42–46). The earlier studies on this topic did not use physiologic markers to confirm the phase of the menstrual cycle. This, in addition to small study numbers and the use of untrained subjects, may be the reason that the results of the earlier studies were often conflicting. More recent studies have utilized physiologic markers to verify the phase of the menstrual cycle (43). DeSouza's study measured multiple performance variables, including VO_2max, time to fatigue, lactate levels, heart rate, and minute ventilation, in eight eumenorrheic and eight amenorrheic runners during submaximal and maximal exercise at various phases of the menstrual cycle. The results demonstrated that exercise performance in female athletes is not changed by menstrual status or phase (43).

The menstrual cycle phase may have an effect on thermoregulation. The core body temperature of a female is 0.4°C higher during ovulation and remains elevated throughout the luteal phase. In a study by Kawahata the threshold for sweating was reported to increase after ovulation (47). Other studies have demonstrated no difference in the onset of sweating with relationship to menstrual cycle phases (48–50). Whether the increased core body temperature of women during the second half of their menstrual cycle affects their thermoregulatory abilities during exercise remains unknown. Several studies have found no difference in rectal temperature, heart rate, exercise tolerance, or sweat rate while exercising in hot, dry conditions during various phases of the menstrual cycle (33,51–52). Avellini and colleagues found that once women were acclimated to exercising in hot, humid conditions, there was no difference in exercise tolerance, rectal temperatures, or sweating thresholds between women in the preovulatory and postovulatory phases (53).

Oral contraceptive pills (OCP) change the menstrual cycle primarily by preventing monthly ovulation. Female athletes take OCPs for a variety of reasons, including contraception, dysmenorrhea, and menstrual dysfunction (oligomenorrhea, amenorrhea). Invariably, athletes are interested in knowing whether OCPs will change their performance. Although research on the newer and more widely used triphasic preparations is limited, it appears that taking OCPs does not significantly alter performance in the majority of women (44,45). Of course, as with any medication, the benefits and risks should be evaluated and monitored on an individual basis.

The Prepubescent Female Athlete

Before puberty, girls and boys are similar in terms of physical capacity, body composition, strength, red blood cell mass, and thermoregulatory ability (9,11,14,22,23) (Table 8–2). Prepubescent boys have slightly higher anaerobic capacities than girls (22) and have the same or slightly higher aerobic capacity than their female counterparts (9,22). A study comparing the cardiovascular responses to exercise of twenty-four 7- to 9-year-old boys and girls found few differences between genders

TABLE 8–2. *Physiologic parameters important to exercise: prepubescent girls compared to prepubescent boys and adult females*

Physiologic parameter	Girls as compared to boys	Girls as compared to adult females
Aerobic capacity	Similar or slightly less	Less
Anaerobic capacity	Slightly less	Less
Percent body fat	Similar	Less
Strength	Similar	Less
Hemoglobin/hematocrit	Similar	Less
Thermoregulation	Similar	Less effective

(54). In contrast, a study of 12-year-old boys and girls found that peak oxygen uptake during exercise was significantly higher in boys (55).

Percent body fat, height, and weight are similar in boys and girls before puberty (14,23). Peak body fat in males occurs at approximately 11 years of age and then decreases. In contrast, females reach peak body fat after puberty (23).

Muscular strength is similar in boys and girls until puberty (23). In 11- to 12-year-old girls, strength is estimated to be 90% of that of 11- to 12-year-old boys. Once girls reach 15–16 years of age, their strength is estimated to be only 75% of that of same-age males (9). Individual muscle cell size in girls peaks when they are approximately 10.5 years old, and large strength gains are seen just before the growth spurt prior to puberty. The maximal growth rate of muscle cells in boys begins at this age and lasts into their twenties with large strength gains occurring about one year after the growth spurt (22–23).

Hemoglobin, hematocrit, and red blood cell mass are similar in prepubescent girls and boys (9,11). At puberty these measurements are comparable to the values found in adult females. Hemoglobin, hematocrit, and red blood cell mass continue to increase in males until they are 17 to 23 years old (9).

Young athletes are at a thermoregulatory disadvantage when exercising in very hot or very cold environments compared to adult athletes. Girls and boys appear to be similar in their thermoregulatory abilities, though research in this area is limited. However, more research has been conducted on the thermoregulatory abilities of girls compared to adolescent and adult women. Girls generate more heat during exercise, have a larger BSA to weight ratio, initiate sweating at higher core body temperatures, and sweat at a slower rate than adolescent or adult women (56). These differences require girls to rely more on convection to dissipate heat than on evaporation (heat loss through sweating). When the ambient temperature exceeds the skin temperature, a large BSA is a disadvantage because the body more readily gains heat from the environment. Under these conditions, evaporation of sweat becomes the only means of dissipating heat. The smaller evaporative capacity of girls, combined with their increased heat production, places them at greater risk of suffering heat illness when exercising in hot climates. Girls shunt more blood to their peripheral circulation when exercising in hot conditions than women do. This enhances heat loss through increased cutaneous vasodilation but secondarily results in a lower venous return and stroke volume, which limits exercise tolerance (22). Additionally, it is important to remember that children take longer than adolescents and adults to acclimate to hot climates and increase their core body temperature more rapidly when they are dehydrated (57).

MUSCULOSKELETAL INJURIES

Sport Injury Rates

Injury on the athletic field is a disruption of an athlete's pursuit for fitness, sport, and competition. Attempts are continually being made to identify key risk factors that are involved in the pathogenesis of sports injuries. Risk factors can be classified into two categories. Extrinsic factors are those that are related to the types of sport activity, the manner in which a sport is played, the environmental conditions, and/or the equipment used to play a sport. Intrinsic factors are the factors that are individual and include both physical and psychosocial characteristics (58).

Early studies assessing injury rates supported the notion that sports injuries sustained by female athletes were no different than those of men (59,60). Early studies of the first female military cadets helped to support that many performance variables between men and women resulted from improper conditioning for young women (61–63). These performance variables could improve with appropriate conditioning for young women, narrowing the gap of differences between men and women. Therefore it was thought that sport injury was largely dictated by the type of sport one plays and by individual fitness and conditioning levels, not by one's gender.

Injury prevention continues to be a goal in sports medicine. This is a challenge, in part owing to the difficulty of controlling studies with numerous variables and a poor understanding by clinicians and scientists of the interrelatedness of such variables. However, studies support the following observations:

1. A history of previous injury is a strong risk factor for recurrent injury (58,64).
2. Women report injuries differently than men (65).
3. Within the military population, men accomplish tasks with fewer injuries and diseases compared to women, and with less apparent stress (63).
4. Women may be capable of equal efficiency and aerobic metabolism (63).
5. There are female differences in upper body strength, power, and endurance and lesser but significant differences in lower extremities for the same values compared to men (66).
6. A greater number of knee injuries are reported among women participating in sports than among men (67–70).
7. There is an increase in noncontact anterior cruciate ligament injuries in women as compared to men (71–73).
8. Ankle sprains may occur more commonly in females (74).
9. Physical fitness may be an independent risk factor for injury (65).

The increase in noncontact anterior cruciate ligament injuries in women has come under much review, with much speculation and numerous theories to date. There is currently no conclusive evidence to support a reason for this increased injury rate. Examining injury risk factors is complex, especially as they relate to gender. A review of the intrinsic and extrinsic factors that may play a role in the increase in noncontact anterior cruciate ligament injuries has been previously published (75). The following will address some of the intrinsic and extrinsic factors that may relate to gender differences in sport injuries.

Multiple joint laxity, or hypermobility, has long been implicated as a risk factor for injury. Hypermobility is most commonly defined by specific tests of joint motion. A laxity scale is defined, giving each joint motion a numerical value. Several scales have been formulated to date, utilizing different joints for their scale (knees, elbows, wrists, fingers, back) (76,77). Hypermobility syndrome is said to be present if an individual has three or more positive laxity tests together with joint or muscle symptoms (78,79). A relationship between joint hypermobility and acute injury to the knee and/or ankle joint has been sought in the past. Nicholas (80) reported that football players with joint hypermobility were more at risk for knee injuries. This finding has not been substantiated in further studies (81–84). Diaz and colleagues (85) correlated a modified laxity scale with musculoskeletal injuries in a military population. These authors concluded that lax individuals (those with three out of five laxity scores) had more musculotendinous injuries than those who were not lax. The above studies centered more on acute musculoskeletal complaints. However, hypermobile joints or an increased laxity scale has been most implicated in the creation of overuse injuries, particularly in females. Their role in patellofemoral pain, overuse injuries about the foot and ankle, including posterior tibialis tendinitis and shoulder laxity syndromes, has been poorly defined to date. Breighton and colleagues (77) thought that musculoskeletal symptoms are positively related to mobility scores, as judged by laxity scales. This relationship is most evident for females. Women demonstrate more laxity than men using laxity scales (85–88). Whether this laxity syndrome is strongly correlated with unique female cyclical hormones has yet to be determined.

There is increasing evidence, however, that certain musculoskeletal disease states may be more common in women. These include arthritic disorders (arthritis and arthralgias), which are 60–80% more common in women (89–91). Within this group, identifiable disease states include osteoarthritis, rheumatoid arthritis, and systemic lupus erythematosus. All are more commonly reported in women. Fibromyalgia is not well understood but is typically associated with muscle pain and joint and muscle swelling. This is more commonly diagnosed in women, typically in the third to fifth decades of life.

Another type of laxity that is defined specifically for the knee is an increase in the measurement in the anterior posterior tibiofemoral motion. This is most commonly measured by using an instrumented arthrometer. Arthrometer measurements of anterior posterior motion in knees has been reviewed in normal male and female basketball players (92), normal knees in the population (93), athletic knees before and after exercise (94,95), anterior cruciate ligament (ACL) intact and ACL deficient knees (84), and athletes across different sports (95). All of the above-mentioned studies revealed no apparent relationship between knee laxity, gender, and acute knee injury. Using a more sophisticated type of knee arthrometer measurement, a recent study has revealed a difference in knee laxity between female athletes and male athletes and between female athletes and male and female controls (96).

Risk Factors for Injury in the Female Athlete

Intrinsic Factors

The role of a female's unique cyclical hormones and their possible effect on disease states and injury is being increasingly discussed and investigated. The hormonal effect on soft tissues, particularly the role of estrogen, is not well understood. Several recent studies have tried to uncover the relationship between ligament biology and hormones (97–99). It is well known that the hormone relaxin, found in females during the last trimester of pregnancy, is largely responsible for the ligamentous relaxation that enables the pelvis to accommodate passage of the fetus during birth. The effect of this relaxation on the pelvic ligaments has been implicated as a reason for potential relaxation of other ligaments in a female's body, leading to the possibility of ankle sprains and other ligamentous injuries during late pregnancy (100). Ligament tissue, specifically the epiligament of the medial collateral ligament, may be susceptible to sex-related hormones, particularly estrogen (97). Investigating further the possible relationship between the role of the female's unique cyclical hormones and ACL injury, researchers have sought a relationship between an acute ACL injury and the phase of menstrual cycle. Two studies to date, both with small databases, have found a clustering of ACL injuries in a specific menstrual phase. However, one study noted it in the luteal phase of menstrual cycle (101), while another found it in the follicular phase (102). This relationship continues to be investigated.

Anatomic limb variation, specifically the angle that the femur makes with the tibia at the knee level (the Q angle), is an often quoted explanation for injuries of the lower extremity in females. Anatomic limb variation has been implicated as responsible for the increased rate of noncontact ACL injuries in women. There are no data to support this to date. A single retrospective study reviewing one sports medicine clinic's experience concluded that there was no apparent relationship between standing tibiofemoral alignment, Q angle, and knee injuries (in particular ACL injuries) in a series of female basketball players (71). A variation in limb alignment has been given the name *miserable malalignment syndrome* (Fig. 8–1). Miserable malalignment is a combination of lower extremity features that includes increased anteversion of the femoral head. With increased anteversion the femur must internally rotate to maintain satisfactory coverage of the femoral head in the bony socket of the pelvis. The limb accommodates for this rotation by externally rotating the tibia to keep the foot pointing straight ahead while walking. The foot accommodates leg rotation with increased pronation to accommodate foot placement to the ground surface. This above discussion may be an oversimplification of a complex limb rotation, but it is helpful in understanding the interrelationship of the different limb components. Miserable malalignment typically involves anteversion of the femoral head, external rotation of the tibia, and a pronated foot. Other features can include an increased Q angle, tibiofemoral valgus, tibia varus, and a hypermobile patella. These anatomic features, alone or in combination, have been blamed for a variety of overuse syndromes in the lower legs of active people, in particular women. Most clinicians have

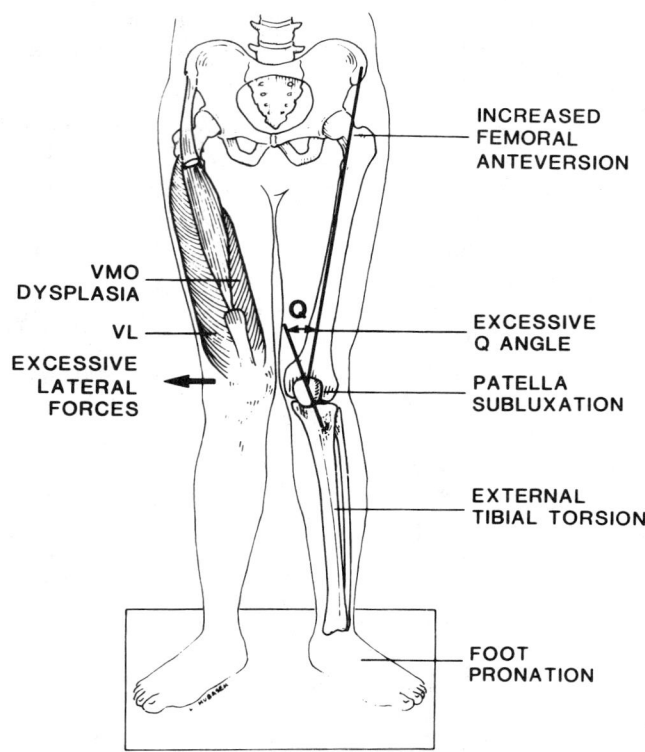

FIG. 8–1. Lower extremity features of miserable malalignment syndrome: increased femoral anteversion, external tibial torsion, foot pronation, along with increased Q-angle and VMO dysplasia/hypoplasia create lateral forces that may sublux and tilt the patella (VL, vastus lateralis; VMO, vastus medialis obliquus). (Adapted from Ireland ML. Special concerns of the female athlete. In: Fu FH, Stone DA, eds. *Sports injuries: mechanism, prevention, and treatment,* 2nd ed. Baltimore: Williams & Wilkins, 1994:153–187.)

supported this speculation, though few population studies to date have looked closely at this relationship. Therefore, the causes of increased musculoskeletal complaints in this type of leg alignment remain speculative only.

One of the most discussed reason in the orthopedic literature for ACL failure in bilateral knee injury and the ACL reconstructed knee has been the dimensions of the intracondylar notch of the knee (the inverted U-shaped space in the middle of the knee through which the ACL runs). The exact role, if any, that notch size plays in creating an ACL tear remains speculative. Whether size or gender is the determining factor in such injuries needs further study before answers are known (103–106).

Extrinsic Factors

Increased friction between a shoe and a playing surface has been implicated as a cause of injury in both knees and ankles (107). A Norwegian study looking at their team handball players revealed that the friction rate of certain shoes on certain materials, particularly a court shoe on a green turf, showed a higher friction rate. This increased friction rate correlated with a higher incidence of noncontact ACL injuries (108). However, if one were to implicate the shoe surface interface as a primary factor in noncontact ACL injuries, this would need to encompass a variety of sports and playing surfaces, including gymnastics (bare foot on a rubber mat), alpine skiing (fixed foot position on a ski), basketball (court shoe on a wooden surface), and soccer (cleated shoe on grass).

Recent focus has investigated the role of neuromuscular function, muscle recruitment, and modifications of training as important components in knee injury risk. An earlier study that tried to identify major injury mechanisms responsible for ACL injuries and then modify those mechanisms was indeed able to show a reduction of ACL injuries over a two-year period (109). More recently, Huston and Wojtys (96) have hypothesized that the female athlete has a quadricep dominant knee. This quadracep dominant knee might be responsible for increased quad activation, resulting in increased anterior tibial translation with certain activities. The role that training may play in changing muscle pattern recruitment has come under recent review. For example, women volleyball players have been shown to have adduction moments decrease on jump landings after 6 weeks of intense training emphasizing plyometrics (110). This is felt to be favorable to the biomechanics of the limb in jump landing, thereby decreasing the possibility of injury.

Common Musculoskeletal Problems in the Female Athlete

Patellofemoral Pain Syndrome

Patellofemoral pain syndrome (PFPS) is a global term that is used to describe anterior knee pain that originates in the extensor mechanism (that being the bony patella and its femoral groove), the surrounding muscles (most specifically the quadracep muscle), and the tendinous attachments of the quadracep and patella tendon. The patella also has a complex weave of static restraints, including the retinacular structures that restrain passive motion. PFPS typically refers to pain without documented joint instability. Central in the treatment of patellofemoral pain is balancing the movement of the patella in its trochlear groove. Indeed, PFPS without X-ray malalignment may represent subtle malalignment that is not detectable with our standard imaging techniques. This subtle malalignment results in an imbalance within the static soft tissue structures of the retinaculum or within the quadracep muscle itself, in either recruitment or absolute strength. This imbalance can secondarily lead to pain. Important elements to include with treatment of PFPS are the following:

1. Rehabilitation, in particular a quadricep muscle-strengthening program, is widely recognized as useful for treating patellofemoral disorders (111,112). A quadricep-strengthening program emphasizing eccentric, closed chain activities is central to a rehabilitative scheme for the patellofemoral joint.
2. Rehabilitation should emphasize a program resulting in a balanced lower extremity. The entire lower leg kinematic chain should be assessed for flexibility as well as strength, of both the proximal and distal portions of the limb. Particular attention should be addressed to external hip rotators and balancing of the pelvis, as this muscle group is complementary to the quadricep muscle and is frequently weak in patients with patellofemoral pain syndrome.
3. Trying to balance or centralize the patella with the use of patella braces and/or tape techniques may be useful for selected patients but must be an adjunct to full treatment.
4. Patella retinacular tightness is assessed by examining medial lateral translation and with referral to physical therapy for patella mobilization and stretching if tight patella restraints are identified (113).
5. Overpronation control of the foot with a semirigid orthosis helps to control rotatory alignment of the limb, decreasing overuse issues of the foot and the joints proximal to the foot.

Stress Fractures

Stress fractures can be thought of as an overuse injury to bone. Bone is living tissue and can successfully accommodate stress or undergo failure in response to increased loading. The ultimate result of increased load can be viewed as a continuum from normal remodeling to fatigue and bone exhaustion. The end stage of failure to respond to increased load would be a frank fracture on X-ray.

Special attention must be given to the developing and mature woman in considering stress phenomena of bone. Estrogen's effect on bone is well documented (114–116). The association of stress fractures and menstrual irregularities has been observed (117,118). A careful menstrual history, as well as a dietary history, are mandatory for the complete evaluation of any stress fracture or stress phenomenon of bone in women and girls.

Stress injury to bone and stress fractures have been noted to occur more commonly in females. This relationship increases in the presence of disordered eating, menstrual irregularities, and low bone density (119,120). Although the complex interaction between mechanical loading, nutritional, and hormonal factors on bone health is not well understood, it is appreciated that any change in intensity, duration, or frequency of the menstrual cycle associated with increased training should be a cause of concern (121).

Shoes

Foot pain, in particular the necessity of wearing a shoe for doing most sports, can be a significant deterrent to keeping a person active. Much footwear, particularly athletic footwear, has been designed for the male population. The female athletic shoe is commonly based on a male foot, being a male shoe that is scaled down by decreasing all key internal dimensions in fixed proportions. The average female foot has a different shape than a male foot, however, often being narrower relative to length with a narrower heel compared to the fore foot. As length increases, fore foot width increases, but heel width rarely increases significantly. This often presents a dilemma for women who are trying to find a well-fitted athletic shoe. They find that shoes are often too loose in the hindfoot, particularly for women with bigger feet (size 8 or larger). Women who have a wide forefoot and narrow hindfoot may try to compromise by having a shoe fit in the hindfoot, creating snugness in the forefoot region. Careful attention to athletic shoe selection will help a woman avoid injury and minimize the forces that can complicate foot problems (122).

Shoulder Pain

Shoulder pain in women athletes may be divided into three general categories. The first is shoulder laxity with secondary impingement of the subacromial soft tissue structures. The second is laxity with recurrent instability. The third is impingement of the subacromial structures without laxity. Contributing factors to the prevalence of these conditions in women athletes include poor upper body strength, short upper extremities, and faulty technical skills in sports mandating upper extremity skills. Whether upper ligamentous laxity is a contributing factor in these shoulder problems remains speculative. Key to the treatment of shoulder issues is an appropriate diagnosis and a directed rehabilitation program. Rehabilitation should focus on strengthening of the rotator cuff musculature and the scapular stabilizers, which improves shoulder mechanics (123). Paying attention to training techniques and rehabilitation techniques is paramount. Proper warmup, shoulder-strengthening activities, and a paced addition of training activities for the upper extremities are imperative for the avoidance of overuse injuries of the shoulder soft tissue structures. Whether one uses free weights or health club machines, it is important to recognize the limitations of this equipment in regard to one's body size. Equipment needs to be sized appropriately for women's bodies, particularly smaller bodies. Isotonic exercise equipment frequently places the hands in the starting position behind the vertical plane of the ears. This can force the proximal humerus anteriorly in the glenoid space. These machines should not be used repetitively by athletes with shoulder instability unless care is taken to keep the shoulder from experiencing this repeated anterior force.

The frozen shoulder syndrome, also termed adhesive capsulitis, is an inflammation of the periarticular shoulder structures. This syndrome results in marked limitation of shoulder motion, particularly forward elevation. Often, this syndrome occurs in the face of a relatively trivial trauma or without an obvious cause. A repetitive activity can be the precipitating event, but frequently, the event does not seem significant enough to create such severe secondary inflammation marked with pain and limited motion. The frozen shoulder syndrome is most common in women between ages 40 and 60 (124). The pathophysiology of this condition is not well known, with adhesions being found both inside and outside the capsule. Some believe that it represents a type of dystrophy. It is often associated with systemic medical conditions such as arteriosclerotic heart disease, epilepsy, pulmonary disorders, thyroid conditions, and diabetes. The frozen shoulder syndrome typically improves with time, though its course can be quite prolonged, lasting several months or more.

Musculoskeletal Conditions of the Lumbar Spine

Spondylolysis is a stress reaction in the pars interarticularis. This is an area of the posterior arch of the lumbar spine. It is seen in athletes who repetitively place their spine in a hyperextended position, including gymnasts, skaters, dancers, and football linemen. Unlike other stress fractures of bone, this stress reaction has not been directly related to low bone mineral density in women. Its occurrence is almost equal in males and females participating intensely in sports that require hyperextension and/or flexion of the spine (125).

Much of the recommendation for treatment depends on the findings on radiographic imaging. The combination of normal X-rays and a positive bone or SPECT scan suggests an early stress reaction in bone. Rest from sport with brace protection utilizing a lumbar orthosis for 3 months is appropriate (126). In the symptomatic athlete with a radiographic defect that is already present, it is important to distinguish between a new and a chronic lesion. Chronic lesions can be treated symptomatically with a period of rest until acute symptoms subside. A brace may be useful in this but can be used intermittently for symptomatic treatment only. Chronicity of a lesion can be assessed by sclerosis at the margins of the radiographic lesion. If needed, thin-sliced axial tomographic views of the lumbar region can help to assess sclerosis. A fracture is considered new if it has a positive bone scan and no previous X-ray evidence of a fracture with no widening or sclerosis at the fracture margins. This perhaps is the most controversial to treat, as there is debate on how aggressive one should be with new fractures. These fractures do have the potential to heal (127,128). Aggressive treatment may include 6 months away from a sport with use of low back orthosis for the first 3 months. Successful treatment would be achieving a pain-free state, with or without radiographic bony healing. In all cases the program is coupled with a rehabilitation program to increase the strength and flexibility of the back and abdominal muscles. Though back extensor muscles are important to strengthen, the hyperextended position should be avoided. Extension exercises to the neutral position, if pain free, are encouraged.

If a pars defect is present on both sides of the vertebral body, instability of the spinal elements can occur with forward slipping of the spine on the vertebrae below the injured pars. This forward slipping is called a spondylolisthesis. There is not unanimous opinion on continued sports participation with this problem. Most orthopedists believe that if the slippage is less than 25% of the anterior posterior width of a vertebrae (Grade I spondylolisthesis) and the athlete is asymptomatic, the athlete can participate in sports, including contact sports. If slippage progresses, activities must be stopped. Most physicians think that an athlete with Grade II or greater slip should not participate in contact sports. Slippage can progress during the menarcheal years of young females and must be followed closely in developing females.

Adolescent idiopathic scoliosis is most prevalent in female adolescents. This is a structural curvature of the spine presenting on or about the onset of puberty. Adolescent idiopathic scoliosis has a female-to-male distribution of 3.6 to 1 for curves greater than 10° (129). Curves are progressive during the rapid growth of early teenage years. Curves less than 20° are usually no obstacle to full athletic participation. Athletic activity does not increase the progression of the curve. It is likely that participation in sports will help to develop lumbar and thoracic spine muscular strength. This is viewed as advantageous to those with scoliosis. Depending on the age of the patient, particularly those who are premenarcheal, bracing is often recommended for those with curves between 20° and 40°. Brace-free time for athletic participation is usually permitted (130). Severe curves, typically those greater than 40°, frequently require surgical intervention.

Arthritic Disorders

Arthritic disorders are the most frequent reason for decreasing physical activity in previously active people in our aging population. Arthritis can attack any joint; however, osteoarthritis (age-related arthritis) frequently affects large weight-bearing joints, including knees and hips. Most patients with arthritis are women. Arthritic disorders (arthralgias and arthritis) include more than 100 different illnesses; they are 60–80% more common in women (89–91). Osteoarthritis, a subdivision of arthritis, is 1.5–4 times more common in women than in men. Rheumatoid arthritis is 2–3 times more common in women of all ages. Ninety percent of lupus patients are women; the disease is three times more common among African-Americans. Fibromyalgia is a chronic musculoskeletal condition characterized by diffuse pain at specific tender points. Up to 90% of all identified fibromyalgia patients are women.

Arthritis clearly is a major women's health issue; in particular, it is a problem for aging Americans. The etiology and pathophysiology of arthritis are not well understood. Most preventative and palliative measures are aimed at patient education, weight loss, and appropriately directed exercise programs.

MEDICAL CONCERNS OF THE FEMALE ATHLETE

Sport and physical activity for girls and women have numerous psychologic and health benefits (131) and should be encouraged. There are a number of special medical concerns of the female athlete, however, of which physicians and other professionals working with the female athlete should have an increased awareness. The medical concerns that will be addressed include the problems of the female athlete triad, iron deficiency anemia, and pelvic floor dysfunction in the female athlete.

The Female Athlete Triad

In 1992 the American College of Sports Medicine held a consensus conference on the female athlete triad (132), bringing national attention to the interrelationship and often coexistence of three medical problems associated with the triad: disordered eating, amenorrhea, and osteoporosis. It is now apparent that the problems encountered in the female athlete triad are more global and have been recognized as potentially serious problems in female athletes worldwide.

Despite the increased awareness of the triad, the often-associated medical problems continue to be under reported, denied, or not recognized. Physicians and health professionals working with female athletes should have an understanding of the triad problems and their interrelationship (133,134). Women with one component of the triad should be screened for the other components (132–134).

Although much is still unknown about the true prevalence of the female athlete triad, a triad profile has emerged. The female athlete triad appears to be more prevalent among young, highly competitive athletes competing in appearance or endurance sports that emphasize low body weight, including gymnasts, figure skaters, dancers, distance runners, divers, and swimmers, though athletes of all sports are potentially at risk (132–135).

Disordered Eating in Female Athletes

In an attempt to lose or maintain weight or to achieve a lean appearance, many female athletes resort to a number of disordered eating behaviors. The internal and/or external pressures placed on young athletes to achieve a certain body weight or thin physique are thought to underlie the development of these disorders (132,134), though many athletes have predisposing risk factors (133,134).

The athlete with disordered eating behaviors often has inadequate caloric intake to meet the demands of her sport. A number of medical problems, including menstrual dysfunction and bone loss, may result from this negative energy balance often associated with weight loss (132–134). Diminished athletic performance often results. A vicious cycle is often begun, and psychologic problems, including depression, and more serious medical problems can result that may even lead to death (136–138).

TABLE 8–3. *Diagnostic criteria for anorexia nervosa*

1. Refusal to maintain body weight at or above a minimally normal weight for age and height (e.g., weight loss leading to maintenance of body weight less than 85% of that expected or failure to make expected weight gain during period of growth, leading to body weight less than 85% of that expected)
2. Intense fear of gaining weight or becoming fat, even when underweight
3. Disturbance in the way one's body weight or shape is perceived, undue influence of body weight or shape on self-evaluation, or denial of the seriousness of the current low body weight
4. In postmenarcheal females, amenorrhea, that is, the absence of at least three consecutive menstrual cycles (A woman is considered to have amenorrhea if her periods occur only following administration of hormone, such as estrogen.)

Specific type:
Restricting types: During the current episode of anorexia nervosa, the person has not regularly engaged in binge eating or purging behavior (self-induced vomiting or the misuse of laxatives, diuretics, or enemas).
Binge eating and purging types: During the current episode of anorexia nervosa, the person has regularly engaged in binge eating or purging behavior (self-induced vomiting or the misuse of laxatives, diuretics, or enemas).

Data from American Psychiatric Association. *Diagnostic and statistical manual of mental disorders,* 4th ed. Washington, DC: American Psychiatric Association, 1994:544–545.

TABLE 8–4. *Diagnostic criteria for bulimia nervosa*

1. Recurrent episodes of binge eating. An episode of binge eating is characterized by both of the following:
   a. Eating in a discrete period (e.g., within any 2-hour period) an amount of food that is definitely larger than most people would eat during a similar period of time and under similar circumstances
   b. A sense of lack of control over eating during the episode (e.g., a feeling that one cannot stop eating or control what or how much one is eating)
2. Recurrent, inappropriate compensatory behavior to prevent weight gain, such as self-induced vomiting; misuse of laxatives, diuretics, or other medications; fasting; or excessive exercise
3. The binge eating and inappropriate compensatory behaviors both occur, on average, at least twice a week for three months.
4. Self-evaluation is unduly influenced by body shape and weight.
5. The disturbance does not occur exclusively during episodes of anorexia nervosa.

Specific type:
Purging type: During the current episode of bulimia nervosa, the person has regularly engaged in self-induced vomiting or the misuse of laxatives, diuretics, or enemas.
Nonpurging type: During the current episode of bulimia nervosa, the person has used other inappropriate compensatory behaviors, such as fasting and excessive exercise, but has not regularly engaged in self-induced vomiting or the misuse of laxatives, diuretics, or enemas.

Data from American Psychiatric Association. *Diagnostic and statistical manual of mental disorders,* 4th ed. Washington, DC: American Psychiatric Association, 1994:549–550.

The female athlete with disordered eating behaviors more typically can be seen falling somewhere along the disordered eating continuum or spectrum and will less commonly fit the criteria for anorexia nervosa or bulimia nervosa as defined by the American Psychiatric Association's *Diagnostic and Statistical Manual of Mental Disorders*, 4th edition (*DSM IV*) (139) (Tables 8–3 and 8–4). The diagnostic category of Eating Disorder Not Otherwise Specified (EDNOS) acknowledges the existence of a variety of eating disturbances, such as individuals who binge eat infrequently (139) (Table 8–5). More research is needed, however, in methods of early recognition, identifying prevalence, comorbidity and recommended treatment for individuals (athletes and nonathletes) along the disordered eating continuum.

The concept of a continuum of preoccupation with weight progressing on to eating disorders has been well accepted in the psychiatric literature (140). This continuum model has been described as a continuum of vulnerability based on a number of risk factors rather than dieting per se (140). On this continuum, normal eating behaviors can be seen as progressing on to abnormal eating patterns, including occasional fasting; restricting food intake; self-induced vomiting; use of laxatives, diet pills, and/or diuretics; and overexercising to lose weight.

TABLE 8–5. *Diagnostic criteria for eating disorder not otherwise specified*

The "Eating Disorder Not Otherwise Specified" category is for disorders of eating that do not meet the criteria for any specific eating disorder. Examples include the following:
1. For females, all of the criteria for anorexia nervosa are met except that the individual has regular menses.
2. All of the criteria for anorexia nervosa are met except that, despite significant weight loss, the individual's current weight is in the normal range.
3. All of the criteria for bulimia nervosa are met, except that the binge eating and inappropriate compensatory mechanisms occur at a frequency of less than twice a week or for a duration of less than 3 months.
4. The regular use of inappropriate compensatory behavior by an individual of normal body weight after eating small amounts of food (e.g., self-induced vomiting after the consumption of two cookies).
5. Repeatedly chewing and spitting out, but not swallowing, large amounts of food.
6. Binge-eating disorder: recurrent episodes of binge eating in the absence of the regular use of inappropriate compensatory behaviors characteristic of bulimia nervosa.

Data from American Psychiatric Association. *Diagnostic and statistical manual of mental disorders,* 4th ed. Washington, DC: American Psychiatric Association, 1994:550.

On the extreme end of the spectrum lie the more severe eating disorders of anorexia nervosa and bulimia nervosa.

Sundgot-Borgen (135) has made an attempt to better identify this group of athletes with disordered eating patterns into a subclinical eating disorder: anorexia athletica (Table 8–6). Her criteria are modified from those proposed by Puglise and colleagues (141). Some athletes with anorexia athletica also meet the criteria of EDNOS. According to Sundgot-Borgen (135), athletes with anorexia athletica usually indicate that they need to lose weight for reasons related to their sport or recommendations from a coach. The proposed diagnostic criteria for anorexia athletica have not been added to the DSM IV criteria for eating disorders, however, and requires further study. It is not known whether further subtyping of athletes with disordered eating will aid in the detection, prevention, and treatment of these disorders.

No widely accepted validated measurement tool has been developed for screening athletes with disordered eating in various sports. However, the weight questionnaire (142) has been found to be reliable and has been validated for athletes in weight-controlled sports, such as rowing and wrestling. The Eating Disorder Inventory (EDI) and the Eating Attitude Test have been tested for reliability and validity but not in athletes. O'Connor and colleagues (143) found that response distortion was high in a group of 25 collegiate gymnasts using the EDI-2. In this study, the gymnasts did not differ significantly from controls on the EDI-2; however, those that had elevated scores on the Drive for Thinness Subscale (DFT) were more likely to report having disruptions in their menstrual cycle for 3 months or more. DFT scores were negatively related to energy intake and whole body bone mineral density. O'Connor and colleagues concluded that DFT scores may be useful in identifying gymnasts at risk for problems associated with eating disorders (143). Further research is needed to develop a valid and reliable instrument that detects individuals who are at risk for disordered eating in athletes.

As we discussed, most studies assessing the prevalence of eating disorders in athletes have found the prevalence to be higher among athletes in sports in which aesthetics and a lean physique are emphasized. However, in addition to different measurement tools utilized in screening athletes for disordered eating, there has been inconsistency in the populations investigated, differences in methodology used, and limited numbers in many of the subgroups studied, making it difficult to draw conclusions as to true prevalence. There is a need for longitudinal epidemiologic studies using validated measures to better define the prevalence of disordered eating in athletes of various sports, age groups, ethnic groups, and competitive levels.

Well-designed preventive efforts in junior and senior high school students have failed to reduce the prevalence or incidence of eating disorders (144). Targeting potentially high-risk groups has been emphasized in the prevention of disordered eating (145), such as athletes who are at risk.

There is a lack of information on preventive programs assessing educational efforts toward the prevention of disordered eating in athletes. However, preliminary data have shown that education does appear to help reduce the reported prevalence of disordered eating behaviors in the female athlete (146).

TABLE 8–6. *Diagnostic criteria for anorexia athletica*

*	Weight loss (>5% of expected bodyweight)
(*)	Primary amenorrhea
(*)	Menstrual dysfunction (primary amenorrhea, secondary amenorrhea, and oligomenorrhea)
(*)	Gastrointestinal complaints
*	Absence of a medical illness or affective disorder explaining the weight reduction
(*)	Distorted body image
*	Excessive fear of becoming obese
*	Restriction of food (<1200 kcal/day)
(*)	Use of purging methods (self-induced vomiting, use of laxatives and diuretics)
(*)	Binge eating
(*)	Compulsive exercise

* Absolute criteria = all need to be met; (*) relative criteria = need to meet one or more

Data from Sundgot-Borgen J. Eating disorders in female athletes. *Sports Med* 1994;17:176–188.

The following guidelines may help to provide guidance in the prevention of disordered eating in the athlete population:

1. Education: Information regarding the potential health consequences and awareness of symptoms and signs of disordered eating should be disseminated to coaches, athletic trainers, physicians, peers, parents, and athletes.

2. Psychological counseling: Food is never the problem; it is only a symptom of an underlying problem. The prognosis is worse for individuals who have struggled with disordered eating for a longer time. It is important to refer to a psychologist early on if disordered eating is suspected, preferably one with expertise in eating disorders in the athletic setting.

3. Nutritional guidance: It is important that the athlete have available sound nutritional guidance, ideally by a registered dietician or physician. It is not recommended that the coach give specific dietary recommendations for weight loss to the athlete. If there is a weight concern, this should be addressed by the health care team that works with the athlete.

4. Medical examinations: A yearly medical examination for the young athlete, screening for disordered eating and related problems, is recommended.

5. Dispelling myths: A common myth among athletes and coaches is that weight loss is the same as body fat loss and that lower body fat improves athletic performance. Weight loss results in loss of both lean body mass and fat content, and loss of lean body mass initially often predominates loss of fat. More research is needed to assess the relationship of body composition and performance.

6. Elimination of weigh-ins: Weigh-ins, especially if monitored by the coach, are frequently reported as a trigger for the development of pathogenic weight-controlling behaviors, especially in the vulnerable athlete (147). Group weigh-ins, public weigh-ins, and singling athletes out for weigh-ins should be discouraged. Coaches should not be the individual monitoring the athlete's weight and making recommendations for weight loss.

Psychotherapy is a key component in the treatment of the athlete with significant disordered eating behaviors. Medications may be helpful in conjunction with psychotherapy, especially in the bulimic athlete. The selective serotonin reuptake inhibitors have offered promising results in reducing binge eating and self-induced vomiting (148,149).

Amenorrhea

Primary amenorrhea (or delayed menarche) is the absence of menses by 16 years of age in a girl with secondary sexual characteristics (150). Secondary amenorrhea is the cessation of menstrual periods for three or more consecutive menstrual cycles after menarche (150,151). Although there are more data on the association of secondary amenorrhea and decreased bone mineral density (BMD) in the athlete (116,152–155), there is also evidence that delayed menarche is associated with an increased incidence of scoliosis and stress fractures (117,156).

The energy availability hypothesis provides the most widely accepted mechanism to date that explains the suppression of reproductive function in amenorrheic athletes. Cross-sectional studies have demonstrated that women with athletic amenorrhea present with a reduction in luteinizing hormone (LH) pulse frequencies (157). More recent studies support the hypothesis that LH pulsatility depends on energy availability (dietary energy intake minus exercise energy expenditure) in women (158–160). Strenuous training in and of itself may not be a sufficient stimulus to disrupt the reproductive hormone secretion unless it is accompanied by dietary restriction (159,160). Loucks and colleagues have recently demonstrated that LH pulsatility is disturbed less by exercise energy expenditure than by dietary energy restriction (160). There may exist a specific threshold whereby further negative energy balance signals the inhibition of hypothalamic GnRH neuronal activity.

Laughlin and Yen (161) have shown that the hormone product leptin of the obesity gene may play a role in the reproductive status of female athletes. A diurnal pattern of 24-hour leptin levels was present in normal cycling athletes and controls and was absent in amenorrheic athletes. This study provides additional evidence supporting the interrelationship between energy and diet in the reproductive system.

Treatment protocols for athletic amenorrhea need to take into account energy balance issues in counseling athletes about prevention and treatment of amenorrhea and potential consequences on bone health, and energy deficits need to be corrected. If the athlete is significantly underweight (<20% ideal weight), efforts to gain weight may help in the resumption of menses and preservation of BMD.

Dueck and colleagues (162) have reported the effect of a 15-week diet and intervention program on energy balance, hormonal profiles, body composition, and menstrual function of an amenorrheic endurance athlete. With a reduction of training of one day per week and addition of a sport nutrition beverage with 360 kcal/day, the athlete experienced a transition from negative to positive energy balance, increasing body fat and LH, and decreasing cortisol. This case study illustrates how nonpharmacologic treatment of athletic amenorrhea can contribute to a positive energy balance and may improve reproductive function.

Ensuring adequate calcium and vitamin D should be part of prevention and treatment of osteoporosis in all individuals. Calcium recommendations should be followed as recommended by the NIH Consensus Conference (163). The female athlete has greater calcium needs than the male athlete. A calcium intake of 1200–1500 mg/day is recommended for young female athletes with menstrual dysfunction and/or disordered eating, as well as 400–800 IU/day of vitamin D.

There is controversy about the benefits of estrogen replacement therapy in the young athlete with exercise-associated amenorrhea. Cummings has demonstrated an increase in BMD of the lumbar spine (8.0% +/− 1.2%) and femoral neck (4.1% +/− 0.3%) in eight amenorrheic women runners (ages 24–34 years) who were followed for 24–30 months on hormone replacement therapy (either Premarin 0.625 mg or estradiol transdermal patch, 50 μg daily with medroxyprogesterone acetate 10 mg qd, 14 days per month) in his retrospective study (164). Control women, who were not taking replacement therapy, had nonsignificant decreases at each site.

Warren and colleagues, by, contrast, found no changes in BMD of the spine, foot, and radius in women with hypothalamic amenorrhea (mean age 22) randomized to hormone replacement therapy (Premarin 0.625 mg qd cycling with medroxyprogesterone acetate 10 mg qd, 10 days per month) for two years (compared to those who were given a placebo) (165). The subjects were then randomized in a crossover protocol into treatment versus no treatment for one year. Eighteen subjects had completed two years of treatment. No differences were noted in the bone density of the amenorrheic athletes who received placebo or hormone replacement, except in those with weight gain.

There is some evidence that there may be a dose-related effect of estrogen on bone (166). There is conflicting data, however, regarding whether or not there is a protective effect of the use of the oral contraceptive pill (OCP) on stress fracture development in the female athlete. Studies in athletes supporting a protective effect include those by Barrow and Saha (118), Lloyd and colleagues (167), and Myburgh and colleagues (168). Most of the studies assessing the effect of OCP use in stress fractures have been cross-sectional or retrospective, and much controversy still exists in this area.

Hergenroeder and colleagues (169) found that OCP therapy for 12 months resulted in an increased lumbar spine and total body BMD in young women (14–24 years of age) with hypothalamic amenorrhea versus controls in a randomized controlled clinical trial. Some, but not all, of the subjects were athletes. Controls received placebo or medroxyprogesterone acetate (10 mg/day for 12 days per month) for 12 months.

In contrast, Keen and Drinkwater studied the BMD of former amenorrheic athletes who had been evaluated 8 years previously and found that there was no significant improvement in vertebral bone density in the athletes with a history of amenorrhea or oligomenorrhea who either had regained menses or had been on oral contraceptive pills for many years, a result suggesting that the bone loss is irreversible (170).

Seeman and colleagues (171) found that OCP were associated with an increase in lumbar spine bone density (but not proximal femur) in amenorrheic women with anorexia nervosa, a result suggesting that the spine may be more sensitive to effects of estrogen than the femur. Kreipe and colleagues (172) found that OCP in the presence of persistently low body weight (<20% ideal) was of limited benefit for BMD and apposition.

Osteopenia and Osteoporosis in the Female Athlete

Osteoporosis in adult women has been defined by the World Health Organization (173) as BMD values greater than 2.5 standard deviations (SD) below the young adult mean value (t-score), with osteopenia or low bone mass defined as BMD values between 1.0 and 2.5 SD below the young adult mean value. Normal BMD is defined as values not more than 1.0 SD below the young adult mean value. Severe osteoporosis (or established osteoporosis) is a BMD value more than 2.5 SD below the young adult mean in the presence of one or more fragility fractures.

The primary contributing cause for premenopausal osteoporosis in the young athletic women is a decrease in ovarian hormone production and a hypoestrogenemia resulting from hypothalamic amenorrhea (116,152–154,174). Rencken and colleagues (174) have demonstrated that extended periods of amenorrhea may result in low bone density at multiple skeletal sites (lumbar spine, femoral neck, femoral shaft, trochanter, intertrochanteric region, Ward's triangle, and tibia), including those individuals who are subject to impact loading during exercise. Body weight combined with months of amenorrhea and age of menarche predicted bone density of the lumbar spine. Body weight and duration of amenorrhea predicted BMD at the femoral neck, trochanter, intertrochanteric region, and tibia. Weight alone predicted BMD at the femoral shaft and tibia. Weight and age predicted lumbar BMD of eumenorrheic athletes. These results suggest that treatment for amenorrheic athletes should involve changes resulting in the resumption of normal menses, including nutrition and weight gain.

Kanis and colleagues (175) have suggested using a BMD cutoff value in adult women for the purposes of osteoporosis prevention, since treatments cannot increase low bone mass to biomechanically normal values. For adult postmenopausal women a cutoff of >1 SD below the average of young normals has been suggested to be a reasonable treatment threshold (175), but other factors need to be considered besides BMD alone, including safety and efficacy of the interventions. Ettinger and colleagues (176) and others caution against using BMD values alone as indicators for treatment.

Guidelines have not been established as yet for the young female athlete with osteopenia or osteoporosis related to athletic amenorrhea and/or disordered eating. As in postmenopausal women, BMD values should aid the clinician in preventive and treatment protocols but not be the sole criterion for intervention. Preventive efforts to normalize menses and energy balance, including proper nutrition and weight gain in some, are appropriate interventions when osteopenia and osteoporosis are detected. There is a lack of large, prospective longitudinal studies assessing the effects of hormone replacement therapy or OCP on BMD and fracture risk in the young athlete. Further research is needed in this area.

In the postmenopausal female there are additional options for the prevention and treatment of osteoporosis. In addition to estrogen replacement therapy, alendronate and risedronate (both bisphosphonates), raloxifene (a selective estrogen receptor modulator), and calcitonin have been approved for treatment of postmenopausal osteoporosis. There is a lack of studies that have evaluated these treatments in the premenopausal female athlete with osteoporosis related to hypothalamic amenorrhea. Alendronate (fosamax), in particular, is not recommended for women of childbearing age, owing to potential teratogenic effects. In addition, alendronate has a very long half-life (several years), and the long-term effects on growing bone (such as in adolescence) is not known.

Miacalcin (nasal calcitonin) is used primarily for postmenopausal vertebral osteoporosis. Drinkwater and colleagues (177), however, have shown that 24 months of nasal spray calcitonin was effective in preventing bone loss in amenorrheic athletes with osteopenia and resulted in small but significant gains in the lumbar spine and proximal femur. More prospective longitudinal studies are needed that follow female athletes with a history of amenorrhea and osteopenia on nasal calcitonin.

There is a need to quantify loads generated from specific types of exercise at clinically important skeletal sites to better identify the optimal exercise program for an individual. Activities that deliver high loads to specific skeletal sites appear to be more osteogenic than lower loads that are generally distributed. These high loads may even offset the effects of low reproductive hormones in some (178–180). Including higher-impact activity may elicit the overload that is needed to stimulate bone remodeling.

Muscle strength has been reported to predict between 15–20% variance in BMD at the hip, spine, and radius (181). Snow (180) has shown that hip abductor strength independently predicted femoral neck BMD and that grip strength independently predicted lumbar spine and radius BMD in premenopausal women. These results have implications with regard to exercise programs in the prevention of osteoporosis. Weight lifting or exercises that use resistance to strengthen muscles may be an important addition to optimize BMD and integrity. Further research is needed to better elucidate the mechanisms involved in bone remodeling in athletes of varying exercise regimes.

Iron Deficiency and Iron Deficiency Anemia

Iron deficiency and iron deficiency anemia are more common in women than in men (athletes and nonathletes). The prevalence of iron deficiency is 9% in adolescent girls and 11% in women of childbearing age, and that of iron deficiency anemia is 2% and 5%, respectively (182). Although it has not been shown that the prevalence of iron deficiency anemia in female athletes is greater than that in the general population, a number of studies have demonstrated chronically low serum ferritin levels in endurance athletes, especially in long-distance runners (183–188).

Causes of iron deficiency and iron deficiency anemia include low dietary iron intake, menstrual bleeding, gastrointestinal bleeding, intravascular hemolysis, and loss of iron through sweat and urine (189). Pseudoanemia, often referred to as sports anemia, is a physiologic anemia due to an expanded plasma volume with a normal red cell mass. This type of anemia is a normal physiologic response to endurance exercise and need not be treated with iron supplementation.

Most studies in the female athlete conclude that a low ferritin level with anemia (iron deficiency anemia) can lead to a significant detriment of athletic performance. However, a low ferritin level in the absence of anemia (iron deficiency alone) has not been consistently associated with a decrease in athletic performance. For iron deficiency anemia, iron supplementation is beneficial to the female athlete. Athletes with a low ferritin level with hemoglobin in the low-normal range may also be responsive to iron supplementation (190). Careful follow-up of the ferritin to assess response to treatment is recommended. Iron supplementation in the absence of anemia is not warranted.

Routine screening of all female athletes by assessing serum ferritin has not been found to be cost effective. However, screening some high-risk athlete groups, such as endurance athletes, especially those with a history of nutritional deficiency, a history of anemia, or symptoms of fatigue and decreased performance, may prove beneficial.

Stress Urinary Incontinence in the Female Athlete

There has been an increased recognition of stress urinary incontinence in young women participating in sports and physical activity. Stress urinary incontinence is the involuntary loss of urine during physical activity. Although this problem is not uncommon in young female athletes, it is underreported and undertreated. The major functions of the pelvic floor muscles are supportive and sphincteric and contribute to the maintenance of continence by increasing intraurethral pressure and stabilization of the supportive endopelvic fascia during contraction of these muscles. The main support for the pelvic viscera to diminish the constant strain on the suspensory mechanism is provided by the levator ani muscle. In stress urinary incontinence, despite normal pelvic floor muscle support, leakage may result from an alteration of the urethral sphincteric unit. It is the increased intra-abdominal pressure seen in certain sports that may place a women at risk for stress urinary incontinence, especially if the increased pressure is chronic and repetitive.

The prevalence of urinary incontinence in women of any age ranges from 10% to 58%. Nygaard and colleagues (191) studied varsity nulliparous athletes (mean age 19.9 years) and found that 28% noted urine loss while participating in their sport. Jumping activities, high-impact landings, and running produced the highest prevalence of urinary incontinence. In regular exercising adult women (mean age of 38.5 years), Nygaard and colleagues found that 47% reported some degree of urinary incontinence (192). High-impact exercises (running and aerobics) resulted in more episodes of incontinence than low-impact exercise. A significant number of women altered their exercise or even stopped exercising owing to the incontinence. Stress urinary incontinence was also found to be more prevalent in physical education students who trained more than three times per week (30%) as compared to sedentary students (10%) (193). This was primarily noted with jumping, landings, and running.

Identifiable risk factors for pelvic floor dysfunction in women (194) include age (most studies support increasing age as a risk factor), gender (females > males), and parity (increasing parity > nulliparous), with vaginal delivery shown to contribute to neuromuscular damage to the pelvic floor in some instances. Other risk factors that have not been as well studied include smoking, obesity, menopause, restricted mobility, urogenital surgery, heavy physical activity, and high-impact sports.

A risk classification to the pelvic floor by sport has been developed by Bourcier and Juras (195) for high-risk sports, including track and field, gymnastics, basketball, and other impact sports. Jogging, tennis, skiing, and skating are classified as having moderate risk to the pelvic floor; swimming, rowing, and cycling are classified as having no risk to the pelvic floor.

There is a lack of knowledge about the natural course of urinary incontinence in the female athlete. Nygaard and colleagues (196) conducted a retrospective cohort study of 104 middle-aged women who had competed for the United States in both high-impact (gymnastics and track and field) and low-impact (swimming) sports at the Summer Olympics between 1960 and 1976. They found that there was no difference in the self-reported prevalence of stress or urge incontinence in these women. A stepwise regression analysis (including sport, age, and parity) revealed that only body mass index was significantly associated with incontinence risk. The long-term effect on women participating in even higher-impact physical activities, such as female military parachutists, as well as other extreme sports is not known and needs further study.

Because women athletes do not usually volunteer this history, the presence and frequency of urinary leakage during physical activity should be assessed by the physician during the preparticipation sport exam and other encounters with the female athlete, especially those involved in higher-impact sports. A physical exam should include a pelvic exam with an evaluation of the pelvic floor muscles by an examiner who is experienced in assessing pelvic floor dysfunction.

Treatment initially includes behavioral therapy, in most instances, which is probably sufficient for most female athletes who experience stress urinary incontinence. Behavioral therapy averages 6–12 weeks. The ultimate aim of pelvic training for female athletes is the isolated recruitment of the levator ani effectively. Kegel exercises, kegel exercises with biofeedback, vaginal cones, and electrical stimulation are the most common behavioral therapies used for urinary incontinence.

Pharmacologic agents may be used as well and include estrogen replacement (usually oral contraceptive pills in the young hypoestrogenic woman), imipramine hydrochloride, and alpha-mimetics (pseudoephedrine hydrochloride, phenylpropanolamine hydrochloride).

Physicians working with female athletes should have an increased sensitivity to the problem of stress urinary incontinence and be able to counsel, assess, and treat or refer the patient for appropriate management.

SUMMARY

Participation in sport and exercise has many psychological and physical benefits and should be encouraged in girls and women of all ages. However, the dramatic increase in participation of women in sports, especially since the advent of Title IX, has enhanced our awareness of some of the medical and orthopedic problems that may result. The unique anatomy and physiology of women has been reviewed, and the intrinsic and extrinsic variables that may contribute to sports injury in the female athlete were discussed. The problems of disordered eating, amenorrhea, and premature osteoporosis are significant medical concerns that should be recognized and treated early. Special attention should be given to the calcium and iron needs of the female athlete, as well as to the importance of maintaining a positive energy balance. To provide the most effective health care for our growing population of female athletes, more research involving longitudinal, prospective studies are needed in the prevention and treatment of the medical and orthopedic problems specific to the female athlete.

REFERENCES

1. Hargreaves J. *Sporting females: critical issues in the history and sociology of women's sports.* London: Routledge, 1994:209.
2. Twin SL. *Out of the bleachers.* Old Westbury, NY: The Feminist Press, 1979:xvi–xvii.
3. Lutter JM. History of women in sports: societal issues. *Clin Sports Med* 1994;13:263–279.
4. Oglesby CA. *Women and sport: from myth to reality.* Philadelphia: Lea & Febiger, 1978:3–13.
5. Guttmann A. *Women's sports: a history.* New York: Columbia University Press, 1991:211–213.
6. NCAA Research Staff. *Participation statistics report 1982–1996,* February 1997.
7. NCAA. Division I Graduation Rates Report, 1997.
8. O'Toole ML, Douglas PS. Fitness: definition and development. In: Shangold MM, Mirkin G, eds. *Women and exercise: physiology and sports medicine,* 2nd ed. Philadelphia: FA Davis Co, 1994:3–26.
9. Sanborn CF, Jankowski CM. Physiologic considerations for women in sport. *Clin Sports Med* 1994;13:315–327.
10. Sady SP, Freedson PS. Body composition and structural comparisons of female and male athletes. *Clin Sports Med* 1984;3:755–777.
11. Berg K. Aerobic function in female athletes. *Clin Sports Med* 1984;3:779–789.
12. Puhl JL. Women and endurance: some factors influencing performance. In Drinkwater, BL, ed. *Female endurance athletes.* Champaign, IL: Human Kinetics, 1986:41–58.
13. Griffin LY. The female athlete. In: DeLee JC, Drez D, eds. *Orthopedic sports medicine: principles and practice* (Vol 1). Philadelphia: WB Saunders, 1994:356–373.
14. McKeag DB, Hough DO, Zemper ED. Conditioning and training programs for athletes/non-athletes. In: McKeag DB, Hough DO, Zemper ED, eds. *Primary care sports medicine.* Dubuque, IA: Brown & Benchmark, 1993:120–125.
15. Davis JA, Brewer J. Applied physiology of female soccer players. *Sports Med* 1993;16:180–189.
16. Mirkin G. Nutrition for sports. In: Shangold MM, Mirkin G, eds. *Women and exercise: physiology and sports medicine,* 2nd ed. Philadelphia: FA Davis Co, 1994:102–125
17. Wilmore JH. Alterations in strength, body composition and anthropometric measurements consequent to a 10-week weight training program. *Med Sci Sports* 1974;6:133–138.
18. Hoffman T, Stauffer RW, Jackson AS. Sex difference in strength. *Am J Sport Med* 1979;7:265–267.
19. Baechle TR. Women in resistance training. *Clin Sports Med* 1984;3:791–808.
20. Heyward VH, Johannes-Ellis SM, Romer JF. Gender differences in strength. *Res Q* 1986;57:154–159.
21. Blank S, Puhl JL. Effect of isokinetic strength training on muscle fiber composition and fiber size in men and women [Abstract]. *Med Sci Sports Exerc* 1982;14:112.
22. Bar-Or O. The prepubescent female. In: Shangold MM, Mirkin G, eds. *Women and exercise: physiology and sports medicine,* 2nd ed. Philadelphia: FA Davis Co, 1994:129–140.
23. Thomas CL. Factors important to women participants in vigorous athletics. In: Strauss R, ed. *Sports medicine and physiology.* Philadelphia: WB Saunders, 1979:304–319.
24. Ebben WP, Jensen RL. Strength training for women: debunking myths that block opportunity. *Physician Sportsmed* 1998;26:86–97.
25. Wells C. Physiological differences and similarities. In: Wells C, ed. *Women, sport, and performance: a physiological perspective.* Champaign, IL: Human Kinetics, 1985:19–34.
26. Cureton KJ, Sparling PB. Distance running performance and metabolic responses to running in men and women with excess weight experimentally equated. *Med Sci Sports Exerc* 1980;12:288–294.
27. Helgerud J, Ingjer F, Stromme SB. Sex differences in performance-matched marathon runners. *Eur J Appl Physiol Occup Physiol* 1990;61(5–6):433–439.
28. Drinkwater BL. Women and exercise: physiological aspects. *Exerc Sport Sci Rev* 1984;12:21–51.
29. Bergh U, Thorstensson A, Sjodin, B, et al. Maximal oxygen uptake and muscle fiber types in trained and untrained humans. *Med Sci Sports Exerc* 1978;10:151–154.
30. Fahey TD. Endurance training. In: Shangold MM, Mirkin G, eds. *Women and exercise: physiology and sports medicine,* 2nd ed. Philadelphia: FA Davis Co, 1994:73–88.
31. Speechly DP, Taylor SR, Rogers GG. Differences in ultra-endurance exercise in performance-matched male and female runners. *Med Sci Sports Exerc* 1996;28(3):359–365.
32. Bam J, Noakes TD, Juritz J, et al. Could women outrun men in ultramarathon races? *Med Sci Sports Exerc* 1997;29:244–247.
33. Frye AJ, Kamon E. Responses to dry heat of men and women with similar aerobic capacities. *J Appl Physiol* 1981;50:65–70.
34. Siegel AJ. Medical conditions arising during sports. In: Shangold MM, Mirkin G, eds. *Women and exercise: physiology and sports medicine,* 2nd ed. Philadelphia: FA Davis Co, 1994:261–281.
35. Wyndham CH, Morrison JF, Williams CG. Heat reactions of male and female Causcasians. *J Appl Physiol* 1965;20:357–364.
36. Dill DB, Yousef MK, Nelson JD. Responses of men and women to two-hour walks in desert heat. *J Appl Physiol* 1973;35:231–235.
37. Haymes EM. Physiological responses of female athletes to heat stress: a review. *Physician Sportsmed* 1984;12:45–59.
38. Stephenson LA, Kolka MA. Hermoregulation in women. *Exerc Sport Sci Rev* 1993;21:231–262.
39. Nunneley SA. Physiological responses of women to thermal stress: a review. *Med Sci Sports Exerc* 1979;10:250–255.
40. Armstrong LE, Maresh CM. The induction and decay of heat acclimatisation in trained athletes. *Sports Med* 1991;12:302–312.
41. Shapiro Y, Pandolf KB, Avellini BA, et al. Physiological responses of men and women to humid and dry heat. *J Appl Physiol* 1980;49:1–8.
42. Shangold MM. Sports and menstrual function. *Physician Sportsmed* 1980;8:66–70.
43. DeSouza MJ, Maguire MS, Rubin K, et al. Effects of menstrual phase and amenorrhea on exercise responses in runners. *Med Sci Sports Exerc* 1990;22:575–580.
44. Grucza R, Pekkarinen H, Titov EK, et al. Influence of the menstrual cycle and oral contraceptives on thermoregulatory responses to exercise in young women. *Eur J Appl Physiol Occup Physiol* 1993;67:279–285.
45. Lebrun CM. The effect of the phase of the menstrual cycle and the birth control pill on athletic performance. *Clin Sports Med* 1994;13:419–441.
46. Shangold MM. Gynecologic concerns in exercise and training. In: Shangold MM, Mirkin G, eds. *Women and exercise: physiology and sports medicine,* 2nd ed. Philadelphia: FA Davis Co, 1994:223–233.
47. Kawahata A. Sex differences in sweating. In: Yoshimura M, Ogata K, Ito S, eds. *Essential problems in climatic physiology.* Kyoto, Japan: Nankodo, 1960:169–184.
48. Sargent F, Weinman KP. Eccrine sweat gland activity during the menstrual cycle. *J Appl Physiol* 1966;21:1685–1687.
49. Senay LC. Body fluids and temperature responses of heat-exposed women before and after ovulation with and without rehydration. *J Physiol (London)* 1973;232:209–219.
50. Wells CL, Horvath SM. Heat stress responses related to the menstrual cycle. *J Appl Physiol* 1973;35:1–5.
51. Wells CL, Horvath SM. Responses to exercise in a hot environment as related to the menstrual cycle. *J Appl Physiol* 1974;36:299–302.
52. Horvath SM, Drinkwater BL. Thermoregulation and the menstrual cycle. *Aviat Space Environ Med* 1982;53:790–794.
53. Avellini BA, Kamon E, Krajewski JT. Physiological responses

of physically fit men and women to acclimation to humid heat. *J Appl Physiol* 1980;49:254–261.
54. Turley KR, Wilmore JH. Cardiovascular responses to submaximal exercise in 7- to 9-yr-old boys and girls. *Med Sci Sports Exerc* 1997;29:824–832.
55. Armstrong N, Welsman JR, Kirby BJ. Peak oxygen uptake and maturation in 12-yr olds. *Med Sci Sports Exerc* 1998;30:165–169.
56. Drinkwater BL, Kuppart IC, Denton JE, et al. Responses of prepubertal girls and college women to work in the heat. *J Appl Physiol* 1977;43:1046–1053.
57. Bar-Or O. Climate and exercising child: a review. *Int J Sports Med* 1980;1:53–56.
58. Lysens R, Steverlynck A, van de Auweele Y, et al. The predictability of sports injuries. *Sports Med* 1984;1:6–10.
59. Calvert R. *Athletic injuries and deaths in secondary schools and colleges, 1975–1976*. National Center for Education Statistics, Department of Health, Education and Welfare. Washington, DC: U.S. Government Printing Office, 1975–1976.
60. Haycock CE, Gillette JV. Susceptibility of women athletes to injury: myths versus reality. *JAMA* 1976;236:163–165.
61. Tomasi LF, Peterson JA, Pettit GP. Women's response to army training. *Physician Sportsmed* 1977;5:32–37.
62. Lenz HW. Women's sports and fitness programs at the US Naval Academy. *Physician Sportsmed* 1979;7:41–50.
63. Protzman R. Physiologic performance of women compared to men. *Am J Sports Med* 1979;7:191–194.
64. Milgrom C, Shlamkovitch N, Finestone A, et al. Risk factors for lateral ankle sprain: a prospective study among military recruits. *Foot Ankle* 1991;12:26–30.
65. Jones BH, Bovee MW, Harris J III, Cowan DN. Intrinsic risk factors for exercise related injuries among male and female army trainees. *Am J Sports Med* 1993;21:705–710.
66. Hoffman T, Stauffer RW, Jackson AS. Sex difference in strength. *Am J Sports Med* 1979;7:265–267.
67. Shively RA, Grana WA, Ellis D. High school sports injuries. *Physician Sportsmed* 1981;8:46–50.
68. Zelisko JA, Noble HB, Porter M. A comparison of men's and women's professional basketball injuries. *Am J Sports Med* 1982;10:297–299.
69. Ferretti A, Papandrea P, Conteduca F, Mariani PP. Knee ligament injuries in volleyball players. *Am J Sports Med* 1992;20:203–207.
70. Lindenfeld TN, Schmitt DJ, Hendy MP, et al. Incidence of injury in outdoor soccer. *Am J Sports Med* 1994;22:364–371.
71. Gray J, Taunton JE, McKenzie DC, et al. A survey of injuries to the anterior cruciate ligament of the knee in female basketball players. *Int J Sports Med* 1985;6:314–316.
72. Ireland ML, Wall C. Epidemiology and comparison of knee injuries in elite male and female United States basketball athletes [Abstract]. *Med Sci Sports Exerc* 1990;22:S82.
73. Arendt E, Dick R. Knee injury patterns among men and women in collegiate basketball and soccer. *Am J Sports Med* 1995;23:694–701.
74. Harrer MF, Berson L, Hosea TM, et al. Lower extremity injuries; females versus males in the sport of basketball [Abstract]. 1996 American Orthopaedic Society for Sports Medicine, Orlando, FL.
75. Arendt EA. Anterior cruciate ligament injuries in women. *Sports Med Arthroscopy Rev* 1997;5:149–155.
76. Carter C. Wilkinson J. Persistent joint laxity and congenital dislocation of the hip. *J Bone Joint Surg Br* 1964;46:40–45.
77. Breighton P, Solomon L, Soskolne CL. Articular mobility in an African population. *Ann Rheum Dis* 1973;32:413–418.
78. Biro F, Gewanter HL, Baum J. The hypermobility syndrome. *Pediatrics* 1983;72:701–706.
79. Gedalia A, Person DA, Brewer EJ Jr, Giannini EH. Hypermobility of the joints in juvenile episodic arthritis/arthralgia. *J Pediatr* 1985;107:873–876.
80. Nicholas JA. Injuries to knee ligaments: relationship to looseness and tightness in football players. *JAMA* 1970;212:2236–2239.
81. Godshall RW. The predictability of athletic injuries: an eight year study. *J Sports Med* 1975;3:50–54.
82. Kalenak A, Morehouse CA. Knee stability and knee ligament injuries. *JAMA* 1975;234:1143–1145.
83. Moretz JA, Walters R, Smith L. Flexibility as a predictor of knee injuries in college football players. *Physician Sportsmed* 1982;10:93–97.
84. Grana WA, Muse G. The effect of exercise on laxity in the anterior cruciate ligament deficient knee. *Am J Sports Med* 1988;16:586–588.
85. Diaz MA, Estevez EC, Guijo PS. Joint hyperlaxity and musculoligamentous lesions: study of a population of homogeneous age, sex and physical exertion. *Br Soc Rheumatol* 1993;32:120–122.
86. Klemp P, Stevens JE, Isaacs S. A hypermobility study in ballet dancers. *J Rheumatol* 1984;11:692–696.
87. Larsson L-G, Baum J, Mudholkar S. Hypermobility: features and differential incidence between the sexes. *Arthritis Rheum* 1987;30:1426–1430.
88. Wiesler ER, Hunter DM, Martin DF, et al. Ankle flexibility and injury patterns in dancers. *Am J Sports Med* 1996;24:754–757.
89. Heiwick CG, Lawrence RC, Pollar RA, et al. Arthritis and other rheumatic conditions: who is affected now, who will be affected later. *Arthritis Care Res* 1995;8:203–211.
90. Gabiel SE. Update on the epidemiology of the rheumatic diseases. *Curr Opin Rheumatol* 1996;8:96–100.
91. Lawta RG. The connective tissue diseases and the overall influence of gender. *Int J Fertil Menopausal Stud* 1996;41:156–165.
92. Weesner CL, Albohm MJ, Ritter MA. A comparison of anterior and posterior cruciate ligament laxity between female and male basketball players. *Physician Sportsmed* 1986;14:149–154.
93. Daniel D, Malcolm L, Losse G. Instrumented measurement of ACL disruption. [Abstract] *Orthopaedic Trans* 1983;7:585–586.
94. Skinner HB, Wyatt MP, Stone ML, Hogdon JA, Barrack RL. Exercise related knee joint laxity. *Am J Sports Med* 1986;14:30–34.
95. Steiner ME, Grana WA, Chillag K, Schelberg-Karnes E. The effect of exercise on anterior posterior knee laxity. *Am J Sports Med* 1986;14:24–29.
96. Huston LJ, Wojtys EM. Neuromuscular performance characteristics in the elite female athletes. *Am J Sports Med* 1996;24:427–435.
97. Hart DA, Roux L, Frank C, Shrive N. Sex hormone influences on rabbit ligaments in vivo and in vitro [Abstract]. 1996 42nd Annual Meeting of the ORS, Atlanta, GA.
98. Sciore P, Smith S, Frank CB, Hart DA. Detection of receptors for estrogen and progesterone in human ligaments and rabbit ligaments and tendons by RT-PCR [Abstract]. 1997 43rd Annual Meeting of the ORS, San Francisco, CA.
99. Slaughterbeck JR, Narayan RS, Clevenger C, et al. Effects of estrogen level on the tensile properties of the rabbit anterior cruciate ligament (ACL) [Abstract]. 1997 43rd Annual Meeting of the ORS, San Francisco, CA.
100. Lutter JM, Lee V. Exercise in pregnancy. In: Pearl AJ, ed., *The athletic female*. Champaign: Human Kinetics, 1993:81–86.
101. Wojtys EM, Huston LJ, Lindenfeld TN, Hewett TE, Greenfield LVH. Association between the menstrual cycle and anterior cruciate ligament injuries in female athletes. *Am J Sprots Med* 1998;26:614–619.
102. Myklebust G, Maehlum S, Holm I, Bahr R. A prospective cohort study of anterior cruciate ligament injuries in elite Norwegian team handball. *Scand J Med Sci Sports* 1998;8(3):149–153.
103. Souryal TO, Freeman TR. Intercondylar notch size and anterior cruciate ligament injuries in athletes: a prospective study. *Am J Sports Med* 1993;21:535–539.
104. LaPrade RF, Burnett QM II. Femoral intercondylar notch stenosis and correlation to anterior cruciate ligament injury: a prospective study. *Am J Sports Med* 1994;22:198–203.
105. Muneta T, Takakuda K, Yamamoto H. Intercondylar notch width and its relation to the configuration and cross-sectional area of the anterior cruciate ligament. *Am J Sports Med* 1997;25:69–72.
106. Shelbourne KD. A prospective study determining the relationship of the intercondylar notch width and the incidence of anterior cruciate ligament tears [Abstract]. 1997 AAOS 46th Annual Meeting, San Francisco, 1997;488:250.
107. Heidt RS Jr, Dormer SG, Cawley PW, et al. Differences in friction and torsional resistance in athletic shoe-turf surface interfaces. *Am J Sports Med* 1996;24:834–842.

108. Myklebust F, Hegerman M, Strand T, et al. Friction tests between handball floors and different types of shoes [Abstract]. Scandinavian Foundation Medical Science Sports, Oslo, Norway, 1992:53.
109. Griffis ND, Vequist SW, Yearout KM. Injury prevention of the anterior cruciate ligament [Abstract]. American Orthopaedic Society for Sports Medicine, 20th Annual Meeting, Abstract No. 13, Traverse City, MI, June 19–22, 1989.
110. Hewett TE, Stoupe AL, Nancy TA, Noyes FR. Plyometric training in female athletes. *Am J Sports Med* 1996;24:765–766.
111. Molnar TJ. Patellofemoral rehabilitation. In: Fox JM, Del Pizzo W, eds. *The patellofemoral joint.* New York: McGraw-Hill, 1993:291–304.
112. Steinkamp LA, Dillingham MF, Markel MD, et al. Biomechanical considerations in patellofemoral joint rehabilitation. *Am J Sports Med* 1993;21:438–444.
113. Arendt EA, Teitz CC. The lower extremities. In: Teitz CC, ed. *The female athlete.* Rosemont, IL: AAOS Monograph Series, 1997:45–59.
114. Arendt E. Osteoporosis in the athletic female: amenorrhea and amenorrheic osteoporosis. In: Pearl AJ, ed. *The athletic female.* Champaign, IL: Human Kinetics, 1993:41–59.
115. Cann CE, Cavanaugh DJ, Schurpfiel K. Menstrual history is the primary determinant of trabecular bone density in women. *Med Sci Sports Exerc* 1988;20:559.
116. Drinkwater BL, Bruemner B, Chestnut CH. Menstrual history as a determinant of current bone density in young athlete. *JAMA* 1990;263;545–548.
117. Warren MP, Brooks-Gunn J, Hamilton LH. Scoliosis and fractures in young ballet dancers. *N Engl J Med* 1986;314:1348–1353.
118. Barrow GW, Saha S. Menstrual irregularity and stress fractures in collegiate female distance runners. *Am J Sports Med* 1988;16:209–216.
119. Loucks AB. Effects of exercise training on the menstrual cycle: existence and mechanisms. *Med Sci Sports Exerc* 1990;22:275–280.
120. Nattiv A, Yeager K, Drinkwater B, et al. The female athlete triad. In: Agostini R, Titus S, eds. *Medical and orthopedic issues of active and athletic women.* Philadelphia: Hanley & Belfus, 1994:169–174.
121. Shangold M, Rebor RW, Wentz AC. Evaluation and management of menstrual dysfunction in athletes. *JAMA* 1990;263:1665–1669.
122. Frey C. Shoes. In: Teitz CC, ed. *The female athlete.* Rosemont, IL: AAOS Monograph Series, 1997: 63–74.
123. Wilk K, Arrigo C, Andrews J. Current concepts in the rehabilitation of the athlete's shoulder. *J South Orthop Assoc* 1994;3:205–215.
124. Ott J, Clancy W, Wilk K. Soft tissue injuries of the shoulder. In: Andrew J, Wilk K, ed. *The athlete's shoulder.* New York: Churchill Livingston 1994:241–259.
125. Jackson D, Wiltse L, Circione R. Spondylolysis in the female gymnast. *Clin Orthop* 1976;117:68–73.
126. Gerbino P, Micheli L. Back injuries in the young athlete. *Clin Sports Med* 1995;14:571–590.
127. Micheli L. Back injuries in gymnasts. *Clin Sports Med* 1985;4:85.
128. Steiner ME, Micheli LJ. Treatment of symptomatic spondylolysis and spondylolisthesis with the modified Boston brace. *Spine* 1985;10:937–943.
129. Weinstein S, Buckwalter J. In:Weinstein S, Buckwalter SA, eds. *Turek's orthopaedics,* 5th ed. Philadelphia: Lippincott, 1994:447–485.
130. Benson D, Wolf A, Shoji H. Can the Milwaukee brace patient participate in competitive athletics. *Am J Sports Med* 1977;5:7–12.
131. Harris S, Casperson CJ, Defriese GH. Physical activity counseling for healthy adults as a primary preventative intervention in the clinical setting. *JAMA* 1989;261:3590–3598.
132. Yeager K, Agostini R, Nattiv A, et al. The female athlete triad. *Med Sci Sports Exerc* 1993;25:775–777.
133. Nattiv A, Agostini R, Drinkwater B, et al. The female athlete triad: the interrelatedness of disordered eating, amenorrhea and osteoporosis. *Clin J Sport Med* 1994;13:405–418.
134. ACSM position stand on the female athlete triad. *Med Sci Sports Exerc* 1997;29:i–ix.
135. Sundgot-Borgen, J. Eating disorders in female athletes. *Sports Med* 1994;17:176–188.
136. Herzog DB, Copeland PM. Eating disorders. *N Engl J Med* 1985;313(5):295–303.
137. Palla B, Litt IF. Medical complications of eating disorders in adolescents. *Pediatrics* 1988;81:613–623.
138. Ratnasuriya RH, Eisler I, Szmukler GI, et al. Anorexia nervosa: outcome and prognostic factors after 20 years. *Br J Psychiatry* 1991:158:495.
139. American Psychiatric Association. *Diagnostic and statistical manual of mental disorders,* 4th ed. Washington DC: American Psychiatric Association, 1994.
140. Garfinkel P, Kennedy SH, Kaplan A. Views on classification and diagnosis of eating disorders. *Can J Psychiatry* 1995;40:445–456.
141. Puglise MT, Lifshitz F, Grad G, et al. Fear of obesity: a cause of short stature and delayed puberty. *N Engl J Med* 1983; 309:513–518.
142. Steen SN, Brownell KD. Current patterns of weight loss and regain in wrestlers: has the tradition changed? *Med Sci Sports Exerc* 1990;22:762–768.
143. O'Conner PJ, Lewis RD, Kirchner EM. Eating disorder symptoms in female college gymnasts. *Med Sci Sports Exerc* 1995;27:550–555.
144. Killen JD, Taylor CB, Hammer LD, et al. An attempt to modify unhealthful eating attitudes and weight regulation practices of young adolescent girls. *Int J Eat Dis* 1993;13:369.
145. Yager J. Eating disorders review. In: Yager J, ed. Carlsbad, CA: Gurze Books, 1996;7:1–3.
146. Sundgot-Borgen J. Unpublished data presented at the American College of Sports Medicine Annual Meeting, Orlando, FL, 1998.
147. Sundgot-Borgen J. Risk and trigger factors for the development of eating disorders in female elite athletes. *Med Sci Sports Exerc* 1994;26.
148. Fluoxetine Bulimia Nervosa Collaborative Study Group. Fluoxetine in the treatment of bulimia nervosa: a multicenter, placebo-controlled, double-blind trial. *Arch Gen Psychiatry* 1992;49:139–147.
149. Goldstein DJ, Wilson MG, Thompson VL, et al. Long-term fluoxeting treatment of bulimia nervosa. *Br J Psychiatry* 1995;166:660–666.
150. Shangold MM, Rebar RW, Wentz AC, et al. Evaluation and management of menstrual dysfunction in athletes. *JAMA* 1990;263:1665–1669.
151. Loucks AB, Horvath SM. Athletic amenorrhea: a review. *Med Sci Sports Exerc* 1985;17:56–72.
152. Cann CE, Martin MC, Genant HK, et al. Decreased spinal mineral content in amenorrheic women. *JAMA* 1984;251:626–629.
153. Drinkwater BL, Nilson K, Ott S, et al. Bone mineral content of amenorrheic and eumenorrheic athletes. *N Engl J Med* 1984;311:277–281.
154. Marcus R, Cann C, Madvig P, et al. Menstrual function and bone mass in elite women distance runners. *Ann Intern Med* 1985;102:158–163.
155. Bachrach LK, Guido D, Katzman D, et al. Decreased bone density in adolescent girls with anorexia nervosa. *Pediatrics* 1990;86:440–447.
156. Bennell KL, Malcolm SA, Thomas SA et al. Risk factors for stress fractures in track and field athletes: a twelve month prospective study. *Am J Sports Med* 1996;24(6):810–818.
157. Loucks AB, Mortola JF, Girton L, et al. Alterations in the hypothalamic-pituitary-ovarian and the hypothalamic-pituitary-adrenal axis in athletic women. *J Clin Endocrinol Metab* 1989;68:402–411.
158. Loucks AB, Heath EM. Dietary restriction reduces luteinizing hormone pulse frequency during waking hours and increases LH pulse amplitude during sleep in young menstruating women. *J Clin Endocrinol Metab* 1994;78:910–915.
159. Williams NI, Young JC, McArthur JW, et al. Strenuous exercise with caloric restriction: effect on luteinizing hormone secretion. *Med Sci Sport Exerc* 1995;27:1390–1398.
160. Loucks AB, Verdun M, Heath EM. Low energy availability, not stress of exercise, alters LH pulsatility in exercising women. *J Appl Physiol* 1998;84:37–46.
161. Laughlin GA, Yen SSC. Hypoleptinemia in women athletes:

161. absence of a diurnal rhythm with amenorrhea. *J Clin Endocrin Metab* 1997;82:318–321.
162. Dueck CA, Matt KS, Manore M, et al. Treatment of athletic amenorrhea with a diet and training intervention program. *Int J Sport Nutr* 1996;6(1):24–40.
163. NIH consensus conference. Optimal calcium intake. *JAMA* 1994;272:1942–1948.
164. Cummings DC. Exercise associated amenorrhea, low bone density, and estrogen replacement therapy. *Arch Intern Med* 1996;156:2193–2195.
165. Warren MP, et al. Osteopenia in hypothalamic amenorrhea: a three year longitudinal study. Paper presented at the Annual Meeting of the Endocrine Society, Anaheim, CA, 1994.
166. DeCherney A. Bone sparing properties of oral contraceptives. *Am J Obstet Gynecol* 1996;174:15–20.
167. Lloyd T, Triantafylou SJ, Baker ER, et al. Women athletes with menstrual irregularities have increased musculoskeletal injuries. *Med Sci Sports Exerc* 1986;18:374–379.
168. Myburgh KH, Hutchins J, Fataar AB, et al. Low bone density is an etiologic factor for stress fractures in athletes. *Ann Intern Med* 1990;113:754–759.
169. Hergenroeder AC, Smith EO, Shypailo R, et al. Bone mineral changes in young women with hypothalamic amenorrhea treated with oral contraceptives, medroxyprogesterone, or placebo over 12 months. *Am J Obstet Gynecol* 1997;176:1017–1025.
170. Keen AD, Drinkwater BL. Irreversible bone loss in former amenorrheic athletes [Editorial]. *Osteoporos Int* 1997;7:311–315.
171. Seeman E, Szmukler GI, Formica C, et al. Osteoporosis in anorexia: the influence of peak bone density, bone loss, oral contraceptive use and exercise. *J Bone Miner Res* 1992;7:1467–1474.
172. Kreipe RE, Hicks DG, Rosier RN, et al. Preliminary findings on the effects of sex hormones on bone metabolism in anorexia nervosa. *J Adolesc Health* 1993;14:319–324.
173. World Health Organization (WHO) Study Group. *Assessment of fracture risk and its application to screening for postmenopausal osteoporosis.* Technical Report Series, 843. Geneva, Switzerland: WHO, 1994.
174. Rencken ML, Chestnut CH, Drinkwater BL. Bone density at multiple skeletal sites in amenorrheic athletes. *JAMA* 1996;276:238–240.
175. Kanis JA, Melton LJ, Christiansen C, et al. The diagnosis of osteoporosis. *J Bone Miner Res* 1994;9:8.
176. Ettinger B, Miller P, McClung MR. Use of bone densitometry results for decisions about therapy for osteoporosis. *Ann Intern Med* 1996;125:623.
177. Drinkwater BL, Healy NL, Rencken ML, et al. Effectiveness of nasal calcitonin in preventing bone loss in young amenorrheic women [Abstract]. *J Bone Miner Res* 993;8(suppl):S264.
178. Wolman RL, Clark P, McNally E, et al. Menstrual state and exercise as determinants of spinal trabecular bone density in female athletes. *Br Med J* 1990;301:516.
179. Slemenda CW, Johnston CC. High intensity activities in young women: site specific bone mass effects among female figure skaters. *J Bone Miner Res* 1993;20:125.
180. Snow CM. Exercise and bone mass in young and premenopausal women. *Bone* 1996;18:51S–55S.
181. Snow-Harter C, Bouxsein ML, Lewis BT, et al. Muscle strength as a predictor of bone mineral density in young women. *J Bone Miner Res* 1990;5:589–595.
182. Looker A, Dallman P, Carroll M, et al. Prevalence of iron deficiency in the United States. *JAMA* 1997;27:973–976.
183. Ehn L, Calmark B, Hoglund S. Iron status in athletes involved in intense physical activity. *Med Sci Sports Exerc* 1980;12:61–64.
184. Clement B, Asmundson RC. Nutritional intake and hematological parameters in endurance runners. *Physician Sportsmed* 1982;10:37–41.
185. Dickson D, Wilkinson R, Noakes T. Effects of ultra-marathon training and racing on hematologic parameters and serum ferritin levels in well-trained athletes. *Int J Sports Med* 1982;3:111–117.
186. Colt E, Heyman B. Low ferritin levels in runners. *J Sports Med Phys Fitness* 1984;24:13–17.
187. Lampe J, Slavian J, Apple F. Poor iron status of women runners training for a marathon. *Int J Sports Med* 1986;7:111–114.
188. Balaban E, Cox J, Snell P, et al. The frequency of anemia and iron deficiency in the runner. *Med Sci Sports Exerc* 1989;21:643–648.
189. Nickerson H, Holubets M, Weiler B, et al. Causes of iron deficiency in adolescent athletes. *J Pediatr* 1989;114:657–663.
190. Garza D, Shrier I, Kohl H 3d, et al. The clinical value of serum ferritin tests in endurance athletes. *Clin J Sport Med* 1997; 7:46–53.
191. Nygaard IE, Thompson FL, Svengalis SL, et al. Urinary incontinence in elite nulliparous athletes. *Obstet Gynecol* 1994;84:183–187.
192. Nygaard I.E., DeLancey JOL, Arnsdorf L, et al. Exercise and incontinence. *Obstet Gynecol* 1990;75:848.
193. Bo K, Maehlum S, Oseid S, et al. Prevalence of stress urinary incontinence among physically active and sedentary female students. *Scand J Med Sci Sports* 1989;11:113.
194. NIH Consensus Development Panel. Urinary incontinence in adults. *JAMA* 1989;261:2685–2690.
195. Bourcier AP, Juras JC. Nonsurgical therapy for stress incontinence. *Urol Clin North Am* 1995;22:613–627.
196. Nygaard IE, et al. Abstract presented at the Annual Scientific Meeting of the American Urogynecologic Society, Tucson, Arizona, 1997.

CHAPTER 9

The Disabled Athlete

Brian C. Halpern, Rosemarie Boehm, and Dennis A. Cardone

INTRODUCTION

Athletes become involved with sports for the therapeutic, recreational, and motivational benefits. Participation in this group includes athletes with disabilities, representing an expanding number of sports enthusiasts. This growth is fueled by the extraordinary accomplishments of the disabled athletes themselves, as well as federal legislation mandating equal access and equal opportunity for persons with disabilities.

The Federal Rehabilitation Act of 1973 prohibited the exclusion of "otherwise qualified" individuals who have disability from participation in federally funded programs (1). The Americans with Disabilities Act (ADA) of 1990, which took effect in 1992, expanded the Federal Rehabilitation to ensure that these rights are upheld in the private sector (1). The ADA proceeded to define a person with a disability as an individual who has a physical or mental impairment that substantially limits one or more of his or her major life activities; a record of an impairment, such as that which may appear in a preparticipation examination form or a physician's notes or charts; or a perception by the public that an impairment limits a major life activity (1). Types of disabilities include cerebral palsy, amputation, blindness, spinal cord injury and paralysis, spina bifida, mental retardation, and les autres. Les autres ("the others") is the official term for locomotor disabilities such as arthritis, osteogenesis imperfecta, muscular dystrophy, and multiple sclerosis.

About the time the ADA was instituted, the U.S. Census Bureau estimated 48.9 million people in the United States as disabled (2). This represented about 19.4% of the population, but defining disability became problematic. The bureau delineated a subset population of 24.1 million (9.6%) as severely disabled, defining this group in a government report as "unable to perform one or more activities, or as having one or more specific impairments, or as a person who used a wheelchair or who was a long term user of crutches, a cane, or a walker" (2). Today, the number of disabled Americans who are involved in athletic competitions in the United States is rapidly increasing, and an even greater number are involved in recreational and leisure sports.

At the same time, the World Health Organization defined impairment as any loss or abnormality of psychological, physical, or anatomic structure or function. It defined a disability as any restriction or lack (resulting from an impairment) of an ability to perform an activity in the manner or within the range that is considered normal for a human being. A handicap was a disadvantage for a given individual, resulting from an impairment or a disability that limits or prevents the fulfillment of a role that is normal (depending on age, sex, and social and cultural factors) for that individual. In 1994 the NCAA proceeded to define impaired student-athletes as those who are confined to a wheelchair; those who are deaf, blind, or missing a limb; those who have only one of a paired set of organs; or those who may have behavioral, emotional, and psychologic disorders that substantially limit a major life activity (1).

HISTORY

The first recorded venture of a sport for the disabled was the World Games for the Deaf held in Paris during 1924. Twenty years later, in the early 1940s, the Stoke-Mandeville wheelchair games were held in England. Sir Ludwig Guttman used the games as a means of rehabilitating paraplegic war veterans after World War II. In 1948 in the United States the National Wheelchair Basketball Association was formed to govern the sport of wheelchair basketball, and in 1956 the National

---

B. C. Halpern: The Hospital for Special Surgery, New York, New York 10021.

R. Boehm and D. A. Cardone: Department of Orthopedic Surgery, Columbia Presbyterian Medical Center, New York, New York 10032.

Wheelchair Athletic Association (NWAA) was formed to allow opportunities for disabled athletes in sports other than basketball. The NWAA, which has changed its name to Wheelchair Sports USA, promotes participation in recreational and competitive sports to athletes with permanent disabilities that affect mobility.

By the 1960s formal venues for competitive games were organized, with the first paraplegic and first wheelchair Olympics in Rome following the 1960 Olympics (3). Four hundred athletes from 23 countries participated (4). The first U.S. team to compete internationally was at these Rome games. The event was given its name, the Paralympic Games, which actually means "next to" or "parallel." Since then, the Paralympic Games have been held every Olympic year, usually in the same country that hosts the Olympic games. These Paralympic games provide competition for elite disabled athletes, following their theme, "Triumph of the Human Spirit" (4).

The last Paralympics was hosted in Atlanta in 1996. It was the largest Paralympics to date, hosting over 3500 athletes and support staff from 104 countries (4). The U.S. team consisted of athletes from Wheelchair Sports USA, Disabled Sports USA, the U.S. Cerebral Palsy Athletic Association, the U.S. Association for Blind Athletes, the Dwarf Athletic Association of America, and Special Olympics International. A total of 317 U.S. athletes brought home a total of 157 medals, leading all countries (4).

Special Olympics International, which was established in 1968, promotes exercise and participation in sports for mentally retarded individuals 8 years of age and older. It offers year-round training and competition in more than 24 Olympic-type sports. Competitions are arranged on local, state, and international levels. There are accredited Special Olympic programs in more than 143 countries, with Special Olympic chapters established in all 50 states of the United States. Athletes are assigned to divisions and compete against those of equal abilities. In keeping with its theme, "Let me win. But if I cannot win, let me be brave in the attempt," Special Olympics does not keep track of records or the number of medals an athlete or country accrues. In the summer the athletes participate in sports as diverse as softball, track and field, soccer, volleyball, equestrian events, cycling, power lifting, tennis, and golf. Winter sports include cross-country and alpine skiing, skating, basketball, gymnastics, and bowling. For athletes with severe handicaps the Special Olympics has established the Special Olympics Motor Activities Training Program. This program emphasizes training and participation over competition (5).

Disabled Sports USA (DS/USA), is a national nonprofit, tax-exempt organization that was founded in 1967 by disabled Vietnam veterans. It is a member of the U.S. Olympic Committee and provides year-round sports and recreation to children and adults with disabilities. It serves individuals with physical disabilities that restrict mobility, including amputations, paraplegia, quadriplegia, cerebral palsy, head injury, multiple sclerosis, muscular dystrophy, spina bifida, stroke, and visual impairments. Under the authority of the U.S. Olympic Committee, DS/USA sanctions and conducts winter and summer competitions in 11 sports, including Nordic and alpine skiing, track and field, standing and sitting volleyball, power lifting, swimming, cycling, sailing, table tennis, lawn bowling, and archery. DS/USA also conducts training camps for novice and advanced athletes in these sports. In addition, DS/USA coordinates the U.S. Disabled Volleyball Team, a national team composed entirely of ambulatory disabled athletes, and the Alpine Junior Elite Team, the nation's top junior disabled ski racers, ranging in age from 12 to 17 (6).

For individuals with neuromuscular impairment the Cerebral Palsy International Sports and Recreation Association was formed in 1978, and the U.S. Cerebral Palsy Athletic Association was founded in 1985. These groups offer sporting opportunities to athletes with cerebral upper motor neuron lesions, including cerebral palsy, as well as those with acquired brain injury and stroke (7).

The U.S. Association for Blind Athletes was created in 1976 to provide opportunities for athletic participation for the blind and visually impaired (4). The Dwarf Athletic Association of America was formed in 1985 to develop, promote, and provide high-quality amateur-level athletic opportunities for dwarf athletes in the United States. It serves the estimated one quarter million Americans who are dwarfs (having a height less than 4'10") due to chondrodystrophy or related causes (4). The American Athletic Association of the Deaf was formed in 1945 originally to promote sports for adult deaf athletes and has expanded to include the younger athlete in recent years (4).

Individuals with physical disabilities face many personal, social, cultural, and vocational challenges (8). Sports are often pursued as a means of self-discipline, competitive spirit, and camaraderie. They help to develop strength, coordination, and endurance, benefiting the mental, physical, spiritual, and social aspects of the human being. Studies have shown that disabled athletes have higher self-esteem, are better educated, and express more satisfaction and happiness with life than disabled nonathletes (3). A sedentary lifestyle can place the disabled individual at greater risk for development of cardiopulmonary disease, adult-onset diabetes, and hypertension, just as in the able-bodied (9). Most recent studies have shown a decrease in depressive symptomatology in disabled athletes who regularly participated in aerobic activity as compared to a control group of inactive adults with physical disability (8). Those who exercised regularly, regardless of their disability, had increased aerobic capacity as measured by VO_2max, decrease in somatic symptoms, and improvement in positive affect (8).

THE PREPARTICIPATION PHYSICAL EXAM

The preparticipation physical exam (PPE) is the mainstay of prevention and promotion of safe participation in athletic endeavors, both training and competition (10). It is traditionally performed annually for most athletes and should be completed before the initiation of any athletic activity. The Special Olympics does require athletes to be medically cleared before participating in Special Olympic events. The primary objectives of any PPE are to detect any condition that may predispose the athlete to injury, to detect any conditions that may be life-threatening or disabling, and to meet legal and insurance requirements (10). The PPE for the disabled athlete should be comprehensive, and the physicians conducting them should be aware of common problems associated with athletes as well as those associated with different disabilities. The often-used station method of examination should be avoided because of the decreased mobility of some athletes with disabilities. If possible, the PPE should be performed by physicians who have provided longitudinal care and know the baseline status of the athlete.

As with any PPE, the medical history is the cornerstone of the medical evaluation (10). A complete history can identify 75% of problems affecting athletes (10). In certain cases the history may need to be obtained from a family member or another person who is familiar with the athlete. It should include a detailed summary of previous injuries and illnesses, risk factors for injuries and illnesses, and current medications. Does the athlete have a history of seizures? Cardiopulmonary disease? Renal disease? Alantoaxial instability (in athletes with Down syndrome)? Menstrual problems? Has the athlete had previous heat stroke or heat exhaustion? Fractures or dislocations? Does the athlete get dizziness, chest pain, or shortness of breath when he or she works out? Is there any use of recreational or ergogenic drugs? What prosthetic devices or special equipment does the athlete use during sports participation? At what levels of competition has the athlete previously participated? Has the athlete ever been medically disqualified?

The physical exam should include blood pressure and pulse, visual acuity, and complete cardiovascular, musculoskeletal, and neurologic examinations.

Lab tests and radiographs are not routinely necessary but must be considered on an individual basis. Uncertainty still exists as to the value of cervical spine radiographs in screening for alantoaxial instability in athletes with Down syndrome. Screening has been performed for possible catastrophic neck injury. In 1983 Special Olympics International mandated obtaining lateral neck radiographs in athletes with Down syndrome before they may participate in any Special Olympics event and restricting certain activities in individuals with radiographic evidence of instability. The American Academy of Pediatrics had previously supported this recommendation but has since retired this policy statement. Further research studies need to be done before more definitive recommendations can be made. If screening radiographs are performed and are normal, it is not necessary to routinely repeat the screening unless it is required for the participation in an athletic event. If the initial films are abnormal, follow-up radiographs should be performed every 2–3 years (11).

If the athlete cannot be cleared for a particular sport or event in which he or she wishes to participate, most athletes can be redirected to another sport (10).

THE WHEELCHAIR ATHLETE

Many individuals use a wheelchair either because of congenital or acquired spinal cord injury. In the United States there are an estimated 1 million people with spinal cord injury or neurologic impairment (2), and the number is rising each year. Motor vehicle accidents account for a large percentage of these injuries; falls, violence, and sports also contribute. Paraplegia and quadriplegia are impairment or loss of function in the spinal cord due to damage to the neural elements within the spinal canal (12). Paraplegia results from a spinal cord injury below the first thoracic vertebra (13), and quadriplegia is a result of a spinal cord injury in the cervical area. "The degree of impairment is determined by the neurologic level and completeness of injury" (12). In 1985 Curtis and colleagues conducted a survey of 210 wheelchair athletes that found that 65% of the athletes had spinal cord injuries, 12% had polio/postpolio syndrome, 9% had congenital disorders, 3% were amputees, and 10% had neuromuscular and musculoskeletal disorders (14). In a similar study, the greatest percentage of participants were congenitally disabled rather than disabled as a result of injury (15).

Classification

The classification of wheelchair athletes with spinal cord injuries is by severity of disability and is based on the level of spinal cord involvement and the extent of injury. In the United States there are two commonly used classification systems. The first (Fig. 9–1) is the system used by the National Wheelchair Athletic Association (NWAA), and the second (Fig. 9–2) is the three class system used by the National Wheelchair Basketball Association (NWBA). These two systems are readily applicable to individuals with spinal cord injury, but flexibility and compromise are necessary in classifying difficult cases, such as athletes with incomplete spinal injury,

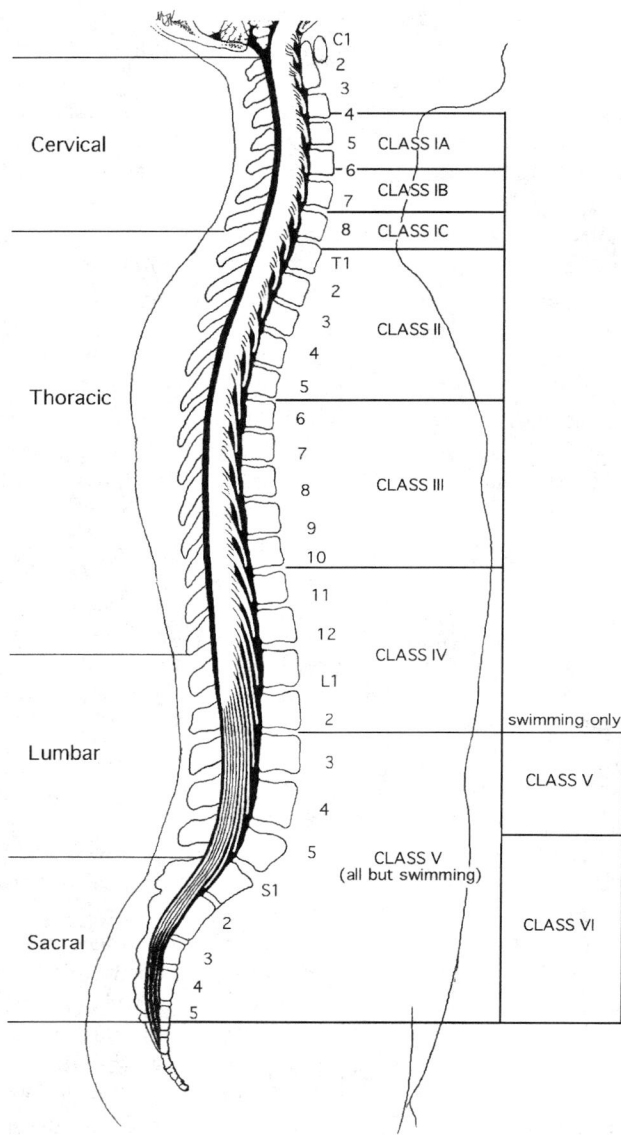

FIG. 9–1. National wheelchair athletic association classification system.

amount of muscle available. In turn, the degree to which the effective muscle mass can be utilized may, as in able-bodied people, influence the maximal oxygen uptake (Vo_2max) (17). The maximum rate at which an individual can consume oxygen (Vo_2max) is an important determinant of peak power output and of maximal sustained output or physical work capacity of which an individual is capable. Generally, in progressing from quadriplegics to high-level paraplegics to low-level paraplegics, there is an increase in the functional muscle mass and therefore a potential for increased O_2 utilization and work output during exercise. In the highest spinal cord lesions, that is, those with the smallest muscle mass, peripheral fatigue often occurs before the cardio-

poliomyelitis, multiple sclerosis, cerebral palsy, and muscle or connective tissue disorders (16). For children the NWAA supports its junior division for children 6–18 years of age. The system (Table 9–1) is divided into four age groups with three neurologic impairment levels. Classification of the athletes is performed by physicians and physical therapists who have been specifically trained and certified.

Exercise Physiology

Individuals in wheelchairs must depend on their upper body for strength, movement, and exercise. In spinal cord injuries the level of injury will determine the

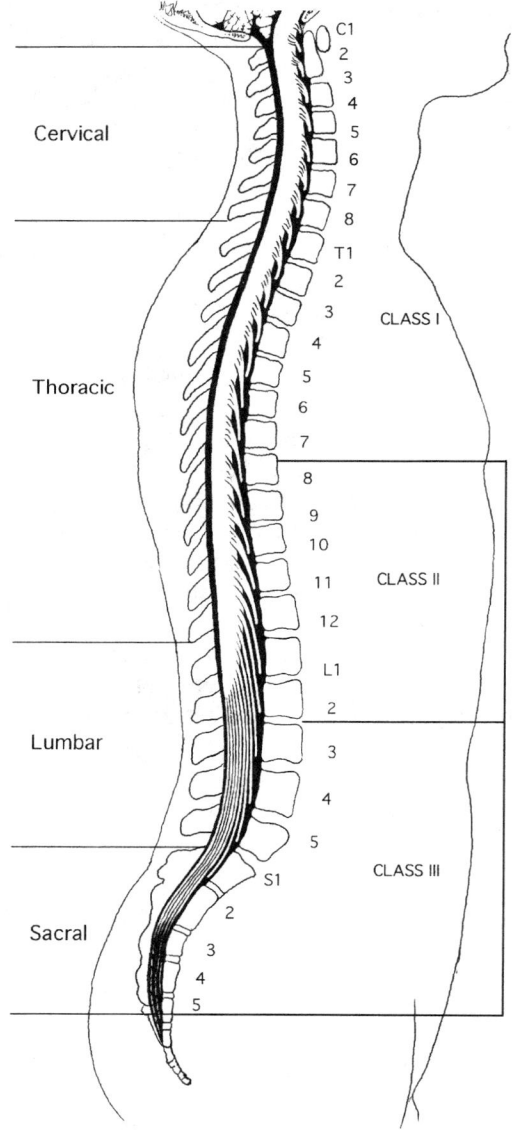

FIG. 9–2. National wheelchair basketball association classification system.

TABLE 9–1. *NWAA Junior Division classification system*

Age group	Disability group		
	Class 1	Class 2	Class 3
A (6–8 years)	NWAA adult classes 1a–1c	NWAA adult classes 2 & 3	NWAA adult classes 4–6
B (9–12 years)	Cervical spinal level impairment	Thoracic level impairment (T1–T10)	Impairment below T10 level (includes amputees)
C (13–15 years)	Cervical spinal level impairment	Thoracic level impairment (T1–T10)	Impairment below T10 level (includes amputees)
D (16–18 years)	Cervical spinal level impairment	Thoracic level impairment (T1–T10)	Impairment below T10 level (includes amputees)

vascular system reaches its limit of pumping capacity. In these individuals O_2 demand is not likely to exceed O_2 delivery (12).

Determining VO_2max for an athlete or individual allows measurement of maximal aerobic capacity. Most of the published research on the aerobic capacity of wheelchair athletes has been done in the laboratory on ergometers. The three types of ergometers that are most often used are the arm cycle ergometer; a wheelchair ergometer, which is usually a specially designed wheelchair; and a regular wheelchair used on a motor-driven treadmill (18). It is clear that the protocol used and the type of ergometer can have a great effect on the measured levels (18). Using a wheelchair on a motor-driven treadmill may require extra energy to keep the wheelchair on a straight course as well as to stabilize the trunk at higher elevations of the treadmill (18).

In terms of mechanical efficiency, an individual who is running requires approximately 1 kcal of energy per kilogram of body weight per kilometer of distance traveled. An individual who is cycling is more efficient, requiring less than one third that energy output. This increased efficiency is because of a level center of gravity instead of the up-and-down change of running. Wheelchair athletes also travel a level path; however, the muscles of the upper body are much less efficient than the muscles of the lower limbs. For example, a cycle ergometer allows 23% mechanical efficiency, an arm crank ergometer allows 18% efficiency, and a wheelchair ergometer allows only 8% efficiency.

In a review of the literature, previous comparisons have shown that the mean VO_2max obtained by wheelchair athletes is only comparable to that achieved by sedentary able-bodied athletes (19). Studies have shown that there is a wide range of VO_2max values among wheelchair athletes, suggesting that many have not reached their potential. Published VO_2max values range from ~16 mL/kg/min to ~50 mL/kg/min with a mean of ~37 mL/kg/min. The highest VO_2max values are seen in individuals with the lowest spinal cord lesion level (18). In strength and endurance events male paraplegic athletes were able to show a progressive increase in VO_2max as their level of performance in competition increased (19).

Wheelchair athletes have a 10–25% reduced cardiac output and a 15–30% lower stroke volume compared to able-bodied athletes performing similar upper body exercise, but Davis and Shephard observed significant increase in peak left ventricular stroke volume and cardiac output in previously untrained paraplegics after 16 weeks of aerobic training (20). Stroke volume is significantly responsive to training as well as deconditioning. It has become apparent that individuals who train intensely in their wheelchairs are able to develop greater peak power than those who use their wheelchairs only for activities of daily living (21). And that the energy requirements for activities of daily living alone are not sufficient to increase VO_2max (21).

These studies show that while there may be a physiological limit to the peak aerobic capacity that wheelchair athletes can obtain, wheelchair exercise training can substantially improve upper body cardiovascular fitness. This physiologic limit is even more evident in the quadriplegic athlete and may be affected by multiple factors such as hypokinetic circulation, disrupted autonomic reflexes, and thermoregulatory dysfunction. Hypokinetic circulation is a dysfunctional syndrome of inadequate hemodynamic responses to increased metabolic demands (12). Below the level of the spinal cord lesion, there is no active muscle pumping, which leads to venous pooling, decreases venous return, and limits cardiac preload and myocardial performance. This in turn decreases stroke volume and cardiac output during exercise. Quadriplegics are frequently hypotensive while exercising in the upright position, most likely because of vasodilatation in exercising muscles with lack of compensatory sympathetic vasoconstriction (12). Disrupted autonomic reflexes are also known as sympathetic decentralization. An interruption of efferent sympathetic outflow results in the separation of the peripheral sympathetic nervous system from control by the cardiovascular centers of the brain (12). Positive cardiac chronotropy and inotropy as well as catecholamine production are profoundly impaired (12). This leads to a significantly lower maximal heart rate in quadriplegics as well as reducing their cardiac output. Interestingly, paraplegics have been found to have maximal heart rates similar to those of able-bodied individuals. Thermoregulatory dysfunction also results in a decreased stroke volume during physical activity. In spinal cord–injured athletes, a lack of neural control of skin blood flow leads to increased blood collecting in the skin to maintain adequate heat loss during exercise.

When blood pressure measurements were done on wheelchair and able-bodied individuals, their resting blood pressures were within normal limits. After maximal physical exertion, repeat blood pressures were typically lower in the wheelchair athletes than in able-bodied individuals (22). In the same study, paraplegics were found to have a reduced capacity to sweat below the level of their injury. When the arterial-venous O_2 was measured, no difference was found between wheelchair athletes and able-bodied athletes. This is an indication that O_2 extraction in the peripheral muscles is normal and that regional blood flow to the working muscles is intact (23).

In a 1997 study of moderate wheelchair exercise, the results showed an increase in hematocrit immediately following exercise, a markedly increased plasma creatine kinase immediately after exercise, reaching a peak at 24 hours postexercise, myoglobin that gradually increased to its highest value at 72 hours postexercise, and a lactate dehydrogenase that reached its peak value immediately postexercise. The increase in hematocrit is probably due to hemoconcentration caused by dehydration. This study strongly suggested that wheelchair propulsion causes some level of muscle damage under certain conditions (24).

As wheelchair sports are increasing in popularity, individuals are becoming more knowledgeable about exercise. Wheelchair racing likely depends on strength and techniques at least as much as it does on a high oxygen uptake (22). Training methods are becoming more specific and more effective, and it is likely that we will see increasing physiologic responses in wheelchair athletes in the near future.

Prevention and Treatment of Injuries

Wheelchair athletes are involved in a wide range of recreational and competitive sports. Time involved includes practice as well as competition. The average sports participation reported is 4.35 ± 1.76 days per week, and training ranges from 0 to over 25 hours per week, the most common being 6–10 hours per week (14). An association between the number of hours spent training and the number of injuries has been reported as well as an increased number of injuries with increased number of different sports participated in (14). The five highest injury risk sports for wheelchair athletes in descending order of risk are track, basketball, road racing, tennis, and field events. Swimming has also been reported as a high-risk sport. The upper extremities, particularly the shoulder and wrist, are most frequently involved in injuries, followed by the lower extremities and then the head and spine. The types of injuries that were found in a year-long survey of elite wheelchair athletes were strains (48%), abrasions (22%), contusions (10%), blisters (6%), fractures (6%), sprains (4%), lacerations (2%), and illnesses (2%) (25). Most injuries in the elite population are minor. Ferrara, in his study of the injury patterns of elite wheelchair athletes, defines injury as a loss of participation in games or practice for one or more days due to an injury or illness, or an injury in which a fracture or dislocation/subluxation occurred but the athlete was able to continue participation (25). Time lost is defined by the National Athletic Injury Reporting System (26) as a minor injury if time lost is 7 or fewer days, a significant injury if it is 8–21 days, and a major injury if it is 22 days or more. Most wheelchair athletes do report at least one injury during their sports participation history, and they have the same types and frequencies of injuries as able-bodied athletes. However, time lost and recovery time as a result of injury are greater for disabled athletes (25). Explanations for this include a delayed healing process with spinal cord injuries and a more conservative rehabilitation program.

The most common mechanisms of injury are overuse and repetitive stress and falls from direct impact with either another chair or other objects (25). A percentage of injuries reported are non-sport-related injuries that occur during wheelchair transfer (25). Major injuries, such as fractures or trauma leading to further disability, are rare. But physicians and therapists working with these athletes must remember that skeletal osteopenia and osteoporosis in disabled athletes are not uncommon, and smaller trauma may result in major injuries. Also, with their neurologic impairment and loss of sensation, a major injury may be overlooked in the wheelchair athlete, whereas in an able-bodied athlete, pain will be an indication of serious injury.

Skin injuries that are common to wheelchair athletes include abrasions, lacerations, blisters, and pressure sores. Abrasions and lacerations are secondary to the equipment used by the athletes or to falls. The athlete's hands, fingers, and arms come into contact with brakes or sharp edges on the wheelchair or can be trapped between wheels. Treatment includes suturing as needed, keeping the area clean and dry, and watching closely for signs of infection. Prevention involves filing off sharp edges on the wheelchair, removing hazardous parts, wearing protective guards or clothing, and cambering wheels. Blisters of hands and fingers are quite common and are caused by friction, shear forces, and irritation from repeated contact with the wheelchair push rim.

Blisters also commonly form on the athlete's back secondary to friction and sweat between the back and the upholstery or seat posts of the chair. The blister may be drained with a sterile needle. The roof of the blister is preserved to act as a barrier to infection and continued trauma until a resistant epidermal layer can be formed. The overlying skin should be protected with petroleum jelly and a tape or gauze dressing; even duoderm is very effective. Preventive measures include gradual toughening of the skin and callus formation, taping of hands and fingers, wearing protective gloves, using a padded seat, and wearing a dry shirt (14,15,25).

Pressure sores are primarily a problem of spinal cord–injured athletes. These athletes have elevated skin pressures over the sacrum and ischial tuberosities for extended periods during training, competition, and normal daily activity. Sports wheelchairs are designed so that the knees are higher than the buttocks, resulting in even more increased pressure over the sacrum and ischial tuberosities. The triad of pressure, shear, and moisture leads to breakdown of the skin and pressure sore formation. These areas of the body become the weight-bearing surfaces while the person is in the wheelchair, and unrelieved pressure causes a decrease in blood supply to the skin in that area. Training can be modified to prevent additional pressure damage and to allow healing. Local wound care includes relief of pressure at the site, bio-occlusive dressings, electric stimulation to increase blood flow to the area, and monitoring for signs of infection. Preventive measures include adequate cushioning and padding for the buttocks and other bony prominences, frequent pressure relief and weight shifting, good nutrition and hygiene, and wearing clothing that absorbs moisture and decreases friction. Frequent skin checks need to be made by coaches, trainers, and medical staff (14,15,25). Redness and blistering are early warning signs of increased pressure.

Wheelchair athletes have an increased incidence of soft tissue injuries, especially of the upper extremities. Injuries sustained include ligamentous injuries, overuse injuries of tendons and muscles, and overexertion without warm-up. These result in strains, sprains, bursitis, and tendinitis. Many injuries are recurrent and can become chronic. Muscle-tendon imbalance can be a source of increased injuries. Wheelchair athletes predominantly use the extensor muscle groups of their upper extremities in wheelchair locomotion. These muscles often increase in strength and size disproportionately to the opposing muscle groups. The result is muscle imbalance and decreased flexibility. Wheelchair propulsion can result in overuse syndromes of the wrist and elbow, with improper push techniques increasing the frequency and severity of overuse as well as causing acute sprains and strains of the soft tissue around these joints. Sprains of the interphalangeal joints and the metacarpal joint of the thumb are seen in injuries of contact with the push rim or tire of the wheelchair. The hands and fingers are subject to direct trauma resulting from wheelchair collisions. Wheelchair athletes may also have unusual stresses across joints, tendons, and muscles secondary to altered body mechanics to compensate for their disabilities (14,15,25). The treatment of soft tissue injuries in wheelchair athletes involves the same principles and practices as in able-bodied athletes. Prevention of soft tissue injuries includes a warm-up period and a cooldown for each workout, a progressive stretching and strengthening program, protection of old injuries with tapping and splinting, padding of the upper extremity, rest, and proper treatment of recurrent injuries. (3,14,15,25).

Wheelchair athletes place a constant demand on their shoulders for propulsion, and the upper extremities become their weight-bearing joints. During training and sports participation the stress across the shoulder is increased far beyond that required by activities of daily life. This leads to a high incidence of shoulder injuries, especially rotator cuff impingement syndrome. Chronic overuse, lack of proper warm-up and stretching, poor flexibility, muscular imbalance, lack of postural control, repetitive overhead arm positioning, and fatigue may contribute to this (9). When compared to able-bodied athletes, wheelchair athletes have a significantly higher ratio of shoulder abduction to adduction strength. The ratio becomes even greater in wheelchair athletes with impingement. This imbalance allows the humeral head to migrate superiorly, causing a relative decrease in the subacromial space. Weak scapulothoracic stabilizers can also contribute to the problem. The shoulder rarely gets rest and recovery time because of the demands of wheelchair propulsion. Prevention and treatment include strengthening of shoulder adductors, internal/external rotators and scapulothoracic stabilizers, modification of training programs and daily activities to minimize shoulder impingement positions, and posture training. If the impingement is causing acute pain, ice, nonsteroidal anti-inflammatory drugs, and corticosteroid injection in the subacromial space can be used.

Peripheral nerve entrapment syndromes are quite common in manual wheelchair users. Carpal tunnel syndrome appears to be the most common peripheral nerve entrapment seen, with estimates ranging from 49% to 75% of these wheelchair users. While its prevalence in the athletic population is quite high, it does not appear to be any greater than that in the general paraplegic population (27). Wrist extension posturing during wheeling and transferring, as well as isometric and isotonic contractions of the finger flexors that travel within the carpal tunnel, results in increased carpal tunnel pressure. This, along with repetitive pressure from the wheelchair on the volar soft tissues overlying the carpal tunnel, contributes to carpal tunnel syndrome. Recent studies have shown that, despite earlier beliefs, nerve conduction abnormalities in wheelchair athletes were not related to the amount of training or competing but were related to the number of years with their disability (28). Ulnar neuropathy is also seen in the same population. It is most prevalent at the wrist, in Guyon's canal, and less commonly noted at the distal flexor aspect of the cubital tunnel. Ulnar neuropathy at the wrist is mainly due to prolonged compressive forces from the wheelchair in this region. Entrapment of the ulnar nerve at the distal aspect of the cubital tunnel is caused by the repetitive contractions of the flexor carpi ulnaris muscle required by the wheelchair athlete, prolonged elbow flexion, and repetitive pressure on this area when the forearm rests against the wheelchair armrest.

Prevention includes wearing padded gloves, especially with padding over the heel of the hand, padding over the push rim, gradual toughening of the skin of the palms, and keeping equipment in good condition. Treatment includes change in wheeling and transfer techniques, wrist splints, 150 mg of vitamin B6 per day, nonsteroidal anti-inflammatory drugs, a slowly progressive rehabilitation program, and local and systemic use of corticosteroids. Finally, surgical decompression is reserved for resistant cases.

Thermoregulation is the body's ability to maintain a particular temperature. It is often impaired in spinal cord–injured athletes because of skeletal muscle paralysis and a loss of autonomic nervous system control. This results in the inability to respond to changes in heat or cold in the individual's environment. The higher and more complete the spinal cord injury, the greater the thermoregulatory impairment (29). Spinal cord–injured individuals have a higher core temperature in the heat and a lower core temperature in the cold. Because of this, they have even been referred to as partial poikilotherms (29). The result of the thermoregulatory dysfunction can be hyperthermia or hypothermia.

The risk of hyperthermia and its consequences is great in wheelchair athletes who perform strenuous exercise in a hot environment. Normal autonomic responses for heat dissipation, including sweat gland secretion, redistribution of cardiac output, and vasodilatation in cutaneous vessels, is impaired. Arm sweating can be unaffected in paraplegics and some lower-level quadriplegics. Spinal cord–injured athletes also must rely on their arms alone for movement to dissipate heat through evaporative losses, whereas in able-bodied athletes, evaporative heat loss can be enhanced by movement of all four extremities. Dehydration can cause additional effects to the hyperthermia, causing a linear increase in core temperature with increasing dehydration (16). Many medications, such as those used for bladder dysfunction, pain, and depression, can adversely affect sweating and thermoregulation. Prevention includes minimizing exposure to the heat and direct sunlight, planning training and competition in the early morning or evening hours, acclimatization to the environment, fluid replacement of more than 1 L/h, appropriate clothing, and use of cooling towels or spraying water over the body surfaces to assist with heat convection (3). The athlete may need to be forced or reminded to increase fluid intake during training and competition, because thirst has been shown to be an inadequate stimulus to maintain hydration (16). Signs and symptoms of heat illness include fatigue, weakness, lightheadedness, headache, myalgia, vomiting, and, in severe cases, progressive neurologic impairment. Treatment includes removing the athlete's clothing, moving the athlete to a cooler environment, external cooling, and oral and/or intravenous fluids. More severe cases may require respiratory and circulatory support, with transport to an emergency facility.

Hypothermia also poses a great risk to the spinal cord–injured athlete. These athletes have a loss of normal autonomic regulatory response to cold, an impaired circulation secondary to reduced skeletal muscle mass and activity, and an inability to shiver. In contrast to hyperthermia, hypothermia generally becomes a problem after completion of a competition or training session. Once the athlete finishes the race or session, heat production stops, and shivering may not occur, but the skin remains vasodilated and saturated with sweat, allowing heat loss to continue. In cold, damp, windy conditions the slower athletes, those who spend 3–5 hours on a race course, are more vulnerable to the hypothermia during the race because they generate less heat. The athlete may also fail to recognize early signs of hypothermia, such as cold extremities, because of a lack of sensation below the level of the spinal cord lesion. Certain medications and medical conditions can predispose the athlete to problems with temperature regulation in the cold. Prevention includes appropriate clothing, which should be layered, providing both insulation and a wind barrier, removing wet clothing and replacing it with dry clothes, taking a warm shower, wrapping in insulated blankets, and adequate fluid replacement. Signs and symptoms include confusion with slurred speech or amnesia, apathy, or clumsiness. More severe hypothermia can lead to coma and cardiac or respiratory failure. Treatment includes the same measures that are used for prevention. More severe cases require transfer to a medical care facility rather than attempting to rewarm on the field (30).

Athletes with spinal cord injuries or other neurologic disorders often have bladder dysfunction or neurogenic bladders. These athletes frequently use indwelling catheters or intermittent catheterization, which can lead to urinary stasis. This puts the athlete at increased risk of infection. Inaccessible bathrooms, positioning in the racing chair, and inadequate hydration produce an environment that is favorable for bacterial overgrowth and subsequent infection. Preventive measures include adequate hydration, ensuring regular bladder emptying, and using proper antiseptic techniques with catheters (31).

The above environmental / physical conditions can lead to autonomic hyperreflexia. This is an acute generalized sympathetic hyperactivity response seen in spinal cord–injured athletes with lesions above the midthoracic (T6) level. It is usually a self-limited response to certain stimuli, including bladder distention, catheterization, urinary tract infection, bowel or bladder obstruction, exposure to hot or cold temperatures, pressure sores, sunburn, and thrombophlebitis. The classic syndrome of autonomic hyperreflexia is subjectively characterized by tightness in the chest, flushing and sweating above the level of their spinal cord lesion, headache, pins and needles in the innervated areas, gooseflesh, shivering, anxiety, and nasal stuffiness. Objective findings include paroxysmal hypertension, bradycardia, cardiac irregularities, dilated pupils, visual disturbances, aphasia, hyperthermia, and alterations in gastrointestinal motility. It may be missed if presentation is mild. Treatment involves removing the athlete from physical activity, emptying bowel and bladder, relief of any obstruction, and monitoring blood pressure. If symptoms persist, an atropinelike substance can be given to block sympathetic outflow. Immediate transfer to a medical facility may be necessary. If hyperreflexia remains unrelieved, it may lead to death (16,32).

Within the past few years, the practice of self-induced autonomic hyperreflexia has gained attention. This intentional induction, also known as boosting, is done for performance enhancement to provide a competitive advantage for the athlete (32). A study of this technique in elite wheelchair athletes showed that overdistending their bladder or sitting in their wheelchair for an extended period of time immediately before the race resulted in autonomic hyperactivity. The boosting effect was a decrease in race time with an improvement in race performance. The mechanisms for this are not fully understood yet, but significantly higher oxygen utilization and cardiac and pulmonary effects were found. Boosting is currently being compared to the use of stimulants in athletes and is considered an ergogenic aid. Although unintentional episodic bouts of autonomic hyperreflexia are common, the threshold for episodes can be lowered by repeated stimulations, causing a continuous dysautonomic state, which may become a medical emergency (32). Concerns include not only the risks and dangers of the procedure but also the disadvantage at which nonboosting athletes are placed.

The overall prevention of injuries in wheelchair athletes should include training as part of a regular sports participation program. Training should emphasize strength, conditioning, and, most important, flexibility.

Educational strategies geared toward proper equipment and techniques, common injuries, and preventive measures should be used. Finally, the value of the health care team, including physicians, physical therapists, athletic trainers, and nutritionists, as well as the coaches and support staff, cannot be overlooked.

THE ATHLETE WITH CEREBRAL PALSY

Cerebral palsy (CP) is a developmental disorder of motor function that is present from infancy or early childhood, due to a nonprogressive cerebral disorder. Impairment of voluntary motor control is the hallmark of CP. It may be secondary to hypoxia and/or ischemia or to events before birth. The more commonly encountered conditions are spastic diplegia (affecting the legs), hemiplegia (affecting the arm and leg on the same side), and heterogeneous extrapyramidal syndromes. About one half of all CP athletes compete in wheelchairs, and about half are ambulatory. In addition to movement disorders, athletes with CP may have associated disorders, including perceptual motor problems, learning disabilities, seizures, visual dysfunction, deafness, and mental retardation.

Classification

The Cerebral Palsy International Sports and Recreation Association has developed an eight-level classification system that is based on the athletes' baseline neurologic characteristics and places similar athletes together. There are eight classes: four wheelchair and four ambulatory. The classes range from class I, athletes with severe spasticity or athetosis who do not have the neurologic potential to propel a manual wheelchair, to class VIII, athletes with a minimal degree of impairment (7).

Exercise Physiology

Research pertaining to the fitness and training of individuals with cerebral palsy is limited. While many depend on a wheelchair for ambulation and some of the available wheelchair data can be extrapolated to them, they have unique characteristics in their functional performance. The majority of children with spastic diplegia are eventually able to ambulate, but the skill is delayed and differs from a normal gait (33). They often spend twice as much energy walking at the same velocity as an able-bodied individual. The increase in energy expenditure is related to the degree of disability. An increased displacement of the center of gravity caused by poor motor control, decreased range of motion, and loss of balance is partly responsible for the reduced mechanical efficiency and increased energy requirements (34). In addition to decreased mechanical efficiency, reduced metabolic capacity at the muscle level may also lead to fatigue and increased energy demands in individuals with CP. Decreased strength and muscular endurance levels have been identified as limiting factors in functional performance (35). A study of children with CP versus nondisabled children showed comparable oxygen uptake and oxygen pulse values at rest but significantly higher values for children with CP at slow walking speeds. This is not surprising, since oxygen pulse increases with increasing work loads, as does oxygen uptake. The most economical walking speed was significantly slower for children with CP (34).

CP athletes may have increased muscle tone, a velocity-dependent resistance to passive muscle stretch, a loss of selective muscle control, deficient equilibrium reactions, and/or relative imbalance of muscle forces across the joints of the lower extremity (33). Individuals may have fluctuating cerebral spasticity, which is affected by many factors, including fatigue. Because of these factors, strength training has been controversial in the past, the argument being that strength training may increase spasticity. In a limited number of studies, strength has been shown to increase through the use of progressive resistance exercises. It may simply be very important in using a strength-training program to carefully monitor the balance of tone to be sure there is positive improvement (7).

Prevention and Treatment of Injuries

Injuries in this group vary depending on ambulation status. Patellofemoral pain is one common presenting complaint. Progressive tightening of the hamstrings and quadriceps muscles leads to a shortened stride length and increased forces across the patellofemoral joint. The condition is more resistant to treatment than in able-bodied athletes. Chronic proximal patellar tendinitis is also common because of the tension on quadriceps mechanism.

Hip abnormalities are common. Muscle tightness and imbalances across the hip can lead to the development of coxa valga and acetabular dysplasia. In more severe cases hip subluxation and dislocation occur. The athlete may initially present with hip pain when running or jumping.

Stress fractures, especially of the lower extremities, may develop because of muscle and stress imbalances and inappropriate training. They are more likely to occur at sites proximal to a brace or prosthesis.

Ankle and foot deformities that are seen in athletes with CP include equinas deformity, equinovarus deformity, and valgus deformity. Frequently, these require surgical repair or bracing. If left untreated, metatarsalgia, ankle instability, calluses, and pressure sores may result.

CP athletes often have inadequate motor control and lack of coordination and balance. Hand-to-eye coordination is impaired. Catching, throwing, and controlling equipment such as racquets, bats, and golf clubs can be difficult. A variety of ball games can be used to improve coordination. Protective gear, such as helmets for athletes with impaired balance, should be used when appropriate.

Prevention of musculoskeletal injuries includes a stretching program, a warm-up and cooldown for each workout, adaptive equipment, well-fitting and functioning braces when needed, and educating athletes, coaching staff, and medical staff to the unique problems encountered by athletes with CP. Strengthening, though still somewhat controversial, should be done with traditional programs to increase muscle strength as well as to increase flexibility and range of motion.

THE ATHLETE WITH MULTIPLE SCLEROSIS

Multiple sclerosis (MS) is a progressive demyelinating disease that produces lesions in the white matter of the central nervous system. It affects more than 300,000 Americans, with a peak age of onset between 20 and 30 years of age. It is considered to be one of the most challenging of all neurologic diseases to diagnose. With the chronic nature of the disease, it has a profound social and economical impact, affecting people during their active years of life. With its progressive degenerative component, MS often worsens over time regardless of the treatment. Physical symptoms range in severity and include ataxia, muscular weakness, fatigue, spasticity, sensory dysfunction, and a hypersensitivity to temperature increases.

Classification

Although there is no specific classification of MS athletes for competition, the International Federation of Multiple Sclerosis Society has developed a Minimal Record of Disability. The primary purpose of this scale is to describe the effects of the disease on ambulation.

Exercise Physiology

Individuals with MS commonly report that weakness and fatigue can interfere with activities of daily living and that previously achieved levels of activity are no longer possible. The measurement of muscle function is sometimes complicated by the presence of weakness, spasticity, ataxia, and incoordination in the athlete with MS. Fatigue also becomes a limiting factor in the measurement. In a study of voluntary progressive exercise, fatigue occurred more rapidly in athletes with MS than in control subjects, though it was of the same relative magnitude. Also found were significantly less metabolic changes in MS than in controls at the same relative exercise intensity. This indicates that fatigue is probably unrelated to metabolism and more likely due to peripheral factors such as chronically decreased physical activity, deconditioning, and decreased strength. Before beginning the study, the individuals with MS had noted muscle weakness. It appears that individuals with MS are capable of improving performance through training. Although maximal aerobic capacity is partially influenced by the level of neurologic impairment, there is encouraging evidence that regular exercise can result in documentable cardiorespiratory adaptations, even in those with a considerable degree of impairment. Whether these changes in exercise ability will translate into functional improvement is still unknown (36–38).

A problem that individuals with MS often encounter is a hypersensitivity to increases in temperature. There has been a documented sudden deterioration of function with very small rises in body temperature. This poses a problem to athletes with MS who wish to increase their physical activity.

THE ATHLETE WITH POLIO/POSTPOLIO SYNDROME

Poliomyelitis is an acute viral infection, the only sites of pathology being the brain and spinal cord. The incidence of the disease peaked in the mid-1950s in the United States, before the development of the vaccine. Since that time, the incidence of the disease has been at an all-time low, but a postpolio syndrome (PPS) has been described, characterized by muscle fatigue and decreased endurance, often accompanied by weakness, fasciculations, and atrophy in selective muscles. This syndrome occurs many years after the original viral infection.

Acute and chronic responses to strength and resistant training as well as aerobic exercise have been looked at in athletes with PPS. A group of symptomatic athletes with PPS significantly increased isometric and isokinetic extensors after a 6-week training program. In the 6 months following this study, without continuation of the exercise, the subjects were able to maintain their strength through daily activities. Thus a short course of resistance exercises may be valuable in achieving improvements in muscle function as well as increase in general activity level (39). In a comparison of oxygen uptake and associated cardiopulmonary function, individuals with PPS were found to have significantly decreased values. The significantly reduced oxygen uptake may account for the fatigue of which individuals with PPS often complain during physical activity. Increased demand on a reduced muscle mass with decreased blood flow hastens muscle fatigue. In a study implementing a 16-week aerobic exercise program, a significant increase in oxygen uptake was found in a group of symptomatic exercising individuals with PPS compared to a control group. It is felt that the most beneficial training program for athletes with PPS is an aerobic program of moderate intensity performed initially in short intervals with intervening recovery periods. This has been shown to increase oxygen uptake by 15–20% (39).

THE BLIND ATHLETE

There is a broad spectrum of vision impairment. Some athletes are completely blind; others may perceive light, dark, and shadows. A wide range of sports activities and recreational and leisure resources are available for blind athletes. Using companions, Braille books, clap sticks, beeping balls, and guide rails, blind athletes can compete in sports, including bicycling, skiing, golf, bowling, baseball, chess, scuba, water skiing, gymnastics, and horseback riding.

In 1981 the United States Association of Blind Athletes adopted a three-class system for classifying athletes according to their visual abilities. The categories are B1, B2, and B3. B1 includes those who may or may not have light perception but are unable to recognize hand motions at any distance. B2 includes those who are able to recognize hand motions, have measurable Snellen visual acuity up to and including 20/600, or have tubular visual fields limited to less than 5°. B3 includes those who have visual acuity better than 20/600 up to 20/200 or who have tubular visual fields limited from 5° to 20° (40).

THE ATHLETE WITH A LIMB AMPUTATION

Athletes with limb amputations compete with various assistive devices, orthoses, and prostheses. Team physicians need to be aware of regulations concerning their use in different sports. In track events, for example, prostheses are permitted, but crutches and canes are prohibited.

Classification

For amputees there are 12 categories made up of combinations of conditions: loss of one or both legs, loss of leg above or below the knee, loss of one or both arms, loss of arm above or below the elbow, and so on (3). This amputee-based classification system was developed by the U.S. Amputee Athletic Association.

Prevention and Treatment of Injuries

Some of the common injuries of amputees include low back pain, skin trauma, bursitis, knee injuries, and injuries to the sound limb.

Lower-extremity amputee athletes often develop low back pain. Excessive lumbar spine lateral flexion and extension compensates for the lack of lower-extremity joint flexion at prosthetic sites. This can result in an imbalance in back musculature and a functional scoliosis. Specific muscle-strengthening and stretching programs can be both preventive and therapeutic.

Prostheses can cause skin breakdown, abrasions, blistering, and skin rashes. Prevention includes adjustment of prosthetic fit and alignment, as well as use of protective pads.

Amputees may develop bursitis as a result of socket irritation. Common sites include the prepatellar, infrapatellar, and pretibial bursae in below-knee amputees and the ischial and trochanteric bursae in above-knee amputations. Treatment involves modification of the prosthesis.

Hyperextension knee injuries can result from the body's forward momentum moving over a fixed prosthesis and the residual limb.

Impact injuries, such as bruising over bony prominences, can result from forces transmitted through the prosthesis to the residual limb.

Amputee runners place unusual stresses, including increased weight, on the sound limb. Injuries include plantar fasciitis, stress fractures, and overpronation of the feet. Altered hip flexion leads to chronic hamstring injuries in both lower extremities.

THE DEAF ATHLETE

Communication is the primary problem for deaf athletes. Colored lights, light dimmers, touch, and hand signals facilitate participation. In some cases the vestibular apparatus is involved, affecting balance and coordination. Activities requiring sharp turns, spins, cuts, or balance can be difficult. Talking directly to the deaf athlete who reads lips is an important communication tool.

THE ATHLETE WITH ARTHRITIS

Under the broadest definition of disability, arthritis is the most prevalent chronic disease in the United States, with an estimated 40 million (one in seven) Americans having the disability, most of them elderly. It has been classified as the leading cause of activity limitation among Americans (2). It limits everyday activities, such as dressing, climbing stairs, getting into and out of bed, and walking, for about 7 million Americans.

According to the 1996 Surgeon General's report on physical activity and health, "For people with arthritis, regular physical activity is necessary to maintain normal muscle strength, joint structure and joint function" (41). Aquatic therapy has been found to be a very helpful therapeutic intervention, increasing joint range of motion and reducing pain while minimizing joint stresses.

SNOW SKIING FOR THE DISABLED

Snow skiing for the physically disabled is one sport that has seen tremendous growth in the past few years. Many individuals—those with cerebral palsy, multiple sclerosis, muscular dystrophy, visual and hearing impairments, spina bifida, spinal cord injuries, and amputations—can participate with adaptive equipment and techniques (42).

Blind and visually impaired athletes require minimal adaptive equipment and usually become proficient skiers. Early in the learning process a ski bra, in which a hook is attached to the tip of one ski and an eyelet to the other, can be used. This helps with muscular imbalance. The most important aspect of skiing for the blind is the guide or instructor who communicates to the athlete through voice and touch. The use of bright orange ski bibs for all blind skiers, instructors, and guides is recommended for safety on the mountain (42).

Just as with these blind athletes, adaptive equipment has made a tremendous impact on the sport for other disabled athletes. Three-tracking is the most widely known method of adaptive skiing. It was developed for amputees with one sound limb and two functional arms, as well as those with polio, traumatic injuries, and hemiplegia who may have limited use of one leg. The athlete uses one full-length ski and two short outrigger skis. Four-track skiing uses four separate skis, two full-length skis, and two outriggers. This was developed for those who need additional support, such as those with CP, MS, or muscular dystrophy. Sit-skiing and monoskiing are methods of skiing for athletes who use a wheelchair. These adaptive skis essentially contain a chassis with an attached downhill ski. It holds the skier tightly in place, giving him or her control as well as support and cushioning. Short, adjustable outriggers are used for help in balance, control, turning, and stopping.

In terms of injuries sustained by disabled skiers, data collected thus far suggest that the disabled skier is at no greater risk of injury, both in terms of actual incidence and severity, than able-bodied skiers.

WORLD T.E.A.M. SPORTS

We hope that this chapter increases medical personnel's awareness and understanding of the participation of disabled athletes in the sporting world. This theme is also reflected in a relatively new organization entitled World T.E.A.M. (The Exceptional Athlete Matters) Sports. Its charge is to create, encourage, promote, and develop opportunities for persons with physical and/or mental disabilities to enable participation in lifetime sporting activities. These are enhanced by the integration of disabled and able-bodied athletes together. Many grass-roots programs have already been instituted, but two global events are of significant note.

AXA World Ride '95 was an 8-month cycling event around the world that included hundreds of cyclists in different stages of the ride. Highlighted were five disabled athletes who completed the entire journey of 13,000 miles through 16 countries. Ninety-six injuries were recorded; the following were the top four in order of frequency: abrasion, pressure sores, gastroenteritis, and strains and sprains. The other event, the Viet Nam Challenge, was completed in January 1998. This enabled approximately 80 disabled and able-bodied athletes to cycle from Hanoi to Ho Chi Minh City (1200 miles in 16 days). Evident throughout this ride was the concept that "disabled" does not mean "unable." All individuals are truly exceptional athletes. Through sports and recreation we can bring the communities of the world together.

SPORTS ORGANIZATIONS

Achilles Track Club
9 East 89th Street
New York, NY 10128
(212) 354-0300

American Athletic Association of the Deaf
3607 Washington Blvd, Suite 4
Ogden, UT 84403-1737
Office(tty) (810) 393-7916
e-mail: aaadeaf@aol.com

Arthritis Foundation
Arthritis Answers hotline
1-800-283-7800
Internet: www.arthritis.org

Disabled Sports USA
451 Hungerford Drive
Suite 100
Rockville, MD 20850
(301) 217-9838
e-mail: dsusa@dsusa.org
Internet: http://www.dsusa.org/dsusa/dsusa.html

Dwarf Athletic Association of America
418 Willow Way
Lewisville, TX 75067
(972) 317-8299
e-mail: jfbda3@aol.com

National Wheelchair Basketball Association
2850 North Gary Ave
Pomona, CA 91767
(909) 596-7733

U.S. Association for Blind Athletes
33 N. Institute Street
Colorado Springs, CO 80903
(719) 630-0422
e-mail: usaba@usa.net
Internet: http://www.usaba.org

U.S. Cerebral Palsy Athletic Association
200 Harrison Avenue
Newport, RI 02840
(401) 848-2460
e-mail: uscpaa@mail.bbsnet.com

U.S. Olympic Committee
Disabled Sports Service Department
One Olympic Plaza
Colorado Springs, CO 80909-5760
(719) 578-4958 or 4818
e-mail: mark.shephard@usoc.org
Internet: http://www.olympic.usa.org

Wheelchair Sports USA
3595 East Fountain Blvd
Suite L-1
Colorado Springs, CO 80910
(719) 574-1150
e-mail: wsusa@aol.com

WORLD T.E.A.M. SPORTS
1919 South Blvd
Suite 100
Charlotte, NC 28203
(704) 344-9030
e-mail: wts@internetmci.com
Internet: www.worldteamsport.org

REFERENCES

1. Nichols AW. Sports medicine and the Americans with Disabilities Act. *Clin J Sports Med* 1996;6(3):190–195.
2. Rimmer JH, Braddock D, Pitetti KH. Research on physical activity and disability: an emerging national priority. *Med Sci Sports Exerc* 1996;28(8):1366–1372.
3. Bielak KM. *The handicapped athlete: the Hughston Clinic sports medicine book.* Baltimore, MD: Williams & Wilkins, 1995: 106–111.
4. U.S. Olympic Committee, Disabled Sports Services, Colorado Springs, CO.
5. Special Olympics International, Washington, DC.
6. Challenge Magazine, Disabled Sports USA, Summer 1997.
7. Richter KJ, Gaebler-Spira DG, Mushett CA. Sport and the person with spasticity of cerebral origin. *Dev Med Child Neurol* 1996; 38:867–870.
8. Coyle CP, Santiago MC. Aerobic exercise training and depressive symptomatology in adult with physical disabilities. *Arch Phys Med Rehabil* 1995;76:647–652.
9. Nyland J, et al. Shoulder rotator torque and wheelchair dependence differences of National Wheelchair Basketball Association players. *Arch Phys Med Rehabil* 1977;78:358–363.
10. American Academy of Family Physicians, et al. *Preparticipation physical evaluation,.* 2nd ed. Minneapolis: The Physician and Sportsmedicine, 1997.
11. American Academy of Pediatrics. Atlantoaxial instability in Down syndrome: subject review. *Pediatrics* 1995;96(1):151–154.

12. Figoni SF. Exercise responses and quadriplegia. *Med Sci Sports Exerc* 1993;25(4):433–441.
13. Davis GM. Exercise capacity of individuals with paraplegia. *Med Sci Sports Exerc* 1993;25,4:423–432.
14. Curtis KA, Dillon DA. Survey of wheelchair athletic injuries: common patterns and prevention. *Paraplegia* 1985;23:170–175.
15. Ferrara MS, et al. The injury experience of the competitive athlete with a disability: prevention implications. *Med Sci Sports Exerc* 1992;24(2):184–188.
16. Schaefer RS, Proffer DS. Sports medicine for wheelchair athletes. *Am Fam Physician* 1989;239–245.
17. Gass GC, Camp EM. The maximum physiological responses during incremental wheelchair and arm cranking exercise in male paraplegics. *Med Sci Sports Exerc* 1984;16(4):355–359.
18. Rotstein et al. Aerobic capacity and anaerobic threshold of wheelchair basketball players. *Paraplegia* 1994;32:196–201.
19. Hooker SP, Wells CL. Aerobic power of competative paraplegic road racers. *Paraplegia* 1992;30:428–436.
20. Davis GM, Shephard RJ. Cardiorespiratory fitness in highly active versus inactive paraplegics. *Med Sci Sports Exerc* 1988;20(5):463–468.
21. Wicks JR, et al. Arm cranking and wheelchair ergometry in elite spinal cord–injured athletes. *Med Sci Sports Exerc* 1983;15(3):224–231.
22. Cooper RA, Horvath SM, Bedi JF, et al. Maximal exercise response of paraplegic wheelchair road racers. *Paraplegia* 1992;30:573–581.
23. Van Loan MD, et al. Comparison of physiological responses to maximal arm exercise among able-bodied, paraplegics, and quadriplegics. *Paraplegia* 1987;25:397–405.
24. Ide M, Ogata H, Kobayashi M, Wada F. Muscle damage occuring in wheelchair sports people. *Spinal Cord* 1997;35:234–237.
25. Ferrara MS, Davis RW. Injuries to elite wheelchair athletes. *Paraplegia* 1990;28:335–341.
26. Ferrara MS, Buckley WE, McCann BC, Limbard TJ, Powell JW, Robl R. The injury experience of the competitive athlete with a disability: prevention implications. *Med Sci Sports Exerc* 1992;28:184–188.
27. Jackson DL, et al. Electrodiagnostic study of carpal tunnel syndrome in wheelchair basketball players. *Clin J Sports Med* 1996;6(1):27–31.
28. Boninger ML, et al. Upper limb nerve entrapments in elite wheelchair racers. *Am J Phys Med Rehabil* 1996;75:170–176.
29. Sawka MN, Latzka WA, Pandolf KB. Temperature regulation during upper body exercise: able-bodied and spinal cord injured. *Med Sci Sports Exerc* 1989;21(5, Supplement):S132–S140.
30. Armstrong LE, et al. Local cooling in wheelchair athletes during exercise stress. *Med Sci Sports Exerc* 1995;27(2):211–216.
31. Wilson PE, Washington RL. Pediatric wheelchair athletes: sports injuries and prevention. *Paraplegia* 1993;31:330–337.
32. Harris P. Self-induced autonomic dysreflexia ("boosting") practiced by some tetraplegic athletes to enhance their athletic performance. *Paraplegia* 1994;32:289–291.
33. Damiano DL, Kelly LE, Vaughn CL. Effects of quadriceps femoris muscle strengthening on crouch gait in children with spastic diplegia. *Physical Therapy* 1995;75, 8:658–671.
34. Rose J, Haskell WL, Gamble JG. A comparison of oxygen pulse and respiratory exchange ratio in cerebral palsied and nondisabled children. *Arch Phys Med Rehabil* 1993;74:702–705.
35. O'Connell DG, Barnhart R, Parks L. Muscular endurance and wheelchair propulsion in children with cerebral palsy or myelomeningocele. *Arch Phys Med Rehabil* 1992;73:709–711.
36. Kent-Braun JA, Sharma KP, Weiner MW, Miller RG. Effects of exercise on muscle activation and metabolism in multiple sclerosis. *Muscle Nerve* 1994;17:1162–1169.
37. Ng AV, Kent-Braun JA. Quantitation of lower physical activity in persons with multiple sclerosis. *Med Sci Sports Exerc* 1997;29(4):517–523.
38. Ponichtera-Mulcare JA. Exercise and multiple sclerosis. *Med Sci Sports Exerc* 1993;25(4):451–465.
39. Birk TJ. Poliomyelitis and the post-polio syndrome: exercise capacities and adaption: current research, future directions, and widespread applicability. *Med Sci Sports Exerc* 1993;25, 4:466–472.
40. Makris VI, et al. Visual loss and performance in blind athletes. *Med Sci Sports Exerc* 1993;25, 2:265–269.
41. Surgeon General. *Physical Activity and Health*. Springfield, VA: National Technical Education Service, 1996.
42. Laskowski ER. Snow skiing for the physically disabled. *Mayo Clin Proc* 1991;66:160–172.

BIBLIOGRAPHY

Bayley JC, Cochran TP, Sledge CB. The weight-bearing shoulder. *J Bone Joint Surg* 1987;69-A:676–678.

Bhambhani YN, Holland LJ, Eriksson P, Steadward RD. Physiological responses during wheelchair racing in quadriplegics and paraplegics. *Paraplegia* 1994;32:253–260.

Bhambhani YN, Holland LJ, Steadward RD. Maximal aerobic power in cerebral palsied wheelchair athletes: validity and reliability. *Arch Phys Med Rehabil* 1992;73:246–252.

Bhambhani YN, Holland LJ, Steadward RD. Anaerobic threshold in wheelchair athletes with cerebral palsy: validity and reliability. *Arch Phys Med Rehabil* 1993;74:305–311.

Botvin Madorsky JG, Curtis KA. Wheelchair sports medicine. *Am J Sports Med* 1984;12(2):128–132.

Botvin Madorsky JG, Madorsky AG. Scuba diving: taking the wheelchair out of wheelchair sports. *Arch Phys Med Rehabil* 1988;69:215–218.

Burnham RS, et al. Shoulder pain in wheelchair athletes: the role of muscle imbalance. *Am J Sports Med* 1993;21(2):238–242.

Burnham RS, Steadward RD. Upper extremity peripheral nerve entrapments among wheelchair athletes: prevalance, location, and risk factors. *Arch Phys Med Rehabil* 1994;75:519–524.

Calmels P, et al. Medical activity during an international sporting competition for the physically disabled: Saint-Etienne World Handicapped Sport Championships. *Disabil Rehabil* 1994;16(2):80–84.

Chatard JC, et al. Physiological aspects of swimming performance for persons with disabilities. *Med Sci Sports Exerc* 1992;24(11):1276–1282.

Chawla JC. Sport for people with disability. *Br Med J* 1994;308:1500–1504.

Corcoran PJ, et al. Sport medicine and the physiology of wheelchair marathon racing. *Orthop Clin North Am* 1980;11(4):697–716.

Coutts KD, McKenzie DC. Ventilatory thresholds during wheelchair exercise in individuals with spinal cord injuries. *Paraplegia* 1995;33:419–422.

Coutts KD, Rhodes EC, McKenzie DC. Maximal exercise responses of tetraplegics and paraplegics. *J Appl Physiol: Respirat Environ Exercise Physiol* 1983;55(2):479–482.

Coutts KD, Stogryn JL. Aerobic and anaerobic power of Canadian wheelchair track athletes. *Med Sci Sports Exerc* 1987;19(1):62–65.

Curtis KA, et al. Development of the wheelchair user's shoulder pain index (WUSPI). *Paraplegia* 1995;33:290–293.

Dykens EM, Cohen DJ. Effects of Special Olympics International on social competence in persons with mental redardation. *J Am Acad Child Adolesc Psychiatry* 1996;35(2):223–229.

Ferrara MS, Buckley WE, Messner DG, Benedict J. The injury experience and training history of the competitive skier with a disability. *Am J Sports Med* 1992;20(1):55–60.

Gass GC, Camp EM. Effects of prolonged exercise in highly trained traumatic paraplegic men. *J Appl Physiol* 1987;63(5):1846–1852.

Gellman H, et al. Carpal tunnel syndrome in paraplegic patients. *J Bone Joint Surg Am* 1988;70-A, 4:517–519.

Glaser RM, et al. Physiological responses to maximal effort wheelchair and arm crank ergometry. *J Appl Physiol: Respirat Environ Exercise Physiol* 1980;48(6):1060–1064.

Harrison RJ, Alfano SI. Pharmaceutical services at the 1995 Special Olympics World Games. *Am J Health-Syst Pharm* 1996;53:2198–2199.

Hoeberigs JH, Debets-Eggen HBL, Debets PML. Sports medical experience from the International Flower Marathon for disabled wheelers. *Am J Sports Med* 1990;18(4):418–421.

Hutzler Y. Physical performance of elite wheelchair basketball players in armcranking ergometry and in selected wheeling tasks. *Paraplegia* 1993;31:255–261.

Kaplan SL. Cycling patterns in children with and without cerebral palsy. *Dev Med Child Neurol* 1995;37:620–630.

Laplaza FJ, Root L. Femoral anteversion and neck-shaft angles in hip instability in cerebral palsy. *J Pediatr Orthop* 1994;14(6):719–723.

Laskowski ER, Murtaugh PA. Snow skiing injuries in physically disabled skiers. *Am J Sports Med* 1992;20(5):553–557.

Lovell ME, Thomas AF, Shakesby R, Mcneilly P. Social adjustment and rehabilitation in international competitors with spinal injuries sustained in military service. *Disabil Rehabil* 1997;19(3):92–96.

McCann BC. Thermoregulation in spinal cord injury: the challenge of the Atlanta Paralympics. *Spinal Cord* 1996;34:433–436.

McCormick DP, Niebuhr VN, Risser WL. Injury and illness surveillance at local Special Olympic games. *Br J Sports Med* 1990;24, 4:221–224.

Mello MT, et al. Correlation between K complex, periodic leg movements (PLM), and myoclonus during sleep in paraplegic adults before and after an acute physical activity. *Spinal Cord* 1997;35:248–252.

Pitetti KH. Introduction: exercise capacities and adaptations of people with chronic disabilities: current research, future directions, and widespread applicability. *Med Sci Sports Exerc* 1993;25(4):421–422.

Reynolds J, et al. Paralympics-Barcelona 1992. *Br J Sports Med* 1994;28(1):14–17.

Rose J, et al. Muscle pathology and clinical measures of disability in children with cerebral palsy. *J Orthop Res* 1994;12(6):758–768.

Rotstein A, Sagiv M, Ben-Sira D, et al. Aerobic capacity and anaerobic threshold of wheelchair basketball players. *Paraplegia* 1994;32:196–201.

Shephard RJ. Benefits of sport and physical activity for the disabled: implications for the individual and for society. *Scand J Rehab Med* 1991;23:51–59.

Tanji JL. The preparticipation exam: special concern for the Special Olympics. *The Physician and Sportsmedicine* 1991;19(7):61–68.

Tun CG, Upton J. The paraplegic hand: electrodiagnostic studies and clinical findings. *J Hand Surg* 1988;13A:716–719.

Valliant PM, et al. Psychological impact of sport on disabled athletes. *Psychological Rep* 1985;56:923–929.

Veeger HEJ, Yahmed MH, Van Der Woude LHV, Charpentier P. Peak oxygen uptake and maximal power output of Olympic wheelchair-dependent athletes. *Med Sci Sports Exerc* 1991;23,10:1201–1209.

Zwiren LD, Bar-Or O. Responses to exercise of paraplegics who differ in conditioning level. *Med Sci Sports Exerc* 1975;7, 2:94–98.

PART III
Psychosocial Issues

CHAPTER 10

Drug Abuse in Athletes

Gary Alan Green and Bassil Aish

INTRODUCTION

While there is the assumption that the association between athletes and drugs (especially drugs that influence performance) is a recent phenomenon, the present epidemic is merely one leg in a race that began thousands of years ago. It seems that the desire to find a substance that makes one stronger and faster is an innate human trait. A corollary of this trait is that it is accompanied by an equally strong desire to control the substances that athletes are legally allowed to use. The International Olympic Committee (IOC) has adopted a list of prohibited classes and methods of doping, which are listed in Table 10–1. This chapter will explore drugs that are found in each class; they will be used as examples, because it would be impossible to discuss all of the potential drugs of abuse in one chapter.

A less formal classification that has also been used to categorize drugs of abuse by athletes utilizes the underlying reason for use. In this system drugs are classified as ergogenic, recreational, or therapeutic drugs. Ergogenic drugs are used by athletes with the sole purpose of increasing their performance and gaining a competitive advantage. Most of the drugs in this chapter fall into this category. Recreational drugs are taken by athletes to alter their mood, escape life stresses, and the like; their reasons, prevalence, and patterns of use are similar to those of their nonathlete peers. Finally, therapeutic drugs are substances prescribed by a physician for the alleviation of a specific medical condition. The advantage of this system is that it addresses the desired effect of the drug, which is important in designing specific prevention and treatment strategies for the various drugs. The downside is that a single drug may be considered in any one of the three categories, complicating decisions relating to sanctions by sports organizations seeking to control drug (especially ergogenic) abuse. Overall, the importance of this system is that it addresses the fact that it is not the substance itself that is the problem, but how the substance is used by a particular athlete.

Although the drugs differ, most ergogenic substances follow a similar pattern of use: initial use by elite athletes, skepticism by the medical community, increasing use and abuse, and finally the development of testing procedures and sanction. With all drugs the questions that need to be answered are as follows:

1. What is the drug?
2. Does it work?
3. Is it safe?

Sports medicine specialists will undoubtedly be questioned by athletes, trainers, coaches, and officials about the drugs that are covered in this chapter, along with new and emerging substances. This chapter provides a framework that can be used to provide the answers to these difficult questions for the drugs that are discussed and for new substances that may emerge.

ANABOLIC-ANDROGENIC STEROIDS

Anabolic steroid use, which was once confined to elite male "power" sports, can now be found in nearly every sport at all levels. Although new ergogenic drugs seem to appear each week, anabolic steroids are important because they provide an excellent example of the relationship between drugs and sports.

Anabolic steroids include testosterone or testosterone-like synthetic substances that result in both anabolic (increasing protein synthesis) and androgenic (enhancement of male secondary sexual characteristics) effects. While athletes consume anabolic steroids for their ana-

---

G. A. Green: UCLA Division of Sports Medicine, and Pepperdine University, Los Angeles, California 90095–1683.

B. Aish: UCLA Department of Family Medicine/Sports Medicine, Los Angeles, California 90095–1683.

TABLE 10-1. *IOC list of prohibited classes and methods*

I. Classes of prohibited substances
   A. Stimulants
   B. Narcotics
   C. Anabolic agents
   D. Diuretics
   E. Peptide and glycoprotein hormones and analogues (and their releasing factors)
II. Prohibited methods
   A. Blood doping
   B. Pharmacologic, chemical, and physical manipulation
III. Classes of drugs subject to certain restrictions
   A. Alcohol
   B. Marijuana
   C. Local anesthetics
   D. Corticosteroids
   E. Beta-blockers
   F. Specified beta-2 agonists

From Catlin DH, Hatton CK. Use and abuse of anabolic and other drugs for athletic enhancement. *Adv Intern Med* 1990;36:381–405.

bolic properties, it is primarily the androgenic aspect that is responsible for adverse effects. It is important to realize that although it may be possible to create a 100% anabolic compound *in vitro,* all anabolic steroids have both anabolic and androgenic properties to some degree and are properly referred to as anabolic-androgenic steroids (AAS). AAS can also be divided according to their solubility, the 17 alpha alkylated compounds, which are water soluble (and can be taken orally), and the oil-soluble 17 beta esterified AAS, which are given via the parenteral route. Some common injectable and oral AAS are listed in Table 10-2.

It is thought that AAS were originally developed in the 1930s and were first used medically to restore a positive nitrogen balance to starvation victims in World War II (1). After the war there were reports that German troops had been given AAS to increase aggressiveness (2). Steroids were introduced to the sports world in the 1950s with reports of use by Soviet male and female athletes and have been a part of athletics ever since (3).

Although AAS have been on the sports scene for over 40 years, accurate data on their use have been difficult to obtain. Numerous studies have attempted to investigate their prevalence in a variety of age levels, but all have been hampered by many factors, including the lack of an adequate denominator and the limitations surrounding self-report surveys. The best these studies can provide is an estimation of AAS usage at any one point in time.

One of the better studies involving both athletes and nonathletes was performed by Buckley and colleagues in 1988 (4). They surveyed twelfth-grade male students from 150 high schools nationwide, received 3403 responses (response rate: 50%), and found that 6.6% used or had used AAS. One of the alarming findings in this study was that 35% of AAS users were not involved in a school-sponsored sport. This clearly demonstrated that AAS use was no longer confined to elite athletes. Although the primary reason given for use was performance enhancement, 27% stated that they took AAS for appearance (4). Another worrisome finding was that over one third of the users reported beginning AAS use at the age of 15 or younger.

In 1997 Yesalis and coworkers published a comprehensive review of AAS use in students aged 12–18 from 1989 to 1996 by compiling data from three nationwide, multiyear surveys (5–9). According to this survey, 4.9% of males and 2.4% of females admitted to using AAS at least once. On the basis of 1995 estimates of high school students, this translates to 375,000 adolescent males and 175,000 adolescent females involved in AAS use. An increasing trend in the use among junior high and high school females since 1991 was noted (5).

Perhaps the most comprehensive survey of AAS among athletes has been conducted by the National Collegiate Athletic Association (NCAA). The 1997 installment of Substance Use and Abuse Habits of College Student-Athletes surveyed 13,914 male and female athletes across 33 sports at 637 Division I, II, and III institutions (10). The study found that only 1.1% admitted to using AAS in the preceding 12 months. Although football players had a comparatively high rate of 2.2%, male water polo players actually had the highest rate of any sport: 2.8%. Sports such as men's baseball and women's field hockey had rates approaching 2%, again demonstrating that AAS use is not limited to football players at the NCAA level. Given the Buckley and Yesalis data, it is not surprising that of the NCAA athletes who reported AAS use, 26% began in junior high school and 25% reported initial use at the high school level. One additional finding in this study was that AAS users were many times more likely than AAS nonusers to use other ergogenic drugs, including human growth hormone

TABLE 10-2. *Common injectable and oral anabolic-androgenic steroids*

Injectable	Oral
Testosterone	Methyltestosterone
Testosterone propionate	Metandienone
Testosterone enantate	Oxandrolone (Anavar)
Testosterone cipionate	Stanozolol
Nandrolone decanoate	Danazol
Nandrolone phenpropionate	Fluoxymesterone
Methandrostenolone (Dianabol)	Oxymetholone (Anadrol)
Methenolone (Primabolin)	

From Council on Scientific Affairs of the AMA. Medical and nonmedical uses of anabolic-androgenic steroids. *JAMA* 1990;264:2923–2927.

(hCG), epitestosterone, clenbuterol, erythropoietin, and nutritional supplements.

In the population of male competitive bodybuilders, two surveys of AAS use revealed prevalence rates of 54% and 38%, respectively (11,12). Delbeke and colleagues in 1994 used gas chromatograph/mass spectroscopic analysis of urine and found a 58% positive rate for AAS among a population of bodybuilders (13). Another group with a high rate of AAS use is weight lifters. This became such a problem that in 1992 the International Weightlifting Federation eliminated all previously recognized weight lifting records, believing that they were all achieved with the aid of anabolic-androgenic steroids. The federation then instituted stringent testing procedures and penalties (14,15), and subsequent urine testing for AAS in 1993 revealed an 8% prevalence among weight lifters (13).

The proposed mechanism by which AAS increase muscle mass has been somewhat controversial. At the cellular level AAS are bound by cytoplasmic proteins and transported to the nucleus. This activates DNA-dependent RNA polymerase and results in the production of messenger RNA for protein synthesis (16). AAS may also have an anticatabolic effect that occurs by attenuating the effects of cortisol. It has been postulated that this results from AAS displacing cortisol from receptors, allowing the athlete to recover more quickly and train at a higher level (17). There is also a theory that AAS act by increasing the motivation of athletes through heightened levels of aggressiveness (17–19).

For many years there was a debate within the medical community as to whether AAS actually "work," that is, whether they increase muscle mass. There have been numerous studies in male athletes that support both improvement (20–24) and no significant improvement in strength (25–28). Some of this discrepancy can be explained by meta-analysis of 30 studies of AAS performed between 1966 and 1990. This revealed that only 16 studies were properly randomized, used placebos, and made objective measurements of strength and percent of change in strength and were thus included in the meta-analysis. The study concluded that while anabolic androgenic steroids may slightly enhance muscle strength in previously trained athletes, results for low steroid dosages could not be generalized to athletes using megadose regimens.

Bhasin and colleagues in 1996 examined the use of suprapshysiologic dosages of testosterone in a well-controlled, randomized, placebo study (29). The investigators found statistically significant strength gains ($p < 0.5$) over a 10-week period in 43 men who were given 600 mg/week of testosterone. The greatest increases were observed when testosterone was given in conjunction with strength training, though some gains were seen in the group that was given testosterone only. While the dose of testosterone used in this study was higher than in previous work, it still does not approach the extremely high doses in multiple combinations that some athletes employ.

To summarize the literature as to whether AAS are effective, one of the best sources is still the 1984 position statement by the American College of Sports Medicine (30). They concluded that in the presence of an adequate diet, AAS can contribute to increases in body weight and lean body mass. Also, the gains in muscular strength that are achieved through high-intensity exercise and proper diet can occur by increased use of AAS in some individuals. Finally, AAS do not seem to increase aerobic power.

Regarding the therapeutic uses for AAS, it is believed that true medical indications account for fewer than 3 million prescriptions per year (31). Currently approved indications include refractory anemias, hereditary angioedema, palliation in advanced breast carcinoma, replacement therapy in hypogonadal males, constitutional growth delay in conjunction with human growth hormone, and wasting syndromes associated with HIV infection. Given these relatively few indications and the fact that several studies have revealed that many users obtained AAS from health care professionals (4,10), AAS were added to Schedule III of the Controlled Substances Act in 1990. It was hoped that this would somewhat reduce the use of AAS.

As we mentioned above, athletes use AAS in amounts that far exceed the recommended therapeutic dosages. In addition, athletes frequently use combinations of AAS, so-called stacking or cycling, in a pyramidal manner to saturate receptors and achieve maximal effect (32). One example of a 2-month drug history of a bodybuilder can be seen in Table 10–3 (33).

Any discussion of adverse consequences of AAS in athletes is complicated by the fact that most reports of side effects involve the use of AAS in physiologic dosages given over long periods of time. This is a far different scenario than athletes using suprapshysiologic dosages over a relatively short period of time. Much of the information about adverse events has been garnered through anecdotal case reports. Given that caveat, the side effects regarding AAS can be divided according to general effects, sex-specific effects, effects relating to

TABLE 10–3. *Two-month history of AAS use by a bodybuilder*

Drug	Dose	Therapeutic dose
Dianabol	75 mg sc QOD	5 mg sc QD
Primabolin	150 mg sc QOD	
Anavar	20 mg po QD	2.5–10 mg po QD
Anadrol	100 mg po QD	5–10 mg po QD

From Tennant F, Black DL, Voy RO. Anabolic steroid dependence with opioid type features: *N Engl J Med* 1988; 319:578.

impurities, psychosocial effects, and effects on immature athletes.

General effects include alterations in the gastrointestinal tract and cardiovascular system. The liver is specifically targeted with the development of hepatocellular dysfunction, peliosis hepatis, and hepatocellular carcinoma (34). Hepatic effects are increased with the use of the 17-alpha alkylated compounds, which are consumed orally and thus undergo first pass metabolism in the liver. Cardiovascular effects can be severe in that AAS are atherogenic by increasing total cholesterol and LDL cholesterol while decreasing HDL cholesterol. When this is combined with the fact that AAS can also increase blood pressure (29), it is not surprising that AAS have been associated with cases of myocardial infarction (35,36) and cerebrovascular accidents (37). Finally, regarding the musculoskeletal system, AAS have been linked to spontaneous tendon rupture and should always be suspected in cases of unusual tendon injury (38,39).

The sex-specific effects of AAS occur because mature men have a much greater daily production rate of testosterone than mature women: 2.5–11 mg versus 0.25 mg, respectively (40). AAS in men function as weak androgens, and users can develop oligospermia, azoospermia, and gynecomastia (30). On the other hand, women experience the virilizing effects of AAS and hormonal alterations that include decreased levels of LH, FSH, estrogens, and progesterone. Women can also develop abnormal menses, male pattern alopecia, hirsutism, clitoromegaly, and deepening of the voice, the latter three possibly being irreversible (41).

Because AAS are often purchased on the black market, they may contain impurities that are responsible for adverse effects, especially with parenteral use. There have been case reports of AAS use being responsible for the development of infection and abscesses (42), as well as the contraction of HIV and hepatitis B following the use of shared needles (43).

There has been a great deal of interest in both the scientific and lay communities in the association between AAS and psychosocial effects. In 1994 Choi and Pope evaluated 37 athletes (23 users, 13 nonusers) and noted statistically significant increases in fights, verbal aggression, and physical aggression toward their significant others when on AAS (44). This confirms previous work in this area that found an increase in frank psychotic behavior while on AAS (45).

Although not much research has been devoted to the adverse effects of AAS in sexually immature athletes, there are potential considerations in this area. Given that several studies demonstrate significant use of AAS in junior high and high school (4,5,10,46), there is good reason to be concerned about the use of AAS in a growing skeleton. Although there are reports of AAS causing premature closure of the epiphyses (30), there are doubtless other areas that require further study.

Perhaps the most chilling "study" of AAS in athletes involved the recently published review of the previously classified, highly secret documents about the systematic use of AAS by the former German Democratic Republic (GDR) (47). Franke and Berendonk describe 30 years of AAS administration to thousands of athletes (often without consent), including minors of both sexes, for the purposes of performance enhancement. While some may legitimately argue that it is unethical to discuss data that were obtained from uninformed subjects, these documents do provide information about the serious adverse consequences of AAS as taken by athletes. The data reveal side effects that included severe liver damage, gynecomastopathy requiring surgery, polycystic ovarian syndrome, and arrest of body growth in adolescents. In addition, there were reports of three deaths related to AAS use, one of which occurred from complications related to liver damage and bile duct obstruction. It is especially reprehensible that the documents describe the concealment of severe medical and surgical complications incurred by "subjects" from the use of high doses and/or prolonged use of AAS. In addition, the article described precise strategies to evade detection by drug testing.

The experience of the GDR is important in considering how the will to win can be ultimately corrupted and developed into an organized, state-sponsored pattern of drug abuse. The long history of AAS in sports serves as a template for understanding the pattern associated with other ergogenic drugs and why this is an ongoing problem in sports. AAS and sports have now been associated for almost 50 years and are a lesson in the cat-and-mouse game of drug testing and drug use. At the present time improved testing for synthetic AAS has led to increasing use of testosterone by athletes. In addition, athletes have turned to testosterone precursors, such as the nutritional supplements DHEA and androstenedione, to increase testosterone. Owing to these practices, the detection of exogenous testosterone use through analysis of the testosterone:epitestosterone ratio is rapidly becoming obsolete. Newer testing strategies, such as carbon isotope testing, will need to be developed to combat the use of AAS in the next century.

HUMAN GROWTH HORMONE (hGH)

The rise of AAS was naturally accompanied by increasingly sophisticated methods to detect its use among elite athletes. This led athletes engaged in power sports to seek alternatives to AAS, and one of the key substances that emerged was human growth hormone. hGH is a polypeptide composed of 191 amino acids and is the most abundant component of the anterior pituitary (48). The average daily production rate of hGH in adult males is 0.4–1.0 mg with 5–10 mg being stored in the pituitary.

The history of hGH began in the same manner as

that of many other ergogenic substances: from the field of animal husbandry. Animal breeders in the 1930s discovered that livestock given a crude extract of species-specific pituitary glands developed increased muscle mass, decreased body fat, and an accelerated growth rate. In the 1950s it was found that these extracts stimulated production of somatomedins, which in turn resulted in increased growth. It was not until 1961, however, that the development of radioimmunoassay allowed hGH to be measured. This permitted small amounts of hGH to be extracted from cadaveric pituitary glands and provided to growth hormone–deficient patients. The breakthrough in hGH occurred in 1985 when the first synthetic hGH preparation could be made via recombinant DNA technology; this led to a huge increase in hGH availability. At least three products are currently available: somatrem and two formulations of somatropin. However, an amendment to the Food, Drug and Cosmetic Act makes nonindicated use or possession with intent to distribute any form of hGH a federal offense (48). Because hGH is produced via recombinant DNA, it is nearly identical to endogenous hGH and therefore cannot be detected by traditional urine testing.

The suspicion of hGH use by athletes has been present since at least 1983 when random urine specimens reportedly discovered high levels at the World Track and Field Championships in Helsinki. Although it is thought to be widely used among football players and bodybuilders, accurate prevalence data are difficult to obtain. The 1997 NCAA survey on drug use in athletes revealed that 3.1% of 13,000 athletes admitted to using hGH in the previous year (10). This is puzzling in that only 1.1% admitted to using AAS during the same period and raises questions about self-report surveys. There is a tremendous amount of misinformation among athletes, and they may become confused by the many nutritional supplements that claim to increase growth hormone. While it is difficult to believe that hGH use is more prevalent than AAS at the NCAA level, the use of hGH is nevertheless a real problem at the international level. This was amply demonstrated in 1998 at the Pan-Pacific Swimming Championships in Australia when a Chinese swimmer was found to have several vials of hGH while going through customs.

Most of the work on hGH's mechanism of action has been done on children who suffer from hypopituitarism. Administration of hGH to growth hormone-deficient children results in a positive nitrogen balance and the stimulation of skeletal and soft tissue growth (49). Metabolic effects include reduction of glucose and protein metabolism, stimulation of lipid mobilization from adipose tissue, and a net anti-insulin effect. This last effect most likely results by inhibiting the cellular uptake of glucose. It is important to note that there have been no well-controlled clinical trials demonstrating improvements in strength or endurance in healthy adults with normally functioning pituitary glands.

Although there have been studies of human growth hormone's effect on muscle, the data are conflicting (50–52). A series of animal experiments by Goldberg (53) concluded that hGH increased the basal metabolic rate of protein synthesis but that this was also determined by the amount of muscular work. Thus it has been difficult to determine hGH's ability to increase contractile elements and improve the performance of normal muscle in humans (48,49). Nonetheless, it does appear that the use of hGH in adults with acquired growth hormone deficiency does result in increased lean body mass, decreased fat mass, and increased basal metabolic rate (54).

At this point there are relatively few therapeutic indications for hGH. These include increasing the stature in hGH-deficient or growth-retarded children (55), use in growth failure with chronic renal failure, and acceleration of wound healing in selected populations. In addition, there has been interest in expanding the use of hGH in other areas, such as attenuating some of the changes associated with normal aging (56).

The therapeutic dose of hGH in deficiency states is 0.3 mg/kg/week, given in divided doses either daily or three times per week intramuscularly. While there is little information about dosing regimens in athletes, there have been reports of athletes consuming 20 times the dosage recommended for deficiency states (4), perhaps up to 20 mg/day. hGH is not inexpensive; it is estimated that for an athlete desiring a minimal ergogenic effect, the cost of an 8-week supply of hGH would be approximately $1000–1500 (4).

The issue of adverse reactions with hGH is a difficult area for discussion. Observations of side effects of growth hormone have been made in patients with acromegaly, a disease of excessive growth hormone production. The problem is that the symptoms of acromegaly occur in patients with relatively small increases in hGH that are compounded over many years to decades. Patients with acromegaly may have daily production rates of hGH as low as 1.9 mg/day, slightly over the normal rate of 0.4–1 mg/day. This is in contradistinction to an athlete taking 20 mg/day over a relatively short time period. It is difficult to determine whether the severe effects of acromegaly would apply to an athlete in this situation. Nevertheless, complications of acromegaly include diabetes, arthritis, myopathy, and typical coarsening in the face, hands, and feet (49). Additional effects include fluid retention, arthralgias, gynecomastia, and possibly carpal tunnel syndrome (57).

There have also been anecdotal reports of adverse reactions to hGH, including the well-publicized case of professional football player Lyle Alzado, who attributed his central nervous system lymphoma in part to the use of massive amounts of hGH. In addition, Creutzfeldt-

Jakob disease, caused by a slow virus, has occurred from the use of hGH derived from cadaveric pituitary glands (58). While the use of recombinant hGH should eliminate the possibility of Creutzfeldt-Jakob, athletes may obtain hGH from black market sources in which the purity or source is unknown. This highlights the dangers of obtaining drugs in this manner, especially in the case of a substance that is given parenterally.

While the relatively high cost and intramuscular route of administration may deter hGH use, its inability to be detected by traditional urine drug testing and perceived ergogenic benefits make hGH a popular drug for athletes. The IOC has made the development of a reliable testing procedure for hGH a priority for the coming year. Until that time, the sports medicine clinician should rely on clinical suspicion based on history and potential adverse effects and should educate athletes about the potential problems associated with hGH use.

BLOOD DOPING AND ERYTHROPOIETIN

While athletes engaged in power sports have experimented with AAS and growth hormone to increase strength, endurance athletes have searched for ways to increase aerobic capacity. It has been known for quite some time that aerobic capacity is dependent on the amount of oxygen that can be delivered to exercising muscle. To this end, athletes have attempted various methods of increasing the oxygen carrying capacity of the blood, mainly by boosting hemoglobin. While some of these methods are legal and ethical (e.g., training at altitude, iron supplements), there have also been unscrupulous attempts to increase Vo_2max.

One of the earliest methods of increasing red blood cell mass was through the process of blood doping (59). Reports in the medical literature describe the infusion of 2000 mL of freshly transfused blood from matched donors to armed forces personnel in 1947 (60). Subsequent well-conducted studies confirmed a direct correlation between increased red blood cell mass and Vo_2max (61). Follow-up examination of blood doping in elite runners as compared to controls confirmed an improvement in maximal oxygen consumption, increased total exercise time, and increased hemoglobin concentration (62).

The advent of improved methods of blood storage permitted athletes to artificially increase red blood cell mass by extracting autologous blood, concentrating the red blood cells, then reinfusing them after reequilibration had occurred. Alternatively, athletes could obtain the same results with a transfusion of matched donor packed red blood cells. For a variety of reasons this type of blood doping had limited popularity and probably peaked in the 1984 Olympics when several U.S. cyclists admitted to blood doping during the Olympic Games. While autologous blood doping does not represent a prohibited substance, it is an example of a prohibited method under the IOC (59). Despite its prohibition, what limited the appeal of blood doping was the difficulty involved in transfusions, the need for proper storage, the incidence of transfusion reactions, and the risk of infectious complications using donor blood. Finally, the development of erythropoietin in the late 1980s rendered blood doping little more than a historical footnote.

Erythropoietin (EPO) is a sialic acid–containing hormone that enhances erythropoiesis by stimulating the formation of proerythroblasts and release of reticulocytes from the bone marrow. It is mainly secreted by the kidneys, and serum levels of EPO are inversely related to the number of circulating red blood cells (63). The direct physiologic effects were further supported by Eschbach and Winearls in 1987, demonstrating the efficacy of recombinant human erythropoietin (r-HuEPO). R-HuEPO stimulates red cell production within days, and effects can be seen for as long as 3–4 weeks (64). Theoretically, r-HuEPO can increase Vo_2max by 10% (64). In data reported at the International Olympic Committee World Congress on Sports Science, marathon runners showed a 10% increase in exercise endurance during a 6-week test after administration of r-HuEPO (65).

Issues regarding use of EPO use as an ergogenic aid came to the forefront with the unexplained deaths of 18 Dutch and Belgian cyclists between 1987 and 1990 (66). A theory on their deaths was that the possible use of erythropoietin in combination with the dehydration often seen in endurance athletes produced severely increased blood viscosity. This resulted in vascular thrombosis in the cardiovascular or cerebral circulation. Suspicions about the use of EPO in professional cyclists were further confirmed by the confiscation of large amounts of EPO from several cycling teams during the 1998 Tour de France race. Other associated adverse effects include hyperkalemia, iron deficiency, and risks associated with the administration of intravenous medications.

Erythropoietin has been used in conjunction with other performance-enhancing substances. In the NCAA data from 1997, 2.5% of anabolic steroid users reported concomitant use of erythropoietin (10); however, exact estimates of usage are difficult to make because testing methods are limited. The reasons for this are that the quantity of r-HuEPO excreted in the urine is small, it is rapidly metabolized, and its effects (up to 6 weeks) greatly outlast its detectability. An assay that uses antibody identification of exogenous EPO but does not bind endogenous EPO is currently in the testing phase (67).

Erythropoietin use poses a serious dilemma for the sports medicine physician because of its difficulty of detection and potentially serious complications. Athletes should be informed of the high-risk nature of erythropoietin use and of the relative paucity of data on the use of erythropoietin in combination with other ergogenic substances. In addition, most endurance athletes have relatively low hematocrits due to an expanded plasma volume, and it is unclear what happens when this physiologic response to exercise is altered.

SYMPATHOMIMETIC AMINES

Athletes seek ergogenic effects from a variety of compounds. These include the type found on the black market, such as AAS and growth hormone, but also relatively easy-to-find sympathomimetic amines. Sympathomimetic drugs act either directly or indirectly on the sympathetic nervous system, mimicking the effects of naturally occurring catecholamines. Their action is largely dependent on the selectivity of the receptors on which they act: alpha, beta 1, or beta 2. These effects and examples of drugs in each class are summarized in Table 10–4 (68). Owing to these varied effects, sympathomimetic amines are an example of drugs that can be used for ergogenic, recreational, or therapeutic purposes and are a challenge to sports organizations.

Alpha effects predominantly result in smooth muscle contraction, that is, vasoconstriction. Beta 1 effects include stimulation of intracellular cAMP, increased heart rate, and increased cardiac contractility with the resultant increase in stroke volume. Beta 2 effects include smooth muscle relaxation, bronchodilation, and stimulation of skeletal muscle (68). Examples of sympathomimetic amines include those commonly found in over-the-counter cold medications, such as phenylpropanolamine, phenylephrine, pseudoephedrine, and ephedrine. Other sympathomimetics include the beta-agonists albuterol, bitolterol, orciprenaline, rimiterol, and clenbuterol.

The use of sympathomimetics to improve athletic performance is not a new phenomenon. Gladiators purportedly used sympathomimeticlike stimulants in 600 B.C. in the Circus Maximus to ward off fatigue (69). The discovery of epinephrine in 1899 allowed researchers to better study and understand the effects of sympathomimetic amines on performance. While studies on horses and livestock demonstrated improvements in cardiorespiratory function with sympathomimetic amines (70–74), research on humans has provided somewhat mixed results. Despite experiments demonstrating increases in cardiorespiratory function (75), significant increases in athletic performance have not been well substantiated (76–78). Regardless, sufficient data were presented to place sympathomimetic amines on the IOC's list of banned substances. There was concern (later proved unfounded) that the inclusion of professional hockey players in the 1998 Winter Olympics would result in disqualifications due to these substances. The most famous case involving sympathomimetic amines remains Rick DeMont, the U.S. swimmer who lost his gold medal because of a positive test for ephedrine in 1972.

Are sympathomimetic amines used by athletes to improve performance? The NCAA 1997 survey of substance use and abuse reported that 3.5% of athletes had used ephedrine in the preceding 12 months (10). (Note that ephedrine was not banned by the NCAA at that time.) This was three times greater than the number who admitted using anabolic steroids during the same time period. Of significance is that 50% of those using ephedrine stated that their main reason for use was to improve athletic performance. Interestingly, men's skiing and wrestling had the greatest usage rate: 18.8% and 10.4%, respectively. According to the survey, ephedrine use did not begin in college; over 40% reported their initial use at the high school level or earlier (10).

Sympathomimetics are widely available for a variety of therapeutic uses, including nonemergent treatment of allergic reactions, asthma, hypotension, atrioventricular block, nasal congestion, and allergic rhinitis (79). Adverse reactions depend on the primary effect of the

---

TABLE 10–4. *Alpha, beta 1, and beta 2 receptor effects*

Alpha 1

Vascular smooth muscle contraction
Increase in skeletal muscle tone
Pupillary dilator muscle contraction (dilates pupils)
Pilomotor smooth muscle contraction (erects hair)
Glycogenolysis
Weak positive ionotrope (increase force of heart contraction)
Increase in blood pressure
Increase ion total peripheral resistance
Examples: phenylephrine, methoxamine, ephedrine

Beta 1

Strong positive ionotrope (increase force of heart contraction)
Strong positive chronotrope (increase rate of heart contraction)
Activation of lipolysis
Increase in blood pressure
Examples: norepinephrine, dobutamine, prenalterol, epinephrine*

Beta 2

Promotion of smooth muscle relaxation (respiratory, uterine, vascular)
Promotion of potassium uptake in skeletal muscle
Activation of glycogenolysis
Seak positive ionotrope
Moderate positive chronotrope
Examples: albuterol, terbutaline, metaproterenol, clenbuterol

* Significant crossover receptor effects.
From Weiner N. Norepinephrine, epinephrine, and the sympathomimetic amines. In: Gilman AG, Goodman LS. *Pharmacological basis of therapeutics,* 7th ed. New York: Macmillan, 1985:145–180.

drug (alpha, beta 1, or beta 2) and include anxiety, palpitations, tremulousness, epigastric distress, insomnia, and sometimes drowsiness (79). There has also been increased concern among recreational drug abuse specialists about pseudoephedrine, which can be synthesized to the highly addictive drug methamphetamine. Finally, many of the sympathomimetic amines are available as "diet" drugs and have the potential for abuse in sports such as wrestling and women's gymnastics in which weight control is an issue and among athletes with issues regarding body image.

A particular beta 2 agonist, clenbuterol, deserves special consideration because of its proposed anabolic as well as sympathomimetic effects. Available since 1977 in Europe and Mexico for the treatment of asthma, its use resulted in the disqualification of six Olympic athletes in the 1992 Barcelona Olympics. Athletes' interest in the anabolic effects of clenbuterol, a beta 2 agonist used in the treatment of asthma, was a surprise to many in the field of drug abuse.

Most of the data on the anabolic effects of clenbuterol are derived from animal studies. Livestock treated with clenbuterol demonstrated increased muscle mass and decreased fatty deposits (80). Rats demonstrated reduced muscle wasting (81) and decreased net bone loss (82) when treated with clenbuterol. Clenbuterol appears to affect skeletal muscle in three ways: (1) inducing a true hypertrophy rather than hyperplasia, (2) shifting muscle fiber type from type 1 slow-twitch fibers to type 2 fast-twitch fibers, and (3) increasing the glycolytic capacity of the muscle as a whole (83,84). Animal studies seem to indicate that these effects occur in dosages far above the typical "therapeutic" dose of clenbuterol that is used in bronchodilation. It also seems that for clenbuterol to have an anabolic effect, it must be taken by the oral, rather than inhaled, route. While the adverse reactions reported with clenbuterol are those typically encountered with a beta 2 agonist, there are no data on side effects at the higher dosages used by athletes.

Sympathomimetic amines are detectable with current drug-testing methods and are banned by the IOC. The exceptions are inhaled beta-agonist drugs when they are used for the treatment of specific conditions, such as asthma. Except for ephedrine, the NCAA does not prohibit the use of sympathomimetic amines or beta-agonists. However, all organizations do strictly bar the use of clenbuterol. There has been debate about the exception made for inhaled beta-agonists and that these may in fact represent an ergogenic aid. The data so far have been inconclusive regarding the ergogenic and anabolic effects of inhaled beta-agonists on nonasthmatic users (84,85), and these are allowed so that asthmatics may compete fairly and safely. Ongoing investigation suggests the existence of subclasses of beta-agonists with anabolic, "nutrition partitioning" properties (86), and insofar as these effects extend to inhaled substances, changes to the current standards may need to be enacted.

COCAINE

Athletes are not immune from the temptations of recreational drugs that are available in the general population. This became quite apparent following the increased accessibility and usage of cocaine in the 1970s and 1980s. The mixture of sports and cocaine became so widespread that the *New York Times* in 1987 declared, "Cocaine has probably joined rotator-cuff injuries, torn ligaments and broken bones as a potential occupational hazard for athletes" (87). This statement reflected data from the 1985 NCAA survey on drug use, which revealed that a staggering 17% of NCAA athletes reported having used cocaine in the previous year. Given these statistics, it was not surprising that 1986 saw the cocaine-related deaths of Cleveland Browns football player Don Rogers and Maryland basketball player Len Bias.

Cocaine is a naturally occurring alkaloid derived from the leaves of the erythroxylon coca plant (88). Archaeologists have discovered evidence that cocaine use dates back to at least 3000 B.C. (89). It was purportedly used by the ancient Incas as both a reward and a stimulant to runners who carried messages between villages (90). Cocaine is easily absorbed and can be taken by several routes, including intravenous, intranasal, and pulmonary. Since the discovery of cocaine, it has enjoyed cyclical peaks in popularity, the extended current epidemic being one such episode. The major difference in the 1990s is the development of "crack" cocaine, a cheap form of purified free alkaloid cocaine that can be ignited and inhaled to produce a rapid effect, similar to intravenous injection. The combination of low cost with a quick, intense high is particularly addictive.

The prevalence of cocaine use among athletes seems to be declining. The 1997 NCAA survey of drug use and abuse demonstrated that cocaine use within the past 12 months was 1.5% (10). According to the study, reported cocaine use was independent of ethnic origin, sport, or gender. The study also revealed that cocaine was primarily a recreational drug among athletes in that only 3.9% reported using cocaine to improve athletic performance. Cocaine use also begins before college, with 45% reporting their initial use in high school or earlier.

The effects of the drug are many (89). At its most basic level, cocaine acts by increasing the release and blocking the reuptake of norepinephrine from neurons. This increased availability of norepinephrine and epinephrine leads to euphoria, hypertension, and tachycardia and lowers the threshold for seizures and ventricular arrhythmias. Cocaine may also cause hyperglycemia, hyperthermia, and increased peripheral reflex speed (91). Additionally, the practice of smoking crack cocaine can damage the lungs and cause bronchiolitis obliterans (89). Of course, intravenous cocaine use carries the attendant risks of infection, such as hepatitis B and HIV infection. The only current therapeutic use for cocaine is in topical anesthesia.

Concern about health effects is a potential area for educating and preventing athletes from using cocaine. Adverse reactions on which athlete education can be based include ventricular dysrhythmias, coronary vasospasm, myocardial infarction, psychosis, depression, seizures, and death. Athletes may be interested in the fact that a higher incidence of myocardial events have been reported with the combined use of cocaine and anabolic-androgenic steroids over time (92).

Cocaine clearly demonstrates that athletes are not immune from recreational drug use and that drug education is imperative. Despite the obvious, sometimes fatal effects of cocaine, its use continues in the athletic population. This was demonstrated by the 1997 arrest of professional baseball player Tony Phillips for the use of cocaine. Cocaine can be a difficult problem to recognize, as the NCAA Drug Survey demonstrated. Most athletes do not use cocaine with their teammates, and only 1% reported that their coaches were aware of their use (10). As long as cocaine is available in the general population, it will continue to plague athletics.

ALCOHOL

There is little debate that alcohol is the most heavily used drug in athletes (10,93–95). It is also the leading cause of social, legal, and personal problems in this population. This information can be confirmed through studies or by a casual glance at the daily sports page. The 1997 NCAA study revealed that 80% of athletes surveyed had consumed alcohol in the previous year with 40% admitting to drinking more than six drinks at a sitting (10). Again, this illustrates that involvement in sports does not provide immunity from recreational drug use and that athletes reflect the pattern of the general population. Alcohol abuse is the leading drug problem in the United States and is responsible for at least 200,000 deaths per year (96). The general properties of alcohol are well known and are beyond the scope of this chapter. This section will focus on alcohol as it specifically applies to athletes.

Alcohol has been a part of human existence for thousands of years. It has even been considered an ergogenic aid at times and was known as the "elixir of life" in the Middle Ages (97). While there still remains some controversy about the health benefits of low-dose alcohol in the prevention of heart disease, the deleterious effects of alcohol on athletic performance are well known. The American College of Sports Medicine (ACSM) issued a position statement with regard to alcohol and exercise that summarized the literature on this subject (98). It states that the acute ingestion of alcohol has a deleterious effect on many psychomotor skills, including reaction times, hand-eye coordination, accuracy, balance, and complex coordination. In addition, alcohol does not substantially influence physiologic parameters such as VO_2max, respiratory dynamics, or cardiac function. Alcohol also does not improve muscular work and decreases athletic performance. The ACSM position paper also states that acute alcohol ingestion may impair temperature regulation during prolonged exercise in a cold environment. Finally, long-term use of alcohol can be toxic to striated muscle in a dose-dependent fashion (99). Overall, it is quite clear that alcohol has negative ergogenic effects.

With the use of alcohol being extremely prevalent in both the athletic and general population, research has attempted to delineate whether there are any differences in consumption patterns. Several comparison studies have examined this question among intercollegiate athletes (99–102). While the research revealed that most college athletes drink alcohol at rates similar to those of their nonathlete peers, some important differences were discovered. Nattiv and colleagues found that athletes tend to consume more drinks at a sitting than nonathletes and to drink in more of a binge manner (102). There was also the disturbing trend found in Leichliter and colleagues' study that not only did athletes appear to drink more than their nonathlete peers, but the self-identified team leaders from the athlete cohort drank significantly more than other athletes in the study (101).

Further information from these studies revealed that athletes also were more likely to engage in other forms of risk-taking behavior, such as riding in a car with an intoxicated driver. The athletes tended to have other risky habits as compared to their nonathlete peers, including not wearing seat belts, not using motorcycle or bicycle helmets, having unprotected sex, and having multiple sexual partners, and were more likely to engage in physical fights (102). It is clear to anyone who has worked with collegiate athletes that these latter behaviors are magnified and can have disastrous consequences when combined with the use of alcohol. The fact that athletes tend to binge drink can have long-term consequences as well. A 1997 study of men (average age: 52) found that drinking more than six beers at a session was associated with an increase in all-cause mortality (103).

The challenge for health care professionals is trying to determine which athletes are at risk for alcohol problems. As is illustrated above, the consumption of alcohol is a somewhat normative behavior in the collegiate athlete population. It can be extremely difficult to ascertain which athletes are either at risk, or have a current problem with alcohol. For a variety of reasons athletic organizations do not test for alcohol. The exceptions are the

TABLE 10–5. *The CAGE questionnaire*

1. Have you ever felt you needed to **C**ut down on your alcohol intake?
2. Have you felt **A**nnoyed by criticism about your alcohol intake?
3. Have you experienced **G**uilt about your alcohol intake?
4. Have you had an early morning or **E**ye opener drink?

"Yes" answers to two or more of the CAGE screening questions should alert the examiner to the need for further evaluation.

From Buchsbaum DG, et al. Screening for alcohol abuse using the CAGE scores and likelihood ratios. *Ann Intern Med* 1991;115:774–777.

NCAA and the IOC, which test for alcohol but only in the shooting events. However, international federations may perform breath or blood alcohol levels in suspicious cases of acute intoxication. While it can be fairly difficult to recognize a person with alcohol problems, one clue is the persistent use of alcohol in the face of serious negative consequences. These consequences can be of a physiologic, psychologic, legal, or social nature.

A great deal of effort has been directed at the early identification of alcohol problems in order to prevent alcoholism and associated problems, such as drunk driving. Several measures have been designed to help assess alcohol problems including the Perceived Benefit of Drinking Scale, the Children of Alcoholics Test, and the Michigan Alcoholism Screening Test (104). Perhaps the simplest and quickest screening tool is the CAGE questionnaire, which consists of four questions; it is summarized in Table 10–5 (105).

Once the identification is made, professionals with experience in the treatment of alcohol problems should be utilized. Education and prevention, however, continue to be the key to limiting the devastating effects that are associated with alcohol abuse.

MARIJUANA

While there is considerable debate among sporting organizations regarding limitations and sanctions about marijuana use, it is quite clear that marijuana use is prevalent among athletes in nearly all sports (10,93). There are almost daily reminders of this in the newspaper accounts of professional athletes possessing and using marijuana. One of the more notable stories of 1998 was during the Winter Olympics at Nagano, when a Canadian snow boarder was asked to forfeit his gold medal after testing positive for (and admittedly using) marijuana. Following an appeal, the IOC later reinstated his medal on a technicality. Of note was the IOC's position that while illegal, marijuana was unlikely to have enhanced athletic performance.

Marijuana is a naturally occurring cannabinoid containing the active ingredient Δ^9-tetrahydrocannabinol (THC). It has been used by many cultures for centuries for its mind-altering properties (106). It has been estimated that over 43 million Americans have tried marijuana, and at least 17 million are regular users (107). The 1997 study of NCAA athletes' substance use reported that over 25% of athletes had used marijuana within the past 12 months, and over half of those reported continued use (10). Remarkably, over 70% of those athletes who reported use stated that their use began in high school or before. When asked their main reason for use, 61% reported that it was for recreational or social purposes, 34% reported that it made them feel good, and 0.6% reported that their main reason for use was improved athletic performance (10).

Other investigators have reported similar prevalence among athletes. Kokotailo and colleagues reported marijuana utilization to be 11% among male college-level athletes within 30 days of the survey and 4% among female athletes (94). Nattiv and Puffer reported a marijuana utilization rate of 20% in college athletes (108), and Nattiv, Puffer, and Green, in a multicenter trial, found similar results (102). Most of these studies reflect that when it comes to marijuana use, athletes are similar to their nonathlete peers. This fairly high prevalence is evidence of the widespread availability and use of marijuana in this age group.

Physiologically, THC affects a variety of organ systems. Cardiovascular actions include tachycardia, which can be blocked by beta-blockers, and increased supine systolic blood pressure (97). The CNS is affected by impaired motor coordination, decreased short-term memory, difficulty concentrating, and decline in work performance (97). Effects on the male reproduction system include decreased plasma testosterone levels, gynecomastia, and oligospermia. Overall, marijuana has negative effects on exercise by reducing both attainable $V_{O_2}max$ and maximal exercise performance, as well as inhibiting sweating, which may lead to an increase in core body temperature (109).

THC is approved in the United States as an antiemetic, antiglaucoma agent, an analgesic for refractory pain, and an appetite stimulant. The latter is mostly in conjunction with chemotherapy, management of metastatic disease, or wasting associated with HIV infection. Although medical THC is a schedule I drug, several states have attempted to make it easier for patients to obtain marijuana for medicinal purposes.

Secondary to its high deposition in lipid, THC can be detected by gas chromatography/mass spectroscopy for as long as 4 weeks or more after exposure. While passive inhalation of marijuana may result in a positive test, sporting organizations generally set limits at 12–15 ng/mL to avoid this scenario. Marijuana is listed as an illegal substance and is banned and tested for by the NCAA. Marijuana is listed under the IOC's class of substances that are subject to certain restrictions, meaning that it can be tested for at the request of the IOC, a National Governing Body, and/or an International Federation. Proponents of maintaining the current policy cite marijuana's lack of performance-enhancing effects, although some have argued that it may aid in sports that require great steadiness and concentration (110). Those who support testing and sanctions cite the fact that marijuana is an illegal drug in most countries, the fact that athletes are often seen as role models, and the potential long-term adverse effects of the drug. Regardless of these controversies, marijuana's use in both the general population and among athletes makes it incumbent on the sports medicine practitioner to be aware of its use and effects on the social, psychological, and performance parameters of athletes.

SMOKELESS TOBACCO

Smokeless tobacco use dates back to at least 1492 when it was introduced to Christopher Columbus by Native Americans and brought to Europe (111). Its popularity increased in the 1600s and 1700s as smokeless tobacco gained notoriety for medicinal and stimulant purposes. It continued to gain appeal in the 1800s as plug tobacco and snuff were popularized in the United States (111). Popularity among athletes has concomitantly grown, and smokeless tobacco is now commonly seen on the field or in the dugout in the arena of sport (112).

While smokeless tobacco use may be overshadowed by the study of more popularized ergogenic substances, the relatively high use of smokeless tobacco among athletes is undisputed in the medical literature. Nattiv, Puffer, and Green, in a study of nearly 2,300 college athletes, found that 17% of athletes reported smokeless tobacco use within the past 12 months, compared with 5% among nonathlete controls (102). Anderson and colleagues found even higher results, with 27% of college athletes reporting use within the past 12 months and half of those reporting regular use (113). Forman and colleagues (93) and Kokotailo and colleagues (94) have found similar rates of usage among collegiate athletes, and a study of professional baseball reported that 34% of professional baseball players used smokeless tobacco on a regular basis (112). The 1997 NCAA survey (10) reported that 22.5% of all athletes used smokeless tobacco, with a 45% rate among the collegiate baseball players surveyed. Of interest, fewer than 1% reported performance enhancement as their main reason for consumption (10), and fewer than 10% of major league baseball players who use smokeless tobacco reported that its use resulted in either improved concentration or performance (114). This is supported by the literature, which reveals neither neuromuscular performance enhancement nor changes in reaction time with the use of smokeless tobacco (112).

On the basis of its mechanism of action, smokeless tobacco acts as a short-acting stimulant (115). Nicotine, the active ingredient, readily crosses the blood–brain barrier and binds acetylcholine receptors at autonomic ganglia, the adrenal medulla, and neuromuscular junctions and in the central nervous system. Stimulation of central nicotinic receptors results in release of acetylcholine, norepinephrine, dopamine, serotonin, vasopressin, growth hormone, and ACTH. At low doses this results in sympathetic discharge with increases in heart rate and blood pressure. While these effects are significant, tolerance develops to the hemodynamic effects (115).

Although smokeless tobacco is often portrayed as an innocuous form of tobacco, it does carry significant health risks. This was recently illustrated by professional baseball player Brett Butler's diagnosis of tonsillar cancer. Smokeless tobacco affects the oral cavity and is associated with a 50-fold increase in oral carcinomas, 240% incidence of dental caries, increased incidence of significant gingival disease, and the development of leukoplakia. In addition, smokeless tobacco causes increased myocardial oxygen demand, increased sodium load (added for flavoring), and addiction (111). While most athletes would not consider using cigarettes, smokeless tobacco can yield serum nicotine levels in the same range as cigarette dependent smokers (116).

As with any addictive substance, controlling the use of smokeless tobacco is a difficult task. There are ongoing studies using nicotine replacement systems to aid in cessation programs. Educating athletes on the health consequences of its use and dispelling fallacies regarding its benefits may help to reduce the use of smokeless tobacco in sport. Several sports organizations have taken steps to eliminate smokeless tobacco during competition. The NCAA has passed the most far-reaching ban and prohibits the use of smokeless tobacco by athletes, coaches, and officials during all competitions. The intent of a ban is to discourage athletes from using smokeless tobacco, as well as to reduce the potential for negatively influencing children.

MISCELLANEOUS SUBSTANCES

Mesocarb

N-phenylcarbomoyl-3-B-phenylisopropyl-sydnonimine, or mesocarb, has been used since the 1970s as a psycho-stimulating drug in the treatment of asthenic conditions (117). Its role as an ergogenic drug deserves consideration in two areas: its effect on circulating dopamine levels and its effects on testosterone production.

Fredholm, after confirming its psycho-stimulatory effects, examined its effect on dopamine and found no increase in dopamine secretion. There was, however, a marked increase in dopamine reuptake inhibition (118). In a further study of its psychostimulatory effects, Mashkovskii and colleagues showed increased levels of circulating catecholamines secondary to oral consumption of mesocarb in a dose-response fashion (119).

As mesocarb use grew, examination of its effect on the hypothalamic-pituitary-gonadal axis were undertaken. Specifically, its effects on LH and serum testosterone were examined. Although much of the work on mesocarb has been done using rat models, when doses of 10 and 20 mg/kg were ingested, they resulted in decreased LH and testosterone levels (117). When mesocarb was taken in combination with theophylline, the stimulatory effects remained, but the effects on the hypothalamic-pituitary-gonadal axis were not present (117).

In summary, given the dopaminergic and catacholaminergic qualities of mesocarb, a performance-enhancing function in athletics may exist. However, human performance outcome studies, as well as examination of adverse effects in human subjects, will be required to better understand its effects and use as an ergogenic aid.

Bromantan

At the 1996 Atlanta Olympics, IOC drug testing revealed a small number of athletes with urine drug tests that were positive for a substance known as Bromantan. At that time there were only four animal and two human studies on Bromantan, all in the Russian literature. In 1995 Sergeeva and colleagues found increased time to exhaustion in exercising rats treated with oral Bromantan (120). In 1993 Sedov and Lukicheva, using factory workers as human subjects, reported that oral Bromantan was associated with a higher physiologic tolerance to an environment of high heat and carbon monoxide (121). In 1995 Badyshtov and colleagues studied the thermoprotective effects of Bromantan at various levels of overheating and found a smaller rise in core body temperature in subjects treated with oral Bromantan (122).

If Bromantan has performance-enhancing properties, the Russian literature suggests two mechanisms. The first suggests that Bromantan's effect on the central nervous system by modulation of dopamine, serotonin, or norepinephrine could effect perception of pain and fatigue. The second cites a direct thermoprotective effect by enhancing heat dissipation (120,122). In 1998 Vigil, Catlin, and Puffer examined both core body temperature and performance outcomes in response to Bromantan therapy using a placebo-controlled rat model and found differences between Bromantan and placebo groups that were substantial enough to warrant subsequent investigation (123). No known side effects of the drug have been cited in the literature to date. Bromantan and the related compound carphedon are currently banned by the IOC.

Creatine Monohydrate

Creatine has become one of the most widely used performance-enhancing supplements for short-term high-intensity exercise and increasing overall mass. Participants in ball sports (e.g., football and baseball) and strength-oriented athletes are often noted as frequent users of creatine. This supplement is discussed in detail in two chapters of the companion volume of this series (124,125).

Androstenedione

In the search for more "natural" anabolic-androgenic support, athletes have been turning to testosterone precursors in an attempt to increase naturally occurring testosterone. If more of the precursors are available, then perhaps more testosterone will be available and the athlete might realize the anabolic-androgenic effects of increased testosterone. The most visible of these is androstenedione ("andro"), which practically became a household word when it was disclosed that Mark McGwire was taking this supplement during his record-breaking home run season of 1998.

Androstenedione is a precursor to testosterone that is produced by the adrenal glands and the gonads. It is converted to testosterone by the action of 17-β-hydroxysteroid dehydrogenase by most tissues. However, this conversion can also lead to increased estrogen levels. Thus, increasing androstendione may lead to an increase in both testosterone and estrogen. One unit of androstendione does not lead to one unit of testosterone, so large amounts of the precursor must be ingested to affect an increase in testosterone. When reading studies of any precursor supplement, researchers must consider the dosage and dosing schedule, and in many projects the amount ingested is relatively low.

There are other anabolic-androgenic supplements available over the counter. For example, androstenediol and dhea (dehydroepiandrosterone) also are potentially converted to testosterone. The 19-nor products (19-norandrostenedione and 19-norandrostenediol) are both precursors of nandrolone. These are all sold as nutritional supplements and are significant because most of the highly publicized positive drug tests reported by the NCAA (personal communication, NCAA) and other sporting organizations over the past two years are secondary to supplements, specifically the 19-norandro products.

Much of the support for the use of androstenedione is based on an early report on two women whose testosterone levels tripled in response to treatment but returned back to normal in only a few hours (126). Recently, five papers have been published that, on the surface, only confuse the issue because two of them show increases in testosterone while three of them fail to show any increase. Although the use of these supplements has exceeded well done scientific studies, there are a few recent studies in the medical literature. Because this is a new area of study, results have been variable and difficult to interpret.

Wallace et al. (127) compared androstenedione and dehydroepiandrosterone (DHEA) versus a placebo. Strength-training subjects ingested 100 mg/day for 12 weeks. Blood, body composition, and performance variable were assessed pre-, mid-, and post-study. While there were small increases in strength and lean mass in the experimental groups, the differences were not statistically different from the placebo group. King et al. (128), in a randomized control trial, looked at acute (i.e., single-dose) and long-term responses to androstenedione ingestion (300 mg/day). Blood data [testosterone, estrogen, leutenizing hormone (LH), follicle-stimulating hormone (FSH), liver function, lipids], muscle (fiber cross sectional area), body composition, and strength were studied in strength-training men. Although acute ingestion led to increases in serum androstenedione, no changes were seen in LH, FSH, or free or total testosterone. Chronic use showed the same pattern, yet estradiol and estrone both increased significantly. Neither increases in strength nor changes in muscle fiber were different between the groups. HDL-cholesterol declined over the eight-week project in the supplement group only. This was followed by Earnest and co-workers (129), who looked at the acute response to a 200-mg dose and showed that testosterone was elevated in the 90 minutes after ingestion. The subjects of Ballantyne and colleagues (130) ingested 200 mg/day of androstendione (versus a placebo) for two days, and their blood was sampled for three days total in this double-blind crossover trial. Exercise increased testosterone with no difference between the supplement and the placebo. However, androstendione did show transient increase in estradiol. Finally, Leder and co-workers (131) randomized subjects to a 100 mg/day, 300 mg/day of androstenedione or placebo groups in their week-long project. Blood was sampled repeatedly on days 1 and 7, while a single sample of blood was drawn on days 2 through 6. On day 7, testosterone was elevated in the high dose group while estradiol was elevated in both experimental groups. Areas under the curve for the 7-day plots of testosterone and estradiol again showed significantly elevated testosterone in the high-dose group and estradiol in both groups.

On the surface, it would appear that the recent literature is equivocal on the use of androstenedione. However, as with any hormone study, a closer look at the data is called for. Changes in blood levels of any hormone can be due to increased production or decreased elimination, and none of these studies addressed the turnover question other than to point out the short half-life of the compounds in question. Another way to look at differences is the actual levels reported. Is the "elevated" group really elevated, or was the control level low to being with? This opens the door to the question of nonresponders. With many supplements, if the subject has normal levels of a variable, then little or no response may be seen. However, if the subject is low on the variable of interest, then any elevation just might be significant. That appears to be the case here. In the studies that show some effect of androstenedione, the free testosterone levels reported by Earnest (129) were on the order of 25% below that of King (128). In Leder (131), the only group that showed a significant increase in testosterone was the 300 mg/day group. Their initial levels were over 40% below that reported by King, and their peak levels were the same as reported by King. Similar comparisons with the other papers reporting a nonresponse are possible. Therefore, the question of the effectiveness of androstendione seems to depend on the initial level of testosterone. Remember, the initial report (126) was on women.

There are at least five other factors to be considered when interpreting the literature. First, it is well accepted that anabolic-androgenic steroids are most effective in experienced weight lifters (23,30). As such, the experience of the subjects in weight training should be considered. Untrained subjects (such as those studied by King) might be expected to gain strength from beginning a weight-training program, and possible additive effects of a supplement might be lost in the initial gain in strength. The reports of Wallace and of Earnest used subjects already participating in a training program that included resistance exercise. Second, the general feeling on strength gain is that initial gains in strength are the result of increased recruitment of muscle fibers in parallel. Later gains in strength are associated with an increase in fiber area and overall muscle mass. The shift from recruitment to hypertrophy should be expected to be quite variable from one person to the next. Thus, the length of any training study should be questioned. An eight-week study (as in King) might be too brief to realize any real effects on muscle mass. Third, aging has well-known effects on skeletal muscle and the hormonal mileau. Young subjects were studied in all but studies but that by Wallace, who used men 40–60 years of age. Fourth, the method of analysis needs to be scrutinized. All these recent studies reported blood levels of testosterone and precursors. Androstenedione has a very short half-life and could be rapidly metabolized to testosterone. Peak levels of testosterone from androstenedione ingestion occur quickly and last only a short time (the half-life of testosterone is only 60–80 minutes). Blood sampling would need to be timed to the peak level of response. Urine sampling might be the better method for such brief and transient changes in testosterone. Finally, the ingestion schedule (and its interaction with detection schedule) should be critiqued. Would a single dose per day (Leder, Earnest, King, Ballantyne) or twice per day (Wallace) be sufficient to chronically elevate testosterone levels to make any real influence on skeletal muscle when the higher levels of testosterone are only for a short time? Also, consider the length of time the subjects ingested the precursor. It is difficult to come to a conclusion when the duration of supplement use was only one dose (Earnest), two days (Ballantyne), one week (Leder), eight weeks (King), or three months (Wallace).

Another concern is the decrease in HDL-cholesterol that King (128) noted as well as the consistent reporting of increases in estradiol and its consequences (e.g., gynocomastia, cardiovascular disease, breast cancer). Also, all studies demonstrate an increase in serum androstenedione and elevations that have been linked to prostate and pancreatic cancer (see King, page 2027). Thus, on closer scrutiny, it appears that androstenedione is only effective at bringing testosterone levels in men with low initial levels up to the levels seen in men with normal testosterone. And there might be health consequences to long-term use that have yet to be proven.

From a very practical standpoint, there have been many positive tests for both nandrolone metabolites and increased testosterone: epitestosterone ratio across nearly all sports, not just those normally associated with anabolic-androgenic steroid use. Athletes need to be alerted to the possibility of a positive drug test from these supplements, because androstenedione, androstenediol, DHEA, 19-norandrostenedione, and 19-norandrostenediol are banned by most sports organizations. It is impossible to determine from urine testing whether nandrolone metabolites came directly from nandrolone (19-nortestosterone) or from the 19-norandrostenedione supplements, both of which are banned by most sports organizations.

In general, ignorance of supplements has not been accepted by sports authorities as a defense for a positive drug test. Supplements are not subject to the same FDA regulations as are pharmaceuticals, and enforcement of labeling requirements has been lax. To avoid testing positive, all athletes should check with their institution or sports authority before ingesting any supplement.

CONCLUSION

This chapter has explored some of the common drugs of abuse by athletes at the current time. It is a given in this field that while the actual substances most certainly will change, the reasons for using them will not. It is incumbent on the sports medicine practitioner to be cognizant of changing trends so that athletes can be educated about effects and adverse reactions. This subject is complicated not only because of changing drugs, but also by the large incentives for athletic success and the addictive nature of many of the drugs.

In addition, the banned lists of sports governing bodies frequently change, and the team physician needs to be aware of which drugs in the pharmacopoeia are allowed in competition. The best advice that can be given to athletes who are subject to drug testing is that they should always check with their trainer, physician, coach, or sports organization before taking any substance, especially over-the-counter supplements. Nutritional supplements can contain banned substances, are poorly regulated, and have questionable purity. As was stated by the U.S. Olympic Committee, "the presence of a prohibited substance in the urine constitutes an offense, irrespective of the route of administration or the manner in which the prohibited substance came to be in the urine" (132).

REFERENCES

1. Loughton SV, Ruhline RO. Human strength and endurance responses to anabolic steroids and training. *J Sports Med Phys Fitness* 1977;17:285–296.
2. Cowart V. Steroids in sports: after four decades, time to return these genes to bottle? *JAMA* 1987;257:421–427.
3. Wadler G, Hainline B. *Anabolic steroids: drugs and the athlete.* Philadelphia, FA Davis, 1989:195.
4. Buckley WE, et al. Estimated prevalence of anabolic steroid use among male high school seniors. *JAMA* 260:3441–3445, 1988.
5. Yesalis CE, et al. Trends in anabolic-androgenic steroid use among adolescents. *Arch Pediatr Adolesc Med* 1997;151:1197–1205.
6. Johnston L, O'Malley P, Bachman J. *National survey results on drug use from the monitoring the future study.* Vol 1: *1989–1995* (NIH publication 96–4139). Washington, DC: National Institute on Drug Abuse, U.S. Department of Health and Human Services, 1996.
7. Kann L, Warren CW, Harris WA, et al. Youth risk behavior surveillance: United States, 1995. *MMWR CDC Surveill Summ* 1996;45:1–84.
8. National Institute on Drug Abuse. *National household survey on drug abuse, 1992* (Publication ADM 92-1887). Washington, DC: U.S. Dept of Health and Human Services, 1992.
9. DuRant R, Escobedo L, Heath G. Anabolic-steroid use, strength training, and multiple drug use among adolescents in the US. *Pediatrics* 1995;96:23–28.
10. 1997 *NCAA Study of Substance Use and Abuse Habits of College Student-Athletes.* Presented to the NCAA Committee on Competitive Safeguards and Medical Aspects of Sports, September 1997.
11. Tricker R, O'Neill LMR, Cook D. The incidence of anabolic steroid use among competitive bodybuilders. *J Drug Educ* 1989;19:313–325.
12. Landstrom M, Nilsson AL, Katzman PL, et al. Use of anabolic-androgenic steroids among bodybuilders: frequency and attitudes. *J Intern Med* 1990;227:407–411.
13. Delbeke FT, Desmet N, Debackere M. The abuse of doping agents in competing body builders in Flanders (1988–1993). *Int J Sports Med* 1995;16:66–70.
14. Marshall E. The drug of champions. *Science* 1988;242:183–184.
15. *Los Angeles Times* 1992 Nov 23:C8.
16. Windsor RE, Dumitru D. Anabolic steroid use by athletes. *Postgrad Med* 1988;84(4):37–49.
17. Haupt HA. Anabolic steroids and growth hormone. *Am J Sports Med* 21(3):468–474, 1993.
18. Pope HG, Katz DL. Psychiatric effects of anabolic steroids. *Psychiatr Ann* 1992;22:24–29.
19. Choi PYL, Parrott AC, Cowan DA. High dose anabolic steroids in strength athletes: effects upon hostility and aggression. *Human Psychopharmacol* 1990;5:349–356.

20. Ariel G. The effect of anabolic steroid upon skeletal muscle contractile force. *J Sports Med Phys Fitness* 1973;13:187–190.
21. Berg A, Keul J. Der einfluss von anabolen substanzen auf das verhalten der freien serumanimosauren von normalperson and scwerathleten in rule and bei korperarbeit. *Oester Z Sportsmed* 1974;4:11–18.
22. Hervey GR, Knibbs AV, Burkinshaw L, et al. Effects of methandienone on the performance and body composition of men undergoing athletic training. *Clin Sci* 1981;60:457–461.
23. Stamford BA, Moffatt R. Anabolic steroid effectiveness as an ergogenic aid to experienced weight trainers. *J Sports Med Phys Fitness* 1974;14:191–197.
24. Ward P. The effect of an anabolic steroid on strength and lean body mass. *Med Sci Sports Exerc* 1973;5:227–282.
25. Hervey GR. Are athletes wrong about anabolic steroids? *Br J Sports Med* 1975;9:74–77.
26. Johnson LD, et al. Effects of anabolic steroid treatment on endurance. *Med Sci Sports Exerc* 1975;7:287–289.
27. Loughton SV, Ruhline RO. Human strength and endurance responses to anabolic steroids and training. *J Sports Med Phys Fitness* 1977;27:285–296.
28. Stromme SB, Men HD, Aakvaag A. Effects of an androgenic anabolic steroid on strength development and plasma testosterone levels in normal males. *Med Sci Sports Exer* 1974;6:203–208.
29. Bhasin S, et al. The effects of supraphysiologic doses of testosterone on muscle size and strength in normal men. *N Engl J Med* 1996;335:1–7.
30. American College of Sports Medicine. *Stand on the use of anabolic-androgens steroids in sports.* Indianapolis: American College of Sports Medicine, 1984.
31. Elashoff JD, Jacknow AD, Shain SG, Braunstein GD. Effects of anabolic-androgenic steroids on muscular strength. *Ann Intern Med* 1991;115:387–393.
32. Council on Scientific Affairs of the AMA. Medical and nonmedical uses of anabolic-androgenic steroids. *JAMA* 1990;264:2923–2927.
33. Tennant F, Black DL, Voy RO. Anabolic steroid dependence with opioid type features: *N Engl J Med* 1988;319:578.
34. Overly WL, et al. Androgens and hepatocellular carcinoma in an athlete. *Ann Intern Med* 1984;100:158.
35. McNutt RA, et al. Acute myocardial infarction in a 22 year old world class weight lifter using anabolic steroids. *Am J Cardiol* 1988;62:164.
36. Huie MJ. Acute myocardial infarction occurring in an anabolic steroid user. *Med Sci Sports Exerc* 1994;26(4):408–413.
37. Frankle MA, et al. Anabolic androgenic steroids and a stroke in an athlete: case report. *Arch Phys Med Rehabil* 1988;69:632–633.
38. Kramhoft M, Solgaard S. Spontaneous rupture of the extensor policis longus tendon after anabolic steroids. *J Hand Surg* 1986;11(1):87.
39. Back BR, et al. Triceps rupture: a case report and literature review. *Am J Sports Med* 1987;15(3):285–289.
40. Wadler GI, Hainline B. *Anabolic steroids: drugs and the athlete.* Philadelphia: FA Davis Co, 1989:58.
41. Aiache AE. Surgical treatment of gynecomastia in the body building. *Plast Reconstr Surg* 1989;83(1):61–66.
42. Maropis C, Yesalis CE. Intramuscular abscess: another anabolic steroid danger. *Phys Sportsmed* 1994;22(1):105–108.
43. Sklarek H, et al. AIDS in a bodybuilder using anabolic steroids [Correspondence]. *N Engl J Med* 1984;311:1701.
44. Choi PYL, Pope HG Jr. Violence toward women and illicit androgenic-anabolic steroid use. *Annals Clin Psychiatry* 1994;6(1):21–25.
45. Pope HG, Katz DL. Affective and psychotic symptoms associated with anabolic steroid use. *Am J Psychiatry* 1988;145(4):487–490.
46. Bahrke MS, Wright JE, Strauss RH, Catlin DH. Psychological moods and subjectively perceived behavioral and somatic changes accompanying anabolic-androgenic steroid use. *Am J Sports Med* 1992;20:717–724.
47. Franke WW, Berendonk B. Hormonal doping and androgenization of athletes: a secret program of the German Democratic Republic government. *Clin Chem* 1997;43(7):1262–1279.
48. Haupt H. Anabolic steroids and growth hormone. *Am J Sports Med* 1993;21(3):468–474.
49. Macintyre JG. Growth hormone and athletes. *Sports Med* 1987;4:129–142.
50. Ahren K, et al. Cellular mechanism of the acute stimulatory effect of growth hormone. In: Pecile, Muller, eds. *Growth hormone and related polypeptides: proceedings of the 3rd International Symposium, Milan, 1975.* Amsterdam: Excerpta Medica, 1975.
51. Goldberg AL. Work induced growth of skeletal muscle in normal and hypophysectomized rats. *Am J Physiol* 1967;213(5):1193–1198.
52. Kostyo JL, Reagan CR. The biology of growth hormone. *Pharmacol Therap* 1976;2:591–604.
53. Goldberg AL. Relationship between growth hormone and muscle work in determining muscle size. *J Physiol* 1969;216:655–666.
54. Salomon F, Cuneo RC, Hesp R, et al. The effects of treatment with recombinant human growth hormone on body composition and metabolism with growth hormone deficiency. *N Engl J Med* 1989;321:1797–1803.
55. Underwood LE. Report of the conference on uses and possible abuses of biosynthetic human growth hormone. *N Engl J Med* 1984;311:606–608.
56. Van Vliet G, et al. Growth hormone treatment for short stature. *N Engl J Med* 1983;309:1016–1022.
57. Recombinant human growth hormone. *Med Lett* 1994;36(930):77–78.
58. Koch TK, et al. Creutzfeldt-Jakob disease in a young adult with idiopathic hypopituitarism: Possible relation to the administration of cadaveric human growth hormone. *N Engl J Med* 1985;313:731–733.
59. Catlin DH, Hatton CK. Use and abuse of anabolic and other drugs for athletic enhancement. *Adv Intern Med* 1990;36:381–405.
60. Pace N, Lozner EL, Consolazio WV, et al. The increase in hypoxia tolerance of normal men accompanying the polycythemia induced by transfusion of erythrocytes. *Am J Physiol* 1947;148:152–163.
61. Kline HG. Sounding board: blood transfusion and athletics. *N Engl J Med* 1985;312:854–856.
62. Buick FJ, et al. Effect of induced erthrocythemia on aerobic work capacity. *J Appl Physiol* 1980;48:636–642.
63. Ersley AJ, et al. The biogenesis of erythropoietin. *Exp Hematol* 1980;8(Suppl 8):1–13.
64. Goldingay R. Potential for abuse of recombinant erythropoietin. *Sports Med Dig* 1989;11(11):5.
65. Spence M. Doctors concerned about side effects of chemical erythropoietin. *The Olympian* 1990:61.
66. Adamson JW, Vapnek D. Recombinant erythropoietin to improve athletic performance. *N Engl J Med* 1991;324:698–699.
67. Drug tester needles the Olympics. *Wall Street Journal Interactive Edition* 1998 May 8.
68. Weiner N. Norepinephrine, epinephrine, and the sympathomimetic amines. In: Gilman AG, Goodman LS. *Pharmacological basis of therapeutics*, 7th ed. New York: Macmillan, 1985:145–180.
69. Wadler G, Hainline B. *Anabolic steroids: drugs and the athlete.* Philadelphia: FA Davis Co, 1989:3.
70. Rose RJ, Allen JR, Brock KA. Effects of clenbuterol hydrochloride on certain respiratory and cardiovascular parameters in horses performing treadmill exercise. *Res Vet Sci* 1983;35:301–305.
71. Rose RJ, Evans DL. Cardiorespiratory effects of clenbuterol in fit thoroughbred horses during a maximal exercise test. In: Gillespie JR, Robinson N, eds. *Equine exercise physiology*, Vol. 2. Davis, CA, ICEEP Publications, 1987:117–131.
72. Short CE, Maylin GA, Collier MA. Responses to submaximal exercise in standardbred horses with and without medication. *Equine Pract* 1990;12:23–28.
73. Slocombe RF, et al. Respiratory mechanics of horses during stepwise treadmill exercise tests, and the effect of clenbuterol pretreatment on them. *Aust Vet J* 1992;69:221–225.
74. Thompson JR, McPherson EA. COPD in the horse 2: therapy, *Equine Vet J* 1983;15:207–210.

75. DeMeersman R, et al. The effects of a sympathomimetic drug on maximal aerobic activity. *J Sports Med* 1986;26:251–257.
76. Ivy JL, et al. Role of caffeine and glucose ingestion on metabolism during exercise. *Med Sci Sports Exerc* 1978;10:66.
77. Sidney KH, Lefoe NM. The effects of Tedral upon athletic performance: a double blind cross-over study. Quebec City International Congress of Physical Activity Sciences, 1976.
78. DeMeersman R, Getty D, Schawefer DC. Sympathomimetics and exercise enhancement: all in the mind? *Pharmacol Biochem Behav* 1987;28:361–365.
79. Lombardo JA. Stimulants and athletic performance: amphetamines and caffeine. *Phys Sportsmed* 1986;14(11):128–139.
80. Spann C, Winter ME. Effect of clenbuterol on athletic performance. *Ann Pharmacother* 1995;29:75–78.
81. Maltin CA, Delday MI, Hay SM, Baillie GS. Denervation increases clenbuterol sensitivity in muscle from young rats. *Muscle Nerve* 1992;14:188–192.
82. Zeman RJ, et al. Clenbuterol, a beta 2 receptor agonist, reduces net bone loss in denervated hindlimbs. *Am J Physiol* 1991;261:E285–E289.
83. Matlin CA, Delday MI, Reeds PH. The effect of a growth promoting drug, clenbuterol, on fiber frequency and area in hind limb muscles from young male rats. *Biosci Rep* 1986;6:293.
84. Zeman RJ, Ludemann R, Easton TG, et al. Slow to fast alterations in skeletal muscle fibers caused by clenbuterol, a beta2 receptor agonist. *Am J Physiol* 1988;254:E726.
85. Yang YT, McElligott MA. Multiple actions of beta-adrenergic agonists on skeletal muscle and adipose tissue. *Biochem J* 1989;261:1.
86. Freidl KE, Moore RJ. Ergogenic aids: clenbuterol, ma huang, caffeine, L-carnitine and growth hormone releasers. *National Strength and Conditioning Association Journal* 1992;14:35.
87. Goodwin M. In sport, cocaine's here to stay. *New York Times* 1987 May 3:Sect. 5:1.
88. Cantwell JD, Rose FD. Cocaine and cardiovascular events. *Phys Sportsmed* 1986;14(11):77–82.
89. Warner EA. Cocaine abuse. *Ann Intern Med* 1993;119:226–235.
90. Kunkel DB. Cocaine then and now: part I. *Emerg Med* 1986;June 15:125–138.
91. Cregler L, Mark H. Special report: medical complications of cocaine abuse. *N Engl J Med* 1986;315:1495–1500.
92. Welder AA, Melchert RB. Cardiotoxic effects of cocaine and anabolic-androgenic steroids on the athlete. *J Pharm Toxicol Methods* 1993;29:61–68.
93. Forman ES, Dekker AH, Javors JR, Davison DT. High-risk behaviors in teenage male athletes. *Clin J Sports Med* 1995;5:36–42.
94. Kokotailo PK, et al. Substance use and other health risk behaviors in collegiate athletes. *Clin J Sports Med* 1996;6:183–189.
95. Meilman PW, et al. Beyond performance enhancement: polypharmacy among collegiate users of steroids. *J Am Coll Health* 1995;44:98–104.
96. Milhorn HT. The diagnosis of alcoholism. *Am Fam Phys* 1988;37(6):175–183.
97. Gilman AG, Goodman LS, Rall TW, Murad F, eds. *Goodman and Gilman's the pharmacologic basis of therapeutics*, 7th ed. New York: Macmillan, 1985.
98. American College of Sports Medicine. Position statement on the use of alcohol in sports. *Med Sci Sports Exerc* 1982;14:ix–x.
99. Urbano-Marquez A, et al. The effects of alcoholism on skeletal and cardiac muscle. *N Engl J Med* 1989;320:409–415.
100. Brewer RD, et al. The risk of dying in alcohol-related automobile crashes among habitual drunk drivers. *N Engl J Med* 1994;331:513–517.
101. Leichliter JS, Meilman PW, Presley CA, Cashin JR. Alcohol use and related consequences among students with varying levels of involvement in college athletics. *College Health* 1998;46:257–262.
102. Nattiv A, Puffer JC, Green GA. Lifestyles and health risks of collegiate athletes: a multi-center study. *Clin J Sports Med* 1997;7:262–272.
103. Kauhanen J, Kaplan GA, Goldberg DE, Salonen JT. Beer bingeing and mortality. *Br Med J* 1997;4(3):846–851.
104. Secretary of Health and Human Services. *Ninth special report to the U.S. Congress on alcohol and health* (NIH publication no. 97-4017). Washington, DC: U.S.Government Printing Office, 1997.
105. Buchsbaum DG, et al. Screening for alcohol abuse using the CAGE scores and likelihood ratios. *Ann Intern Med* 1991;115:774–777.
106. Tashkin DP, Gong H, Fligiel SEG. How the lungs are affected by marijuana smoke. *J Respir Dis* 1987;8(11):87–107.
107. Powell DR. Does marijuana smoke cause lung cancer? *Primary Care Cancer* 10:15, 1987.
108. Nattiv A, Puffer JC. Lifestyles and health risks of collegiate athletes. *J Fam Pract* 1991;33:585–590.
109. Renaud AM, Cormier Y. Acute effects of marijuana smoking on maximal exercise performance. *Med Sci Sports Exerc* 1986;18(6):685–689.
110. Catlin DH, Murray TH. Performance-enhancing drugs, fair competition, and Olympic sport. *JAMA* 1996;276(3):231–237.
111. Glover ED, Edmundson EW, Edwards SW, Schroeder KL. Implications of smokeless tobacco use among athletes. *Phys Sports Med* 1986;14(12):95–105.
112. Bergert N. The dangers of smokeless tobacco. *Sports Med Digest* 1989;11(6):1–8.
113. Anderson WA, Albrecht RR, McKeag DB. Second replication of a national study of the substance use and abuse habits of college student-athletes. Report to NCAA, Mission, KS, 1993.
114. Connolly GN, Orleans CT, Kogan M. Use of smokeless tobacco in major-league baseball. *N Engl J Med* 1988;318(19):1281–1284.
115. Benowitz NL. Pharmacologic aspects of cigarette smoking and nicotine addiction. *N Engl J Med* 1998;319(20):1318–1330.
116. Edwards SW, Glover ED, Schoeder KL. The effects of smokeless tobacco on heart rate and neuromuscular reactivity in athletes and nonathletes. *Phys Sports Med* 1987;15(7):141–146.
117. Dimitrov TG. Effect of mesocarb. *Clin Pharmacol* 1993;15(3):189–192.
118. Fredholm BB. Adenosine and central catecholamine neurotransmission. In: *Adenosine: receptors and modulation of cell function*. Washington, DC: Oxford Press, 1985:91–104.
119. Mashkovskii MD, Altshuler RA, Avrutskii G, Aleksandrovskii YA, Smulevich RL. Experimental and clinical study of Syndocarb: a new psychostimulant. *Zh Nevrol Psikhiatr Im S S Korsakova* 1971;11:1704–1709.
120. Sergeeva SA, Krapivin SV, Losev AS, Morosov IS: Correlated interconnection between pharmacokinetic and dynamic development of the pharmacologic effects of bromantane. *Biull Eksp Biol Med* 1995;119(3):305–308.
121. Sedov AV, Lukicheva TA. Experimental rationale for the use of drugs to increase the resistance of the human body to the combined action of carbon monoxide and hyperthermia. *Med Tr Prom Ekol* 1993;9–10:10–11.
122. Badyshtov BA, Losev AS, Makhnycheva AL, et al. Study of heat-protective effects of bromantane at various levels of overheating. *Vopr Med Khim* 1995;41(2):54–57.
123. Vigil D, Catlin DH, Puffer JC. Thermoprotective effect of Bromantan. Unpublished data.
124. Williams MH, Branch JD. Ergogenic aids for improved performance. In: Garrett WE, Kirkendall DT, eds. *Exercise and sport science*. Philadelphia: Lippincott Williams & Wilkins, 2000:373–383.
125. Volek JS. Enhancing exercise performance: nutritional implications. In: Garrett WE, Kirkendall DT, eds. *Exercise and sport science*. Philadelphia: Lippincott Williams & Wilkins, 2000:471–485.
126. Mahesh VB, Greenblatt RB. The in vivo conversion of dehyroepiandrosterone and androstenedione to testosterone in humans. *Acta Endocrinol* 1962;41:400–406.
127. Wallace MB, Lim J, Cutler A, Bucci L. Effects of dehydroepiandrosterone vs. androstenedione supplementation in men. *Med Sci Sports Exerc* 1999;31:1788–1792.
128. King DS, Sharp RL, Vukovich MD, Brown GA, Reifenrath TA, Uhl NL, Parsons KA. Effect of oral androstenedione on serum testosterone and adaptations to resistance training in young men. *JAMA* 1999;281:2020–2028.
129. Earnest CP, Olson MA, Broeder CE, Breuel KF, Beckham SG. In vivo 4-androstene-3,17-dione and 4-androstene-3β,17β-diol

supplementation in young men. *Eur J Appl Physiol* 2000;81: 229–232.
130. Ballantyne CS, Phillips SM, MacDonald JR, Tarnopolsky MA, MacDougall JD. The acute effects of androstenedione supplementation in healthy young males. *Can J Appl Physiol* 2000;25.
131. Leder BZ, Longcope, C, Catlin DH, Ahrens B, Schoenfeld DA, Finkelstein JS. Oral androstenedione administration and serum testosterone concentrations in young men. *JAMA* 2000;283: 779–782.
132. 1998 U.S. Olympic Committee on Drug Control, Colorado Springs, CO.

CHAPTER 11

Drug Testing in Sports

Richard T. Ferro and Douglas B. McKeag

INTRODUCTION

Despite our many technological advances, it appears that the unethical agendas of a significant proportion of athletes and athletic programs, as well as our society's tendency to value winning above almost all else, continue to mandate drug testing in sports. Many who support drug testing believe that it remains a necessary evil and that it is athletes' responsibility as society's role models to live up to a high ethical standard. They argue that the relative decline in positive drug test results, then, stands as an affirmation that the sentinel effect is working (1).

On the other hand, there are those who view drug testing in athletics as an unnecessary invasion of Fourth Amendment rights and as an ineffective tool for its purported use: identifying those who use drugs to gain an unfair advantage in athletic competition (2–5). They argue that drug use and doping procedures in this age of big-money sports have risen to a new level (6). Some believe that drug testing will always be one step behind the latest ergogenic breakthrough and that the large sums of money that are spent on its development and implementation would be better spent on prevention programs (4).

The use of drugs to enhance athletic performance can no longer be perceived as just the result of scientists working behind the scenes to further the Cold War political agendas of their governments. Instead, the use of ergogenic aids is a by-product of a new era of profitable athletic competition, in which self-proclaimed drug gurus help athletes to circumvent established drug-testing procedures to gain a performance advantage (7). Accordingly, the knowledge and use of effective ergogenic aids by athletes at all levels appear to be more pervasive than ever before.

The purpose of this chapter is not to present or dispute the moral and ethical concerns raised by drug testing in sports or in our society at large. Ultimately, those are issues that can be understood only within the context of the generation, society, political, and religious environments from which one evolves. Instead, we will explore the development of drug-testing procedures in our society and examine the policies, technological aspects, and problems faced in trying to create fair and level playing fields (8).

ORIGINS OF DRUG TESTING IN SPORTS

Since the ancient Olympic games, athletes have used a variety of drugs in their quest for enhancement of athletic performance, from the ingestion of mushrooms that contained muscarine to the consumption of bread laced with opium (9,10). By the 1800s the extensive use of ergogenic substances such as caffeine, nitroglycerin, amphetamines, strychnine, and ephedrine was reported, making it quite obvious that a win-at-any-price attitude had been well established in athletics long before the modern professionalization of sports (9,10).

One of the first reported drug-induced deaths in an athlete occurred in 1886 (11). Apparently, an English cyclist trying to enhance his performance died from an overdose of the drug trimethyl (probably a form of ether) (12). Since the rebirth of the Olympic Games, ergogenic drug use has continued to flourish in the athletic arena, especially after the synthesis of testosterone in 1935 (13). However, it was not until the death of Danish cyclist Kurt Enemar Jensen at the 1960 Summer Olympic Games in Rome that a considerable antidoping movement was initiated (14). The fact that Jensen and

---
R. T. Ferro: Department of Community and Family Medicine and Division of Orthopaedic Surgery, Duke University Medical Center, Durham, North Carolina 27710.
D. B. McKeag: Department of Family Medicine, Indiana University School of Medicine, and National Institute of Fitness and Sport, Indianapolis, Indiana 46202-5102.

two of his fellow teammates became ill after ingesting amphetamine and Roniacol (a cough syrup) for performance enhancement stunned many. Jensen ultimately died, and his two teammates were admitted to an Italian hospital in critical condition. These incidents helped to generate considerable antidoping sentiment and began the cascade of significant worldwide antidoping legislation. A gradual evolution in collective thinking also began; drug use for performance enhancement was no longer considered just a matter of personal choice. Instead, it became an unethical act that clearly carried significant health risks and that directly influenced others to use ergogenic drugs to compete equitably (9,15).

In response to the growing antidrug use sentiment, the European sports governing body held a convention in 1963 to address the problem of drug use in sports. During this conference a definition of doping was established that would subsequently be adopted by the International Olympic Committee (IOC) and the Federation Internationale de Medicine Sportive in October 1964 (16,17). Doping was then defined as "the administration to, or the use by, a competing athlete of any substance foreign to the body or any physiological substance taken in abnormal quantity or by an abnormal route of entry into the body, with the sole intention of increasing in an artificial and unfair manner his performance in competition" (16). The term *doping* may have originated from several sources. The Kafir tribe of southeast Africa would use dop, a brandy made from grapes, as a stimulant for ceremonial dances. The term may also have been derived from the Dutch "doop" meaning viscous opium juice, which later became "dope" or any stupefying substance (9). In the late 1800s the term *doping* was placed into the English dictionary to refer to a mixture of opium and other narcotics (10,18).

Although no official drug testing program was established at the Tokyo Olympiad in 1964, a questionnaire was given to athletes that indicated a high prevalence of drug use (17). In addition, spot checks revealed that several Olympic cyclists were receiving injections of unidentified substances. Since many of these athletes refused to cooperate with the IOC members, a petition was sent to IOC president Avery Brundage denouncing the use of drugs by Olympic athletes (10). As a result Belgium and France enacted antidoping laws in 1965. In this same year sensitive gas chromatography testing techniques were first used to monitor drug abuse in the Tour of Britain cycling race, resulting in the disqualification of three cyclists (11,15). Sadly, these countermeasures would not prevent more tragedies associated with the use of ergogenic drugs in sports. In 1967 Tommy Simpson, a notable British cyclist, died during the thirteenth day of the Tour de France. At the time of his death a vial of amphetamine was found in his possession (11). The following year amphetamine abuse was believed to play a major role in the deaths of cyclist Yves Mottin and soccer player Jean-Louis Quadri (11).

In the face of a growing antidoping movement the IOC established a Medical Commission in 1967, which would be responsible for the oversight of all issues relating to medicine and the use of drugs. The Subcommittee on Doping Control and Biochemistry, under the direction of Manfred Donike, was specifically established "to safeguard the health of the athletes, and to ensure respect for the ethical concepts implicit in fair play, the Olympic Spirit and medical practice" (19). The program encompassed research into the use and detection of performance-enhancing drugs. The subcommittee developed an extensive plan that resulted in the establishment of both a list of banned substances and the development of a formal drug-testing protocol. The original list has been modified over the years to include the broad categories of stimulants, narcotics, anabolic agents (including beta-2 agonists), diuretics, peptide and glycoprotein hormones, and other classes of restricted substances (see Appendix 11-1).

Although the drug-testing program officially started with the 1968 Winter Olympic Games in Grenoble, screening for only a relatively small number of stimulants and narcotics was actually performed, owing to the limitation of analytic techniques at the time. Comprehensive screening using more sensitive equipment (gas chromatographers with nitrogen-specific flame alkali detectors) to test for a broader range of drugs did not begin until the 1972 Munich Summer Games (18–20). The IOC, all accredited international testing facilities, and most sports testing bodies have used gas chromatography/mass spectrometry (GC/MS) to identify and confirm all positive drug screens since then (11). Despite the widespread abuse of anabolic androgenic steroids (AAS), testing for these substances and their metabolites was delayed until 1976. This occurred because of the lack of a practical method to rapidly screen a large number of samples for AAS and because the metabolites of AAS were still not well documented at the time (11,20). A radioimmunoassay technique was finally developed in 1975 that could more rapidly screen a large number of specimens (21). This development, along with improvements in GC/MS methods, allowed testing for AAS at the 1976 Montreal Olympic Games, when they were officially added to the IOC list of banned substances.

Unfortunately, despite the deep level of commitment given to antidoping programs, these testing techniques could not differentiate endogenous from exogenous testosterone, and only eight athletes tested positive for AAS at the Montreal Olympic Games. By most athletes' accounts, that number was greatly erroneous and was believed to be due to the fact that the underground steroid users continued to stay a few steps ahead of the testing techniques by switching from other exogenous forms to pure testosterone (11,22). To confound matters further, finding abnormal concentrations of an endogenous steroid is generally insufficient evidence to presume the use of an exogenous substance (23).

Meanwhile drug testing done on U.S. athletes in 1980 indicated that up to 20% may have tested positive if the Moscow Olympic Games had not been boycotted (11). To curtail the prohibited use of AAS, continued research determined that the administration of exogenous testosterone would result in a testosterone to epitestosterone ratio (T/E) of greater than or equal to 6:1 (24). Subsequently, at the 1983 Pan American Games held in Caracas, Venezuela, 15 American male athletes tested positive for AAS, and at least 12 more withdrew from competition, presumably worried about potential disqualification due to AAS use (25). Analytic techniques continued to improve such that by the 1984 Los Angeles Games, it was feasible for all samples to be tested for the elevation of the T/E ratio by GC/MS, with a resultant T/E ratio greater than 6:1 considered to be evidence of exogenous AAS use (20). In fact, at the 1984 U.S. Olympic Trials, an additional 86 athletes tested positive for AAS use because of these advanced analytic techniques and the increased drug screening efforts of the United States Olympic Committee (USOC) (11).

Around 1982, when the T/E test was first introduced, there were several notable methods of circumventing drug tests that East German athletes, and presumably others, used. These included the technique described as the "precompetition bridging program," in which an athlete would switch from specific cycles of exogenous AAS to (the more difficult to detect) testosterone in the last few weeks, depending on the retention times of the various steroid preparations used (26). Their T/E ratio would then be carefully monitored, and testosterone administration would be adjusted accordingly so as not to go above the 6:1 ratio. Additionally, in 1982 VEB Jenapharm, the East German state-owned facility, began producing preparations of testosterone and epitestosterone propionate, presumably to beat the doping-control system since there was no apparent pharmaceutical use for epitestosterone at the time (27). Thus by coadministration of epitestosterone with testosterone, the athletes would effectively normalize their T/E ratio. So began the sophisticated version of a chemical hide-and-seek game, which continues today. Just as newer drug testing technology was invented, it seemed as though either a new undetectable substance or a new way to obtain a falsely negative test appeared.

It was not long after the considerable antidoping movement and establishment of international legislative groups that other sports organizations fell in line, creating their own, often unique, drug-testing policies and banned substances lists (summarized in Table 11-1) (28).

Numerous drug-related incidents, scandals, and tragedies rocked the NCAA and the many other professional and nonprofessional organizations. These incidents spurred a variety of important changes in their drug-testing policies and procedures. The growing antidrug sentiment was steadily fueled by the media attention given to the continued drug abuse in sports and society.

In 1982 the National Football League (NFL) began formally drug testing its players in training camps. By 1987 the NFL expanded this testing to include AAS. After considerable media attention was given to numerous anecdotal reports and testimonials concerning the NFL's questionable drug-testing practices, there was an outcry for stricter enforcement (29–30). Subsequently, despite considerable opposition, the NFL's drug-testing protocol was further amended in 1990 to include random drug testing every 6 weeks, in addition to the previously scheduled testing done at preseason camp, the scouting combine sessions and for "reasonable cause" (31–33).

In September 1983 the National Basketball Association (NBA) and the National Basketball Players Association instituted an innovative Anti-Drug Agreement designed to eliminate the use of illegal drugs in the NBA. The program was unique for its time because it provided and stressed education and rehabilitation over clear, predetermined penalties for illicit drug use, including permanent dismissal from the NBA. Additionally, it encouraged players who had problems with drugs to voluntarily come forward to seek treatment. It did this by not imposing penalties of any kind (e.g., lost salary) on the first-time treatment seeker, as long as the player abided by the terms of the prescribed care. Furthermore, it not only provided counseling and medical assistance at the expense of the team, but it also expressly guaranteed confidentiality outside the organization. It is not difficult to understand why the concept and policies inherent in this Anti-Drug Agreement have been embraced by so many (34).

In February 1984 the NCAA felt substantial pressure from the ethical, legal, and medical concerns surrounding the use of drugs by athletes to propose its own drug-screening program to member institutions. The NCAA's desire to avoid significant health risks and "to preserve the appearance of fair and equitable competition provided by the members of the NCAA" was published in a set of guidelines known as Proposition 30 (4). In 1985 the NCAA sponsored a Michigan State University study on the prevalence of college athlete drug use (35). It revealed a significant amount of drug use among college athletes and became the driving force behind the NCAA's approval of the drug-testing program in 1986 (36). Ironically, Proposition 30 was accepted in 1986, only several months before the well-publicized death due to "crack" cocaine of Len Bias, one of the best college basketball players at the time (37). Initially, the NCAA instituted its own drug-testing program at championships, certified postseason football

TABLE 11–1. *Major sports organizations and their drug testing policies*

Organization	Testing policy	Banned substances	Banned methods	Who gets tested	When tests are done	Penalty for positive test
U.S. Olympic Committee (USOC) National Anti-Doping Program One Olympic Plaza Colorado Springs, CO 80909–5780 800-233-0393 www.olympicusa.org	Provides a list of banned substances and methods to National Governing Bodies (NGBs); administers tests at Olympic and Pan American Games and trials, USOC-sponsored competitions and if mutually agreed upon, at NGB events	Stimulants, narcotics, anabolic agents (including β-2 agonists), diuretics, designer drugs, peptide and glycoprotein hormones and analogues, marijuana and subject to certain restrictions: alcohol, local anesthetics, corticosteroids, β-blockers	Doping, pharmacological, chemical or physical manipulation by, for example, catheterization, urine substitution, tampering, or inhibition of renal excretion	First four competitors in the finals, a random selection of others at Olympic, Pan American and NGB events both in and out of competition; all prospective team members at Olympic and Pan American trials	In competition: 1 hour following competition, upon determination of final results, or at other times, within 1 hour of notification; No advance notice: within a reasonable amount of time after being notified	For violations with (1) anabolic agents (including β-2 agonists), stimulants, cocaine, diuretics, β-blockers, peptide hormones, narcotics, designer drugs and prohibited substances not covered in number 2 below: 2 years for first offense, life ban for second; (2) Caffeine, ephedrine, pseudoephedrine, phenylpropanolamine, norpseudoephedrine etc. (i.e., sympathomimetic amines) and all other banned substances or practices: a maximum of 3 months for the first offense, 2 years for the second offense, or a life ban for the third offense; forfeiture of any medals won; team disqualification, if violating athlete is on a team
The National Football League (NFL) 280 Park Avenue New York, NY 10017–1216 212-450-2000 www.nfl.com	Provides a list of banned substances and administers drug test to all prospective and current NFL players	Cocaine, marijuana, amphetamine and its analogues, opiates, and phencyclidine (PCP)	None	Rookies who have not been tested 4 months before their pre-employment test, draft eligible players, veterans desirous of signing a new NFL contract, and all players under contract with an NFL club	Before employment with an NFL club; once during preseason (between May 1 and August 20); randomly every 6 weeks; upon determination by Medical Advisor or Medical Director; and for all of the above, within 24 hours of notification	Mandatory participation in a three-stage intervention program; payment of a percentage of salary, suspension for consecutive games without pay, notification of the NFL and NFLPA or banishment for 1 year to life depending on stage, failure to comply with treatment plan, and number of positive test violations within a stage
The National Basketball Association (NBA) 645 Fifth Avenue New York, NY 10022–5986 212-826-7000 www.nba.com	Anti-Drug Agreement between the NBA and the NBA's Player Association provides for educational and rehabilitation programs and sets clear, predetermined penalties for violators	Heroin, cocaine, and illegal drugs	None	Any player but only when reasonable cause is established such as the belief that a player may have engaged in the illegal use, possession or distribution of illegal drugs; any player who voluntarily comes forward to seek treatment; rookies	Involuntary selection for reasonable cause: four times during a 6-week period at random times and without any prior notification; rookies: randomly before employment during regular training camp, randomly three times during each rookies first year in the NBA	Players who voluntarily come forward for use, possession or distribution of illegal drugs: first time: counseling and medical assistance at the expense of the club, continued pay and no penalty of any kind as long as terms of prescribed treatment are complied with; for second time: suspension without pay during period of counseling and medical assistance and no further penalty; for third time: permanent dismissal from NBA; for players who do not voluntarily come forward and are convicted or plead guilty to a crime involving the use, possession or distribution of heroin or cocaine: immediate and permanent dismissal from the NBA

Organization	Program	Drugs tested	Who is tested	When testing occurs	Consequences
Major League Baseball (MLB) Office of the Commissioner 350 Park Avenue New York, NY 10022–6022 212-339-7800 www.majorleaguebaseball.com	Conducts centralized, regular, random, testing of certain major and minor league employees; program includes evaluation, education, counseling, and rehabilitation	All illegal drugs and all controlled substances including steroids or prescription drugs for which the individual in possession does not have a prescription. Tests are done for cocaine, marijuana, amphetamines, opiates and phencyclidine (PCP)	MLB owners, executives, field managers, umpires, trainers, players with guaranteed contracts containing drug testing clauses or who have known drug involvement, amateur entry level players, all staff, or anyone else involved with the game	Four times per season; off-season if necessary; announced for major league players; for remainder of career of major league players admitting to or detected using banned drugs; unannounced for randomly selected minor league players, amateur entry level players, and all other personnel	Initial positive test, admission of drug use, or identification of use through other means result in required participation in MLB's Employee Assisted Program (EAP) as well as recommended treatment or rehab; discipline (not specified by MLB) will result for refusing to be tested or enter into EAP, evading or altering testing, or not cooperating with EAP treatment or rehab; immediate discipline (not specified by MLB) will result for second and any subsequent violation of MLB drug policy, for sale or distribution of illegal drugs or controlled substances, or conviction of a drug-related offense
National Collegiate Athletic Association (NCAA) 6201 College Boulevard Overland Park, KS 66211–2422 913-339-1906 www.ncaa.org	Provides a list of banned substances to member institutions; administers tests at NCAA individual and team championships, postseason bowl events, and nonchampionship events	Stimulants, anabolic agents, substances banned for specific sports, diuretics, street drugs, and peptide hormones and analogues	Blood doping, pharmacological, chemical, or physical manipulation	Student athletes and nonrecruited student athletes on the basis of position, athletics, financial aid status, playing time, randomly or any combination thereof; student athletes who become ineligible; student athletes who test positive in conjunction with drug testing administered by other athletic organizations	Year round in Division I and II sports; may occur before, during or after NCAA championships and postseason bowl games; championship events: after established cool down period after event and within 1 hour of notification or the next morning if competition begins at 9 P.M. or later; on-campus nonchampionship events: at scheduled times and dates; ineligible athletes: at any time during period of ineligibility and at a mandatory exit test before the last month of their minimum period of eligibility; athletes who test positive at other athletic organizations: at scheduled times and dates	For a first offense, loss of eligibility for participation in regular-season and postseason competition in all sports for 365 days from the time of the positive drug test, until the athlete tests negative, and until eligibility is restored; this period must include a minimum of one full season of competition (e.g., if the athlete tests positive in the middle of a season, ineligibility will last until the middle of the season of the following year); for a second offense, loss of eligibility for regular-season and postseason competition in all sports; for the use of a "street drug," after eligibility is restored, the athlete will lose a minimum of one additional full season of competition in all sports

Source: Modified from Gall SL, Duda M, Giel D, Rogers CC. Who tests which athletes for what drugs? *Phys Sports Med* 1988;16:155–161.

games, and bowl contests (4,38). In December 1986 the NCAA randomly selected 10 games from the 18 Division I postseason bowls, which included the five major bowl games. Approximately 36 members from each team were selected, including the 22 starters. Overall, more than 700 players from 20 universities underwent urinalysis, which resulted in a number of players being banned from postseason play. The most noteworthy case involved Brian Bosworth, an all-American linebacker from the University of Oklahoma, who was banned because he tested positive for anabolic steroids (39). The NCAA's testing program has since evolved into a tightly controlled system that includes scheduled and random testing at both championship and nonchampionship events (40).

Before 1984 the IOC rules prohibited only drugs that could be definitively identified by analytical techniques. However, after the 1984 American cyclists' blood-doping scandal this policy was revised, and a Category II, Prohibited Methods, was created. In 1987 the drug probenecid was detected in the urine samples of U.S. weight lifters and found to effectively inhibit the urinary excretion of several compounds, including AAS (9). Subsequently, Category II was expanded to include pharmacologic, chemical, and physical manipulation of urine, such as the use of probenecid, adulterants, and catheterization, respectively. In 1989 an additional class of Category I prohibited substances was created to accommodate growth hormone (GH) and human chorionic gonadotropin (hCG) abuse (9). Category III currently includes classes of drugs that are subject to certain restrictions, such as approval before competition.

Although the reported and actual positive test results often vary greatly, there have been relatively few positive drug tests for banned substances, including AAS, at the Olympic Games. The few positive tests in the face of known drug abuse are due to a variety of reasons, including superior circumvention techniques and inadequate drug-screening capabilities. Even though our capacity to detect a greater number of banned substances has steadily improved, there are numerous known substances (e.g., endogenous steroids, hCG, hGH, dihydrotestosterone), unknown substances and metabolites, and doping methods that allow athletes to circumvent present testing procedures and threaten the ideals inherent in fair competition (19). Some of these more widely used ergogenic substances and doping methods and the challenges they present to ergogenic substance detection will be discussed in more detail later in this chapter.

ISSUES IN DRUG TESTING

Intent of Drug Testing

Drug testing of athletes has become an accepted practice before they are allowed to compete in high school sports, during college and professional training camps and sports events, and after winning an Olympic medal; yet controversy continues to surround its practice (4,38,40–42). The basic premise behind most governing sports organizations' policies is that mandatory drug testing is necessary, not only to ensure a level playing field, but also to eradicate substance abuse (43–46). Numerous legal arguments for drug testing have been purported, including protecting athletes' health and safety, deterring drug use among athletes, identifying athletes with drug-related problems so that proper medical attention can be given to them, and ensuring compliance with rehabilitation programs (43). Questionable arguments to uphold drug testing athletes have been to prevent them from being perceived as drug users, because they are role models representing their respective institutions, and to protect the image and economic viability of the athletic programs involved (47,48).

Legal Issues

A certain amount of controversy has been caused by the seemingly individualistic nature in which some organizations enforce their policies (4,38,41,49). Nonetheless, three legal issues have typically been involved in evaluating the constitutionality of random drug testing (42). The first issue is that drug tests may violate athletes' Fourth Amendment rights against unreasonable searches and seizures and invasion of privacy. In this regard, some might view a visually monitored urine collection as a significant invasion of personal privacy. Others may cite the relative infrequency of drug use in their sport, sex, and/or age group as grounds for an unreasonable search (35,50,51). The second issue concerns whether a drug test violates athletes' Fifth Amendment rights against self-incrimination by forcing athletes to provide testimony (in this case urinalysis) against themselves (52). The final issue relates to whether or not drug testing violates athletes' Fourteenth Amendment rights to equal protection under the law. Categorizing these individuals as athletes and then mandating urinalysis for them but not for nonathletes may be in violation of their Fourteenth Amendment rights, especially when one considers that the drugs being tested for, such as marijuana, may have nothing to do with performance enhancement (41,42).

One recent example illustrating the constitutional issues involved in drug testing athletes is the case *Vernonia (Oregon) School District 47J v. Acton* (1995), which was heard before the U.S. Supreme Court. In this case a seventh grader, James Acton, and his parents refused to sign a drug-testing consent form, and he was thereby prohibited from participating in the school's athletic programs. The Actons argued that the drug test would violate James's Fourth and Fourteenth Amendment rights (53). The school district argued that the express purpose for random drug testing was to prevent high school student-athletes from using drugs, to protect their health and safety, and to provide drug users with assistance programs (44).

The Supreme Court ignored discussion of Fifth and Fourteenth Amendment rights and based its decision on issues related to the Fourth Amendment (42). In weighing privacy issues, the Court attempted to find a balance between the relative encroachment of a specific athlete's privacy and the health and safety of student-athletes in general. First, the Court deemed that drug testing is a minimal intrusion on student-athletes' privacy. One of the numerous reasons given for this decision was that athletes' expectations of privacy are lessened because they voluntarily choose to associate with a team. In doing so, they subject themselves to a diminished degree of privacy, as when they are required to change, shower, and use the restroom in a communal and open environment (53). Second, the Court ruled that the Vernonia school district demonstrated a need to deter drug use among its student athletes and to provide a safe learning environment (44). The Court strengthened Vernonia's role in drug testing by citing the doctrine of *in loco parentis,* by which educators are allowed to dispense a small degree of parentlike supervision or discipline to students (42). Third, the Court decided that impartiality was ensured through the use of a random drug-testing policy, which would not allow subjective intrusion of privacy and which increased the efficacy of the program. Fourth, the Court found the random drug-testing policy to be reasonable, because it believed the policy to be an effective and minimally intrusive means by which to deter drug use among student-athletes (44). In essence, since the school district demonstrated that there was significant drug abuse among its student-athletes, then there were compelling interests of health and safety for these individuals to undergo random drug tests, which outweighed their legitimate privacy interests (53). The final decision handed down by the Supreme Court ruled in favor of allowing mandatory drug testing for these student-athletes.

Many other legal issues are involved in the drug testing of athletes. There are concerns that such testing procedures reject the fundamental tenet of presumption of innocence until proven guilty (43,54). By rejecting this ideal, drug testing shifts the burden of proving innocence entirely to athletes. A drug dealer who is caught selling narcotics is presumed innocent until proven guilty and given a fair trial, whereas an athlete or prospective employee who voluntarily consents to a drug test is often irrefutably guilty, regardless of the accuracy, reliability, quality controls, or procedures of the medical laboratory (55). Thus these athletes must prove their innocence every time they are made to give a urine sample (43). Other serious concerns involve whether athletes who submit to drug testing receive adequate protection under the basic principles of fairness and due process in testing (54,56). Faults that have been found in the procedural process have included a lack of informed consent, no compulsory disclosure of evidence on the part of the prosecution, no right to cross-examine prosecution witnesses, failure to assure neutral hearing officers, failure to allow athletes to be present at hearings pertaining to their case, a lack of unbiased representation, failure to give adequate notification to athletes who test positive, and insufficient policies in regard to appealing a positive drug test (38,54,56).

Thus many of the basic rights of due process afforded to other individuals are denied to athletes, although they often have much greater monetary rewards and public reputations at stake. Therefore to ensure against the propensity to ignore their individual rights, athletes should be afforded an appropriate appeals process in which they can explain extenuating circumstances, dispute false-positive results, and correct inaccuracies in their testing (56).

DRUG TESTING POLICY

In developing a formal drug-testing policy, a number of important steps must be undertaken. One of the most significant components is to devise an inclusive written policy, which should be distributed to all athletes who are affected by the program. The policy should specify the purpose(s) for testing; the selection of athletes to be tested; a detailed list of banned substances; the type of specimen to be obtained; the protocol for collecting, handling, and transporting the sample, including a detailed chain of custody; the consequences of a positive test; and a description of the appeal process (57,11). To avoid legal complications, present drug testing policies are often developed to fit within existing state and federal constitutional constraints (57). Despite this fact, a number of problems are faced during the implementation of a fair and effective drug-testing program; these include the accuracy and reliability of tests for performance-enhancing substances, the internal and external chain of custody, the logistics of obtaining and transporting a large number of athletes' urine samples, the financial means to establish and continually update testing laboratories, the enforceability of sanctions for testing positive, the need to update banned substances lists and rules and properly notify athletes of these changes, and the need for conferring proper informed consent (38,58,59).

Informed Consent

In distributing and reviewing the drug testing policy with the athlete, the consent form should explicitly state what the athlete is consenting to by signing the form.

The form should also specify that the athlete has received, has read, and understands the most current drug-testing policy. The form should also state who has access to the supposedly confidential tests and under what circumstances this information is shared. The form should also specify whether the athlete must inform the organization and/or physician about current drug or medication use and should be explicit as to what types of drugs need to be reported (i.e., banned, illicit, prescription, over-the-counter). Since most policies require the athlete to legally consent to drug testing in order to participate, the form should also explain what sanctions are imposed should the athlete refuse to sign. It should also specify that the athlete understands the consequences for testing positive. Additionally, the form may contain clauses that require the athlete to waive state, federal, and other legal rights, including the right to sue the organization (38,45). Table 11–1 lists the policies of the major sports organizations that drug test their athletes.

Furthermore, the drug-testing policy must be written and conveyed at a comprehension level commensurate with that of the athlete being tested. The formal drug-testing policy espoused by the institution should also accurately reflect the actual drug-testing procedures. Thus, by ensuring that athletes understand the drug-testing policy and give their true informed consent, an institution can better guarantee fair and ethical treatment of athletes, effective deterrence against drug use, reductions in ignorance-related positive tests, and protection from burdensome legal disputes over athletes' constitutional rights (38). Ultimately, a drug-testing policy should be set up to protect the health of the athletes from the hazards of drug use.

Scheduling Policy

After reviewing the drug-testing policy, athletes should explicitly understand when and how they may be tested. When drug testing was first initiated in many sports organizations, it was done only at major competitions. However, this practice has evolved because drug testing can be most effective only if done in an unannounced, year-round manner. This approach is now in practice in most organizations during competition and training periods (22,60). To further increase the efficacy of their drug-testing policies, most organizations have adopted either a short notice or no advance notice (NAN) drug-testing protocol. As these sports organizations increased their number of short and NAN, out-of-competition (OOC) tests in the early 1990s (to as high as 83% of all those performed in the case of the NCAA), the number of positive tests for banned substances dramatically increased (22,61). To make their drug-testing policies more economically feasible, the short and NAN testing usually screens only for anabolic agents, masking agents (e.g., probenecid and epitestosterone), and diuretics, while the scheduled competition testing also encompasses other classes of banned substances, including stimulants and illicit drugs (22). In an attempt to help make international drug-testing policy more financially practical, some have suggested that only the top 30 athletes in each event should be ranked and tested in a year-round OOC manner. These top 30 athletes would then be subject to testing at any time and at any place, and no world records could be set by athletes outside this monitored group (58). A summary of when athletes are tested by the major sports organizations is included in Table 11–1.

Chain of Custody

To process large numbers of specimens while keeping the clinical techniques within the forensic practices of evidence handling, a strict chain of custody was established (17). This concept pertains to the establishment of absolute accountability for every specimen collected and tested. The chain of custody starts from the time the specimen is collected and continues with its transfer to the laboratory, all the while clearly documenting who collected it, when it was collected, how and when it was sent to the laboratory, who received it at the laboratory, who processed it there, how it was stored, and how the results were returned to the person(s) authorized to receive them. All of these steps require detailed verification, from the label on the urine collection containers to the final reports. The goal is to minimize the number of people who have access to the athletes' specimens, test samples, and documentation and to eliminate opportunities to tamper with the samples. To achieve this, all areas associated with any part of this process must be well secured with access limited to authorized individuals only. Since many successful appeals have centered on chain of custody discrepancies such as alleged sabotage and switching of samples, precautionary steps must be able to prevent substitution, dilution, or other tampering with athletes' urine samples (45,62–64). It is no wonder that chain of custody procedures and documentation have become one of the most important links to prove the irrefutability of positive tests. These procedures are necessary not only to fight off legal challenges, but, more important, to protect the innocent from being falsely accused. Therefore ensuring the authenticity of athletes' specimens and their test results is an essential component of any successful drug testing program (59).

The collection protocols used by the NCAA and the USOC are almost identical to that created by the IOC. The sample identity is known only to the governing bodies (65). During Olympic competition the athlete is usually notified of the mandatory test immediately after competing by a Doping Control Escort. The athlete then has 1 hour to report to the Doping Control Station.

However, no matter whether it is a random, short-notice NCAA drug screen or an OOC, NAN USOC mandatory drug test, once the athlete arrives at the drug-testing station, the steps in the collection protocol are fairly uniform. If a specimen is incomplete or inadequate, the competitor is required to remain in the collection station under observation until a sample of adequate volume, pH, and specific gravity is obtained (66). Failure to follow these procedures, including failure to appear within the 1-hour time period without justification, failure to provide an adequate urine specimen, or refusal to provide a urine specimen, will result in the athlete's being subject to the same actions and consequences as if he or she had used a banned substance (8,11,65,66). A summary of specimen collection procedures at the Olympic Games is found in Table 11–2.

Once at the laboratory the "A" sample is analyzed, as the strict chain of custody procedures are clearly documented. If the athlete's "A" sample is found to contain a banned substance (utilizing the methods described later in this chapter), the urine from the "A" bottle is then reanalyzed to ensure the accuracy of the results. If the "A" sample tests positive for a banned substance a second time, the proper officials are notified, and they notify the athlete and his or her representing organization. The athlete or a representative then has the option to observe the "B" sample testing, which is done as soon as possible and varies depending on the organization (anywhere from 24 hours to 45 days) (8). Since the results are deemed positive only if the "B" sample is also found to contain a banned substance(s), only then will the proper sanctioning authorities be notified. Before sanctions are imposed, most drug-testing policies allow for a fair hearing in accordance with prespecified rules and regulations on appeals. The athlete is given a chance to explain any extenuating circumstances before punitive action is taken. However, the athlete may waive this right and voluntarily accept the penalty to be imposed (8,18,27).

To help protect the athletes from false positive results, many organizations allow only IOC-accredited laboratories to perform their drug testing. There are currently 25 IOC-accredited laboratories in the world, and two of them are in the United States: one at UCLA, the other at Indiana University Medical Center (55,67). Both of these are also the only labs that are fully accredited by the NCAA.

Consequences of a Positive Test

The sanctions imposed for testing positive vary according to the governing organization, the substance found, the athlete's previous history of positive tests, and the sport in which the athlete was competing. The most punitive measures are imposed for doping with drugs that are known to be more effective at improving athletic performance, such as AAS, beta-blockers, and amphetamines (22). Table 11–1 summarizes the policies adopted by some of the sports organizations that test U.S. athletes. The policies vary greatly in their approach to detection and penalties for those testing positive. Over the last few years, there has been a significant push for more uniform sanctions and enforcement among the various national and international sports governing bodies. Therefore, organizations such as the IOC have recommended that all sanctions imposed on an athlete by one be given reciprocity by all others (58).

In addition to temporary or permanent ineligibility or exclusion during competition, USOC/IOC penalties are as follows: For anabolic agents (including beta-2 agonists), stimulants, diuretics, beta-blockers, narcotics, designer drugs, and peptide and glycoprotein hormones and their analogues, athletes are subject to a 2-year suspension for the first offense and a lifetime ban for the second offense. For sympathomimetic amines, such

TABLE 11–2. *Summary of in-competition specimen collection procedures at the Olympic Games*

Under the direct supervision of a Doping Control Officer the athlete is required to:

1. Report to the Doping Control Station no later than 1 hour after notification.
2. Provide appropriate identification to a Doping Control Officer. The athlete's signature and time of arrival are then recorded on the Doping Control Notification/Signature Form.
3. Declare any substances taken in the preceding 2 weeks.
4. Select a collection vessel and visually check that it is empty and clean.
5. Urinate a minimum of 100 mL (amount required may vary) in the collection vessel under the observation of the Doping Control Officer.
6. Select a urine control kit and pour approximately two thirds into bottle A and one third into bottle B, leaving a few drops in the collection vessel. The Doping Control Officer will then ensure that the urine pH is >5 and <7.5, and that the urine specific gravity is ≥1.010 (or ≥1.005 if by refractometer).
7. Verify that the code numbers from the numbered security seals that were applied to the bottles are identical to those recorded on the Doping Control Notification/Signature Form.
8. Sign the Doping Control Notification/Signature Form signifying that the entire procedure was performed according to the stated rules and that:
   - the specimen submitted was sealed in their presence
   - all the numbers match and
   - they are aware that all specimens are subject to analysis.
9. The athlete can then leave the Doping Control Station.

Modified from U.S. Olympic Committee. National Anti-Doping Program policies and procedures. Colorado Springs, CO: USOC Drug Control Administration; and Landry GL, Kokotailo PK. Drug screening in the athletic setting. *Curr Probl Pediatr* 1994;24:344–359.

as ephedrine, pseudoephedrine, and phenylpropanolamine, as well as caffeine and all other banned substances or practices; there is a maximum penalty of 3 months suspension for the first offense, 2 years for the second offense, and a lifetime ban for the third offense (8,68). If an athlete who tests positive for a prohibited substance is part of a team, then the entire team is subject to disqualification and forfeiture of any medals won (68). Some National Governing Bodies (NGB) and International Sports Federations (ISF) have different penalties from those of the IOC for certain substances. When there is a discrepancy in the sanctions to be employed, the penalties of the athletes' respective NGB or ISF will take precedence and be applied over those of the IOC (68). Thus Ross Rebagliati, a Canadian who won a gold medal in the men's snowboard giant slalom at the 1998 Nagano Winter Olympics had his medal repealed and was suspended for testing positive for marijuana. Even though the IOC considered marijuana only a "drug subject to certain restrictions" and did not ban it outright, the fact that the International Ski Federation did ban the use of marijuana made the IOC impose the penalties. However, the discrepancy between the IOC's and International Ski Federation's policies on marijuana opened the ruling to arbitration. Therefore the Canadian Olympic Association objected to the ruling on his behalf, while Rebagliati further claimed that he had passively inhaled marijuana smoke. The International Court of Arbitration for Sport (ICAS) then overturned the ruling, stating that there was no proper agreement between the IOC and the International Ski Federation over testing procedures. Therefore Rebagliati was reinstated and was allowed to keep his medal (69). To avoid any future confusion or embarrassment, the IOC has since placed marijuana on its banned list (70).

DOCTOR-PATIENT RELATIONSHIP

The doctor-patient relationship must not be undermined in enacting a drug-testing program. The treating physician should not be involved in the selection process for drug screening. Furthermore, the physician should not be involved in the communication of test results to third parties, including coaches and athletic directors. All medical information obtained from an athlete must be considered absolutely confidential unless the athlete or the athlete's legal guardian authorizes the release of that information (11).

DRUG-TESTING METHODOLOGY

The overall purpose of drug-testing methodologies is to distinguish a substance, sometimes at picogram and nanogram per milliliter levels, from the extensively diverse mixture of substances that are found in urine. Thus, in using any measuring device such as a mass spectrometer, the goal is to try to enhance the signal produced by the substance of interest to distinguish it from the noise inherent in the urine milieu (27). However, given the rapid turnaround time needed for this type of analysis in competitive sports and the serious consequences of a positive result, testing must be done as exactly, yet as efficiently, as possible. Therefore one of the primary objectives of lab officials, who are trying to detect the intake of banned substances, is to create a single screening method that is able to detect and quantitate the maximum number of substances at one time (18,71,72). As will become apparent, this has been achieved to a degree for most, but not all, of the classes of banned substances. In a sense, this is due in large part to the properties of urine.

Urine has many advantages as a medium for drug testing. It is easily obtainable, is not as invasive as obtaining a blood sample, and may contain large concentrations of drugs along with their metabolites (71,73,74). However, urine also has many disadvantages as a medium for drug testing. It can easily be adulterated, diluted, and substituted. Urinary drug concentrations may vary depending on dose, route of administration, time elapsed since administration, urine flow, pH, and metabolism. The analysis of urine reveals the presence or absence of banned substances and/or their metabolites but not the amount, time, duration, or purpose of use (73,74). In most of the following techniques the athlete's urine sample has to be preprocessed to prepare it for the appropriate testing technique. These preparation techniques, though essential, are beyond the scope of this chapter.

Drug Testing Procedure

Drug-testing procedures for urine samples are usually divided into screening tests and confirmatory tests (45,74–76). Screening tests are set up to maximize sensitivity or to limit the number of false negative results, whereas confirmatory tests are designed to maximize specificity or to limit the number of false positive results. (11,18,28,45,65,74) Common screening tests include radioimmunoassays, enzyme immunoassays, fluorescence polarization immunoassays, and thin-layer chromatography (73). Since these screening methods may be susceptible to cross-reactivity or other errors, once a banned substance has been identified by one of these preliminary tests, a second more specific method is used to confirm the results. Common confirmatory tests include gas chromatography, gas chromatography-mass spectrometry, and high-performance liquid chromatography, although these tests could also be used for screening (45,73,76). Other confirmatory tests include gas chromatography/high resolution mass spectrometry, tandem mass spectrometry, and combinations of the above, for instance, high-performance liquid chromatography/tandem mass spectrometry (77).

Radioimmunoassay

A radioimmunoassay (RIA) is performed by mixing an animal antibody to the drug (e.g., erythropoietin) being tested for with the sample to be tested and a radiolabeled ligand or tracer molecule, usually I^{125} (78). Upon mixing with the sample, the antibody will bind to the drug. When this in turn is mixed with the radiolabeled ligand, the ligand competes with the free drug in the sample to bind to the antibody. Upon equilibrium of the mixture, the amount of drug in the sample equals the amount of radioactive ligand that has not been bound to the antibody (73).

Enzyme Immunoassay

The most common enzyme immunoassay (EIA) is the enzyme-multiplied immunoassay technique (EMIT) (45). While similar to RIA because it is also based on an equilibrium antigen-antibody process, EMIT measures the enzymatic activity of glucose-6-phosphate dehydrogenase (G6PD), instead of radiolabeled antibodies. First, the enzyme G6PD is combined with the drug to be assayed, forming an enzyme-drug conjugate. This enzyme-drug mixture is then combined with the urine sample, an antibody to the drug, nicotinamide adenine dinucleotide (NAD), and a substrate for the enzyme. Upon mixing, the free drug in the sample and that bound to G6PD compete for binding sites on the antibody. The more free drug is in the sample, the less the drug-enzyme conjugate will bind to the antibodies. Therefore more drug-enzyme conjugate will be available to react with the substrate, resulting in greater enzyme activity, ultimately resulting in a conversion of NAD to NADH. Thus the presence of more enzyme product, or higher levels of NADH, directly correlates with a higher concentration of free drug in the sample (73,79).

Fluorescence Polarization Immunoassay

In a fluorescence polarization immunoassay (FPIA), antibodies are mixed with a tracer or chemical labeled with fluorescein and the sample. As in both RIA and EIA, competition for antibody-binding sites occurs between the free drug in the urine sample and the tracer. Samples with a low drug concentration will generate more tracer binding, which results in more polarization of fluorescence. Samples with a high drug concentration will generate less tracer binding, which results in less polarization of fluorescence (73).

Thin-layer Chromatography

In thin-layer chromatography (TLC) a pretreated urine specimen is placed on a gel-covered plate that has first been coated with different chemicals and that has one end resting in a solvent mixture (73). A small amount of the urine sample is placed at the end of the gel-covered plate closest to the solvent (80). The compounds in the urine sample move up the gel-covered plate at different rates because larger molecules move up the plate more slowly than smaller ones as they are attracted to the different coatings. In this manner the sample is separated into its components. Once this process is complete, the plate is removed and stained. Depending on the substances in the urine, chemical reactions occur, producing different-colored spots. Chromatographic analysis consists of comparing these spots to those of a control sample (80). Certain colors or patterns will indicate the presence or absence of one or more substances.

Each of the screening tests has advantages and disadvantages, which are summarized in Table 11–3 (11, 74,81,82).

In any of the confirmatory tests, urine samples must first undergo a number of steps as alluded to previously, which can include extraction, derivatization, evaporation, and hydrolysis. The sample is then separated into its components, using the methodologies described below. Through the process of mass spectrometry (MS), these components are then identified by matching their mass spectral patterns to those of reference compounds (67).

Gas Chromatography

In gas chromatography (GC) the chemicals in an extracted urine sample are vaporized in an oven and then carried by a gas (e.g., helium or nitrogen) over a heated separation column (67,73,83). The vaporized compounds in the sample tend to move along the column at their own relative speed, grouping together and separating from the other compounds in the sample (83). These chemical components then leave the column at distinct times. The rate at which these groups travel over a particular column medium can be measured and used for their identification (84). As they exit, they are subjected to a detector, and a recorder is set up to monitor the amount of compound(s) in the substance (80). The identification of the substance is based on its retention time in the separation column and its signal strength. Common detectors are flame ionization detectors and nitrogen phosphorus detectors. Nitrogen phosphorus detectors monitor compounds that contain a nitrogen or phosphorous atom (65).

TABLE 11-3. Advantages and disadvantages of preliminary screening tests

Method	Advantages	Disadvantages
Radioimmunoassay (RIA)	• Nominal personnel requirements • Objective results • Small sample requirements • Minimal sample preparation • Limited equipment required	• Radioactive isotope • Special atomic energy license required • Heterogeneous assay • Labor intensive • May cross-react with molecules similar in structure to substance being tested for thereby causing false positives
Enzyme immunoassay (EIA)	• Nominal personnel requirements • Objective results • Adaptation to batch or random access analyzers • Uniform procedures • Short analysis time • Minimal sample preparation • Limited equipment required	• Reagents expensive • Not specific for single drugs • May cross-react with molecules similar in structure to substance being tested for • Batch to batch variation in antibody reagents
Fluorescence polarization immunoassay (FPIA)	• Very sensitive • Objective results • Minimal sample preparation • Limited equipment required	• Limited capability • More expensive than other immunochemical methods
Thin-layer chromatography (TLC)	• Low equipment cost • Limited equipment required • Rapid analysis • Simultaneous determination of several drugs and metabolites	• Skill dependent; requires much training and experience in interpretation • Labor intensive • Low sensitivity • Sample pretreatment • Subjective interpretation of results • Nonreproducible raw data • Considered inadequate and obsolete for drug abuse screening

Modified from U.S. Olympic Committee. National anti-doping program policies and procedures. Colorado Springs, CO: USOC Drug Control Administration; Kapur B. Drug testing methods and interpretations of test results. In: Macdonald S, Roman P, eds. Drug testing in the workplace. New York: Plenum Press, 1994; Substance-Abuse Testing Committee. Critical issues in urinalysis of abused substances: report of the substance-abuse testing committee. Clin Chem 1988;34:605-632; Finkle BS. Drug-analysis technology: overview and state of the art. Clin Chem 1987;33:13B-17B.

Gas Chromatography/Mass Spectrometry

In gas chromatography/mass spectrometry (GC/MS) a sample is initially subjected to gas chromatography as described above. However, after the chemical compounds undergo GC and leave the detector, they are bombarded by electrons in a vacuum. The electrons transfer a charge to the molecules, some acquiring enough energy to fragment into their constituent ions (65,80). The ions travel through a strong magnetic field, which causes them to separate according to mass and charge. An ion detector then monitors the mass, charge, and abundance of the ions. A mass spectrum of fragment masses and charges versus relative abundance is produced from this information (65). Each chemical compound produces a specific mass spectrum and can be identified by that pattern (73). Ultimate confirmation is made when the test substance's pattern is matched to that of a reference compound's, stored as a "molecular fingerprint" in a mass spectral library (17,85). GC/MS can provide the mass spectra for all of the fragments in a given substance, which is referred to as a full scan. In selected ion monitoring (SIM) mode GC/MS, only some fragments characteristic of a substance are scanned. Full-scan mode GC/MS is more specific than SIM mode GC/MS, while SIM mode GC/MS is more sensitive than full-scan mode GC/MS (82,83). Thus, with the advent of GC/MS a test that was both highly sensitive and specific was created.

High-Performance Liquid Chromatography

High-performance liquid chromatography (HPLC) utilizes a process similar to GC, but substances do not have to be vaporized, and the medium that carries the substance over the separation column is a liquid instead of a gas (73,74). Furthermore, the column is usually at room temperature or slightly higher (74). The detector that is commonly used with HPLC is an ultraviolet (UV) absorbance detector, which adds specificity by allowing the choice of a wavelength characteristic of the substance being sought (65). HPLC is used for substances that are hard to volatilize or are heat labile (74). HPLC is very sensitive; however, MS is still necessary to confirm the identity of each substance.

Gas Chromatography/High Resolution Mass Spectrometry

A more selective confirmatory technique such as gas chromatography/high resolution mass spectrometry (GC/HRMS) can extend the limits of detection (77). This technique is useful when low limits of detection are necessary, as in attempting to confirm the presence of anabolic steroids in urine (67). Some substances have very similar mass-to-charge ratios (m/z) and therefore produce very similar spectral patterns, which can be extremely difficult to differentiate using standard GC/MS (77). In GC/HRMS the differences between similar substances are effectively magnified, leading to better identification. Thus, the advantage of GC/HRMS is the high degree of differentiation and therefore detection of substances similar in molecular structure but varying in m/z (67,77,86).

Tandem Mass Spectrometry

In tandem mass spectrometry (MS/MS) two mass filters are joined, and selected product parent ions from the first analyzer are collided with neutral gas molecules in the collision chamber of the second analyzer, producing daughter ions (87). These collision-induced daughter ions are then monitored, and a highly specific ion spectrum is produced that enables technicians to identify compounds even in complex mixtures (77,87). However, the stability of the spectra produced by MS/MS has been questioned. Besides the absence of large MS/MS spectral libraries, a number of problems still need to be resolved with this confirmatory method before more widespread use is accepted (27). The advantages and disadvantages of the confirmatory tests are summarized in Table 11–4.

TABLE 11–4. *Advantages and disadvantages of confirmatory tests*

Method	Advantages	Disadvantages
Gas chromatography (GC)	• Reliable • Sensitive analysis • Reproducible results • Objective results • Simultaneous determination of several drugs and metabolites • Can be automated	• Samples must be run one at a time • Labor intensive • Limited capacity • Sample preparation, i.e., the need to derivatize nonvolatile substances • Expertise required • High maintenance
High-performance liquid chromatography (HPLC)	• Highly sensitive analysis • Objective results • Simultaneous determination of several drugs and metabolites • Highly reproducible retention times, offering greater specificity • Can be automated • Less sample preparation than GC	• Similar to GC • Slower and less sensitive than GC
Gas chromatography/mass spectrometry (GC/MS)	• Highly specific and sensitive analysis • Objective results • Computerized mass spectral libraries make identification easy • Can be automated • Preferred method for legal defense	• Costly equipment • Complex instrumentation • High level of skill necessary to operate and interpret data • Compounds in a mixture with similar mass spectra are not discernible
Gas chromatography/high-resolution mass spectrometry (GC/HRMS)	• Greater degree of differentiation and detection of substances similar in molecular structure but with varying mass to charge ratios • Objective results • Can be automated	• Relatively large instruments • Costly equipment • Costly maintenance • High degree of expertise required to operate • Extensive sample preparation
Tandem mass spectrometry (MS/MS)	• Extremely sensitive analysis • Objective results • Can be automated	• Stability of the spectra produced is debated • Absence of MS/MS libraries

Modified from Cowan DA, Kicman AT. Doping in sport: misuse, analytical tests, and legal aspects [Editorial]. *Clin Chem* 1997;43:1110–1113; Kapur B. Drug testing methods and interpretations of test results. In: Macdonald S, Roman P, eds. *Drug testing in the workplace.* New York: Plenum Press, 1994; Bowers LD. Analytical advances in detection of performance enhancing compounds. *Clin Chem* 1997;43:1299–1304; Substance-Abuse Testing Committee. Critical issues in urinalysis of abused substances: report of the substance-abuse testing committee. *Clin Chem* 1988;34:605–632.

METHODOLOGIES BY DRUG GROUP

The topic of what drugs athletes use and how these are employed has been written about extensively (9–10,13,22,28,40,88) (see Chapter 9). Instead, in this chapter we will discuss drugs in terms of the methods that are used to detect them. The classes of drugs banned by the IOC provide a convenient framework from which to explain these methods because (1) the IOC bans the largest number of substances, (2) testing is usually conducted on drugs with similar properties, and (3) an attempt is made to test the greatest amount of drugs at one time for efficient doping control.

Stimulants, Narcotics, Beta-blockers and Beta-2 Agonists

Stimulants, narcotics, beta-blockers, and beta-2 agonists share many characteristics: (1) they can be excreted into urine as unconjugated free drug or conjugated as glucuronides or sulfates, (2) they are weakly basic and volatile, (3) almost all of them have functional groups that can be derivatized to improve their gas chromatographic behavior, (4) they contain nitrogen in the amine group, and (5) their physiological effects are produced by high dosages (with the exception of clenbuterol, salbutamol, and terbutaline) (71,72). Despite extensive metabolism of this group of drugs, large quantities of unconjugated drug are still excreted in urine (71).

Stimulants, narcotics, and beta-blockers are screened and confirmed by the combination of two complementary methods: For the parent compound and unconjugated metabolites, GC is done after a single-step extraction, followed by detection with a nitrogen-specific detector and/or MS. For the conjugated metabolites, GC is done after hydrolysis, extraction, derivatization, and then detection by MS (71). The derivatization process for beta-2 agonists is different from that for the rest of the compounds in this group. To obtain better sensitivity and a more specific fragmentation pattern of beta-2 agonists, it is recommended that they be derivatized to form cyclic boronates (72). Because of their low therapeutic doses, beta-2 agonists are better detected by SIM mode GC/MS (72). More than 100 stimulants, narcotics, beta-blockers, and beta-2 agonists can be screened and confirmed 24 hours after administration of a therapeutic dose by the combination of these two methods and the modifications for beta-2 agonists (71).

The IOC has set guidelines for the testing of doping substances that contain nitrogen, such as stimulants and narcotics. If they are excreted in free form, the IOC minimally requires screening to be done by GC with a NPD and a "capillary column, cross-linked with a moderate polarity phase" (8). If they are excreted as conjugates, the IOC minimally requires "GC screening after hydrolysis and extraction at pH 9.5, derivatization, [and] cross-linked capillary column detection" with an NPD or by SIM (8). For beta-blocking agents the IOC minimally requires screening by GC and/or GC/MS (8). In all cases, as was previously emphasized, analysis by MS is required for definite identification (8).

Anabolic Androgenic Steroids

There are many challenges in the detection of AAS in urine, including the low concentrations of anabolic steroid metabolites (μg/L range), the large number of known steroids (at least 7000) and their metabolites that need to be screened for, the fact that steroids of similar molecular structure exist in urine at concentrations 1000 times higher than the banned substances that are being sought, their poor volatility and thermal lability, and the close structural similarity of this entire class of drugs (77,85). Because of these challenges, SIM mode GC/MS is the most common methodology used for the detection of doping with exogenous and endogenous AAS (89).

For exogenous AAS, screening is based on identifying the parent drug and/or metabolite(s). The chromatographic relative retention time and the mass spectrum of the sample are compared to the relative retention times and mass spectra of reference compounds to find the identity of the metabolite or parent drug (67,89). For reference the main urinary metabolites of almost all known AAS have been characterized, synthesized, and identified by their GC retention times and full or selected mass spectra (67,89). If the concentration of urinary exogenous AAS is too low and prevents analysis by MS, then a comparison of characteristic ion ratios can be made (89). A low concentration of exogenous AAS can also be better detected by a selective detection technique such as GC/HRMS. SIM mode HRMS screens for exogenous AAS and full-scan mode HRMS confirms their presence (77).

Detection of doping with endogenous AAS is more complex because analysis by GC/MS does not differentiate between endogenous and exogenous testosterone (77,90). As was previously discussed, the presence of a T/E ratio greater than 6:1 in an athlete's urine is considered proof of doping with endogenous AAS unless there is evidence that this ratio is caused by a physiologic or pathologic condition (8). Administration of endogenous AAS increases the concentration of testosterone and decreases that of epitestosterone, thereby elevating the T/E ratio (27). Since there have been cases of athletes with T/E ratios that are naturally higher than 6:1, other markers of endogenous testosterone administration are being sought (77,89). One method has measured the carbon isotope ratio $^{13}C/^{12}C$ in urine samples (67,77,90). The carbon isotope ratio is lower in exogenous testosterone than in endogenous testosterone. Furthermore, carbon isotope ratios for endogenous testosterone and its metabolites decrease after administration with exogenous testosterone (90). This method proved comparable to use of the T/E greater than 6:1 test in the detection of doping with testosterone. However, the large amount of sample necessary for analysis and high equipment costs hinder its present practical application (90).

Since most AAS are excreted as glucuronides or sulfate metabolites in urine, HPLC/MS/MS has been used to directly detect the sulfate and glucuronide conjugates of endogenous AAS (77,89). Urinary testosterone glucuronide and epitestosterone glucuronide concentrations increase upon administration of the parent compounds (89). However, approximately 33% of the cases of T/E ratios that are higher than 6:1 have been shown to be the result of very high concentrations of epitestosterone sulfate and low concentrations of epitestosterone glucuronide (77). In some people a T/E ratio greater than 6:1 will not occur with testosterone administration (90). Though the T/E ratio of 6:1 as a limit for the detection of endogenous AAS has been verified as realistic, ultimate proof of endogenous AAS administration is sought by GC/MS under stringent protocols (89).

A method of detection for both endogenous and exogenous AAS has recently been developed. AAS can now be identified by their retention time, ultraviolet-visible (UV-vis) spectra, and mass spectra. This is accomplished through the use of HPLC with a UV-vis photodiode array detector that is coupled with a particle beam MS detector (85). The advantages of each type of detector are maximally utilized to find lower concentrations of AAS. Thus, the coupling of the UV-vis photodiode array detector and particle beam MS detector provide quantitative and qualitative measurements in a single experiment (85).

The IOC has minimum drug-testing methodology requirements for the detection of doping with AAS, which vary depending on the manner of their excretion. If they are excreted in free form, the IOC minimally requires "extraction at pH 9.0, derivatization and detection" by SIM. (8) If they are excreted as conjugates, the IOC minimally requires "enzymatic hydrolysis, extraction, trimethylsilylation and detection by" SIM (8). Again, definite identification of anabolic steroid free form or conjugates is done by analysis with MS. In addition, a T/E ratio greater than 6:1 must be corroborated by previous and subsequent tests along with endocrine examinations before a sample is declared positive for AAS use (8). If no previous tests are available, the athlete has to submit to unannounced testing once a month for at least 3 months before the sample is declared positive (8).

Diuretics

Diuretics as a class are made up of compounds with varying molecular structures and physicochemical properties. Diuretics can be classified by their mechanism and primary site of action in the nephron, by their chemical structure and nature of their functional groups, and by their potency (91). Most diuretics are to some extent excreted in urine unchanged, ranging from 4–12% for a compound like triamterene to 99% for acetazolamide (92). Extraction of the drugs from urine has been achieved by targeting the chemical nature of their functional groups, which can be classified as basic, neutral, weakly acidic, or strongly acidic (93). The most widely used techniques to isolate unadulterated diuretics from urine are liquid-liquid extractions. The most effective manner to extract a wide range of diuretics is comprised of alkaline extraction (pH 9.5) with ethyl acetate, using sodium chloride to promote the effect of salting-out (92).

After extraction the most efficient method to screen for diuretics in urine is liquid chromatography combined with ultraviolet absorbance detection (LC-UV) (92). LC methods involve the separation of compounds by gradient elution, in which various phases of chemicals wash out the diuretics at different pH levels. The resulting chromatogram has peak shapes indicating the diuretic used. UV spectra that facilitate identification are then produced by monitoring these wavelengths using photodiode array detectors (18).

The most widely used method to screen for diuretics in urine is GC/MS after methylation (92). However, LC-UV is more efficient than GC/MS because it does not necessitate this time-consuming derivatization of the sample (92). LC-UV is also a more comprehensive screening technique for diuretics than GC/MS. Nonetheless, the great distribution of many GC/MS instruments and the high degree of standardization of the GC/MS technique contribute to its greater use as a screening method for diuretics in urine (92). Currently, the IOC's minimum requirements for the detection of doping with diuretics are "extraction and derivatization, [then] GC with nitrogen specific detection" by SIM or by HPLC (8).

Peptide and Glycoprotein Hormones

Detection of adrenocorticotropin, human growth hormone (hGH), chorionic gonadotropin (hCG), erythropoietin (EPO), and their releasing factors by immunoassay has been well established but is not accepted as definitive proof of administration (71,77). On the other hand, the production of multiply charged ions from peptides and proteins has been facilitated by electrospray (ES) ionization and extends the mass range of the mass spectrometer. Thus the generation of ions directly from

TABLE 11-5. *Advantages and disadvantages of confirmatory tests for specific drug groups*

Method	Advantages	Disadvantages
High-performance liquid chromatography/tandem mass spectrometry (HPLC/MS/MS) For analysis of AAS (77,89)	• Directly detects the sulfate and glucuronide conjugates of steroids • Provides a powerful tool to investigate stage II metabolism of AAS • Little or no sample preparation required • Extremely sensitive analysis • Objective results • Simultaneous determination of several drugs and metabolites • Can be automated • Less sample preparation than GC	• Deuterated internal standards required for sulfate and glucuronide conjugates of testosterone and epitestosterone • Samples must be run one at a time • Labor intensive • Limited capacity • Expertise required • High maintenance • Absence of HPLC/MS/MS libraries
High-performance liquid chromatography with ultraviolet visible-particle beam mass spectrometry (HPLC with UV-vis-PB MS) For analysis of AAS (85)	• Identification of substances based on retention time, UV-vis spectra, and mass spectra • Qualitative and quantitative information provided from a single experiment • UV-vis photodiode array detector better for quantitative analysis due to greater sensitivity, reproducibility, and wide linear dynamic ranges when compared with particle beam MS detector • Highly sensitive analysis • Objective results • May provide simultaneous determination of several drugs and metabolites • Retention times may be highly reproducible, offering greater specificity • Can be automated • Less sample preparation than GC	• Samples must be run one at a time • Labor intensive • Limited capacity • Sample preparation, i.e., the need to derivatize nonvolatile substances • Expertise required • High maintenance
Liquid chromatography with ultraviolet absorbance detection (LC-UV) For analysis of diuretics (92)	• No derivatization required for sample • More comprehensive screening than GC/MS (since some diuretics cannot be methylated and therefore cannot be analyzed by GC/MS) • UV detection using diode arrays improves selectivity for identification of substances after LC separation • Objective results	• Less selective than GC/MS • Samples must be run one at a time • Labor intensive • Limited capacity • Sample preparation, though involving less steps, is still necessary • Expertise required • High maintenance
Enzyme-linked immunosorbent selective assay (ELISA) NordiTest For analysis of hGH (94)	• Highly sensitive analysis ensures that endogenous forms of hGH are determined as well as commercially available hGHs • Allows possibility of urinary hGH measurements without preparation of sample (no concentration, no dialysis) • Tested for specificity and did not cross-react with similar types of structurally related hormones or urine compounds • Nominal personnel requirements • Objective results • Adaptation to batch or random access analyzers • Uniform procedures • Short analysis time • Limited equipment required	• Detection of doping with hGH is still not definitive with this test • Cannot be used for in-competition testing (because strenuous effort increases hGH levels) • Batch-to-batch variation in antibody reagents
Blood testing For analysis of EPO (97–99)	• Results are known within 1 hour • More sensitive than any other method currently available for detection of doping with EPO	• With currently available blood tests, certainty rate of detecting doping with EPO is only 80% • Certainty rate is unacceptable in court • More invasive than urine testing • Levels of hematocrit which indicate doping with EPO have not been set by ISFs or IOC

liquids may make it possible to confirm administration of peptide hormones by MS, although the reproducibility of this method must be established (77).

One test that detects urinary hGH is the enzyme-linked immunosorbent selective assay (ELISA) NordiTest (94). Despite this and other immunoassays that can detect urinary hGH, there are no IOC-approved urine tests for the detection of doping by recombinant hGH (95). There are many reasons for this. The major component of both hGH and recombinant hGH is a single-chain peptide of 191 amino acids stabilized by two disulfide bonds; therefore current immunoassays cannot reliably differentiate between exogenous and endogenous hGH (95). Also, the concentration of hGH in urine is 1000-fold lower than it is in blood (61). Furthermore, since hGH is secreted in pulses and is relatively short lasting, a urine test based only on augmented hGH would be inaccurate, especially since exercise tends to increase hGH secretion (94–96). In fact, at the 1992 Barcelona Olympics, short bouts of intense exercise, such as a 400-m dash, were shown to increase levels of hGH dramatically (94).

It has been suggested that specific ratios of the many insulinlike growth factors (IGF) could lead to a more sensitive and specific confirmatory urine test of doping with somatropin (one form of recombinant hGH) (77,95). Administration of somatropin decreases the serum concentration of IGF-binding protein 2 (IGFBP-2) and subsequently increases the ratios of IGF-I/IGFBP-2 and IGFBP-3/IGFBP-2 (95). Unfortunately, since the presence of these markers in urine is greatly reduced, current testing based solely on urinalysis is not yet reliable. However, three-ion SIM mode ES ionization HPLC/MS has successfully detected 10 fmol of IGF-1, proving that detection of hGH markers is possible (77).

Although ES ionization HPLC/MS has been used to screen for hCG in urine, the quantitative and qualitative identification data have not been well established (77). Therefore the IOC minimal drug-testing methodology for the detection of doping with hCG currently consists of "a validated immunoassay to detect and quantitate hCG" and "for confirmation, a second different immunoassay" (8).

Charge differences have been observed between native and recombinant human EPO (rHuEPO) and have been used to detect it in urine samples (77). This may lead to an HPLC/MS method for the detection of exogenous EPO in urine, but there is currently no sensitive and specific method for the detection of exogenous EPO in urine (77,78). ELISA and RIA have been successful in detecting EPO concentrations in urine; however, the analysis was long (2 days for RIA), difficult, and expensive (78). Other problems in the identification of rHuEPO in urine are that EPO is present at picomolar levels and that EPO and rHuEPO have similar structures: one polypeptide chain of 166 amino acids with two disulfide bonds and four polysaccharide chains, with the exception that rHuEPO has "heterogeneous carbohydrate moiety" (78). Because of these problems and the fact that EPO is more easily detectable in blood, biathlon participants in the 1998 Nagano Winter Olympics were actually required to undergo blood tests for the detection of rHuEPO (69). Despite this, the USOC does not currently have any plans to administer blood testing to U.S. athletes (Personal communication with Amy Krasikov, representative, USOC Drug Education Program, April 17, 1998).

Major advances in analytical technology occurred in 1983 when benchtop quadrupole GC/MS instruments were used to screen all urine samples and again at the 1996 Olympic Games in Atlanta when GS/sector MS systems were used at moderate mass resolution to screen all of the urine specimens for anabolic agents (77). However, the most recent major departure from previous analytical methodology occurred at the 1998 Nagano Winter Olympics when athletes had to submit to blood testing to detect for EPO. Introduced by the IOC and ISFs for winter sports, blood testing for rHuEPO may become a commonplace component of the IOC's doping control program. In fact, the vice-president of the IOC Medical Commission, Dr. Jacques Rogge, has stated that the IOC is prepared to introduce blood testing in the 2000 Sydney Olympic Games if it deems that this is necessary (97). Since rHuEPO increases hematocrit, acceptable levels have been set by the ISFs that are currently conducting blood testing. The International Ski Federation uses hemoglobin levels set at 16.5 g/dL for women and 18.5 g/dL for men as limits. The International Cyclist Union uses a 50% hematocrit limit (approximately 16.5 g/dL) for men (98). In these tests, 4 mL of blood is drawn, hemoglobin levels are analyzed, and results are usually available within an hour (99). In terms of reliability, the tests that are currently available can prove that someone has taken rHuPO with a certainty rate of 80% (97). The advantages and disadvantages of confirmatory tests for specific drug groups are summarized in Table 11–5.

FLAWS, LIMITATIONS, AND SOURCES OF ERROR

False Positives and False Negatives

Despite the aura of scientific exactness, drug-testing methods are not immune to flaws. Two major flaws in drug testing are false positives and false negatives. False positives occur when the test results indicate that the banned substance is present when it actually is not. False negatives occur when the tests results indicate that the banned substance is not present when it actually is. Both false positives and false negatives occur for many reasons and depend on the type of screening or confirmatory test(s) conducted. False positives are more dependent on the specificity of the drug detection method, while false negatives are more dependent on the sensitivity of the drug detection method. False negatives may be caused by a method's limits of detection (LOD). The LOD of the test may be too high, or the absolute quantity of the drug may be too low (74). The LOD is often purposefully set at a point that may allow a few individuals who are using banned substances to test negative rather than having even one athlete who is not using banned substances to falsely test positive. Additionally, a unique flaw surrounds the positive test. A positive test indicates only that the banned substance, its metabolite, or a marker was found. From a positive test, it is often difficult to determine the banned substance's form; when or how much was taken; whether it was used socially, therapeutically, misused or abused; and whether the person was exposed voluntarily or involuntarily (5,45,71,74,83). An analytic true positive can simultaneously be a false indicator for illicit use of a banned substance (100). This occurs when the test results indicate that the banned substance is present but the person who tested positive did not intentionally take the substance and was exposed by other means. For example, a true positive occurs when clostebol (an AAS) is found in an athlete and is confirmed by GC/MS. The test result is simultaneously a false positive because it is discovered that the athlete is not illicitly using clostebol but instead had eaten beef from cattle treated with clostebol (74,100).

As was discussed previously, screening and confirmatory tests are used for their distinct advantages in detecting banned substances. However, each of these different methods is susceptible to producing the most serious mistake: a false positive result. For instance, immunoassays are susceptible to cross-reactivity, which occurs when other substances in the urine cross-react with testing reagents, thereby producing false positive results (45). Common substances that have been shown to cause false positive results in immunoassays are asthma medications, allergy medications, Alka Seltzer Plus, Sudafed, herbal teas, and poppy seeds (5,74, 101).

Although GC/MS is considered the best overall testing method, this technique may also produce false positive and false negative results (102). Furthermore, confirmatory analysis by GC/MS will not correct for false negatives that are produced by the initial screening test used (45). False positive results in GC/MS may occur for a number of reasons. First, it is possible, though unlikely, for substances to have the same mass spectrum, GC retention times, and structure as in the case of the D- and L-isomers of methamphetamine (100). Second, in SIM mode GC/MS, a substance and an interferant could have similar three-ion mass spectra and GC retention times (100). The major fragmentation patterns for each substance would occur at areas along their respective molecules that are similar to each other. For example, the derivatives (after di-trimethylsilyl derivatization) of the nandrolone metabolite (19-norandrosterone) and vitamin E metabolite (alpha-tocopheronolactone) have similar GC retention times and three ion mass spectra (at m/z 405,420,422). Thus ingestion of vitamin E could produce false positive results for nandrolone. Third, a derivative of one drug can be converted into another's during the GC/MS process (100). For example, the carbethoxyhexafluorobutyryl (CB) chloride derivative of ephedrine converts into the CB methamphetamine derivative at high GC injection port temperatures. Thus ephedrine could cause a false positive for methamphetamine. False negative results in GC/MS may occur in two steps of the overall process. First, competition for derivatization agents may interfere with the derivatization of a banned substance, causing smaller amounts of it to be derived and ultimately producing a false negative (100). Second, another substance that separates with the targeted substance may interfere with its ionization (100). If either substance is present in greater concentration than the other in the ionization chamber, the ionization beam can become saturated, and some of the target drug may not be ionized or reach the detector. Thus, the detected concentration of the target drug may be decreased. This type of interference is easily apparent in full-scan mode GC/MS but not very apparent in SIM mode GC/MS (100).

Certain substances within the IOC's classes of banned substances tend to be more susceptible to producing false positives and false negatives than others. The following examples may be due to an incorrect analysis or interpretation of test results, faults in the instrumentation used, faults inherent in the type of screening method used, and faults in the preparation of the sample for analysis (103,76,100).

Stimulants

In the stimulant class, false positives for cocaine and amphetamines are more apt to occur. For example, consumption of Health Inca or Mate de Coca tea (not available in the United States) may lead to passive ingestion of cocaine because both have been found to contain small amounts of the drug (104). In addition, false positives may occur for cocaine if a person is passively exposed to it through skin absorption (105). However, casual exposure is rarely sufficient to produce benzoylecgonine levels greater than 300 ng/mL, which is the current limit for this metabolite of cocaine (76,105). In the case of amphetamines the possibility for false positives occurs because several different compounds can be converted into amphetamines in the human body (74,76). For instance, the simultaneous administration of desipramine and amantadine has been shown to cause a false positive for amphetamines in FPIA (106). However, over-the-counter (OTC) drugs containing phenethylamines (e.g., ephedrine and pseudoephedrine) are the most common source of false positives for amphetamines in some immunoassays (105). Other common pharmaceutical preparations that may cause false positives include Eldepryl (selegiline), which metabolizes into the L-forms of methamphetamine and amphetamine; chlorpromazine and promethazine, which are phenothiazine derivatives (and cause false positives in the EMIT II immunoassay); Contact; Sudafed; and Vicks' Nasal Inhaler, which was known to cause false positives for the D-isomer of methamphetamine (5,76,103,105). In addition, the passive inhalation of methamphetamine smoke from cigarettes laced with this substance may cause a false positive result (105).

Narcotics

In the class of narcotics heroin, morphine, and codeine are the substances that are most susceptible to false positives. The presence of morphine or codeine in urine samples could indicate heroin use. Definitive proof of heroin administration is the presence of its direct urinary metabolite, 6-monoacetylmorphine (76,105). However, since codeine is also used extensively in cough medicine and is converted 24 hours after administration into morphine, interpretative expertise is necessary to determine what substance was taken (74,76). Additionally, the ingestion of poppy seeds may cause a false positive test for the opiates morphine, codeine, and heroin (45,100,105,107). However, a morphine-to-codeine ratio of less than 2 or a urinary level of greater than 1000 ng/mL of morphine with no codeine detected (less than 25 ng/mL) cannot be explained by the ingestion of poppy seeds alone and may indicate morphine, codeine, or heroin abuse (105). Furthermore, dextromethorphan, a common OTC drug, may also lead to a false positive test for narcotics. Dextromethorphan is converted into dextrophan, the D-isomer of L-levorphanol, a banned narcotic drug (71). Thus, distinguishing between banned and allowable narcotics can be problematic (76).

Anabolic Androgenic Steroids

AAS also have a potential for false positives. As we have discussed, the sheer number of known steroids (more than 7000), their common metabolic pathways, their similar molecular structures, and the creation of common metabolites complicate the interpretation of results and can cause false positives (85,76). For example, nandrolone (19-nortestosterone) is metabolized into norandrosterone and noretiocholanolone, which are detectable months after administration (45). However, norandrosterone is also a metabolite of noretisterone, which is found in many contraceptive pills (45,76). Thus ascertaining which substance was the origin of the norandrosterone metabolite can be difficult. False positives may arise over the T/E ratio that is used as a screening cutoff for the detection of testosterone administration. Since the T/E ratio differs according to race and sex and between individuals, it can lead to false positives. This is one of the main reasons why the IOC requires additional endocrinologic testing if someone is found to have a T/E ratio above the 6:1 limit (8,76).

Diuretics

There are numerous flaws associated with the tests for the detection of diuretics. They can range from a lack of knowledge about specific metabolites of these substances to the potential for false positives and negatives. For example, spironolactone is completely metabolized into canrenone. However, because canrenone is a metabolite of many substances, its presence in urine does not indicate the actual compound ingested (76). Another example involves acetazolamide, which renders urine alkaline. Alkaline urine is known to mask the excretion of weak basic compounds, such as many stimulant drugs. This could obviously lead to false negative tests for these substances (76). This is one of the many reasons why these substances are banned.

Peptide and Glycoprotein Hormones

The potential for false positives in the detection of peptide and glycoprotein hormones can occur as a result of the testing method used. Most are detected by immunoanalysis, and antibodies that are designed for one may cross-react with similar hormones and lead to false positives. Another drawback in the testing of peptide hormones is that no internationally acceptable reference standards exist for some of them. Therefore results from one lab or method are not easily compared to those from another (76).

Marijuana

A false positive for marijuana use may result from inhaling secondhand smoke, which introduces small amounts of cannabinoids into the body (5,45,108). Unknowingly ingesting marijuana-laced food can also result in a positive test for one of the THC metabolites in urine (105). Several studies have been run that confirmed THC levels for people who were passively exposed to marijuana in different ways. To avoid this type of false positive, a screening cutoff concentration of 50 ng/mL has been recommended (the currently available level of sensitivity is at least 20 ng/mL) (45,105). A person who does not use marijuana and inhales secondhand smoke or passively ingests small quantities in tea, spaghetti sauce, or brownies should not test positive if this cutoff is used (105). Furthermore, ibuprofen, naproxen, and other substances have been shown to produce false positive results for cannabinoids, particularly with the use of immunoassays (5,109). A summary of some substances that may cause false positives is included in Table 11–6.

Reliability

Finally, another serious flaw in drug testing has to do with the scope of existing drug-testing technology. All

TABLE 11–6. *Substances that may cause false positive test results for banned substances*

Substance	May cause false positive results for this banned substance	IOC drug class
• Steroid-treated meats and poultry (54,100)	Clostebol Methyltestosterone Nortestosterone Testosterone Trenbolone	AAS
• Contraceptive pills containing noretisterone (45,76) • Vitamin E metabolite (α-tocopheronolactone) (100)	Nandrolone	AAS
• Chlorpromazine • Ephedrine (105): Bronkaid, Collyrium with Ephedrine, Pazo Suppository, Wyanoids Suppository, Vatronol Nose Drops, herbal teas and medicines containing ma huang (Chinese ephedra): Action Caps, Bishop's Tea, Breathe Easy Herbal Decongestant Tea, Brigham Tea, Chi Powder, Energy Rise, Ephedra, Excel, Free Herbal "Energy Tablets," Joint Fir, Mexican Tea, Miner's Tea, Mormon Tea, Popotillo, Quick Shot Vitamin B-12, Squaw Tea, Super Charge, Teamster's Tea • Famprofazone • Phenylpropanolamine: ARM, Allerest, Alka-Seltzer Plus, Contac, Dexatrim, Dietac, 4–way Formula 44, Naldecon, Novahistine, Arnex, Sine-Aid, Sine-Off, Sinutab, Triaminic, Triaminicin, Sucrets Cold Decongestant • Promethazine • Pseudoephedrine (105): Actifed, Ambenyl-D, Anamine, Afrin Tablets, Afrinol, Co-Tylenol, Deconamine, Dimacol, Emprazil-A, Fedahist, Fedrazil, Histalet, Isoclor, Lo Tussin, Nasalspan, Novafed, Nucofed, Poly-Histine, Pseudo-Bid, Pseudo-Hist, Rhinosym, Ryna, Sudafed, Triprolidine, Tussend, Chlorafed, Chlor-Trimeton-DC, Disphoral, Drixoral, Polaramine Expectorant, Rondec • Simultaneous administration of desipramine and amantadine (106) • Vicks' Nasal Inhaler (5,76,103,105)	Amphetamines	Stimulants
• Health Inca Tea (104) (not available in U.S.) • Mate de Coca Tea (not available in U.S.) • Passive exposure	Cocaine	Stimulants
• Ephedrine (carbethoxyhexafluorobutyryl (CB) chloride derivative) (100) • Eldepryl (selegiline) • Famprofazone • Passive inhalation of crystal meth smoke	Methamphetamine	Stimulants
• Codeine (74,76) • Poppy seeds (45,100,105,107)	Heroin Morphine	Narcotics
• Dextromethorphan (76)	L-levorphanol (narcotic)	Narcotics
• Ibuprofen (5,74,109) • Naproxen (5,74,109) • Passive ingestion • Secondary smoke inhalation	Marijuana	Classes of drugs subject to certain restrictions

of the drug-testing methodologies are based on the fact that confirmation is achieved by comparison with standards or controls, that is, the known relative retention times, gas chromatographic spectra, ultraviolet spectra, mass spectra, or other quality of the substance being sought. What if the substance that is being used to enhance athletic performance is not known? With advances in the fields of chemistry, molecular biology and genetic engineering, coupled with greater monetary incentives, it should not be difficult to concede that there are rogue laboratories and scientists producing "designer drugs" that cannot be detected in competition because they are not yet known to exist. Their metabolism and effects are rumored to be precisely tailored to escape the specificity and sensitivity of current detection methods. Thus a potential flaw and continual threat is for the doping control community to be lulled into a false sense of technological superiority over those who resort to doping.

To further protect against inadvertent false positives, many organizations, such as the IOC, have created minimum urine drug levels for some of their banned substances. Because of the strict standards for accredited IOC labs, concern for false positive results at Olympic-sponsored events have been minimized (11). However, at the types of testing facilities that are bound to be used by organizations such as high schools, there is great inconsistency in the degree to which both false negative and, most important, false positive results are produced (110). Many states do not even have set standards that regulate the accuracy of drug tests (55). In fact, one study reports that when the drug use among the population being tested is only 2.4%, then a lab's 2% false positive rate translates into a 50.4% false accusation rate for certain substances (55). While IOC laboratories ultimately set the standard for drug testing in sports, even they have not gone without criticism. Surprisingly, in 1989 it was reported that 25% of the certified IOC laboratories did not pass routine proficiency tests (111).

CIRCUMVENTION TECHNIQUES

There have been numerous anecdotal reports of how athletes have escaped detection by using any one of various circumvention techniques. Since most doping control systems are currently based on the analysis of urine, one of the most obvious ways to avoid being caught is to substitute drug-free urine for urine containing banned substance(s). In fact, there are companies that offer drug-free urine and urine "purifying" products with which to beat urine tests (74). To escape detection, athletes have employed elaborate means, including catheterizing themselves to put drug-free urine directly into their own bladders and hiding "clean" urine in condoms, containers, animal bladders, and intravaginal pouches. To help prevent cheating, collection of urine specimens should always be done under the direct observation of a doping control officer who has been trained in the techniques used to circumvent drug testing. However, there are times when even this deterrent is not used, as in the testing of high school athletes (53).

Catheterization and Urine Substitution

Despite monitored testing, it has been rumored that one of the U.S. female sprinters participating in the 1988 Olympic Games used her fingernail to puncture a hole in a "bladder" of clean urine that was allegedly concealed in her vagina. If the story is accurate, she provided drug-free urine at an appropriate body temperature (112). Not that this is a new technique; it has been done countless times before. One of the more notorious incidents occurred earlier in this decade when three world-class female German track athletes were banned from international competition after being caught producing three chemically identical urine samples (113). Apparently, these women had placed the drug-free urine into specialized intravaginal pouches, which they used to falsely produce the mandatory specimens. They did this through a well-practiced technique whereby they would give the appearance of urinating by squeezing the specialized pouch with their pelvic muscles. If they had given drug-free urine from different sources, instead of all using the same source, they probably would have never been caught (113).

There are numerous underground stories of athletes easily beating the doping prevention system by voiding their own urine and then being catheterized so that drug-free urine can be infused into their bladders. Even with a doping control escort at the athlete's side and direct visual monitoring until a urine sample is produced, it is still technologically feasible to have unadulterated urine inserted into an athlete before testing. While the IOC and NCAA do specifically prohibit such urine manipulation, a review of their drug-testing policies does not mention any procedures other than the visual monitoring that could detect surgical or similar means of substituting urine.

Timed Abstinence

One of the most commonly used circumvention techniques is to adjust the administration of banned substance according to the known detection or retention times (9). An illustration of this method, also referred to as timed abstinence, is for an athlete to cycle on a drug to obtain the desired training effect, then cycle off the drug in time to escape detection (5). In fact, with the continual development of new forms and modes of use, retention times have shortened from months with drugs such as oil-based AAS to days or purportedly even hours with the new "designer" AAS (67,89). Furthermore, short-acting sublingual drugs, such as testosterone cyclodextrin, could be used close to competition without significant increases in testosterone or a T/E ratio over accepted limits. Thus athletes can switch from AAS with longer retention times to shorter-acting sublingual or transdermal AAS closer to competition. In this manner significant performance enhancement can be obtained without testing positive (67). This can be a very effective circumvention technique if athletes are tested only on known dates or are infrequently tested on a random, short-notice basis, as is done by the NCAA (9).

Choice of College

Most high school athletes will never be tested. Owing in part to the improved drug-testing policies of the NCAA, many learn to use banned ergogenic substances before matriculation to college, where they may be tested. In this way they get the increases in size, speed, and strength without risking the possible loss of scholarships or incurring other penalties, if any, for drug use. Once in college, many athletes are still never tested unless they make it to an NCAA championship. Thus choosing a college that does not have mandatory testing can also be used as a circumvention method.

Urine Dilution

Another technique is to ingest large amounts of fluid to dilute the urine drug concentration below the detection limits (5). Drinking large quantities of water before voiding, or "water-loading," is thought to play a role in avoiding the detection of doping with a number of substances, including caffeine (5,9,114). Furthermore, to increase the effectiveness of this technique, athletes may try to discard their first urine after a competition, rapidly rehydrate, and then delay urination as long as possible so as not to exceed the drug's maximum urine limit (9). Specific gravity is supposed to detect the urine dilution caused by water loading, but the measurement range is limited and has not always been very effective (74). Measuring urine creatinine levels has also been examined as a possible water-loading detection method but has likewise shown limited success (74,114).

Adulterants

Another method that is used to circumvent drug tests is to add adulterating agents to urine that can produce false negative results. Common, known adulterating agents that have been used to try to produce false negative results include sodium chloride (table salt), vinegar, liquid bleach, liquid soap, liquid Drano, Visine eye drops, ascorbic acid (vitamin C), ammonia-based cleaners, lemon juice, golden seal tea, vinegar, and whole blood anticoagulated with EDTA, as well as other household products (5,73–74,115). Much of the effect of these substances appears to be attributable either to a change in pH, resulting in interference with screening tests, or direct chemical degradation (115). Thus the immediate measurement of pH, specific gravity, and temperature, as well as monitored urination and improved analytic techniques, should be used to prevent or detect attempts at adulteration of samples. However, especially in cases in which direct observation of urination is not required, the athlete should be asked to provide another specimen under direct observation if tampering with the urine samples is suspected (73).

Designer Drugs and Masking Agents

One of the most disturbing and clandestine ways of circumventing doping tests is through the use of designer drugs and masking agents. The development of designer drugs by scientists to aid elite athletes in avoiding detection has occurred for years. Accordingly, some scientists affirm that all cheaters need do is "'rearrange one carbon atom and, although the compound will have exactly the same effect, we won't be testing for it'" (116). By continually using drugs that either are undetectable or are not yet officially banned, a significant proportion of elite and professional athletes will always remain a step ahead of present-day testing techniques. A prime example is the remarkably swift emergence of elite Chinese swimmers and runners, who shattered many world records earlier in this decade. They eluded numerous drug tests given to them over a period of several years, despite the strong suspicion of doping that surrounded their success. It was not until the 1994 Asian Games when 11 Chinese medal winners tested positive for a derivative of testosterone that these suspicions were put to rest (58). There have also been stories involving the scientific institutes that propelled elite East German athletes to world record status with the use of ergogenic substances, including AAS, without fear of testing positive. In fact, 20 former East German swimming coaches confirmed that their athletes had used ergogenic drugs for years, successfully eluding all testing (58). It was not until after the unification of Germany and the dissolution of their doping institutes that an elite East German swimmer tested positive for drugs (117). A relatively recent illustration of the continued development and use of designer drugs involves those being sold on the black market by former members of the Soviet sports doping community. Allegedly, many of these drugs are capable of producing false negative drug tests. One example is Cealabolil, a testosterone derivative that contains large amounts of the mineral silica, which may assist in eluding detection. Unfortunately, underground reports have linked this drug to the development of heart failure and to the deaths of at least three renowned powerlifters (112).

Masking agents provide another possible means of circumventing drug tests. There are many known masking agents; one of the more notable examples is the uricosuric and renal tubular transport blocking agent probenecid (118). It was originally found in the urine of U.S. weight lifters at the Pan American Games in 1987 (119). Subsequently, it was shown to inhibit the excretion of AAS and was therefore added to the IOC's banned drug list in the fall of 1987 (8,11,118,120). Human chorionic gonadotrophin is another ergogenic aid that can be used as a masking agent for AAS. It stimulates testosterone and epitestosterone production in men and may mask evidence of testosterone administration by lowering the T/E ratio (77,121). As was discussed previously, epitestosterone can also be used to rapidly lower a T/E ratio that is high because of testosterone doping (120,121). The IOC has banned the use of epitestosterone and set 200 μg/L as a cutoff for its detection (67). Bromantan is yet another masking agent (and a stimulant) that is known to alter the T/E ratio. First detected in a Russian athlete at the 1996 Summer Olympic Games in Atlanta, Bromantan has since been banned by the IOC (8,19). Moreover, diuretics have been another common source for masking agents. Banned as a class by the IOC, they can mask doping by increasing urine volume or by increasing urinary pH, ultimately reducing the concentration of a banned substance in urine (11,92,120).

Finally, even if athletes test positive for banned substances, there are still legal loopholes that have been exploited in the past to invalidate the results. Most of the successful major legal challenges to positive drug test results have centered on chain of command issues (54). It is one of the most crucial, if not the most crucial, components of an organization's drug-testing policy. If an organization that is drug testing cannot assure its athletes of protection against tampering and privacy of results, then it leaves itself open to litigation and jeopardizes the reputation, monetary rewards, and well-being of the athletes that it is supposed to protect (49). Most of these cases have focused not so much on proving athletes' innocence beyond a reasonable doubt as on placing a reasonable doubt about the validity of the chain of command by highlighting flaws in the system or citing steps in the process that are open to potential tampering. It is no wonder that the previously discussed strict chain of command procedures have been so enthusiastically adopted by most organizations. The ICAS was created in 1994 to further ensure impartiality and provide a fair appeals process for athletes who may have been improperly accused, while helping to decrease the amount of litigation, expenses, and false appeals.

COST OF TESTING

Since the IOC is the only organization that bans a large amount and variety of substances, the cost of testing for all of the IOC-banned substances was used as a benchmark. There are only two IOC-approved laboratories that conduct doping tests in the United States: in Indianapolis and Los Angeles. An estimate for the cost of testing for substances banned by the IOC at the Los Angeles lab ranged from $85 to $100 (U.S.) per sample (Personal communication with Tom Callahan, UCLA Olympic Analytical Laboratory). In fact, the costs charged for drug testing are now the major financial support that allows continued research and development of doping methods at IOC labs. While there are many commercial laboratories that conduct drug screening tests for the government and private industry, the quality of the tests and the ability to detect all of the substances that are banned by the IOC vary. Those that can provide detection for such substances charge and discount by volume; that is, the cost per sample varies depending on the number of samples to be tested. In one lab the cost per sample to run what was termed an IOC profile of testing was $195.00 (U.S.). That same lab offered other types of profiles, such as an anabolic steroid profile, which ranged from $60 to $85 (U.S.) per sample. A collegiate profile, which would test for marijuana, cocaine, stimulants, and opiates would range from $24 to $40 (U.S.) per sample.

CONCLUSION

In the future many changes will need to be made to current drug-testing policies if they are to effectively prevent the use of prohibited ergogenic substances. This most surely means an increasing reliance on more invasive techniques, including blood testing. Since these practices will increase the degree of invasiveness and further impinge on the constitutional rights of athletes and others, they will undoubtedly create additional medical, legal, moral, and religious concerns. The controversy surrounding basic rights and drug testing will continue, as the good of the many may in fact outweigh the rights of the not so few athletes who choose to use drugs to artificially enhance their athletic performance. In an age when genetic engineering and cloning loom in the background, the only certainty in the future of drug testing in sports may be that technology will continue to dominate as new drugs of abuse, newer methods of detection, and ingenious methods of evasion are developed.

It would be unrealistic to believe that our present methods of detection are even close to foolproof. Numerous testimonies by athletes who have successfully evaded the doping control system demonstrate otherwise (83). In fact, our present methods of detection may be perceived as "a vain attempt to preserve what is beautiful and admirable in sports" (22). However, studies indicate that drug testing can be an effective means for deterring drug use, especially with the use of intensive, year-round, OOC, NAN testing (1,102,122). Though education and rehabilitation programs remain an integral part of present drug deterrence policies, collectively they still do not prevent athletes from using banned substances. To truly be effective, the doping control community needs to be as tenacious in its commitment to prevent drug use as society is in rewarding the win-at-all-costs philosophy in sports. This might entail the creation of penalties for using banned ergogenic aids that are as offensive and intolerable as their use. For instance, if a track and field athlete is caught using ergogenic substances at the Olympic Games, not only would the athlete be banned for life from the sport for the first offense, but the athlete's country would also be completely eliminated from the competition. This means that athletic programs and the sports governing bodies need to be more vehemently committed to terminating drug use, which naturally would include increased financial resources, a higher priority on education and prevention, and unified enforcement of sanctions. Unfortunately, it seems that there are significant athletic interests that allow individuals to gain supraphysiologic advantages from drug use and do not want stricter penalties or enforcement. Instead, they prefer the false appearance that all athletes are competing on a level playing field.

We must weigh the increased monetary costs of extensive doping control programs against the cost to society if we do not attempt to level the playing fields, by refusing to accept the use of drugs or other methods to gain unfair advantages in sport. Sadly, the ultimate cost of drug testing may be paid by the men and women who hold to the ideals of fair competition without the use of banned substances or doping methods.

The science of drug testing is continually evolving, and there are significant technologies on the horizon that may make it possible to detect biological markers of lifetime drug use. However, it is uncertain whether drug-testing procedures will ever be comprehensive enough to prevent those wishing to circumvent the process. The only constant in this biochemical playing field is that it may never be level. Therefore we cannot and should not rely on or expect science to cure what is a societal ill.

REFERENCES

1. Fuentes RJ, Davis A, Sample B, Jasper K. Sentinel effect of drug testing for anabolic steroid abuse. *Journal of Law Medicine, and Ethics* 1994;22:224–230.
2. Anonymous. Courting controversy (Supreme Court's decision on junior and high school random drug testing). *Sports Illustrated* 1995;83:11.
3. Louria DB. Technologic cornucopias, the Bill of Rights, and slippery slopes. *NJ Med* 1993;90:44–46.
4. Albrecht RR, Anderson WA, McKeag DB. Drug testing of college athletes: the issues. *Sports Med* 1992;14:349–352.
5. DeCew JW. Drug testing: balancing privacy and public safety. *Hastings Center Report* 1994;24:17–23.
6. Yesalis CE, ed. *Anabolic steroids in sport and exercise.* Champaign, IL: Human Kinetics, 1993.
7. Duchaine D. *Underground body opus militant weight loss and recomposition.* Carson City, NV: Xipe Press, 1996.
8. U.S. Olympic Committee. *National anti-doping program policies and procedures.* Colorado Springs, CO: USOC Drug Control Administration.
9. Catlin DH, Hatton CK. Use and abuse of anabolic and other drugs for athletic enhancement. *Adv Intern Med* 1991;36:399–424.
10. Puffer JC. The use of drugs in swimming. *Clin Sports Med* 1986;5:77–89.
11. Landry GL, Kokotailo PK. Drug screening in the athletic setting. *Curr Probl Pediatr* 1994;24:344–359.
12. Voy R. *Drugs, sports and politics: the inside story about drug use in sport and its political cover-up, with a prescription for reform.* Champaign, IL: Leisure Press, 1991:6.
13. Hoberman JM, Yesalis CE. The history of synthetic testosterone. *Sci Am* 1995;272:76–81.
14. Beckett AH, Cowan DA. Misuse of drugs in sport. *Br J Sports Med* 1979;12:185–194.
15. Beckett AH, Tucker GT, Moffat AC. Routine detection and identification in urine of stimulants and other drugs, some of which may be used to modify performance in sport. *J Pharm Pharmacol* 1967;19:273–294.
16. Barnes L. Olympic drug testing: improvements without progress. *Phys Sports Med* 1980;8:21–24.
17. Beckett AH. Use and abuse of drugs in sport. *J Biosoc Sci Suppl* 1981;7:163–178.
18. Park J, Park S, Lho D, et al. Drug testing at the 10th Asian Games and 24th Seoul Olympic Games. *J Anal Toxicol* 1990;14:66–72.
19. Cohen RW. Doping control in the '96 Olympics. *J Med Assoc Ga* 1997;86:33–36.
20. Catlin DH, Kammerer RC, Hatton CK, et al. Analytical chemistry at the Games of the XXIIIrd Olympiad in Los Angeles, 1984. *Clin Chem* 1987;33:319–327.
21. Brooks RV, Firth RG, Sumner NA. Detection of anabolic steroids by radioimmunoassay. *Br J Sports Med* 1975;9:89–92.
22. Catlin DH, Murray TH. Performance-enhancing drugs, fair competition, and Olympic sport. *JAMA* 1996;276:231–237.
23. Bowers LD, Segura J. Anabolic steroids, athletic drug testing, and the Olympic Games [Editorial]. *Clin Chem* 1996;42:999–1000.
24. Brooks RV, Kicman AT, Nanjee NSE, Sothan GJ. Detection of the administration of testosterone. Abstract 1305 in Proceedings of the 12th International Congress of Clinical Chemists, Rio de Janeiro, 1984.
25. Koszuta LE. Medical care and drug testing at the Pan American Games. *Phys Sports Med* 1987;15:157–161.
26. Franke WW, Berendonk B. Hormonal doping and androgenization of athletes: a secret program of the German Democratic Republic government. *Clin Chem* 1997;43:1262–1279.
27. Cowan DA, Kicman AT. Doping in sport: misuse, analytical tests, and legal aspects [Editorial]. *Clin Chem* 1997;43:1110–1113.
28. Gall SL, Duda M, Giel D, Rogers CC. Who tests which athletes for what drugs? *Phys Sports Med* 1988;16:155–161.
29. Demak R, Kirshenbaum J. The NFL fails its drug test: the league's drug program misleads the public and can be unfair to the players. *Sports Illustrated* 1989;71:40–41,43,46–48,50.
30. Cowart VS. Road back from substance abuse especially long, hard, for athletes. *JAMA* 1986;256:2645–2649.
31. Duda M. Drug testing challenges college and pro athletes. *Phys Sports Med* 1984;12:109–118.
32. Ferstle J. Evolution and politics of drug testing. In: Yesalis CE, ed. *Anabolic steroids in sport and exercise.* Champaign, IL: Human Kinetics, 1993.
33. National Football League. *National football league policy and*

program for substances of abuse. Orlando, FL: Drug Program Agents Meeting, 1998.
34. NBA, NBAPA. *The anti-drug program of the National Basketball Association and the National Basketball Players Association.* New York: NBA Publishing Ventures, 1996.
35. Anderson WA, Albrecht RR, McKeag DB, et al. A national survey of alcohol and drug use by college athletes. *Phys Sports Med* 1991;19:91–104.
36. MacKnight W. Drug testing in intercollegiate athletics. *Seton Hall Sport Law* 1995;5:529–551.
37. Lamar JV. The penalty flag has been thrown for drug use among athletes. *Time* 1986;52:55.
38. Albrecht RR, Anderson WA, McGrew CA, et al. NCAA institutionally based drug testing: do our athletes know the rules of this game? *Medicine and Science in Sports and Exercise* 1992; 24:242–246.
39. Wolff C. Bosworth barred from bowl for steroids. *New York Times* 1986 Dec 26:D7.
40. Albrecht RR. Impact of medical issues on sports participation: drug use. *Sports Medicine and Arthroscopy Review* 1995;3: 95–100.
41. NF. Introduction: drug screening for athletes: do the means justify the ends? *Curr Probl Pediatr* 1994;24:334.
42. Carpenter L. The Supreme Court's view of drug testing high school athletes. *Strategies* 1996;9:13–15.
43. Covell KS, Gibbs A. Drug testing and the college athlete. *Creighton Law Review* 1989/1990;1–18.
44. Arnold TL. The constitutionality of random drug testing of student athletes makes the cut . . . but will the athletes? *Journal of Law and Education* 1996;25:190–198.
45. Uzych L. Drug testing of athletes. *Br J Addiction* 1991;86:25–31.
46. Gregus DR. The NFL's drug-testing policies: are they constitutional? *Entertainment and Sports Lawyer* 1993;10:1–4,25–28.
47. *Bally* v. *Northeastern University,* 403 Mass. 713, 532 N.E.2d 49, 51 (1989).
48. *O'Halloran* v. *University of Washington,* 679 F. Supp. 997 (W.D. Wash. 1988).
49. Dougherty RJ. Controversies regarding urine testing. *J Subst Abuse Treat* 1987;4:115–117.
50. Leeson TA. The drug testing of college athletes. *Journal of College and University Law* 1989;Fall:325–341.
51. Ross CT. Oregon: U.S. Supreme Court upholds constitutionality of random, suspicionless drug-testing for high school athletes. *Sports and the Courts* 1995;16:2–5.
52. Curran WJ. Compulsory drug testing: the legal barriers. *N Engl J Med* 1987;316:318–321.
53. York DR. *Vernonia School District 47J* v. *Acton:* suspicionless drug testing of student-athletes held reasonable under the Supreme Court's balancing test. *J Contemporary Law* 1996;22: 281–292.
54. Hoxha TM. Atlanta '96 and athletes' rights: an update on drug testing and the International Olympic Committee. *Entertainment and Sports Lawyer* 1996;14:7–10.
55. Lockard DW. Protecting medical laboratories from tort liability for drug testing: the amorphous concept of duty. *J Leg Med* 1996;17:427–455.
56. Panner MJ, Christakis NA. The limits of science in on-the-job drug screening. *Hastings Center Report* 1986;16:7.
57. Uzych L. Athletes, drug testing and the law. *Ann Sports Med* 1990;5:105–106.
58. Jacobs JB, Samuels B. The drug testing project in international sports: dilemmas in an expanding regulatory regime. *Hastings International and Comparative Law Review* 1995;18:557–589.
59. Willette RE. Chain of custody. In: Segura J, de la Torre R, eds. *First international symposium: current issues of drug abuse testing.* Boca Raton, FL: CRC Press, 1992.
60. Cowart VS. Random testing during training, competition may be only way to combat drugs in sports. *JAMA* 1988;260:3556–3557.
61. NCAA drug-testing results, year-by-year. *NCAA News* 1996; 33:July 8:2.
62. Cowart VS. Drugs at Seoul: what message did we get? *Physician and Sportsmedicine* 1988;16:118.
63. Higdon H. Beyond a shadow of a doubt. *Runner's World* 1989; January:41.
64. Higdon H. Did RIA or didn't she? *Runner's World* 1989; January:42.
65. Merdink J, Woolley B. Drug testing: history, philosophy, and rationale. In: Tricker R, Cook DL, eds. *Athletes at risk: drugs and sport.* Dubuque, IA: WC Brown, 1990.
66. Sample RHB, Baenziger JC. Forensic and technical aspects of drug testing in athletics. *Sports Med Training Rehab* 1993; 4:257–274.
67. Catlin DH, Hatton CK, Starcevic SH. Issues in detecting abuse of xenobiotic anabolic steroids and testosterone by analysis of athletes' urine. *Clin Chem* 1997;43:1280–1288.
68. Speltzer S, ed. *U.S. Olympic Committee drug education handbook.* Colorado Springs, CO: USOC National Anti-Doping Program, 1996.
69. Anonymous. Winter Olympics medical scans. *Phys Sports Med* 1998;26: from http://www.physsportsmed.com.
70. Anonymous. Plus: Olympics; marijuana becomes banned substance. *New York Times* 1998 Apr 28:Sports Desk, from http://archives.nytimes.com/archives/search/fastweb?search.
71. Hemmersbach P, de la Torre R. Stimulants, narcotics and β-blockers: 25 years of development in analytical techniques for doping control. *J Chromatogr B: Biomed Appl* 1996;687:221–238.
72. Solans A, Carnicero M, de la Torre R, Segura J. Comprehensive screening procedure for detection of stimulants, narcotics, adrenergic drugs, and their metabolites in human urine. *J Anal Toxicol* 1995;19:104–114.
73. Eskridge KD, Guthrie SK. Clinical issues associated with urine testing of substances of abuse. *Pharmacotherapy* 1997;17: 497–510.
74. Kapur B. Drug testing methods and interpretations of test results. In: Macdonald S, Roman P, eds. *Drug testing in the workplace.* New York: Plenum Press, 1994.
75. Fields L, Lange WR, Kreiter NA, Fudala PJ. A national survey of drug testing policies for college athletes. *Med Sci Sports Exerc* 1994;26:682–686.
76. Segura J. Doping control in sports medicine. *Ther Drug Monit* 1996;18:471–476.
77. Bowers LD. Analytical advances in detection of performance enhancing compounds. *Clin Chem* 1997;43:1299–1304.
78. Choi D, Kim M, Park J. Erythropoietin: physico- and biochemical analysis. *J Chromatogr B: Biomed Appls* 1996;687:189–199.
79. Kelly KL. EMIT enzyme immunoassays in testing for drugs of abuse. In Segura J., de la Torre R, eds. *First international symposium: current issues of drug abuse testing.* Boca Raton, FL: CRC Press, 1992.
80. Donald K. *The doping game.* Brisbane, Australia: Boolarong Publications, 1983.
81. Substance-Abuse Testing Committee. Critical issues in urinalysis of abused substances: report of the substance-abuse testing committee. *Clin Chem* 1988;34:605–632.
82. Finkle BS. Drug-analysis technology: overview and state of the art. *Clin Chem* 1987;33:13B–17B.
83. McBay A. Drug-analysis technology: pitfalls and problems of drug testing. *Clin Chem* 1987;33:33B–40B.
84. Greenblatt DJ. Urine drug testing: what does it test? *N Engl Law Review* 1988–89;23:651–666.
85. Mesmer MZ, Satzger RD. Determination of anabolic steroids by HPLC with UV-vis-particle beam mass spectrometry. *J Chromatograph Sci* 1997;35:38–42.
86. Mueller RK, Grosse J, Lang R, Thieme D. Chromatographic techniques: the basis of doping control. *J Chromatogr B: Biomed Appl* 1995;674:1–11.
87. Shipe JR. Mass spectrometry instrumentation in the 1990s. In: Shipe JR, Savory J, eds. *Drugs in competitive athletics: proceeding of the first international symposium held on the islands of Brioni, Yugoslavia 29 May–2 June 1988.* Oxford, England: Blackwell Scientific Publications, 1991.
88. Potteiger JA, Stilger VG. Anabolic steroid use in the adolescent athlete. *J Athl Training* 1994;29:60–62;64.
89. Ayotte C, Goudreault D, Charlebois A. Testing for natural and synthetic anabolic agents in human urine. *J Chromatogr B: Biomed Appl* 1996;687:3–25.

90. Aguilera R, Becchi M, Casabianca H, et al. Improved method of detection of testosterone abuse by gas chromatography/combustion/isotope ratio mass spectrometry analysis of urinary steroids. *J Mass Spectrom* 1996;31:169–176.
91. Warnock DG. Diuretic agents. In: Katzung BG, ed. *Basic and Clinical Pharmacology.* Norwalk, CT: Appelton & Lange, 1989.
92. Ventura R, Segura J. Detection of diuretic agents in doping control. *J Chromatogr B: Biomed Appl* 1996;687:127–144.
93. Ventura R, Segura J, de la Torre R. Potential of HPLC for screening and confirmation of diuretics. In: Shipe JR, Savory J, eds. *Drugs in competitive athletics: proceeding of the first international symposium held on the islands of Brioni, Yugoslavia 29 May-2 June 1988.* Oxford, England: Blackwell Scientific Publications, 1991.
94. Saugy M, Cardis C, Schweizer C, et al. Detection of human growth hormone doping in urine: out of competition tests are necessary. *J Chromatogr B: Biomed Appl* 1996;687:201–211.
95. Kicman AT, Miell JP, Teale JD, et al. Serum IGF-I and IGF binding proteins 2 and 3 as potential markers of doping with human GH. *Clin Endocrinol* 1997;47:43–50.
96. Flanagan DE, Taylor MC, Parfitt V, Mardell R, Wood PJ, Leatherdale BA. Urinary growth hormone following exercise to assess growth hormone production in adults. *Clin Endocrinol.* 1997;46:425–429.
97. Korporaal G. Athletes may be blood-tested. *Sydney Morning Herald* 1997 Oct 24:1, from http://www.smh.com.au/daily/content/971024/pageone/pageone9.html.
98. Martin DT, Ashenden M, Parisotto R, Pyne D, Hahn AG. Blood testing for professional cyclists: what's a fair hematocrit limit? *Sportscience News* 1997;Mar–Apr, from http://www.sportsci.org/news/news9703/AISblood.html.
99. Magnay J. Drawing blood in the war against drug cheats. *Sydney Morning Herald* 1997 Aug 22:1, from http://www.smh.com.au/daily/content/970822/pageone/pageone9.html.
100. Wu AHB. Mechanism of interference for gas chromatography/mass spectrometry analysis of urine for drugs of abuse. *Ann Clin Lab Sci* 1995;25:319–329.
101. Winek CL, Elzein EO, Wahba WW, Feldman JA. Interference of herbal drinks with urinalysis for drugs of abuse. *J Anal Toxicol* 1993;17:246–247.
102. Coombs RH, Ryan FJ. Drug testing effectiveness in identifying and preventing drug use. *Am J Drug Alcohol Abuse* 1990;16:173–184.
103. Smith-Kielland A, Olsen KM, Christophersen AS. False-positive results with Emit II amphetamine/methamphetamine assay in users of common psychotropic drugs. *Clin Chem* 1995;41:951.
104. Siegel RK, ElSohly MA, Plowman T, et al. Cocaine in herbal tea [Letter]. *JAMA* 1986;255:40.
105. El Sohly MA, Jones AB. Drug testing in the workplace: could a positive test for one of the mandated drugs be for reasons other than illicit use of the drug? *J Anal Toxicol* 1995;19:450–458.
106. Merigian KS, Browning RG. Desipramine and amantadine causing false-positive urine test for amphetamine [Letter]. *Ann Emerg Med* 1993;22:160–161.
107. McCutcheon JR, Woods PG. Snack crackers yield opiate-positive urine. *Clin Chem* 1995;41:769–770.
108. Cone EJ, Johnson RE. Contact highs and urinary cannabinoid excretion after passive exposure to marijuana smoke. *Clin Pharmacol Therapeut* 1986;40:247–256.
109. Moyer TP. Laboratory medicine: marijuana testing: how good is it? *Mayo Clinic Proc* 1987;62:413–417.
110. Barnum DT, Gleason JM. The credibility of drug tests: a multistage Bayesian analysis. *Industrial & Labor Relations Review* 1994;47:610–621.
111. Cowart VS. Athlete drug testing receiving more attention than ever before in history of competition. *JAMA* 1989;261:3510.
112. Anonymous. Notes from the underground. *Muscle Media 2000* 1996;55:109–114.
113. Johnson WO, Vershoth A. Testy times in Germany. *Sports Illustrated* 1992;76:51–52.
114. Kapur BM. Drug testing methods and clinical interpretations of test results. *Bull Narc* 1993;45:115–154.
115. Schwarzhoff R, Cody JT. The effects of adulterating agents on FPIA analysis of urine for drugs of abuse. *J Anal Toxicol* 1993;17:14–17.
116. Block G. Financial rewards proposed for major competitions. *Swimnews Online* 1997 July, http://www.swimnews.com/Mag/1997/JulMag97/wscaconf.shtml.
117. Hersh P. China's swimming success raises specter of East Germany. *Chicago Tribune* 1993 Nov 16:1.
118. *Physician's Desk Reference,* 48th ed. Montvale, NJ: Medical Economics Data Production Company, 1994:1408.
119. Cowart VS. On to 1988 Olympics . . . with lessons learned. *JAMA* 1987;258:2485–2486.
120. MacAuley D. Drugs in sport. *Br J Med* 1996;313:211–215.
121. Honour JW. Steroid abuse in female athletes. *Curr Opin Obstet Gynecol* 1997;9:181–186.
122. Borack JI. An estimate of the impact of drug testing on the deterrence of drug use. *Military Psychology* 1998;10:17–25.

APPENDIX 11–1: BANNED SUBSTANCES FOR MAJOR SPORTS ORGANIZATIONS

This list contains examples of the drugs that are prohibited by the major sports organizations in the United States and is not intended to be comprehensive. Many substances that are not in this list are banned under "related substances." Additionally, the most updated list of banned substances should be obtained from the organization of interest, as changes continuously occur. See Table 11–1 for contact information.

Generic name	Example	IOC	USOC	NCAA	NBA	MLB
Stimulants		×	×	×		
Amfepramone	Apisate	×	×			
	Tenuate	×	×			
	Tepanil	×	×			
Amfetaminil	AN-1 (Germany)	×	×			
Amineptine	Survector (Europe)	×	×			
Amiphenazole	Dapti	×	×	×		
	Daptizole	×	×	×		
	Amphisol	×	×	×		

Generic name	Example	IOC	USOC	NCAA	NBA	MLB
Amphetamine	Delcobese	×	×	×		
	Obetrol	×	×	×		
	Benzedrine	×	×	×		
Bambuterol		×				
Bemegride	Megimide	×	×	×		
Benzphetamine	Didrex	×	×	×		
Bromantin	Bromantin	×	×	×		
Caffeine		no >12 µg/mL	no >12 µg/mL	no >15 µg/mL		
Carphedon		×	×			
Cathine (no >5 µg/mL for IOC)	(Norpseudoephedrine)	×	×			
	Adiposetten N (Germany)	×	×			
Chlorphentermine	Pre Sate	×	×	×		
	Lucofen	×	×	×		
Clobenzorex	Dinintel (France)	×	×			
Clorprenaline	Vortel	×	×			
	Asthone (Japan)	×	×			
Cocaine	Methyl-benzoylecgonine	×	×	×	×	×
Cropropamide	(component of "Micoren")	×	×	×		
Crothetamide	(component of "Micoren")	×	×	×		
Desoxyephedrine	Vicks Inhaler	×	×			
Diethylpropion				×		
Diethylpropion HCL	Tenuate	×	×	×		
	Tepanil	×	×	×		
Dimetamfetamine	Amphetamine	×	×			
Dimethylamphetamine				×		×
Doxapram				×		
Ephedrine (no >5 µg/mL for IOC)	Tedral	×	×	×		
	Bronkotabs	×	×	×		
	Rynatuss	×	×	×		
	Primatene	×	×	×		
Etafedrine	Mercodal	×	×			
	Decapryn	×	×			
	Nethaprin	×	×			
Ethamivan	Emivan	×	×	×		
	Vandid	×	×	×		
Ethylamphetamine				×		×
Etilamfetamine	Apetinil (Netherlands)	×	×			
Fencamfamine	Envitrol	×	×	×		
	Altimine	×	×	×		
	Phencamine	×	×	×		
Fenetylline	Captagon (Germany)	×	×			
Fenproporex	Antiobes Retard (Spain)	×	×			
	Appetizugler (Germany)	×	×			
Formoterol		×				
Furfenorex	Frugal (Arg.)	×	×			
	Frugalan (Spain)	×	×			

Generic name	Example	IOC	USOC	NCAA	NBA	MLB
Isoetharine HCL	Bronkosol	×	×			
	Bronkometer	×	×			
	Numotac	×	×			
	Dilabron	×	×			
Isoproterenol	Isuprel	×	×			
	Norisodrine	×	×			
	Metihaler-ISO	×	×			
Meclofenoxate	Lucidril	×	×	×		
	Brenal	×	×	×		
Mefenorex	Doracil (Arg.)	×	×			
	Pondinil (Switz.)	×	×			
	Rondimen (Germany)	×	×			
Mesocarbe	Mesocarb	×	×			
	Mesocarbi	×	×			
	Sydnocarb (Europe)	×	×			
Metaproterenol	Alupent	×	×			
	Metaprel	×	×			
Methamphetamine	Desoxyn	×	×	×	×	
	Met-Ampi	×	×	×	×	
Methoxyphenamine	Orthoxicol Cough Syrup	×	×			
Methyl-ephedrine (no >5 µg/mL for IOC)	Tzbraine	×	×			
	Methep (Germany, G.B.)	×	×			
Methylphenidate				×		
Methylphenidate HCL	Ritalin	×	×			
Morazone	Rosimon-Neu (Germany)	×	×			
Nikethamide	Coramine	×	×	×		
Pemoline	Cylert	×	×	×		
	Deltamine	×	×	×		
	Stimul	×	×	×		
Pentetrazol/Pentylenetetrazol	Leptazol	×	×	×		
Phendimetrazine	Phenzine	×	×	×		
	Bontril	×	×	×		
	Plegine	×	×	×		
Phenmetrazine	Preludin	×	×	×		
Phentermine				×		
Phentermine HCL	Apidex-P	×	×			
	Fastin	×	×			
	Ionamin	×	×			
Picrotoxine	Cocculin	×	×	×		
Pipradol	Meratran	×	×	×		
	Constituent of Alertonic	×	×	×		
Prolintane	Villescon	×	×	×		
	Promotil	×	×	×		
	Katovit	×	×	×		
Propylhexedrine	Benzedrex Inhaler	×	×			
Pyrovalerone	Centroton	×	×			
	Thymergix	×	×			
Reproterol		×				
Selegiline	Eldepryl	×	×			
	Plurimen (Spain)	×	×			
	Deprenyl	×	×			

Generic name	Example	IOC	USOC	NCAA	NBA	MLB
Strychnine	Movellan (Germany)	×	×	×		
And Related Substances		×	×	×		
Over-the-counter medications containing prohibited substances		×	×			
Desoxyephedrine	Vicks Inhaler	×	×			
Pseudoephedrine (no >10 µg/mL for IOC)	Actifed	×	×			
	Ambenyl-D	×	×			
	Anamine	×	×			
	Afrin Tablets	×	×			
	Afrinol	×	×			
	Co-Tylenol	×	×			
	Deconamine	×	×			
	Dimacol	×	×			
	Emprazil-A	×	×			
	Fedahist	×	×			
	Fedrazil	×	×			
	Histalet	×	×			
	Isoclor	×	×			
	Lo Tussin	×	×			
	Nasalspan	×	×			
	Novafed	×	×			
	Nucofed	×	×			
	Poly-Histine	×	×			
	Pseudo-Bid	×	×			
	Pseudo-Hist	×	×			
	Rhinosym	×	×			
	Ryna	×	×			
	Sudafed	×	×			
	Triprolidine	×	×			
	Tussend	×	×			
	Chlorafed	×	×			
	Chlor-Trimeton-DC	×	×			
	Disphoral	×	×			
	Drixoral	×	×			
	Polaramine Expectorant	×	×			
	Rondec	×	×			
Phenylpropanolamine (no >10 µg/mL for IOC)	ARM	×	×			
	Allerest	×	×			
	Alka-Seltzer Plus	×	×			
	Contac	×	×			
	Dexatrim	×	×			
	Dietac	×	×			
	4-way Formula 44	×	×			
	Naldecon	×	×			
	Novahistine	×	×			
	Arnex	×	×			
	Sine-Aid	×	×			
	Sine-Off	×	×			
	Sinutab	×	×			
	Triaminic	×	×			
	Triaminicin	×	×			
	Sucrets Cold Decongestant	×	×			
	and related products	×	×			
Propylhexedrine	Benzedrex Inhaler	×	×			

Generic name	Example	IOC	USOC	NCAA	NBA	MLB
Ephedrine	Bronkaid	×	×	×		
	Collyrium with Ephedrine	×	×	×		
	Pazo Suppository	×	×	×		
	Wyanoids Suppository	×	×	×		
	Vatronol Nose Drops	×	×	×		
	Herbal teas and medicines containing ma huang (Chinese ephedra)	×	×	×		
Ma huang (herbal ephedrine)	Action Caps	×	×	×		
	Bishop's Tea	×	×	×		
	Breathe Easy Herbal Decongestant Tea	×	×	×		
	Brigham Tea	×	×	×		
	Chi Powder	×	×	×		
	Energy Rise	×	×	×		
	Ephedra	×	×	×		
	Excel	×	×	×		
	Free Herbal "Energy Tablets"	×	×	×		
	Joint Fir	×	×	×		
	Mexican Tea	×	×	×		
	Miner's Tea	×	×	×		
	Mormon Tea	×	×	×		
	Popotillo	×	×	×		
	Quick Shot Vitamin B-12	×	×	×		
	Squaw Tea	×	×	×		
	Super Charge	×	×	×		
	Teamster's Tea	×	×	×		
Narcotics		×	×			
Alphaprodine	Nisentil	×	×			
Anileridine	Leritine	×	×			
	Apodol	×	×			
Buprenorphine	Buprenex	×	×			
Dextromoramide	Palflum	×	×			
	Jetrium	×	×			
	D-Moramid	×	×			
	Dimorlin	×	×			
Diamorphine	Heroin	×	×	×	×	×
Dipipanone	Pipadone	×	×			
	Diconal	×	×			
	Wellconal	×	×			
Ethoheptazine	Panalgin (Italy)	×	×			
Levorphanol	Levo-Dromoran	×	×			
Methadone HCL	Dolophine	×	×			
	Amidon	×	×			
Morphine (no >1 µg/mL for IOC)	Cyclimorph 10	×	×		×	×
	Duromorph	×	×		×	×
	MST-Continus	×	×		×	×
Nalbuphine	Nubain	×	×			
Pentazocine	Talwin	×	×			
Pethidine	Demerol	×	×			
	Centralgin	×	×			
	Dolantin	×	×			
	Dolosal	×	×			
	Pethold	×	×			

Generic name	Example	IOC	USOC	NCAA	NBA	MLB
Phenazocine	Narphen	×	×			
Meperidine	Demerol	×	×			
	Mepergan	×	×			
And Related Compounds, i.e.,		×	×			
Hydrocodone	Hycodan	×	×			
	Tussionex	×	×			
	Vicodin	×	×			
Opiates					×	
Oxycodone	Percodan	×	×			
	Tylox	×	×			
Oxymorphone	Numorphan	×	×			
Hydromorphone	Dilaudid	×	×			
Tincture Opium	Paragoric	×	×		×	×
Anabolic agents		×	×	×		
Androstenedione	Androsten	×	×	×		
Bolasterone	Vebonol	×	×	×		
Boldenone	Equipoise	×	×	×		
Clostebol	Steranobol	×	×	×		
Dehydrochlormethyl Testosterone	Turinabol	×	×	×		
Dehydroepiandrosterone (DHEA)		×	×	×		
Dihydrotestosterone	Stanolone	×	×	×		
Dromostanolone		×	×	×		
Fluoxymesterone	Android F	×	×	×		
	Halotestin	×	×	×		
	Ora-Testryl and	×	×	×		
	Ultradren	×	×	×		
Gestrinone		×	×	×		
Mesterolone	Androviron	×	×	×		
	Proviron	×	×	×		
Metandienone	Danabol	×	×	×		
	Dianabol	×	×	×		
Metenolone	Primobolan	×	×	×		
	Primonabol-Depot	×	×	×		
Methandrostenolone	Dianabol	×	×	×		
Methyltestosterone	Android	×	×	×		
	Estratest	×	×	×		
	Metandren	×	×	×		
	Virilon	×	×	×		
	Oreton Methyl	×	×	×		
	Testred	×	×	×		
Nandrolone	Durabolin	×	×	×		
	Deca-Durabolin	×	×	×		
	Kabolin	×	×	×		
	Nandrobolic	×	×	×		
Norethandrolone	Nilevar	×	×	×		
Oxandrololone	Anavar	×	×	×		
Oxymesterone		×	×	×		
Oxymetholone	Anadrol	×	×	×		
	Anapolon 50	×	×	×		
	Adroyd	×	×	×		

Generic name	Example	IOC	USOC	NCAA	NBA	MLB
Stanozolol	Winstrol	×	×	×		
	Stromba	×	×	×		
Testosterone	Malogen	×	×	×		
	Malogex	×	×	×		
	Delatestryl	×	×	×		
Related compounds, i.e.,		×	×	×		
Danazol		×	×	×		
Danocrine		×	×	×		
Dehydroepiandrosterone (DHEA)		×	×	×		
Zeranol		×	×	×		
Clenbuterol		×	×	×		
Growth hormone		×	×	×		
Human chorionic gonadotrophin		×	×	×		
Beta-2 agonists (only inhaling of these is allowed)		×	×	with restrictions		
Salbutamol	Albuterol	×	×			
	Ventolin Inhaler	×	×			
	Proventil Inhaler	×	×			
Salmeterol	Serevent	×	×			
Terbutaline	Brethaire	×	×			
Salbutamol/Ipratropium	Combivent	×	×			
Diuretics		×	×	×		
Acetazolamide	Diamox	×	×	×		
	AK-ZOL	×	×	×		
	Dazamide	×	×	×		
Amiloride	Midamor	×	×			
Bendroflumethiazide	Naturetin	×	×	×		
Benzthiazide	Aquatag	×	×	×		
	Exna	×	×	×		
	Hyrex	×	×	×		
	Marazide	×	×	×		
	Proaqua	×	×	×		
Bumetanide	Bumex	×	×	×		
Canrenone	Aldadiene	×	×			
	Aldactone (Germany)	×	×			
	Phanurane (France)	×	×			
	Soldactone (Switzerland)	×	×			
Chlormerodrin	Orimercur (Spain)	×	×			
Chlorothiazide				×		
Chlortalidone	Hygroton	×	×	×		
	Hylidone	×	×	×		
	Thalitone	×	×	×		
Diclofenamide	Daranide	×	×			
	Oratrol	×	×			
	Fenamide	×	×			
Ethacrynic Acid	Edecrin	×	×	×		
Flumethiazide				×		
Furosemide	Lasix	×	×	×		

Generic name	Example	IOC	USOC	NCAA	NBA	MLB
Hydrochlorothiazide	Esidrix	×	×	×		
	Hydro-Diuril	×	×	×		
	Oretic	×	×	×		
	Thiuretic	×	×	×		
Mannitol (IV only)	Osmitol	×	×			
Mersalyl	Salyrgan	×	×			
Methyclothiazide				×		
Metolazone				×		
Polythiazide				×		
Quinethazone				×		
Spironolactone	Alatone	×	×	×		
	Aldactone	×	×	×		
Torsemide	Demadex	×	×			
Triamterene	Dyrenium	×	×	×		
	Dyazide	×	×	×		
Trichlomethiazide				×		
Related substances		×	×	×		
Peptide and glycoprotein hormones and analogues		×	×			
Chorionic gonadotrophin (HCG–human chorionic gonadotrophin)		×	×	×		
Corticotrophin (ACTH)		×	×	×		
Growth hormone (hGH, somatotrophin)		×	×	×		
Erythropoietin (EPO)		×	×	×		
All the respective releasing factors of the above-mentioned substances		×	×	×		
Blood doping		×	×	×		
Intravenous administration of blood, red blood cells, or related red blood products, including EPO		×	×	×		
Pharmacologic, chemical, and physical manipulation		×	×	×		
Substances and methods that alter integrity and validity of urine samples used in testing: catheterization, urine substitution and/or tampering, inhibition of renal excretion (e.g., by Probenecid and related compounds, Bromantin), & epitestosterone (no >200 ng/mL for IOC) administration		×	×	×		
Substances subject to certain restrictions		×	×			
Alcohol		×	×	for rifle		
Marijuana		×	×	×	×	×

Generic name	Example	IOC	USOC	NCAA	NBA	MLB
Local anesthetics		×	×			
Corticosteroids		×	×			
Beta-blockers		×	×	for rifle		
Street drugs				×		
Mescaline						×
Psilocybin						×
Diethylamide (LSD)						×
THC (tetrahydrocannabinol)		×	×	×	×	×
Phencyclidine (PCP)					×	×
Controlled substances (U.S.)						×
Dihydromorphine						×
Methaqualone						×
Tilidine						×
Fenethylline (fenethylline hydrochloride)						×
Acetylmethadol						×

CHAPTER 12

Eating Disorders

J. Sundgot-Borgen

Some female athletes and nonathletes do not consider training or exercise sufficient to accomplish their idealized body shape or level of thinness. Therefore, to meet their goals, a significant number of them diet and use harmful though ineffective weight-loss practices such as restrictive eating, vomiting, laxatives, and diuretics to meet their goals (1). *Eating disorders* is the common term for such behaviors. Eating disorders can result in short- and long-term morbidity, decreased performance, amenorrhea, and mortality. In the author's experience, signs and symptoms of eating disorders in competitive and elite athletes are often ignored. In some sports disordered eating seems to be regarded as a natural part of being an athlete (2). It has been claimed that female athletes are at increased risk for developing eating disorders because of the focus on low body weight as a performance enhancer, comments from coaches or important others, and the pressure to perform (3,4). Nevertheless, symptoms of eating disorders are more prevalent among elite athletes than among nonathletes (3,5–7). This article discusses the nature of eating disorders among elite female athletes.

DEFINITIONS

Eating disorders are characterized by disturbances in eating behavior, body image, emotions, and relationships. Athletes constitute a unique population, and special diagnostic considerations should be made in working with this group (8,–10). Despite similar symptoms, subclinical cases are easier to identify in athletes than in nonathletes (3). Since athletes, at least at the elite level, are evaluated by their coaches every day, changes in behavior and physical symptoms may be observed.

J. Sundgot-Borgen: Department of Sports Medicine, The Norwegian University of Sport and Physical Education, Oslo, Norway.

However, symptoms of eating disorders in competitive and elite athletes are too often ignored or not detected by coaches. One reason for this is lack of knowledge about symptoms and developed strategies for the eating-disordered athlete.

Tables 12–1 and 12–2 summarize the DSM-IV (11) diagnostic criteria for anorexia nervosa and bulimia nervosa. These new criteria formalize overlapping conventions for subtyping anorexia nervosa into restricting and binge-eating/purging types on the basis of the presence or absence of bingeing and/or purging (i.e., self-induced vomiting or the misuse of laxatives or diuretics). Most eating-disordered athletes move between these two subtypes. However, it is the author's experience that chronicity leads to an accumulation of eating-disordered athletes in the binge-eating/purging subgroup.

The Eating Disorders Not Otherwise Specified category refers to disorders of eating that do not meet the criteria for any specific eating disorder. This category acknowledges the existence and importance of a variety of eating disturbances.

PREVALENCE OF EATING DISORDERS AMONG ATHLETES

Estimates of the prevalence of the symptoms of eating disorders and clinical eating disorders among female athletes range from less than 1% to as high as 75% (3,12,13). The prevalence of anorexia nervosa in female elite athletes (1.3%) is similar to the range reported among nonathletes (14), whereas bulimia nervosa (8.2%) and subclinical eating disorders (8%) seem to be more prevalent among athletes than nonathletes (3). The prevalence of eating disorders in men has been unknown until recently. A recent Norwegian study reported the prevalence of eating disorders to be as high as 8% among male elite athletes and 0.5% in a matched group of men (7). Eating disorders are significantly more frequent among female athletes competing in aesthetic

TABLE 12-1. *Diagnostic criteria for anorexia nervosa*

A. Refusal to maintain body weight at or above a minimally normal weight for age and height (e.g., weight loss leading to maintenance of body weight less than 85% of that expected or failure to make expected weight gain during period of growth, leading to body weight less than 85% of that expected)
B. Intense fear of gaining weight or becoming fat, even though underweight
C. Disturbance in the way in which one's body weight or shape is experienced, undue influence of body weight or shape on self-evaluation, or denial of the seriousness of the current low body weight
D. In postmenarcheal females, amenorrhea, that is, the absence of at least three consecutive menstrual cycles (A woman is considered to have amenorrhea if her periods occur only following administration of hormone, e.g., estrogen.)

Specify type:
Restricting type: During the episode of anorexia nervosa the person has not regularly engaged in binge-eating or purging behavior (i.e., self-induced vomiting or the misuse of laxatives, diuretics, or enemas).
Binge eating/purging type: During the current episode of anorexia nervosa the person has regularly engaged in binge eating or purging behavior (i.e., self-induced vomiting or the misuse of laxatives, diuretics, or enemas).

From American Psychiatric Association. *Diagnostic and statistical manual of mental disorders,* 4th ed. Washington, DC: American Psychiatric Association, 1994.

TABLE 12-2. *Diagnostic criteria for bulimia nervosa*

A. Recurrent episodes of binge eating. An episode of binge eating is characterized by both of the following: (1) eating, in a discrete period of time (e.g., within any 2-hour period), an amount of food that is definitely larger than most people would eat during a similar period of time in similar circumstances and (2) a sense of lack of control over eating during the episode (e.g., a feeling that one cannot stop eating or control what or how much one is eating).
B. Recurrent inappropriate compensatory behavior to prevent weight gain, such as self-induced vomiting; misuse of laxatives, diuretics, or other medications; fasting; or excessive exercise
C. Occurrence of both the binge eating and inappropriate compensatory behaviors, on average, at least twice a week for 3 months
D. Self-evaluation that is unduly influenced by body shape and weight
E. Occurrence of the disturbance not exclusively during episodes of anorexia nervosa

Specify type:
Purging type: The person regularly engages in self-induced vomiting or the misuse of laxatives, diuretics, or enemas.
Nonpurging type: The person uses other inappropriate compensatory behaviors, such as fasting or excessive exercise, but does not regularly engage in self-induced vomiting or the misuse of laxatives, diuretics, or enemas.

From American Psychiatric Association. *Diagnostic and statistical manual of mental disorders,* 4th ed. Washington, DC: American Psychiatric Association, 1994.

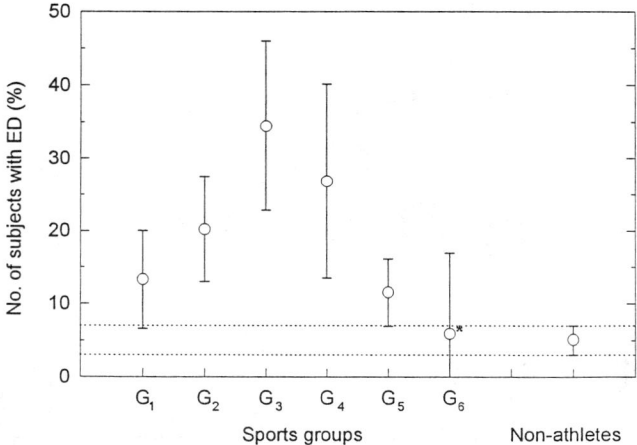

FIG. 12-1. Prevalence of eating disorders in female elite athletes representing technical sports ($n = 98$), endurance sports ($n = 119$), aesthetic sports ($n = 64$), weight-dependent sports ($n = 41$), ball games ($n = 183$), power sports ($n = 17$), and nonathletes ($n = 522$). The data are shown as mean and 95% confidence intervals.

and weight-class sports than among other sport groups in which leanness is considered less important (Fig. 12-1).

RISK FACTORS FOR THE DEVELOPMENT OF EATING DISORDERS

The etiology of eating disorders is multifactorial (15,16). Because of additional stress associated with the athletic environment (4), however, female elite athletes appear to be more vulnerable to eating disorders than the general female population. Furthermore, recent studies suggest that specific risk factors for the development of eating disorders occur in some sport settings. One retrospective study indicates that a sudden increase in training load may induce a caloric deprivation in endurance athletes, which in turn may elicit biologic and social reinforcements leading to the development of eating disorders (3). However, longitudinal studies with close monitoring of a number of sport-specific factors (volume, type, and intensity of the training) in athletes representing different sports-specific factors (clothing, weight classes, physical and psychological demands, rules, subjective judging, and coaching behavior) are needed to answer questions about the role played by different sports in the development of eating disorders. Female athletes with eating disorders have been shown to start sport-specific training at an earlier age than athletes without eating disorders (3). Another factor to consider is that if female athletes start sport-specific training at a prepubertal age, they might not choose the sport that will be most suitable for their adult body type.

From subjective experience athletes have reported that they developed eating disorders as a result of what they call a traumatic event, such as the loss or change of a coach, an injury, illness, or overtraining or illness that left them temporarily unable to continue their normal level of exercise (3,15,17). An injury can curtail the athlete's exercise and training habits. As a result, the athlete may gain weight owing to less energy expenditure, which in some cases may develop into an irrational fear of further weight gain. Then the athlete may begin to diet to compensate for the lack of exercise (10).

Pressure to reduce weight has been the common explanation for the increased prevalence of eating related problems among athletes. However, the important factor may not be dieting per se, but rather the situation in which the athlete is told to lose weight, the words used, and whether or not the athlete received guidance. The various reasons for the development of eating disorders reported by eating-disordered high-level athletes are presented in Table 12–3. In addition to the pressure to reduce weight, athletes are often pressed for time, and they have to lose weight rapidly to make or stay on the team. As a result they often experience frequent periods of restrictive dieting or weight cycling (3). Weight cycling has been suggested as an important risk or trigger factor for the development of eating disorders in athletes (3,18).

On the other hand, some authors have argued that specific sports attract individuals who are anorectic before commencing their participation in sports, at least in attitude if not in behavior or weight (10,19). It is this author's opinion that the attraction-to-sport hypothesis might be true for the general population, but athletes do not achieve the elite level if the only motivation is weight loss. Therefore, this hypothesis could probably rather be true for lower-level athletes.

Most researchers agree that coaches do not cause eating disorders in athletes, although through inappropriate coaching, the problem may be triggered or exacerbated in vulnerable individuals (4). In most cases, then, the role of coaches in the development of eating disorders in athletes should be seen as a part of a complex interplay of factors.

To sum up, there is no hard evidence for sport-specific risk factors for eating disorders. The use of longitudinal quantitative and qualitative studies is clearly needed.

MEDICAL ISSUES

For both athletes and nonathletes eating disorders may cause serious medical problems and can even be fatal. Whereas most complications of anorexia nervosa occur as a direct or indirect result of starvation, complications of bulimia nervosa occur as a result of binge-eating and purging (10). Hsu (20), Johnson and Connor (21), and Mitchell (22) provide information on the medical problems encountered in eating-disordered patients. Anorexia nervosa patients have a standard mortality rate up to six times higher than that of the general population, while mortality is rather unknown among bulimic patients (23). Death is usually attributable to fluid and electrolyte abnormalities, or suicide (24). Mortality in bulimia nervosa is less well studied, but deaths do occur, usually secondary to the complications of the binge-purging cycle or suicide.

Mortality rates of eating disorders among athletes are not known. However, a number of deaths of top-level athletes in the sports of gymnastics, running, alpine skiing, and cycling have been reported in the media. Five (5.4%) of the female elite athletes diagnosed in the Norwegian study (3) reported suicide attempts.

Long-term Health Effects of Eating Disorders

The long-term effects of body weight cycling and eating disorders in athletes are unclear. Biologic maturation and growth have been studied in girl gymnasts before and during puberty, suggesting that young female gymnasts are smaller and mature later than females from sports that do not require extreme leanness, such as swimming (25,26). However, it is difficult to separate the effects of physical strain, energy restriction, and genetic predisposition to delayed puberty.

Besides increasing the likelihood of amenorrhea and stress fractures, early bone loss may inhibit achievement of normal peak bone mass. Thus athletes with frequent or longer periods of amenorrhea may be at high risk of sustaining fractures. Longitudinal data on fast and

TABLE 12–3. *The various reasons for the development of eating disorders reported by eating-disordered athletes*

Reason	Number of eating-disordered athletes	Percentage
Prolonged periods of dieting	29	37
New coach	23	30
Injury/illness	18	23
Casual comments	15	19
Leaving home/failure at school/work	8	10
Problem in relationship	8	10
Family problems	5	7
Illness/injury to family members	5	7
Death of significant others	3	4
Sexual abuse (by coach)	3	4

Multiple answers were allowed. 15% did not give any specific reason.

From Sundgot-Borgen J. Risk and trigger factors for the development of eating disorders in female elite athletes. *Med Sci Sports Exerc* 1994;4:414–419.

gradual body weight reduction and cycling in relation to health and performance parameters in different groups of athletes are clearly needed.

The nature and the magnitude of the effect of eating disorders on athletic performance are influenced by the severity and chronicity of the eating disorder and the physical and psychological demands of the sport. No studies have appeared looking at specific tests and the results of shorter or longer periods of disordered eating. Nevertheless, loss of endurance due to dehydration impairs exercise performance (27). Norwegian female elite athletes reported increased fatigue, anger, or anxiety when attempting to rapidly lose body weight (17).

Identifying Athletes with Eating Disorders

Most individuals with eating disorders do not realize that they have a problem and therefore do not seek treatment on their own. Athletes might consider seeking help only if they experience that their performance level is leveling off.

TABLE 12-4. *Physical symptoms and psychological and behavioral characteristics of athletes with anorexia nervosa or anorexia athletica*

Significant weight loss beyond that necessary for adequate sport performance	Anxiety, both related and unrelated to sport performance
Amenorrhea or menstrual dysfunction	Avoidance of eating and eating situations
Dehydration	Claims of "feeling fat" despite being thin
Fatigue beyond that normally expected in training or competition	Resistance to weight gain or maintenance recommended by sport support staff
Gastrointestinal problems (constipation, diarrhea, bloating, postprandial distress)	Unusual weighing behavior (excessive weighing, refusal to weigh, negative reaction to being weighed)
Hyperactivity	Compulsiveness and rigidity, especially regarding eating and exercise
Hypothermia	Excessive or obligatory exercise beyond that required for a particular sport
Bradycardia	Exercising while injured despite prohibitions by medical and training staff
Lanugo	Restlessness—relaxing is difficult or impossible
Muscle weakness	Social withdrawal
Reduced bone mineral density	Depression and insomnia
Stress fractures	

Modified after Thompson RA, Trattner-Sherman R. *Helping athletes with eating disorders.* Champaign, IL: Human Kinetics, 1993.

TABLE 12-5. *Physical symptoms and psychological and behavioral characteristics of athletes with bulimia nervosa*

Callus or abrasion on back of hand from inducing vomiting	Binge eating
Dehydration, especially in the absence of training or competition	Agitation when bingeing is interrupted
Dental and gum problems	Depression
Edema, complaints of bloating, or both	Dieting that is unnecessary for appearance, health, or sport performance
Electrolyte abnormalities	Evidence of vomiting unrelated to illness
Frequent and often extreme weight fluctuations (e.g., mood worsens as weight goes up)	Excessive exercise beyond that required for the athlete's sport
Gastrointestinal problems	Excessive use of the restroom
Low weight despite eating large volumes	Going to the restroom or disappearing after eating
Menstrual irregularity	Self-critical, especially concerning body, weight, and sport performance
Muscle cramps, weakness, or both	Secretive eating
Swollen parotid glands	Substance abuse—whether legal, illegal, prescribed, or over-the-counter drugs, medications, or other substances
	Use of laxatives, diuretics, or both that is unsanctioned by medical or training staffs

From Thompson RA, Trattner-Sherman R. *Helping athletes with eating disorders.* Champaign, IL: Human Kinetics, 1993.

In contrast to the athletes with anorectic symptoms most athletes suffering from bulimia nervosa are at or near normal weight, and therefore their disorder is difficult to detect. Hence the team staff must be able to recognize the physical symptoms and psychological characteristics listed in Tables 12-4 and 12-5. It should be noted that the presence of some of these characteristics does not necessarily indicate the presence of the disorder. However, the likelihood of the disorder being present increases as the number of presenting characteristics increases (10).

TREATMENT OF EATING DISORDERS

Eating-disordered athletes seem more likely to accept the idea of going for a single consultation than the idea of committing themselves to prolonged treatment. The treatment of athletes with eating disorders should be undertaken by health care professionals. It is the author's experience that it is easier to establish a trusting relationship when the eating-disordered athlete realizes that the therapist knows the athlete's sport in addition to being trained in treating eating-disordered patients. Therapists who have good knowledge about eating disorders and know the various sports will better understand the athlete's training setting, daily demands, and relationships that are specific to the sport, type of event, and competitive level. Building such a relationship includes respecting the athlete's desire to be lean for athletic performance and expressing a willingness to work together to help the eating-disordered athlete to become lean and healthy. The treatment team needs to accept the athlete's fears and irrational thoughts about food and weight and then present a rational approach for achieving self-management of healthy diet, weight, and training program (28). The various types of treatment strategies have been described in detail elsewhere (10).

It is the author's experience that a total suspension of training during treatment is not a good solution. Therefore unless severe medical complications are present, training at a lower volume and at a decreased intensity should be allowed. In general, to avoid a message of sport performance as more important than health, it is not recommended that athletes compete during treatment. Nevertheless, competitions during treatment might be considered for individuals with less severe eating disorders who are engaged in low-risk sports.

PREVENTION OF EATING DISORDERS IN ATHLETES

In contrast to findings from the general adolescent population (29,30), talking to athletes and coaches about eating disorders and related issues such as reproduction, bone health, nutrition, body composition, and performance prevents eating disorders in that population (17). Therefore coaches, trainers, administrators, and parents should receive information about eating disorders and related issues such as growth and development and the relationship between body composition, health, nutrition, and performance. In addition, coaches should realize that they can strongly influence their athletes. Coaches or others who are involved with young athletes should not comment on an individual's body size or require weight loss in young and still growing athletes. Without further guidance, dieting may result in unhealthy eating behavior or eating disorders in highly motivated and uninformed athletes (31). Early intervention is also important, since eating disorders are more difficult to treat the longer they progress. Therefore professionals working with athletes should be informed about the possible risk factors for the development of eating disorders; early signs and symptoms; the medical, psychological, and social consequences of these disorders; how to approach the problem if it occurs; and what treatment options are available.

WEIGHT LOSS RECOMMENDATIONS

A change in body composition and weight loss can be achieved safely if the weight goal is realistic and based on body composition rather than weight-for-height standards.

1. The weight loss program should start well before the season begins. Athletes must consume regular meals that provide sufficient energy and nutrients to avoid menstrual irregularities, loss of bone mass, loss of muscle tissue, and the compromised performance.
2. The health care personnel should set realistic goals for dieting, rate of weight change, and target range of weight and body fat.
3. Change in body composition should be monitored regularly, including a period after the weight or body fat percent goal has been reached to detect any continued or unwarranted losses or weight fluctuations.
4. Measurements of body composition should be done in private to reduce the stress, anxiety, and embarrassment of public assessment.
5. A registered dietitian who knows the demands of the specific sport should plan individual nutritionally adequate diets. Throughout this process, the role of overall good nutrition practices in optimizing performance should be emphasized.
6. Coaches should never try to diagnose or treat eating disorders, but they should be specific about their suspicions and talk with the athlete who may be eating-disordered about the fears or anxieties the athlete may be having about food and performance. Encourage medical evaluation, and support the athlete.
7. The coach should assist and support the athlete during treatment for eating disorders.

SUMMARY

Many studies have shown an increased prevalence of eating disorders among female athletes compared with the general adolescent population. It is at present unknown whether this increase in prevalence represents an increased risk for developing eating disorders among athletes. Eating disorders in female athletes can easily be missed unless they are specifically searched for. Disordered eating may result in amenorrhea because of energy deficit. If untreated, eating disorders can have long-lasting physiologic and psychological effects and may even be fatal. Treating athletes with eating disorders should be undertaken only by qualified health care professionals. Ideally, these individuals should also be familiar with, and have an appreciation for, the athlete's sport.

REFERENCES

1. Sundgot-Borgen J, Larsen S. Nutrient intake and eating behavior of female elite athletes suffering from anorexia nervosa, anorexia athletica and bulimia nervosa. *Int J Sport Nutr* 1993;3:431–442.
2. Sundgot-Borgen J. Eating disorders, energy intake, training volume, and menstrual function in high-level modern rhythmic gymnasts. *Int J Sport Nutr* 1996;6:100–109.
3. Sundgot-Borgen J. Risk and trigger factors for the development of eating disorders in female elite athletes. *Med Sci Sports Exerc* 1994;4:414–419.
4. Wilmore JH. Eating and weight disorders in female athletes. *Int J Sport Nutr* 1991;1:104–117.
5. Dummer GM, Rosen LW, Heusner WW. Pathogenic weight-control behaviors of young competitive swimmers. *Physician and Sportsmedicine* 1987;5:75–86.
6. Rosen LW, McKeag DB, Hough DO. Pathogenic weight-control behaviors in female athletes. *Physician and Sportsmedicine* 1986;14:79–86.
7. Torstveit G, Rolland CG, Sundgot-Borgen J (1998). Pathogenic weight control methods and self-reported eating disorders among male elite athletes. *Med Sci Sports Exerc* 5[Suppl]:181.
8. Sundgot-Borgen J. Prevalence of eating disorders in female elite athletes. *Int J Sport Nutr* 1993;3:29–40.
9. Szmuckler GI, Eisler I, Gillies C, Hayward ME. The implications of anorexia nervosa in a ballet school. *J Psychiatr Res* 1985;19:177–181.
10. Thompson RA, Trattner-Sherman R. *Helping athletes with eating disorders.* Champaign, IL: Human Kinetics, 1993.
11. American Psychiatric Association. *Diagnostic and statistical manual of mental disorders,* 3rd ed. Washington, DC: American Psychiatric Association, 1987:65–69.
12. Gadpalle WJ, Sandborn CF, Wagner WW. Athletic amenorrhea, major affective disorders and eating disorders. *Am J Psychiatry* 1987;144:9399–9443.
13. Warren BJ, Stanton AL, Blessing DL. Disordered eating patterns in competitive female athletes. *Int J Eat Disord* 1990;5:565–569.
14. Andersen AE. Diagnosis and treatment of males with eating disorders. In: Andersen AE, ed. *Males with eating disorders.* New York: Brunner/Mazel, 1990:133–162.
15. Katz JL. Some reflections on the nature of the eating disorders. *Int J Eat Disord* 1985;4:617–626.
16. Garfinkel PE, Garner DM, Goldbloom DS. Eating disorders implications for the 1990's. *Can J Psychiatry* 1987;32:624–631.
17. Sundgot-Borgen J, Klungland M. The female athlete triad and the effect of preventive work. *Med Sci Sports Exerc* 1998;5[Suppl]:181.
18. Brownell KD, Steen SN, Wilmore JH. Weight regulation practices in athletes: analysis of metabolic and health effects. *Med Sci Sports Exerc* 1987;6:546–560.
19. Sacks MH. Psychiatry and sports. *Ann Sports Med* 1990;5:47–52.
20. Hsu LKG. *Eating disorders.* New York: Guilford Press, 1990.
21. Johnson C, Connor SM. *The etiology and treatment of bulimia nervosa.* New York: Basic Books, 1987.
22. Mitchell JE. *Bulimia nervosa.* Minneapolis: University of Minnesota Press, 1990.
23. Nielsen S, Møller-Madsen S, Isager T, et al. Standardized mortality in eating disorders: a qualitative summary of previously published and new evidence. *J Psychosom Res* 1998;44:413–434.
24. Brownell KD, Rodin J. Prevalence of eating disorders in athletes. In: Brownell KD, Rodin J, Wilmore JH, eds. *Eating, body weight and performance in athletes: disorders of modern society.* Philadelphia: Lea & Febiger, 1992:128–143.
25. Mansfield MJ, Emans SJ. Growth in female gymnasts: should training decrease during puberty? Pediatrics 1993;122:237–240.
26. Theintz MJ, Howald H, Weiss U. Evidence of a reduction of growth potential in adolescent female gymnasts. *J Pediatr* 1993;122:306–313.
27. Fogelholm M. Effects of bodyweight reduction on sports performance. *Sports Med* 1994;4:249–267.
28. Clark N. How to help the athlete with bulimia: practical tips and case study. *Int J Sport Nutr* 1993;3:450–460.
29. Rosenvinge JH, Gresko RB. Do we need a prevention model for eating disorders? *Eating Disorders: The Journal of Treatment and Prevention* 1997;5:110–118.
30. Gresko RB, Rosenvinge JH. The Norwegian School-based prevention model: development and validation. In: Vandereycken W, Noordenbos G, eds. *The prevention of eating disorders.* London: Athlone Press/New York: New York University Press, 1998.
31. Eisenman PA, Johnson SC, Benson JE. *Coaches guide to nutrition and weight control,* 2nd ed. Champaign, IL: Leisure Press, 1990.

CHAPTER 13

Psychological Impact of Injury and Rehabilitation

John Heil and Edmund A. O'Connor

> I had seen the world. But nothing prepared me for what was about to take place on this operating table. I was so sad that I started crying. I tried to suppress my emotions. It was useless. I'm really, really scared. The mind is always the last place to heal.
> — Former NBA basketball player Bill Walton (1)

Virtually all athletes become injured at some point during their careers (2). Athletes engage in rigorous training programs and competitions that make injury a pervasive part of sports participation (3). Approximately 17 million sport injuries occur yearly in the United States (4), and the threat of injury is ever present in sport. The ability to remain injury free and to recover rapidly when injured is important to any athlete's longevity and success.

However, when injury does occur, it will often have a profound effect on the mind, as well as the body, of the athlete. An individual's mental state can cause a reaction in the body, such as muscle tension in reaction to worry. In turn, medical conditions can influence an individual's thinking and emotions, as when depression follows a stroke (5). Behavioral medicine applies behavioral techniques (e.g., relaxation training, self-monitoring of thoughts and feelings) to medical disorders and related problems (e.g., obesity, chronic pain, diabetes, compliance issues).

Sport psychology shares much with behavioral medicine. Both attempt to achieve specific changes in behaviors through programs that are goal oriented, are time limited, and place the client/patient in an active, skill-based role. Sport psychology addresses the relationship between psychological behavior and sport and exercise. The most distinct focus is the applied science of performance enhancement, which deals with areas that assist an athlete in his or her athletic performance. These techniques (e.g., motivation, mental training) can also be applied to address the psychological consequences of sport injury and rehabilitation.

A recent study by Larson, Starkey, and Zaichkowsky (6) found that 47% of the 482 athletic trainers they questioned believed that every injured athlete suffers psychological trauma. Almost 90% of the athletic trainers surveyed reported that it was important to treat the psychological aspect of an athletic injury. Among those who did refer patients, 8.2% of their caseload warranted a psychological referral.

The degree of psychological impact injury has on an individual depends on a number of mediating psychosocial factors, including personality, self-esteem, locus of control, motivation and achievement orientation, the importance of sport in the athlete's life, injury history, and psychological coping skill strategies. Situational factors also come into play, including the nature and severity of injury, the time of the season the injury occurs, role ambiguity, interpersonal team dynamics, and the social support networks available to the athlete (6–9). Other stress-related psychological reactions to injury include loss of identity, shattered hopes and dreams, separation and loneliness, fear of reinjury, anxiety and uncertainty, physical inactivity, unrealistic expectations regarding return to preinjury levels of performance, and diminished self-confidence (10,11).

Given the numerous factors that contribute to the impact of injury and rehabilitation, individual reactions across individuals will vary. Some athletes perceive the consequences of injury to be a disaster, while others simply take it in stride depending on the type of injury, personality characteristics, and motivational orientation (12). Because athletes are so dependent on their physical skills and because their identities are so wrapped up in their sport, injury can be a tremendously threatening experience (13).

Psychological rehabilitation can significantly benefit

J. Heil: Lewis-Gale Clinic, Valley View Medical Center, Roanoke, Virginia 24012.

E. A. O'Connor: Pain and Headache Rehabilitation Programs, Grand Rapids, Michigan 49503.

athletes by cultivating a better understanding of rehabilitation, building an increased sense of responsibility and control over their recoveries (14), and guiding them in the transfer of sport skills to rehabilitation. This will enable the athlete to move from recovering athlete to performing athlete while building confidence that they can perform at or above their pre-injury levels of performance.

PSYCHOLOGICAL RESPONSE

Minor aches and pains are a routine part of sport and are accepted by a majority of athletes as part of the game. More serious injury, however, can take its toll emotionally on one athlete, while others remain positive and rehabilitate quickly. Rod Woodson of the Pittsburgh Steelers, for example, tore his anterior cruciate ligament (ACL) in the 1995 season opener and returned just $4\frac{1}{2}$ months later to play in the Super Bowl (15). During the 1997 season, Jerry Rice of the San Francisco 49ers worked to return to professional football only $3\frac{1}{2}$ months after major reconstructive knee surgery that repaired his torn ACL, torn posterior medial capsule, and strained medial collateral ligament (MCL) (15). Others may respond in a maladaptive fashion (e.g., anxiety) that can delay the healing process so that they return to their sport at a later date, if at all. "My knee's shot. My knee's shot. There goes my whole career. It's over. I'm through" (16, p. 37). This quote, from Minnesota Vikings defensive tackle Keith Millard after he went down with an injury against the Tampa Bay Buccaneers, illustrates this adverse reaction. Marybeth LaFontaine, wife of NHL player Pat LaFontaine, described Pat's reaction after his fifth career concussion: "He was very emotional. I would walk into a room and he would be crying. He cried a lot. . . . He wouldn't leave the house for a week. He wouldn't change his clothes, wouldn't shower. It was all the classic signs of depression" (17, p. 73). The most frequent problems noted by athletic trainers were stress and anxiety, anger, treatment compliance problems, depression, problems with attention and concentration, and exercise addiction (6). Other problems may include weight control issues and substance abuse. Despite the range of potential complications, all athletes appear to experience similar stresses due to injury and undergo a common affective cycle during the course of rehabilitation.

Stresses of Injury

The stresses of injury are many and varied (Table 13–1). They influence physical, emotional, and social well-being, as well as underlying self-concept. Ultimately, the impact of injury is the net effect of the stress of the injury itself and the athlete's coping resources.

These multiple factors can lead to psychological distress, which may have a negative impact on the injured athlete's response to rehabilitation in the form of lowered confidence in recovery, reduced adherence to rehabilitation protocols, decreased effort in physical therapy, increased anxiety, and intensified pain (14). Low to moderate levels of psychological distress (e.g., some depression and anxiety) are natural when injury occurs and will often resolve as the athlete copes with his or her situation. However, negative reactions that significantly impair daily functioning in rehabilitation or other areas (e.g., school, social relationships, or work) may require additional professional attention. Possible antecedents of psychological difficulties include negative expectations, lack of social support, pain and the inability to manage it effectively, and functional disability (14). Psychological problems are most common among athletes who have been seriously injured and require a lengthy, potentially painful rehabilitation. This is often due to the significant pain, extended removal from sport, lengthy and difficult rehabilitation, and prominent concerns about a full recovery.

TABLE 13–1. *The stresses of injury*

Physical well-being
- Physical injury
- Pain of injury
- Physical rigors of treatment and rehabilitation
- Temporary physical restriction
- Permanent physical changes

Emotional well-being
- Psychological trauma at injury occurrence
- Feelings of loss and grief
- Threats to future performance
- Emotional demands of treatment and rehabilitation

Social well-being
- Loss of important social roles
- Separation from family, friends, and teammates
- New relationships with treatment providers
- Necessity of depending on others

Self-concept
- Loss of sense of control
- Dealing with altered self image
- Threat to life goals and values
- Necessity for decision making under stressful circumstances

Pain

Pain is an integral part of the athletic experience both in sport performance and in injury. The athlete must learn while healthy to differentiate performance pain from injury pain and, when injured, to discriminate between benign pain and harmful pain. The athlete also must deal with the distraction of minor aches and pains, the extreme pain of acute injury at its occurrence, the recurring pain of overuse injury, and the persistent pain of unresolved injury.

Pain is a complex biopsychosocial experience. It begins as a biological event (nociception) that gives rise to psychological awareness (perception). From this follows a search for the meaning of the pain based on cognitive and affective interpretations, which then serves as a guide for a behavioral response to the pain.

Pain is a term that is used to describe many things. It is the meaning attributed to pain that will determine the athlete's emotional, psychological, and behavioral response to pain. For example, pain experienced during rehabilitation may be interpreted in one of two ways. An athlete who views this pain as a sign of working hard and pushing his or her body to the limit will gain a sense of accomplishment and reinforcement from the work she or he is doing. On the other hand, an athlete who views this pain as damaging will decrease his or her effort and risks slowing his or her rehabilitation progress.

The Affective Cycle of Injury

Athletes' emotional reactions to injury are complex and resist simple understanding. Traditional theories suggest that recovery is a one-time, linear progression through a set of stages [e.g., Kubler-Ross (18); Rotella (19)]. However, this model has not withstood empirical scrutiny (20). The common shortcoming of the early stage theories and the more recent empirically driven cognitive appraisal models is that they are single-discipline "psychology only" perspectives on injury. In contrast, injury is best viewed from a multidisciplinary perspective.

A pragmatic resolution of the stage theory question begins with a shift in focus from the psychological to the physical functional process of injury rehabilitation. From this medically grounded perspective, injury and recovery are readily conceivable as a series of stages. One such model that is firmly rooted in the physical aspects of rehabilitation, but is also psychologically minded, is that of orthopedic surgeon J. Richard Steadman (21). Each of the following stages is conceived of as eliciting interrelated physical and psychological demands:

1. Preinjury
2. Immediate postinjury
3. Treatment decision and implementation
4. Early postoperative/rehabilitation
5. Late postoperative/rehabilitation
6. Specificity
7. Return to play

For more information on this model, see Steadman (21).

The way in which these physical functioning stages are in turn linked to the psychology of injury is reflected in the affective cycle of injury (22). This model proposes that emotional recovery from injury is cyclical with a relative balance of distress and coping. It is useful to envision an embedded set of cycles: a macrocycle (which spans the recovery process), minicycles (which are linked to the medical process of injury and rehabilitation), and microcycles (which reflect the ups and downs of daily living). This approach links emotional response to the course of physical functional recovery.

This model describes three styles of response: distress, denial, and determined coping. *Distress* recognizes the inherently disrupting and disorganizing impact of injury on emotional equilibrium. It includes shock, anger, bargaining, anxiety, depression, guilt, isolation, humiliation, preoccupation, and helplessness. Certain levels of distress are normal, but the magnitude needs to be assessed to determine how appropriate it is relative to the severity of the injury. Chicago Bears running back Rashaan Salaam, following a broken right fibula that ended his 1997 season, illustrated emotional distress: "When you get hurt, it's unbearable, man. Not just the physical part. We've learned to take the pain. It's mental. To work every day for months, and in a second it's gone. Now I'm lying here on some bench, knowing my season's over. It's a sick feeling" (23, p. 74).

Denial includes a sense of disbelief as well as varying degrees of outright failure to accept the severity of injury or its consequences. Denial may be reflected in the athlete's rather weak assurances to health providers, teammates, and others about plans to quickly return to top form. Given the specifics of its occurrence, it may serve an adaptive purpose (e.g., an initial method of coping to provide the athlete time to accept the reality of the situation) or may interfere with rehabilitation progress (e.g., lack of adherence to treatment). Denial is most common at the time of injury but may also occur in conjunction with treatment setbacks and at transitions such as slow, gradual progressions during the rehabilitation process. Denial may also be evident when the athlete perceives rehabilitation progress to be more favorable than do treatment providers.

The best approach to denial is to give the athlete a positive and adaptive future focus. Systematic goal setting can effectively challenge denial while simultaneously reducing the risk of poor limit setting and risk of reinjury. More obvious forms of denial are best addressed by the treatment team directly working with the athlete in a tactful and supportive manner. For more on denial, see Heil (24).

Determined coping implies varying degrees of acceptance of the severity of the injury and its impact on the athlete's short-term and long-term goals. It is characterized by the purposeful use of coping strategies and resources in working through the process of recovery. Udry (25) found that athletes recovering from knee surgery used instrumental coping (i.e., attempts to alleviate the source of stress or discomfort through activities such as finding out more about a health condition and/or listening to the advice of health care providers) most frequently throughout rehabilitation. Ninety percent of the athletes reported coping by "driving through" rehabilitation (10). This included responses such as maintaining or resuming activities of daily living, setting and working toward and accomplishing goals, and focusing on rehabilitation and training. This method of coping was also associated with increased adherence to rehabilitation.

Distress and denial will tend to dominate the athlete's emotions in the early stages of injury, with a general trend toward determined coping as rehabilitation proceeds. Because each stage in the injury and rehabilitation process presents new challenges to the athlete, periods of increased distress and denial may occur, even during otherwise successful rehabilitation. Setbacks in the treatment process and pain flare-ups are the most likely triggers of a shift from determined coping to distress or denial. However, shifts from one affective phase to another can occur at any time, and rarely will one phase dominate 24 hours a day. Specific events or experiences may cause an abrupt shift in emotional response, such as reviewing game films that show any injury. Generally, an athlete's emotional well-being will vary predictably with her or his subjective sense of progress through rehabilitation.

ASSESSMENT

In contrast to the general medical patient, the athlete is both uniquely challenged by injury and particularly well prepared to cope with it. An athlete's advantages typically include a goal orientation, fondness for physical training, strong motivation to return to optimal functioning, and willingness to tolerate pain. The athlete likely has more experience than the nonathlete in coping with injury. But there are disadvantages for the athlete as well. Return to normal daily functioning is simply not good enough for the athlete, who obviously needs a longer recovery to meet the demands of sport. The athlete experiences a greater loss with injury and a potentially greater threat to self-esteem than does the nonathlete, owing to the athlete's identification with sport. The relative balance of the positive and negative factors associated with injury will determine the speed and effectiveness of rehabilitation.

The psychological status of the injured athlete is of concern to all treatment providers. Because chronicity of injury and psychological complications are mutually reinforcing, the benefit of early identification is great. Bridges (26) developed a checklist to enhance the early identification of rehabilitation problems. The Sports Medicine Injury Checklist (27) (Table 13-2) extends

TABLE 13-2. *Sports medicine injury checklist*

Acute phase
___ Failure of pain to respond to routine management strategies
___ Failure of athlete to comply with recommended rehabilitation program
___ Rehabilitation setbacks
___ Emotional distress (depression, irritability, confusion, guilt, withdrawal)
___ Irrational fear or anxiety in specific situations in the otherwise well-adjusted athlete (may be seen as avoidance of feared situation)
___ Overly optimistic attitude toward injury and recovery
___ Persistent fatigue
___ Sleep problems
___ Gross overestimate or underestimate of rehabilitation progress by athlete

Chronic phase

Current factors
___ Persistence of pain beyond natural healing
___ Odd descriptions of pain
___ Inconsistency in "painful" behavior or reports of pain
___ Failed attempt(s) at return to play
___ Performance problems following return to play
___ Inability to identify realistic goals for recovery
___ Recent stressful life changes in sport situation
___ Stressful life circumstances (within the last year)
___ Depression (including changes in sleep, appetite, energy, and libido)
___ Strained relationships with coaches, teammates, or friends
___ Personality conflicts between treatment providers and athlete
___ Poor compliance with scheduled visits and medication use
___ Additional medical treatment sought by athlete without consulting current treatment providers (including emergency room visits)
___ Iatrogenic problems
___ Repeated requests for pain (especially psychoactive) medication
___ Evidence of illicit drug use (recreational or ergogenic)

History
___ Multiple surgeries at pain site
___ Chronic pain in the same or another physiological system (may be resolved)
___ Family members with chronic pain
___ Problematic psychosocial history (behavior problems in school; vocational, marital, or legal problems; history of physical or sexual abuse)
___ Problematic psychological history (repeated or prolonged psychosocial adjustment problems, alcohol/drug problems, eating disorders)

From Heil J. Early identification and intervention with injured athletes at risk for failed rehabilitation. Workshop conducted at the annual meeting of the Association of the Advancement of Applied Sport Psychology, Nashua, NH, October 1988.

the work of Bridges (26) by identifying factors that are of particular relevance to athletes. The checklist is best considered simply as a guide to inquiry and evaluation that ensures a comprehensive diagnostic approach. The physician and sports medicine team provide the first line of psychological intervention with injured athletes. The Sports Medicine Injury Checklist provides these practitioners with a tool to identify possible psychological difficulties throughout the rehabilitation process.

The acute phase section of the checklist allows the user to identify potential difficulties in the immediate postinjury period. An athlete's failure to comply with the rehabilitation regimen, persistent difficulties in pain management, and obvious emotional distress are the most reliable early indicators of rehabilitation problems. Signs of anxiety demonstrated only in conjunction with specific performance situations suggest fear of reinjury. When either physical or psychological difficulties become evident, the athlete's input on how rehabilitation is progressing needs to be sought. When the athlete's perspective on injury differs substantially from objective medical opinion, problems are in the making.

Prolonged or repeated difficulties with rehabilitation and pain inevitably lead to the development of psychological difficulties. The chronic phase section of the checklist is designed to provide a more detailed review of the athlete's psychological status. The assessment of current factors relies significantly on observation of the athlete's behavior. However, the provider will need to consult with the athlete on items such as identifying realistic goals for recovery and distinguishing between benign pain and pain that signals injury. It may also be necessary to consult with the coaching staff on issues such as performance problems and interpersonal relationships.

Knowledge of the athlete's personal history helps treatment providers to place other observations in perspective. As a general rule, a history of difficulty in adapting to psychological stressors is predictive of present difficulties. Because of their intrusive nature, questions about history should be presented with sensitivity to the athlete's privacy.

PSYCHOLOGICAL TREATMENT

When injury occurs, it is useful for the athlete to think of rehabilitation as part of the game that she or he must play well to succeed. The objectives of psychological intervention with athletic injury are as follows:

1. Facilitation of the rehabilitation process
2. Maintenance of emotional balance
3. Mobilization of existing coping resources
4. Promotion of a sense of self-efficacy
5. Enhancement of mental readiness for performance

As medical recovery is speeded (by advances in sports medicine), there is correspondingly greater pressure for swift psychological recovery. Quick physical recovery and mental readiness for return to play involve more than simple compliance by the athlete; they demand vigorous physical effort and mental tenacity (21). Psychological management of the injured athlete involves education, goal setting, social support, and mental training. Goals define the task, and education provides an understanding of how to proceed with that task. Mental training and social support are the coping resources the athlete may use to remain on task in the face of adversity. Putting these key elements together points the athlete toward optimal recovery from sport injury.

This approach defines a performance-enhancement model of intervention that emphasizes skill-based approaches to treatment. It projects rehabilitation as a sports performance challenge and encourages the use of psychological skills already developed for sport performance.

Education

The primary goal of education is to help the athlete understand in detail the process underlying injury and rehabilitation. The athlete cannot give optimal effort to something she or he does not understand. Injury is an opportunity for learning about the body and physical performance. The sport emphasis is simply shifted from performance skills to health and safety. Essential injury management skills, such as differentiating pain and injury, can be refined. This enhanced understanding of the body's limits gained through rehabilitation can play an important role in preventing future injury. Athletes who address physical performance from the perspectives of skill development and health maintenance improve their chances for longevity and success in sport. In addition, attempts to alleviate stress or discomfort by gathering information about the injury and listening to the advice of health care providers was the strategy most frequently used by athletes recovering from knee surgery (25). This method of coping was also associated with higher rates of adherence to rehabilitation.

In general medical practice, compliance with medication use and with prescribed independent activities is known to be poor; treatment providers use medical terminology and provide brief explanations that patients often simply do not understand. This confusion may be compounded by the stress of injury and a poor understanding of medical practice on the part of the athlete. The antidote to this is the treatment provider's consistent, systematic attention to education and explicit efforts to determine whether the athlete understands the information provided.

Following an injury, its cause and physical consequences should be described in terms that the athlete can understand. Treatment providers should give the athlete a sense of how the injury will heal and specific information about methods of rehabilitation and how they aid healing. Providers should also describe the timetable of rehabilitation and the expectations they have of the athlete. Special concerns such as anticipated plateaus in progress and tolerance of pain may need to be addressed.

Goal Setting

Most athletes are familiar with goal setting as part of their sport training; application of this skill will reinforce the idea that rehabilitation is an aspect of sport performance in which their competitive skills may be applied. It can also increase the athletes' feelings of familiarity, predictability, and control over their injuries while improving their confidence and reducing their anxiety about rehabilitation (14). Involving the athletes in the goal-setting process improves their motivation (28) by establishing an implicit statement of commitment, and identifying treatment as a collaborative process. Additional guidelines for setting goals are described below.

Goals Should Be Specific and Measurable

The athlete must know exactly what to do and be able to determine whether gains are made. This is usually accomplished by behavioral performance criteria (e.g., when and how long ice should be applied) rather than effort or general goals (e.g., "Be sure to use ice when you need it").

Goals Should Be Stated in Positive Language

Knowing what to do guides behavior, whereas knowing what to avoid creates a focus on errors without providing a constructive alternative (e.g., after a back injury, when sitting, say, "Maintain an erect posture with your head in a neutral position," not "Don't slouch").

Goals Should Be Challenging but Realistic

Overly difficult goals set up failure and pose a threat to the athlete. The lower the athlete's self-confidence, the more important success becomes and the greater the importance of setting attainable goals. Easy goals, however, will not adequately challenge the athlete to achieve optimal progress. Athletic trainers report that setting realistic goals is one of the most important techniques trainers need to learn to enhance their work with injured athletes (6).

Short-, Intermediate-, and Long-Term Goals Should Be Integrated

A comprehensive program links day-to-day rehabilitation with expectations for return to play and with season and career goals. The short-term goals will build a plan of action to achieve intermediate goals, which in turn will build a plan of action for the achievement of long-term goals. Having a clear timetable for completion provides a check as to whether recovery is on course.

Outcome Goals Should Be Linked to Performance Goals

Performance goals (e.g., stretching the knee through pain to the point of tension, then relaxing) define the pathway to outcome goals (e.g., regaining normal range of motion). In competitive sport outcomes are influenced by a variety of factors, many of which may be beyond the athlete's control. Performance goals focus the athlete on factors most readily controlled, enhancing achievement. Outcome goals are highly motivating, connecting the athlete to the reason for the intense grind of rehabilitation (e.g., return to the starting lineup by state championships).

Sport Goals Should Be Linked to Life Goals

Identification of sport and rehabilitation as life learning experiences helps the athlete to put sport in a broader perspective. This is especially important for athletes whose return to sport is doubtful.

Goals Should Be Monitored and Evaluated

Feedback must be provided to assess goals. Goals should be modified on the basis of progress. To be effective, goals need to remain in the athlete's mind. This may be achieved by posting them in an easily seen place.

The process of setting, monitoring, and refining goals clarifies communication between the athlete and the sports medicine team and maintains a performance enhancement orientation to injury rehabilitation.

Social Support

Social support buffers the effects of stress on health and enhances the prospects for recovery of those who are ill or injured. Those who possess a strong sense of social support demonstrate greater self-efficacy, lower anxiety, better interpersonal skills, and more risk-taking behavior (29), as well as better compliance (30,31). The sport psychology literature consistently notes the benefits of social support in helping to cope with injury (32,33). Athletes themselves recognize its importance and advise coaches and sports medicine teams to provide positive support and empathy (10). On the other end of the spectrum, pressure or confrontation regarding injury is distressing and potentially detrimental (34).

Support is most effectively provided by a network of individuals. The three segments of the injured athlete's support system are the sport team, the sports medicine team, and family and friends; each has a unique role to play. Support needs to be developed and nurtured as part of an ongoing program rather than simply as a reaction to crisis. Specific recommendations offered for treatment providers include being a willing listener, acknowledging both effort and mastery of rehabilitation tasks, and balancing the use of technical appreciation acknowledgment of good performance) and technical challenge (encouragement to meet performance goals) (35).

Unfortunately, the injured athlete often tends to be separated from the team and loses this source of support at a time when it is most important. Their athletic identities make up a large part of the personal identities of dedicated athletes. When an injured athlete is removed from the sport environment, feelings of depression, worthlessness, helplessness, decreased confidence, doubt in the ability to recover, and increased anxiety may follow. This may decrease motivation, slowing rehabilitation (14).

Continuing team contact decreases isolation, offers emotional support, and carries numerous other benefits. Attending practice and games keeps the athlete current with changes in plays and team strategies. It helps the athlete stay in touch with the rhythm of the season and continues established relationships with team members. It also gives the athlete an opportunity for continued visual learning, which can be supplemented by formal mental training. Continued involvement with the team has been reported to provide a feeling of being needed and a sense of security (i.e., reassurance that the coach has not given up on the injured athlete) (36,37).

Social support is most needed and least available with injury requiring surgery and lengthy rehabilitation. The athlete is taken out of the sport system, limiting the opportunity for contact with coaches and fellow athletes. Visits by coaches and teammates to athletes who are hospitalized for surgery are quite valuable, especially when family is not conveniently located. When more intense interventions are necessary, injury support groups and peer modeling should be considered (38,39). The effects of social support, though intangible, are significant.

Mental Training

Mental training has been used widely to improve sport performance and is equally effective in helping the athlete to meet the challenges of rehabilitation. Mental training methods typically include some combination of relaxation training, mental imagery, self-talk, concentration training, biofeedback, and hypnosis. A series of mental training interventions are described below.

Continued Performance Enhancement Training

The importance of maintaining continuity of physical training during injury is widely recognized. Continued mental training is a natural extension of this principle; it helps the athlete maintain a performance oriented mind-set and facilitates mental readiness for return to play. The athlete may use the down time of injury to learn these skills at a time when they are particularly useful or to continue established mental training regimens.

The athlete can maintain fundamental arousal and attentional control, as well as psychomotor skills (40), by mentally rehearsing sport-specific techniques as if she or he were still playing. This can be facilitated through review of films or videotapes of prior performances. By attending team meetings, practices, and competitions, athletes can rehearse sport skills in real time by projecting themselves into the performance situation as it unfolds before them.

Rehabilitation Rehearsal

Rehabilitation rehearsal may address any aspect of the rehabilitation process, from coping with pain and anxiety immediately following injury through rehabilitation and return to competition. Rehearsal scenarios are built from images. Images are best experienced by using all of the senses (i.e., sights, sounds, kinesthetic feel, tastes, and scents) to vivify the imagination and to give rise to an "inner theater." Within this inner theater any of life's experiences can be rehearsed, evaluated, and refined; a broad range of mental skills may be practiced, from positive self-talk, to preparation routines, to emotions such as confidence and enthusiasm, to specific performance skills.

Rehearsal typically begins with a relaxation procedure that calms the athlete and enables him or her to focus intently on the mastery or coping imagery. Mastery imagery rehearses a favorable process and outcome, such as rehabilitation occurring without any problems. Coping imagery has the athlete rehearsing and applying coping techniques to anything from day-to-day hassles, to critical transition points, to rehabilitation setbacks. Both styles build confidence, a characteristic that can greatly enhance the speed of recovery. Picabo Street returned to skiing one year after ACL reconstruction and won Olympic gold at Nagano. Most skiers believe that it takes two years to recover from that type of surgery, but Street stated, "When it comes to physical challenges, I rarely doubt myself" (41).

Healing Imagery

Surgent (42) suggested that the mind can facilitate the healing process. Hall (43), Achterberg (44), AuBuchon

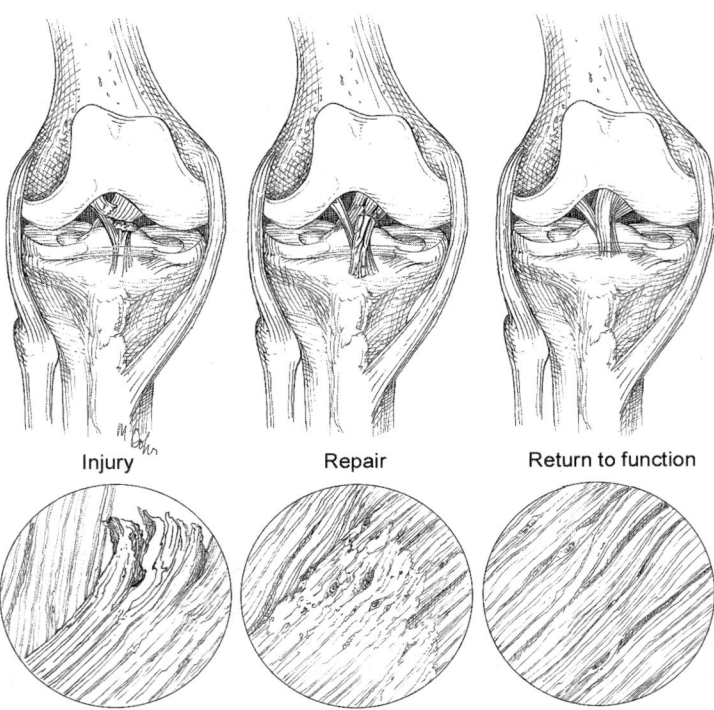

FIG. 13-1. Healing progression of an ACL injury.

(45), and Post-White (46) have provided evidence supporting the positive effects of imagery on the immune system.

Anxiety can increase pain and produce a physiologic state that hinders healing by increasing muscle tension and reducing blood flow to the injured area (14). The most likely and frequent benefit of healing imagery appears to be the reduction of anxiety. Control of the image is important, since images that anticipate reinjury and those that recall the injury can negatively affect recovery (47,48).

Preliminary research with athletes shows that spontaneous use of positive imagery is greatest among those who recover most quickly (48). This includes images of the healing process itself as well as images of healed injury. It is useful to provide the athlete with pictures, drawings, or diagrams of the injury and the stages of healing so that a vivid image of the healing process may be created. The images may be a realistic visualization of strong muscle or bone, or they may be powerful and meaningful symbols of a treatment modality or the injured area. See Figure 13-1 for an illustrated example of the healing progression of an ACL injury.

Biofeedback

Biofeedback is a self-regulation technique in which auditory or visual feedback provides information about biologic functions that is not usually available to a person's awareness (49), such as muscular activity or peripheral temperature. Electromyographic biofeedback applications with injury include muscular relaxation (reduction in muscle tension), muscle reeducation (increase in muscular activity with sensory motor deficits), and discrimination training (relaxing one muscle while the other is activated). Using muscular feedback to reduce tension can speed recovery. For example, it can teach the athlete to decrease muscular guarding and bracing, which commonly are seen in injury and can increase pain, diminish performance, and increase injury risk.

Mental Training for Pain Management

Playing with pain is often expected and encouraged in sport. Pain is also a compelling and common aspect of rehabilitation. The key question is, When does pain move beyond simply limiting performance and signal imminent injury? After an injury, the most important question regarding pain is its status as benign or, alternatively, as a signal of danger.

The familiar arena of competition may be a useful metaphor to incorporate into the rehabilitation setting (50). Having athletes compete against themselves or others for recognition (e.g., posting outstanding progress) in rehabilitation may give them a familiar setting to apply their sport skills and can provide the incentive to tolerate pain. Stress inoculation training (51), setting specific goals for tolerance (52,53), and distraction with a purposeful task (54) also increase pain tolerance.

TABLE 13–3. *Cognitive pain control strategies*

Strategy	General	Sport
External focus of attention	Listening to music; focusing on the horizon	Concentrating on the ball; attending to environmental cues that are related to sport performance
Pleasant imaginings	Imagining relaxing on the beach; imagining being at a favorite place or with a favorite person	Imagining the feeling of having performed well; imagining celebrating with others following a victory
Neutral imaginings	Thinking of a routine activity such as walking up the steps, or imagining nonemotive events	Imagining calmly dressing before or after a competition or practice.
Rhythmic cognitive activity	Counting backward from 100; repeating a neutral mantra or self-affirmation	Coordinating breathing with activity; making repetitive performance or pain coping self-affirmations
Pain acknowledging	Imagining generalized feelings of anesthesia; imagining pain being moved away from an area of the body through circulation of the blood; observing pain with a sense of emotional detachment	Imagining lactic acid buildup as inducing numbness without pain; perceiving pain as a positive sign of effort
Dramatized coping	Seeing oneself in pursuit of a heroic task in which tolerance of pain is associated with personal triumph	Imagining pain experienced during rehabilitation as occurring in conjunction with outstanding athletic achievement

Adapted with permission from "Overall and Relative Efficacy of Cognitive Strategies in Attenuating Pain." Paper presented by Dennis Turk and Ephren Fernandez at the 94th Annual Convention of the APA in Washington, DC, August 25, 1986.

These results illustrate that the general rehabilitation enhancement concepts presented earlier, and the cognitive pain control strategies presented in Table 13–3, may also specifically enhance the tolerance of pain.

Mental Training for Fear of Reinjury

Fear of reinjury can limit the athlete's tendency to return to play too soon or to take inappropriate risks. However, it is also a potential distraction that may slow rehabilitation, seriously inhibit performance following return to play, and increase the likelihood of reinjury. Jacksonville Jaguars quarterback Mark Brunell, after a series of injuries, had a decline in his performance during the 1997 season. Following a game against the Tennessee Oilers in which he put up his best numbers of the 1997 season, he stated, "The difference is that I never thought about my body. Every player will tell you that if you have your health, you can play to your fullest" (55).

As with pain, the athlete must learn to determine whether fear is relatively benign or dangerous. In addressing fear, the sports medicine professional should do the following:

1. Normalize the athlete's response; that is, let the athlete know that it is normal to experience some fear.
2. Reassure the athlete that fear itself is not the problem, though how fear is dealt with can be a problem.
3. Emphasize the adaptive value of fear in setting safe limits.
4. Reframe the arousal component of fear as the body becoming energized and ready for performance.
5. Clarify the current status of injury, identifying safe limits for performance as clearly as possible.
6. Reassure the athlete of the benign nature of pain within appropriate limits.
7. Encourage the use of mental training approaches as appropriate (e.g., refocusing techniques to concentrate on performance, not fear).

THE REFERRAL PROCESS

Psychological reactions to athletic injury may require more intensive or specialized treatments than are available from the sports medicine team. Common referral issues include depression, anxiety, substance abuse, and disordered eating. Less common but potentially important are compliance issues, persistent pain, and conflicts with coaches, treatment providers, and others. Psychological intervention is essential when significant adjustment problems exist premorbidly or as a consequence of injury. When and how vigorously referral should be recommended will be influenced by the severity and urgency of the problem and by how significantly it is interfering with rehabilitation or the patient-athlete's sport and personal life.

Professionals who are qualified to treat injured athletes will have a doctorate in clinical, counseling, or sport psychology. Certification by the Association for the Advancement of Applied Sport Psychology identifies professionals who are trained in performance-enhancement techniques. When bona fide psychological disorders are apparent (e.g., major depression, posttraumatic anxiety, eating disorder, or substance abuse), re-

TABLE 13-4. *Referral information: National organizations*

The United States Olympic Committee (USOC) Sport Psychology Registry. Contact: Kirsten Peterson, Ph.D.; Address: Sport Psychology Program, USOC Sport Science and Technology, One Olympic Plaza, Colorado Springs, CO 80909; Telephone: (719) 578-4722; E-mail: kpeterson@usoc.org; Web page: http://www.psyc.unt.edu/apadiv47/usoc.htm.

Association for the Advancement of Applied Sport Psychology. Web page (for a listing of certified consultants): http://www.aaasponline.org and follow the link at the top of the page.

ferral should be to a licensed psychologist or counselor, ideally one who specializes in the treatment of athletes. The U.S. Olympic Committee maintains a registry of sport psychologists. Table 13–4 provides referral contact information.

Psychological referral is a process that includes preparation, actual referral, and follow-up with the athlete and psychologist. In explaining to the athlete the reason for the referral, emphasize the performance enhancement potential of sport psychology and the inherently stressful nature of injury. The purpose of treatment can be described as helping to apply the mental skills of sport performance to rehabilitation to speed recovery. Further explanation is needed where the athlete shows signs of a significant psychological disorder in dealing with injury. Simply stating that psychological treatment will help with problems with pain (or sleep or feeling on edge) is often sufficient. Describing previous referrals and success associated with them is reassuring and encourages follow-through by the athlete. It should also be noted that this is an opportunity for the athlete to speak with someone confidentially about worries and concerns associated with sport injury or other life situations. This helps to mentally prepare the athlete by letting him or her know what to expect, and it also expresses understanding and support of psychological treatment.

The simplest way to ensure follow-through is to immediately, in the athlete's presence, schedule an appointment with the psychologist. By also scheduling a follow-up with the athlete soon after she or he meets with the psychologist, the sports medicine team member will limit the athlete's fear of being dumped or ignored. This also provides an opportunity to review the athlete's experience with the psychologist, facilitating coordination of care and reinforcing the psychological treatment plan.

TOPICS OF SPECIAL INTEREST

A full and thorough review of the psychology of sport injury is beyond the scope of this chapter. *Psychology of Sport Injury* (22), *Psychological Approaches to Sports Injury Rehabilitation* (14), and *Psychological Bases of Sport Injuries* (56) are resources for more detailed information. Additional topics that are relevant to sport injury and rehabilitation are presented briefly with suggested readings for more information.

Psychological Antecedents to Injury

Multiple factors, including muscle imbalances, high-speed collisions, overtraining, physical fatigue, and psychological factors, have been found to play a role in injury risk (2). Among psychological factors, stress level in particular has been identified as an important precursor to athletic injury (7). As stress increases, so does the occurrence of injury. This is likely due to concentration disruption (57) or increased muscle tension (58), which commonly occur in reaction to stress. This stress-injury relationship is strongest among athletes who have minimal social support and a low level of coping skills (8,59).

Personality characteristics and attitudes inherent in sport also play a role. Rotella and Heyman (33) and Heil (27) have identified attitudes such as "Act tough and give 110%" and "If you're hurt, you're worthless" to predispose athletes to injury (Fig. 13–2).

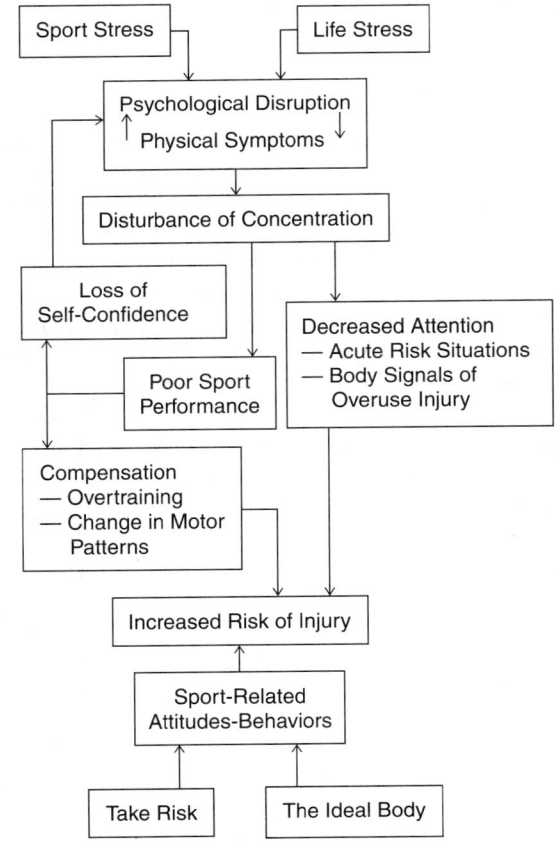

FIG. 13-2. Psychology and injury risk.

Remarkable Feats of Pain Tolerance

Remarkable feats of pain tolerance have been reported in military (60) and athlete populations. Heil (61) hypothesizes that this is associated with the following elements: the expectation that pain can and will be tolerated; a strong achievement-driven goal orientation, absorption in the work in progress whereby performance relevant perceptions predominate over pain, a survival context (literal or metaphorical), and the anticipation of a positive outcome in conjunction with the implicit assumption of limited pain duration.

Suggested readings for more information on pain management in rehabilitation include Heil (61,62) and Chapter 14 in this text.

Compliance

Poor compliance merits special attention because of its relative frequency, its potential for leading to treatment complications, and its tendency to occur in conjunction with psychological adjustment problems (63). Noncompliance is most easily observed in treatment attendance but may also be evident in lack of effort and/or follow-through (e.g., home exercise). In many cases poor adherence is a sensitive early indicator of psychological problems due to injury or other life circumstances (22).

When there is poor adherence, the treatment providers should first look for issues such as scheduling problems, financial concerns, or poor understanding for the rational of treatment. More in-depth exploration may be needed to determine whether the athlete understands the connection between short-term goals of rehabilitation and long-term goals of recovery, has sufficient trust and confidence in the rehabilitation team, feels confident in his or her ability to achieve the goals that have been set, or is experiencing psychological adjustment problems (related to pain, fear of reinjury, or other issues) (22).

Overcompliance may be a problem as athletes overdo prescribed physical rehabilitation protocols and ignore recommended limits on daily activities. Warn the athlete that these behaviors risk treatment setbacks and reinjury, emphasize the prescribed amount, and support consistency and accuracy in goal attainment. Develop a flare-up plan to help athletes cope with treatment setbacks and redirect the athlete's desire and energy for more work at rehabilitation into mental training (22).

Substance Abuse

Premorbid

Athletes have been identified to be at risk for alcohol and drug problems (64). They may use drugs and alcohol to manage the emotional ups and downs associated with athletic competition. The most common substances abused by athletes include alcohol, marijuana, and mushrooms (psilocybin) (14). Legal and illicit substances carry a host of effects that lead to an increased risk of injury. For example, a blood alcohol level as low as 0.04 can impair motor skills, with coordination and judgment impairment evident at the 0.05 level (65). For more information, consult *Anabolic Steroids in Sport and Exercise* (66) and *Drugs and the Athlete* (67).

Reactive

In efforts to cope with injury and rehabilitation athletes may develop a substance abuse problem (14). Athletes may attempt to self-medicate with alcohol or drugs to deal with not only pain but also depression, anxiety, pain, anger, and other emotional sequelae of injury (64). The short term-benefits of these substances is overshadowed by the long-term physical and psychological consequences of their use.

The reliance on medication to manage pain can inadvertently result in physical and psychological dependence (64). Paradoxically, narcotic analgesic use can actually increase the amount of pain experienced until the patient is fully withdrawn from the drug. This risk of medication abuse, when coupled with the proven effectiveness of nonpharmacologic pain management strategies, illustrates the need to focus on and provide nonpharmacologic alternatives beyond the acute injury period.

Readers are encouraged to review *Athletes at Risk: Drugs and Sports* (64) and *Alcohol and Sport* (68), as well as Chapter 10 in this text.

Eating Disorders

Premorbid

Athletes are uniquely at risk for eating disorders because of the sport community's emphasis on low body fat composition and enhanced athletic performance (69). Athletes are often asked to lose weight in an effort to perform better and attempt to do so through dieting, often leading to disordered eating. Disordered eating behaviors that fall short of full-blown clinical syndromes can undermine performance and lead to serious medical and physical consequences. Amenorrhea is linked to bone mineral density loss and related complications such as stress fractures (70–72) and dehydration.

Reactive

Disordered eating problems may occur when previously active athletes are rendered inactive because of injury (14,73). Their demanding physical activities may have previously burned off a high caloric intake, but now they are unable to do so. A failure to modify diet to correspond with calorie expenditure can result in a significant weight gain. In an effort to control their weight, athletes may begin to restrict their food intake or engage in pathogenic weight-loss measures. Other athletes may change their eating pattern as a result of depression or overeat in an effort to feel better about their situation. Weight gain can cause further detriment to their physical condition, inhibiting their rehabilitation and return to sport.

An excellent resource for weight control is *Weight Loss Through Persistence* (74). The reader is also referred to *Helping Athletes with Eating Disorders* (63) and Chapter 12 in this text.

Severe Injury

Career-ending Injury

Injury plays a significant role in the closing of athletic careers. The greater the athlete's commitment, achievement, and rewards for success and the more abrupt and unanticipated the ending of a sport career, the greater the adjustment. In addition to the loss of physical function and of the highly prized sport experience, the patient may suffer from the loss of his or her athletic identity. Counseling of the athlete who suffers career-ending injury should address three issues: the trauma of the injury, the loss of the athletic career, and reorientation to a new lifestyle.

Catastrophic Injury

Catastrophic injury includes trauma that results in permanent functional disability, typically damage to the head and spinal cord, and other injuries of comparable severity. The psychological impact of catastrophic injury involves the immediate trauma of the injury, the continuing trauma of hospitalization and treatment, the loss of sport activity, the loss of the ability to engage in ordinary activities, and the disruption of long-term life plans (e.g., social and career). Referral to a qualified psychologist is recommended to help the athlete deal with each of these issues.

Sport participation does not necessarily have to end following disability. Sport offers the same benefits to the person who is disabled as to the one who is not (75). There are opportunities for the casual recreational athlete who wants and needs an outlet for physical activity. The seriously committed athlete has the opportunity to pursue competitive excellence through specially organized sport activities. For more information, consult *Disability and Sport* (76) and Chapters 9 and 16 in this text.

Fatal Injury

Fatal injury creates an emotional shock wave throughout the athlete's social sphere and leaves a legacy of sadness with family, teammates, and friends. Counseling is tremendously beneficial in helping them cope with their loss, limiting the worst of the long-term consequences of fatal injury on the survivors (77).

For more information on serious injury, the reader is referred to Zernacchia, Reardon, and Templin (78) and *Psychology of Sport Injury* (22).

SUMMARY

Sport injury and rehabilitation create numerous psychological stressors for the athlete. Responses can range from determined coping and remarkable recovery to severe cases of depression and anxiety. Typically, athletes will cycle through a range of emotional responses throughout rehabilitation. The Sports Medicine Injury Checklist is a useful tool to assess the psychological status of the injured athlete and identify those who may need a referral for psychological intervention. For the majority of athletes, however, education, goal setting, social support, and mental training will sufficiently enhance their rehabilitation and return to sport.

The central goal of rehabilitation from a sport injury is to guide the patient in thinking and acting like an athlete (79). Conceptualizing the patient as an athlete casts rehabilitation in a positive and upbeat light, defined by the work ethic of athleticism: personal dedication, goal orientation, challenging practice regimens, pain tolerance, and striving to move to a higher level of performance. Ten principles of sport psychology that may guide the athlete in transferring his or her mental skills to rehabilitation follow (80):

1. Know the game — "Knowledge is power"
2. Goal-directed thinking — "A road map to recovery"
3. Focused attention — "Mental tenacity"
4. Emotional intensity — "Bringing heart to rehabilitation"
5. Precise skill execution — "Goodness of form"
6. Training intensity — "Overloading without overdoing"
7. Performance over pain — "Mastering the mind/body relationship"
8. Playing the edges — "Calculated risk taking"
9. Mental toughness — "Courage in adversity"
10. Striving for personal best — "Self-actualization"

REFERENCES

1. Walton B, Wojciechowski G. *Nothing but net: just give me the ball and get out of my way.* New York: Hyperion 1994:10.
2. Weinberg RS, Gould D. *Foundations of sport and exercise psychology.* Champaign, IL: Human Kinetics, 1995.
3. Kraus JF, Conroy C. Mortality and morbidity from injuries in sports and recreation. *Annu Rev Public Health* 1984;5:163–192.

4. Booth W. Arthritis Institute tackles sports. *Science* 1987;237:846–847.
5. Robinson RG, Lipsey JR, Price TR. Diagnosis and clinical management of post-stroke depression. *Psychosomatics* 1985;26(10):769–778.
6. Larson GA, Starkey C, Zaichkowsky LD. Psychological aspects of athletic injuries as perceived by athletic trainers. *Sport Psychol* 1996;10(1):37–47.
7. Anderson MB, Williams JM. A model of stress and athletic injury: prediction and prevention. *J Sport Exerc Psychol* 1988;10:294–306.
8. Smith RE, Smoll FL, Ptacek JT. Conjunctive moderator variables in vulnerability and resiliency research: Life stress, social support, coping skills, and adolescent sport injuries. *J Pers Soc Psychol* 1990;55:360–370.
9. Wiese-Bjornstal DM, Smith AM, LaMott EE. A model of psychologic response to athletic injury and rehabilitation. *Athletic Training: Sports Health Care Perspectives* 1995;1:17–30.
10. Gould D, Udry E, Bridges D, Beck L. The psychology of ski racing injury rehabilitation: final report. Paper presented as part of US Olympic Committee Sports Science and Technology Grant Project, March 1996.
11. Petitpas A, Danish SJ. Caring for injured athletes. In: Murphy SM, ed. *Sport psychology interventions.* Champaign, IL: Human Kinetics, 1995:255–281.
12. Rotella RJ, Heyman SR. Stress, injury, and the psychological rehabilitation of athletes. In: Williams JM, ed. *Applied sport psychology: personal growth for peak performance,* 3rd ed. Mountain View, CA: Mayfield, 1997:409–428.
13. Petrie G. Injury from the athlete's point of view. In: Heil J, ed. *Psychology of sport injury.* Champaign, IL: Human Kinetics, 1993:17–23.
14. Taylor J, Taylor S. *Psychological approaches to sports injury rehabilitation.* Gaithersburg, MD: Aspen Publishers, 1997.
15. Silver M. Final push. *Sports Illustrated* 1997;87(24):72–78.
16. Lieber J. Deep scars. *Sports Illustrated* 1990;75(5):36–44.
17. Montville L. Can't quit now. *Sports Illustrated* 1997;87(22):73–79.
18. Kubler-Ross E. *On death and dying.* New York: Macmillan, 1969.
19. Rotella RJ. Psychological care of the injured athlete. In: Kuland DN, ed. *The injured athlete.* Philadelphia: Lippincott, 1982:213–224.
20. Brewer BW. Review and critique of models of psychophysiological adjustment to athletic injury. *J Appl Sport Psychol* 1994;6:87–100.
21. Steadman JR. A physician's approach to the psychology of injury. In: Heil J, ed. *Psychology of sport injury.* Champaign, IL: Human Kinetics, 1993:25–31.
22. Heil J. *Psychology of sport injury.* Champaign, IL: Human Kinetics, 1993:33–48.
23. King P. The inner game: a morning after. *Sports Illustrated* 1997;87(13):74.
24. Heil J. The injured athlete. In: Y Hanin, ed. *Emotion in sport.* Champaign, IL: Human Kinetics, 2000:245–265.
25. Udry E. Coping and social support among injured athletes following surgery. *J Sport Exerc Psychol* 1997;19:71–90.
26. Bridges JK. Try comprehensive case management to curb chronicity during rehabilitation. *Back Pain Monitor* 1987;5(11):145–147.
27. Heil J. Early identification and intervention with injured athletes at risk for failed rehabilitation. Workshop conducted at the annual meeting of the Association of the Advancement of Applied Sport Psychology, Nashua, NH, October 1988.
28. Kyllo LB, Landers DM. Goal setting in sport and exercise: a research synthesis to resolve the controversy. *J Sport Exerc Psychol* 1995;17:117–137.
29. Sarason IG, Sarason BR, Pierce GR. Social support, personality, and performance. *J Appl Sport Psychol* 1990;2(2):117–127.
30. Duda JL, Smart AE, Tappe MK. Predictors of adherence in the rehabilitation of athletic injuries: an application of personal investment theory. *J Sport Exerc Psychol* 1989;11(4):367–381.
31. Fisher AC, Domm NA, Wuest DA. Adherence to sports-injury rehabilitation programs. *Physician and Sportsmedicine* 1989;16(7):47–51.
32. Danish S. Psychological aspects in the care and treatment of athletic injuries. In: Vinger PE & Hoerner EF, eds. *Sports injuries: the unthwarted epidemic,* 2nd ed. Littleton, MA: PSG, 1986:121–146.
33. Rotella RJ, Heyman SR. Stress, injury and the psychological rehabilitation of athletes. In: Williams JM, ed. *Applied sport psychology: personal growth to peak performance.* Palo Alto, CA: Mayfield, 1986:343–364.
34. Hankins P, Gipson M, Foster M, et al. Psychosocial factors in sports injury diagnosis and rehabilitation: the case of women's intercollegiate volleyball. Paper presented at the first International Olympic Committee World Congress on Sport Sciences, Colorado Springs, CO, October 1989.
35. Richman JM, Hardy CJ, Rosenfeld LB, Callanan RAE. Strategies for enhancing social support networks in sport: A brainstorming experience. *Appl Sport Psychol* 1989;1:150–159.
36. LaMott EE, Petlichkoff LM. Psychological factors and the injured athlete: is there a relationship? Paper presented at the annual meeting of the Association for the Advancement of Applied Sport Psychology, San Antonio, TX, September 1990.
37. Weise DM, Weiss MR, Yukelson DP. Sport psychology in the training room: a survey of athletic trainers. *Sport Psychol* 1991;5(1):15–24.
38. Wiese DM, Weiss MR. Psychology rehabilitation and physical injury: implications for the sportsmedicine team. *Sport Psychol* 1987;1(4):318–330.
39. Flint F. Seeing helps believing: modeling in injury rehabilitation. In: Pargman D, ed. *Psychological bases of sport injuries.* Morgantown, WV: Fitness Information Technology, 1993:183–198.
40. Hecker JE, Kaczor LM. Application of imagery theory to sport psychology: some preliminary findings. *J Sport Exerc Psychol* 1988;10:363–373.
41. Layden T. Picabo Street. *Sports Illustrated* 1998;88(5):123.
42. Surgent FS. Using your mind to beat injuries. *Running & FitNews* 1991;January:4–5.
43. Hall HR. Hypnosis and the immune system: a review with implications for cancer and the psychology of healing. *Amer J Clin Hypn* 1983;25(3):92–103.
44. Achterberg J. Enhancing the immune function through imagery. Paper presented to the Fourth World Congress on Imagery, Minneapolis, May 1991.
45. AuBuchon B. The effects of positive mental imagery on hope, coping, anxiety, dyspnea, and pulmonary function in persons with chronic obstructive pulmonary disease: tests of a nursing intervention and a theoretical model. Paper presented to the Fourth World Congress on Imagery, Minneapolis, May 1991.
46. Post-White J. The effects of mental imagery on emotions, immune function and cancer outcome. Paper presented to the Fourth World Congress on Imagery, Minneapolis, May 1991.
47. Grunert BK, Devine CA, Matloub HS, et al. Flashbacks after traumatic hand injuries: prognostic indicators. *J Hand Surg* 1988;13a(1):125–127.
48. Ievleva L, Orlick T. Mental links to enhanced healing: an exploratory study. *Sport Psychol* 1991;5(1):25–40.
49. Schwartz MS. *Biofeedback: a practitioner's guide.* New York: Guilford 1987.
50. O'Connor EA. The effect of competition on acute pain tolerance. Unpublished dissertation. Chicago, IL: Illinois Institute of Technology, July 1998.
51. Whitmarsh BG, Alderman RB. Role of psychological skills training in increasing athletic pain tolerance. *Sport Psychol* 1993;7:388–399.
52. Ladouceur R, Carrier C. Awareness and control of pain. *Percept Mot Skills* 1983;56:405–406.
53. Stevenson MK, Kanfer FH, Higgins JM. Effects of goal specificity and time cues on pain tolerance. *Cogn Ther Res* 1984;8(4):415–426.
54. Heck SA. The effect of purposeful activity on pain tolerance. *Am J Occup Ther* 1988;42(9):577–581.
55. King P. Inside the NFL: back in the groove. *Sports Illustrated* 1997;87(21):88.
56. Pargman D, ed. *Psychological bases of sport injuries.* Morgantown, WV: Fitness Information Technology, 1993.
57. Williams JM, Tonymon P, Anderson MB. The effects of stressors and coping resources on anxiety and peripheral narrowing. *J Appl Sport Psychol* 1991;3:126–141.

58. Nideffer RM. The injured athlete: psychological factors in treatment. *Orthop Clin North Am* 1983;14(2):373–385.
59. Hanson SJ, McCullagh P, Tonymon P. The relationship of personality characteristics, life stress, and coping resources to athletic injury. *J Sport Exerc Psychol* 1992;14:262–272.
60. Beecher HK. Pain in men wounded in battle. *Ann Surg* 1946;123(1):96–105.
61. Heil J. Understanding remarkable feats of acute pain tolerance. Poster presented at the 13th annual scientific meeting of the American Pain Society, Miami Beach, FL, 1994.
62. Heil J. Pain management: what price the gain? *Performance Edge* 1995;5(2):3–8
63. Dishman RK. Exercise adherence: its impact on public health. Champaign, IL: Human Kinetics, 1988.
64. Tricker R, Cook DL. *Athletes at risk: drugs and sports.* Dubuque, IA: Wm C Brown, 1990.
65. Corry JM, Cimbolic P. *Drugs: facts, alternatives, decisions.* Belmont, CA: Wadsworth, 1985:171.
66. Yesalis CE. *Anabolic steroids in sport and exercise.* Champaign, IL: Human Kinetics, 1993.
67. Wadler GI, Hainline B. *Drugs and the athlete.* Philadelphia: FA Davis Co, 1989.
68. Stainback, RD. *Alcohol and sport.* Champaign, IL: Human Kinetics, 1997.
69. Thompson RA, Sherman RT. *Helping athletes with eating disorders.* Champaign, IL: Human Kinetics, 1993:22.
70. Drinkwater BL, Nilson K, Chestnut CH, et al. Bone mineral context amenorrheic and eumenorrheic athletes. *N Engl J Med* 1984;311:277–281.
71. Marcus R, Cann C, Madvig P, et al. Menstrual function and bone mass in elite women distance runners. *Ann Intern Med* 1985;102:158–163.
72. Shangold M, Rebar RW, Wentz AC, Schiff I. Evaluation in management of menstrual dysfunction in athletes. *JAMA* 1990;263:1665–1669.
73. Thompson RA, Sherman RT. *Helping athletes with eating disorders.* Champaign, IL: Human Kinetics, 1993:145–146.
74. Kirschenbaum D. *Weight loss through persistence.* Oakland, CA: New Harbinger Publications, 1994.
75. Asken MJ. Sport psychology and the physically disabled athlete: interview with Michael D. Goodling, OTR/L. *Sport Psychol* 1989;3:166–176.
76. Depauw KP, Gavron SJ. *Disability and sport.* Champaign, IL: Human Kinetics, 1995.
77. Henschen KP Heil J. A retrospective study of the effect of an athlete's sudden death on teammates. *Omega* 1992;25(3):217–223.
78. Zernacchia RA, Reardon JP, Templin DP. Sudden death in sport: managing the aftermath. *Sport Psychol* 1997;11(2):223–235.
79. Heil J, Wakefield C, Reed C. Patient as athlete: A metaphor for injury rehabilitation. In: Hays K, ed. *Integrating exercise, sports, movement and mind: therapeutic unity.* New York: The Haworth Press, 1998:21–39.
80. Heil J. The psychology of sport injury: a review and critique. Paper presented at the International Society of Sport Psychology, IX World Congress of Sport Psychology meeting, Innovations in Sport Psychology: linking Theory and Practice, Israel. July 1997.

CHAPTER 14

Pain and Injury in Sport

Stephan R. Walk

If people were asked to list the professionals on the subject of human pain and injury who come to mind, it is quite likely and perhaps appropriate that most would number physicians first and sociologists last. While the sociology of medicine has made this fact less obvious (1–3), it is an objective of this chapter to both summarize and explicate the value of sociologic inquiry into what appear to be principally medical and radically individual concerns. The following will attempt to make this case by reviewing two developing areas of sociologic research into the pain and injury of athletes. Specifically, one area of inquiry centers on the relationship between the social structures of sport and the routine acceptance of pain and injury by athletes. The second area of research examines elements of athletic subcultures that both foster and reward athlete pain and injury. In general, sociologic study of pain and injury among athletes has involved a critical examination of the social structures and cultural elements of sport, particularly those that lead to compromised health and well-being.

This chapter will begin with an explication of the case for the sociologic study of pain and injury in sport. This will be followed by a summary of studies of sports organizations that have normalized not only risk taking, pain, and injury among athletes, but also the provision of medical care to athletes. Next, a summary of research that has examined the health-related attitudes, values, practices, and beliefs of athletes, coaches, and athletic trainers will be presented. The final section will offer suggestions for mitigating the force of the social and cultural elements of sport that perpetuate health compromises among athletes.

THE STUDY OF PAIN AND INJURY IN THE SOCIOLOGY OF SPORT

A fundamental premise of sociology is that human societies are phenomena that are qualitatively different from the sum of their individual members (4). Social groups and institutions are therefore studied by using theories that focus on their structures, patterns of interaction, and dominant cultural systems (5). Since a given social group will both constrain some behaviors and encourage others, sociologists focus critical attention on how prevailing norms, value systems, and common practices are established and maintained. Attention is then paid to how these elements of group culture influence its overall structure, that is, whether they lead to social change or work to maintain the existing order. In particular, sociologists are concerned with how dominant elements of culture are connected to social inequalities and social power.

A cursory examination of sport in the United States reveals that it possesses an elitist, hierarchical structure. Sport persists in being male-dominated in all areas, including participants (6,7), coaches and administrators (8), and athletic trainers (9). Mass participation in sport is reserved for children living in communities with sufficient resources, some children having very limited opportunities to experience a diversity of sports offerings (10). While the total number of sports participants among youth ages 5–17 is estimated at over 22 million (7), these numbers drop dramatically during early adolescence (11), leaving most as permanent nonparticipants. Successive levels of sport are accompanied by increases in the intensity of competition and ever-growing requirements of worklike dedication among athletes. Youths who continue their involvement confront a progressively narrowing structure of opportunities and have nearly a 100% chance of being cut from a sport. As Leonard (7) observed, of the 1.9 million participants in high school football, basketball, baseball, and ice hockey in 1994, just over 90,000 played their sport in

S. R. Walk: Division of Kinesiology and Health Promotion, California State University, Fullerton, California 92834-6870.

college, and only 3,155 of the latter advanced to the professional ranks.

These very basic structural and cultural characteristics of sport seldom appear as the context for discussions of athletic injury. In the majority of medical literature injury and pain are discussed as biomedical problems that transcend sociocultural issues (12). Occasionally, studies of sport injury discuss "psychosocial factors" as among other "risk factors" accounting for incidences of injury (13–17). As seen in the following quote from a recent book on sports injury epidemiology, however, the development of quantitative epidemiologic techniques suggests that such risk factors are increasingly being seen as background variables, in favor of direct causal "mechanisms" and "inciting events":

> An inciting event is more obviously (or visually) related to injury than a risk factor and may be viewed as a precipitating factor associated with the definitive onset of an injury. For example, the inciting event for an anterior shoulder dislocation in a football quarterback may be a tackle during a windup phase of a throwing maneuver, and the injury mechanism could be an abduction/external rotation force. The quarterback may have been predisposed to this injury by his history of previous shoulder dislocation (i.e., intrinsic risk factor) and an enabling factor such as wet field conditions, which resulted in the athlete slipping and being tackled (13).

While those who study the epidemiology of sports injuries would welcome the systematic collection of such information, most sociologists would find the above account lacking. Rather than conceptualizing injury and pain in terms of cases that are reducible to anatomies, personalities, and mechanisms, sociologic inquiry will tend to locate explanations for injury in the social context in which they take place. In the above example omitting a discussion of the sociocultural constitution of football, particularly the violent ethos that animates players, coaches, and spectators, makes it an incomplete account indeed. The fact that defensive players receive encouragement and rewards for delivering hard blows to quarterbacks, the fact that football helmets are often used as weapons (18), the fact that the quarterback in question may have been subtly or directly encouraged to hide injury and play in pain and/or with a previously existing injury and/or in conditions that increase the likelihood of injury, the fact that the player's institution may not provide adequate medical care or information, and the fact that the player may be risking permanent pain and disability are some of the items that sociologists attempt to place in the foreground in the study of injury in sport. Moreover, that these conditions of play are often taken for granted in football is precisely the reason they are of interest to sociologists of sport.

In general, sport has been the site of values, beliefs, and routine practices in which rewards are earned through socially approved violence, bodily sacrifice, and publicly displayed indifference to pain (19). Such behavior becomes the subject of keen sociologic attention when it becomes normalized among certain groups. Indeed, observations of athletes reveal how they become ever more immersed in the institution of sport, how they increasingly assume primarily athletic identities, and how they come to accept sport's value systems and core beliefs. Eventually, the routines and belief systems of sport are seen as commonsense ways of thinking and behaving, and deviance from them may invite ridicule (20). For example, athletes, coaches, and spectators often belittle athletes who are seen as unwilling to play aggressively. Nevertheless, while the violent and painful characteristics of sport often seem inevitable or natural, closer examination reveals that they are ultimately rooted in human collective decisions that could be otherwise.

Unlike the risk factors that are identified in epidemiologies, the deeply rooted beliefs and practices in sport can, at best, be understood only partially by reducing them to quantitative variables. As will be seen below, surveys are effective at identifying general attitudes, but they tend to miss crucial elements of pain and injury as they take on meaning to athletes. Furthermore, since norms, value systems, and practices in sport are socially constructed, that is, learned through language and other processes of social interaction (21), the study of sports language and the employment of ethnographic techniques have become standard tools for their analysis. The most commonly used ethnographic techniques include interviews and/or participant observations, which involve extensive immersion of the researcher in the routines and practices of sport organizations. These methods allow the researcher to understand how athletes and others involved in sport attach meaning to their own actions and the actions of others.

Indeed, the study of pain turns out to be an excellent illustration of the usefulness of such techniques. In what is perhaps the classic study demonstrating how pain is a product of social and cultural constructions, Zborowski (22) found that the ways in which people experienced and expressed pain in a veterans' hospital varied along ethnic and cultural lines. In general, he found that people learn how to interpret their own pain and express it to others by virtue of the values and beliefs specific to their cultures. As subsequent social analysts have revealed (12), both the experience and expression of pain are imbued with meanings that are embedded in deeply held belief systems that are resistant to change. People learn that pain may be expressed to some audiences and not others and that responses of others to expressions of pain will vary considerably.

Just as the behavior of athletes becomes normalized through memberships within athletic subcultures, we may expect that the delivery of institutionalized medical services to athletes has also become routinized. Research has shown, for example, that the orientation of medical professionals to patients may differ for reasons related to the stereotypes they hold of patients, as well as to the difficulties encountered in managing their complaints (23,24). Zborowski's *People in Pain* discovered that physicians and other medical staff found members of certain ethnic and cultural groups (i.e., ones similar to their own) preferable to others, resulting in differences in decisions about medication and other treatments. As Encandela (12) suggested, it is important to study how pain is conceptualized and responded to by institutionalized medicine, focusing in particular on routines and categories of pain sufferers. Hence, identifying the operative pain- and injury-related beliefs and practices that prevail among sports medicine personnel is also of interest to sociologists of sport. This is particularly important because pain is routine in sport, pain is perhaps the quintessential subjective experience (25), and pain reports must first be believed to be assessed and treated.

Accordingly, the following will center on two mutually reinforcing topics of study in the sociology of sport: the social structures and interaction patterns in sport organizations and their relationship to pain and injury and the values, beliefs, attitudes, and practices of members of sport organizations that are brought to bear on issues of risk-taking, pain, and injury among athletes.

PAIN AND INJURY AND THE SOCIAL STRUCTURES OF SPORT

Most of the pain and injury research in the sociology of sport has attempted to explain the social structural and cultural factors that are at work in the acceptance of sport injury by athletes. With a few exceptions this research has been conducted within the past ten years, has focused primarily on intercollegiate sport, and therefore must be seen as parts of a growing body of literature. This section will summarize theoretical and limited empirical work that examines whether the process of accepting sport injury and pain as natural is related to the structural characteristics of elite sports organizations. Moreover, it asks whether athletes are encouraged by their sports organizations to conceptualize their injuries and pain in ways that lead them to minimize their implications and serve organizational interests.

One of the earliest studies to address these questions was conducted by Kotarba (26) in his book *Chronic Pain: Its Social Dimensions*. He interviewed current and former professional athletes about their pain and injuries and made several interesting discoveries. First, he found that professional athletes followed the principle "Play with pain, talk injury," which suggested that athletes were to accept pain as part of sport and talk about injury only to carefully selected audiences to ensure the security of their jobs. Second, Kotarba found that athletes formed exclusive athletic subcultures, partially founded on the need to keep their injuries and pain secret from coaches, management, the media, and spectators. Third, he found that the athletes who felt the greatest need to hide injuries were those whose status in the organization was marginal. Finally, while visibly serious injuries (e.g., broken bones) did not require secrecy, athletes felt the need to conceal less obviously serious yet painful injuries, such as muscle pulls, even though they probably should have resulted in discontinuing play. Although athletic trainers often agreed to surreptitiously help such athletes with their injuries, the medical facilities that they used were often too visible for athletes to risk being discovered. Athletes therefore pursued outside, sometimes questionable, medical services and information via networks of fellow athletes.

Kotarba's analysis revealed some of the organizational structures that form in and around the pain and injury of professional athletes. First, professional athletic organizations emphasize productivity and performance and most often employ athletes for less than 4 years. Reflective of the hierarchic structure of sport, most athletes within such organizations are highly transitory. Players realize the odds they have beaten to earn their positions and thereby believe that subordinating their health and well-being is worth the chance for what is often a short and sometimes lucrative career. Implicit in these attitudes is that to move up in sport hierarchies, one should be increasingly willing to sacrifice the body. Although intuitively, it would seem logical for teams to attempt to maintain athlete health, injury within professional sport only obviates the eminent replaceability of athletes. As a result, athletes tend to form closed societies that essentially insulate them from proper medical care and information and/or compromise the quality of the medical consultations they receive.

Following on Kotarba, Nixon (27) modified a more general area of social theory termed "social network analysis" for the study of what he termed "sportsnets" (i.e., sports networks), a name that he used to describe large athletic organizations such as those in colleges and universities. Nixon theorized that the structural characteristics of sportsnets make athletes vulnerable to messages that encourage them to play with pain or injuries. His network analysis was intended to identify relations among individuals, roles, and organizational units within sportsnets, focusing particular attention on the nature of these relationships. Specifically, Nixon argued that, since their primary function is the production of winning teams, sportsnets continually work to minimize uncertainties in the pursuit of their objectives. Injuries to key players often generate such uncertainties. A standard medical response to an injury always threatens to counsel the discontinuation of play and is therefore among a number of destabilizing factors. As a result, the sportsnet may work to insulate its members from more conservative medical decisions that might be made in other contexts.

Nixon believed the sportsnet structure to be essentially conspiratorial in that it is characterized by a set of working ideologies in which risk, pain, and injury are made to seem normal and natural. These ideas dominate what is presented to athletes as a support system, which includes other athletes, coaches, administrators, athletic trainers, and physicians, all of whom have simply normalized the treatment of injuries and pain. Athletes are thus oriented to returning to participation as soon as possible, rather than to restoring their overall health, since that is the primary orientation of those surrounding them. More generally, according to Nixon, members of sportsnets share the same beliefs and tend to discredit or insulate themselves from those who would question these beliefs. Moreover, since athletes know the consequences of injury within the sportsnet, in particular its bearing on playing time, status on the team, and athletic identity, they are encouraged to hide injuries from influential and connected members of the sportsnet and thereby risk health and well-being.

On the basis of his observations about social relationships and information in sportsnets, Nixon conducted a study on the interactions of college student athletes with others in their sportsnets, including coaches, teammates, and athletic trainers (28). He found little support for the notion that these others within the sportsnet act in collusive ways to subvert athlete help seeking with respect to their injuries. Instead, he found that the receptivity of athletic trainers to the health problems of athletes played a key role in whether they decided to hide their injuries and pain. Indeed, other studies in the athletic training literature have found that the receptivity of athletic trainers plays an important role in maintaining their contact with health care personnel (29–31).

A study by Walk (32) based on interviews with student athletic trainers (SATs) at a large NCAA Division I institution found similar results. He discovered that, among health care personnel in intercollegiate sport, interning SATs were used frequently and were in many cases on the front lines in delivering medical services in intercollegiate sports programs. SATs spent considerable amounts of time in exclusive interactions with athletes—indeed more than other members of sportsnets—and functioned as essentially underpaid or unpaid labor for their institutions. Moreover, these students witnessed the comprehensive scope of activities related to intercollegiate sport, including practices, competitions, and team travel, in addition to their performance of health care services. For these and other reasons, SATs had conflicting alliances in their work—namely, alliances with their supervising medical staffs and alliances with their peer students (athletes and student athletic trainers). While student trainers wished to obtain professional credentials as health care workers, they also maintained social relationships of various sorts with athletes. Walk concluded that this web of relationships alone, in addition to the myriad others that characterize intercollegiate athletic programs, lent itself to a diversity of attitudes, beliefs, and practices that had a bearing on athlete health and well-being. Walk concluded that, although Nixon's social network analysis may provide a good theoretical starting point, the machinations of large athletic programs are not very well captured in the notion of a conspiratorial alliance dominated by a universally endorsed ideology.

Unfortunately, few additional studies have been conducted that have been able to test the usefulness of Nixon's sportsnet model. There is, moreover, some disagreement in the literature as to the most appropriate way to theorize the activities within sportsnets in light of both theoretical and empirical considerations (32–34). While we do not yet fully understand the complex social contexts of athlete-health behaviors, particularly across very different institutions, it seems clear that structural factors have a bearing on unnecessary athlete pain and injury. This is particularly the case if these factors work to discourage athletes from seeking help and insulate them from receiving proper medical attention and information. Future research must target these issues and study them across a number of different settings.

HEALTH-RELATED VALUES, ATTITUDES, AND BELIEFS IN SPORT

It is manifestly obvious to most athletes early in their careers that injuries are common in sports, especially at elite levels. What must an athlete come to believe about the goals of sport, the limits of their own bodies, and the role of health care services, in the course of routinely accepting injuries and playing in pain? How do others within the sport context go about normalizing the risks and witnessing various forms of suffering? Moreover, in what ways does the context of elite-level sport influence the delivery of medical services? Answers to these questions lie in the cultural elements that are part of the socialization of athletes, including value systems, norms of behavior, and personal beliefs. The following will summarize inquiry into the basic ethical values of sport, surveys on pain and injury attitudes of athletes and coaches, and interview-based studies of both athletes and student athletic trainers.

Athletes and the Sport Ethic

Hughes and Coakley (35) observed that sport is dominated by a central set of ethical principles that define what it means to be a "real athlete." In the course of discussing attention paid to "deviant athletes," they contended that a number of the problems in sport relate not to underconforming to sport's ethical principles, but rather to overconforming to them. That is, too often athletes are overcommitted to their achievement in sport and are willing to exhaust almost everything in the pursuit of their goals. The first ethical principle identified by Hughes and Coakley states that being an athlete "involves making sacrifices for the game," which means that athletes are to subordinate their own interests to those of their teams, sponsoring institutions, and sport. The second principle states that being an athlete "involves striving for distinction," suggesting that "[t]rue athletes seek to improve, to get better, to come closer to perfection." Hughes and Coakley observed, in this regard, that much of sports science is devoted to enhancing performance, rather than to enhancing the athlete's overall welfare, and thereby contributes to the search for perfection. Reflective of the dominant themes identified by Kotarba and Nixon, the third principle states that "being an athlete involves accepting risks and playing through pain." This applies both to extreme physical and psychological forms of stress and pain, the overcoming of which testifies to the athlete's "moral courage." Finally, Hughes and Coakley observed that athletes are to refuse "to accept limits in the pursuit of possibilities," and indeed athletes who do not accept this view are often ostracized or given "corrective" advice.

To what extent do those in the sport culture accept and promote these ethical principles with respect to pain and injury? A study by Nixon attempted to assess the extent to which injury- and pain-legitimizing ideas have become part of popular discourse in sport (36). He undertook a content analysis of 22 years of *Sports Illustrated* magazine to identify how issues of pain, injury, disability, and rehabilitation were referred to and discussed by athletes, journalists, doctors, athletic trainers, coaches, retired athletes, management, and others. Reminiscent of Kotarba's research, Nixon found that the majority of comments on health issues were connected to the security of athlete jobs, organizational rationalizations about the inevitability and necessity of injury, the expectations and values of key socializing agents within sport, and the explicit acceptance of the necessity of pain and injuries as part of sport participation.

Since he found that most of the injury-related comments in *Sports Illustrated* came from either athletes or journalists, Nixon noted the thematic differences between these two groups. While journalists tended to rationalize injuries and pain with reference to organizational demands, athletes tended to connect these elements of sport to their sense of character and masculinity and cited their trust in medical personnel to provide them with sound advice. Overall, these key figures in popular sport culture indicated that the rewards of advancement to elite ranks in sport are partly an exchange for the acceptance of risk, pain, and injury. Nixon concluded that, although athletes provide rational explanations for health-jeopardizing actions, a "culture of risk" pervades popular discourse about sport, a culture that seldom provides support for, and often criticizes, athletes who choose health over continued participation.

Surveys of Coaches, Students, and Student Athletes

Nixon's identification of an injury- and pain-accepting popular sports culture set the stage for a series of surveys of athletes and coaches. First, Nixon used six themes he identified in *Sports Illustrated* to construct a questionnaire on the pain and injury beliefs of coaches (37). He found that male and female coaches of both male and female athletes possess paradoxical views about the risk, pain, and injury of athletes. Specifically, while coaches agreed with several injury-legitimizing ideologies (e.g., "No pain, no gain"), they also stated that they sympathized and were concerned about the welfare of athletes. While Nixon recommended caution in generalizing from his results, as it reflected the views of the coaches at a single university, he suggested that a number of sportsnet members may express views in public that do not conform to their actual behavior and practices with athletes. Overall, Nixon pointed to a "risk-pain-injury paradox," in which athletes are driven to their limits by those who also genuinely care about them and who want them to avoid risks.

Nixon has also conducted surveys of college student-athletes focusing on the degree to which they have experienced and normalized pain and injury. The first study focused on how well sports pain and injury attitudes are explained by gender, race, and variables related to the athlete's status on the team (38). While he found very modest support for his race and sports status hypotheses, his most notable finding was a more frequent experience with, and higher normative acceptance of, injuries among male versus female athletes. However, he also found evidence to suggest that the *female* athletes in the study had experienced as many injuries as their male counterparts, though male athletes tended to have more serious injuries that involved surgery and long-term disability. Of some note was the fact that nearly 70% of the athletes in the study had been seriously injured, almost all of them reported playing while hurt, nearly half said that they received pressure from coaches to play while hurt, and over 40% reported being pressured by athletic trainers to play while hurt.

In a second study, Nixon surveyed both college students from introductory sociology classes and student athletes about the levels of pain that would lead them to seek medical care (expressed pain thresholds) both in daily life and in sport (39). Among the athletes in the study, Nixon found a picture that was similar to the one in his previous study with respect to the high numbers of athletes who had sustained serious injuries and who played while hurt. However, he did not find differences between men and women, whether athletes or nonathletes, on expressed pain thresholds. He did, however, find a relationship between higher pain threshold levels among college students who were involved in friendship networks with male athletes. This was true of both men and women, suggesting that males tend to have tolerant orientations to pain.

Again, a set of general patterns has emerged in terms of the sources of pressure for athletes to play with pain and injury. Specifically, a number of members of the sport culture have adopted and continually reinforce a sport ethic in which pain and injury are essential elements of elite sports participation. Coaches and athletes, however ambivalently, may tend to reflect these more general principles, and an injurious and painful atmosphere may prevail among male athletes or among those who develop their pain and injury beliefs among male athletes.

Interview and Ethnographic Research on Pain and Injury in Sport

As was mentioned earlier, while survey research is useful in identifying general patterns of attitudes and beliefs, interview and ethnographic studies are useful in identifying how people make their behavior meaningful. Since the survey research summarized above linked the acceptance of pain and injury to male athletes, a brief examination of the historical origins of the association between pain and injury and masculinity might be a useful pretext for the interview and ethnographic research discussed below.

Conceptions of the human body that developed in late 19th and early 20th century biology and medical practices associated frailty, irrationality, and vulnerability with girls and women and strength, rationality, and protective roles with boys and men. Additionally, rapid industrial development significantly diminished the importance of manual labor and left few outlets for the display of male physicality. Educators and others saw school-based sport and physical education as essential sites for the preservation and development of masculinity, in that they both emphasized the strength of men and worked to prevent weakness and effeminacy (40). Moreover, early modern sport in the United States identified masculinity with bodily objectification, stoicism in the face of pain, and sacrifice in the service of manliness (40,41). Studies of the role of sport in the development and maintenance of gender identity have consistently found an instrumentalist conception of the body in the socialization of male athletes (41,42). In other words, the body is seen as a weapon in male athletic subcultures, particularly those in violent sports.

Among the first studies in the sociology of sport to specifically relate masculinity with pain and injury was a case study conducted by Curry (43). He looked at the process by which a collegiate wrestler normalized injury in the process of being socialized into his athlete role. Over the course of three in-depth interviews, Curry was able to identify the key life events and significant people to which the wrestler pointed in the development of his identity. His early, or primary, socialization was characterized by the fulfillment of what Curry called "masculinity needs" and involved strong athletic expectations and direct teaching of sports values by his father. His father taught him that injuries were routine, insignificant, an indicator of being tough, and part of the important distinction between masculinity and femininity. Additionally, during childhood, his injuries presented opportunities to receive special attention as an athlete. During the secondary socialization period, that is, with age and a developing history of sports injury, the athlete gained a sense of accomplishment by being presented with, and overcoming, a series of increasingly more serious injuries. Curry called this a "professionalization" period, in which the athlete identified himself completely with his athlete role, sacrificed his health to remain functional, and played through injury. Finally, as his career approached its end, the athlete was confronted with ever more risky competitions and felt pressure to simply ignore his injuries.

In a study of 16 male athletes, Young, White, and McTeer found similar themes (44). The former rugby and football players in the study were asked about their experiences with injury and described their earliest memories of athletic injury, the effects of sport on their overall health, their self concepts, and their relationships with others in sport. Because all of the athletes had suffered serious injuries that resulted in long-term disabilities and chronic pain, the researchers asked specific questions about these experiences. Similar to the athlete in Curry's study, they found that all of the athletes connected their early attractions to sport to their relationships with their fathers. Moreover, they found that the athletes attached particular importance to the opportunities they had to express dominance through masculinity displays. One was considered masculine to the degree that one was willing to experience pain, play while injured, or inflict pain on others. However, while pain was a validation of masculinity, succumbing to injury was not. Athletes attempted to hide pain; found it unwelcomed by teammates, coaches, and others; and distanced themselves from injuries by describing them in depersonalized ways (e.g., by referring to injured parts rather than to the self as a whole). Overall, the researchers found the athletes to be generally unreflective about their injuries and pain, suggesting an uncritical acceptance of this aspect of their sports experiences.

Much of the literature in the area of pain and injury has involved study and analysis of male sport subcultures, particularly those attached to violent sports characterized by high rates of injury and aggression (19).

Maintaining one's status within these subcultures has required that one be clearly seen on the masculine side of a set of masculine/feminine dualisms that include being "active" rather than "passive," "hard" rather than "soft," and "strong" rather than "weak" (45). However, there are indications that these dualisms are beginning to break down. Although female athletes have been shown to be less likely to engage in behaviors that might harm others (46), there is mounting evidence that they are increasingly accepting the pain- and injury-legitimating ethos of masculine sport.

Young and White interviewed female former athletes who had suffered serious injuries in sport and who had long-term pain and disabilities (47). Given their previous study of male athletes, they found a number of similarities in the ways in which the women discussed their pain and injuries. Specifically, the women were influenced early by male role models, were quite willing to expose themselves to risk and reinjury, and attempted to distance themselves from their injuries in their language and other behaviors. Young and White concluded that, although they differed in the degree to which they embraced masculine ideologies, the men and women coped with their pain in similar ways. Moreover, like men, women adopted these coping strategies for their pain and injury to demonstrate their courage and character, to cement ties with teammates, to earn playing time, and to cope with the demands of their sports.

Hence, while the tendency to accept pain and injury may be rooted in the values and practices of male athletic subcultures, there is some evidence to suggest that women's athletic subcultures are emulating those of men. Disturbingly, it appears that few athletes are encouraged to question their sport-related health problems either during or after the end of their careers. Further examinations of the early socialization practices of both male and female athletes, particularly the activities of male role models, might be particularly useful in showing how these attitudes develop. Additionally, a further look into the sources of ambivalence among athletes about injuries and pain might be undertaken to examine whether athletes possess accurate information on the long-term consequences of their injuries. Perhaps most significantly, it might be expected that what is often called the male model of sport will continue to be followed by the growing numbers of programs of girl's and women's sport.

Studies of Athletic Trainers in Sport

In his book on chronic pain, Kotarba found athletic trainers functioning as bridges among athletes, coaches, physicians, administrators, and others, suggesting that health care professionals in sport often find themselves in mediating roles (26). He noted that athletic trainers seemed committed to resisting the interests of coaches and others by not allowing athletes to play with what they believed were medically prohibitive injuries. While Kotarba found that athletes often concealed serious injuries from athletic trainers, he also found that the athletic trainers tended to like to work with athletes who did not frequently complain about pain and injury, given their extremely busy schedules. Indeed, the trainers made distinctions between athletes they referred to as "gamers" versus "nongamers." Gamers were athletes who were tolerant of injury, who seldom complained about pain, and who evidenced a strong commitment to achievement within their sports. "Nongamers," on the other hand, constantly complained and frequently sought the trainer's services.

Such findings are troubling, in that they suggest that athletic trainers and other sports medicine personnel may stereotype athletes and potentially ignore serious injuries and pain. Moreover, it suggests that medical staffs may normalize high pain tolerance levels and permit medically inadvisable risk taking among athletes as a result of their immersion in the athletic subculture. Walk's study of student athletic trainers in an intercollegiate athletic program (32) found attitudes and behavior similar to those in Kotarba's work but also noted that the provision of medical care in a large athletic organization was a vast and complicated enterprise.

First, student athletic trainers in Walk's study reported a wide range of athlete behaviors with respect to health and to the use of medical services, ranging from those who were quite knowledgeable, health-conscious, and competent users of athletic training facilities to others who apparently knew little about the functioning of their own bodies, displayed comprehensively unhealthy lifestyles, and were variously uncompliant with the school's medical professionals. SATs also described how they, along with their professional supervisors, identified "head cases," a term for athletes who were alleged to be faking injuries. Indeed, they noted a pattern in which competitive losses, poor individual performances, and difficult practices were consistently related to high numbers of reported, and allegedly faked, injuries. Even though the SATs accommodated them, such "head cases," and those similar to Kotarba's "nongamers," presented substantial difficulties to the medical staff's attempts to provide athletic training services to large numbers of athletes.

SATs in Walk's study also reported that they were concerned and frustrated by athletes who persisted in playing with injuries and pain after being informed of their risks of long-term disability. This was especially true of athletes with chronic injuries (e.g., *female* gymnasts and swimmers), since their injuries required rest to which the athletes would not agree. Instead, such athletes were constant fixtures in the training room and continually complained about pain. The apparent result of these circumstances was that these athletes' complaints were normalized by the medical staff to such a degree that new and serious medical problems were occasionally overlooked. In other words, the staff could not differentiate a pain report that related to a new, serious condition against the backdrop of routine pain reports among these athletes. This latter problem may illustrate evidence of a kind of social inflation of pain tolerance levels among athletes on a team and their normalization among medical staff. Moreover, if the athletes are women stereotyped as "head cases," their more socially acceptable expressions of emotion may have more serious consequences for them than for male athletes.

The study of the experiences and beliefs of sports medicine personnel is obviously in its infancy, and there are many questions to be answered. Although there is ample evidence to support the contention that athletes participate in social structures and cultural systems that foster the acceptance of risk taking, pain, and injury, the role of physicians and other allied health care workers in these processes is unclear. As with the study of the structures of sports organizations, new studies must focus not only on the practices and beliefs in institutionalized sports medicine, but also on the nature of the relationships among health care personnel and athletes. Moreover, research must focus on the relative amounts of power over decision making among all those involved in athlete health care, including coaches, athletic trainers, physicians, parents, and, alas, the athletes themselves.

RECOMMENDATIONS

While sociologists have accused physicians and others of overmedicalizing health issues, sociologists may be accused of oversocializing them. Indeed, it might be observed that, much like public roadways, sports are simply places where accidents happen. Furthermore, it might be added that, while sport may be injurious, painful, sometimes violent, and often exploitative of athletes, it shares these features with other elements of society, such as high-risk, high-stress occupations. However, acknowledging these facts does not eliminate the clearly preventable and changeable aspects of sport that result in athlete health compromises.

Indeed, there is some evidence of increasing popular concern with these issues. The *Kansas City Star,* in an October 1997 critique of the NCAA, suggested that health care services for college athletes are, at best, inconsistent across institutions and, at worst, woefully inadequate (48). In making this case, the *Star* pointed to incidents of athlete deaths and long-term disabilities they alleged could have been prevented. The *Star's* investigation concluded that there is a lack of a consistent policy for medical safeguards across NCAA institutions, a lack of basic medical training among coaches, and insufficient resources for the acquisition of medical supplies and equipment and the hiring of certified athletic trainers. They suggested the NCAA institute a requirement for a specific ratio of certified athletic trainers to athletes, require coaches to undergo CPR training, and include a review of health care services as part of NCAA institutional certification processes.

While these policies might be good starting places, they will only marginally change the elements that have been identified in the literature summarized in this chapter. On the basis of the studies reviewed herein, five recommendations might be made. First, the link between the hierarchic structure of sport and health-compromising behaviors seems clear, particularly in terms of the limited opportunities and brief careers of athletes. While these hierarchies exist in commercialized, professional sports, over which little social control may be exercised, they are also seen in youth sports programs and at publicly funded high schools and universities. Since only 5% of high school athletes and fewer than 1% of college athletes will advance to higher levels in their sports (7), the purposes of these programs must more explicitly identify health and well-being among their objectives. Should these programs continue to pursue high-intensity, competitive objectives, they must become more reflective about and accountable for their definitions of courage and discipline. For example, despite protestations based on traditional ideas about masculinity, athletes should never receive support from coaches for inflicting injuries on other players. Likewise, instead of rewarding athletes for their sacrifices in returning to play before they are healthy, institutions might commend athletes for the commitment needed to complete a successful rehabilitation, perhaps even rewarding an athlete for prudently discontinuing his or her participation. Since both bodily sacrifice and disciplined rehabilitation have educational values, the healthier option should be emphasized.

Second, it is insufficient to simply prepare coaches to administer first aid or CPR, that is, to react to athlete health problems. Coaches must, in addition, be prepared to act with other sports medicine professionals in promoting athlete health. This includes not only the use of sound practice drills, techniques, and conditioning programs, but also dietary guidelines and lifestyle habits that can be sustained throughout a lifetime. Furthermore, coaches must be rewarded by their institutions not only for competitive achievements in their sports but also for maintaining the health and well-being of their athletes. Seldom do high school, college, or university sports programs qualify their championships by listing the team's injury rates. In general, these efforts must be communicated not only to coaches, but also to a number of key figures throughout sport. These points are especially important for coaches and parents who are involved in youth programs, given the research identifying the importance of early socialization of athletes.

Third, influential figures in sports medicine and elsewhere must be less willing to simply treat health problems and be more willing to publicly critique the values and practices in sport that equate serious health compromises with achievement. Such critiques imply the redefinition of sport-related masculinity and athletic identity. The near-universal glorification of the acts of sacrifice by athletes, such as those of Kerri Strug in the 1996 Olympic Gymnastics Finals, suggests that such critiques will meet with social resistance. Nevertheless, the numbers of athletes who are willing to emulate health-compromising behavior appears to be growing, particularly among female athletes participating in sports modeled on the values and practices of men's programs. Moreover, the research agendas and technologies of sports science must increasingly be scrutinized to the extent that they are uncritically geared to producing to ever-greater performance goals in athletes (34), rather than contributing to the well-being of athletes. These critiques might also target such issues as the length of competitive seasons, the special problems of overuse injuries, dietary and weight control disorders, psychological problems among athletes, and the untested claims of producers of athletic equipment and dietary supplements.

Fourth, the roles of athletic trainers in sports programs appear to be critical in the establishment and maintenance of athlete help seeking that will ensure the timely identification and treatment of injuries. Given the continuing and perhaps intensifying social support of highly competitive athletic programs, it appears that athletic trainers must be stalwart in their efforts to avoid being co-opted by the competitive agendas of sports organizations, to maintain open information channels with athletes, and to continually earn their trust. This includes avoiding the tendency to stereotype athletes as malingerers or to demonstrate preferences for those identified as "gamers." It also includes an awareness of the potential to underestimate health problems by normalizing high pain tolerance levels among athletes. Crucially, institutions must also demonstrate their commitment to athlete health and well-being by supplying athletic training staffs with salaries and resources commensurate with the importance of their positions. Furthermore, it appears that many college and university athletic programs are using student athletic trainers to deliver a substantial portion of their on-site medical care. Student athletic trainers in these positions must also be given ample institutional support to both successfully complete their educational programs and do their clinical rotations well.

Finally, athletes and those responsible for them must receive factual information about the risks and benefits of participation in their sports. This includes not only epidemiologic information but also facts about their chances of advancing to higher levels in their sports. Moreover, athletes must believe that the organizations for which they compete are genuinely interested in their health and well-being. They must also perceive that the medical treatment they receive is not tainted by the competitive interests of their institutions. Athletes who receive subtle or direct messages that indicate that they are expected to play with prohibitive injuries should have clear channels to report and redress these problems. More generally, athletes should be informed participants in sports programs as well as competent users of sports medical services in their institutions.

REFERENCES

1. Cockerman WC. *Medical sociology,* 2nd ed. Englewood Cliffs, NJ: Prentice Hall, 1982.
2. Brown P, ed. *Perspectives in medical sociology.* Belmont, CA: Wadsworth, 1989.
3. Lorber J. *Gender and the social construction of illness.* Thousand Oaks, CA: Sage, 1997.
4. Bourdieu P, Wacquant JD. *An invitation to reflexive sociology.* Chicago: University of Chicago Press, 1992:7–11.
5. Harris J. Suited up and stripped down: perspectives for sociocultural sports studies. *Soc Sport J* 1989;6:335–347.
6. Seefeldt VD, Ewing ME. Youth sports in America: an overview. *Research Digest: President's Council on Physical Fitness and Sports* 1997;2:11.
7. Leonard WM. The odds of transitioning from one level of sports participation to another. *Soc Sport J* 1996;13:288–299.
8. Women's Sport Foundation. Women's sports facts. 1998; March 10: http://www.lifetimetv.com/WoSport/stage/RESLIB/html/women_sfitnessfacts.html
9. Arnold BL, Van Lunen BL, Gansneder BM, et al. 1994 athletic trainer employment and salary characteristics. *J Athl Training* 1996;31(3):215–218.
10. Seefeldt, V. Recreating recreation and sports in Detroit, Hamtramck, and Highland Park: final report to the Skillman Foundation. Detroit: The Skillman Foundation, 1995.
11. Seefeldt V, Ewing ME, Walk S. An overview of youth sports programs in the United States. Paper commissioned by the Carnegie Council on Adolescent Development. New York: Carnegie Corporation of New York, 1995.
12. Encandela JA. Social science and the study of pain since Zborowski: a need for a new agenda. *Soc Sci Med* 1993;36,6:783–791.
13. Caine GC, Caine DJ, Lindner KJ. The epidemiologic approach to sports injuries. In: Caine GC, Caine DJ, Lindner KJ, eds. *Epidemiology of sports injuries.* Champaign, IL: Human Kinetics, 1996:1–13.
14. Bramwell ST, Masuda M, Wagner NN, Holmes TH. Psychosocial factors in athletic injuries: development of the Social and Athletic Readjustment Rating Scale (SARRS). *J Hum Stress* 1975; June:6–20.
15. Taerk GS. The injury-prone athlete: a psycho-social approach. *J Sports Med* 1977;17:187–194.
16. Cryan PD, Alles WF. The relationship between stress and college football injuries. *J Sports Med* 1983;23:52–58.
17. Bond JW, Miller BP, Chrisfield PM. Psychological prediction of injury in elite swimmers. *Int J Sports Med* 1988;9:345–348.
18. Gelberg JN. The lethal weapon: how the plastic football helmet changed the game of football, 1939–1994. *Bull Sci Tech Soc* 1995;15(5–6):302–309.
19. Messner M. When bodies are weapons: masculinity and violence in sport. *Int Rev Soc Sport* 1990;25:203–218.
20. Donnelly P, Young K. The construction and confirmation of identity in sport subcultures. *Soc Sport J* 1988;5:223–240.
21. MacAloon J. An observer's view of sport sociology. *Soc Sport J* 1987;4:103–115.

22. Zborowski M. *People in pain*. San Francisco: Jossey-Bass, 1969.
23. Goffman E. *Asylums: essays on the social situation of mental patients and other inmates*. Garden City, NY: Doubleday, 1961.
24. McKinlay JB, Potter DA, Feldman HA. Non-medical influences on medical decision-making. *Soc Sci Med* 1996;42:769–776.
25. Scarry E. *The body in pain*. New York: Oxford University Press, 1985.
26. Kotarba JA. *Chronic pain: its social dimensions*. Beverly Hills, CA: Sage, 1983.
27. Nixon HL II. A social network analysis of influences on athletes to play with pain and injuries. *J Sport Soc Issues* 1992;10:127–135.
28. Nixon HL II. Social pressure, social support, and help seeking for pain and injuries in college sports networks. *J Sport Soc Issues* 1994;18:340–355.
29. Fisher AC, Mullins SA, Frye PA. Athletic trainers' attitudes and judgments of injured athletes' rehabilitation adherence. *J Athl Training* 1993;28,1:43–47.
30. Fisher AC, Hoisington LL. Injured athletes' attitudes and judgments toward rehabilitation adherence. *J Athl Training* 1993;28, 1:48–54.
31. Fisher AC, Scriber KC, Matheny ML, Alderman MH, Bitting LA. Enhancing athletic injury rehabilitation adherence. *J Athl Training* 1993;28,4:312–318.
32. Walk SR. Peers in pain: the experiences of student athletic trainers. *Soc Sport J* 1997;14:22–56.
33. Roderick M. The sociology of risk, pain, and injury: a comment on the work of Howard L. Nixon, II. *Soc Sport J* 1998;15:64–79.
34. Nixon HL II. Response to Martin Roderick's comment on the work of Howard L. Nixon, II. *Soc Sport J* 1998;15:80–85.
35. Hughes R, Coakley J. Positive deviance among athletes: the implications of overconformity to the sport ethic. *Soc Sport J* 1991; 8:307–325.
36. Nixon HL II. Accepting the risks and pain of injury in sport: mediated cultural influences on playing hurt. *Soc Sport J* 1993;10:183–196.
37. Nixon HL II. Coaches' views of risk, pain, and injury in sport, with special reference to gender differences. *Soc Sport J* 1994;11:79–87.
38. Nixon HL II. Explaining pain and injury attitudes and experiences in sport in terms of gender, race, and sports status factors. *J Sport Soc Issues* 1996;20:33–44.
39. Nixon HL II. The relationship of friendship networks, sports experiences, and gender to expressed pain thresholds. *Soc Sport J* 1996;13,78–86.
40. Crosset T. Masculinity, sexuality, and the development of early modern sport. In: Messner M, Sabo D, eds. *Sport, men and the gender order*. Champaign, IL: Human Kinetics, 1990:45–54.
41. Sabo D, Panepinto J. Football ritual and the social reproduction of masculinity. In: Messner M, Sabo D, eds. *Sport, men and the gender order*. Champaign, IL: Human Kinetics, 1990:115–126.
42. Messner MA. *Power at play: sports and the problem of masculinity*. Boston: Beacon Press, 1992.
43. Curry TJ. A little pain never hurt anyone: athletic career socialization and the normalization of sports injury. *Symbolic Interaction* 1993;16(3):273–290.
44. Young K, White P, McTeer W. Body talk: male athletes reflect on sport, injury, and pain. *Soc Sport J* 1994;11:175–194.
45. Bryson L. Challenges to male hegemony in sport. In: Messner M, Sabo D, eds. *Sport, men and the gender order*. Champaign, IL: Human Kinetics, 1990:173–184.
46. Nixon HL II. Gender, sport, and aggressive behavior outside of sport. *J Sport Soc Issues* 1997;21,4:379–391.
47. Young K, White P. Sport, physical danger, and injury: the experiences of elite women athletes. *J Sport Soc Issues* 1995;19(1):45–61.
48. Money games: inside the NCAA. Part 4: Dying young. *Kansas City Star*. 1997 Oct 8: http://www.kcstar.com/ncaa/part4.html.

CHAPTER 15

Gender: Its Relevance to Sports Medicine

Cynthia A. Hasbrook

INTRODUCTION

The purpose of this chapter is to provide a sociologic analysis of how gender is bound up in patterns of human physical activity and inactivity and is subsequently associated with health and health-related outcomes of activity and inactivity. More specifically, we will identify and explore how the gendered nature of physical activity excludes some individuals from participation, discourages and eventually eliminates others who had participated, and circumscribes, in ways that can negatively affect health, the nature of involvement for those who continue to participate. We begin by defining gender relative to physical activity.

DEFINING GENDER

Gender has been conceptualized as a thing; a possession of the individual; a binary, dichotomous, categorical variable that can assume one of two values (male or female, masculine or feminine) (1,2). On the basis of such a definition, gender has often been conceptualized and researched as difference: difference between males and females, girls and boys, men and women; difference on any number of variables from levels of sport participation, to physiologic capacities for exercise, to physical skill acquisition and execution.

Gender has also been defined as a social structural factor and a basis for social inequality in sport. When gender is conceptualized in this manner, the focus has often been limited to girls' and women's lack of sport-related opportunities, rewards, and authority and how to achieve equity. Gender-related problems associated with boys' and men's sport participation tend to be overlooked (3).

Gender is now understood to be far more complex and greater in scope. Gender is not a clear-cut, absolute, one-or-the-other construct. Indeed, there is often more difference within the categories male and female, masculine and feminine, than between them. Gender is not simply a variable or a social role; it cannot simply be reduced to a collection of psychological traits or physiologic or anatomic differences. Gender is accomplished at the individual, relational, and structural levels. Gender permeates every aspect of social life and organization. Importantly, gender operates in concert with and is dependent on other determinants of social position (class, race and ethnicity, age, sexuality, and physical ability/disability) to shape individual identities and behavior and to direct social interactions and relationships of everyday life. Social organizations are gendered—from the family, corporate America, and government in which divisions of labor are along gender lines to education and sport (1,4). For example, displays of physical competence and involvement in competitive sports are prominent social expectations of boys and men that influence their status and daily social interactions and relationships (1,5,6). Sport and the demonstration of physical prowess, aggression, and dominance are of great importance in the achievement of masculine identities and serve as markers of masculinity (4,7,8). Historically, sport has been a male preserve founded on biologic and medical ideologies of the male body as strong, powerful, and physically superior and the female body as weak, frail, vulnerable, and inferior (9–11).

This chapter is premised on such an understanding of gender and on the acknowledgement that it is the social construction or human invention of gender, not assumed biologic gender differences, that provides a more critical, adequate, and insightful understanding of gender in relation to physical activity, health, and health-related outcomes. Finally, it is important to note from the outset that while gender is recognized to operate in conjunction with class, race and ethnicity, age,

---

C. A. Hasbrook: Department of Human Kinetics, University of Wisconsin–Milwaukee, Milwaukee, Wisconsin 53201.

and physical ability/disability, there is currently little published physical activity and sport research that has examined gender in relation to these other important social factors.

GENDER AND EXCLUSION FROM PHYSICAL ACTIVITY

According to the 1996 Surgeon General's report on physical activity and health (12), there are numerous and well-documented positive health and health-related outcomes of regular moderate physical activity, including reduced risk for coronary heart disease, hypertension, colon cancer, and diabetes; reduced symptoms for depression and anxiety; and aid in controlling weight and building and maintaining healthy bones, muscles, and joints. Yet almost half of young people aged 12 to 21 do not engage in regular, vigorous physical activity, and 14% are sedentary. Further, young girls and women are twice as likely to be inactive as young boys and men (12). In 1994–1995 approximately 50% of all boys and 66% of all girls enrolled in high school did not participate in athletics (13). Observational data from sociologic studies of youth suggest that gender has much to do with these patterns of physical activity and inactivity.

It is well documented that elementary school boys from varying class, racial, and ethnic backgrounds who demonstrate low levels of physical skill are accorded less social status among peers, often being severely chastised for their lack of physical skill, and effectively excluded from participation in physical play, games, and sport (5,6,14–17). More specifically, the masculinity of such boys is often placed in question, ridiculed, and threatened by peers' verbal taunts of "sissy," "homo," and "fag." Research also indicates that, regardless of class, racial, and ethnic background, elementary school girls' physical skills and physical activity involvement are often denounced by male peers as inferior (6,17,18). Often, the femininity of girls who demonstrate superior physical skill and participate in sport is threatened and questioned by peers who accuse them of being "tomboys" or of looking or acting like boys (6,18).

There is also limited evidence to suggest that girls from lower-income and/or particular racial and ethnic backgrounds grow up in families in which parents place greater importance on sport participation for their sons than for their daughters. Hmong girls reported that their parents viewed physical activity as acceptable for older boys but "childish" for older girls (19). As Yates (20) has noted, sport and physical activity are not typically valued or recognized in the cultures of Asian immigrants, especially for girls. In a survey of more than one thousand parents, African-American parents were more likely than Caucasian parents to view sport participation as of greater importance for sons than for daughters (21).

Gender matters deeply to children. Young children work hard at creating clearly visible "appropriately" gendered selves because such accomplishment is crucial to being accepted as a competent member of one's peer group (16). When boys lack what is viewed as an appropriate level of physical skill or when girls demonstrate superior physical ability, their gender identities and social acceptance and status may be threatened. Not surprisingly, many children respond to such threat by learning to avoid physical activity (5,6,14,18,22) and consequently may not experience the positive health and health-related outcomes of regular physical activity. However, not all children respond to such threat by avoiding physical activity. Indeed, greater numbers of young girls are participating in sport and appear to be successfully managing this apparent gender identity dilemma of being female but engaging in sport (23). Eventually, though, as many of these girls reach adolescence, they drop out of sport.

Gender and Elimination From Physical Activity

Numerous studies in the United States and Britain note a longstanding pattern of adolescent girls losing interest in and dropping out of vigorous physical activity and sport (21,24–28). There is no such commensurate drop in boys' participation rates. The reasons for the existence of this longstanding pattern among adolescent girls and its absence among adolescent boys are gender related.

Athletic participation has long been an important basis for social status and popularity among high school boys (29–32). Yet, among high school girls athletic participation generally has not been viewed as a basis for status and popularity (31,32). Rather, "being in the leading crowd" has been reported as the number one basis for female popularity in high school (31). Indeed research indicates that many adolescent girls feel pressured to conform to mainstream or traditional notions of femininity and believe that participation in vigorous physical activity and sport is unfeminine (25,27,28). While athletics serve many boys as an arena for social status from elementary school on, appearance and relationships with boys become of primary importance to many girls during adolescence (18). Therefore it is not difficult to understand why large numbers of adolescent girls but not boys tend to drop out of vigorous physical activity and sport. Unfortunately, there are no longitudinal studies that reveal whether adolescent girls who drop out of vigorous physical activity and sport return to it at a later time in their lives and experience the health and health-related benefits associated with such participation.

GENDER AND THE CIRCUMSCRIPTION OF PHYSICAL ACTIVITY INVOLVEMENT

The following section reviews the literature that describes how gender circumscribes the nature of physical activity involvement and discusses how various sports are gender typed, resulting in the likely channeling of many girls and boys and young men and women into "gender-appropriate" sports. The discussion then turns to the differing sets of gender-related expectations and requirements of these "gender-appropriate" sports and to how such expectations and requirements lead to negative health and health-related practices and outcomes.

The Gender Typing of Physical Activity and Sport

Various sports are generally viewed as more appropriate for one gender than for the other. For example, girls' and women's participation in wrestling or football is often frowned upon, and boys' and men's participation in figure skating or ballet is often discouraged. Girls and women are often encouraged to pursue dance, gymnastics, figure skating, or tennis, while boys and men are often encouraged to play basketball or football or wrestle. Sport sociologists draw upon the classic work of Eleanor Metheny (33) to help explain this phenomenon. According to Metheny, there are "female-appropriate" sports in which participants use their bodies in aesthetically pleasing ways (gymnastics, dance) or use light instruments to overcome light objects (tennis, golf). "Female-inappropriate" sports are those in which participants use their bodies as instruments of physical power and force to overcome or subdue opponents (contact sports such as football and wrestling). Conversely, "male-appropriate" sports are those in which participants display power, force, strength, aggression, and the ability to overcome opponents. "Male-inappropriate" sports are those emphasizing aesthetically pleasing movement. Sociologic studies provide consistent empirical evidence of the gender typing of physical activity and sport across age and gender groups.

Bailey (22) reports that among preschool children, playing with dolls, dressing up, skipping and dancing, and picking flowers are viewed as appropriate activities for girls, while baseball, basketball, fighting, hockey, karate, and soccer are accepted as activities for boys. Studies of elementary school age children (15–18) all note how various forms of physical activity are viewed as more appropriate for one gender than for the other. Jump rope and small group circle games, often involving singing and dancing, are considered appropriate for girls but inappropriate for boys. Sports such as baseball, basketball, football, and wrestling are thought appropriate for boys but inappropriate for girls. College students identify gymnastics as a sport that is "appropriate" for females but inappropriate for males, while they identify basketball as an "appropriate" sport for males but not for females (34). Older men and women identify several sports, including marathon running, the shot put event in track and field, and basketball, as more appropriate for men than women and ballet as more appropriate for women than men (35).

The gender typing of sport may appear to hold little relevance for sports medicine until one considers that such typing may create difficult conditions for girls and boys who are involved in "gender-inappropriate" sports, such as the lack of peer support and acceptance. In addition, the gender typing of sport often leads to the channeling of boys into "masculine" sports in the hopes that it will aid in the development of manhood and prevent weakness and effeminate behavior and girls into "feminine" sports that emphasize and promote grace, delicate movement, and feminine appearance. Once in these "gender-appropriate" sports, participants face a number of expectations that can affect health and health-related outcomes of their sport involvement. These expectations are often gender-related and associated with what sport sociologists term "the sport ethic" (36).

"Gender-Appropriate" Sports and the Sport Ethic

Research indicates that within competitive sports there exists a "sport ethic." This ethic represents a collection of beliefs and values that shape expectations about what it really means to be a competitive athlete. These expectations include sacrificing for "the game," striving for distinction, accepting risks and playing through pain, and accepting no limits in the pursuit of possibilities (36). While athletes accept or embrace these expectations to differing degrees, this set of expectations and especially the practices they promote are important to consider with respect to "gender-appropriate" sports such as ballet, figure skating, football, gymnastics, synchronized swimming, and wrestling. The focus here is on two specific sets of practices promoted by the sport ethic: body weight control and playing with pain and injury.

"Gender-Appropriate" Sports, the Sport Ethic, Body Weight Control, and Negative Health Outcomes

Body weight control in the form of weight gain, weight loss, and/or weight maintenance practices is considered a necessary aspect of the training and conditioning methods of competitive athletes. Among all sports and athletes it is generally accepted that one major and nongendered reason for weight control practices is the achievement and maintenance of a body weight that allows for maximum physical performance. There are, however, also gendered reasons for the existence of weight control practices. In "male-appropriate" sports requiring the demonstration of power and force, such as football, substantial weight gain is often expected and demanded of athletes in certain playing positions. Yet a sport ethic embracing substantial weight gain for female athletes in any sport is relatively unheard of and inconsistent with the value placed on female slenderness in U.S. society. In "female-appropriate," aesthetically pleasing sports such as figure skating, gymnastics, and synchronized swimming, in which bodily appearance is believed to affect the judges' performance ratings, athletes are expected to be thin so as to enhance the aesthetic qualities of their performance (37–40). Cosmetic thinness or the necessity of maintaining a low body weight for purposes of enhancing bodily appearance and aesthetic appeal is not an aspect of the sport ethic within "masculine sport." However, this is not to suggest that male athletes do not practice weight loss. For example, in sports in which there are weight classes or weight restrictions, such as wrestling, weight loss that allows a competitor to wrestle in a lower weight class (and consequently often against a smaller opponent) is practiced as a means of gaining a competitive advantage (41).

Expectations of body weight control among athletes can lead to negative health-related practices that in turn may lead to negative health outcomes. Such negative health-related practices may include the use of substances such as steroids to enhance body-building efforts; self-induced vomiting; using diet pills, diuretics, or laxatives; and overexercising (42–50).

The prevalence of pathogenic weight control methods of losing weight among athletes is uncertain. However, adolescent girls and young women are approximately ten times more likely than adolescent boys and young men to develop anorexia or bulimia (51), and adolescent girls and young women who are involved in sport are more prone to use pathogenic weight control methods than the normal population (42,43,49,50). There is also some evidence to suggest that female athletes in sports in which aesthetic appeal is important, such as diving, gymnastics, ballet, figure skating, and body building, may be at higher risk for developing disordered eating patterns or eating disorders (52). Osteoporosis, amenorrhea, and disordered eating are health outcomes associated with female athletes who become preoccupied with body weight and engage in excessive training and conditioning regimes to control it (53–56).

"Gender-Appropriate" Sports, the Sport Ethic, Pain and Injury, and Negative Health Outcomes

In addition to gender-linked expectations of body weight control among athletes, the expectation that athletes should play with or through pain and injury is anchored in notions of masculinity. Playing with or through pain and injury is a major facet of the sport ethic (36). Data show that as boys and young men participate in competitive sport, particularly violent, contact, "masculine" sports, they learn to accept physical risk, pain, and injury as normal, everyday aspects of the game (57). Indeed, playing with or through pain; hiding, denying, or ignoring pain; and inflicting pain on others are required and rewarded practices among male contact sport athletes (8,57,58). Data also show that women athletes accept pain and injury as a natural part of competitive sport and an "indication of a player's ability and an affirmation of her commitment to her team and her sport" (59, p. 79). There is a crucial distinction to be made between why male and female athletes accept the sport ethic of physical risk, pain, and injury, and this distinction illustrates the essentialness of gender, in particular masculinity, in understanding the sport ethic of physical risk, pain, and injury.

The endurance of pain and injury and its infliction upon others has historically been associated with masculinity (60). Male athletes who show their pain or drop out of competition because of injury report being ridiculed and having their masculinity and dedication to sport questioned by teammates, coaches, the public, and the media (57,58). The athletic *and* gender identities of male athletes are bound up in the sport ethic of physical risk, pain, and injury. While a female athlete's dedication to her sport may be questioned if she refuses to play with or through pain and injury, her gender identity is not threatened because the endurance of athletic pain and injury is not an expectation of femininity. This may serve as at least a partial explanation for why some female athletes have been found to accept physical risk, pain, and injury to a lesser degree than male athletes (61,62).

The health and health-related outcomes of playing through or with pain and injury are to a great extent self-evident. It is important to note here that there is speculation and some evidence to suggest that chronic pain among female athletes may not receive the serious attention that it often warrants. Walk (63) suggests that frequent reports of chronic pain among female athletes in cross-country, gymnastics, and swimming may become normalized, dismissed as psychological rather than physiologic, and/or ignored by athletic training staff personnel because of its invisible nature. Such chronic pain is often associated with overuse injuries and repetitive motion traumas that are invisible, and sports medicine personnel may more often be drawn to the more visible and acute injuries suffered by males in more violent, contact sports (63, p. 53).

SUMMARY AND CONCLUSIONS

Gender is bound up in that which is physical. Understanding gender as a social construction or human invention that permeates every aspect of social life affords a more critical and adequate means to understanding gender and what it has to do with physical activity, health, and health-related outcomes. Considering gender as not only a dimension of individual identity, but also as an aspect of social relations (status and popularity) and social organizations such as competitive sport, provides a framework for understanding young people and their physical activity or inactivity. Gender is relevant to sports medicine because it clearly plays a role in explaining why children, adolescents, and young adults are discouraged or steered away from, drop out of, or are channeled into sports in which a sport ethic of gender-linked expectations of weight control and playing through and with pain and injury may lead to negative health practices and outcomes.

REFERENCES

1. Connell RW. *Gender and power*. Stanford, CA: Stanford University Press, 1987.
2. West C, Zimmerman D. Doing gender. *Gender & Society* 1987;1:125–151.
3. Coakley J. *Sport in society: Issues and controversies*, 6th ed. Boston: McGraw-Hill, 1998.
4. Lorber J. *Paradoxes of gender*. New Haven, CT: Yale University Press, 1994.
5. Adler P, Kless SJ, Adler P. Socialization to gender roles: popularity among elementary school boys and girls. *Sociol Educ* 1992; 65:169–187.
6. Hasbrook CA, Harris O. Wrestling with gender: physicality and masculinity(ties) among inner-city first and second graders. *Men and Masculinities* 1999;1:302–318.
7. Messner MA, Sabo DF. *Sport, men, and the gender order: critical feminist perspectives*. Champaign, IL: Human Kinetics, 1990.
8. Messner MA. *Power at play: sports and the problem of masculinity*. Boston: Beacon Press, 1992.
9. Crosset T. Masculinity, sexuality, and the development of early modern sport. In: Messner MA, Sabo D, eds. *Sport, men, and the gender order*. Champaign, IL: Human Kinetics, 1990.
10. Vertinsky P. Body shapes: the role of the medical establishment in informing female exercise and physical education in nineteenth-century North America. In: Mangan JA, Park R, eds. *From fair sex to feminism: sport and the socialization of women in the industrial and post-industrial eras*. London: Frank Cass, 1987.
11. Vertinsky P. *The eternally wounded woman: women, exercise and doctors in the late nineteenth century*. Manchester, England: Manchester University Press, 1990.
12. U.S. Department of Health and Human Services. *Physical activity and health: a report of the Surgeon General*. Atlanta, GA: U.S. Department of Health and Human Services, Centers for Disease Control and Prevention, National Center for Chronic Disease Prevention and Health Promotion, 1996.
13. National Federation of State High School Associations. *The National Federation of State High School Associations handbook, 1995–96*. Kansas City, MO: NFSHSA, 1995–1996.
14. Best R. *We all have scars*. Bloomington: Indiana University Press, 1983.
15. Davies B. *Frogs and snails and feminist tales*. Sydney, Australia: Allen & Unwin, 1989.
16. Davies B. Lived and imaginary narratives and their place in taking oneself up as a gendered being. *Aust Psychol* 1990;25:318–332.
17. Ignico AA. The influence of gender-role perception on activity preferences of children. *Play & Culture* 1990;3:302–310.
18. Thorne B. *Gender play*. New Brunswick, NJ: Rutgers University Press, 1993.
19. Jaffee L, Ricker S. Physical activity and self-esteem in girls: the teen years. *Melpomene: A Journal of Women's Health Research* 1993;12(3):19–26.
20. Yates PD. A case of mistaken identity: interethnic images in multicultural England. In: Spindler G, Spindler L, eds. *Interpretive ethnography of education*. Mahwah, NJ: Lawrence Erlbaum Associates, 1987.
21. Wilson Sporting Goods. *The Wilson report: moms, dads, daughters and sports*. River Grove, IL: Author, 1988.
22. Bailey KR. *The girls are the ones with the pointy nails*. London, Ontario: Althouse Press, 1993.
23. Watson T. Women athletes and athletic women: the dilemmas and contradictions of managing incongruent identities. *Sociological Inquiry* 1987;57:431–446.
24. American Association of Univeristy Women Education Foundation and the Wellesley College Center for Research. *How schools shortchange girls*. Washington, DC: Author, 1992.
25. Cockerill S, Hardy C. The concept of femininity and its implications for physical education. *British Journal of Physical Education* 1987;8(4).
26. Orenstein P. School girls. *Young women, self-esteem, and the confidence gap*. New York: Doubleday, 1994.
27. Hendry L. *School, sport and leisure*. London: Lepus Books, 1978.
28. Scranton S. *Shaping up to womanhood: gender and girls' physical education*. Philadelphia: Open University Press, 1992.
29. Coleman JS. Athletics in high school. *Ann Am Acad Political Soc Sci* 1961;338:33–43.
30. Eitzen DS. Athletics in the status system of male adolescents: a replication of Coleman's "the adolescent society." *Adolescence* 1975;10:267–276.
31. Thirer J, Wright SD. Sport and social status for adolescent males and females. *Sociol Sport J* 1985;2(2):164–171.
32. Chandler TJL, Goldberg AD. The academic all-American as vaunted adolescent role-identity. *Sociol Sport J* 1990;7(3):287–293.
33. Metheny E. *Connotations of movement in sport and dance*. Dubuque, IA: William C. Brown, 1965.
34. Kane MJ, Snyder E. Sport typing: the social "containment" of women in sport. *Arena Review* 1989;13:77–96.
35. Ostrow AC, Dzewaltowski DA. Older adults' perceptions of physical activity participation based on age-role and sex-role appropriateness. *Res Q Exer Sport* 1986;57(2):167–169.
36. Hughes R, Coakley J. Positive deviance among athletes: the implications of overconformity to the sport ethic. *Sociol Sport J* 1991;8(4):307–325.
37. Caldwell M. Eating disorders and related behavior among athletes. In: Cohen GL, ed. *Women in sport: issues and controversies*. Thousand Oaks, CA: Sage, 1993:158–167.
38. Johns D. Fasting and feasting: paradoxes of the sport ethic. *Sociol Sport J* 1998;15(1):41–63.
39. Taub DE, Benson RA. Weight concerns, weight control techniques, and eating disorders among adolescent competitive swimmers: the effect of gender. *Sociol Sport J* 1992;9(1):76–86.
40. Thompson RA. Management of the athlete with eating disorders: implications for the sport management team. *Sport Psychol* 1987;1:114–126.
41. Steen SN, Brownell KD. Patterns of weight loss and regain in wrestlers: has the tradition changed? *Med Sci Sports Exerc* 1990;22:762–768.
42. Black DR, Burckes-Miller ME. Male and female college athletes: use of anorexia nervosa and bulimia nervosa weight loss methods. *Res Q Exerc Sport* 1988;59:252–256.
43. Clark N, Nelson M, Evans W. Nutrition education for elite female runners. *Phys Sportsmed* 1988;16(3):124–136.
44. Dummer GM, Rosen LW, Heusner WW, et al. Pathogenic weight control behaviors of young competitive swimmers. *Phys Sportsmed* 1987;15(5):75–86.
45. Hsu G. *Eating disorders*. New York: Guildford Press, 1990.
46. Hui YH. *Principles and issues in nutrition*. Monterey, CA: Wadsworth Health Series, 1995.
47. Rosen LW, McKeag DB, Hough DO, Curley V. Pathogenic weight-control behavior in female athletes. *Phys Sportsmed* 1986;14(1):79–83.
48. Rosen LW, Hough DO. Pathogenic weight control behaviors of female college gymnasts. *Phys Sportsmed* 1988;16(9):141–145.
49. Sundgot-Borgen J. Risk and trigger factors for the development of eating disorders in female elite athletes. *Med Sci Sports Exerc* 1994;26:414–419.

50. Thornton JS. Feast or famine: eating disorders in athletes. *Phys Sportsmed* 1990;18(4):116, 118–122.
51. Waldron I. Gender and health related behavior. In: Gochman D, ed. *Health behavior: emerging research perspectives.* New York: Plenum Press, 1988:193–208.
52. Plaisted V. Gender and sport. In: Summers TMJ, ed. *Sport psychology theory, applications and issues.* New York: John Wiley & Sons, 1995:538–574.
53. Barr SI. Relationship of eating attitudes to anthropometric variables and dietary intakes of female collegiate swimmers. *J Am Diet Assoc* 1991;91:976–977.
54. Rucinski A. Relationship of body image and dietary intake of competitive ice skaters. *J Am Diet Assoc* 1989;89:98–100.
55. Wichmann S, Martin DR. Eating disorders in athletes: weighing the risks. *Phys Sportsmed* 1993;21(5):126–135.
56. Wilmore JH. Eating and weight disorders in the female athlete. *Int J Sport Nutr* 1991;1:104–117.
57. Curry T. A little pain never hurt anyone: athletic career socialization and the normalization of sports injury. *Symbolic Interaction* 1993;16(3):273–290.
58. Young K, White P, McTeer W. Body talk: male athletes reflect on sport, injury, and pain. *Sociol Sport J* 1994;11:175–194.
59. Theberge N. "It's part of the game": physicality and the production of gender in women's hockey. *Gender & Society* 1997;11(1):69–87.
60. Connell R. A very straight gay: masculinity, homosexual experience and the dynamics of gender. *Amer Sociol Rev* 1992;57:735–751.
61. Nixon HL. Accepting the risks of pain and injury in sport: mediated cultural influences on playing hurt. *Sociol Sport J* 1993;10(2):183–196.
62. Young K, White P. Sport, physical danger, and injury: the experiences of elite women athletes. *J Sport and Social Issues* 1995;19(1):45–61.
63. Walk SR. Peers in pain: the experiences of student athletic trainers. *Sociol Sport J* 1997;14(1):22–56.

CHAPTER 16

Disability and Sport: A Sociological Analysis

Sharon R. Guthrie and Shirley Castelnuovo

Two weeks after the close of the Olympics in Atlanta, Georgia, in 1996, the Summer Paralympics took place. Many different types of sports were offered, including archery, athletics, basketball, bocce, cycling, equestrian events, fencing, goalball, judo, powerlifting, shooting, soccer, table tennis, tennis and volleyball (1). Among the 4000 athletes competing were amputees, dwarfs, the visually impaired, and those with cerebral palsy and spinal cord injuries. The remarkable nature of this event, which dates back to 1960 in Rome[1] can be appreciated only within a sociohistoric perspective, which demonstrates the ongoing struggle that people with disabilities have had to face in becoming recognized as capable of athletic achievement.

A wheelchair basketball game played by war veterans at a California naval station in 1945 has been identified at the first athletic event for individuals with disabilities in the United States. During that same year the first disability sport organization, the American Athletic Association for the Deaf, was founded. Before the 1940s, disability sport would have been labeled an oxymoron. Indeed, organized sport competition for people with disabilities, and general acceptance thereof, is a relatively recent phenomenon.

The fact that the year 1945 was also the year that saw the end of World War II is not coincidental. Disability scholars have noted that between World War I and World War II, greater national attention was given to the issue of disability. Although there have always been people with disabilities, the large number of veterans returning home with war-related impairments after service to their country increased the concern of both their families and the government regarding their social and medical treatment. Moreover, the dominant cultural perspective of disability, which had undergone many transformations through history, was again shifting.

HISTORICAL PERCEPTIONS OF DISABILITY

Humans and societies reveal themselves in the ways in which they conceptualize and respond to perceived difference, regardless of whether these differences are associated with gender, ethnicity, age, class, or sexual orientation. Disability, like all socially constructed categories of difference, has produced widely varying perspectives, reflecting both the ethos of a particular time period and the ongoing ambivalence and consternation among able-bodied people toward those who do not conform, either in appearance or behavior, to prescriptive norms. As might be expected, these differing perspectives have resulted in diverse societal responses to disability, ranging from cruelty and disregard to tolerance, special education, medical rehabilitation, and even veneration.

For example, during the ancient Greek and Roman periods, disability was associated with evil, impurity, and humanity's relationship with the gods. Those born with physical and mental impairments often faced intolerance, abandonment, and infanticide. In contrast, those who acquired their disability in battle, which was considered a heroic act supported by the gods, were revered (2,3).

During the medieval period the influence of Christianity caused a shift in thinking about disability, one

---

[1] Although the first Paralympics occurred in Rome in 1960, these games were actually founded by Sir Ludwig Guttman over 50 years ago at Stoke Mandeville Hospital in Aylesbury, England. Guttman wished to establish a connection between the Paralympic Games and the Olympic Games, thus making them more socially distinctive. He achieved his goal; since 1960 the Olympics have shared the same country, and, more recently, they have shared the same city. In fact, current bidding for the Olympic Games includes consideration for the Paralympics (19).

S. R. Guthrie: Department of Kinesiology and Physical Education, California State University, Long Beach, California 90840.
S. Castelnuovo: Department of Political Science, Saddleback College, Mission Viejo, California 92692–3635.

that was grounded in ethics rather than superstition. Physical impairments became viewed as forms of suffering that were an inevitable part of God's plan for human life on earth. Consequently, prayer, an acceptance of religious explanation, and charity were emphasized. Although this ethicospiritual discourse fostered care of the disabled by families and charitable patrons, people with disabilities remained marginal in society, that is, without any social function or identity as a distinct group (4).

During the 18th century Enlightenment period the Christian charity discourse on disability was replaced by a medical model, which emphasized description and categorization rather than a spiritual explanation. Education and reeducation of people with disabilities were also emphasized; for example, Abbé de l'Epée (1712–1789) and Valentin Haüy (1745–1822) developed sign language for deaf-mutes and initiated education for the blind, respectively. Owing to these early and ongoing efforts, by the end of the 19th century there were educational institutions for people with visual and hearing impairments and orthopedic institutions for correcting what were considered bodily infirmities.

The 19th century experienced a further expansion of the medical perspective on disability, which was followed by a similar but more rehabilitative approach in the 20th century. The belief in rehabilitation of disability was propelled by the large number of men who suffered bodily impairments during World War I. Prostheses were developed, and with them the ideals of replacement, substitution, and compensation materialized. Moreover, because notions of normalcy and rehabilitation intersected those of equality and equal opportunity, it was felt that physical differences should be mitigated as much as possible so that each person could have an equal chance to succeed in life. According to disability scholars Ingstad and Whyte, although earlier eras viewed those with disabilities as exceptional in some way, albeit oftentimes negatively,

> the modern intention (or pretension) is that they are ordinary and should be integrated into ordinary life and work. Infirmities do not raise metaphysical problems so much as technical ones to be taken in hand and administered by social workers, vocational trainers, and medical and legal specialists. The assumption is that we master all the outcomes; every condition can be treated and adjusted, though not all can be cured (5).

This medical-rehabilitative paradigm is still prominent at the beginning of the 21st century, as are the trends toward social reform, increased governmental concern, and progressive inclusion and acceptance of individuals with disabilities. Today, people with disabilities compete in a variety of sports and competitions at international, national, and local levels and experience far more support for their athletic endeavors than in the past. Amid these advancements, however, it is important to remember that the full participation and social integration of individuals with disabilities, whether in sport or elsewhere, are still far from being facts of life.

It is also noteworthy that the anecdotal accounts of people with disabilities indicate that the medical-rehabilitative norms, although pervasive and seemingly humanitarian, have not completely eradicated older perceptions of disability as representing a curse of the devil and other evil spirits. Two disabled women reveal the darker side of their interactions with the able-bodied world as follows:

> It is the knowledge that each entry into the public world will be dominated by stares, by condescension, by pity and by hostility.

> I was a freak, an outsider, an "other" and the world made it very clear that I owed them an explanation (6).

Robert Murphy, a well-known cultural anthropologist, is another person who experienced aversion from the able-bodied world. He began speaking and writing about the vilification of the disabled after he found that his acquired disability—paraplegia, which later developed into quadriplegia—became his dominant public persona, demolishing his status as a white male academic. In fact, his status as "disabled" became a more significant identifier than his age, occupation, and ethnicity, or even gender. As a disabled person he experienced loss of status, avoidance, fear, and hostility; he also was treated as if he were asexual (7).

Murphy believed that because gender expectations are more rigorous for men in general, disabled men feel a greater sense of overall failure as humans if they are born or become disabled. Indeed, the "normal" sexually attractive male body is supposed to convey masculinity, as well as physical strength, speed, and stamina. This shape, as Murphy and others have noted, is achieved by diet, exercise, and sometimes steroids and is driven by a zealous moral fervor that worships youth, virility, and successful participation in sport. These idealized male bodies are the ones that appear on the playing field on Super Bowl Sunday, as well as in mass-mediated interscholastic and college sporting events. Physically disabled bodies, particularly those that are visually obvious, radically contravene this American male ideal. Therefore, males with such disabilities are without any guarantee that they will be assigned a valued position in society. According to Murphy, their only hope is to normalize themselves by adopting roles that reestablish their masculine identities (e.g., becoming athletes in the Paralympics).

Other writers and scholars claim that gender expectations fall equally hard on females with disabilities (1,6,8–10). Contemporary women, just like men, are supposed to "normalize" themselves in terms of physical fitness and physical appearance, which are both associated with sexual attractiveness. They, more often than men, however, are primarily defined by their physical appearance.

Thus, regardless of disabled/nondisabled status, females are more likely than males to believe that physical beauty is a critical, if not *the* critical, factor in their achieving success and happiness in life.

INTERSECTION OF DISABILITY LEGISLATION AND SPORT

Although this normalizing perspective can certainly dampen one's self-acceptance, it has positively influenced legislation, which in turn has led to the advancement of sporting opportunities for people with disabilities in the United States. Disability legislation emerged from the Civil Rights movement with its emphasis on equality of opportunity and inclusion of minority groups in the societal whole. Its foundation was the Civil Rights Act of 1964, which addressed discrimination on the basis of race but also provided the legal basis for disability rights law.

The enactment of several laws influencing the physical activity and mobility potentials of people with disabilities followed thereafter. For example, in 1967 the Amended Elementary and Secondary Education Act provided training programs in physical education and recreational opportunities for people with disabilities. In 1968 the Architectural Barriers Act was passed, which dealt with issues such as building and street access. In 1973 the Rehabilitation Act mandated that all programs receiving federal money, which included most universities and about one half of all private businesses, could not discriminate against an otherwise qualified person solely on the basis of handicap. The Education of All Handicapped Children Act, passed in 1975, required instruction in physical education as part of special education. In 1978 the Amateur Sports Act recognized athletes with disabilities as part of the Olympic movement and the U.S. Olympic Committee. In 1990 Congress passed the Americans with Disabilities Act, which broadened federal antidiscrimination protection to cover all businesses in employment, public services, and public accommodations. Sport and recreational programs, while not specifically named, were interpreted as public services. This legislation also required businesses to make accommodations for people with disabilities whether or not the businesses currently employ such individuals.

The intersection of the Civil Rights movement with the disability rights movement is evident in the legislative language of these laws, particularly the Amateur Sports Act. This act makes specific reference to facilitating sporting opportunities for disabled individuals, females, and ethnic minorities. However, disability researchers have consistently noted that far more men than women participate in elite disability sport, as well as in recreational sport and physical activity programs (1,10). Moreover, Caucasians with disabilities are more frequent participants than people of color. Much of this has to do with the sociopolitical and economic resources available to certain groups of individuals, as well as to this country's history of sexism, classism, and racism, which affects notions of self-identity and socially acceptable activity.

As was mentioned, however, the legal leverage is in place for action to occur. As different groups within the disabled community identify their own needs, individuals who are disabled as well as being female and/or a member of a minority group may very well use this legislation to provide more sporting and recreational options for their specific groups.

ELITE DISABILITY SPORT: A BLESSING OR A CURSE?

Sporting opportunities for individuals with disabilities fall into two general categories: international, national. and regional competitions for elite athletes (e.g., the Paralympics, which is the equivalent of Olympic international competition, the World Games for the Deaf, the Paralympics for Persons with Mental Handicaps, the Boston Marathon, collegiate sport) and recreational sport and physical activities (e.g., Special Olympics International, leisure sport and exercise) that are available primarily at the local level. Although physical activity in both categories offers many physical, psychological, and social benefits to people with disabilities, elite disability sport receives far more attention. Undoubtedly, this is because the competitors are participating in one of America's most prized cultural practices and dramatic spectacles.

Competitions for elite athletes with disabilities follow able-bodied sport and Olympic protocol. As such, they promote equality of opportunity and inclusion, as well as providing positive images of the athletic capabilities of people with disabilities to the able-bodied world. The message projected is that physical disability does not have to represent negative difference, vulnerability, and an inability to fit into able-bodied society—that people with disabilities can be just like those in the dominant group.

In this regard, disabled elite athletes, like their ablebodied counterparts, affirm quintessential American values—in particular, the view that competition is the best means of identifying and rewarding outstanding skills as well as distinguishing the wheat from the chaff. The problematic results of this ideology include the reification of athletic elitism and winning-at-all-costs attitudes and behaviors. The former restrict mass participation; the latter often result in a loss of bodily and mental integrity associated with overtraining, denial of injury, eating disorders, and substance abuse.

Although most Americans who follow and participate in sport are aware of these problems, athletic elitism and winning at all costs are considered part and parcel of elite sport and touted, by many able-bodied and disabled people alike, as demonstrating "survival of the fittest" at its best. Moreover, the integration of people with disabilities into the public mainstream, whether or not a particular mainstream domain has structural and ideological flaws, is considered progressive humanitarianism. Efforts that are underway to expand disability sport and integrate athletes with disabilities into the Olympic Games and other national and international contests reflect such perspectives.[2]

They are also reflected in the decision in a recent court case involving Casey Martin, a 23-year-old golfer with a circulatory leg disorder. Martin's lawyers argued that Casey could not walk an 18-hole round and therefore needed a golf cart to compete in the PGA and Nike tours. "We're seeking an equal opportunity for Mr. Martin to demonstrate his abilities," they claimed (11). Federal District Court Judge Thomas Coffin ruled that Martin could play PGA and Nike tours with the aid of a golf cart and that the controllers of professional sports were responsible for accommodating the needs of disabled athletes in pro sport.

This case marks the first time the Americans with Disabilities Act, designed to expand opportunities for persons with disabilities in public accommodations, has been applied to athletes in a major U.S. sport. The battle to secure the rights of athletes with disabilities is not yet over, however. Although the Martin ruling was recently upheld by an appeals court when challenged by the PGA, the Federal Court of Appeals for the Seventh Circuit recently held that Ford Olinger, who has a degenerative hip condition, could not use a golf cart in the United States Open. In Olinger's case, walking was determined to be an essential part of golf competition. Thus two appeals courts have arrived at disparate conclusions regarding the use of gold carts by pro golfers with disabilities. Unless the Supreme Court resolves this issue, golfers playing in the states of the Ninth Circuit will be allowed to use golf carts while those playing in the states of the Seventh Circuit will not.

Although the Olinger ruling may be considered a setback for disability rights, the Martin case is undoubtedly viewed by many people, both those with and without disabilities, as a tremendous victory—one indicating that the consciousness of American society is evolving in a humanitarian direction. These people look forward to celebrating the time when people with disabilities receive more opportunities to become symbols of victory against all odds—the epitome of the American success story—and thus send a message of hope and self-responsibility. In a world in which disability is often viewed as a failure of bodily or rational control, athletes with disabilities can become American heroes.

It should be noted, however, that there are those in both the disabled and nondisabled communities who view efforts to expand elite disability sport and to integrate people with disabilities into able-bodied sport with mixed emotion. Susan Wendell, a disabled feminist scholar, is an example. Although she admits that disabled athletic heroes may be inspiring to others with disabilities and comforting to able-bodied people because they reaffirm the possibility of overcoming bodily vulnerability and dependency, their athletic success may also give the false impression that anyone can transcend a disability.

Wendell reminds us that disabled sport heroes usually have extraordinary social, economic, and physical resources that are not available to most people with their same disabilities. In addition, many people with disabilities are not capable of performing physical heroic feats because, as she says:

> many (perhaps most) disabilities reduce or consume the energy and stamina of people who have them and do not just limit them in some particular kind of physical activity. Amputee and wheelchair athletes are exceptional, not because of their ambition, discipline and hard work, but because they are in better health than most disabled people can be (12).

Wendell argues that while images of the disabled athletic hero may reduce the "otherness" of a few disabled people, these images also create an ideal that the majority cannot meet, which in turn may increase the sense of otherness so many disabled people already feel. Indeed, elite disability sport, like able-bodied sport, reinforces the American obsession with body culture, which contributes to the idealization of hard, lean bodies—bodies that many people, whether or not they have a disability, are not able to achieve because of their genetics and socioeconomic factors.

The icon status of such bodies was evident in the photographic presentation of Olympic athletes in special editions of *The New York Times Magazine*, *Vanity Fair*, and *Life Magazine* before the 1996 Olympics. We can anticipate the integration of photos of elite disabled athletes in future collections. Unfortunately, such presentations may contribute to a social construction of disability that is even less accepting of diverse bodies than the one we have today. The highlighting of such images, particularly in a culture in which few alternative images are presented, conveys a negative message to the majority of disabled women and men: They must normalize themselves to be socially acceptable and sexually desirable; otherwise, they are too harsh a reminder of human frailty and the fragility of bodily ideals.

Thus, although it is possible that focusing on the similarities between disabled and able-bodied people, in

---

[2] Although efforts have increased to integrate disabled individuals into the Olympic Games beyond exhibition events, which they have been participating in since the 1984 Winter and Summer Games, the IOC did not pass a 1997 proposal for inclusion (19).

effect making disability less noticeable in comparison to other human qualities, will lead to assimilation on an individual basis and thus gradual social change, we do not believe, nor does Wendell, that this strategy directly challenges "able-bodyism." Moreover, in some cases assimilation, even on an individual or small-scale level, may not be forthcoming because of a lack of resources or political resistance from able-bodied people; clearly, not all Americans support the integration of minority groups into the dominant culture.

Another problem with the hyperfocus on elite disability sport is that it can lead to a disregard for participation in recreational sport and other forms of physical activity, which are of tremendous importance in enhancing physical and psychological health. These nonelite activities can also serve the majority of disabled individuals who do not have the requisite athletic bodies and skills for high-level competition. Contesting the restrictive body-beauty norms associated with elite athleticism requires placing at least an equal emphasis on physical activity designed for nonconforming yet valued bodies. Moreover, it requires an emphasis on developing self-confidence and a sense of control over one's internal and external environment. Each of these qualities has been found to be enhanced with regular participation in sport and exercise, regardless of skill and competitive level.

We have documented these self-change processes in our ongoing research with women with disabilities. It seems that when a woman empowers herself at the bodily level there is a profound change in her self-structure and overall identity. Another study has confirmed these benefits for men as well (13).

RECREATIONAL SPORT AND PHYSICAL ACTIVITY FOR PEOPLE WITH DISABILITIES

Extensive research over the past century has demonstrated that participation in sport and other forms of physical activity contributes to enhanced physical self-perceptions. Moreover, these perceptions of the physical self have been found to generalize to more global aspects of the self (e.g., self-esteem, self-confidence). In this section we discuss the findings of our research involving women with disabilities, which are largely consistent with the results of other similar studies (13–14).

As we mentioned previously, the dominant paradigm associated with disability in contemporary American society is medical-rehabilitative; as a result, most research studies have been attempts to understand the biology of physical and mental impairments and to discover the best programs and technology for remediation and compensation, if not cure. As might be expected, sociologic analyses of disability, particularly those associated with sport and physical activity, are more difficult to find. Studies that do exist point in the same direction: People with disabilities derive a variety of benefits from regular involvement in physical activity, both competitive and noncompetitive, and these changes extend beyond the physical health dimension. The problem seems to be making sport and exercise accessible and accommodating for the majority of disabled people.

In our work with women with diverse disabilities ($N = 162$), the majority ($n = 101$, 62%) were participating in some form of sport or exercise on a regular basis (i.e., at least three times per week for at least 20–30 minutes), while 23% ($n = 37$) claimed that they were physically active but only sporadically. Thus, among this sample, only 15% ($n = 24$) were completely inactive at the time of the study and had never participated regularly in any form of physical activity. Moreover, of the 24, only five claimed that they had no interest in participating in physical activity and did not intend to alter their behavior in the near future.[3]

The high level of physical activity among these women may have to do with the fact that a large percentage of them were college students or college-educated professionals; researchers have consistently found a positive relationship between exercise adherence and education among able-bodied populations. While it is good news that these women are physically active, it is equally noteworthy that physical activity seems to result in positive self-change. These perceived changes were categorized into the following thematic categories.

Empowerment

All of the women who had or were participating in competitive sport on a regular basis ($n = 43$) reported that they felt strengthened, both psychologically and physically, as a result; 93% of those who had no athletic experience but were exercising regularly ($n = 58$) also perceived such benefits. Subthemes within the broader empowerment category included the following:

1. Improved body image (i.e., feelings about and evaluation of the body)
2. Improved physical self-efficacy (i.e., the belief that one has the requisite skills to accomplish a physical task such as a sport or exercise skill)
3. Increased sense of psychological hardiness (i.e., the feeling that one can overcome obstacles when they

---

[3] The women in our study, ranging in age from 20 to 72, had a variety of disabilities, including those associated with acquired brain injury, hearing, vision, communication, learning, physical mobility, and other (e.g., diabetes, AIDS). A person with a disability was defined in accordance with American Disability Act criteria: an individual who has a condition that substantially limits one or more major life activities. There was a fairly equal mix of congenital and acquired disabilities. Subjects had lived with their disabilities from less than 6 months to over 50 years. The population included African-American/Black ($n = 22$), Hispanic ($n = 16$), Asian American ($n = 19$), Native American ($n = 8$), Caucasian ($n = 76$), multiracial ($n = 14$), and other ($n = 7$).

arise and viewing them as a challenge or learning opportunity)
4. Enhanced feelings regarding sexual identity
5. Improved global self-esteem
6. The perception that by being physically active, one is deconstructing society's negative messages regarding what women with disabilities should be capable of doing in the physical realm.

The last benefit was mentioned most often by those with obvious physical disabilities (e.g., spinal cord injuries) as opposed to learning disabilities and most often in relation to sport participation as opposed to exercise training alone.

Therapeutic Value of Sport and Exercise

The vast majority (73%) of the women who had engaged in regular physical activity at some point in their lives ($n = 118$) reported that it had served an important therapeutic function. Most often, they experienced the following benefits:

1. Improved physical and psychological health and fitness
2. A sense of expanded independence from limitation of the disability
3. Regained sexual interest
4. Stress reduction and increased episodes of positive affect
5. Improved spatial and bodily awareness
6. A sense of freedom from social constraints associated with having a disability
7. Becoming more outgoing socially because of not feeling so awkward and self-conscious in physical movement
8. Enhanced perception of the bodies and physical capacities of others with similar disabilities.

Integration of Mind-Body-Spirit

Most of the women who were physically active or had been physically active in the past also noted an improved awareness of the mind-body-spirit connection and that engaging in regular physical activity helped them to integrate these elements of their being. More specifically, they mentioned gaining a better understanding of how physical health and fitness intersect mental and spiritual health and becoming more motivated to change attitudes and behaviors to improve overall wellness (e.g., diet, social support).

This study is entirely consistent with our previous research demonstrating that regular physical activity, whether it be sport or exercise, helps to enhance body image and self-esteem among diverse groups of women (15–18). It certainly seems to be the case that when a woman empowers herself at the bodily level, there is a profound change in her self-perception. Our findings also indicate a twofold problem, however: Not all people with disabilities engage in regular physical activity because of perceived and actual barriers, and many people with disabilities do not have the energy or stamina for physical activity because of limiting health conditions.

The barriers that were reported to be the most limiting by those who did not regularly participate in physical activity, prioritized from high to low, were as follows:

1. Fear of injury
2. Lack of energy or stamina
3. Lack of self-discipline
4. Lack of time because of family or work
5. Lack of knowledgeable instructors
6. Lack of money
7. Lack of company to exercise with
8. Lack of people who are similar to the respondent (e.g., those who have disabilities at the exercise facility)
9. Discouragement from others because of disability.

Of these nine, three were categorized as environmental barriers (lack of time, lack of knowledgeable instructors, lack of money), three were self-related (lack of energy or stamina, lack of self-discipline, fear of injury), and three were socially-related (discouragement from others because of disability, lack of similar people, lack of company). Thus it is clear that while regular physical activity should be made available and encouraged, not all people with disabilities believe that they can take part. Moreover, those who do participate, or would like to, feel that they still face external barriers, most of which are modifiable.

SOME THOUGHTS ABOUT THE FUTURE

We believe that providing more opportunities for people with disabilities to participate in physical activity of all types is critical for health reasons as well as sociopolitical reasons. Continued legislation that supports the rights of people with disabilities and change in societal perceptions of disability are needed to accomplish this goal, however.

Although disability legislation and rights have progressed in the United States, inaccessible facilities, lack of transportation, inadequate information, and lack of publicity about programs still exist. Such limitations are often more constraining than disability itself (1,14). Still, recent legislative and judicial changes have played an important role in fostering a more enabling physical environment for disabled individuals. We hope that such changes will be sustained and that further improvements will be made in the future.

Because political changes are the direct result of

changes in human consciousness, however, efforts must also be directed toward transforming negative social perceptions of disability. This is not an easy goal, for it requires able-bodied people to confront their fears associated with loss of physical and mental control, aging, and, ultimately, death. It also requires identifying the processes that facilitate positive self-regard among people with disabilities and then providing the venues in which these enhanced perceptions may materialize.

We know from our work and life experience that one's sense of self is developed through physical interaction of the body with the environment. This is the case for individuals who are disabled, as well as those who are able-bodied. Regular exercise and/or participation in sport can appreciably enhance this sense of self. However, if such programs of physical activity are to be successful in transforming the lives of individuals who live with disabilities, they must be designed and provided for the majority of individuals with disabilities, not just a small minority.

This emphasis on physical activity for the disabled majority does not, and should not, preclude the expansion of opportunities for elite disabled athletes, for there are benefits to be achieved in this arena as well. Moreover, because elite sport is a popular public domain and receives much public attention, elite athletes with disabilities are more likely to become positive role models for the world community, including both those with and without disabilities.

We believe that the able-bodied population can learn much from people with disabilities—for example, how one negotiates and comes to terms with a cultural ideology that fuses bodily perfection with success and happiness while living with an imperfect body. In our ongoing research we have found that people with disabilities are often more capable than the able-bodied of comprehending the creative possibilities associated with bodily difference and change, particularly those who are born with disabilities and are least aligned with body-beauty, health, and fitness ideals. These individuals are also more likely to understand the social construction of disability in American society and the fact that difference does not necessarily negate the experience of joy and life satisfaction.

We believe that more exposure to people with disabilities, whether they are doing physical or nonphysical activity, is needed for able-bodied people to gain these insights. Elite disability sport does provide a powerful venue for Americans to discover that disability does not preclude extraordinary athletic skills; moreover, because this form of sport takes place in large public spaces (e.g., the Paralympics), it stands a better chance of becoming a mass-mediated cultural event than do recreational physical activities. Thus able-bodied individuals, through expanded awareness and personal reflection, may come to learn what most of the disabled women in our study seem to know from experience.

Admittedly, disability sport receives far less media coverage and hoopla than does able-bodied sport; in fact, most Americans may not even be aware of the Paralympics, collegiate disability sport, or the fact that disabled Americans have competed in the Olympic Games. However, with the social changes that are occurring today, we predict that there will be increasing awareness, acknowledgement, and support for disability sport coming from able-bodied sectors as time goes on. Moreover, the Martin Olinger decisions will certainly lead to debate within the elite sporting community and the general public about rules of professional sports and whether they should accommodate our nation's constitutional and legislative imperative of equality of opportunity.

Americans should not just have their attention focused on elite disability sport, however. We believe that it would be equally consciousness-raising, if not more so, for the able-bodied population to see, hear, and read about people with disabilities being physically active in health clubs and in recreational sporting contests. Their levels of awareness would be raised even higher if disabled people in large numbers began demanding accommodations in these physical fitness sites with instructors and trainers who are knowledgeable about and sensitive to their issues and concerns. We, along with many others, look forward to that day.

REFERENCES

1. Depauw KP, Gavron SJ. *Disability and sport.* Champaign, IL: Human Kinetics, 1995.
2. Davies E. *Adapted physical education,* 3rd ed. New York: Harper & Row, 1975.
3. Rothchild CS. Prejudice against the disabled and the means to combat it. In: Stebbins, J, ed. *Social and psychological aspects of disability: a handbook for practitioners.* Baltimore, MD: University Park Press, 1968.
4. Ingstad B, Whyte SR, eds. *Disability and culture.* Berkeley: University of California Press, 1995.
5. Ingstad B, Whyte SR, eds. *Disability and culture.* Berkeley: University of California Press, 1995:270.
6. Morris J. *Pride against prejudice: transforming attitudes to disability.* Philadelphia: New Society Publishers, 1991:23,25.
7. Murphy, RF. *The body silent.* New York: Henry Holt, 1987:131.
8. Hillyer B. *Feminism and disability.* Norman: University of Oklahoma Press, 1993.
9. Fine M, Asch A. *Women with disabilities: essays in psychology, culture and politics.* Philadelphia: Temple University Press, 1988.
10. Sherrill C. Paralympic Games 1996: feminist and other concerns—what's your excuse? *Palaestra* 1997;13:32-38.
11. Murphy K. Disabled golfer wins access to cart in pro tours, *Los Angeles Times* 1998 Feb 12:A1.
12. Wendell, S. Toward a feminist theory of disability. *Hypatia* 1989;4(2):104–124.
13. Blinde E, McClung LR. Enhancing the physical and social self through recreational activity: accounts of individuals with physical disabilities. *Adapted Physical Activity Quarterly* 1997;14:327-344.
14. Henderson KA, Bedini LA. I have a soul that dances like Tina Turner, but my body can't: physical activity and women with mobility impairments. *Res Q Exerc Sport* 1995;66(2):151–161.

15. Guthrie SR, Castelnuovo S. Liberating the Amazon: empowering women through feminist education with the martial arts. *Perspectives: Journal of the Western Society of Physical Education of College Women* 1996;15:57–65.
16. Guthrie SR. Liberating the Amazon: feminism and the martial arts. *Women and Therapy* 1995;16:107–120.
17. Guthrie ST, Ferguson C, Grimmett D. Elite women bodybuilders: ironing out nutritional misconceptions. *Sport Psychol* 1994;8(3):271–283.
18. Guthrie S. Defending the self: martial arts and women's self-esteem. *Women in Sport & Physical Activity J* 1997;6(1):1–28.
19. Depauw KP. Sport and physical activity in the life-circle of girls and women with disabilities. *Women in Sport & Physical Activity Journal* 1997;6(2):225–237.

PART IV

General Medical Problems

CHAPTER 17

Sports Dermatology

Thomas N. Helm and Wilma F. Bergfeld

INTRODUCTION

The physician who is interested in sports medicine quickly finds himself or herself confronted by a wide array of dermatologic disorders. Athletes are prone to all of the dermatologic problems that affect the population at large, but because of long hours of practice and hard work the skin diseases may become more troubling at a more rapid rate, and they also may interfere with peak athletic performance. This chapter will outline the most common dermatologic findings that are encountered in the practice of sports medicine and outline treatment approaches (Table 17-1).

INFECTIONS

Herpes Infection

Herpes simplex infection can spread rapidly. This is especially true in wrestlers. If one wrestler has active herpetic lesions and then contacts another wrestler, widespread herpetic lesions may develop. If one of the affected individuals has an underlying skin disease such as atopic dermatitis or Darier's disease, herpetic lesions may be widespread and hemorrhagic. This constellation of findings is known as herpes gladiatorum. Although herpes gladiatorum was treated with hospitalization and intravenous acyclovir in the past, the newer antiviral agents such as valacyclovir (Valtrex), when given at a dosage of 500 mg twice daily, lead to prompt resolution. Use of bland topical emollients as well as cool compresses followed by topical antibiotic ointments (e.g., Polysporin ointment) may be of value.

Localized herpetic infections are also frequent. Skiers are particularly prone to herpes labialis involving the lower lips. Sunburn and exposure to cool winds and chapping of the lips may precipitate an outbreak. Often individuals will report a pins and needles sensation before the onset of clustered vesicles and pustules on an erythematous base (Fig. 17-1). Many times treatment is not necessary, but in widespread cases of primary herpetic gingivostomatitis, treatment with oral agents and meticulous oral hygiene with mouthwashes and dental care is necessary to prevent morbidity and to hasten resolution. When herpes infections occur more than nine times a year, suppressive therapy may be advisable. Famciclovir (Famvir) at a dosage of 250 mg twice daily or valacyclovir (Valtex) at a dosage of 500 mg twice daily may be of value for suppressive therapy.

Tinea Infections

Tinea pedis (athlete's foot) is characterized by redness and itching of the feet. A variety of different clinical manifestations are possible. Some individuals are prone to an interdigital form of maceration with web space fissuring and cracking, most commonly involving the third and fourth web spaces. Other individuals may have predominantly scaling on the bottom of the feet with mild itching, and in other individuals bullous lesions may occur. Bullous lesions may be of abrupt onset and extremely itchy and uncomfortable. Topical imidazole antifungal agents are extremely helpful. Miconazole cream applied twice daily is inexpensive and our first line of therapy, but other products are more potent (oxiconazole, econazole nitrate, ketoconazole).

With cool compresses applied two to three times daily followed by the topical imidazole cream, marked clinical improvement is often seen within 2 or 3 days. Treatment should be continued for at least a week for most of the agents previously mentioned, and many athletes find it beneficial to apply cream once or twice weekly as a prophylactic measure if they have been prone to recur-

---

T. N. Helm: State University of New York at Buffalo, Williamsville, New York 14221.

W. F. Bergfeld: Section of Dermatologic Research, Cleveland Clinic Foundation, Cleveland, Ohio 44195.

TABLE 17-1. Treatment of common skin disorders in athletes

Disease	Treatment
Blisters	Decompress with sterile needle; if needed, apply hydrocolloid or petrolatum dressing
Contact dermatitis	Avoid triggering allergen; topical corticosteroid (e.g., triamcinolone 0.1% cream) 3 times daily for 10 days
Folliculitis	Topical erythromycin or clindamycin gel or pads twice daily for 10 days
Herpes simplex (recurrent autopeak)	Famiclovir 125 mg BID × 5 days; Valacyclovir 500 mg BID × 5 days
Herpes zoster	Valacyclovir 1 mg TID × 7 days; Famciclovir 500 mg TID × 7 days
Seborrheic dermatitis	Shampoos and topical corticosteroids as needed (e.g., ketoconazole, selenium sulfide, or zinc pyrithiamine shampoo and fluocinonide solution applied once or twice daily as needed)
Tinea pedis and corporis	Imidazole antifungal twice daily for 2-4 weeks (e.g., miconazole, sulconazole cream)
Tinea versicolor (pityriasis versicolor)	Selenium sulfide 2½% lotion applied for 10 minutes each day for 1 week; hold oral ketoconazole or itraconazole in reserve
Warts, plantar	Topical salicylic acid plasters (e.g., Mediplast and Transplaster applied daily)
Warts, common	Topical salicylic acid (e.g., occlusal, Duofilm), destructive techniques (e.g., liquid nitrogen cryotherapy)
Xerosis	Frequent use of emollients and lactic-acid-containing lotions (e.g., LacHydrin lotion)

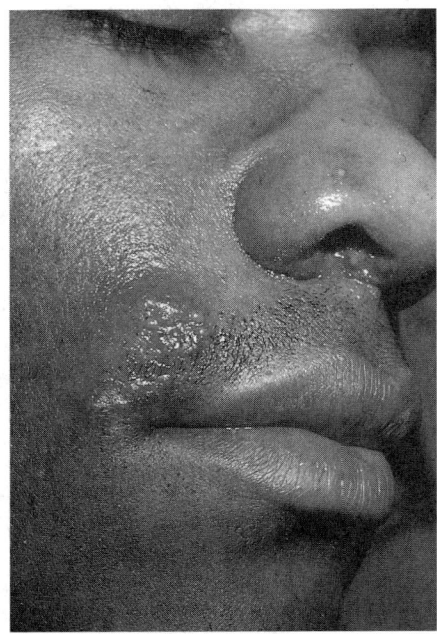

FIG. 17-1. Herpes labialis in a wrestler characterized by cluster vesicles and pustules on an erythematous base.

prompt improvement in widespread or recalcitrant cases. Topical agents are also effective but may be more cumbersome when wide body areas are involved.

Pityriasis Versicolor (Tinea Versicolor)

Pityriasis versicolor is the correct name for what has previously been referred to tinea versicolor. Because pityriasis versicolor is caused by a commensal yeast, it is not appropriate to refer to it as a tinea, which is a term reserved for cutaneous infection by a dermatophyte agent. Pityriasis versicolor may have different presentations in individuals of different skin color (Figs. 17-2 and 17-3). Individuals with a fair complexion may

rences. Using a powder on the feet (e.g., Zeasorb-AF) on a regular basis and wearing cool absorbent cotton socks may also be of value.

Tinea Corporis/Cruris

Tinea corporis may be quite extensive, and we have encountered very widespread examples in wrestlers. Those wrestlers may be disqualified. Rapid treatment is desired. In the past, oral griseofulvin had been the mainstay of therapy, but the newer agents such as oral terfenadine at a dosage of 250 mg daily, itraconazole (e.g., Sporanox) at a dosage of 200 mg daily, or Fluconazole at a dosage of 150 mg daily all lead to rapid and

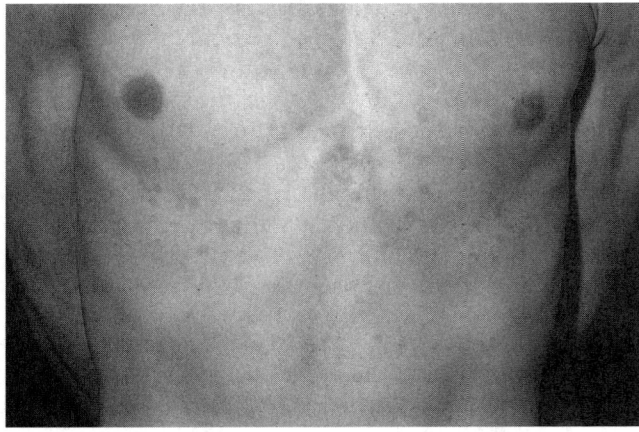

FIG. 17-2. Tinea versicolor in fair-complected individuals may show up as red/brown scaling macules.

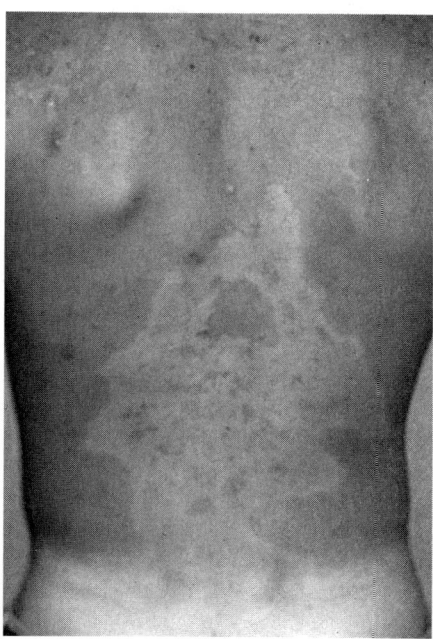

FIG. 17-3. In dark-complected individuals, tinea versicolor may lead to hypopigmentation. This individual also has acne lesions on the upper back exacerbated by contact with his football pads.

have red/brown macular areas on the chest and back. People with darker skin types may develop hypopigmented lesions because the azaleic acid produced by the organism interferes with normal tyrosinase activity. Lesions may be mildly pruritic, but most individuals present for evaluation because of the unsightly appearance and dyschromia. Selenium sulfite 2½% lotion or ketoconazole 2% shampoo applied from the neck to the waist for 10 minutes each day for one week will lead to resolution. Individuals who are prone to recurrence may need to prophylactically treat themselves once a month or more. Topical imidazole antifungal creams (e.g., Spectazole cream) may be given as an adjunctive agent. Individuals should be reassured that this is a benign and self-limited disorder. Unlike vitiligo, areas are hypopigmented rather than depigmented, and this difference can be clearly demonstrated by using a Wood's lamp, in which case vitiligo would have a bone-white appearance, whereas tinea versicolor would have a dull, lighter appearance under examination. In severe or widespread cases oral imidazole agents (e.g., ketoconazole and itraconazole) may be given, but because of the concerns of hepatotoxicity, these agents are not recommended for first-line therapy.

Erythrasma

Erythrasma represents infection by *Corynebacterium minutissium*. Dull, red round plaques are found in intertriginous areas. Under a Wood's lamp a characteristic pink florescence is seen. This is due to a porphyrin by-product produced by the Corynebacterium.

Corynebacterium may also cause a disorder of the plantar surface known as pitted keratolysis, as well as another disorder known as trichomycosis axillaris. In trichomycosis axillaris, concretions develop around hair shafts in the axilla or groin. In pitted keratolysis, small dells are noted on the plantar surface of the feet, and these may be associated with hyperhidrosis and malodor of the feet.

Treatment with erythromycin at a dosage of 250 mg four times daily for one week is curative. Alternatively, topical erythromycin as well as clindamycin may be of benefit. Topical miconazole creams are also of value, and some individuals have suggested that good soap-and-water cleansing with aeration and keeping the areas cool and dry will lead to resolution as well.

Intertrigo

Intertrigo represents maceration of skin surfaces in body folds. Rubbing and heat lead to erosion and ulceration of the skin, and there is often secondary infection with oozing and weeping. Cool compresses followed by an application of a vital dye such gentian violet aqueous solution 1% may be of value. A favorite agent used for compresses is Burrow's aluminum acetate solution (at a concentration of 1:40). After application of the Burrow's compresses, a protective ointment such as zinc oxide protective ointment (USP 10%) can be applied. An imidazole antifungal agent (e.g., Spectazole, Oxistat) may be applied at bedtime.

Warts and Molluscum

Plantar warts can be particularly troubling in athletes. Warts may be painful and interfere with normal function. First-line treatment involves the use of topical salicylic acid plasters. For plantar warts we prefer to use a 40% salicylic acid plaster (e.g., Mediplast) applied each night after paring. Repeated long-term use leads to resolution of many warts. Otherwise, destructive modalities (e.g., cryotherapy) or the application of acids such as nitric acid or loichloracetic acid may be of value. These destructive treatments must be used with caution, however, as scarring or secondary infection may result. Alternatively a non-FDA approved agent known as Cantharone has been very popular in the past. Topical Cantharone is not painful when applied and is a vesicant leading to subepidermal bulla formation. When the bulla heals, the wart will be often desquamated. In other instances excision or laser surgery may be appropriate, but these treatments must be used with caution in athletes because the risk of scarring or secondary infection.

Molluscum contagiosum is a pox virus infection of

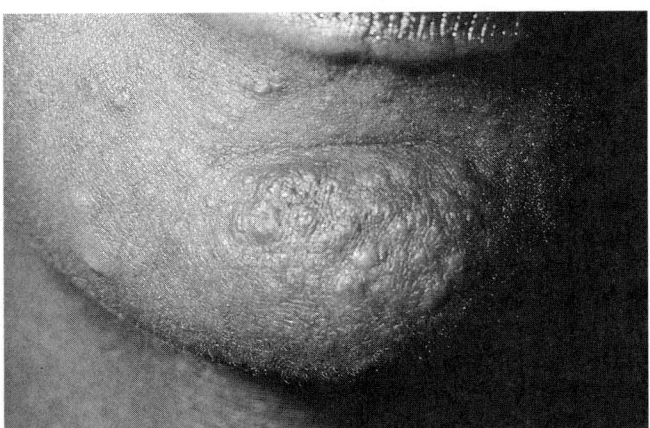

FIG. 17–4. Molluscum contagiosum lesions can spread widely and involve the chin, simulating acne as in this individual. Careful observation will reveal umbilicated flesh-colored lesions that lack inflammation.

the skin. Flesh-colored to pink papules with central umbilication may be found scattered across the body or confined to a localized area. The central umbilication allows for differentiation from folliculitis (Fig. 17–4). Cryotherapy, curettage, and Cantharone application are the treatments of choice.

MECHANICAL AND PHYSICAL PROBLEMS

Sunburn

Athletes practice long hours outside. The sun is especially intense between 10:00 A.M. and 2:00 P.M., and fair-complected individuals should avoid exercising during these hours if possible. The sun contains roughly 100 times more ultraviolet A than ultraviolet B during midday hours, but ultraviolet B is the main culprit that leads to sunburn. Reflection from sand and water may exaggerate the effect of both ultraviolet A and ultraviolet B and is especially important in water sports and for skiers (Fig. 17–5).

Although ultraviolet B is the main culprit for sunburn, ultraviolet A may also cause aging changes in the skin that have been linked with the production of skin cancer. Because skin cancers are so prevalent, it is especially important that athletes use adequate sun protection. Sunscreens of sun protection factor 15 or greater are recommended. Agents that are broad spectrum and contain cinnamates and benzophenones or Parsol 1789 are advisable. Athletes should apply sunscreen a half hour before exercise, and it is very important for athletes to apply sunscreen to areas that are often forgotten, such as the ears and back of the neck. Treatment for sunburn is difficult. Some relief can be obtained with ice cold milk or water compresses and aspirin taken every 2 hours. Prostaglandin inhibitors such as oral ibuprofen are of value also.

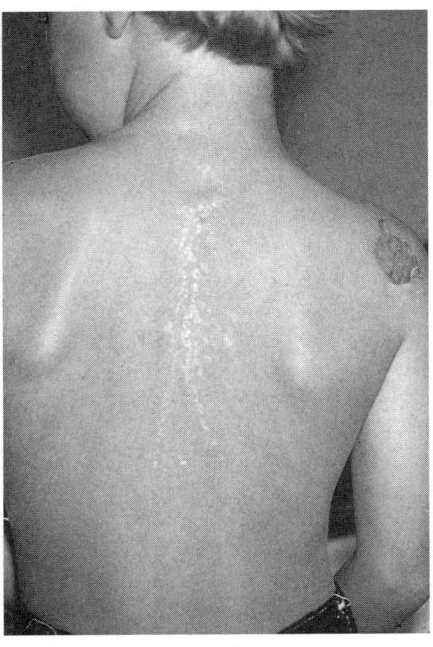

FIG. 17–5. Widespread sunburn may be accompanied not only by erythema but also by blister formation, as in this second-degree sunburn involving the back.

Frostbite

Frostbite commonly involves the ears, cheeks, fingers, and toes. The frozen body part becomes pale and indurated, but affected individuals may not have pain or discomfort. With rewarming, erythema and edema develop, and there may be blister and gangrene formation. Rapid rewarming in a water bath between 100°F and 110°F is the treatment of choice for frostbite. When the skin is pink in color and has normal texture, the affected area has been adequately thawed.

Blisters and Corns

Blisters and corns are the most commonly encountered dermatoses seen in athletes. Blisters develop when shearing forces lead to a dissolution of keratinocytes within the epidermis or in a subepidermal location. Many blisters do not require treatment, but if blisters are large or impede performance, they may be drained by prepping the skin with alcohol or betadine and gently opening the blister roof in a small area by using either a sterile number 11 blade or Iris scissors. The blister roof should not be removed in its entirety, but the collapsed blister roof should be left intact over the denuded underlying skin. We prefer to use a petrolatium dressing and a telfa nonabsorbent pad held in place by gauze wrap or an elasticized gauze (e.g., Elastoplast). Other agents that are more expensive but also help include the use of hydrocolloid dressings (e.g., Duoderm or Actiderm patches).

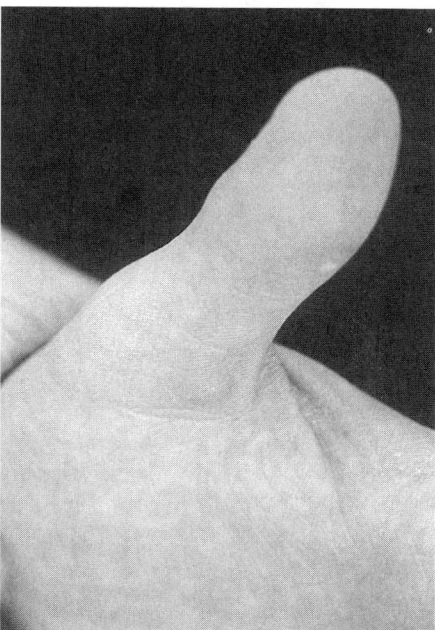

FIG. 17-6. Bowler's callus. Calluses are seen after long hours of bowling involving the thumb at sites of contact with the bowling ball.

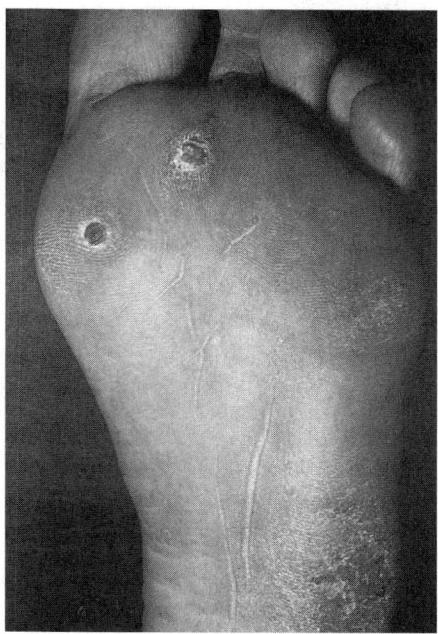

FIG. 17-7. Calluses in runners commonly involve the ball of the foot.

Corns are painful collections of hyperkeratosis in areas of repeated injury or friction. They may be pared by using a sterile scalpel, or gentle debridement with a pumice stone may be of value. Whereas corns may cause discomfort, calluses are a more diffuse hyperkeratosis and actually may be protective. Many athletes prize the calluses as marks of virtuosity and of long hours of practice (Figs. 17-6 and 17-7). Novice athletes are more likely to run into difficulties with blisters in the rapid development of calluses.

Tennis Toe

Tennis toe represents a subungual hematoma precipitated by rapid starting and stopping. Rapid pressure in sports that involve starting and stopping such as racquet sports (e.g., tennis, squash, and racquetball) may lead to rupture of a subungual longitudinal capillary with resultant hemorrhage. The hemorrhage may be painful but many times goes unnoticed. Individuals notice a dark discoloration under the nail and become concerned that they may have a pigmented lesion such as a melanoma. A subungual hematoma will grow out over time, and clipping the nail or removing a small portion of the nail plate will show that the pigment is housed entirely within the nail. If pigment involves the proximal nail fold or there are different colors or history of precursor nevus, biopsies are mandatory to exclude the possibility of melanoma. Many individuals with lentiginous melanoma will be given an erroneous history of trauma; therefore history cannot entirely distinguish between subungual hemorrhage in a suspicious pigmented lesion.

Talon Noir

Analogous to tennis toe, talon noir represents subcorneal petechiae due to rapid starting and stopping. Basketball and other sports involving rapid starting and stopping may cause rupture of capillaries in the papillary dermis and resultant hemorrhage into the stratum corneum. No treatment is required; if individuals are concerned, the affected area may be pared.

Jogger's Nipples

The nipples do not form calluses, as do other parts of the body. After extreme exercise the nipples may become sore. This is most commonly encountered when individuals use jerseys or tops made of synthetic materials that contain polyester or other abrasive materials. The nipples may become reddened, and there may be bleeding, which may lead to the question and concern of an underlying tumor (Figs. 17-8 and 17-9). The symmetry provides reassuring evidence of a benign process.

Signs of Virtuosity

Some changes may represent signs of extreme training or endurance. For example, surfer's nodules are connective tissue nodules that are seen in infrapatellar locations and are accompanied by overlying epidermal hyperpla-

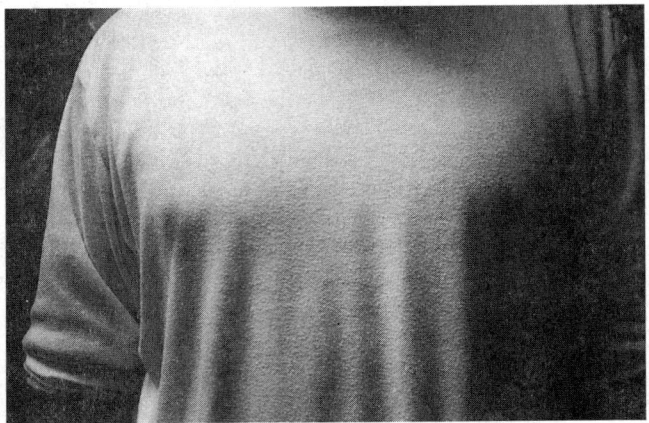

FIG. 17–8. Bleeding from the nipples after a 15-kilometer race.

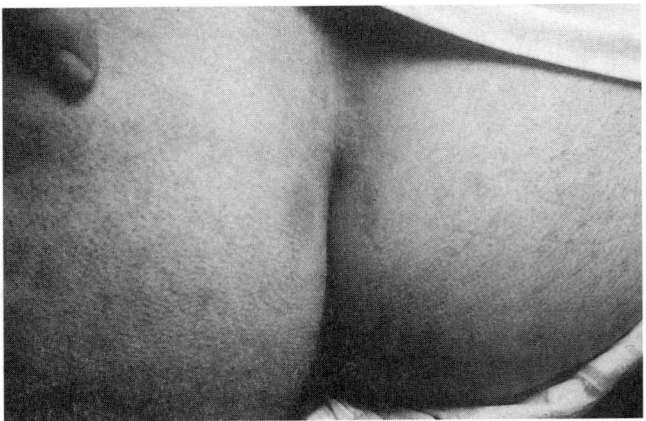

FIG. 17–10. Brown lichenified plaques symmetrically distributed on the buttocks near the intergluteal areas from running and not having appropriate underlying padding.

sia. They are caused by long hours paddling on a surfboard but are of no major consequence. If they become painful, excision may be necessary. Trap shooters may develop areas of atrophy on the cheek where they undergo repetitive injury, and rowers may develop lichenification of the intergluteal area (Fig. 17–10). Novice skiers who have endured long hours of training on a mogul field may develop ecchymoses on the palms; practiced in-season skiers are less likely to have mogul skier's palm because of training and minimization of unnecessary force in pole planting.

EXACERBATIONS OF UNDERLYING CONDITIONS

Acne

Acne is a condition due to plugging of a pilosebaceous unit. Inflammatory lesions commonly develop in areas of pressure. Athletes are prone to develop acne in areas where helmets occlude the skin or where pads apply pressure. Treatment with an aqueous-based 2.5% benzyl peroxide gel in the morning and a topical retinoil at bedtime (e.g., Retin-A or Differm Gel) is typical first-line therapy. The shoulders are commonly involved in athletes. Folliculitis can also be precipitated by occlusion from tight-fitting clothing (Figure 17–11).

Other

Psoriasis, lichen planus, and discoid lupus erythematosus all may undergo what is known as the isomorphic

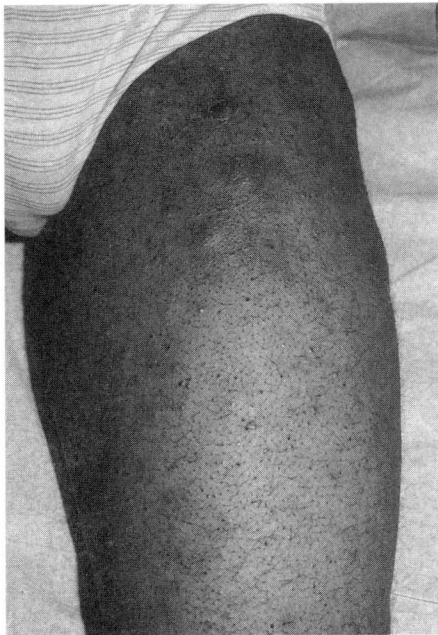

FIG. 17–11. Prolonged rubbing with tight-fitting padded pants used in football may precipitate folliculitis lesions.

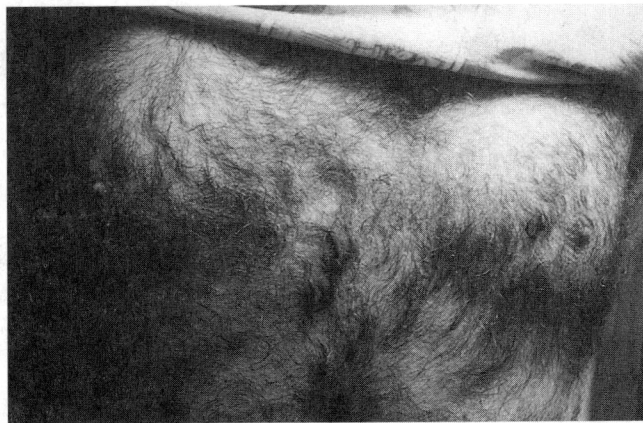

FIG. 17–9. The nipples are red and inflamed with no abnormalities other than superficial erosion.

phenomenon (e.g., Koebner's phenomenon). Areas of friction or rubbing may lead to spreading of an underlying dermatosis. Treatment of the dermatosis with topical steroids will likely lead to resolution. Contact dermatitis may be encountered in athletes. Adhesives and rubber products are common culprits. Thiuram and mercapto mix may be found in hockey gloves and athletic shoes. Patch testing may help to delineate these allergens. We have encountered increasing numbers of athletes with shoe dermatitis.

CONCLUSION

Skin problems are commonly encountered in athletes and can be easily addressed by the team physician in most instances. Familiarity with the dermatologic problems of athletes is extremely important in achieving prompt resolution.

BIBLIOGRAPHY

Basler RS. Acne mechanica in athletes. *Cutis* 1992;50:125–128.
Becker TM. Herpes gladiatorum: a growing problem in sports medicine. *Cutis* 1992;50:150–152.
Belongia EA, Goodman JL, Hollard ES, et al. An outbreak of herpes gladiatorum at a high school wrestling camp. *N Engl J Med* 1991;325:906–910.
Bergfeld WF, Elston D. Skin problems of athletes. In: Fu FH, Stone D, eds. *Sports injuries*. Baltimore, MD: Williams & Wilkins, 1994:781–795.
Bergfeld WF, Helm TN. Skin disorders in athletes. In: Grana WA, Kalenak A, eds. *Clinical sports medicine*. Philadelphia: WB Saunders, 1991:110–118.
Bergfeld WF, Helm TN. The skin. In: Strauss RH, ed. *Sports medicine and physiology*. Toronto: WB Saunders, 1991:117–131.
Bergfeld WF, Taylor JS. Trauma, sport, and the skin. *Am J Ind Med* 1985;403–413.
Cohen PR, Eliezri YD, Silvers DN. Athlete's nodules: sports related connective tissue nevi of the collagen type (collagenomas). *Cutis* 1992;50:131–135.
Cortese TA, et al. Treatment of friction blisters. *Arch Dermatol* 1968;97P:717.
Doller J, Strother S. Turf toe. *J Am Podiatr Med Assoc* 1978;68:512.
Exum WF, Scott MJ. Trap shooter's stigma. *Cutis* 1992;50:110.
Farber GA, et al. Football acne. *Cutis* 1977;20:356.
Gibbs R. Tennis toe. *Arch Dermatol* 1973;107:918.
Herring KM, Ritchie DH. Friction blisters and sock fiber composition: a double blind controlled study. *J Am Podiatr Med Assoc* 1990;80:63.
Izumi AK. Pigmented palmar petechiae (black palm). *Arch Dermatol* 1974;109:261.
Levine N. Dermatologic aspects of sports medicine. *J Amer Acad Dermatol* 1980;3:415–424.
Levit F. Jogger's nipples (letter). *N Engl J Med* 1977;198:1127.
Sedar JI. Treatment of blisters in the running athlete. *Arch Podiatric Med Foot Surg Sports Med* 1978[Suppl 1];290–334.
Sheard C. Simple management of plantar clari. *Cutis* 1992;50:138.
Sher RK. Joggers' toe. *Int J Dermatol* 1978;17:719.
Swinehart JM. Mogul skier's palm: traumatic hypothenar ecchymoses. *Cutis* 1992;50:117–118.
Toback A, Korson R, Krusinski PA. Pulling boat hands: a unique dermatosis from coastal New England. *J Am Acad Dermatol* 1985;12:649–655.
Tomecki KJ. Mikesell JF. Rower's rump. *J Am Acad Dermatol* 1987;16:890.
Yaffee H. Talon nor. *Arch Dermatol* 1971;104:452.

CHAPTER 18

Infectious Mononucleosis in Athletes

Warren B. Howe

All physicians who treat athletes will eventually be forced to deal with the dilemmas posed by the occurrence of infectious mononucleosis (IM) in the population they serve; most will need to do so frequently. In the United States this viral illness has its peak incidence between the ages of 15 and 25 years, precisely the period when organized sports activity is an important part of life for many people. The folklore attached to the disease, such as tales of severe or protracted disability associated with it, often trigger exaggerated emotional responses on the patient's, parents', or coach's part when the diagnosis is made. Although IM is usually straightforward in its manifestations, it can occasionally present very atypically and sometimes with alarming or life-threatening symptoms, making diagnosis difficult and therapeutic decisions critical. When it occurs, the disease can be responsible for significant time loss from sports participation and even longer periods of reduced effectiveness in the sporting activity after the athlete returns to play. Because of the splenomegaly that accompanies most cases and fear of enhanced susceptibility to spontaneous or traumatic splenic rupture, athletic participation may be proscribed for what may seem to the athlete to be endless lengths of time, even after the symptoms seem otherwise resolved, putting great stress on the physician-athlete relationship and sometimes on that of the coach and team physician as well. For these reasons IM is not a simple matter for the sports physician, and it ought to be thoroughly understood.

PATHOPHYSIOLOGY

IM is caused by the Epstein-Barr virus (EBV), one of the human herpesviruses. Initial infection occurs in nasopharyngeal mucosal cells, where viral replication followed by cell lysis and viral liberation occurs. B-lymphocytes then become infected, but in contrast to the infection in mucosal cells, the virus is not replicated and released, but its genome is carried in the B-cell throughout the body. Infected B-cells continue to reproduce despite harboring the virus. They produce a number of polyclonal antibodies, including the heterophil antibody, detection of which is important in the laboratory diagnosis of IM, and various autoantibodies that may play a part in some of the clinical manifestations and complications of IM. The presence of the EBV genome in the B-cell creates surface antigens on the cell membrane, which are recognized and reacted to by the host. In a two-pronged defense, cytotoxic T-cells attack the virus-infected cells, their work being facilitated by IgM and IgG antibodies against viral capsid antigen (VCA), and later EB nuclear antigen (EBNA). The IgM antibodies are transient, while the IgG antibodies persist for life. Although this defense terminates the clinical effects and manifestations of the infection, the EBV genome persists in latent form within B-cells permanently. This is similar to the way in which other herpesviruses behave, but unlike, for instance, the herpes simplex virus, reactivation of the latent EBV is exceptionally rare. There has been considerable speculation about the possible role of EBV in the causation of Burkitt's lymphoma, Asian nasopharyngeal carcinoma, and some other malignancies, but the association has not been specifically characterized or definitively proved.

EPIDEMIOLOGY

Transmission of EBV is by close and probably repeated contact with an individual who is shedding the virus, usually occurring by oral-to-oral exchange in saliva. Virus is shed most frequently by individuals with active IM or by immunocompromised people, but approximately

---

W. B. Howe: Team Physician, Western Washington University, Bellingham, Washington 98226.

15% of seropositive but otherwise normal individuals may be shedding virus at any given time, probably with decreasing incidence as the length of time following primary infection increases. Primary EBV infection occurs when the virus invades a seronegative host and is "recognized" and responded to by the host's immune system. This event results in seroconversion: the appearance of permanent antibodies against EBV that confer lifelong immunity against reinfection. Primary EBV infection is not synonymous with clinical IM, however. The clinical picture associated with primary EBV infection depends on a number of factors, the most important being age at the time of primary infection. Until about age 10, primary EBV infection is usually clinically inapparent. Above age 10, primary EBV infection is much more likely to be manifested as clinical IM: 25–50% of those infected between the ages of 15 and 25 will develop symptomatic disease, females (peak age incidence: 16) and males (peak age incidence: 18) being equally affected. In developing areas of the world and in the lower socioeconomic classes elsewhere, most of the population has undergone primary infection and seroconversion by age 10, while it is delayed in middle and upper socioeconomic classes, giving rise to the observed characteristics of IM occurrence: rare in developing countries, highest incidence in the United States between ages 15 to 25, with a much higher incidence in whites than blacks. Approximately 1–3% of college students develop clinical IM annually. There is no evidence to suggest that athletes are any more susceptible to developing IM than others of their age, but since the peak age incidence of IM corresponds roughly to the peak age of athletic activity in the United States, many athletes at critical points in their careers will be afflicted.

Quarantine is ineffective as a control measure for IM. Studies have shown that even susceptible college roommates of IM patients do not acquire the disease (1,2), and only 6% of patients can recall contact with a known case (3).

SIGNS AND SYMPTOMS

The symptoms of IM develop after a 3- to 5-day prodrome, which is relatively indistinguishable from that of many viral illnesses, consisting of headache, malaise, fatigue, anorexia, and perhaps myalgia. Characteristically, the disease then presents with fever, sore throat, and adenopathy, the latter usually involving the posterior cervical chain initially and then becoming more generalized to include anterior cervical and axillary nodes. Although I have not found it mentioned in the literature, my experience is that epitrochlear adenopathy is significantly correlated with the disease. The pharyngitis is usually severe, accompanied by edema, erythema, lymphoid and tonsillar hyperplasia, and, in many cases, a thick, gray-white tonsillar exudate. Petechiae on the soft palate are common but are not pathognomonic of IM.

Other symptoms are frequently seen in addition to these classic features. Splenomegaly is common: in up to 50–75% of cases clinically (4) and approaching 100% if imaging techniques such as ultrasound are used (5). Hepatomegaly is considerably less common, but many patients will complain of right upper quadrant discomfort even in its absence. Jaundice occurs in about 10% of cases. A maculopapular rash is seen in about 10% of IM patients and in 90% or more of IM patients who are treated with ampicillin. It is thought that the ampicillin-related rash is caused by reaction with one of the IM-associated antibodies (6) and is not a manifestation of ampicillin or penicillin allergy. Periorbital edema is relatively common (7). The frequency and timing of the major physical signs and symptoms seen in IM are displayed in Figure 18–1.

It has long been recognized that IM patients may present various combinations of symptoms and signs, which may be thought of as IM syndromes. The three commonly recognized clinical forms of IM include (a) pharyngeal, or anginose; (b) glandular, and (c) febrile, or typhoidal (8). In pharyngeal IM the illness is most acute, with tonsillar signs predominating. The glandular syndrome is marked by adenopathy and malaise, with less impressive pharyngitis. Typhoidal IM is the most slowly evolving of the three types, with adenopathy appearing only after 2–3 weeks, prolonged fever and malaise, and prominent gastrointestinal symptoms including anorexia, nausea, and vomiting.

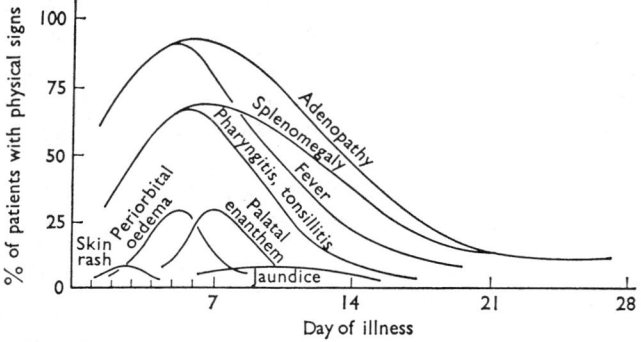

FIG. 18–1. Approximate frequency, timing, and duration of physical signs and symptoms in young adults with infectious mononucleosis. (Reprinted with permission from Finch SC: Clinical symptoms and signs of infectious mononucleosis. In: Carter RL, Penman HG, eds. *Infectious Mononucleosis.* Oxford, England: Blackwell Scientific, 1969.)

Since the presentation of IM can be so variable, it is important to consider it in the differential diagnosis of nonspecific febrile illness affecting a young athlete until it can be ruled out with certainty.

DIAGNOSIS

The diagnosis of IM depends on demonstrating the classic triad associated with the disease: clinical, peripheral blood, and serologic features. The clinical signs and symptoms, which were mentioned above, include fever, malaise, lymphadenopathy, and tonsillopharyngitis. These may develop quickly and almost simultaneously or over a more prolonged period of up to 1–2 weeks.

The frequency and timing of major laboratory abnormalities in IM are displayed in Figure 18–2. A leukocytosis of 10,000–20,000 white blood cells/mm^3 consisting of predominantly lymphocytosis (>50%) is highly characteristic; 10–20% of the lymphocytes will be atypical or variant, sometimes called Downey cells. These are large mononuclear cells, with bizarre shapes, unusual cytoplasmic and nuclear appearance, and variable staining characteristics. Most of these are actually CD8 T-lymphocytes whose production is stimulated by the infection; some are B-lymphocytes infected with EBV. Neutropenia is common, especially early in the course. Significant neutrophilia may indicate presence of sepsis or splenic rupture (3) or signal the need to consider alternative diagnoses. Barring complications, there is usually no significant change in red cell numbers or morphology. Mild thrombocytopenia is not uncommon, affecting up to 50% of patients.

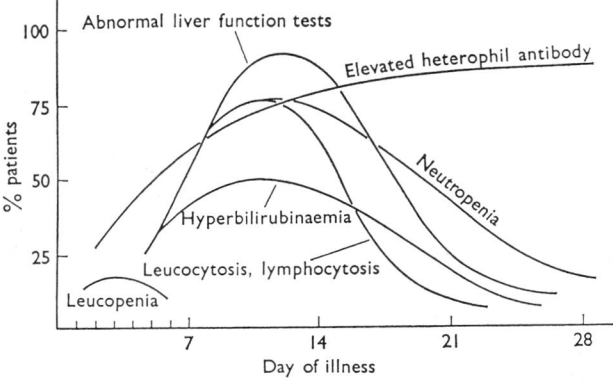

FIG. 18–2. Approximate frequency, timing, and duration of significant laboratory abnormalities and findings in young adults with uncomplicated infectious mononucleosis. (Reprinted with permission from Finch SC: Laboratory findings in infectious mononucleosis. In: Carter RL, Penman HG, eds. *Infectious Mononucleosis.* Oxford, England: Blackwell Scientific, 1969.)

Most IM patients will have abnormalities in liver function tests (4). The aminotransferases (ALT, AST), gamma glutamyl transpeptidase (GGT), lactic dehydrogenase (LDH), and alkaline phosphatase may increase to 2–3 times normal but seldom to the ranges that are seen in acute viral hepatitis A or B. The serum bilirubin may be slightly elevated, but clinical jaundice is unusual. In the absence of certain rare renal complications, kidney function tests remain normal.

Confirmation of IM depends on serologic evidence, the development of which is pictured in Figure 18–3. Most patients with IM (70% in the first week, approaching 95% by the end of the third week) will produce heterophil antibody (HA) (8). This antibody reacts against antigens on erythrocytes of various species—notably sheep, horses and goats—but not with EBV-specific antigens. It also cross-reacts with other antibodies, such as Forssman, serum sickness, and some associated with various malignancies. Paul, Bunnell, and Davidsohn developed a test for IM-associated HA in 1932, preadsorbing serum to be tested with guinea pig kidney cells to remove cross-reactivity before testing for sheep-erythrocyte agglutination (9). This technique forms the basis for the several screening tests for IM that are currently employed in offices and laboratories, which are simple to use, inexpensive, and accurate. If the test is initially negative but clinical suspicion is high, it should be repeated periodically through the first 3 weeks. With these tests, there are only rare false positives, but up to 10–15% of patients with clinical IM will repeatedly test negative for HA (3). Some of these will be found to have an alternative diagnosis (Table 18–1), while others will have HA-negative IM. Although one might question the need to aggressively pursue the diagnosis of what is almost always a self-limited disease in these cases, the prognostic implications of IM for the athlete, especially in terms of return-to-activity considerations, demand that an exact diagnosis be made if possible. Detection of IgM antibodies to VCA or IgG antibodies to EBNA is possible by using immunofluorescent or enzyme-linked immunosorbent assay techniques and should be pursued through reference laboratories in these cases. Consultation with a clinical pathologist in these situations may be very helpful.

The differential diagnosis of IM is listed in Table 18–1. Of these entities the most important are cytomegalovirus (CMV) infections and pharyngitis caused by Group A, beta-hemolytic streptococcal (GABHS) pharyngitis. CMV probably accounts for most HA-negative disease resembling IM and has been described as having milder pharyngitis and more severe hepatitis (10). Two cases of spontaneous rupture of the spleen in association with CMV-mononucleosis have been reported (11). GABHS infection and IM often coexist; the former should be searched for and, if found, treated even if IM

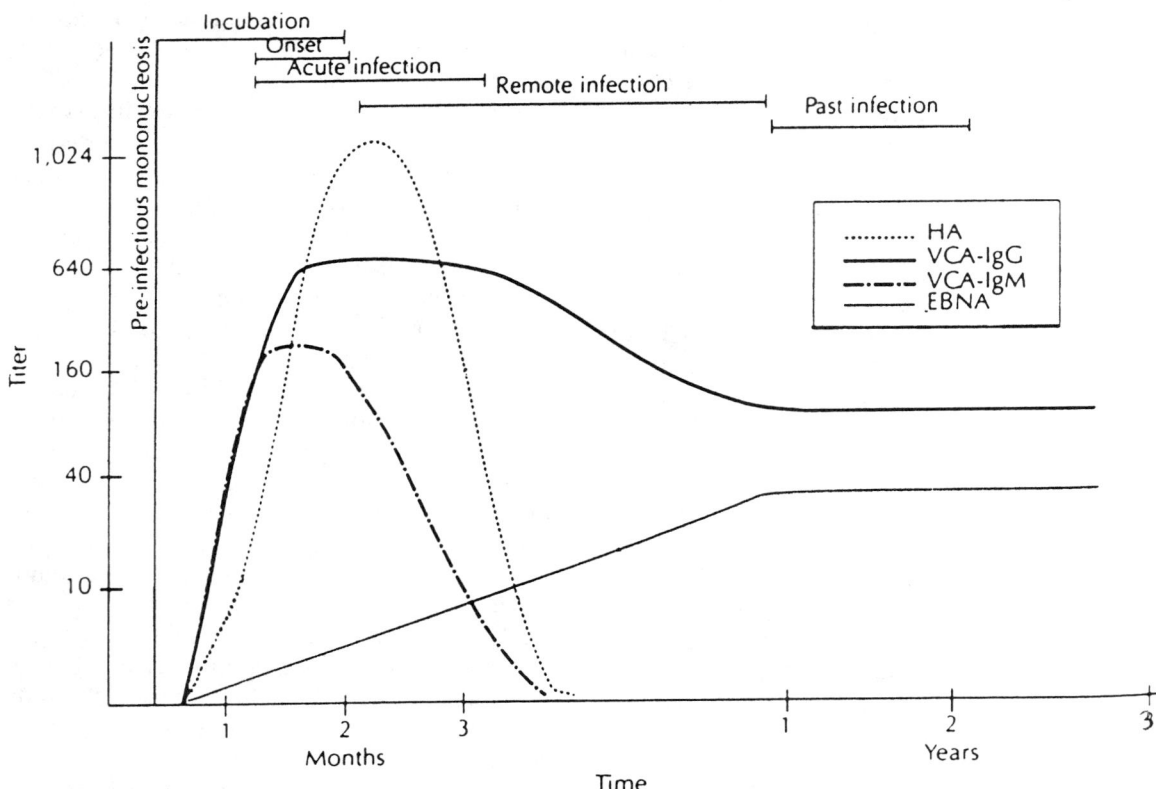

FIG. 18-3. Approximate timing, duration, and magnitude of significant antibody responses in infectious mononucleosis. (HA, heterophil antibody; VCA, viral capsid antigen; EBNA, Epstein-Barr nuclear antigen.) (Modified from Bailey RE. Diagnosis and treatment of infectious mononucleosis. *Am Fam Phys* 1994;49(4):879–888.)

TABLE 18-1. *Differential diagnosis of infectious mononucleosis*

Cytomegalovirus (CMV) infection
Group A, beta-hemolytic streptococcus (GABHS) pharyngitis
Toxoplasmosis
Arcanobacter hemolyticum pharyngitis
Human immunodeficiency virus (HIV)
Viral hepatitis
Roseola
Mumps
Viral URI (adenovirus)
Brucellosis
Diphtheria
Lymphoma/Hodgkin's disease
Tuberculosis
Serum sickness
Drug reaction
Leptospirosis
Subacute bacterial endocarditis (SBE)
Malaria

---

is diagnosed, whether or not the GABHS is thought to be pathologic. The remainder of the conditions listed are of lesser importance and will usually be either easily confirmed or ruled out.

CLINICAL COURSE

The typical case of IM is usually 1–3 weeks in duration, with a prodromal period lasting from 3 to 5 days, followed by the classic manifestations of the disease for up to 15 additional days. A hump-backed course has been described in about 10% of patients, in which severe symptoms of IM develop late, many days after the initial symptoms (12). After resolution of the acute clinical symptoms, vague fatigue and malaise may persist for longer periods, though generally no more than about 6 weeks. Up to 10% of patients may experience such symptoms for even longer, however (13). The elite athlete may require 3–6 months to regain pre-illness performance and fitness levels (10,14).

The occasional association of IM with prolonged symptoms of fatigue has prompted evaluation of EBV infection's possible role in so-called chronic fatigue syndrome (CFS). While it has been found that most patients with this syndrome test positive for EBV antibodies, the same can be said for the vast majority of the population. There is, in fact, no objective evidence that EBV infection is a causative factor for CFS (15).

In general, it appears that the more insidious the development of symptoms, the longer the course of clinical IM is likely to be. The number of days that elapse between symptom onset and establishment of a firm diagnosis of IM seems to correlate directly with the total duration of symptoms to be expected (8). A predominance of gastrointestinal symptoms, which usually correlates with delayed diagnosis, may also herald a prolonged course. Other than these factors, nothing, including extent or seriousness of clinical symptoms, degree of physical signs such as adenopathy or splenomegaly, or magnitude of laboratory abnormality, correlates significantly with a protracted course.

TREATMENT

The treatment of IM is basically supportive. It is important to maintain adequate hydration, even in the face of painful dysphagia caused by pharyngitis. Intravenous fluids, such as lactated Ringer's solution or saline in dextrose, can be administered during the most symptomatic periods and may hasten clinical improvement. Saline gargles or pharyngeal irrigations may provide some symptomatic relief; in my experience harsh chemical gargles are best avoided. Analgesics such as acetaminophen or a nonsteroidal anti-inflammatory will usually suffice for pain and fever control. Codeine may be added for severe pain. Because of the potential for Reye's syndrome and the possibility of adding to the platelet dysfunction that is often associated with IM, aspirin should be avoided. Local anesthetics, such as viscous lidocaine, may be used to decrease pharyngeal pain and, when used before attempting meals, may assist in maintaining hydration and nutrition. Some would recommend the use of stool softeners, particularly if the spleen is clinically enlarged, in an attempt to reduce straining with defecation and the theoretical risk of splenic rupture that increased intra-abdominal pressure may pose.

Rest is appropriate as necessary, but there is no reason to enforce bed rest for IM. In fact, prolonged bed rest, which is known to cause deconditioning, has been associated with prolonged recovery time in IM patients (13).

Antibiotics are indicated only for specific infections by sensitive organisms. The most common of these is GABHS infection, which should be cultured for in all cases of significant pharyngitis and treated when found. Prophylactic antibiotic administration is not appropriate. As was mentioned earlier, the use of ampicillin or amoxicillin in patients with IM will almost certainly cause an impressive, but not clinically serious, rash.

TABLE 18–2. *Possible indications for corticosteroid use in infectious mononucleosis*

Impending airway obstruction
Severe pharyngitis interfering with hydration
Hematologic complications (thrombocytopenia, hemolytic anemia)
Neurologic complications
Myocarditis
Severe splenomegaly
Severe or long-lasting hepatitis
Severe systemic symptoms: fever, malaise, pharyngitis, etc.

The question of whether or not to employ corticosteroid therapy is an important one. There are very little good data to either support or discourage use of these agents. Some clinicians, probably only a minority, use corticosteroids quite liberally, citing observations of early improvement coupled with essentially no side effects resulting from a short course of therapy (16). Others are much more conservative, restricting the use of corticosteroids to very precise and limited indications, on the grounds that their use may adversely affect immune function and the response of the body to EBV, with unknown and potentially adverse short- or long-term consequences (8). One placebo-controlled, double-blind study on the use of corticosteroids in IM showed an improvement in symptoms in the first week that was, however, not statistically significant (17).

A list of possible indications for corticosteroid use appears in Table 18–2; the order reflects my prejudice as to the relative validity of the proposed application and my clinical practice. If the decision is made to use corticosteroids, prednisone is appropriate, with a dosage starting at 40–80 mg per day in one or two doses, or the equivalent, and tapering to discontinuation over 10–12 days. Therapy can be initiated with a parenteral corticosteroid if oral administration is too uncomfortable.

Although acyclovir has been shown to reduce EBV replication and shedding in IM patients, actual clinical benefit appears to be slight, if any (18).

COMPLICATIONS

Although IM is usually a self-limited illness which resolves over about 3 weeks, significant complications do occur. These are listed in Table 18–3. Fortunately, the incidence of such complications is rare, and most will resolve without permanent sequelae if the patient receives prompt and appropriate supportive care.

Splenic rupture is the most feared complication but is rare, occurring only in about 0.1% of cases, most commonly within the first 3 weeks of illness (19). It

TABLE 18-3. *Complications associated with infectious mononucleosis*

Splenic rupture
Otolaryngologic: airway obstruction, coincident GABHS infection, peritonsillar abscess
Hematologic: autoimmune hemolytic anemia, severe thrombocytopenia, granulocytopenia, aplastic anemia
Neurologic: Guillain-Barre syndrome, encephalitis, aseptic meningitis, transverse myelitis, optic neuritis, peripheral neuropathies, seizures
Hepatic: severe hepatitis, hepatic necrosis
Cardiac: nonspecific ECG changes, myocarditis, pericarditis
Dermatologic: urticaria, erythema multiforme
Respiratory: pneumonia
Genitourinary: glomerulonephritis, orchitis

usually occurs spontaneously, although it may also be associated with activity or trauma. The apparent severity of the IM bears no relationship to the risk of splenic rupture. The involved spleen is usually 2–3 times normal size, but rupture may occur in spleens that are not thought to be clinically enlarged. It seems logical that spleen rupture would occur while the organ is rapidly enlarging, since the profuse lymphocytic infiltration that characterizes this phase stretches and weakens the capsule and trabeculae (20). Conversely, one would expect that once enlargement ceases and return to normal size begins, the risk of rupture would decrease quickly. Activities that increase intra-abdominal pressure, such as straining at stool or arising from a bed or chair, have been implicated in causation of rupture, as have episodes of direct trauma, including palpation by an examining physician (14).

The most important symptom of splenic rupture is the sudden onset of abdominal pain in an IM patient, usually localized, at least initially, in the left upper quadrant. Since abdominal pain is an unusual feature of IM, its occurrence should raise suspicion of this complication (21). Pain may radiate to the left shoulder (Kehr's sign) because of irritation of the diaphragm by blood. Signs of hypovolemia and shock usually follow. Following splenic rupture, the peripheral blood smear may show leukocytosis with neutrophilia, a distinctly unusual finding in uncomplicated IM. Imaging studies, most commonly ultrasound, will usually demonstrate the problem definitively.

For the athlete urgent splenectomy is the appropriate and definitive therapy for splenic rupture. Nonoperative treatment has been studied (22,23), but its use requires very careful patient selection and follow-up and would delay return to athletic activity for up to 6 months in contrast to the usual return to full activity 4–8 weeks following splenectomy (24). There is the possibility of increased susceptibility to septicemia after splenectomy; it is most common in children, and the risk is thought to be quite small for adults in the absence of coexisting hematologic disease (25). Nevertheless, it is important to consider immunization of the splenectomized athlete against pneumococcal, Hemophilus and meningococcal disease.

Otolaryngologic complications usually relate to airway embarrassment caused by tonsillar and lymphoid tissue hypertrophy. This is the prime indication for corticosteroid therapy, which is almost always dramatically effective. Emergent tonsillectomy has been used successfully in some cases (26), as has nasotracheal intubation or tracheostomy, but these interventions are rarely necessary. Peritonsillar abscess has been attributed to use of corticosteroid therapy but probably is a complication that is related directly to the IM disease process (27).

Significant hematologic complications in IM are rare, although transient mild thrombocytopenia and neutropenia are not uncommon. Autoimmune hemolytic anemia due to anti-"i" cold agglutinins has been described, as have cases of severe granulocytopenia, thrombocytopenia, and even aplastic anemia. These usually occur late in the course, after the first 3 weeks, and usually respond to corticosteroid therapy (3). Intravenous immune globulin has been suggested for severe thrombocytopenia also (28). Anemia is so uncommon in IM that its occurrence should cause the clinician to think of occult hemorrhage or hemolysis.

Neurologic complications, occurring in 1–2% of cases, are the most common cause of mortality in IM and may be the patient's presenting complaint. Mortality has chiefly been due to Guillain-Barre syndrome with associated respiratory failure or to meningoencephalitis (8). Although a large number of neurologic syndromes have been associated with IM, the prognosis for most is excellent, provided that careful attention to supportive care is maintained.

Almost all patients with IM have demonstrable abnormalities in liver function that are transient, but severe hepatitis or hepatic necrosis has, on occasion, been encountered. It is usually considered an indication for corticosteroid therapy, but some authorities have advised caution with such treatment, noting that in other viral hepatitises corticosteroids may produce a "biochemical whitewash" in which host factors that limit the virus are depressed by the treatment, so that while the laboratory test results seem to improve, actual healing is delayed (8).

Other complications, including cardiac, renal, dermatologic, and respiratory manifestations, are very rare. Nonspecific electrocardiographic abnormalities are seen in up to 25% of patients, but myocarditis and pericarditis are uncommon. Although pneumonia is not infrequent, it is almost always due to aspiration, probably as a result of the disordered pharyngeal mechanics caused by severe inflammation.

CONSIDERATIONS RELATED TO ATHLETES

Is the Course of IM Different in Athletes Than in Nonathletes?

As in many other illnesses or injuries, an athlete's motivation to return to training or competition may accelerate symptomatic improvement after IM. One might speculate that a more fit person would recover more quickly from a disease episode than a less fit individual. One study suggested that IM patients who are allowed activity as desired during the illness improved more rapidly than those kept at bed rest while symptomatic. The same study also hinted that a group of athletes in training at the onset of the disease recovered more rapidly than other students, but the finding was not thought to be significant because of the small sample size (13).

A comparison of two prospective studies (1,2,14) of IM occurring in undergraduate college students is of interest. In these studies, which followed IM seroconversion rates, the ratio of symptomatic to subclinical cases of EBV infection was higher in Yale students (3:1) than in presumably more active West Point cadets (1:3). Does this indicate that well-trained athletes may be relatively resistant to clinical IM, compared to their more sedentary contemporaries?

There does not appear to be any indication that exercise, carried on within self-limits, adversely affects the course of IM. Similarly, there is no evidence that severe or life-threatening complications (with the possible exception of splenic rupture) are either triggered by exercise or more common in those who exercise as tolerated during and after the symptomatic phase of the disease.

Return-to-Play Decisions

The decision as to when to allow an ill or injured athlete to return to training or competition is a multifaceted and often very perplexing one. With IM it is especially difficult because there may be excellent reasons to continue limitation of activity, at least for contact or collision sports, for a considerable period of time after the athlete feels fully recovered.

Contagion is not an issue in deciding whether the athlete is ready for return, despite the fact that recovering IM patients may shed EBV for months, because transmissibility is very low and most of the population that the athlete will encounter is probably already immune to the disease (29).

Viral illnesses, which may include IM, have documented effects on physical performance (29). Muscle strength decrements lasting for some weeks have been demonstrated in convalescing subjects. This may lead to not only diminished performance upon return, but also an increased risk of musculoskeletal injury. Decreases in inspiratory and expiratory airflow rates in subjects who are free of reactive airway disease but recovering from viral illness have also been documented. Acute febrile illness may increase the risk of heat injury during exercise.

Concern about the potential for splenic rupture prompts most concerns about returning the athlete to activity following IM. It is important to remember that a palpable spleen is significantly enlarged but that a nonpalpable spleen may also be significantly enlarged. Rupture may occur in the absence of palpable enlargement and almost always happens within the first 3 weeks of illness, usually spontaneously.

In view of the foregoing, my customary protocol for returning an athlete to training and competition following IM is as presented in Table 18–4. This seems to be an appropriate compromise between absolute safety and avoidance of excessive restriction. It is important that when the athlete returns to activity, the athlete, coaches, and trainers understand the potential dangers involved, particularly the symptoms of splenic rupture, and be prepared to take appropriate action should those symptoms appear. In general, the duration of significant systemic symptoms can guide the rate of return to full activity. Athletes with illness of longer duration should be returned to full function more gradually and over a more prolonged period of time. Obviously, following recovery from IM, more caution is necessary in returning an athlete to contact or collision sports than to sports with a lower risk of direct trauma.

TABLE 18–4. *Returning the athlete to activity after infectious mononucleosis*

1. Confirm the diagnosis (heterophil or EBV-specific antibodies).
2. Bed rest only if and as long as athlete desires.
3. Recall that spleen rupture almost always occurs within the first 3 weeks; use relative restriction during that time.
4. After 3 full weeks, athlete may return to activity if:
   a. feels fine and has no complaints
   b. general clinical examination normal
   c. labs (blood counts, liver functions), if done, are improving
   d. splenomegaly is absent
      - by US (≤13.0 cm) through fourth week
      - clinical exam sufficient after 4 full weeks
5. Impose demand gradually upon return, limiting to approximately 50% intensity in first week, monitoring athlete's objective and subjective responses, and increasing as tolerated thereafter.

REFERENCES

1. Hallee TJ, Evans AS, Neiderman JC, et al. Infectious mononucleosis at the United States Military Academy: a prospective study of a single class over four years. *Yale J Biol Med* 3:182, 1974.
2. Sawyer RN, Evans AS, Niederman JC, et al. Prospective studies

of a group of Yale University freshmen: I. Occurrence of infectious mononucleosis. *J Infect Dis* 1971;23:263.
3. Maki DG, Reich RM. Infectious mononucleosis in the athlete. *Am J Sports Med* 1982;10(3):162.
4. Eichner ER. Infectious mononucleosis: recognition and management in athletes. *Phys Sportsmed* 1987;1;5(12):61.
5. Dommerby H, Strangerup SE, Strangerup M, et al. Hepatosplenomegaly in infectious mononucleosis, assessed by ultrasonic scanning. *J Laryngol Otol* 1986;100:573–579.
6. Levy M. Role of viral infections in the induction of adverse drug reactions. *Drug Saf* 1997;16(1):1–8.
7. Decker GR, Berberian BJ, Sulica VI. Periorbital and eyelid edema: the initial manifestation of acute infectious mononucleosis. *Cutis* 1991;47(5):323–324.
8. Chetham MM, Roberts KB. Infectious mononucleosis in adolescents. *Pediatr Ann* 1991;20(4):206–213.
9. Gray JJ, Caldwell J, Sillis M. The rapid serological diagnosis of infectious mononucleosis. *J Infect* 1992;25(1):39–46.
10. Eichner ER. Infectious mononucleosis: recognizing the condition, reactivating the patient. *Phys Sportsmed* 1996;2;4(4):49.
11. Rogues AM, Duponn M, Cales V, et al. Spontaneous splenic rupture: an uncommon complication of cytomegalovirus infection. *J Infect* 1994;29(1):83–85.
12. Evans AS. Infectious mononucleosis in university (Wisconsin) students. *Am J Hygiene* 1961;71:342–362.
13. Dalrymple W. Infectious mononucleosis: 2. Relation of bed rest and activity to prognosis. *Postgrad Med* 1964;35(4):345–349.
14. Sevier TL. Infectious disease in athletes. *Med Clin North Am* 1994;78(2):389–412.
15. Bailey RE. Diagnosis and treatment of infectious mononucleosis. *Am Fam Physician* 1994;49(4):879–888.
16. Ryan AJ, Evans AS, Hoagland RJ, et al. Infectious mononucleosis in athletes, round table. *Phys Sportsmed* 1978;6(2):41.
17. Collins M, Fleischer G, Kreisberg J, et al. Role of steroids in the treatment of infectious mononucleosis in the ambulatory college student. *J Am Coll Health* 1984;33(12):101–105.
18. Andersson J, Britton S, Ernberg I, et al. Effect of acyclovir on infectious mononucleosis: a double-blind, placebo-controlled study. *J Infect Dis* 1986;153:283–290.
19. Haines JD. When to resume sports after infectious mononucleosis. *Postgrad Med* 1987;81(1):331–333.
20. Ali J. Spontaneous rupture of the spleen in patients with infectious mononucleosis. *Can J Surg* 1993;36(1):49–52.
21. Birkinshaw R, Saab M, Gray A. Spontaneous splenic rupture: an unusual cause of hypovolemia. *J Accid Emerg Med* 1996;13(4):289–291.
22. Guth AA, Pachter HL, Jacobowitz GR. Rupture of the pathologic spleen: is there a role for nonoperative therapy? *J Trauma* 1996;41(2):214–218.
23. Schuler JG, Filtzer H. Spontaneous splenic rupture: the role of nonoperative management. *Arch Surg* 1995;130(6):662–665.
24. Farley DR, Zietlow SP, Bannon MP, et al. Spontaneous rupture of the spleen due to infectious mononucleosis. *Mayo Clin Proc* 1992;67(9):846–853.
25. Gordon MK, Rietveld JA, Frizelle FA. The management of splenic rupture in infectious mononucleosis. *Aust N Z J Surg* 1995;65(4):247–250.
26. Stevenson DS, Webster G, Stewart IA. Acute tonsillectomy in the management of infectious mononucleosis. *J Laryngol Otol* 1992;106(11):989–991.
27. Ganzel TM, Goldman JL, Padhya TA. Otolaryngologic clinical patterns in pediatric infectious mononucleosis. *Am J Otolaryngol* 1996;17(6):397–400.
28. Cyran EM, Rowe JM, Bloom RE. Intravenous gammaglobulin treatment for immune thrombocytopenia associated with infectious mononucleosis. *Am J Hematol* 1991;38(2):124–129.
29. Noffsinger J. Physical activity considerations in children and adolescents with viral infections. *Pediatr Ann* 1996;25(10):585–589.

CHAPTER 19

Blood-Borne Pathogens in Sports

Christopher McGrew

Blood-borne pathogens are defined as disease-causing microorganisms that can be transmitted through blood contact. Many have been identified, but the focus in sports medicine is on the human immunodeficiency virus (HIV) and hepatitis B virus (HBV). This chapter discusses current practical issues involving primarily these two diseases. There is also a brief discussion of hepatitis C, although its relevance in athletics is not clear at this time.

There are 40,000–50,000 new HIV infections diagnosed each year in the United States, and nearly 100% of these patients become chronically infected. HIV infects millions of individuals worldwide, the highest numbers being in Africa, the United States, and Asia. In 1996 approximately 40,000 HIV-related deaths occurred in the United States (1). Since 1995 (when there were approximately 50,000 deaths) the mortality rate has been steadily declining.

Approximately 300,000 new cases of HBV are diagnosed each year in the United States, and 5–10% of these patients become chronically infected. Currently, there are approximately 1 million to 1.5 million chronic HBV carriers in the United States. An estimated 5,000–10,000 deaths annually are attributed to HBV (2).

Both HIV and HBV are transmitted through sexual contact, parenteral exposure to blood and blood components, contamination of infected blood into open wounds or mucous membranes, and perinatally from an infected mother to fetus or infant.

In the general population, as in health care, HBV is transmitted far more readily than HIV. This may be due to several factors. Blood contains only hundreds to thousands of infectious particles of HIV per milliliter, in contrast to hundreds of millions of particles of HBV.

C. McGrew: Department of Orthopaedics and Rehabilitation, University of New Mexico, Albuquerque, New Mexico 87131-5296.

HIV is less durable than HBV in its resistance to inactivation by drying or exposure to air. Both viruses are inactivated by a variety of chemicals. In the case of HBV the chronic carrier who is E-antigen positive represents the greatest concern for transmission. There is no evidence of transmission via other routes, such as aerosol or casual household contact. Tears, sweat, saliva, and sputum and respiratory droplets have not been implicated in infection transmission; therefore blood becomes the pertinent topic for discussion in athletics.

The overwhelming majority of new infections for both HIV and HBV in the total U.S. population come from the well-recognized routes of sexual intercourse and sharing of intravenous needles.

Approximately 150,000 new cases of hepatitis C (HCV) infection are diagnosed each year in the United States, and 50–75% of these patients become chronically infected (3). Data from 1995 suggest that there are approximately 3.5 million chronic HCV carriers in the United States (4). Information on transmission remains incomplete for HCV. Some similarities exist with HBV. HCV is probably transmitted by exposure to blood and blood components, but whether transmission occurs through other routes remains unclear. Blood transfusion and needle sharing among intravenous drug users efficiently transmit the virus, but transmission rarely arises from occupational exposure in the health care setting. (5).

Transmission of HIV during sporting activity has not been validly documented. One alleged case of HIV transmission supposedly occurred in 1990 between soccer players in Italy (6). This case lacks sufficient documentation to be considered a true case of transmission through athletic activity (7). There has been one valid report (based on epidemiologic documentation) of transmission of HBV during sports. This involved a group of high school-aged sumo wrestlers in Japan, and it was reported in 1982 (8). No reports of HCV transmission during sports have emerged.

The risk of transmission in the sports arena has

been investigated for HIV in only a few circumstances, American football receiving the most attention. Initially, the risk of transmission on the football field in both the National Football League and National Collegiate Athletic Association (NCAA) had been conservatively estimated at a rate of less than one transmission per million games (9,10). These risk estimates were based on the prevalence of HIV in players, the number of significant bleeding incidents per game, and the transmission rate in health care settings for needle sticks with typical hollow-bore needles. However, typical blood exposures in American football and in other athletic events involve superficial blood spattering on intact or nonintact skin or mucous membrane. Blood spattering is not comparable to deep needle sticks, and therefore one would expect that these estimates, although representing a minute chance of transmission, actually overestimate the true risk. In a different study using a set of data involving a lower transmission risk, Brown and colleagues reported a different way of calculating potential risk that estimated a transmission rate of less than one per 85 million game contacts (11). No published estimates are available for potential HBV transmission in the athletic arena. By extrapolating from the HIV estimates previously mentioned, one can substitute the risk of transmission by parenteral exposure of HBV in the health care setting (approximately 15–30%) into the calculations that were used in estimating the potential for HIV transmission. This is compared to HIV transmission rate at 0.3% by parenteral exposure. This extrapolation rate yields a rate that is 20–100 times greater for HBV than for HIV. Therefore the chance is of 1 HBV infection transmitted for every 10,000–50,000 games. When the lower risk formula reported by Brown and colleagues is used, extrapolation of HBV data gives an estimate of one transmission in 850,000 to 4.25 million game contacts. Again, it should be noted that using parenteral route transmission rates overestimates the potential for infections in the athletic arena. A more realistic rate would be calculated by using data for transmission via mucocutaneous exposure (12).

It is not known how many athletes infected with HIV are participating in organized sports. A 1993 survey of athletic trainers at NCAA institutions revealed that there were 12 schools that had athletes with AIDS/HIV infection, but only in four of those institutions were the athletes participating in intercollegiate sports (13). Other than this information from the NCAA, there are no published reports of the prevalence of HIV in the athletic population.

In general terms, patients with HIV and/or HBV infection usually have years of good health during which they may need guidance on many issues, including sports participation. Regular moderate exercise is beneficial to the general health of the HIV-infected athlete. Exercise can be continued throughout the course of the disease, and it plays an important role in disease management while also improving the quality of life (14). Unfortunately, there are no data concerning the effects of high-intensity training competition at an elite level. Studies of the effects of exercise on the immune system in the general population have shown mixed results. Regular exercise may be protective against certain upper respiratory infections and improve certain immune system parameters; on the other hand, overtraining may increase the susceptibility of certain groups of athletes to upper respiratory tract infections. There is no evidence in the HIV-infected population that overtraining increases the susceptibility to the characteristic opportunistic infections.

The first priority in the HIV-infected athlete is to ensure that he or she comes under the care of a physician who is knowledgeable in the rapidly changing area of management of HIV infection as well as the demands of exercise in sports competition. Variables to consider in deciding on the level of continued athletic participation or competition include the athlete's current state of health and the status of the HIV infection, the nature and intensity of the HIV infection, the athlete's current drug regimen, and the potential contribution of stress from athletic competition.

Calabrese and LaPierre have suggested the following empirical guidelines to participation competition (14):

1. Before initiating a new exercise program, a complete physical exam is advisable.
2. Healthy asymptomatic athletes may continue in competition exercise without restriction but should avoid overtraining.
3. Athletes with AIDS-related complex may continue to train but not exhaustively and not for competition.
4. Athletes with frank AIDS may remain physically active and continue training on a symptom-related basis but should avoid strenuous exercise and reduce or stop training during acute illness.

In general, acute HBV infections may be viewed like any other viral infection. Decisions about exercise are made according to clinical signs and symptoms such as fatigue, fever, or organomegaly. There is no evidence that intense training is harmful to the asymptomatic HBV-infected patient, in either the acute or the chronic stage. In the presence of clinical manifestations (signs, symptoms, or laboratory evidence of organ impairment) activities should be curtailed to reduce the duration, intensity, and frequency of exercise (15,16).

Much of the research on exercise and HIV has focused on CD4 (lymphocyte) levels, which appear to increase with exercise (17). Viral load (quantitative measurement of HIV RNA) gives an indication of the amount of current viral activity and has been shown to correlate with disease progression. Research is needed to determine the usefulness of this lab test in evaluating the effective exercise on the HIV-infected athlete.

The consensus of published guidelines suggests that athletes do not require routine tests for blood-borne pathogens (18–22). The two main points underlining the rationale for this consensus of recommendations are as follows:

1. From a public health standpoint, testing would have to be justified as to its likelihood of preventing transmission on the athletic field. As was previously discussed, the likelihood of transmission is infinitesimally small in the athletic arena. Therefore it is impossible to show how testing would prevent disease.

2. The frequency of testing would be indefinite. For example, an athlete with a negative test before the season would not be guaranteed of having a negative test 6 weeks later, given the lag time for positive tests for blood-borne pathogens.

Voluntary testing of athletes should always be encouraged and offered for both active and nonactive athletes, as well as the general population. Those who have risk factors, such as a history of multiple sex partners, sexual contact with high-risk individuals, sexually transmitted diseases, intravenous drug abuse, or blood transfusion before 1985 deserve testing and education primarily to deal with personal health issues, not necessarily because of their risk to other competitors.

Blood-borne pathogen education for the athlete should be first emphasized safe behavior off the field, as this is where the risk is greatest. The sports medicine provider has an ample opportunity to work with the younger age population, such as adolescents and young adults, which is one of the fastest-growing groups of blood-borne pathogen-infected individuals. Many of the routine interactions with this group, including preparticipation physicals, sporting event coverage, and office evaluation of injuries provide opportunities for education.

It is important for sports medicine providers to dispel any misconceptions about the risk on the athletic field and to emphasize that there are more realistic dangers, such as sharing needles when using illicit ergogenic substances as well as unprotected intercourse.

Responsibilities of the athletic health care team include typical hygiene issues and infection control measures. In athletic health care, as elsewhere, good hygiene practices make good sense from a public health standpoint. The following guidelines arise from modifications of universal precautions and body substance isolation protocols (20):

1. Pre-event preparation includes proper care for existing wounds, abrasions, cuts, or weeping wounds that may serve as a source of bleeding are as important an entry for blood-borne pathogens. These wounds should be covered with an inclusive dressing that will withstand the demands of competition. Likewise, care providers with any healing wounds or dermatitis should have these areas adequately covered to prevent transmission to or from a participant. Athletes may be advised to wear more protective equipment to protect high-risk areas such as elbows and hands.

2. The necessary equipment and/or supplies important for compliance with universal precautions should be available for caregivers. These supplies include appropriate gloves, disinfectant bleach, antiseptics, designator receptacles for soiled equipment and/or uniforms, bandages and/or dressings, and a container for appropriate disposal of needles, syringes, or scalpels.

3. When an athlete is bleeding, the bleeding must be stopped, and the open wound must be covered with a dressing sturdy enough to withstand the demands of activity before the athlete may continue participation in practice or competition. Immediate aggressive treatment of open wounds or skin lesions that are deemed to have potential risk for transmissions of disease is imperative. Participants with active bleeding should be removed from the event as soon as is practical. Return to play is determined by appropriate medical staff personnel. Any participant whose uniform is saturated with blood, regardless of the source, must have that uniform evaluated by appropriate medical personnel for potential infectivity and change, if necessary, before returning to participation.

4. During an event early recognition of uncontrolled bleeding is the responsibility of the officials, athletes, coaches, and medical personnel. In particular, athletes should be aware of their responsibilities to report a bleeding wound to the proper personnel.

5. Personnel managing an acute blood exposure must follow the guidelines for universal precautions. Sterile latex gloves should be worn for direct contact with blood or body fluids containing blood. Gloves should be changed after treating each individual participant, and after glove removal hands should be washed.

6. Any surface that is contaminated with spilled blood should be cleaned in accordance with the following procedures. With gloves on, the spill should be contained in as small an area as possible. After blood is removed, the surface area should be cleaned with an appropriate decontaminate.

7. Proper disposal procedures should be practiced to prevent injuries caused by needles, scalpels, and other sharp instruments or devices.

8. After each practice or game any equipment or uniforms that are soiled with blood should be handled and laundered in accordance with the hygienic methods that are normally used for treatment of any soiled equipment or clothing before subsequent use.

9. All personnel involved with sports should be trained in these infection control measures

REFERENCES

1. *MMWR* 1997 Feb 28;46(8):165–169.
2. Protection against viral hepatitis: recommendations of the Immunization Practices Advisory Committee (ACIP). *MMWR* 1990 Feb 9;39(RR-2):1–26.
3. Dolan PJ, Skiba RM, Pagen RC, Kilgore WR III. Hepatitis C: prevention and treatment. *Am Fam Physician* 1991;43(4):1347–1360.
4. Gumber SC, Chopra S. Hepatitis C: a multi-faceted disease. Review of extra hepatic manifestations. *Ann Intern Med* 1995;123:615–620.
5. Wormser G, Forseter G, Jowene C, et al. Hepatitis C infection in the health care setting: 1. Low risk from parenteral exposure to blood of human immunodeficiency virus adaptations. *Am J Infect Control.* 1991;12:237–242.
6. Torre D, et al. Transmission of HIV via sports injury. *Lancet* 1990;335:1105.
7. Goldsmith M. When sports and HIV share the bill smart money goes on common sense. *JAMA* 1992;267:1311–1314.
8. Kashiwagi S. Outbreak of hepatitis B in members of a high school sumo wrestling club. *JAMA* 1982;1248:213–214.
9. Dick R, Worthman A. Frequency of bleeding and HIV transmission in intercollegiate athletics. *Med Sci Sports Exerc* 1995;5(Suppl.):S13.
10. Brown L, Drotman P. What is the risk of HIV infection in athletic competition? (Abstract). Ninth International Conference on AIDS, June 6–11, 1993.
11. Brown L, Drotman P, Chu A, et al. Bleeding injuries in professional football: estimates of the risk of HIV transmission. *Ann Intern Med* 1995;122:271–275.
12. McGrew C. HIV and HBV in sports and medicine. Part II of III. *Sports Med Prim Care* 1995;1:35–37.
13. McGrew C, Dick R, Schniedwind K, Gikas P. Survey of NCAA institutions concerning HIV/AIDS policies and universal precautions. *Med Sci Sports Exerc* 1993;917–921.
14. Calabrese L, LaPierre D. HIV infections: exercise in athletes. *Sports Med* 1993;15:1–3.
15. Nieman D. Exercise in upper respiratory tract infection and the immune system. *Med Sci Sports Exerc* 1994;26:128–139.
16. Eichner R. Infection, immunity and exercise: what to tell patients? *Phys Sportsmedicine* 1993;1:125–135.
17. LaPerreire A, O'Hearn P, Ironson G, et al. Exercise and immune function in healthy HIV antibody positive gay males. In: *Proceedings of the 9th Annual Scientific Sessions of the Society of Behavioral Medicine,* Boston 1988:28.
18. World Health Organization International Federation of Sports Medicine. Consensus statement on AIDS in sports. Geneva, Switzerland: World Health Organization 1989.
19. Canadian Academy of Sports Medicine Task Force on Infectious Disease in sports. HIV as it relates to sports. *Clin J Sports Med* 1993;3:63–65.
20. Guideline 2H Blood-borne pathogens and intercollegiate athletics. In: *NCAA Sports Medicine Handbook,* 1997 ed. Overland Park, KS: NCAA, 1997:24–28.
21. Brown L, et al. HIV/AIDS policies in sports in the National Football League. *Med Sci Sports Exerc* 1994;26:403–407.
22. American Medical Society for Sports Medicine and American Orthopaedic Society for Sports Medicine. Physician's statement on HIV and other blood-borne pathogens in sports. *Clin J Sport Med* 1995;5:199–204.

CHAPTER 20

The Athletic Heart Syndrome

Bryan W. Smith and Mario F. Ciocca

The term *athlete's heart* refers to the multiple physiologic and morphologic adaptations that an athlete's cardiovascular system may undergo as a result of chronic physical training. Some of these adaptations produce findings on physical examination or with cardiac testing that may be confused with a pathologic process. It is important for the physician who takes care of athletes to recognize this benign condition so that the athlete who has these normal training-induced changes avoids unnecessary and expensive testing to rule out heart disease. Conversely, it is important to distinguish athlete's heart from pathologic disease and minimize the risk of sudden cardiac death. The cardiovascular health benefits that the public associates with exercise become overshadowed and questioned when an athlete dies suddenly. Although a rare event, 100 nontraumatic deaths over a ten-year period from 1983 to 1993 were attributed to cardiovascular conditions in high school and college athletes (1).

HISTORICAL PERSPECTIVE

Bergman initially described athlete's heart in animals, finding larger hearts in wild animals than in domesticated animals (2). In the later part of the nineteenth century, Henschen was the first to describe athlete's heart in humans (3). By percussion he discovered enlargement of the heart in cross-country skiers. Henschen concluded that the enlargement was physiologic and based on both dilatation and hypertrophy. His findings, though having been a source of controversy throughout this century, remain true today.

Many researchers refuted Henschen's conclusions. Dietlen and Moritz postulated that strenuous activity might result in a more rapid deterioration of the heart (4). Later, Moritz described athlete's heart as being the result of myocardial failure (5). Before the 1950s there was a general belief that the affected athlete's life expectancy was shorter than normal, although there were no data to support this claim. Contradictory statements continued until as recently as 1972, when Friedberg described athlete's heart as a consequence of overexertion in a rheumatic, syphilitic, or congenitally damaged heart (6).

In the 1930s Kirch published the first reports describing the anatomy of athlete's heart (7,8). He described asymmetric cardiac hypertrophy with enlargement of the right ventricle predominant. Heart weights were observed not to exceed 500 grams. Kirch concluded that the cardiac hypertrophy that he found was due to exercise. Twenty years later, Linzbach's histologic findings demonstrated that physiologically, hypertrophied myocardium was identical to normal myocardium (9). In addition, he concurred with Kirch that 500 grams was the critical weight limit between physiologic and pathologic hypertrophy. However, the hearts that were investigated were from moderately trained athletes. Normal heart weights probably do exceed 500 grams, especially since heart volumes of up to 1700 mL have been reported (10). However, the degree of physiologic hypertrophy is not unlimited, and establishing a critical heart weight may be a crude, rather than absolute, marker (11).

Noninvasive assessment of athlete's heart has undergone refinement over the last century. Shortly after Henschen's findings, in the early 1900s, Moritz was the first to perform radiologic investigation (12). In 1916 Rohrer applied radiography to measure cardiac volume and define cardiac enlargement (13). This was repeated independently by Kahlstorf in 1933 (14). In 1934 Moritz published his investigation on heart size based on planimetric, quantitative evaluation (5). His findings did not correspond with the findings of today and may have been due to a lack of a third radiologic dimension that

---

B. W. Smith and M. F. Ciocca: University of North Carolina at Chapel Hill, Student Health Service, Chapel Hill, North Carolina 27599-7470.

had been achieved through volume assessment (11). In 1933 a quantitative assessment of cardiac function was described by Nylin, who developed an index to describe the relationship between heart volume and stroke volume (15). In 1960 Reindell and colleagues combined spiroergometry with radiographs, which provided the initial method to differentiate physiologic from pathologic enlargement (16).

Electrocardiograms have played a minor role in the definition of athlete's heart. In 1929 Hoogerwerf was the first to provide a description of the electrocardiogram in athletes (17). Many studies followed in the 1950s and 1960s after the introduction of unipolar and precordial leads (18). Because the usual indices of left ventricular hypertrophy on electrocardiograms correlate poorly with anatomic findings in athletes, radiologic techniques remained the method to describe cardiac structure and function until echocardiograms came into use.

In 1972 Rost initiated use of echocardiography in athletes, which revolutionized noninvasive, dynamic evaluation of anatomy and function combined (19). This opened a reexamination of the physiologic adaptations that were defined as athlete's heart. Initial studies that utilized M-mode echocardiography were limited because of errors in the definition of wall thickness.

Through echocardiography Morganroth and colleagues was the first to introduce the idea that there may be cardiac adaptations in power athletes as well as endurance athletes, although later studies refuted this when taking into account the increase in body mass (20–23). They also described an increase in heart volume without an increase in wall thickness in endurance athletes (20). However, these initial results using echocardiograms were limited by the crude quality. Recent echocardiographic studies have shown an increase in wall thickness (24–34). Another early limitation of M-mode echocardiography was the poor right ventricular imaging. This resulted in echocardiographers postulating that athlete's heart was a left ventricular phenomenon only (35). As echocardiography became more sophisticated with two-dimensional viewing, Henschen's initial findings of eccentric hypertrophy in aerobic athletes as well as biventricular enlargement were confirmed (35).

PHYSIOLOGY

Changes that are seen clinically and diagnostically are secondary to the physiologic adaptations to exercise, and therefore it is important to review these. As with skeletal muscle, cardiovascular adaptations are dependent on the type of exercise—dynamic (isotonic) or static (isometric)—as well as the intensity, duration, and frequency of exercise. Simply stated, dynamic exercise involves a change in muscle length against a small change in tension, such as is seen in an aerobic activity such as endurance running. Static exercise involves little or no change in muscle length against high tension, such as is seen in weight lifting. Most exercise consists of a combination of dynamic and static exercise.

To support the metabolic demands of dynamic exercise, oxygen uptake must increase. Oxygen uptake is dependent on cardiac output and the arteriovenous oxygen difference. Therefore an increase in either or both of these parameters will cause an increase in oxygen uptake. However, cardiac output accounts for the majority of the increase in oxygen uptake (36). Cardiac output is the product of heart rate and stroke volume. Since maximal heart rate is not significantly affected by conditioning, an increase in stroke volume is mainly responsible for the concomitant increase in cardiac output. Oxygen uptake can be increased by an increase in the arteriovenous oxygen difference, which is increased by a greater oxygen extraction or increased blood flow to the working muscles. Maximal, dynamic exercise may result in a fourfold increase in cardiac output, a threefold increase in heart rate and arteriovenous oxygen difference, and a twofold increase in stroke volume from resting values (37).

A rapid increase in heart rate is the initial cardiovascular response to dynamic exercise. An increase in stroke volume occurs because of an increase in venous return from the pumping action of skeletal muscle and a decrease in intrathoracic pressure. As exercise continues, there is a progressively shorter diastolic filling time. Therefore the stroke volume increase is maintained by increased contractility and decreased end-systolic volume. Vascular responses that are found during dynamic exercise include an increase in systolic blood pressure and a decrease in diastolic blood pressure. In addition, blood is diverted from the splanchnic system to the exercising muscles and the coronary circulation.

Exercise training may cause adaptations in coronary flow and vascularity. Studies in healthy humans are limited because of the invasiveness of tests that would be required. Therefore, studies have relied mainly on laboratory animals. Exercise training may increase the coronary vascular space relative to the myocardial mass. The increase in coronary vascular space is due to both an increase in the cross-sectional area of vessels and an increase in the total number of capillaries (37).

The cardiovascular response to static exercise differs from dynamic exercise. Only modest increases in oxygen consumption and cardiac output occur. The cardiac output increase is primarily due to an increase in heart rate. During static exercise, blood flow is temporarily reduced to exercising muscle. Upon cessation of contraction there is an oxygen demand resulting in an increase in blood flow to address metabolic requirements. With these demands come transient increases in oxygen uptake and arteriovenous oxygen difference. In contrast to dynamic exercise, performance improvement in static exercise is thought to be secondary to muscle group adaptations rather than cardiovascular adaptations (38).

Alteration in cardiac structure is dependent on the type of training (dynamic versus static) and is determined by the law of Laplace (wall tension = pressure × radius ÷ [wall thickness × 2]). Theoretically, dynamic exercise produces a chronic volume overload, while static exercise produces a chronic pressure overload. Therefore when chronic volume overload occurs, there is an increase in end-diastolic dimension and a proportional increase in septal and free wall thickness to normalize stress. When chronic pressure overload occurs, the heart adapts by increasing septal and free wall thickness to normalize stress.

The time required to gain a physiologic adaptation resulting in a significant increase in maximum oxygen uptake is usually several weeks. To observe a significant training effect, the minimum duration of exercise needs to be 30–60 minutes, three to four times per week, at 60–70% of maximum oxygen uptake (38). Once training is stopped, a decrease in maximum oxygen uptake occurs rapidly over the first 2–3 weeks, followed by a gradual decrease over the next 5 weeks (39).

Morphologic changes occur quickly with initiation of training and regress after cessation of training. Left ventricular end-diastolic diameter achieves a maximum value at 1 week, left ventricular mass significantly increases after 1 week, and an increase in left ventricular posterior wall thickness is seen after 5 weeks (40). When athletes stop training, the left ventricular end-diastolic diameter starts and progressively decreases after 4 days (40). The posterior wall thickness and the left ventricular mass decrease significantly, and the reduction in left ventricular mass appears complete after 3 weeks (41). Also, with cessation of training, training-induced septal wall thickness may decrease 15–33% (42).

CLINICAL EXAMINATION

The physical examination of the athlete can be quite variable and nonspecific. However, a thorough evaluation can help to identify potential conditions associated with sudden death. In many high-performance athletes, particularly endurance athletes, an increase in parasympathetic tone may cause a resting bradycardia. Dynamic training may also cause a decrease in resting blood pressure (43). However, a widened pulse pressure should be viewed carefully, as it may be an indicator of aortic insufficiency.

A comprehensive cardiac exam is essential in athletes. Third and fourth heart sounds, usually associated with pathologic conditions, may be present in athletes and are of no clinical significance as an isolated finding (44). Palpation may reveal a left ventricular impulse that is displaced and prolonged (44). Auscultation should be performed in multiple positions or maneuvers in an attempt to bring out murmurs. Because of the increase in cardiac volume, as many as 30–50% of high-performance athletes may have a grade I–II, midsystolic murmur (44). These are benign flow murmurs and are usually heard in the supine position (owing to an increase in venous return) but often disappear on standing (45). A systolic murmur that increases with standing and valsalva and decreases with squatting has been associated with the obstructive form of hypertrophic cardiomyopathy. This is due to the hypertrophic septum further obstructing the left ventricular outflow tract with the decrease in ventricular volume.

A diastolic murmur may indicate aortic insufficiency, which could be associated with Marfan's syndrome. Additional cardiac findings in Marfan's syndrome may be a systolic click of mitral valve prolapse or frank mitral insufficiency. Physical examination should include a search for other stigmata of Marfan's. These include tall stature, long limbs, long and slender digits, pectus excavatum or carinatum, scoliosis, kyphosis, striae over shoulders or buttocks, myopia, a high arched palate, pes cavus, and hypermobility of joints (46).

ELECTROCARDIOGRAM

The electrocardiogram of athletes can differ greatly from untrained counterparts and may sometimes resemble the electrocardiogram of pathologic conditions (47) (Figs. 20–1 through 20–3). The changes are mainly attributable to aerobic training and are the result of increased vagal tone and physiologic hypertrophy (43). The most frequent finding is a resting sinus bradycardia, which can be as low as 25 beats per minute (44). Sinus pauses greater than 2 seconds are found in more than one third of athletes (48). Other rhythms that are attributable to vagal hypotonia include sinus arrhythmia, wandering atrial pacemaker (see Fig. 20–2), junctional rhythm, and first-degree (see Fig. 20–1) or transient second- or third-degree atrioventricular block. These arrhythmias should disappear with exercise (49). Third-degree atrioventricular block is rare even for athletes, and underlying heart disease should always be ruled out (48).

Another common electrocardiogram finding is high voltage in the left ventricular leads. Usually, in most young athletes this is a factor of body habitus. However, an increase in cardiac mass may be a contributing factor (49). When the Sokolow and Lyon index (R in V5 + S in V1 > 35 mm) is used to define left ventricular hypertrophy in athletes, the incidence of left ventricular hypertrophy has been reported as high as 80% (48) (see Fig. 20–2) Right ventricular hypertrophy has been reported in up to 69% of athletes using the formula of R in V1 plus S in V5 greater than 10.5 mm (48) (see Fig. 20–1).

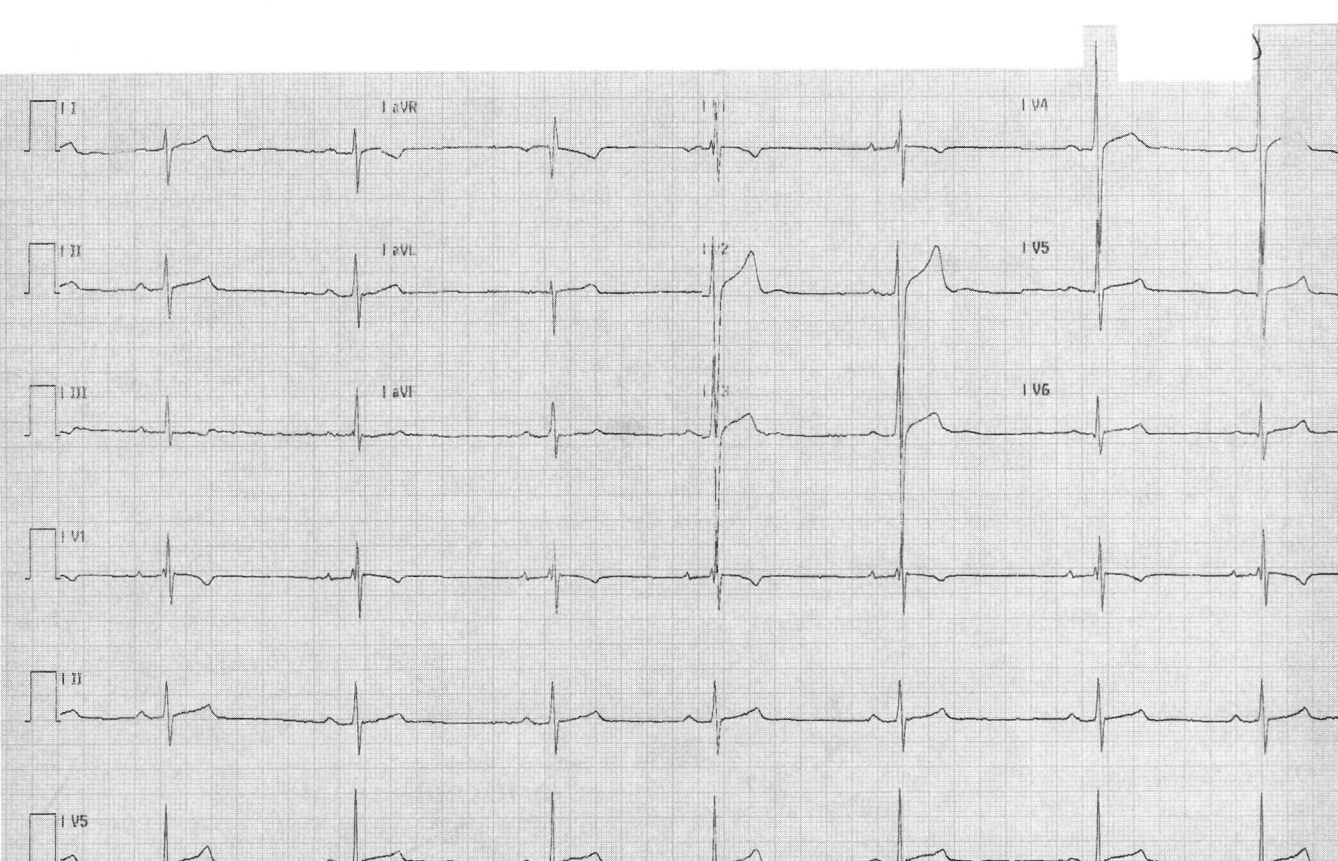

FIG. 20–1. An electrocardiogram in an asymptomatic elite collegiate basketball athlete that displays sinus bradycardia, a first-degree atrioventricular block, right ventricular hypertrophy as defined in the text, right axis deviation, and ST segment elevation in V2 through V4.

Nonspecific changes in the QRS and ST segments as well as P-wave amplitude changes have been attributed to cardiac muscle hypertrophy. Variants that are seen more frequently include a more vertical QRS axis, ST segment elevation (most prominent in V2–V4) (see Fig. 20–1), ST segment depression (less often than elevation), tall, peaked T-waves, inverted T-waves (see Fig. 20–2), biphasic T-waves, and increased P-wave amplitude and notching (44). Changes that are found less often include incomplete right bundle branch block, which appears related to increased muscle mass of the right ventricle, a longer QT interval (see Fig. 20–3), which does not correlate with ventricular arrhythmias, and prominent U-waves (43,44,48). Most of the electrocardiographic changes eventually disappear with cessation of training, and the arrhythmias disappear with exercise.

Atrial fibrillation has been reported more frequently in athletes than in the general population, but other supraventricular arrhythmias and AV node ectopic beats are not more frequent (48). A medical workup of atrial fibrillation is essential, though. A long-term holter monitor, exercise testing, and an echocardiogram are usually indicated to rule out heart disease (50).

As with atrial fibrillation, certain electrocardiographic changes should not be assumed to be secondary to athlete's heart and need to be worked up further. Conditions that are indicated for further workup are listed below, and recommendations for participation in athletic activity can be found in the 26th Bethesda Conference (50). Those with bradycardia, sinus pauses less than 3 seconds, sinus arrhythmia, wandering atrial pacemaker, or junctional rhythm do not require further workup unless they are symptomatic (50). If a sinus pause is greater than or equal to 3 seconds, then a 12-lead electrocardiogram, a 24-hour holter monitor, an exercise test, and an echocardiogram should be performed (50). No further workup of a first-degree atrioventricular block is needed if the QRS complex is normal. An exercise test, a 24-hour holter monitor, and an echocardiogram are indicated if the QRS complex is abnormal or the PR interval is greater than or equal to

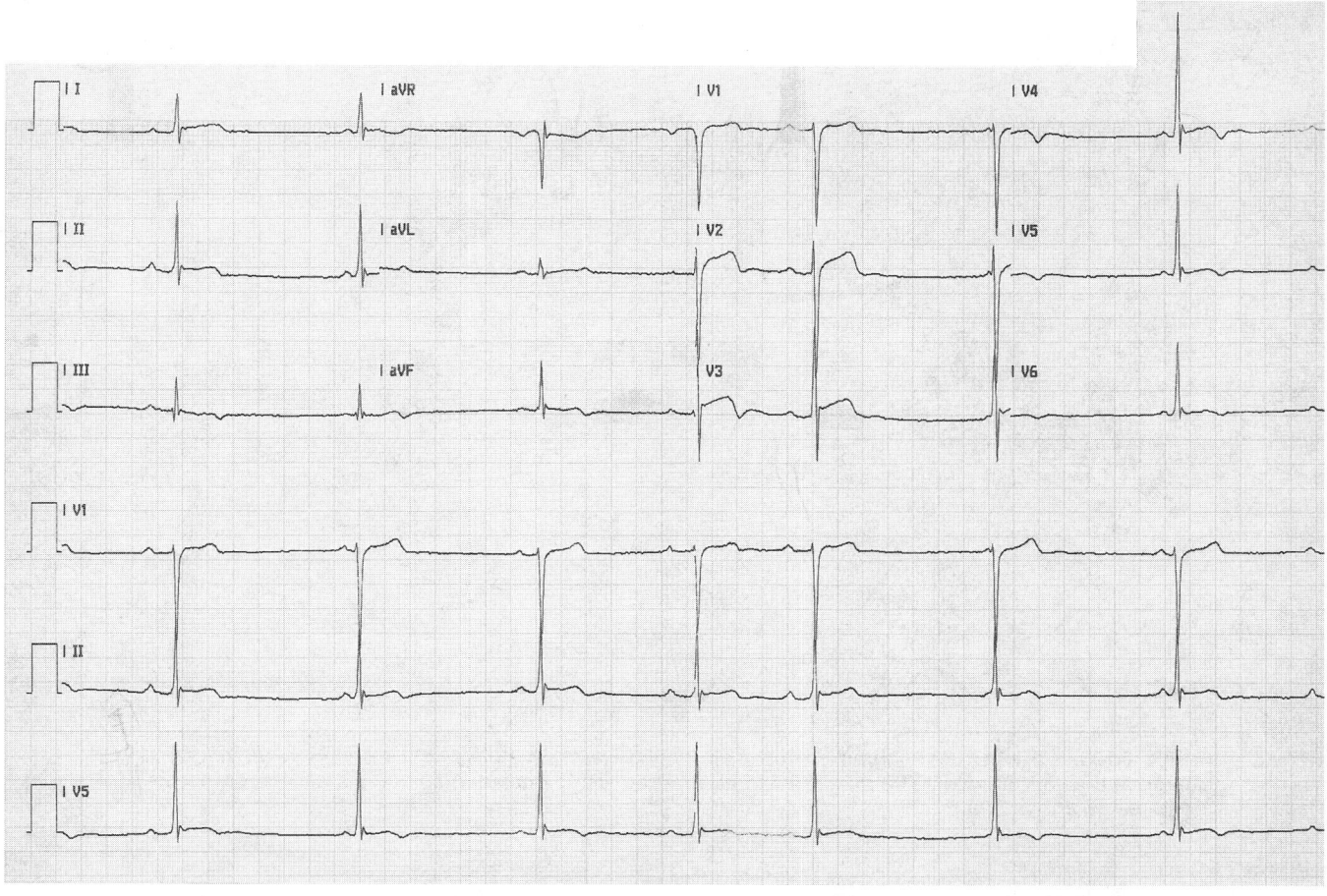

FIG. 20–2. An electrocardiogram in an asymptomatic elite collegiate basketball athlete that displays bradycardia with a wandering atrial pacemaker, left ventricular hypertrophy as defined in the text, ST segment elevation in V2 through V4, biphasic T waves, and T wave inversion.

0.3 seconds (50). The same workup is indicated for a Wenckebach atrioventricular block and a congenital complete heart block. Mobitz type 2 atrioventricular block and acquired complete heart block normally requires cardiac pacing before clearance for athletic activity (50). Those with a prolonged QT interval (QTc greater than 440–450 ms) need to be distinguished from the congenital long QT interval syndromes, as these people are at risk for sudden death with exercise (see Fig. 20–3).

There is limited research on the effects of training as they pertain to cardiac function in the adolescent and prepubertal child. However, with exercise training, male adolescents show similar electrocardiographic changes on sinus node function and atrioventricular conduction, although extreme low sinus rates are not as common as seen in adults (51). Electrocardiograms in aerobically trained, prepubertal males have not shown training-induced changes (52). This may be secondary to the limited duration and intensity of training as well as a lower catecholamine response and a lack of testosterone before puberty (52).

Female athletes may not have the same changes as male athletes. In comparison, women can have a higher heart rate, shortened conduction time, and a longer QT corrected interval (see Fig. 20–3) Other electrocardiographic differences as compared to males include a lesser degree of ST segment elevation and a decreased incidence of incomplete right bundle branch block. The increase in P, Q, and T amplitudes and indices of left, right, and septal hypertrophy are not as large (53).

ECHOCARDIOGRAPHY

With the advent of echocardiography in the early 1970s, structural changes of the heart secondary to chronic conditioning have been more adequately studied. Rost and colleagues were the first to perform an echocardiographic evaluation of athletes (19), and many studies followed (24–34). Most studies, however, have had a

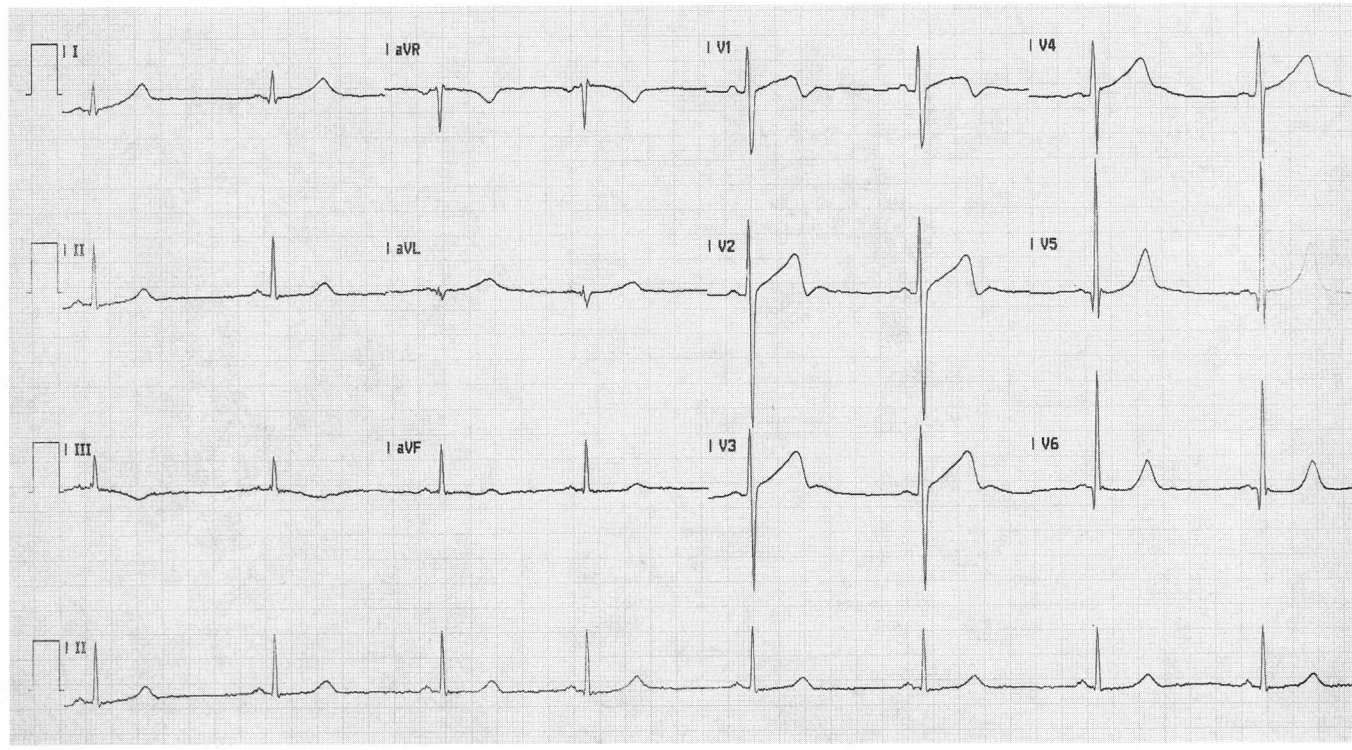

FIG. 20-3. An electrocardiogram in a female collegiate crew athlete that displays a prolonged QT interval (QTc of 500 ms). The prolongation normalized with exercise. Also seen is a sinus bradycardia with sinus arrhythmia.

small number of subjects, who were mainly male, and the data have been mostly cross-sectional (54). In addition, the values for cardiac dimensions are only slightly increased, rarely exceed normal range, and are usually within the methodological error for M-mode echocardiography (55). However, many studies achieve statistical significance and are consistent in the differences, suggesting that they are valid.

A consistently demonstrated feature in dynamic athletes is an increase in end-diastolic diameter (20,25, 26,28,30,31,34,56,57). When body surface area and weight are taken into account, diameter increase is still maintained. However, the increase in size is usually within the normal range, with an average dimension of 54 mm and usually less than 60 mm (55).

Left ventricular wall thickness increases as compensation for the increase in end-diastolic diameter. The increases in septal and posterior wall thickness are not substantial. Pelliccia and colleagues found a wall thickness greater than or equal to 13 mm in fewer than 2% of endurance athletes, and none had a thickness greater than 16 mm (33). The wall thickening is usually symmetrical, with the ratio of septal to free wall lying within the normal range (<1.3) (55). Since end-diastolic diameter and wall thickness are used to calculate mass, there is also an increase in left ventricular mass. This increase is sustained after correction for body weight and surface area. Other dimensions that are increased are the right ventricle (average increase 24%), the left atrium, and possibly the end-systolic left ventricular cavity size (54).

In contrast to the volume load that is seen with dynamic exercise, static exercise produces a pressure load that is responsible for the cardiovascular adaptations. Isometric activities can induce increases of systolic blood pressure greater than 300 mm Hg (54). Athletes training in predominantly isometric activities have an increase in left ventricular wall thickness and cardiac mass without an increase in end-diastolic diameter (28). The hypertrophy is usually mild and less than 13 mm. When corrected for body mass, the increase in mass (based on wall thickness) is normalized (21–23). When isometric and isotonic exercise are combined (as in cycling), there tends to be an increase in end-diastolic diameter with a disproportionate increase in ventricular hypertrophy (30).

Many of the earlier echocardiographic studies have been done primarily on male athletes. Recent evaluation of women reveals that similar adaptations are seen as compared to men. In a study of endurance-trained women, left ventricular end-diastolic diameter was increased and similar to changes in men (34). When corrected for body surface area, the increase in left ventricular cavity size was greater in women than in men. Left ventricular wall thickness was increased but within normal limits and was less than reported in males. No females had a wall thickness in the "gray zone" of 13–15 mm that could be confused with hypertrophic cardiomyopathy (34).

Limited research is available in evaluating cardiovascular adaptations to exercise in prepubertal children. On physical examination there have been no differences in the frequency of carotid bruit, central venous hums, heart murmur, or third or fourth heart sounds between prepubertal athletes and nonathletes (52). Similarly, electrocardiographic findings are sparse except for resting bradycardia (58). Echocardiographic data vary and range from unchanged echocardiograms in athletes to a high percentage of wall and diameter sizes above normal (52,59). This is likely due to the wide variation in skill levels, which decreases the need for optimal training to achieve success.

ATHLETE'S HEART?

Sudden cardiac death may occur in athletes who have been free of cardiovascular symptoms, thereby making it difficult to predict who will suffer a cardiac event (60). These events are rare as compared to a high percentage of athletes who will have potential abnormal findings on physical examination. When an asymptomatic athlete is found to have "abnormal" changes on examination or electrocardiogram, it is important to recognize that they may be consistent with athlete's heart and not necessarily place the athlete in the category of increased risk for sudden death. When an athlete is symptomatic, though, it is important to distinguish athlete's heart from pathologic change.

Since the most common cause of sudden death in the young athlete is hypertrophic cardiomyopathy, the following will concentrate on its distinction from athlete's heart. However, other predisposing conditions should not be forgotten. An important historical point is a family history of sudden death or hypertrophic cardiomyopathy. On physical examination obstructive hypertrophic cardiomyopathy can have a loud systolic murmur that increases with maneuvers that decrease preload. However, the nonobstructive form of hypertrophic cardiomyopathy is the more prevalent form of hypertrophic cardiomyopathy, and therefore a systolic murmur may be soft or absent. This likely explains how these individuals at risk for sudden death are not identified with the traditional screening process.

Electrocardiographic changes that may make you more suspicious for hypertrophic cardiomyopathy include voltage increases, prominent Qs, and deep negative T-waves (61). A recent study recommends performing screening electrocardiograms, but data for this are lacking and may lead to further unnecessary testing (62). Echocardiographic findings of athlete's heart can be confused with hypertrophic cardiomyopathy. The left ventricular wall thickness in athlete's heart is rarely greater than or equal to 13 mm, and the upper limit appears to be 16 mm (33). In hypertrophic cardiomyopathy the average wall thickness is 20 mm, but a few patients may have a wall thickness in the "gray zone" of 13–15 mm (61). For those that fall in this gray zone, further distinction can be made by the contour of wall thickening and the size of ventricular end-diastolic diameter. Those with hypertrophic cardiomyopathy have sharp and abrupt transitions between areas of hypertrophy, the hypertrophy is asymmetric, and the left ventricular end-diastolic dimension is usually less than 45 mm while it is greater than 55 mm in endurance athletes (61). Also, those with hypertrophic cardiomyopathy will show abnormal diastolic filling as compared to trained athletes who have normal diastolic filling (63–64). One method to distinguish the normal training effect from hypertrophic cardiomyopathy is to have the athlete undergo a deconditioning period of several weeks. Serial echocardiograms will demonstrate in time a heart with normal wall thickness in the athlete without hypertrophic cardiomyopathy (42).

SUMMARY

There are many physical examination changes that may be confusing to one who is not familiar with athlete's heart. Predominantly aerobically trained, isotonic athletes undergo an increase in cardiac cavity size, wall thickness, and heart mass. The strength-trained, isometric athletes undergo an increase in cardiac wall thickness and mass, but this is unchanged when adjusted for body mass. Electrocardiographic changes are many and are secondary to cardiac hypertrophy, increased vagal tone, and repolarization variations. Some of these changes may be indistinguishable from pathologic disease. Therefore, electrocardiograms should not be done routinely on asymptomatic athletes, as this may cause unnecessary further testing (65). Radiologic techniques have been used to assess cardiac size, volume, and function. However, two-dimensional echocardiography has allowed distinction of cardiac wall size and cavity size as well as further definition of function. Using echocardiograms, one is more likely to discriminate physiologic changes from changes associated with pathologic disease. However, the current cost of echocardiograms precludes the use of this modality as a screening tool. It has been estimated that prevention of one case of sudden death would cost approximately one billion dollars if the present technology were used as a screen (66).

A physician needs to be able to adequately screen athletes in an attempt to reduce the probability of sudden death. A thorough history and physical examination accompanied by specialized cardiac testing when appropriate should be a preparticipation examination requirement for athletic participation. It is hoped that improved technology will one day be cost-effective so as to be employed as a widespread screening tool. Until then proper recognition of the changes seen with athlete's heart allows avoidance of unnecessary testing and/or inappropriate disqualification.

REFERENCES

1. VanCamp SP, Bloor CM, Mueller FO, et al. Nontraumatic sports death in high school and college athletes. *Med Sci Sports Exerc* 1995;27:641–647.
2. Bergmann R. Uber die herzgrosse freilebender und domestizierter tiere. Inaugural dissertation, Munchen, 1884 (cited by Rost).
3. Henschen S. Skilanglauf und skiwettlauf: eine medizinische sportstudie. *Mitt Med Klin Upsala (Jena)*, 1899 (cited by Rost).
4. Dietlen H, Moritz F. Uber das verhalten des herzens nach langundauerndem und anstrengendem radfahren. *Munch Med Wochenschr* 1908;55:489 (cited by Rost).
5. Moritz F. Grosse und form des herzens bei meistern im sport. *Dtsch Arch Klin Med* 1934;176:455 (cited by Rost).
6. Friedberg C. *Erkrankungen des herzens,* 2nd ed. Stuttgart: Thieme, 1972 (cited by Rost).
7. Kirch E. Anatomische grundlagen des sportherzens. *Verh Dtsch Ges Inn Med* 1935;47:73 (cited by Rost).
8. Kirch E. Herzkraftigung und echte herzhypertrophie durch sport. *Z Krieslaufforsch* 1936;28:893 (cited by Rost).
9. Linzbach A. Struktur und funktion des gesunden und kranken herzens. In: Klepzig H, ed. *Die funktionsdiagnostik des herzens.* Berlin: Springer, 1958:94 (cited by Rost).
10. Medved R, Friedrich V. The largest athlete heart recorded in the literature. *Lijec Vjesn* 1964;86:843 (cited by Rost).
11. Rost R, Hollmann W. Athlete's heart: a review of its historical assessment and new aspects. *Int J Sports Med* 1983;4:147–165.
12. Moritz, F. Uber orthodiagraphische untersuchungen am herzen. *Med Wochenschr* 1902;49:1 (cited by Rost).
13. Rohrer F. Volumenbestimmung an korperhohlen und organen auf orthodiagraphischem wege. *Fortschr Rontgenstr* 1916;24:285 (cited by Rost).
14. Kahlstorf A. Uber korrelationen der linearen herzmasse und des herzvolumens. *Klin Wochenschr* 1933;12:262 (cited by Rost).
15. Nylin G. The relation between heart volume and cardiac output per beat as a measure of cardiac activity. *Svenska Lakartidningen* 1933;10 (cited by Rost).
16. Reindell H, Klepzig H, Steim H, et al. *Herz-krieislaufkrankheiten und sport.* Munchen: Barth, 1960 (cited by Rost).
17. Hoogerwerf S. *Electrokardiographische untersuchungen der Amsterdammer Olympiakampfer.* Berlin: Springer, 1929 (cited by Venerando).
18. Venerando A. Electrocardiography in sports medicine. *J Sports Med Phys Fitness* 1979;19:107–128.
19. Rost R, Schneiderk K, Stegmann N. Vergleichende echokardiographischen untersuchungen am herzen des leistungssportlers und des nichttrainierten. *Med Welt* 1972;23:1088 (cited by Rost).
20. Morganroth J, Maron BJ, Henry WL, et al. Comparative left ventricular dimensions in trained athletes. *Ann Intern Med* 1975;82:521–524.
21. Longhurst JC, Kelly AR, Gonyea WJ, et al. Echocardiographic left ventricular masses in distance runners and weight lifters. *J Appl Physiol* 1980;48:154–162.
22. Longhurst JC, Kelly AR, Gonyea WJ, et al. Chronic training with static and dynamic exercise: cardiovascular adaptation, and response to exercise. *Circ Res* 1981;48[Suppl I]:I171–I178.
23. Pelliccia A, Spataro A, Caselli G, et al. Absence of left ventricular wall thickening in athletes engaged in intense power training. *Am J Cardiol* 1993;72:1048–1054.
24. Roeske WR, O'Rourke RA, Klein A, et al. Noninvasive evaluation of ventricular hypertrophy in professional athletes. *Circulation* 1976;53:286–292.
25. Gilbert CA, Nutter DO, Felner JM, et al. Echocardiographic study of cardiac dimensions and function in endurance-trained athlete. *Am J Cardiol* 1977;40:528–533.
26. Cohen JL, Gupta PK, Lichstein E, et al. The heart of a dancer: noninvasive cardiac evaluation of professional ballet dancers. *Am J Cardiol* 1980;45:959–965.
27. Nishimura T, Yamada Y, Kawai C. Echocardiographic evaluation of the long-term effects of exercise on left ventricular hypertrophy and function in professional bicyclists. *Circulation* 1980;61:832–840.
28. Keul J, Dickhuth HH, Simon G, et al. Effect of static and dynamic exercise on heart volume, contractility, and left ventricular dimensions. *Circ Res* 1981;48[Supp I]: I162–I170.
29. Shapiro LM, Smith RG. Effect of training on left ventricular structure and function:. an echocardiographic study. *Br Heart J* 1983;50:534–539.
30. Fagard R, Aubert A, Staessen J, et al. Cardiac structure and function in cyclists and runners: comparative echocardiographic study. *Br Heart J* 1984;52:124–129.
31. Shapiro LM. Physiological left ventricular hypertrophy. *Br Heart J* 1984;52:130–135.
32. Douglas PS, O'Toole ML, Hiller DB, et al. Left ventricular structure and function by echocardiography in ultraendurance athletes. *Am J Cardiol* 1986;58:805–809.
33. Pelliccia A, Maron BJ, Spataro A, et al. The upper limit of physiologic cardiac hypertrophy in highly trained elite athletes. *N Engl J Med* 1991;324:295–301.
34. Pelliccia A, Maron BJ, Culasso F, et al. Athlete's heart in women: echocardiographic characterization of highly trained elite female athletes. *JAMA* 1996;276:211–215.
35. Rost R. The athlete's heart. *Cardiol Clin* 1992;10:197–207.
36. Clausen JP. Effect of physical training on cardiovascular adjustments to exercise in man. *Physiol Rev* 1977;57:779–815.
37. Schaible TF, Scheuer J. Cardiac adaptations to chronic exercise. *Prog Cardiovasc Dis* 1985;27:297–324.
38. Crawford MH. Physiologic consequences of systematic training. *Cardiol Clin* 1992;10:209–218.
39. Ehsani AA. Loss of cardiovascular adaptations after cessation of training. *Cardiol Clin* 1992;10:257–266.
40. Ehsani AA, Hagberg JM, Hickson RC. Rapid changes in left ventricular dimensions and mass in response to physical conditioning and deconditioning. *Am J Cardiol* 1978;42:52–56.
41. Martin WH III, Coyle EF, Bloomfield SA, et al. Effects of physical deconditioning after intense endurance training on left ventricular dimensions and stroke volume. *J Am Coll Cardiol* 1986;7:982–989.
42. Maron BJ, Pelliccia A, Spataro A, et al. Reduction in left ventricular wall thickness after deconditioning in highly trained Olympic athletes. *Br Heart J* 1993;69:125–128.
43. Wight JN Jr, Salem D. Sudden cardiac death and the 'athlete's heart.' *Arch Intern Med* 1995;155:1473–1480.
44. Huston TP, Puffer JC, Rodney WM. The athletic heart syndrome. *N Engl J Med* 1985;313:24–32.
45. Mills JD, Moore GE, Thompson PD. The athlete's heart. *Clin Sports Med* 1997;16:725–737.
46. Smith BW, MacKnight JM. Marfan's syndrome. In: Fields KB, Fricker PA, eds. *Medical problems in athletes,* 1st ed. Malden, MA: Blackwell Science, 1997.
47. Zeppilli P, Fenici R, Sassara M, et al. Wenckebach second-degree A-V block in top-ranking athletes: an old problem revisited. *Am Heart J* 1980;100:281–294.
48. Zehender M, Meinertz T, Keul J, et al. ECG variants and cardiac arrhythmias in athletes: clinical relevance and prognostic importance. *Am Heart J* 1990;119:1378–1391.
49. Oakley CM. The electrocardiogram in the highly trained athlete. *Cardiol Clin* 1992;10:295–302.
50. Zipes DP, Garson Jr A. Task force VI: arrhythmias. *J Am Coll Cardiol* 1994;24:892–899.
51. Viitasalo M, Kala R, Eisalo A. Ambulatory electrocardiographic findings in young athletes between 14 and 16 years of age. *Eur Heart J* 1984;5:2–6.
52. Rowland TW, Unnithan VB, MacFarlane NG, et al. Clinical manifestations of 'athlete's heart' in prepubertal male runners. *Int J Sports Med* 1994;15:515–519.
53. Storstein L, Bjornstad H, Hals O, et al. Electrocardiographic

findings according to sex in athletes and controls. *Cardiology* 1991;79:227–236.
54. Shapiro LM. Morphologic consequences of systematic training. *Cardiol Clin* 1992;10:219–226.
55. Maron BJ. Structural features of the athlete heart as defined by echocardiography. *J Am Coll Cardiol* 1986;7:190-203.
56. Fagard R, Aubert A, Lysens R, et al. Noninvasive assessment of seasonal variations in cardiac structure and function in cyclists. *Circulation* 1983;67:896–901.
57. Ikaheimo MJ, Palatsi IJ, Takkunen JT. Noninvasive evaluation of the athletic heart: sprinters versus endurance runners. *Am J Cardiol* 1979;44:24–30.
58. Rowland TW, Delaney BC, Siconolfi SF. 'Athlete's heart' in prepubertal children. *Pediatrics* 1987;79:800–804.
59. Allen HD, Goldberg SJ, Sahn DJ, et al. A quantitative echocardiographic study of champion childhood swimmers. *Circulation* 1977;55:142–145.
60. Maron BJ. Triggers for sudden cardiac death in the athlete. *Cardiol Clin* 1996;14:195–210.
61. Maron BJ, Pelliccia A, Spirito P. Cardiac disease in young trained athletes: insights into methods for distinguishing athlete's heart from structural heart disease with particular emphasis on hypertrophic cardiomyopathy. *Circulation* 1995;91:1596–1601.
62. Fuller CM, McNulty CM, Spring DA, et al. Prospective screening of 5615 high school athletes for risk of sudden cardiac death. *Med Sci Sports Exerc* 1997;29:1131–1138.
63. Granger CB, Karimeddini MK, Smith VE, et al. Rapid ventricular filling in left ventricular hypertrophy: I. Physiologic hypertrophy. *J Am Coll Cardiol* 1985;5:862–868.
64. Lewis JF, Spirito P, Pelliccia A, et al. Usefulness of doppler echocardiographic assessment of diastolic filling in distinguishing "athlete's heart" from hypertrophic cardiomyopathy. *Br Heart J* 1992;68:296–300.
65. Maron BJ, Thompson PD, Puffer JC, et al. Cardiovascular preparticipation screening of competitive athletes: a statement for health professionals from the Sudden Death Committee (clinical cardiology) and Congenital Cardiac Defects Committee (cardiovascular disease in the young), American Heart Association. *Circulation* 1996;94:850–856.
66. Feinstein RA, Colvin E, Oh MK. Echocardiographic screening as part of a preparticipation examination. *Clin J Sports Med* 1993;3:149–152.

CHAPTER 21

Exercise-Induced Anaphylaxis and Urticaria

Gregory L. Landry

INTRODUCTION AND TERMINOLOGY

There has been an increasing recognition that exercise can produce a variety of allergy syndromes. Symptoms range from mild urticaria with warmth and flushing to life-threatening laryngeal edema and vascular collapse (1–5). It is important to understand that urticaria, angioedema, and anaphylaxis are different entities that may occur separately or together in the same syndrome. *Urticaria* is the skin rash represented by localized nonpitting edema of the superficial dermis. There are usually well-circumscribed erythematous wheals that often coalesce to form larger wheals. They are almost always pruritic. *Angioedema* is well-demarcated localized edema that involves deeper layers of skin and subcutaneous tissue. *Anaphylaxis* is a life-threatening illness that usually includes upper airway distress and/or hypotension in previously sensitized individuals. Anaphylaxis may occur with or without urticaria or angioedema. *Exercise-induced anaphylaxis* (EIAna) describes a syndrome of large (10- to 15-mm) urticaria, choking, stridor, and sometimes syncope occurring during exercise. At least half of the patients with EIAna are symptomatic with exercise only after ingestion of a specific food. These patients are said to have food-dependent EIAna (Table 21-1). *Exercise-induced urticaria* (EIU) is usually synonymous with *cholinergic urticaria* (CU). CU is the production of small 2- to 4-mm hives with exercise or any activity that warms the body. It is usually not associated with any systemic symptoms. In the unusual case in which CU is associated with respiratory distress and/or hypotension, the diagnosis is *variant EIAna*. EIAna and EIU are often described in the literature as allergic syndromes distinct from *exercise-induced asthma* (EIA), which is manifested by bronchospasm without skin manifestations. In practice, there is considerable overlap between these entities, and exercise may trigger one or a combination of any of these entities. The medical practitioner's recognition of symptoms that are compatible with the diagnosis of EIAna is important because it is associated with hypotension and shock and can be life threatening.

About 40% of patients with EIAna will have classic type EIAna, 50–60% will have what is described as food-dependent EIAna, and 10% or less will have variant EIAna. CU and EIAna are sometimes called forms of the physical urticarias because they are induced by physical environmental changes, even though hives do not occur in EIAna 100% of the time. About 10–20% of all chronic urticarias are physical urticarias.

CHOLINERGIC URTICARIA

Cholinergic urticaria (CU) is characterized by generalized flushing and distinctive, punctate 2- to 4-mm pruritic wheals surrounded by a red flare. The reaction is a result of an increase in core body temperature. Anything that raises body temperature can induce the reaction, such as fever or a hot tub. Anxiety or emotional stress may trigger CU. Classic CU does not produce angioedema, bronchospasm, or hypotension, but these have been reported in the literature (see the discussion of variant EIAna below). Cholinergic stimulation may produce increased lacrimation, salivation, and diarrhea. Some patients with CU have lower airway symptoms or pulmonary symptoms, which produce wheezing and cough, therefore overlapping with EIA. A significant decrease in FEV_1 has been demonstrated during exercise challenge in some patients, but this does not occur in most patients with CU.

CU usually starts between the ages of 10 and 30 and often persists throughout life, though in at least half the patients the symptoms will improve over time. Exercise-induced CU usually comes on 6 minutes into exercise

---

G. L. Landry: Department of Family Medicine, University of Wisconsin-Madison, Madison, Wisconsin 53792-4116.

TABLE 21-1. Classification of exercise-induced syndromes

Type	Precipitant	Urticaria type	Vascular collapse	Respiratory symptoms
CU	Heat, stress, exercise	2–4 mm	rare	Occassional bronchospasm
EIAna	Exercise	10–15 mm	yes	Laryngeal edema
Food-dependent EIAna	Food and exercise	10–15 mm	yes	Laryngeal edema
Variant EIAna	Exercise	2–4 mm	yes	Laryngeal edema

CU, Cholinergic urticaria; EIAna, exercise-induced anaphylaxis
Modified from Volcheck GW, Li JTC. Exercise-induced urticaria and anaphylaxis. *Mayo Clin Proc* 1997;72:140–147.

and worsens over the next 20–25 minutes. The urticaria usually starts on the chest and neck and tends to spread distally. The urticaria usually resolves in 2–4 hours.

Other types of urticaria may occur with exercise that are not CU or EIAna. Cold-induced urticaria occurs only on the body where the skin is exposed to cold. There is localized swelling, erythema, and pruritus. The diagnosis is confirmed by doing an ice water challenge test. Urticaria will erupt when exposed to a cold water-filled test tube.

Aquagenic urticaria will occur in susceptible individuals when the skin is in contact with water. The perifollicular hives are thought to occur because when the sebum comes into contact with water, a toxic substance is produced that stimulates mast cell degranulation.

EXERCISE-INDUCED ANAPHYLAXIS

Exercise-induced anaphylaxis (EIAna) was first described in a case report by Maulitz and colleagues in 1979 (6) and was designated as a distinct syndrome occurring in 16 patients by Sheffer and Austen in 1980 (7). These patients experienced anaphylactic reactions while exercising without any known exogenous allergen. They described fatigue, generalized warmth, pruritus, and erythema with exercise. Soon after onset of symptoms, their skin developed large urticaria (10–15 mm) and angioedema. With a full attack, patients described choking, stridor, dysphagia, abdominal pain, and vomiting. Symptoms lasted 30 minutes to 4 hours. Twelve of the 16 patients reported collapse with brief episodes of loss of consciousness.

The clinical syndrome of EIAna was described in more detail from an epidemiologic study by Wade and colleagues of 199 patients (134 female and 65 male) diagnosed with EIAna (8). Many of the individuals were well-trained athletes. Jogging was the most common precipitating activity, but almost any aerobic athletic activity was associated with EIAna. Typically symptoms occurred 2–3 times per week. The type of environment that tended to precipitate an attack varied in this group. The majority (64%) felt that exercise in a warm environment precipitated an attack; 23% stated that cold environments produced their symptoms. High humidity was a factor for 32% of the patients. Pruritus was the most common early symptom of EIAna, and urticaria, angioedema, and flushing were frequently reported. (Table 21-2). Upper respiratory symptoms occurred in 59%, and 30% had gastrointestinal symptoms. Loss of consciousness occurred in 32%. Since the initial report, nearly 1000 cases have been reported; surprisingly, only one death has appeared in the literature (9).

VARIANT TYPE EXERCISE-INDUCED ANAPHYLAXIS

Variant type EIAna is so named because the urticaria are small (2–4 mm) that develop with exercise, but symptoms progress and can lead to vascular collapse. This type appears to represent only 10% of EIAna. Although the urtica are small, as in CU, they are produced only by exercise and not by passive rewarming.

FOOD-DEPENDENT EXERCISE-INDUCED ANAPHYLAXIS

Food-dependent EIAna occurs in patients who are susceptible to ingestion of a specific food before exercise. At least half of the athletes with EIAna have food-dependent EIAna [54% in patients reported by Wade and colleagues (8)]. Symptoms occur 2–4 hours after ingestion of a particular food, and this is very reproducible. Some athletes with EIAna will become symptomatic with exercise close to any meal, regardless of the type of food ingested. Unlike other allergic syndromes,

TABLE 21-2. Signs and symptoms of EIAna

Symptom	Percentage of cases
Pruritus	92
Urticaria	83
Angioedema	78
Flushing	75
Respiratory symptoms	59
Sweating	43
Syncope	32
Gastrointestinal	30

Modified from Wade JP, Liang MH, Sheffer AL. Exercise-induced anaphylaxis: epidemiologic observations. *Prog Clin Biol Res* 1989;297:175–182.

patients who have a strong history of EIAna after ingestion of a specific food may have negative skin tests to that food. Some patients will have positive tests for multiple foods. Numerous foods have been implicated in EIAna, including celery, wheat, shellfish, cabbage, peaches, chicken, hazelnuts, and apples. Celery was the most frequently offending food in the patients reported by Wade and colleagues; subsequent reports have implicated wheat as the most common offender. Medications have also been reported to precipitate EIAna, including alcohol, aspirin, nonsteroidal anti-inflammatory drugs, antibiotics, and cold remedies. Most patients with this form of EIAna are able to exercise without symptoms as long as the offending agent is avoided and/or exercise is avoided close to a meal.

EPIDEMIOLOGY

The true prevalence of exercise-induced allergy syndromes is unknown. EIAna appears to be a rare entity, but no one has studied large numbers of adult athletes. Of 179 patients with anaphylaxis at the Mayo Clinic, only 7% appeared to have EIAna (10). CU and EIAna appear to be relatively uncommon in Japanese children. In Japan teachers of 11,647 pupils were surveyed in 11 kindergartens, 11 elementary schools, and 5 junior high schools (11). According to the teachers, none of the kindergartners reported had experienced EIAna, and 0.05% of the elementary school children and 0.21% of the junior high children had experienced those symptoms. In a prospective study of 493 high school and university students there were 11.2% who reported symptoms of CU, but only 22% sought medical attention (12). EIAna was not examined in this study.

PATHOPHYSIOLOGY

Most urticarial and anaphylactic responses result from antigen-induced or physical agent-induced release of biologically active materials from IgE-sensitized mast cells and basophils. Antigens may be proteins, polysaccharides, and haptens, while the physical stimuli include exercise, heat, cold, sunlight, and water.

CU appears to result from an exaggerated cholinergic response to body warming or emotional stress. It is thought that body warming or stress can stimulate cholinergic fibers that innervate eccrine sweat glands. The acetylcholine released from these fibers causes mast cell degranulation and histaminemia, which produces the urticaria. Small studies of patients with CU have shown increased histamine levels, and there is general agreement that histamine is the major mediator in CU. Complement activation does not seem to have a role, and studies have not shown increased levels of bradykinin.

Patients with classic EIAna have been shown to have elevated histamine levels when they exercise and are symptomatic. Reproducing symptoms during exercise challenge is not as consistent as with CU even when high exertion occurs. Like CU and EIAna, variant-type EIAna has an associated increase in serum histamine levels. The cause of the histamine release is not known. Since patients with EIAna do not have a response to passive body warming, it has been suggested that an immunoglobulin-antigen complex similar to an IgE-mediated anaphylactic event may provoke the anaphylactic response. The lack of predictability in reproducing EIAna with exercise challenges and the ingestion of specific foods before exercise suggest that a priming phenomenon may be needed for mediator release. In food-dependent EIAna, histamine levels seem to be increased only with the ingestion of food and exercise but not with exposure to either alone. This implies that the interaction with IgE and the food antigen lowers the mast cell threshold to another stimulus such as exercise. The mechanism for this phenomenon is unclear.

A high percentage of athletes with CU and EIAna have an atopic history. The mechanism for the genetic predisposition to atopy is not clear. There are two reports in the literature of familial EIAna. In one family, two siblings with EIAna shared an HLA haplotype A3-B8-DR3 with their atopic father (13).

DIAGNOSIS

The patient's history will usually give the practitioner the diagnosis. The size of the hives, type of pulmonary involvement, and precipitating factors such as food and passive rewarming will help to pin down the diagnosis. Because of overlapping of the syndromes, it may be more practical to simply divide the patients into those with exclusively skin manifestations and those with skin and systemic symptoms. Any patient with systemic symptoms should be treated more aggressively, regardless of the specific diagnosis.

Provocative testing is unnecessary in the majority of cases. It is time consuming, expensive, and risky in patients with a history of systemic symptoms. There are two tests for CU that are not very sensitive (30–40%) but are highly specific. Passive heat challenge produces urticaria in about 30% of patients with CU. If the body core temperature is raised 0.5–1.5°C with a heating blanket, serum histamine levels will increase, and urticaria will be produced. It is usually more convenient and more comfortable for the patient to immerse an extremity in hot (40–42°C) water to produce hives. The methacholine stimulation test is an intradermal injection of acetyl methacholine chloride. This will produce 2- to 4-mm urticaria in patients with CU but not in those with EIAna. Since these tests lack sensitivity, negative tests do not rule out CU.

Consultation with an allergist should be considered for all patients with EIAna. Because of the high percentage of athletes who have food-dependent EIAna, testing for food allergens is desirable in most patients.

TREATMENT

The treatment of acute EIAna is the same as that for any anaphylactic reaction. The drug of choice is subcutaneously administered epinephrine. Intravenous fluids, antihistamines, and oxygen are also helpful if symptoms do not quickly improve with epinephrine. The person who is exercising and develops these symptoms must stop exercising immediately and administer epinephrine as soon as possible. Some athletes report rapid improvement of symptoms if they simply stop exercising. The key to the treatment of most cases of EIAna is prevention.

The symptoms of CU may be so mild that the patient may not require treatment. If treatment is necessary, antihistamines are the medications that are most likely to be helpful. Diphenhydramine is often chosen first because it is over-the-counter and inexpensive. Some practitioners prefer hydroxyzine because of its longer half-life and better efficacy in treating pruritus. Both of these compounds have limited use in individuals who are susceptible to their sedative effects. Some of the individuals who are drowsy on these antihistamines will develop tolerance to the adverse side effects with regular use. Nonsedating antihistamines such as loratadine, cetirizine, and fexofenadine may be just as effective but have not been evaluated in any systematic fashion in CU or EIAna. As with other forms of urticaria, if the H1 blocker is not effective, addition of a H2 antihistamine blocker such as cimetidine, ranitidine, nizatidine, or famotidine may improve control of symptoms. Unfortunately, combination therapy with H1 and H2 blockers has not been studied in CU or EIAna.

PREVENTION

Prevention is most important for patients with the most severe symptoms. Unfortunately, no regimen seems to completely prevent symptoms, but interventions seem to improve most patients symptoms. It is important to identify any coprecipitators such as foods or prescription and over-the-counter medications, including supplements. Keeping a food diary may be necessary to identify the offending food. Most authors recommend avoiding exercise for at least 4–6 hours after eating anything. The lowest-risk time to exercise is usually in the morning after an overnight fast.

As with CU, patients with EIAna will usually benefit from use of antihistamines, either as single agents or with the combination therapy with H1 and H2 antagonists. Antihistamine doses are limited only by sedation. For example, it may take up to 200 mg of hydroxyzine per day in divided doses to reduce symptoms of EIAna.

There are case reports of use of oral cromoglycolate and inhaled cromolyn. On the basis of this limited experience, widespread use cannot be recommended.

An important aspect of treatment is modification of each individual exercise program. If warm and humid days seem to provoke symptoms, then avoiding exercise on those days or reducing the intensity of exercise may be necessary. Some patients may do well to gradually increase their training and will tolerate higher levels of exercise if the exercise load is increased slowly over weeks and months. Patients with EIAna should learn how to self-inject epinephrine in the form of either a epinephrine anaphylaxis kit or Epi-Pen and should carry this with them while exercising. It is also recommended that they wear a medical alert bracelet or necklace. The patient should not exercise alone and should make the person exercising with him or her aware of the possibility of anaphylactic symptoms and knowledgeable about how to help.

REFERENCES

1. Volcheck GW, Li JTC. Exercise-induced urticaria and anaphylaxis. *Mayo Clin Proc* 1997;72:140–147.
2. DuBuske LM, Horan RF, Sheffer AL. Exercise-induced allergy syndromes. In: Weiler JM, ed. *Allergic and respiratory disease in sports medicine.* New York: Marcel Dekker, 1997:253–278.
3. Christodoulou CS, Diaz JD, Charlesworth EN. Exercise-induced urticaria and angioedema. In: Weiler JM, ed. *Allergic and respiratory disease in sports medicine.* New York: Marcel Dekker, 1997:235–251.
4. Terrell T, Hough DO, Alexander R. Identifying exercise allergies: exercise-induced anaphylaxis and cholinergic urticaria. *Phys Sportsmed* 1996;24(11):76–89.
5. Nichols AW. Exercise-induced anaphylaxis and urticaria. *Clin Sports Med* 1992;11(2):303–312.
6. Maulitz RM, Pratt DS, Schocket AL. Exercise-induced anaphylactic reaction to shellfish. *J Allergy Clin Immunol* 1979;63:433.
7. Sheffer AL, Austen KF. Exercise-induced anaphylaxis. *J Allergy Clin Immunol* 1980;66:106–111.
8. Wade JP, Liang MH, Sheffer AL. Exercise-induced anaphylaxis: epidemiologic observations. *Prog Clin Biol Res* 1989;297:175–182.
9. Ausdenmoore RW. Fatality in a teenager secondary to exercise-induced anaphylaxis. *Pediatr Asthma Allergy Immunol* 1991;5:21–24.
10. Yokum MW, Khan DA. Assessment of patients who have experienced anaphylaxis: a 3 year survey. *Mayo Clin Proc* 1994;69:16–23.
11. Tanaka S. An epidemiological survey on food-dependent exercise induced anaphylaxis in kindergartners, schoolchildren and junior high school students. *Asia Pac J Public Health* 1994;7:26–30.
12. Zuberbier T, Althaus C, Chantraine-Hess S, Czarnetzki BM. Prevalence of cholinergic urticaria in young adults. *L Am Acad Dermatol* 1994;31:978–981.
13. Longley S, Panush RS. Familial exercise-induced anaphylaxis. *Ann Allergy* 1985;54:35–38.

CHAPTER 22

The Athlete with Epilepsy

Tom W. Bartsokas

INTRODUCTION

Epilepsy is a group of neurologic disorders characterized by recurrent seizures. For more than 30 years medical authors have debated the appropriateness of various sports and recreational activities for patients who have been diagnosed with epilepsy. Some of the reasons proposed for restriction of activities were based on theoretical conjecture and not founded on actual injury/morbidity statistics. Fortunately, some published reports have identified relative risks inherent for some sports, such as aquatics (1–4), and rational recommendations based on these findings may be offered. For many sports and activities, however, risk from participation remains undocumented (5). The sports medicine practitioner's responsibility, then, is to provide individualized attention to patients with epilepsy. This duty includes confirmation of a proper diagnosis, monitoring of antiepileptic drug therapy, compassionate patient and family counseling and education, and encouragement to pursue a vigorous and healthy lifestyle. The goal of this work is to provide rational information about the prescription of exercise for patients with epilepsy. This chapter summarizes medical literature pertaining to epilepsy and sports and concludes with recommendations for physicians, parents, coaches, and educators.

DEFINITIONS

Central to the terminology of epilepsy is the term *seizure*. Seizures are transient, paroxysmal, and synchronous discharges of populations of neurons in the brain (6). Although considered abnormal, seizures can occur in both normal and abnormal brain tissue. The clinical manifestations of seizures are dependent on the location and population size of the neurons involved in the seizure discharge and the duration of this discharge. Well-known triggers for seizure activity in the brain include sleep, hyperventilation, stroboscopic light stimulation, hypoglycemia, extreme fatigue, psychological stress, hyperthermia, and alcohol withdrawal.

Epilepsy is defined as recurrent seizures and may result from congenital or acquired factors (6). The most frequently known cause of acquired epilepsy is head injury; however, in more than half of patients—especially younger cases—no clear causative factor can be identified. The diagnosis of epilepsy is made, by definition, when a person has had at least two seizures (5). Implicit in this diagnosis is the fact that all reversible causes of seizures have been identified and corrected. Over 10% of the population will have a seizure or a few seizures during a lifetime, whereas epilepsy occurs in 1–2% of the population (6). Seizures are one of the most common neurologic disorders and may occur at any age. The incidence of epilepsy is relatively high in infancy, decreases during childhood, and is at its lowest in adolescence and young adulthood (6). There appears to be a sharp increase in the incidence of epilepsy in the elderly.

Convulsions are episodes of paroxysmal, violent muscular activity that is uncontrolled and unpredictable. When this activity is sustained, the convulsions are termed *tonic;* when this activity is intermittent, they are *clonic*. When these two types of convulsions occur together, they are called *tonic-clonic* or *clonic-tonic-clonic*. Convulsions may or may not accompany a seizure.

CLASSIFICATION OF SEIZURES

Several classifications of seizures have been used in the past, and this created substantial confusion about seizure types (6). In 1981 the International League Against Epilepsy proposed a classification of epileptic seizure

---

T. W. Bartsokas: Bone and Joint Clinic, Franklin, Tennessee 37064.

types based on clinical and electroencephalographic criteria. This system of classification is widely accepted and divides seizures into three major categories: partial, generalized, and unclassified (7).

Partial Seizures

Partial seizures may be either simple or complex (8). If the patient remains fully conscious, the seizure is classified as simple partial. While if the focal discharge involves brain regions subserving awareness or if the seizure spreads widely enough to cause the patient to lose conscious contact, the seizure is classified as complex partial. A simple partial seizure may spread to become a complex partial or even a generalized tonic-clonic seizure (6). Patients with complex partial seizures lose conscious contact regardless of the experience that may precede the seizure. Complex partial seizures usually begin with arrest of motion and a blank stare. Automatisms such as simple hand movements, or alimentary behavior such as tasting movements or swallowing, or verbal utterances may occur either initially or during the seizure. If a complex motor task is under way at the beginning of a seizure, the patient may continue that activity, but the accuracy of the behavior will deteriorate (6). Postictal effects differentiate a complex partial seizure of temporal lobe origin from an absence seizure, because the patient does not have any postictal symptoms in the latter (9). Finally, simple and complex partial seizures may secondarily generalize and produce a tonic-clonic convulsion, but most partial seizures do not secondarily generalize (6).

Generalized Seizures

Generalized seizures cause a spectrum of behavior from the nonconvulsive pattern of simple absence through myoclonus to the fully developed generalized tonic-clonic seizure (10). Convulsions are the most common type of generalized seizures (6). Generalized convulsions were previously known as *grand mal* seizures. These are characterized by loss of consciousness associated with apnea and violent contractions of the musculature of the trunk and extremities. Most generalized convulsions begin with a tonic phase, in which there is sustained contraction of all muscles with extended legs and either flexed or extended arms. This phase usually lasts for several seconds and is followed by a clonic phase, which is characterized by rhythmic contractions of the limbs that may last for up to 1–2 minutes. During a generalized convulsion, respirations cease, salivation increases, heart rate increases, and blood pressure is elevated. The convulsing patient may appear cyanotic. After the violent muscle contractions subside—usually after 2 minutes or so—the patient enters a postictal phase in which breathing resumes and unresponsiveness is replaced by gradual recovery of consciousness. The postictal patient may remain confused and drowsy for several minutes and frequently complains of muscle soreness and headache. The postictal patient characteristically has amnesia for the time of the generalized convulsion.

Another form of generalized seizures, *absences,* usually begin in childhood. These seizures were formerly termed *petit mal.* The prevalence of childhood absence epilepsy is estimated to be 2–8% (11). The clinical picture consists of a sudden interruption of the patient's activities accompanied by a blank stare and slowing of speech. These episodes are usually brief (less than 10 seconds), are not preceded by an aura, and typically are not associated with any lingering postictal effects. During an absence seizure the patient does not react to stimuli and after a few seconds may suddenly resume his/her activities without noticing that an interruption has occurred (12).

Revised Seizure Classification

In 1989 the International League Against Epilepsy acknowledged that an epilepsy syndrome encompasses not only the behavior during a seizure, but also the electroencephalogram (EEG) changes, the patient's mental and motor development, and the family history. This recognition of alterations to patients' quality of life resulted in a revision of the system for classifying seizures (10). An important point to note is that the repertoire of seizure manifestations is limited; therefore similar seizure types may be found as components of several syndromes with widely divergent prognoses. Defining a specific epilepsy syndrome often requires repeated assessment, evaluation of development, and review of responses to treatment (6). A detailed discussion of specific epilepsy syndromes is beyond the scope of this chapter, but realize that syndromes are considered to be either benign or progressive on the basis of the ultimate outcome of intellectual function and survival. Although some syndromic seizures are benign in their impact on intellectual function, lifelong treatment with antiepileptic/anticonvulsant drugs may be required (6). Finally, keep in mind that epileptic seizures do not always constitute a solitary disorder. Patients often suffer from other disorders of motor, cognitive, and/or psychosocial functioning, and these impairments may affect the severity of the epilepsy syndrome. Therefore an appropriate evaluation of a patient with seizures includes both a classification of the type and frequency of seizures and consideration of the unique physical makeup and social milieu of that individual patient.

TREATMENT OF SEIZURES AND EPILEPSY

The principal treatment of seizures is drug therapy. Patients with chronic recurrent seizures, regardless of etiology, should be treated with antiepileptic drugs (AEDs) (6). The aim of therapy is to reduce or achieve remission of the seizures with these medications. With rare exceptions, monotherapy to reduce seizure occurrences is considered the best treatment (6,13). Studies have shown that drug doses and schedules need not be altered when patients participate in physical exercise (14).

The main AEDs that are used to treat patients with epilepsy in the United States are carbamazepine, ethosuximide, gabapentin, lamotrigine, phenobarbital, phenytoin, primidone, and valproate (6). Some benzodiazepines, including clonazepam, diazepam, and lorazepam, are also used to treat seizures. With the exception of clonazepam, the benzodiazepines are used for short-term treatment of acute seizures or status epilepticus and are usually administered parenterally. Clonazepam can be used to treat epilepsy but is not recommended, because most patients develop tolerance to its antiepileptic effect (6).

All AEDs can produce adverse effects, which are numerous and vary considerably from patient to patient. Dose-dependent neurotoxicities are the most common adverse effects of AEDs and limit the amount of drug that may be used. All AEDs cause depression of cortical function, which may lead to symptoms of sedation and decreased concentration. In the context of sports performance, central nervous system depression may cause decreased movement velocity and increased reaction times (15). In addition, some AEDs may cause diplopia, nystagmus, ataxia, and even confusion. Obviously, the adverse effects of AEDs can interfere with the attainment of maximal sports performance and thereby further complicate the issue of compliance with a therapeutic regimen.

Drugs that are administered to children may have unpredictable effects, and barbiturates are well known to cause hyperactivity in children. Depression and psychosis may be caused by AEDs, most effects on behavior appearing to be dose related (6). Mild sensory neuropathy has been reported in 8–15% of patients who are treated with AEDs and seems to require long-term exposure (16). The clinical effect usually is not severe, but loss of deep tendon responses or vibratory sensation at the ankles may occur. Other adverse reactions to AEDs include idiosyncratic effects, such as some forms of hepatotoxicity and aplastic anemia; dose-related leukopenia; dermatologic reactions, such as dose-related exanthema, acne, and alopecia; connective tissue disorders, such as lupus erythematosus, scleroderma, Sjogren's syndrome, and eosinophilic fasciitis; and metabolic effects, such as hyponatremia and altered thyroid function (6). Altered bone metabolism and bone density have been associated with phenytoin, phenobarbital, and caramezepine. These effective AEDs, then, pose an increased risk for the development of osteopenia, osteoporosis, osteomalacia, and fractures. Active patients will benefit from education regarding proper nutrition (especially as this relates to consumption of calcium and vitamin D), encouragement to participate in weight-bearing exercise, and avoidance of alcohol and smoking. In addition, consideration of estrogen replacement therapy in menopausal athletes who have a history of taking phenytoin, phenobarbital, and carbamezepine should be undertaken when not contraindicated.

Surgical treatment is an option for patients who have failed to respond to conventional AED treatment or who have intolerable adverse drug effects, whose seizures have a focal origin, and whose seizures originate in tissue that can be removed without causing disability (17,18). The most commonly performed surgical procedure for uncontrolled epilepsy is temporal lobectomy. Approximately 70% of patients remain seizure free after surgery and an additional 20% are greatly improved (6).

PROGNOSIS OF EPILEPSY

The prognosis for epilepsy is expressed in terms of the morbidity and mortality associated with the disorder. Morbidity may be expressed in the amount of seizures experienced, the type of seizures, and any other functional impairments that exist as comorbid states. To counsel patients with regard to recommended sports and recreational activities, a basic understanding of the prognosis for various forms of epilepsy is advised.

Prognosis for medical control of generalized and partial seizures has improved with better methods for assessment, introduction of new drugs, and more rational use of older agents (19,20). A good outcome—that is, attainment of extended seizure-free periods—is achieved in 60–65% of patients with new-onset seizures treated with a single drug (21). Control is difficult to achieve in patients with epilepsy of longer duration, partial seizures, more seizures before starting treatment, seizures with a known cause, and epileptiform patterns on EEG (22,23). Poor seizure control also is associated with impaired social adjustment, multiple types of seizures with abnormalities on EEG, delay in the start of treatment for more than one year, and frequent seizures (24). Some studies show a five-year remission in at least 70% of patients who were followed for 20 years. Of these patients, 50% were in true remission and were not taking any medication (25).

Patients with complex partial seizures have a less favorable prognosis for control than patients with generalized seizures. Nevertheless, good outcome for patients with complex partial seizures is possible when patients possess normal mentation, experience a short duration of illness, and show a low seizure frequency (26). Indicators for a poor prognosis in patients with complex partial seizures include more than one seizure a day, an aura at the onset of seizures, psychiatric disease, and associated tonic-clonic seizures (6,27).

With respect to mortality, epileptic patients have a shorter life expectancy than average, possibly because of underlying brain damage in some patients (28–31). Most deaths occur with patients in bed, 6–30% happening during sleep. At autopsy few patients had therapeutic blood levels of prescribed AEDs, and 50% had no detectable levels at all. Seizures are not always the cause of death; cardiac arrhythmias are implicated as the terminal event in many instances (32,33). The prevalence of sudden death is between one in 2000 and one in 900 patients with epilepsy (6).

OVERVIEW OF ISSUES RELATED TO SPORTS PARTICIPATION FOR PATIENTS WITH EPILEPSY

A currently accepted axiom is that regular physical exercise is essential to physical and emotional health for all people, including those with chronic medical problems. A review of the medical literature reveals that within the past 25 years authors have been debating the degree to which exercise and sports activities of epilepsy patients should be limited. In an article addressed to physical education instructors in 1973, epilepsy was likened to severely debilitating chronic illnesses, and the recommendation for rest was given (34). For the general public epilepsy evokes feelings of apprehension. This concern probably stems from the complexity of the disorder, the difficulty clinicians have in identifying the cause or site of seizures in most cases, and the unpredictable nature of some seizures. Nevertheless, good evidence exists to support full participation in sports for all individuals with well-controlled epilepsy.

As far back as 1941, Lennox stated, "Physical and mental activity seems to be an antagonist of seizures. Enemy epilepsy prefers to attack when the patient is off guard, sleeping, resting, or idling" (35). In fact, epileptic seizures frequently occur in association with sleep, and many patients have their seizures only at that time (36). In 1968 the American Medical Association and the American Academy of Pediatrics (AAP) published position stands that initiated a change in attitude toward the participation of epilepsy patients in sports. The AAP's recommendations in 1968 included the statement that "As a general principle, every effort should be made to minimize restrictions. With proper medical management, the majority of epileptic children in schools should participate fully in physical education programs" (37). Since 1968 several authors have opined that almost any sport is suitable for epileptic patients who have only one or two seizures a year (38–45).

To give epilepsy patients satisfactory advice about sports, it is necessary to understand various facets of exercise physiology that could affect the disorder. It is well known, for example, that voluntary hyperventilation at rest precipitates spells of absence seizures. Hyperventilation leads to respiratory alkalosis, which is a known seizure-provoking factor for many patients. Physical exercise and its attendant overbreathing do not alter body chemistries in the same way and therefore do not increase the risk of seizures (46). Telemetric monitoring of EEGs was performed during forced hyperventilation and during muscular work (repetitive squatting). These researchers found that EEG abnormalities are elevated during voluntary hyperventilation, while the EEG tends to normalize (lower frequency of background activity and disappearance of seizure discharges) during muscular exercise. Furthermore, Gotze and colleagues reported that if their subjects voluntarily hyperventilated for 10–15 seconds almost immediately after the exercise bout, the EEG abnormalities associated with hyperventilation before exercise were less marked and were delayed in onset. The conclusion of this study, then, was that physical exercise elevates the seizure threshold in adolescent epileptics and thereby reduces the likelihood of seizures (46).

Hypoxia has been linked to causation of seizures (47). Although hypoxia is not a typically occurring phenomenon in sports, one may experience varying levels of hypoxia in mountain-climbing or alpine-skiing events that are held at altitudes above 2000 meters (48). Nevertheless, Dr. Samuel Livingston of the Johns Hopkins Hospital Epilepsy Unit, Baltimore, Maryland, stated in 1971 that "A considerable number of our patients who have traveled into areas of exceedingly high altitude have not experienced a rise in the frequency of their seizures" (41). Dr. Livingston, who was head of a department that treated over 20,000 patients with epilepsy, did not believe that a change in atmospheric pressure is likely to precipitate an epileptic seizure.

Hyperthermia is also known to trigger seizures. While it is true that prolonged exercise at high temperatures and under humid conditions can put people at risk for exertional heat illness syndromes, no documented reports of such heat-stress-induced seizures were identified.

Hyperhydration, which may result from ingestion of large volumes of water or from conditions that cause an extreme loss of serum sodium, is a well-known factor in provoking seizures. Overingestion of hypotonic liquids during prolonged endurance events, such as marathon runs, triathlons, and distance swims, may lead to hyponatremia and thereby trigger seizures (49,50). By encouraging the consumption of isotonic electrolyte replacements before, during, and after events of this nature, one can hope to reduce the risk of seizures in this situation.

SPORT-SPECIFIC CONSIDERATIONS FOR PATIENTS WITH EPILEPSY

Water Sports

Several studies have looked at the risk of drowning and near drowning during swimming. The incidence of death from drowning among people with seizure disorders has been reported to be from 0% to 8% of all deaths from drowning (3,4,51–54). The relative risk of drowning for epileptics has been estimated to be four times greater than that for the general population (2). Two relatively recent reports on the inherent risks of water sports for people with epilepsy concluded that seizure-related drownings represent a small but potentially preventable proportion of all drownings (1,55). These authors suggest that by strict adherence to water safety rules, the risks of swimming and other aquatic activities may be minimized.

As a means of identifying risk factors for drowning in epilepsy patients, Ryan and Dowling performed a retrospective review of medical examiner's investigations into drowning deaths in Alberta, Canada, from 1981 to 1990 (55). Of the 482 deaths from drowning studied, 25 (5%) were considered to be directly related to seizures. Fifteen (60%) of the 25 deaths occurred while the person was taking a bath unsupervised, and only one person (4%) died while taking a shower (55). Two victims fell out of moving boats while having seizures, but neither person had been wearing a personal flotation device (55). Perhaps most troubling was the finding that 19 (83%) of 23 patients who had been prescribed anticonvulsant drug therapy had undetectable or subtherapeutic levels of one or more drugs at autopsy (55). In a similar analysis from the United Kingdom, Kemp and Sibert reviewed coroners' and pediatricians' records from 1988 to 1989 regarding the drownings and near drownings in children under the age of 15 years (1). Of 306 submersion incidents (157 near drownings and 149 drowning deaths) reported, 10 incidents followed an epileptic seizure, and four of these children died (1). As a result of this study, children with epilepsy were found to have a higher incidence of submersion accidents; the risk was estimated to be 7.5 times greater than that in children without epilepsy (1). Noteworthy is the fact that two of the four fatalities in the United Kingdom study occurred in bathtubs, while no child participating in supervised swimming drowned. The dangers of drowning in the bath for patients of all ages with epilepsy are well known and have been highlighted in other studies as well (45). One particularly tragic case that illustrates the hazards of the bath came from Kemp and Sibert's report, in which a nonepileptic infant drowned in the bath when her mother had an epileptic seizure (1). A summary of recommendations for safe participation in water sports appears in Table 22–1 and is derived from several studies addressing this issue (1,14,15,55,56).

Theoretical risks for serious accidents have been proposed for scuba diving with epilepsy. Hyperbaric oxygen, which is used during scuba diving, may be causally linked to seizures, thereby precluding this activity for all patients with epilepsy (56–58). Another consideration given for the exclusion of epilepsy patients from scuba diving is that the safety of a companion diver would also be endangered during a seizure, owing to the need for an unplanned rescue effort and additional underwater time (15).

TABLE 22–1. *Water safety recommendations for patients with epilepsy*

Swimming

Always swim with a friend.
Swim only in pools that are supervised by personnel trained in basic life support (cardiopulmonary resuscitation).
Perform cool-down activities on the land instead of in the water.
Inform supervisory personnel about children's epilepsy.
Avoid swimming in open waterways, such as rivers, lakes, and oceans.
Scuba diving is contraindicated.
Competitive underwater swimming is contraindicated.

Bathing

Shower in an unlocked room.
Supervise the bathing of small children with epilepsy at all times.
If no shower is available, bathe seated in tub, with hand-held shower head and with drain plug out.
Encourage a mother with epilepsy to be accompanied while bathing her baby or toddler.

Boating

All passengers should use floatation devices at all times.
Water skiers should use floatation devices at all times.
Supervisors or partners should be present for boating, sailing, surfing, and wind surfing.

Fishing

Even if fishing from the bank of a body of water, wear a flotation device.
Preferably fish with a companion.

Adapted from Kemp AM, Sibert JR. Epilepsy in children and the risk of drowning. *Arch Dis Child* 1993;68:684–685.

Contact and Collision Sports

In spite of the fact that no clear evidence exists on a possible relationship between repetitive minor head injuries and the provocation of epileptic seizures, some authors believe that participation of epileptic patients in contact sports (e.g., soccer, basketball, racquetball) and collision sports (e.g., rugby, ice hockey, American football, boxing) should be discouraged (48). Nevertheless, several authors have supported the participation of epilepsy patients in sports such as these, since no definite proof of deterioration in the control of epilepsy has emerged from the study of contact and collision sports (41,44,59–61). An experiment on repetitive heading of a soccer ball did not show evidence for resultant brain dysfunction, but speculation on possible transient subclinical cerebral dysfunction was raised (62). In their

1973 report, Livingston and Berman stated, "The performance of body contact sports is, in our opinion, associated with a calculated risk of injury which is the same for all individuals, epileptic and non epileptic. It is true that persons who sustain penetrating injuries to the head are made more susceptible to the development of epilepsy; however, we believe that the relationship of the adverse effect of head injuries on the course of preexisting epilepsy has been completely exaggerated and probably does not exist" (36).

GENERAL RECOMMENDATIONS FOR THE PARTICIPATION OF ATHLETES WITH EPILEPSY

Counseling regarding participation in athletic endeavors for individuals with epilepsy should be based on a careful scrutiny of various characteristics of each patient. Among the factors that merit consideration are the frequency of seizures, the timing of seizures, the type of seizures, drug compliance, and adverse reactions to treatment (14,44). An important factor is freedom from seizures; for if seizures have been controlled for over 2 years, the risk of relapse is the same as the risk of a first seizure (14). Patients who experience frequent seizures, that is, daily to weekly, should not be permitted to engage in body contact sports (44) and should probably be advised to participate in such activities as light impact aerobics. Patients whose seizure attacks occur only in association with sleep should be evaluated and advised in the same manner as individuals who are not subject to seizures at all (44).

When the potential for falling and subsequent serious injury as a result of having a seizure exists, it is wise to recommend avoidance of that specific sport. Examples in this category include parachuting, hang gliding, aviation, tree climbing, mountain climbing, and rope climbing. The American Academy of Pediatrics (63) has also suggested that some gymnastics activities, such as parallel bars and the trampoline, be restricted. Other authors believe that as long as seizures have been suppressed for a prolonged period, gymnasts may train and compete without restriction (45).

Other sports, in which a fall or loss of control may result in less serious injuries, may pose acceptable risks for some patients. Two recent studies have evaluated the risks for injury in patients with epilepsy. Wirrell and colleagues (64) found that accidental injury is common in children with absence epilepsy and that the risk for injury is greatest after the initiation of antiepileptic drug treatment. Their recommendations include aggressive injury prevention counseling throughout the course of treatment and mandatory helmet use for all bicycle-riding patients (64). Taylor and colleagues (65) examined statistics from road traffic accidents over a 3-year period. After adjustment for differences in age, sex, driving experience, and mileage between drivers with epilepsy and those without, there was no evidence of any overall increased risk of accidents in the population of drivers with epilepsy (65). These authors were quick to point out, however, that there was evidence of an increased risk of more severe accidents in the population with epilepsy. Therefore it is vital that both physician and patient have a good understanding of the demands of the activity in question, accepted safety guidelines, the specific diagnosis and its implications, and the social context in which participation questions are being raised. Again, emphasis needs to be placed on promotion of active lifestyles in the vast majority of individuals with epilepsy.

CONCLUSIONS

In spite of the relative safety of most sports and recreational pursuits for people with epilepsy, participation rates in these activities have been found to be much lower in patients than in the general population (66–68). Bjorholt and colleagues (66) observed that patients with epilepsy were treated with an overprotective, "safety-first" attitude by health care personnel, as well as by family, friends, and educators. Despite having good facilities in their surroundings for participation in social, cultural, and physical activities, most patients in this Norwegian study lived a sedentary life and were about half as active as the general population (66). In addition, a considerably reduced maximum oxygen uptake and a pronounced decrease in aerobic capacity with increasing age were identified in patients.

In a study of 136 patients with epilepsy and a matched control group of 145 individuals, Steinhoff and colleagues from the University of Göttingen, Germany, assessed several issues of social and physical activity (68). This clinical study demonstrated a lack of physical fitness in patients, as evidenced by significant differences in aerobic endurance, muscle strength endurance, physical flexibility, and body mass index favoring the control subjects. In addition to the overprotective attitudes of relatives, patients from this German study revealed that health care personnel had contributed indirectly to the avoidance of physical activities (67). Fewer than half of the patients in this study thought themselves sufficiently informed about physical fitness, and 45% had never talked to a doctor about the issue of physical activity and epilepsy. Steinhoff and colleagues conclude their study by stating, "We strongly recommend not only motivating and supporting patients with epilepsy to perform sports and other active leisure-time habits regularly but encourage them by initiating programs with appropriate supervision by sports instructors or social workers" (68).

Despite there being a large number of reports that acknowledge the psychosocial consequences of epilepsy, there has been very little in the way of research that attempts to rectify the situation. Early literature has suggested that children with disabilities, especially chronic medical or biologic disabilities, are more susceptible to the development of psychopathology and negative self-concepts. Dr. Livingston wrote, "I emphasize that the most serious hazard of epilepsy is often not the seizures per se but the associated emotional aberrations that are prone to develop in patients with this disorder" (42).

In 1993 Regan and colleagues published very encouraging results regarding an intervention program that addresses self-concept and education. This Australian group provided a detailed description of the educational components, counseling components, and recreational activities included in their program. An analysis of data collected over 2 years at special camps for children aged 5–18 years revealed significant improvements in subjects' self-concepts, learning regarding epilepsy, and treatment compliance, particularly with long-term medications (69). Further, it was apparent to these investigators that there was a link between knowledge of seizure type for each individual and increased levels of self-esteem. One interesting facet of the Australian program was that teenaged campers participated in vigorous alpine skiing as a means of adopting a positive attitude about pleasurable recreational pursuits.

Lewis and colleagues (70) focused their intervention strategies on the child and his or her family. They concluded that educational programs positively increased children's perceptions of social competency and offered the additional benefit of improved seizure management.

Perhaps traditional means of delivering medical care and supportive counseling to patients with epilepsy need to be supplemented by intense, multidisciplinary intervention strategies in the future. The therapeutic recreation program in Australia is one excellent example that merits attention and expanded study. Individuals with epilepsy require thorough, thoughtful, and progressive evaluations when presenting to sports medicine practitioners. Remember that there are no data to suggest that participation in athletics by an individual with well-controlled epilepsy increases the risk of injury (71). Patients with epilepsy do need to follow certain guidelines when it comes to water sports and bathing (see Table 22-1). Contact and collision sports are not absolutely contraindicated but certainly merit individual consideration. Physical fitness training is well known to benefit normal subjects. Encouragement to maintain active lifestyles should be the mandate for all clinicians advising patients with epilepsy, since several studies have shown a remarkable seizure decrease in approximately two thirds of patients undergoing routine sports (72–74).

REFERENCES

1. Kemp AM, Sibert JR. Epilepsy in children and the risk of drowning. *Arch Dis Child* 1993;68:684–685.
2. Orlowski JP, Rothner D, Lueders H. Submersion accidents in children with epilepsy. *Am J Dis Child* 1982;135:777–780.
3. Pearn J. Epilepsy and drowning in childhood. *Br Med J* 1977;1:1510–1511.
4. Pearn J, Bart R, Yamaoka R. Drowning risks to epileptic children: a study from Hawaii. *Br Med J* 1978;2:1284.
5. Gates JR, Spiegel RH. Epilepsy, sports and exercise. *Sports Med* 1993;15(1):1–5.
6. Willmore LJ, Ferrendelli JA. Epilepsy. In: Dale DC, Federman DG, eds. *Scientific American Medicine*. New York: Scientific American, 1977:1–21.
7. International League Against Epilepsy Commission on Classification and Terminology. Proposal for revised clinical and electroencephalographic classifications. *Epilepsia* 1981;22:489–501.
8. Theodore WH, Porter RJ, Penry JK. Complex partial seizures: clinical characteristics and differential diagnosis. *Neurology* 1983;33:1115.
9. Rocca WA, Sharbrough FW, Hauser WA, et al. Risk factors for complex partial seizures: a population-based case-control study. *Ann Neurol* 1987;21:22.
10. International League Against Epilepsy Commission on Classification and Terminology. Proposal for revised classification of epilepsies and epileptic syndromes. *Epilepsia* 1989;30:389–399.
11. Cavazutti GB. Epidemiology of different types of epilepsy in school-aged children of Modena, Italy. *Epilepsia* 1980;21:57.
12. Dieterich E, Baier WK, Doose H, Tuxhorn I. Longterm followup of childhood epilepsy with absences: epilepsy with absences at onset. *Neuropediatrics* 1985;16(3):149–154.
13. Taylor MP. Improving the outlook for patients with epilepsy. *Practitioner* 1983;227:381–388.
14. van Linschoten R, Backx FJG, Mulder OGM, Meinardi H. Epilepsy and sports. *Sports Med* 1990;10(1):9–19.
15. Cordova F. Epilepsy and sport. *Aust Fam Physician* 1993;22(4):558–562.
16. Shorvon SD, Reynolds EH. Anticonvulsant peripheral neuropathy: a clinical and electrophysiological study of patients on single drug treatments with phenytoin, carbamazepine or barbituates. *J Neurol Neurosurg Psychiatry* 1982;45:620.
17. Gummit RJ. Selection of adult patients for surgical treatment of epilepsy. *Acta Neurol Scand* 1988;117[Suppl.]:42.
18. Gates JR. Presurgical evaluation for epileptic surgery in the era of long-term monitoring for epilepsy. In: Apuzzo MLJ, ed. *Neurosurgical aspects of epilepsy*. Park Ridge, IL: American Association of Neurological Surgeons, 1991.
19. Mattson RH, Cramer JA, Collins JF, et al. Comparison of carbamazepine, phenobarbital, phenytoin, and primidone in partial and secondarily generalized tonic-clonic seizures. *N Engl Med* 1985;313:145.
20. Willmore LJ. Prognosis of epilepsy. In: Evans RW, Baskin DS, Yatsu FM, eds. *Prognosis in neurological disease*. New York: Oxford University Press, 1989:483.
21. Beghi E, Togoni G. Prognosis of epilepsy in newly referred patients: a multicenter prospective study. *Epilepsia* 1988;29:236.
22. Elwes RDC, Johnson AL, Shorvon SD, et al. Early prognosis of epilepsy. *Br Med J* 1982;285:1699.
23. Elwes RDC, Johnson AL, Shorvon SD, et al. The prognosis for seizure control in newly diagnosed epilepsy. *N Engl J Med* 1984;311:944.
24. Holowach J, Thurston DL, O'Leary J. Prognosis of childhood epilepsy. *N Engl J Med* 1972;286:169.
25. Annegers JF, Hauser WA, Elveback LR. Remission of seizures and relapse in patients with epilepsy. *Epilepsia* 1979;20:729–737.
26. Chao D, Sexton JA, Pardo SS. Temporal lobe epilepsy in children. *J Pediatr* 1962;60:686.
27. Schmidt D. Prognosis of chronic epilepsy with complex partial seizures. *J Neurol Neurosurg Psychiatry* 1984;47:1274.
28. Jay GW, Leetsma JE. Sudden death in epilepsy: a comprehensive review of the literature and proposed mechanisms. *Acta Neurol Scand* 1981;82[Suppl.]:1–66.

29. Hauser WA. Mortality in patients with epilepsy. *Epilepsia* 1980;21:399–412.
30. Terrence CF, Wisotzkey HM, Perper JA. Unexpected, unexplained death in epileptic patients. *Neurology* 1975;25(6):594–598.
31. Krohn W. Causes of death among epileptics. *Epilepsia* 1963;4:315–321.
32. Leestma JE, Kalelkar MB, Teas SS, et al. Sudden unexpected death associated with seizures: analysis of 66 cases. *Epilepsia* 1984;25:84.
33. Leestma JE, Walczak T, Hughes JR, et al. A prospective study of sudden unexpected death in epilepsy. *Ann Neurol* 1989;26:195.
34. Simmons RW. Epilepsy: the implications for the teacher of physical education. *Br J Phys Educ* 1973;4(5):75–76.
35. Lennox WG. *Science and seizures*. New York: Harper & Row, 1941:134.
36. Livingston S, Berman W. Participation of epileptic patients in sports. *JAMA* 1973;224(2):236–238.
37. American Academy of Pediatrics Committee on Children with Handicaps. The epileptic child and competitive school athletics. *Pediatrics* 1968;42(4):700–702.
38. Berman W. Sports and the child with epilepsy [Correspondence]. *Pediatrics* 1984;74(2):320–321.
39. Bower BD. Epilepsy and school athletics. *Dev Med Child Neurol* 1969;2:244–245.
40. Kugel R. The epileptic child and school athletics. *Pediatrics* 1968;42:700–702.
41. Livingston S. Should physical activity of the epileptic child be restricted? *Clin Pediatr* 1971;10(12):694–696.
42. Livingston S. Epilepsy and sports [Editorial]. *Am Fam Physician* 1978;17(6):67, 69.
43. Livingston S. Comprehensive management of epilepsy in infancy, childhood, and adolescence. Springfield, IL: Charles C. Thomas, 1972.
44. Livingston S, Berman W. Participation of the epileptic child in contact sports. *J Sports Med* 1974;2(3):170–174.
45. O'Donohoe NV. What should the child with epilepsy be allowed to do? *Arch Dis Child* 1983;58(11):934–937.
46. Gotze W, Kubicki S, Munter M, Teichmann J. Effect of physical exercise on seizure threshold: investigated by electroencephalographic telemetry. *Dis Nervous Syst* 1967;28:664.
47. Laidlaw J, Richens A. *A textbook of epilepsy*, 2nd ed. Edinburgh: Churchill Livingston, 1982.
48. McLaurin RL. Epilepsy and contact sports: factors contraindicating participation. *JAMA* 1973;225(3):285–287.
49. Bennett HJ, Wagner T, Fields A. Acute hyponatremia and seizures in an infant after a swimming lesson. *Pediatrics* 1983;72(1):125–127.
50. Noakes TD, Goodwin N, Rayner BL, et al. Water intoxication: a possible complication during endurance exercise. *Med Sci Sports Exerc* 1985;17:370–375.
51. Adams AI. The descriptive epidemiology of drowning accidents. *Med J Aus* 1966;2:1257–1261.
52. Chun B, Okihiro MM, Hale RW. An analysis of drowning incidents in Oahu, 1960–1970. *Hawaii Med J* 1973;32:92–95.
53. Dietz PE, Baker SP. Drowning: epidemiology and prevention. *Am J Public Health* 1974;64:303–312.
54. MacLachlan J. Drownings, other aquatic injuries and young Canadians. *Can J Public Health* 1984;75:218–222.
55. Ryan CA, Dowling G. Drowning deaths in people with epilepsy. *Can Med Assoc J* 1993;148(5):781–784.
56. Dreifuss FE. Epilepsy and scuba diving. *JAMA* 1985;253:1877–1878.
57. Millington JT. Should epileptics scuba dive? [Correspondence]. *JAMA* 1985;254(22):3182–3183.
58. Ho SU. Seizure disorder in a scuba diver. *JAMA* 1984;252:565.
59. American Academy of Pediatrics Committee on Children with Handicaps. Sports and the child with epilepsy. *Pediatrics* 1983;72(6):884–885.
60. American Medical Association Committee on the Medical Aspects of Sports. Epileptics and contact sports. *JAMA* 1974;229:820–821.
61. Livingston S. Epilepsy and sports. [Correspondence]. *JAMA* 1978;239(1):22.
62. Tysvaer AT, Storli OV. Soccer injuries to the brain: a neurologic and electroencephalographic study of active football players. *Am J Sports Med* 1989;17:573–578.
63. American Medical Association (Joint Statement). Convulsive disorders and participation in sports and physical education. *JAMA* 1968;206:1291.
64. Wirrell EC, Camfield PR, Camfield CS, et al. Accidental injury is a serious risk in children with typical absence epilepsy. *Arch Neurol* 1996;53(9):929–932.
65. Taylor J, Chadwick D, Johnson T. Risk of accidents in drivers with epilepsy. *J Neurol Neurosurg Psychiatry* 1996;60(6):621–627.
66. Bjorholt PG, Nakken KO, Rohme K, Hansen, H. Leisure time habits and physical fitness in adults with epilepsy. *Epilepsia* 1990;31(1):83–87.
67. Clement MJ, Wallace SJ. A survey of adolescents with epilepsy. *Dev Med Child Neurol* 1990;32:849–857.
68. Steinhoff BJ, Neususs K, Thegeder H, Reimers CD. Leisure time activity and physical fitness in patients with epilepsy. *Epilepsia* 1996;37(12):1221–1227.
69. Regan KJ, Banks GK, Beran RG. Therapeutic recreation programmes for children with epilepsy. *Seizure* 1993;2:195–200.
70. Lewis MA, Salas I, de la Sota A, et al. Randomized trial of a programme to enhance the competencies of children with epilepsy. *Epilepsia* 1990;31[Suppl 1]:101–109.
71. Rothner AD. Sports participation in children and adolescents with neurological impairments. *Va Med Q* 1996;123(2):94–97.
72. Eriksen HR, Ellersten B, Gronningaeter H, et al. Physical exercise and electroencephalography in women with intractable epilepsy. *Epilepsia* 1994;35:1256–1264.
73. Nakken KO, Bjorholt PG, Johannesen SI, et al. Effect of physical training on aerobic capacity, seizure occurrence, and serum level of antiepileptic drugs in adults with epilepsy. *Epilepsia* 1990;31:88–94.
74. Denio LS, Drake ME Jr, Pakalnis A. The effect of exercise on seizure frequency. *J Med* 1989;2:171–176.

CHAPTER 23

The Athlete with Asthma or Other Pulmonary Disease

David M. Orenstein

Oxygen delivery to exercising muscle and carbon dioxide removal (to prevent system acidosis) are so important to exercise tolerance that it is one of the many wonders of human physiology that the lungs almost never limit exercise capacity. Certainly in the overwhelming majority of people, athletes and nonathletes, it is the cardiovascular system and peripheral muscles that limit exercise, and there is ample pulmonary system reserve even at exhaustion in all but a very few elite endurance athletes (1–4).

For athletes with pulmonary disorders, the lungs can influence exercise tolerance in important ways, including limiting gas exchange and causing intolerable shortness of breath. These effects can be caused directly by altered organ functioning or indirectly by generalized physical deconditioning because of habitual inactivity. In this chapter I will discuss pulmonary disorders as they influence the athletes who have them, with the majority of the emphasis on asthma.

ASTHMA

Asthma is the most common chronic illness of children and adolescents in developed countries, affecting between 5% and 15% of the population, or some 2.5 million young people in the United States. It is characterized by periodic airways obstruction that is reversible (although not completely so in some patients), either with treatment or spontaneously. The airway obstruction is caused by spasm of bronchial smooth muscle, endobronchial inflammation, or both, and there is increased sensitivity of the bronchi to various stimuli (5). Asthma has a major impact on lifestyle, accounting for a huge amount of missed school; furthermore, 30% of young people with asthma have limited activity, compared with 5% of youngsters without asthma (6).

Exercise-Induced Asthma

Most people with asthma have exercise-induced asthma (EIA), with worsened symptoms during—or especially after—exercise. These symptoms can include cough, chest tightness, chest pain, difficulty breathing, wheezing, or a combination of these symptoms. Not all asthma problems are characterized by wheezing, a fact that causes many cases of EIA to go undiagnosed. The actual incidence of EIA depends in part on the method that is used for diagnosing it, be it questionnaire, field testing, or sophisticated laboratory testing. Published incidences vary from 50% to 80% of those with already recognized asthma (7), but the true incidence is probably closer to 100% (8).

EIA also affects many young people, including athletes, who have no history of asthma. As many as 10–15% of high school (9) and college (10) athletes have been found to have EIA. Elite athletes are not protected from EIA, nor does asthma preclude successful competition at the highest level of sport, as is demonstrated by such well-publicized asthmatic Olympic athletes as Jackie Joyner-Kersee (track and field), Nancy Hogshead (swimming), Bill Koch (cross-country skiing) (11), Tom Dolan (swimming) (12), and Amy Van Dyken (swimming) (13). In 1984, the last Olympic Games for which these data are readily available, 67 of 597 athletes on the U.S. team had EIA, and they accounted for 15 gold medals, 21 silver medals, and 5 bronze medals in wres-

D. M. Orenstein: School of Medicine and School of Education, University of Pittsburgh, and Department of Pediatric Pulmonology, Children's Hospital of Pittsburgh, Pittsburgh, Pennsylvania 15213.

tling, track and field, swimming, and other sports (14,15).

Clinical Presentation

EIA can occur in association with virtually any type of exertion, but it is most likely to happen with relatively vigorous activity that is sustained for 6–8 minutes and conducted in cool, dry environments. Exercise that lasts less than 6 minutes is less asthmagenic (16,17), and exercise lasting longer may also elicit a smaller EIA response (16,17). In fact, with exercise of longer duration, athletes may "run through" their asthma (16,17). Short, extremely strenuous—supramaximal—exercise may also provide a potent stimulus to EIA (18). In the typical case symptoms of chest tightness, cough, or wheeze begin shortly after a 6- to 8-minute bout of exercise and persist for 30–90 minutes before abating spontaneously. In some patients there may also be a recurrence of these symptoms hours later, the *late asthmatic response* (19). Some patients who experience EIA have the interesting, and sometimes useful, phenomenon of the *refractory period*, whereby a second exercise challenge repeated within 30–120 minutes after the first elicits a smaller EIA response than the first (20). The symptoms of EIA correlate with objectively measurable parameters of expiratory air flow, particularly those measures that reflect flow from (and therefore caliber of) the smallest, peripheral, airways (21,22).

It had been thought that different forms of exercise were more or less likely to induce asthma, running being among the most likely and swimming the least likely (23). With our improved understanding of the pathophysiology of EIA, it now appears that many of the apparent differences among various exercise stimuli had more to do with the volume, temperature, and humidity of the inspired air than with the character of the exercise itself (23). There remains, however, an unexplained distinction between swimming and other activities in that, even when controlling for the inspired air conditions and the intensity of the exercise challenge, swimming is less asthmagenic than other forms of exercise (24).

Pathophysiology

It is not clear what makes the airways of people with asthma susceptible to the development of bronchospasm, inflammation, and edema that characterize the asthmatic response to various stimuli while the airways of nonasthmatic people do not develop such responses to those stimuli. However, our understanding of the stimuli and some of the intermediate steps leading toward the airway changes has increased over the past decade (7,23,25,26).

It has been clear for more than 100 years that cold air is more asthmagenic than warm air (23). Experimental evidence has accumulated over the past three decades supporting the role of cold inspired air in the pathogenesis of EIA (27,28). Dry air has also been recognized as more asthmagenic than humidified air (29). The complex interaction of temperature and humidity in determining total respiratory system heat loss has been discussed by a number of different investigators (24,30). More recently, Anderson has postulated that although there are important interactions between the temperature and humidity of the inspired air, it is water loss from the airways that is the principal stimulus for EIA (26). In real life the essential point is that breathing cold, dry air induces EIA in the susceptible airway much more readily than breathing warm, humid air does. This occurs during exercise and not at rest because at rest the upper airways condition the inspired air very efficiently, so the air reaching the intrathoracic airways is warmed to body temperature and fully saturated with water vapor, while the greater minute ventilation employed during exercise overwhelms the ability of the upper airway to carry out its warming and humidifying tasks. In fact, in Deal's important early investigation patients had identical degrees of EIA if they exercised or sat still, provided that the volume, temperature, and humidity of the inspired air were the same between trials (30).

The route through which the environmental stimuli cause airway narrowing probably includes the release of various inflammatory and bronchospastic chemical mediators (23). Among the many studies suggesting the role of inflammatory mediators—especially those of mast cell origin—in the genesis of EIA include those showing that EIA is blocked by cromolyn sodium (31), a mast cell stabilizer that is not by itself a bronchodilator. Other studies have shown elevated circulating levels of histamine, neutrophil chemotactic factor, or both, coincident with EIA (32,33), while still other studies have shown lessened EIA when patients were treated with leukotriene blockers before exercise challenge (34,35).

Treatment and Prevention

Asthma symptoms following exercise typically abate on their own over the ensuing 30–90 minutes but can be relieved much more quickly by the administration of an inhaled beta-agonist bronchodilator such as albuterol (7). Fortunately, EIA can also be prevented in the large majority of patients. Inhalation of either cromolyn sodium (31), nedocromil sodium (a newer agent, similar to cromolyn) (36), a beta-agonist (e.g., albuterol or terbutaline) (37), or both (38) 15 minutes before exercise is almost always successful in blocking EIA if the underlying asthma and airway inflammation are well controlled. The protection lasts about 2 hours for cromolyn alone (7) and 2 hours for terbutaline alone (7). Interestingly, the combination of cromolyn and terbutaline doubles the protection of either agent, giving 4 hours of protection (38). Albuterol alone gives 4 hours of protection (7), and salmeterol protects against EIA for upward of 12 hours (39). In the unusual patient who does not get satisfactory protection from these medications, it is likely that there is ongoing airways inflammation that needs to be controlled, perhaps with inhaled steroids. Unrecognized underlying airway inflammation is the likely explanation for the finding that children with EIA who take one such drug (budesonide) by inhalation for 1–3 weeks have less severe EIA than they had before starting the drug (40) (Fig. 23–1).

Figure 23-2 presents an overall approach to the prevention of EIA.

Asthma Drugs and International Competition

Table 23–1 lists drugs used for asthma, their route of administration, effectiveness, whether they are legal or banned for international competition, and whether their use is prophylactic or therapeutic. In addition, the U.S. Olympic Committee Drug Control Program maintains a hotline (1-800-233-0393) to keep coaches, physicians,

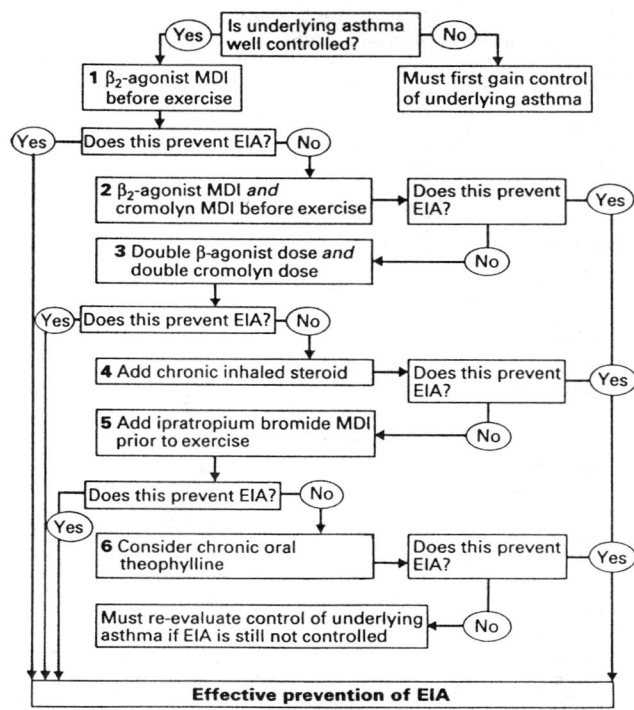

FIG. 23–2. Flowchart for selecting drugs to prevent exercise-induced asthma (EIA). (From Orenstein D. Asthma and sports. In: Bar-Or O, ed. *The Child and Adolescent Athlete,* 1st ed. Oxford, England: Blackwell Science Ltd, 1996:433-454 (Commission IOCM, ed. *Encyclopaedia of Sports Medicine,* Vol. VI); adapted from Morton A, Fitch K. Asthmatic drugs and competitive sport: an update. *Sports Med* 1992; 14(4):228–242.)

and athletes apprised of the latest regulations pertaining to banned drugs.

Nonpharmacologic Measures

Nonpharmacologic steps can also be effective in blunting EIA.

Sport Selection

Not many high school or college athletes will agree to lessening their EIA by switching from cross-country to swimming or archery, but in advising the parents of young asthmatic children who are just starting into sports, the physician can point out that swimming is the least asthmagenic of all sports and that sports calling for short–or less intense and prolonged–exercise are less likely to cause EIA than events asking for a strenuous 6- to 8-minute effort.

Warm-up

Some athletes are able to take advantage of the refractory period (see above) to perform warm-up exercise

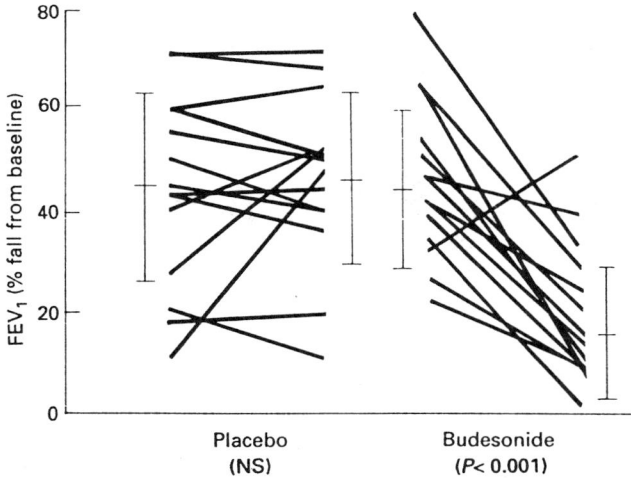

FIG. 23–1. Individual percentage falls in forced expiratory volume in 1 second (FEV_1) induced by exercise before and after 3 weeks of treatment with budesonide aerosol and its placebo. Means and standard deviations are shown. (From Orenstein D. Asthma and sports. In: Bar-Or O, ed. *The Child and Adolescent Athlete,* 1st ed. Oxford, England: Blackwell Science Ltd, 1996:433–454 (Commission IOCM, ed. *Encyclopaedia of Sports Medicine,* Vol. VI); original data from Henriksen J, Dahl R. Effects of inhaled budesonide alone and in combination with low-dose terbutaline in children with exercise-induced asthma. *Am Rev Respir Dis* 1983;128:993–997.)

TABLE 23–1. *Drugs commonly used for exercise-induced asthma; their route of administration; their effectiveness; whether they are legal or banned for intercollegiate and international competition; and whether they are used prophylactically, for treatment, or both*

Medication	Route of administration	Effectiveness in EIA	Legal or banned	Prophylaxis (P) Therapeutic (T)
Cromolyn sodium	Aerosol	Good	Legal	P
Nedocromil sodium	Aerosol	Good	Legal	P
β2-Agonists				
Albuterol	Aerosol	Excellent	Legal	P,T
	Oral	Good	Banned	P,T
Terbutaline	Aerosol	Excellent	Legal	P,T
	Oral	Good	Banned	P,T
Orciprenaline	Aerosol	Excellent	Legal	P,T
Salmeterol	Aerosol	Excellent	Legal	P,T
Clenbuterol	Aerosol	Excellent	Banned	P,T
Theophylline	Oral	Good	Legal	P,T
Ipratropium bromide	Aerosol	Fair	Legal	T
Steroids				
Beclomethasone	Aerosol	?	Legal	P,T
Budesonide	Aerosol	Fair	Legal	P,T
Prednisone	Oral	?	Banned	T
Prednisolone	Oral	?	Banned	T

From Orenstein D. Asthma and sports. In: Bar-Or O, ed. *The Child and Adolescent Athlete,* 1st ed. Oxford, England: Blackwell Science Ltd, 1996:433–454 (Commission IOCM, ed. *Encyclopaedia of Sports Medicine,* Vol. VI); originally adapted from Morton A, Fitch K. Asthmatic drugs and competitive sport: an update. *Sports Med* 1992;14(4):228–242.

45 minutes to 1 hour before competition and thus avoid EIA during the competition. Although the ideal warm-up for blocking EIA has not been discovered, both prolonged submaximal exercise (41) and short sprints (42) have been shown to be protective. Apparently, the warm-up exercise need not itself induce EIA to be protective (41).

Miscellaneous

Particularly for athletes who are exercising in cold air, a scarf or mask around the face serves to warm and humidify inspired air and to blunt EIA (43) (Fig. 23–3).

Diagnosis

In most cases the diagnosis of EIA is not challenging. For example, a young athlete who is known to have asthma and who complains of chest tightness, cough, shortness of breath, or chest pain with—or especially after—exercise can usually and safely be assumed to have EIA and may be treated appropriately (23). In the older patient, in whom coronary artery disease and angina cannot be ignored, more extensive evaluation is warranted, as is also the case for the young athlete whose story is atypical or who does not respond promptly to pre-exercise treatment with albuterol, cromolyn, or both. Oral albuterol syrup or tablets are relatively poor bronchodilators (and have a greater incidence of side effects than the inhaled preparations do), so a history of failure with the oral preparations should not make one question the diagnosis or prevent one from trying the inhaled drug.

Even in the slightly atypical patient—for example,

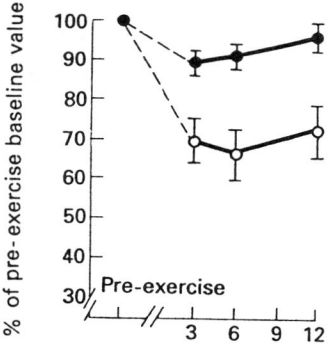

FIG. 23–3. Average FEV_1 while breathing room air, without (open circles) and with (closed circles) a mask at 3, 6, and 12 minutes after exercise, expressed as a percent of baseline value (mean ± SE for 10 subjects). (From Orenstein D. Asthma and sports. In: Bar-Or O, ed. *The Child and Adolescent Athlete,* 1st ed. Oxford, England: Blackwell Science Ltd, 1996:433–454 (Commission IOCM, ed. *Encyclopaedia of Sports Medicine,* Vol. VI); redrawn from Brenner A, Weiser P, Krogh K, Loren M. Effectiveness of a portable face mask in attenuating exercise-induced asthma. *JAMA* 1980;244: 2196–2198.)

one with no previous diagnosis of asthma or one whose symptoms occur *during* exercise—the first diagnostic test might well be a therapeutic trial of preexercise inhaled albuterol (23). Disappearance of the symptoms on this regimen confirms the diagnosis. In many patients pulmonary function testing can be helpful, particularly if it shows evidence of smaller airway obstruction. If that obstruction is reversible in the laboratory with bronchodilator inhalation, the diagnosis of asthma is fairly well established, and therefore the case for EIA is on firm ground. However, if further proof is needed, an exercise challenge can sometimes be diagnostic. The exercise challenge should be intense enough to raise the patient's heart rate to 80% of its maximum and should last 6–8 minutes (16,17). Pulmonary function should be assessed before exercise and again at 3- to 5-minute intervals beginning immediately after exercise and continuing for 20 minutes. Different investigators have recommended different specific parameters of pulmonary function as the best for diagnosing EIA and have required different magnitudes of decrement. A fall of 10–20% in forced expired volume in 1 second (FEV_1) is one commonly used criterion. We like to see such a change (in FEV_1 or maximal midexpiratory flow rate, a parameter that is more sensitive to flow from the peripheral airways) in the face of an unchanged forced vital capacity (FVC), since the preserved FVC reassures us that a postexercise fall is not attributable to fatigue and a poor effort but truly reflects airway narrowing (23). Conducting the exercise test with the subject breathing frigid dry air probably increases the sensitivity of the exercise test (44). In fact, some laboratories have even substituted a cold air challenge for the exercise test, with the patient at rest but employing a minute ventilation comparable to what would be used during exercise (45). Some laboratories also prefer to compare the highest values of the chosen pulmonary function parameters before, during, or after exercise and after bronchodilator administration with the lowest obtained after exercise, rather than simply looking at the fall after exercise (23). We routinely administer albuterol 20 minutes after exercise to increase comfort for the patient who has suffered bronchoconstriction and to increase the sensitivity of the test for the patient who has not had a dramatic decrease in pulmonary function. Whatever method used, there is a large false-negative rate of laboratory testing for EIA (46).

Conditioning

As one might guess from the fact that there have been so many successful athletes with asthma, patients with asthma can become fit with exercise training and derive the same cardiopulmonary benefits from exercise training as their nonasthmatic peers. There are numerous reports in the literature of benefits from exercise programs for patients with asthma, with no apparent harmful effects, particularly if individual sessions are begun with a preventive medication. The benefits of exercise programs have included the subjective—increased ability to participate in activities, improved emotional status, and decrease in intensity of wheezing attacks (23)—and objective, including increased running performance (47), increased aerobic fitness as measured by peak oxygen consumption (48,49), and cardiac stroke volume (49). The effects of improved fitness on the severity of the underlying asthma have been unclear. Early studies, performed before our understanding of the importance of minute ventilation in the initiation of EIA, were likely to conclude that the underlying asthma was better after conditioning because patients suffered less severe EIA for an identical exercise challenge. The fallacy here is that these early investigations did not take into account the fact that the patients' improved fitness meant that an increased anaerobic threshold. In turn, the increased anaerobic threshold meant that an equal workload called forth a smaller minute ventilation and this smaller ventilation presented the upper airway's air conditioning apparatus with an easier task (23). Thus patients had less EIA for a given exercise challenge after conditioning than before. Most (47,50), but not all (51), more recent studies that have provided challenges that were controlled for equal minute ventilation (rather than equal workload on a treadmill or cycle ergometer) have almost all shown equal EIA responses after conditioning than before. That is, exercise conditioning is good for patients with asthma, but lessened underlying airway reactivity is probably not among the benefits. No studies or clinical experienced have suggested any worsening of asthma with conditioning programs.

Not only is the underlying degree of airway reactivity probably not influenced by conditioning, but perhaps more important, the degree of airway obstruction does not predict the degree of overall fitness and exercise tolerance of individuals with asthma. Just one week before Amy van Dyken became the first American woman to win four gold medals in a single Olympics, her FEF_{25-75} (forced expiratory flow between 25% and 75% of vital capacity—a sensitive measure of smaller airways function) was only 35% of predicted (13). Strunk and colleagues (51) and Garfinkel and colleagues (52) showed a poor relationship between airway obstruction and fitness levels among people with asthma, and Garfinkel and colleagues showed in contrast a close relationship between fitness and habitual activity level (52) (Fig. 23-4).

The message seems clear: Athletes with asthma can have a successful and rewarding experience with sports if they are given effective preparticipation medication and if they are encouraged to become fit, just like their nonasthmatic peers.

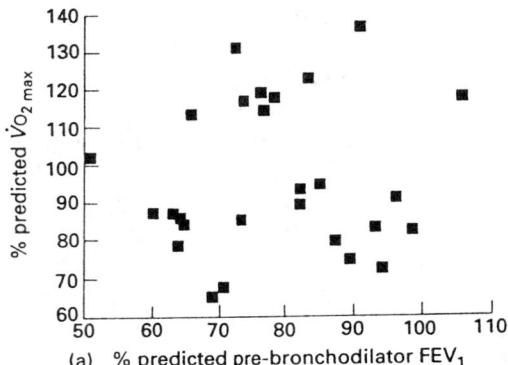
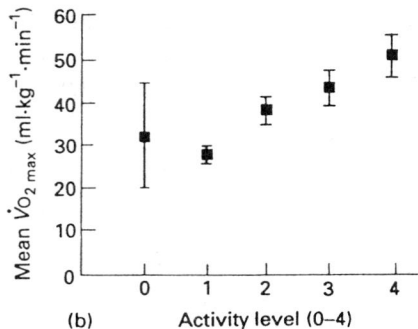

FIG. 23–4. Relationships between fitness and resting pulmonary function (a) and habitual activity level (b) in a group of adults with asthma. There is no relationship between fitness (expressed as percent predicted oxygen consumption, $\dot{V}O_2$) and degree of airway obstruction, whereas there is a relationship between fitness and habitual activity. (From Orenstein D. Asthma and sports. In: Bar-Or O, ed. *The Child and Adolescent Athlete*, 1st ed. Oxford, England: Blackwell Science Ltd, 1996:433-454 (Commission IOCM, ed. *Encyclopaedia of Sports Medicine*, Vol. VI); redrawn from Garfinkel S, Kesten S, Chapman K, Rebuck A. Physiologic and nonphysiologic determinants of aerobic fitness in mild to moderate asthma. *Am Rev Respir Dis* 1992;145:741–745.)

Asthma: Summary

Most patients who are known to have asthma and many with no history of asthma have exercise-induced asthma, with cough, chest tightness, or wheeze during or especially after exercise. In the majority of patients these symptoms can be prevented by inhaled medications taken just before exercise, and patients with asthma can have successful athletic careers. Fitness levels among people with asthma correlate much more closely with habitual activity than with the degree of airway obstruction.

CYSTIC FIBROSIS

Cystic fibrosis (CF) is the most common inherited profoundly life-shortening disease among white populations, with an incidence in North America of one in 3300 live births (53). CF causes progressive airway obstruction, infection, and inflammation, with eventual fibrosis, increasing exercise intolerance, and an early death. Although life expectancy was less than a year or two of age when the disease was first described in 1938, improvements in diagnosis and treatment have increased median survival to 31 years (53). Along with longer survival has come better quality of life, and young CF patients now most often lead a very active life and often participate in sports. In fact, some have completed marathons (54) and Ironman-distance triathlons (2.4-mile swim, 112-mile bike, 26.2-mile run). Fitness levels have been shown to correlate strongly with survival in CF patients (55), so active participation in exercise and sports is to be encouraged. Few special considerations need be made for the athlete with CF.

CF is characterized by thick bronchial mucus, and most patients with CF cough when they exercise. This can be distressing to coaches and spectators and can be uncomfortable to the patient, but it is not dangerous and in fact is helpful in that it helps to clear the airways of the excess mucus. The cough is not contagious, so the coughing CF athlete is not a hazard to teammates or opponents. The child with more advanced disease may have trouble keeping up with his or her peers and may need to stop to catch his or her breath. Even these athletes, though, are not endangering their health and, when possible, should be allowed and encouraged to participate in physical activity as much as possible.

CF sweat contains several times as much salt, drop for drop, as non-CF sweat, and young patients with CF do not have as accurate a thirst drive as non-CF adults or children, so such athletes should be encouraged to drink electrolyte-containing solutions during exercise in the heat (56).

ACKNOWLEDGMENT

Much of the material presented in this chapter appeared in Orenstein DM, Asthma and sports, Chapter 29 of *The Child and Adolescent Athlete* (Bar-Or O, editor), Volume VI of the International Olympic Committee's *Encyclopaedia of Sports Medicine*, 1996, Blackwell Scientific, Oxford.

REFERENCES

1. Johnson B, Saupe K, Dempsey J. Mechanical constraints on exercise hyperpnea in endurance athletes. *J Appl Physiol* 1992;73: 874-886.
2. Johnson B, Beck K. Respiratory system responses to dynamic exercise. In: Weiler J, ed. *Allergic and respiratory disease in sports medicine.* New York: Marcel Dekker, 1997:1–34. (Kaliner M, ed. *Clinical allergy and immunology,* Vol. 11.)
3. Dempsey J, Hanson P, Henderson K. Exercise-induced arterial

hypoxemia in healthy human subjects at sea level. *J Physiol (London)* 1984;355:161.
4. Powers S, Lawler J, Dempsey J, Dodd S, Landry G. Effects of incomplete pulmonary gas exchange on V_{O_2} maximal. *J Appl Physiol* 1989;66:2491–2495.
5. Expert Panel of the National Heart, Lung, and Blood Institute National Asthma Program. Guidelines for the diagnosis and management of asthma. *J Allergy Clin Immunol* 1991;88:425–534.
6. Taylor W, Newacheck P. Impact of childhood asthma on health. *Pediatrics* 1992;90:657–662.
7. Lemanske R, Jr., Henke K. Exercise-induced asthma. In: Gisolfi C, Lamb D, eds. *Youth, exercise, and sport.* Indianapolis: Benchmark Press, 1989:465–511.
8. McFadden E. Exercise-induced asthma: assessment of current etiologic concepts. *Chest* 1987;91:151S–157S.
9. Rupp N, Guill M, Brudno D. Unrecognized exercise-induced bronchospasm in adolescent athletes. *Am J Dis Child* 1992;146:941–944.
10. Rice S, Bierman CW, Shapiro GG, Furukawa C, Pierson WE. Identification of exercise-induced asthma among intercollegiate athletes. *Ann Allergy* 1985;55:790–793.
11. Silvers W. Skiing and other winter sports. In: Weiler J, ed. *Allergic and respiratory disease in sports medicine.* New York: Marcel Dekker, 1997:345–351. (Kaliner M, ed. *Clinical allergy and immunology,* Vol. 11.)
12. General Mills, Inc. Tom Dolan: first American gold medal winner 1996 Atlanta Games (Wheaties box). Minneapolis, MN: General Mills, 1996.
13. Peter M, Silvers W, Thompson F, Weiler J. Case studies of asthma in elite and world-class athletes: the roles of the athletic trainer and physician. In: Weiler J, ed. *Allergic and respiratory disease in sports medicine.* New York: Marcel Dekker, 1997:353–366. (Kaliner M, ed. *Clinical allergy and immunology,* Vol. 11.)
14. Voy R. The U.S. Olympic Committee experience with exercise-induced bronchospasm, 1984. *Med Sci Sports Exerc* 1986;18:328–330.
15. Monahan T. Sidelined asthmatics get back in the game. *Phys Sportsmed* 1986;14(5):61–66.
16. Fitch K. Comparative aspects of available exercise systems. *Pediatrics* 1975;56[Suppl.] (Symposium on Exercise and Asthma):904–907.
17. Godfrey S, Silverman M, Anderson S. The use of the treadmill for assessing exercise-induced asthma and the effect of varying the severity and duration of exercise. *Pediatrics* 1975;56[Suppl.] (Symposium on Exercise and Asthma):893–898.
18. Inbar O, Alvarez D, Lyons H. Exercise-induced asthma: a comparison between two modes of exercise stress. *Eur J Respir Dis* 1981;62:160–167.
19. Speelberg B, Panis E, Bijl D, et al. Late asthmatic responses after exercise challenge are reproducible. *J Allergy Clin Immunol* 1991;87:1128–1137.
20. Edmunds A, Tooley M, Godfrey S. The refractory period after exercise-induced asthma: its duration and relation to the severity of exercise. *Am Rev Respir Dis* 1978;117:247–254.
21. Jones R. Assessment of respiratory function in the asthmatic child. *Br Med J* 1966;2:972–975.
22. Godfrey S. *Exercise testing in children.* Philadelphia: WB Saunders, 1974.
23. Orenstein D. Asthma and sports. In: Bar-Or O, ed. *The Child and Adolescent Athlete,* 1st ed. Oxford, England: Blackwell Science Ltd, 1996:433–454 (Commission IOCM, ed. *Encyclopaedia of Sports Medicine,* Vol. VI.)
24. Bar-Yishay E, Gur I, Inbar O, et al. Differences between swimming and running as stimuli for exercise-induced asthma. *Eur J Appl Physiol* 1982;48:387–397.
25. Makker H, Holgate S. Pathophysiology: role of mediators in exercise-induced asthma. In: Weiler J, ed. *Allergic and respiratory disease in sports medicine.* New York: Marcel Dekker, 1997:136. (Kaliner M, ed. *Clinical allergy and immunology,* Vol. 11.)
26. Anderson S, Daviskas E. Pathophysiology of exercise-induced asthma: the role of respiratory water loss. In: Weiler J, ed. *Allergic and respiratory disease in sports medicine.* New York: Marcel Dekker, 1997:87–114. (Kaliner M, ed. *Clinical allergy and immunology,* Vol. 11.)
27. Wells RJ, Walker J, Hickler R. Effects of cold air on respiratory airflow resistance in patients with respiratory-tract disease. *N Engl J Med* 1960;263:268–273.
28. Strauss R, McFadden E, Ingram R Jr, Jaeger J. Enhancement of exercise-induced asthma by cold air. *N Engl J Med* 1977;297(14):743–747.
29. Bar-Or O, Neuman I, Dotan R. Effects of dry and humid climates on exercise-induced asthma in children and preadolescents. *J Allergy Clin Immunol* 1977;60:163–168.
30. Deal E, Jr., McFadden E, Jr., Ingram R Jr. Hyperpnea and heat flux: initial reaction sequence in exercise-induced asthma. *J Appl Physiol: Respir Environ Exerc Physiol* 1979;46(3):476–483.
31. Godfrey S, Konig P. Inhibition of exercise-induced asthma by different pharmacological pathways. *Thorax* 1976;31:137–143.
32. Anderson S, Bye P, Schoeffel R, et al. Arterial plasma histamine levels at rest and during and after exercise in patients with asthma: effects of terbutaline aerosol. *Thorax* 1981;36:259–267.
33. Lee T, Nagakura T, Papageorgiou N, et al. Mediators in exercise-induced asthma. *J Allergy Clin Immunol* 1984;73:634–639.
34. Manning P, Watson R, Margolskee D, et al. Inhibition of exercise-induced bronchoconstriction by MK-571, a potent leukotriene D4-receptor antagonist. *N Engl J Med* 1990;323:1736–1739.
35. Finnerty J, Wood-Baker R, Thomson H, Holgate S. Role of leukotrienes in exercise-induced asthma: inhibitory effect of ICI 204219, a potent leukotriene D4 receptor antagonist. *Am Rev Respir Dis* 1992;145:746–749.
36. Morton A, Fitch K. Asthmatic drugs and competitive sport: an update. *Sports Med* 1992;14(4):228–242.
37. Woolley M, Anderson S, Quigley B. Duration of protective effect of terbutaline sulfate and cromolyn sodium alone and in combination on exercise-induced asthma. *Chest* 1990;97:39–45.
38. Kemp J, Dockhorn J, Busse W, et al. Prolonged effect of inhaled salmeterol against exercise-induced bronchospasm. *Am J Respir Crit Care Med* 1994;150:1612–1615.
39. Henriksen J, Dahl R. Effects of inhaled budesonide alone and in combination with low-dose terbutaline in children with exercise-induced asthma. *Am Rev Respir Dis* 1983;128:993–997.
40. Reiff D, Choudry N, Pride N, Ind P. The effect of prolonged submaximal warm-up exercise on exercise-induced asthma. *Am Rev Respir Dis* 1989;139:479–484.
41. Schnall R, Landau L. Protective effects of repeated short sprints on exercise-induced asthma. *Allergy Proc* 1980;35:828–832.
42. Brenner A, Weiser P, Krogh K, Loren M. Effectiveness of a portable face mask in attenuating exercise-induced asthma. *JAMA* 1980;244:2196–2198.
43. Orenstein D. Assessment of exercise pulmonary function. In: Rowland T, ed. *Pediatric laboratory exercise testing: clinical guidelines.* Champaign, IL: Human Kinetics, 1993:141–163.
44. Deal E Jr, McFadden E Jr, Ingram R Jr, et al. Airway responsiveness to cold air and hyperpnea in normal subjects and in those with hay fever and asthma. *Am Rev Respir Dis* 1980;121:621–628.
45. Nixon P, Orenstein D. Exercise testing in children. *Ped Pulmonol* 1988;5:107–122.
46. Nickerson B, Bautista D, Namey M, et al. Distance running improves fitness in asthmatic children without pulmonary complications or changes in exercise-induced bronchospasm. *Pediatrics* 1983;71:147–152.
47. Varray A, Mercier J, Terral C, Prefaut C. Individualized aerobic and high intensity training for asthmatic children in an exercise readaptation program: is training always helpful for better adaptation to exercise? *Chest* 1991;99:579–586.
48. Orenstein D, Reed M, Grogan F, Crawford L. Exercise conditioning in children with asthma. *J Pediatr* 1985;106:556–560.
49. Fitch K, Blitvich J, Morton A. The effect of running training on exercise-induced asthma. *Ann Allergy* 1986;57:90–94.
50. Haas F, Pasierski S, Levine N, et al. Effect of aerobic training on forced expiratory airflow in exercising asthmatic humans. *J Appl Physiol* 1987;63:1230–1235.

51. Strunk R, Rubin D, Kelly L, Sherman B. Determination of fitness in children with asthma. *Am J Dis Child* 1988;142:940–944.
52. Garfinkel S, Kesten S, Chapman K, Rebuck A. Physiologic and nonphysiologic determinants of aerobic fitness in mild to moderate asthma. *Am Rev Respir Dis* 1992;145:741–745.
53. FitzSimmons S. *Cystic fibrosis data registry report for 1996.* Bethesda, MD: Cystic Fibrosis Foundation, 1997.
54. Stanghelle JK, Skyberg D. The successful completion of the Oslo Marathon by a patient with cystic fibrosis. *Acta Paediatrica Scandinavica* 1983;72(6):935–938.
55. Nixon P, Orenstein D, Kelsey S, Doershuk C. The prognostic value of exercise testing in patients with cystic fibrosis. *N Engl J Med* 1992;327:1785–1788.
56. Orenstein D. *Cystic fibrosis: a guide for patient and family,* 2nd ed. Philadelphia: Lippincott-Raven, 1997.

CHAPTER 24

Headache and the Athlete

William Primos and Robert Nahouraii

Headache has been a major source of medical concern to the general public and to health professionals, causing pain, lost work and leisure time, and other unaccountable effects on our society. Headaches account for 18.3 million, or 43.2 per 100, physician visits per year (1). Owing to the high prevalence of headache, physicians who care for athletes should be well versed in the diagnosis and treatment of headaches. This chapter contains a presentation of some of the more common causes of headache in the general population followed by a discussion of headaches that are caused by or occur during exercise.

HEADACHE EMERGENCIES

The majority of headaches in the active athlete will be benign, but the physician treating this population should be aware of the signs and symptoms of an acute neurologic process, along with the indications for imaging and treatment (Table 24–1).

The presenting symptoms may include vomiting, diploplia, ataxia, and severe head pain. The headache is often described as "the worst headache of my life." Many of these symptoms result from an acute increase in intracranial pressure, leading to traction on the brainstem, sixth cranial nerve, or posterior fossa contents. If these signs are not addressed quickly, these individuals may experience a loss of cerebral autoregulation and a herniation syndrome.

The examination must include a rapid neurologic examination. The initial evaluation should begin with the assessment of mental status. A patient who is found to be difficult to arouse requires emergency evaluation. The cranial nerve examination may include impairment of upgaze, a sixth cranial nerve palsy, or impairment of cough or gag. The last findings are ominous, as they may indicate lower cranial nerve dysfunction.

Nuchal rigidity may indicate meningeal irritation, either from an infectious process or from hemorrhage. Papilledema cannot be relied on as an important finding, since this can be a late sign. Hyperreflexia and upgoing toes are important upper motor neuron findings that can be assessed rapidly. Traumatic injuries may be seen in the form of hemotympanum, "raccoon eyes," or a significantly depressed skull fracture.

After the rapid assessment of the patient, the question of the need for imaging often occurs. Many of the above signs on physical examination are indications for cranial computed tomography, which at this time is still the study of choice in the acute setting. Computed tomography is sensitive to acute hemorrhage, edema, and fracture. It can be performed quickly, allows easy monitoring of the unstable patient, and is readily available. It also allows a screen for intracranial lesions before lumbar puncture.

At this point, an identified lesion may need medical or surgical intervention. Edema and impending herniation may require intubation and hyperventilation. Osmotic agents or diuretics can reduce intracranial volume while other intervention is planned. Neurosurgical consultation with pressure monitoring for trauma, hemorrhage, and mass lesions can permit the evacuation of hemorrhage, measure intracranial pressure, and accurately guide therapy. Obstructive hydrocephalus may be an indication for ventriculostomy placement and drainage.

TUMOR-RELATED HEADACHE

Headache secondary to a brain tumor can be a cause of early morning, episodic headache due to meningeal irritation or increased intracranial pressure. In adults this has been reported to occur in 40% of new onset tumor diagnoses (2). Generally, one expects progressive

---

W. Primos and R. Nahouraii: Sport Science Center, Charlotte, North Carolina 28211.

TABLE 24-1. Headache emergencies

Signs	Management
Altered mental status	Airway assessment
Nausea	Rapid neurological examination
Vomiting	Cranial computed tomography
Ataxia	Lumbar puncture
Gaze palsies	Surgical intervention
Hyperreflexia	Corticosteroids
Papilledema	Analgesics

worsening of headache over several weeks to months, difficulty with gaze or gaze paresis, dystaxia, and visual field defects.

The sudden worsening of neurologic signs may be due to spontaneous hemorrhage within a tumor, an event in 10% of headache onset (2). Other acute signs that may be present include seizures, hemiparesis, and encephalopathy.

The treatment of tumors may include resection, radiation therapy, chemotherapy, anticonvulsants, and osmotic agents.

MIGRAINES

Migraine headaches are one of the most common types of recurrent headaches. In adolescents and young adults they occur more commonly in females. A recent epidemiologic study found migraine prevalence to be 3% for males and 7.4% for females (3). There is often a family history of migraines in migraine sufferers. These individuals may inherit a predisposition to migraines.

Individuals who experience migraines usually experience two to four attacks of head pain per month. The headache may be preceded by a prodrome that occurs days to hours before the headache. Symptoms of the prodrome may include depression, anorexia, or fluid retention.

There are two general types of migraines: classical migraines, which have a definite aura followed by the headache, and common migraines, which do not have a well-defined aura.

An aura typically begins 5–30 minutes before the headache. Some of the sensory phenomena that may be experienced during the aura include visual disturbances, flashing lights, ringing in the ears, abnormal smells, and paresthesias in the extremities.

The pain of a migraine usually begins as a dull ache and progresses to a severe throbbing sensation. Most commonly, the pain is located on one side of the head or face. The duration of the severe pain may range from 4 hours to several days. Symptoms that may accompany the headache include nausea, vomiting, photophobia, and phonophobia.

After the severe headache subsides, some individuals experience a postdrome with lethargy, drowsiness, and dull pain in the head and neck. The postdrome may last as long as 3 days.

The underlying pathophysiology of migraines is not completely understood. Recent studies have suggested that there are biochemical changes that occur in the brain before a migraine (4). Some of these changes include neuronal depolarization with changes in distribution of potassium, sodium, calcium, and chloride ions; release of excitatory amino acids; changes in neurotransmitter function; and impairment of glycogen mobilization.

Different theories for the actual cause of the headaches have been proposed. Graham and Wolff proposed the vascular theory, which stated that there is an initial vasoconstriction of intracranial vasculature that occurs during the preceding aura. The vasoconstriction is followed by vasodilation, which causes the pain (5). In the neurogenic theory, release of serotonin in the brain results in secretion of neuropeptides. These neuropeptides produce inflammation of intracranial vasculature and the head pain (6).

A variety of activities and substances have been shown to precipitate migraine attacks. Some of the triggers are certain foods, bright or flashing lights, alcohol, emotional stress, and physical exertion. To prevent headaches, individuals may be advised to avoid the specific triggers that cause recurrences.

Pharmacologic treatment of migraines consists of abortive and prophylactic medications (Table 24-2). Abortive medications are taken at the first symptom of a migraine attack. These drugs prevent progression of the headache. Many migraines can be relieved by simple analgesics such as acetaminophen and nonsteroidal anti-inflammatory drugs. Other medications that may be used as abortive therapy include ergot preparations, sumatriptan succinate, and isometheptene mucate with dichloralphenazone.

TABLE 24-2. Migraine therapy

Abortive/analgesic medications	Prophylactic medications
Acetaminophen	Beta-adrenergic blockers (propanolol)
Nonsteroidal anti-inflammatory drugs (ibuprofen, naproxen)	Calcium channel blockers (Verapamil)
Butalbital (Fiorinal)	Tricyclic antidepressants (amitryptyline)
Isometheptene mucate (Midrin)	Anticonvulsants (carbamazepine)
Sumatriptan (Imitrex)	Serotonin uptake inhibitors/antihistamines (cyproheptadine HCl)
Zolmitriptan	
Ergotamine tartrate	

Prophylactic medications may be used if the attacks occur more frequently than twice per month. Prophylactic medications include beta-adrenergic blockers, tricyclic antidepressants, calcium channel blockers, and antiserotonin/antihistaminic medications. Because of their cardiac effects, the use of beta-adrenergic blockers by athletes should be considered only when other therapies have been ineffective.

POSTTRAUMATIC HEADACHES

Athletes and sports participants frequently experience headaches after trauma to the head. Head injuries and concussions are discussed in detail in Chapter 30.

The pathophysiology of posttraumatic headaches can be due to local trauma of the head or muscle injury in the neck. In other cases in which there is no obvious local injury, the pathogenesis of the pain is not definitely known.

There has been research to suggest that the symptoms after mild traumatic brain injury (MTBI) may be due to biochemical changes (7). Many of these changes are similar to the changes found in migraine headaches. Some of the brain alterations that are found in both MTBI and migraine include neuronal depolarization, amino acid and neurotransmitter release, serotonin accumulation, reductions in glucose metabolism, alterations in endogenous opioids, increased intracellular calcium, and changes in magnesium ion concentration. These alterations can cause damage to brain cells and lead to functional deficits and headache (4).

A postconcussion syndrome may occur after a mild head injury. Individuals with postconcussion syndrome may have headache, dizziness, memory and concentration disturbances, fatigue, irritability, depression, and personality changes. The symptoms usually develop within 48 hours of the head injury. These individuals may continue to have problems for months or even years.

Posttraumatic headaches may be primarily muscle contraction/tension headache type or migraine/vascular type.

Trauma-triggered migraines are migraine headaches that result from a blow to the head. They have also been referred to as "footballer's migraine" (8). This headache usually follows a blow to the head or face. The symptoms are similar to those in a classical migraine. The headache is usually preceded briefly by a variety of symptoms, such as flashing lights, blurred vision, visual field defects, speech problems, or paresthesias in the hands. After the neurologic symptoms begin to improve, the headache develops. The headache is a throbbing pain that may last for several hours. There is often associated nausea, vomiting, and photophobia. Recurrences occur after repeated blows to the head or face. These individuals often have a history of migraines not related to trauma and a family history of migraines.

Patients with posttraumatic headache should be closely evaluated to rule out intracranial hemorrhage, since these headaches present in a similar fashion (9). These individuals should be monitored for rising intracranial pressure. Studies such as CT scan are performed for focal neurologic abnormalities, mental status changes, or altered level of consciousness.

Posttraumatic migraines may be treated like nontraumatic migraines with analgesics and abortive medications for the acute attacks and prophylactic therapy such as beta blockers, tricyclic antidepressants, cyproheptadine methysergide, clonidine, and calcium channel blockers.

Headaches that are not migraines but similar to tension headaches may be treated with mild analgesic and nonsteroidal anti-inflammatory medications and muscle relaxers. Biofeedback and muscle relaxation techniques may also be useful.

Athletes with a posttraumatic headache should not be allowed to return to contact sports until all symptoms have resolved (10). Returning to contact sports too soon may lead to a life-threatening condition referred to as *second impact syndrome*. In this condition rapid swelling and herniation of the brain occur after a seemingly minor head injury that was suffered while the individual was experiencing symptoms from a previous concussion.

TENSION HEADACHES

Tension or muscle contraction headaches are headaches that are neither vascular nor inflammatory in origin. The name comes from the belief that the pain originates from contracture of the neck and scalp musculature. However, the pathophysiology of tension headaches is not completely understood. Even though people with tension headaches may have increased muscle contraction, the muscle contraction might not be the cause of the headache pain. The muscle contraction may simply be a consequence of the pain (11). Anxiety or mental stress is often present in tension headache patients, but there is little evidence that anxiety or stress causes muscle tension (12).

These headaches occur in individuals of all ages from adolescence through old age. The pain is often precipitated or worsened by fatigue or stress. The head pain is usually bilateral and in the temporal or occipital regions. It is a steady, dull ache that may be described as feeling like a vise or band around the head. The discomfort usually builds gradually through the day. These headaches can be continuous and may last for weeks, months, or years. There may be associated pain in the posterior neck and shoulders. There may be tenderness of the neck and scalp on exam. Nausea and vomiting are not commonly associated with tension headaches. There is no aura or warning preceding these headaches. Individuals with tension headaches may also experience depression or anxiety.

Tension headaches can be treated with analgesics and nonsteroidal anti-inflammatory medications used in moderation. Other medications that may be useful include muscle relaxants, antidepressant medications, and anxiolytic agents. A variety of nonpharmacologic therapies may also be used in treatment. Some of these include biofeedback, relaxation techniques, and physical therapy. Psychotherapy may also be beneficial to patients who are experiencing depression or anxiety.

NONORGANIC HEADACHES

Many headaches do not fit neatly into one of the above categories or have no organic basis after extensive evaluation. Frequently, the depressed or anxious patient may present with symptoms that are vague, inconsistent, or poorly localized. Headache calendars that document the frequency, duration, and severity of headaches can be helpful before therapy or intervention. Identifying and eliminating stressors can help. Physical therapy and antidepressant therapy may also be useful.

EXERTION-RELATED HEADACHES

Many individuals suffer from headaches that occur only during physical exertion. The symptoms of these headaches are similar to the symptoms of the types of headaches that have been discussed previously in this chapter.

Some exertion-related headaches may be classified as vascular/migraine headaches. To be classified as a sports migraine, the headache should show some of the characteristics of migraine headaches such as an aura before the headache, duration of several hours, unilateral location, throbbing pain, associated nausea and vomiting, and a family history of migraine. An effort migraine is initiated by physical exertion. They often occur after strenuous aerobic exercise such as running in hot conditions. These headaches may also occur with lifting a heavy object. Possible factors in the development of effort migraine headaches include overheating, dehydration, hypoglycemia, and hypoxia (9). It was reported that effort migraine was common among athletes competing in the 1968 Summer Olympic Games in Mexico City (13). It is believed that hyperventilation occurring during exercise or at a high altitude causes hypocapnea that leads to cerebral vasoconstriction, cerebral edema, and hypoxia. Exertion causes elevation of blood pressure with associated headache (14).

Effort migraines may be treated as non-exertion-related migraines with abortive and prophylactic medications. A physical conditioning program, relaxation exercises, and biofeedback may give some protection to individuals with effort migraines. An adequate warm-up period before strenuous exertion may also prevent recurrences or decrease the severity of attacks.

The most common activity-related headache is the effort-exertion headache. This type of headache may be further categorized as either an effort headache or an exertion headache.

An effort headache usually occurs after prolonged aerobic exercise, such as jogging or swimming. These headaches may last for several hours. The pathogenesis of effort headaches is believed to be similar to the mechanisms involved in effort migraines. In both, possible mechanisms involve dehydration, overheating, and fatigue (14–16).

Exertion headaches may also be referred to as benign exertional headaches. These headaches are usually triggered by very intense, short-duration exertion such as heavy lifting or any activity that causes the individual to valsalva. These headaches are usually rapid in onset. The pain may occur in any part of the head. The initial severe pain usually lasts for only a few minutes and is then followed by a dull ache. There have been reports of prolonged exertional headaches lasting for approximately 4 hours (17).

In the management of activity-related headaches, intracranial lesions such as tumors, vascular abnormalities, or Arnold Chiari malformations should be considered in the evaluation. After exclusion of more serious causes of headache, benign exertional headaches can be managed by observation and conservative treatment. Treatment may include anti-inflammatory medications, activity modification, or possibly a general conditioning program (18,19).

REFERENCES

1. Ries PW. *Current estimates from the National Health Interview Survey, United States, 1984.* Washington, DC: National Center for Health Statistics, 1986. (Vital and Health Statistics, Series 10, No. 156 Department of Health and Human Services Publication (PHS) 86-1584.)
2. Cohen ME, Duffner PK. *Brain tumors in children: principles of diagnosis and treatment.* New York: Raven Press, 1994.
3. Linet MS, Stewart WF, Celentano DD, Ziegler D, Sprecher M. An epidemiologic study of headache among adolescents and young adults. *JAMA* 1989;261(15):2211–2216.
4. Packard RC, Ham LP. Pathogenesis of posttraumatic and migraine: a common headache pathway? *Headache* 1997;37:142–152.
5. Graham JK, Wolff HG. Mechanism of migraine headache and action of ergotamine tartrate. *Arch Neurol Psychiatry* 1938;39:737–763.
6. Derman HS. Headaches: diagnosis and treatment. In: Appel S, ed. *Current neurology,* Vol. 14. St. Louis: Mosby, 1994.
7. Hayes RL, Dixon CE. Neurochemical changes in mild head injury. *Semin Neurol* 1994;14:25–31.
8. Mathews WB. Footballer's migraine. *Br Med J* 1972;2:326–327.
9. Atkinson R, Appenzellar O. Headache in sport. *Semin Neurol* 1981;1:334–343.
10. Cantu RC. Guidelines for the return to contact sports after a cerebral concussion. *Phys Sports Med* 1986;14(10):75–83.

11. Pickoff H. Is the muscular model of headache still viable? A review of conflicting data. *Headache* 1984;24:186–198.
12. Ziegler DK, Murrow HG. Headache. In: Joynt RJ, ed. *Clinical neurology,* Vol. 2. Philadelphia: Lippincott-Raven, 1995:1–49.
13. Jokl E. Olympic medicine/sports cardiology. *Ann Sports Med* 1984;1:148–149.
14. Massey EW. Effort headache in runners. *Headache* 1982;22:99–100.
15. Dalessio DJ. Effort migraine. *Headache* 1974;14:53.
16. Williams SJ, Nukada H. Sport and exercise headache: Part 2. Diagnosis and classification. *Br J Sp Med* 1994;28(2):96–100.
17. Diamond S. Prolonged benign exertional headache: its clinical characteristics and response to indomethacin. *Headache* 1982;22:96–98.
18. Dimeff RJ. Headaches in the athlete. *Clin Sports Med* 1982;11(2):339–349.
19. Kunkel RS. Complicated and rare forms of migraine. In: Diamond S, ed. *The practicing physician's approach to headache.* Baltimore: Williams & Wilkins, 1986:76–83.

BIBLIOGRAPHY

Adams RD. *Principles of neurology: headache.* New York: McGraw-Hill, 1993.

Saper J, et al. *Handbook of headache management.* Baltimore: Williams & Wilkins, 1993.

CHAPTER 25

The Athlete with Type 1 Diabetes

Kris Berg

Exercise has long been a part of management for individuals with type 1 or insulin-dependent diabetes. Physical activity provides many benefits for people with type 1 or insulin-dependent diabetes, and for this reason, current medical expertise supports the role of exercise in the management of diabetes (1,2). However, the American Diabetes Association cites the specific enhancement of blood glucose (BG) management in type 2 patients, whereas this benefit is less likely to occur in most people with type 1 diabetes (3).

This chapter focuses on the athlete with type 1 diabetes because athletes are more likely to be younger. Type 2 diabetes does not typically develop until age 40, the rate of incidence increasing with age.

TYPES OF DIABETES

The characteristics of the two major types of diabetes are summarized in Table 25–1. Approximately 90% of the 16 million people with diabetes in the United States have type 2 or non-insulin-dependent diabetes mellitus. Exercise probably offers more medical benefits for those in this majority group than for those with type 1. Although people with type 2 diabetes are prone to hypoglycemia if taking oral hypoglycemic medication or insulin, they are not prone to ketosis. In addition, with exercise, some type 2 patients may be able to control their BG without oral medication or insulin, particularly with significant weight loss.

BENEFITS OF EXERCISE

Consistent maintenance of BG levels reasonably close to normal may reverse the sequelae of poorly controlled diabetes such as retinopathy, nephropathy, microangiopathy, and neuropathy. The Diabetes Control and Complications study substantiated the importance of BG management. In 1400 type 1 patients following a regimen of three or more shots of insulin daily and four or more BG assessments, sequelae previously stated were reduced by about 60%. Patients using this tight pattern of control achieved mean BG values of about 155 mg/dL, equivalent to a HbA_{1c} of 7.2% (4). More recent work shows that lower BG values result in lower glycosylated hemoglobin levels, which should further minimize the incidence and rate of development of sequelae. Because exercise typically causes the BG to drop in controlled patients of both types, exercise is a useful adjunct to the insulin or medication-diet regimen.

Patients with type 1 diabetes appear to be as exercise trainable in most studies as nondiabetics if a reasonable level of health exists so that the vigor and duration of exercise sessions are comparable (5,6). For these reasons exercise appears to offer a number of advantages for people with diabetes in terms of general health as well as diabetes management specifically.

With access to a BG meter, athletes with diabetes should find it easier and safer to exercise. Maintenance of a daily record of BG test results enables both the patient and the physician to keep track of BG control. Periodic measures of glycosylated hemoglobin (HbA_{1c}) can also substantiate BG control for the previous 2–3 months. Table 25–2 summarizes the physical, physiological, and psychological benefits that can occur with exercise in people with diabetes. Details are available elsewhere in the literature (7).

EXERCISE GUIDELINES

BG should be measured before and after exercise. An athlete with diabetes will perform effectively during exercise when BG is normal to moderately elevated (e.g., 100–200 mg/dL) and some insulin is in the blood. This

---

K. Berg: School of Health, Physical Education, and Recreation, University of Nebraska–Omaha, Omaha, Nebraska 68182-0216.

TABLE 25-1. Characteristics of type 1 and type 2 diabetes

Characteristics	Type 1 or insulin dependent	Type 2 or noninsulin dependent
Former terminology	Juvenile onset	Adult onset
Typical age at onset	Before 20	After 40
Family history	Infrequent	Frequent
Appearance of symptoms	Rapid	Slow
Use of insulin	Always	Common but not always required
Production of insulin by pancreas	Absent or partial early after diagnosis	Usually normal or elevated
Proneness to ketoacidosis	Prone	Not prone, rarely occurs
Body fatness	Usually normal or lean	Often obese

facilitates normal substrate utilization rather than an exaggerated use of protein and fat. In moderate and vigorous exercise, limited use of glycogen and glucose impairs performance because they are the primary sources of energy for vigorous activity. Exercise with BG levels above 250 mg/dL tends to further elevate BG as well as possibly lead to ketosis. When BG reaches this threshold level, the lack of insulin stimulates the liver to release glucose via glycogenolysis and slows glucose uptake of tissues. The rise in BG during activity in this metabolic condition is fairly small, but the danger in promoting ketoacidosis exists. If the urinary ketone level is low, exercise is permissible. If the ketone level is moderate to high, exercise should be delayed until the ketone level drops (8).

Low blood insulin levels also stimulate the breakdown of fat through lipolysis. A rise in hormones including the catecholamines, cortisol, growth hormone, and glucagon adds to the effects of insulin shortage and enhances the rise in ketones and glucose. Patients with type 1 diabetes are particularly prone to these effects. The liver converts some of the fatty acids to ketones, leading to ketoacidosis. Severe disturbance in acid-base balance, dehydration, and loss of electrolytes makes for a serious state that may necessitate hospitalization. Consequently, exercising diabetics should have a functional level of insulin in the blood to prevent these changes. Assessment of BG before exercise is essential for this reason. Patients should understand the importance of monitoring ketones when BG exceeds 250 mg/dL.

Exercise an hour or so after a meal or snack is often recommended as a means of minimizing hypoglycemia during activity. If an athlete's practice or contest occurs between meals, supplemental food or reduction in insulin peaking at the time of activity is an effective countermeasure. Guidelines for food intake and insulin are described in Table 25-3. Exercise-induced hypoglycemia actually occurs more frequently in the hours after exercise rather than during activity because of the increased insulin sensitivity of muscle tissue, the increased uptake of BG by muscle, and the small but prolonged rise in metabolism in the hours after exercise.

Skyler and associates recommend BG levels in the range of 60–130 mg/dL before meals, 140–180 mg/dL 1 hour after meals, and 120–150 mg/dL 2 hours after meals (9). If BG remains reasonably close to these values, BG management can be considered adequate.

It is all too common that athletes with diabetes purposely allow the BG to be elevated to high levels to

TABLE 25-2. Benefits of exercise in persons with type 1 diabetes

1. Improved aerobic fitness
    Greater maximal minute ventilation and frequency
    Capacity for greater workload before heavy breathing occurs (i.e., a rise in ventilation or lactate threshold)
    Greater maximal stroke volume and cardiac output
    Less strain on heart at the same submaximal workload (i.e., lower pressure rate product due to reduction in exercise heart rate and blood pressure)
2. Improved ability for tissues to use oxygen
    Greater volume of mitochondria
    Greater activity of mitochondrial enzymes
    More myoglobin
    Enhanced use of fat versus glycogen as a source of muscular energy, which increases the capacity for prolonged exercise and allows a more vigorous work pace to be sustained
3. Greater muscular fitness: increased strength, muscle mass, muscle endurance, and power
4. Increased joint range of motion
5. Reduced risk factors for cardiovascular disease
    Less body fat
    Drop in blood pressure
    Reduced cholesterol and triglyceride
    Improved lipoprotein profile: greater HDL, greater HDL-to-total-cholesterol ratio, less LDL
    Increased maximum oxygen uptake
    Increased fibrinolysis
    Reduced clotting
    Reduced uric acid
    Better ability to tolerate stress
    Increased joie de vivre
6. Improved blood sugar control
7. Reduced insulin or oral medication to regulate blood glucose
8. Improved self-concept and self-image

TABLE 25-3. *Guidelines for pre-exercise snack*

Blood glucose	Guideline
>250 mg/dL	Check ketone level of urine: If absent, exercise without a snack. If moderate or higher, delay exercise until ketone level is low. Use fast-acting insulin to lower blood glucose.
200–250 mg/dL	No snack is needed. If duration exceeds 30 minutes, assess BG.
130–200 mg/dL	Consume 15 g of carbohydrate (one carbohydrate exchange) every half hour.
<130 mg/dL	Consume 30 g of carbohydrate before exercise and 15 g every 30 minutes therafter.

prevent hypoglycemia during practice and games. Athletes may be informed that hypoglycemia resulting from exercise most frequently occurs several hours after activity or even at night. Monitoring BG before exercise and taking a snack based on the BG value may relieve the athlete of worry. Also, anxiety about hypoglycemia during activity may be alleviated by having glucose, dextrose-sugared drinks, or energy bars immediately available on the sidelines or in the training area. It is recommended that BG be measured during practice sessions as well.

BG should be assessed soon after exercise as well as several hours afterward. Metabolism and uptake of glucose from blood remain elevated for hours after an exercise session (10). Hypoglycemia associated with exercise often occurs during this latter period, so a postexercise snack may be needed. Nocturnal hypoglycemia may need to be counteracted by BG checks in the middle of the night, particularly if energy expenditure has been higher than normal or if the activity occurred in the evening. Athletes with diabetes should understand that precontest anxiety mimics symptoms of hypoglycemia, such as muscle weakness, lethargy, trembling, and sweating. Checking BG before competition allows distinguishing between normal pregame jitters and true hypoglycemia. Stress associated with the pregame conditions may elevate BG via catecholamine stimulation of hepatic glycogenolysis. If the athlete eats something as a treatment for symptoms of false hypoglycemia, BG may rise to the point of compromising performance. Ketoacidosis may even be produced, which would inhibit performance owing to decreased blood pH, dehydration, and nausea.

In general, athletes with diabetes must be willing to assess BG more than nonathletes. This may require six or more readings daily to minimize problems.

Exercise should occur after a meal or snack whenever possible. This will minimize the occurrence of hypoglycemia. Hypoglycemia independent of exercise most commonly occurs late in the interval between meals or at the time of a scheduled snack. If exercise is scheduled at this time, a snack before exercise can provide the energy needed. As was stated previously, a BG test before exercise followed by one after the exercise session will indicate whether enough or too many calories of the right type were consumed. The snack should be composed largely of carbohydrates, which can be digested and assimilated rapidly. Protein can be included (e.g., in a sandwich) to sustain the release of glucose for 1–2 hours.

Insulin dosage should be reduced when a training program is started or increased in duration and intensity. In the first several months of an exercise program, a 20–40% reduction is typical (11). In addition to expending more energy, exercise and fat loss increase insulin sensitivity, so less insulin or medication is needed. Additional reductions may not be needed with some athletes because one of the results of aerobic or endurance training is increased utilization of fat during submaximal exercise (12,13) and increased storage of muscle and liver glycogen (14). Skyler and colleagues suggest an insulin dosage for patients with type 1 diabetes in the range of 0.5–1.0 unit/kg of body weight (9). However, highly active individuals such as athletes may need even less, particularly during days of high energy expenditure (15). The insulin that peaks during exercise needs to be reduced as well as the basal insulin dosage (e.g., NPH, lente, ultralente).

The physical activity of athletes may greatly vary with the training stage (e.g., preseason, competitive season) and day of week (e.g., easy versus hard training days, day before a contest, tournament play). Consequently, insulin dose and food intake must be flexible to accommodate these variations. Results of BG monitoring are vital in making effective adjustments.

Strenuous exercise may raise rather than lower BG level. It should not be assumed that exercise always causes BG to drop. Most athletes with diabetes make this assumption. High-intensity exercise, because of increased sympathoadrenal activation, often leads to a rise in BG in athletes with diabetes. This phenomenon appears to occur at exertion levels above 80% VO_2max (16,17). Endurance athletes using interval training at intensities equal to or even surpassing VO_2max often note this disturbing trend. However, the surge in BG typically subsides within several hours after catecholamine degradation and sustained glucose uptake by muscle. The tricky question then arises as to whether or not to administer a bolus of regular insulin to counteract the elevated BG. Because of the heightened insulin sensitivity, glycogen resynthesis, and metabolic rate following exercise, supplemental insulin may produce hypoglycemia. For this reason, if supplemental insulin is used, the dosage should be smaller than when such a rise is not associated with exercise. Furthermore, BG should be monitored at least once within 90 minutes after insulin has been administered to determine the magnitude of change in BG.

During prolonged exercise, such as running a marathon or playing in a daylong athletic tournament, additional BG measurements should be made and extra carbohydrate snacks should be consumed. The dosage of intermediate (e.g., NPH, lente) or long-lasting insulin (e.g., ultralente) should be decreased about 50%, but some insulin is needed to maintain normal metabolism in type 1 patients (1). Additional BG monitoring is helpful in determining dietary alterations.

The insulin injection site should be selected according to the type of exercise performed. The absorption of insulin into blood is enhanced by an increase in local circulation during exercise (2). This brings the injected insulin(s) to a peak effect sooner than normal, which tends to lower the BG faster. To avoid this problem, insulin should not be injected in the thigh before running, cycling, or other leg-predominant forms of exercise. Similarly, the arm or shoulder should not be used as an injection site before activities such as rowing, weight training, and calisthenics. Patients with type 1 diabetes are prone to accidental intramuscular injection of insulin due to lack of subcutaneous fat (18). Concern about injection site has been simplified somewhat by the observation that the most consistent absorption rates of insulin occur when injected into the abdomen. Generally, the farther from the heart, the slower the absorption rate and the longer the time to peak insulin action. Most patients are advised to use the abdomen as the preferred site. If this location is always used and exercise occurs at a similar time on a daily basis, the summative effects of insulin, food, and exercise will provide a fairly consistent BG response. Furthermore, the increased rate of insulin absorption with exercise occurs only in the first hour or two after injection. Most athletes with diabetes would not inject insulin before exercise unless correcting for hyperglycemia or taking the morning dosage. Consequently, for most athletes the injection site may not be particularly critical as long as a consistent pattern is established with insulin, food, and exercise.

Improved BG control can aid weight gain. Elevation of BG indicates an inadequate level of insulin in a type 1 patient. The insulin deficiency retards glucose uptake by the tissues and the synthesis of glycogen. Because glycogen formation is accompanied by water storage, the poorly regulated patient stores less glycogen and water and tends to be chronically dehydrated. Inadequate insulin also slows the uptake of amino acids, which may interfere with the normal rate of protein synthesis and maintenance of skeletal muscle mass.

A shortage of insulin stimulates lipolysis and inhibits fat synthesis by decreasing the rate of glucose uptake into the adipose tissue to produce triglyceride. Consequently, the sum of these effects is that a person with diabetes with chronically elevated BG loses glycogen, body water, protein, and fat. Athletic performance is limited in such patients.

Most young male athletes wish to increase muscle mass. Progressive resistance exercise is effective in producing muscle hypertrophy in those with diabetes as well as nondiabetics, but a second factor promoting weight gain for diabetics is BG management. Tight control minimizes water, fat, and protein loss and helps to maximize the building and maintenance of muscle weight. For some patients this realization may encourage stricter dietary management and BG control.

CONTRAINDICATIONS FOR EXERCISE

Metabolic control should be established before an exercise program is started. As was previously stated, if exercise occurs with a lack of insulin in the blood, the BG will rise during exercise, and ketosis may develop. Newly diagnosed patients or those who are not reasonably well controlled should not begin an athletic training program. The first priority should be to achieve fairly stable BG control. Once control is demonstrated by acceptable BG data and HbA_{1c} level, only then should exercise be introduced. For some athletes this special clearance for exercise may aid motivation to achieve sound BG control. Participation with a parent in a certified diabetes education program is highly recommended.

An exercise electrocardiogram is often warranted for patients older than age 40 or if the duration of diabetes has exceeded 25 years. Patients with diabetes have two to three times the risk for heart and large artery disease as nondiabetics. Silent myocardial ischemia is common in patients who have diabetes for many years (19). Consequently, a functional test of circulation and exercise capacity should be administered for such patients. The results of the test are useful in deciding whether competitive exercise is safe.

Exercise that causes trauma to the feet should be avoided in patients with limited peripheral nerve and blood vessel function. The most common site of vascular insufficiency and peripheral sensory neuropathy is the foot. Patients with these disabilities may injure their feet without perceiving pain. For those with limited peripheral circulation, injuries are slow to heal, and risk of infection is increased. Some sports, such as running, basketball, martial arts, and diving, place considerable trauma on the feet. The athlete as well as the athletic training staff should inspect the athlete's feet daily for superficial wounds, nail care, callus development, and the like. The skin should be kept well lubricated, and callus formation should be minimized.

Patients with retinopathy should avoid strenuous activity that may induce hemorrhage. Contact sports, jumping, scuba diving, weight training, and hanging inverted are not recommended for patients with retinopathy. Systolic blood pressure during activity should be limited to minimize episodes of hemorrhaging. Consequently, limits may need to be set even on nonjarring aerobic exercise such as cycling and swimming, particularly in patients with proliferative retinopathy (20).

SUMMARY

Individuals with type 1 diabetes can and do participate in competitive sport, even at the highest levels of competition. Athletes with diabetes should consistently use exercise in a judicious manner as a basic part of their overall management program. Exercise has a number of physical, physiological, social, and psychological benefits, many of which may directly or indirectly affect BG and consequently patients' long-term health. With appropriate use of glucose-monitoring devices, most patients can and should be regularly active. To minimize metabolic problems, six or more BG assessments daily are advised for athletes with diabetes. For many adolescents with diabetes, participation in sports may remove the common stigma that they are physically limited. Furthermore, regular exercise may motivate some athletes with diabetes to maintain better BG control because of the impact on their capacity to perform.

REFERENCES

1. Berger M, Berchtold P, Cuppers JJ, et al. Metabolic and hormonal effects of muscular exercise in juvenile type diabetics. *Diabetologia* 1977;13:355–365.
2. Vranic M, Berger M. Exercise and diabetes mellitus. *Diabetes* 1979;28:147–163.
3. American Diabetes Association. Exercise and NIDDM. *Diabetes Care* 1990;13:785–789.
4. American Diabetes Association. Implications of the diabetes control and complications trial. *Clinical Diabetes* 1993(July/Aug):41–96.
5. Costill DL, Cleary P, Fink WJ, et al. Training adaptations in skeletal muscle of juvenile diabetics. *Diabetes* 1979;28:812–822.
6. Larsson Y, Persson B, Sterky G, Thoren C. Functional adaptation to vigorous training and exercise in diabetic and nondiabetic adolescents. *J Appl Physiol* 1964;19:629–635.
7. Berg K. Metabolic disease: diabetes mellitus. In: Seefeldt V, ed. *Physical activity and human well being*. Reston, VA: American Alliance of Health, Physical Education, Recreation and Dance, 1986.
8. Leontos C, Dawson L. Special report: highlights of the American Dietetic Association's 75th annual meeting. *Diabetes Spectrum* 1993;6:62–65.
9. Skyler J, Skyler D, O'Sullivan M. Algorithms for adjustment of insulin dosage by patients who monitor blood glucose. *Diabetes Care* 1981;4:311–318.
10. Hagberg JM, Mullin JP, Nagle FJ. Effect of work intensity and duration in recovery O_2. *J Appl Physiol* 1980;48:540–544.
11. A round table: diabetes and exercise. *Phys Sportsmed* 1979;7:49–64.
12. Felig P, Wahren J. Amino acid metabolism in exercising man. *J Clin Invest* 1971;50:2703–2714.
13. Hagenfeldt L, Wahren J. Metabolism of free fatty acids and ketone bodies in skeletal muscle. In: Pernow B, Saltin B, eds. *Muscle metabolism during exercise*. New York: Plenum Press, 1971.
14. Bergstrom J, Hermansen L, Saltin B. Diet, muscle glycogen and physical performance. *Acta Physiol Scand* 1967;71:140–150.
15. Berg K. Blood glucose regulation in an insulin-dependent diabetic backpacker. *Phys Sportsmed* 1983;11:101–104.
16. Kjaer M, Farrell P, Christensen N, Galbo H. Increased epinephrine response and inaccurate glucoregulation in exercising athletes. *J Appl Physiol* 1986;61:1693–1700.
17. Marliss E, Purdon C, Miles P, et al. Glucoregulation during and after intense exercise in control and diabetic subjects. In: Devlin J, Horton E, Vranic M, eds. *Diabetes mellitus and exercise*. Nishimura, Japan: Smith-Gordon, 1992.
18. Frid A, Gunnarsson P, Guntner P, Linde B. Effects of accidental intramuscular injection of insulin on insulin absorption in IDDM patients. *Diabetes Care* 1988;11:41–44.
19. Wallberg-Hendriksson H. Exercise and diabetes mellitus. In: Holloszy J, ed. *Exercise and sport sciences reviews*. Baltimore: Williams & Wilkins, 1992.
20. Vitug A, Schneider S, Ruderman N. Exercise and type 1 diabetes mellitus. In: Pandolf K, ed. *Exercise and sports sciences reviews*. New York: Macmillan, 1988.

CHAPTER 26

Hematological Problems in Athletes

E. Randy Eichner

INTRODUCTION

Blood has long fascinated humankind: It permeates our language as it permeates our bodies. We speak of blood being thick or thin, hot or cold, bad or blue. We tell of blood feuds and blood brothers. For two thousand years, physicians prescribed blood-letting. Plasmapheresis, or blood-washing, is used today to treat certain ailments. And today in sports, alas, we have blood boosting.

Athletes, trainers, and coaches focus on blood and performance. They want to know what hemoglobin level is normal for an athlete and what level it takes to win. They ask about sports anemia. They ponder hematologic aspects of altitude training: how it changes the blood, whether or not it poses a risk of thrombosis. They need to know the risks of competition for athletes with mild bleeding disorders. They are puzzled by low ferritin values—why they happen, what they mean. They want tips on preventing iron-deficiency anemia. They are curious about footstrike hemolysis and how to avoid it. They want to know the sports implications of sickle-cell trait. And they have concerns about blood boosting in sports. These aspects of blood and sports are covered here.

ANEMIA

The finding of a subnormal hemoglobin concentration is common among certain athletes, especially endurance athletes—women more than men. Two problems arise in interpreting such "low" values in athletes. First, normal hemoglobin values are set by testing healthy people from the general population, many of whom are sedentary. As will be covered below, sedentary people tend paradoxically to have *higher* hemoglobin concentrations than athletes. So the normal range for hemoglobin levels in the general population is not normal for all athletes.

The second problem is that anemia is generally diagnosed by finding a low hematocrit or low hemoglobin concentration, but these routine laboratory tests do not gauge the mass of circulating red blood cells. Rather, they reflect the dilution of red cells in blood plasma. So hematocrit or level of hemoglobin is low if the mass of circulating red cells is low—the definition of anemia. But hematocrit or level of hemoglobin is also low when red cell mass is normal but plasma volume is higher than average, as in athletes.

Parenthetically, the habit of defining anemia by level of hematocrit should be dropped, because by modern laboratory methods—electronic blood counters—hematocrit is a calculated value and therefore more prone to error than is the measured concentration of hemoglobin. The usual criterion for the diagnosis of anemia is a hemoglobin concentration under 14 g/dL in a man or under 12 g/dL in a woman. But because mild, undiagnosed iron-deficiency anemia is fairly common among the general population of women (those from whom "normal" laboratory values are determined), a more sensitive yet realistic marker of anemia in women is a hemoglobin concentration under 13 g/dL.

Mild anemia in athletes can be subtle, manifesting itself as fatigue only during all-out exercise. For example, as was reported in a recent benchmark article on exercise as a disease detector, an 18-year-old collegiate basketball star experienced undue breathlessness and fatigue on the court for 2 months and was thought to have exercise-induced asthma before the correct diagnosis of mild anemia (hemoglobin 11 g/dL) was made. The milder the anemia, the more likely it is that strenuous exercise will be the only unmasker (1).

Another key point is that anemia is not a diagnosis, but a sign that something is wrong—a sign of underlying disease. So the potential causes of anemia are many. Before proper therapy can be given to the athlete with anemia, the cause of the anemia must be pinpointed.

E. R. Eichner: University of Oklahoma Health Sciences Center, Oklahoma City, Oklahoma 73111–6657.

Although any athlete can in theory have any anemia—being born with thalassemic trait or hereditary spherocytosis, for example—the three most common causes of anemia (low hemoglobin level) in athletes are sports anemia, iron-deficiency anemia, and footstrike hemolysis. Probably the most common, at least in endurance athletes, is sports anemia.

SPORTS ANEMIA

Athletes, especially endurance athletes, tend normally to have slightly low hemoglobin levels as judged by the norms for the general population. In other words, endurance athletes tend to be diagnosed as "slightly anemic." This has been called sports anemia.

The term *sports anemia,* however, is imprecise, because no one anemia is tied to sports. Worse, *sports anemia* is a misnomer, because most often a slightly low hemoglobin level in an endurance athlete is a false anemia. The red cell mass is not low, but normal. The hemoglobin concentration is decreased because regular aerobic exercise expands the baseline plasma volume, which dilutes the red cell count and hemoglobin concentration. Put another way, the naturally lower hemoglobin level of an endurance athlete is a dilutional pseudoanemia.

This pseudoanemia is surely an adaptation to the loss of plasma—the hemoconcentration—that occurs early in each workout. Vigorous exercise acutely reduces plasma volume by up to 10–20% in three ways. First, the exercise-induced rise in mean arterial blood pressure and muscular compression of venules boosts capillary hydrostatic pressure. Second, the generation of lactic acid and other metabolites in working muscle increases tissue osmotic pressure. These two forces drive an ultrafiltrate of plasma from blood to tissues. Third, some plasma is lost in sweat.

In adapting to the repeated hemoconcentration of aerobic training, the body releases renin, aldosterone, and vasopressin to conserve water and salt. Also, albumin is added to the blood (2). As a result, baseline plasma volume expands. Even a single bout of intense, intermittent exercise can expand the plasma volume 10% within 24 hours (3). As a rule of thumb, the baseline plasma volume may expand by about 5% in recreational walkers or joggers to as much as 15–20% in top endurance athletes (4).

It is common, then, for a top endurance athlete (training at sea level) to have a hemoglobin level that is 1 g/dL or even 1.5 g/dL below the "lower limit of normal." Recognizing this as pseudoanemia depends on knowing the setting (aerobic training) and excluding other anemias, notably iron-deficiency anemia. The baseline plasma volume waxes and wanes quickly in concert with level of exercise, so athletes who train the most have the lowest hemoglobin levels, and when daily workouts are stopped, the hemoglobin level soon rises.

Athletic pseudoanemia is a key part of aerobic fitness. The increase in plasma volume—along with the adaptations of athlete's heart—increases the cardiac stroke volume. This overrides the fall in hemoglobin concentration per unit of blood, so more oxygen is delivered to muscles. Pseudoanemia also lowers the heart rate for a given exercise intensity and increases the ability to shed heat. These changes make for a better athlete. As a benefit, dilutional pseudoanemia is to be desired, not prevented.

IRON-DEFICIENCY ANEMIA

The most common "true" anemia in athletes, as in the general population, is iron-deficiency anemia. Iron-deficiency anemia is not common in male athletes unless they have bled from the nose or gastrointestinal (GI) tract. But it is common in female athletes, who have physiologic depletions of iron and may eat diets that are low in available iron. Surveys suggest that up to 20% of female athletes are low in iron and about 5% have iron-deficiency anemia.

Debated is whether iron deficiency among female athletes is due to their sport. Athletic training, especially endurance training, does tend to lower the serum ferritin level, as reviewed elsewhere (5). But the fall in ferritin from training is not necessarily pathophysiologic; it may reflect only hemodilution and a shift of iron from stores to the functional compartments, hemoglobin and myoglobin.

Because training lowers ferritin level (i.e., iron stores), one might expect trained athletes to be uniquely prone to iron-deficiency anemia. Early studies suggested this to be so, but recent studies, better controlled, suggest that athletes as a group are not uniquely prone to this anemia. An exception may be female distance runners (5).

So the question becomes, Why do some athletes develop iron-deficiency anemia? Controversial is whether athletes can lose enough iron in sweat to cause iron deficiency. A recent study finds that sweat iron loss is modest. In 1 hour of moderate exercise, athletes lost only 6–11% of the iron that is typically absorbed daily. The authors concluded that sweat iron losses would not likely deplete iron stores in men but might do so in female athletes whose diets are low in iron (6).

Only trivial amounts of iron are normally lost in urine. Athletes can get hematuria from diverse causes but not enough hematuria to drain iron stores (7). Nor does footstrike hemolysis drain iron stores. Urinary iron loss in athletes is negligible.

Iron-deficiency anemia in athletes such as female distance runners is generally due to inadequate dietary iron for physiologic needs. Women who lose more than 60 mL of blood per menses are more apt to develop anemia. Pregnancy also drains iron stores. Female athletes lose more iron via sweating than inactive women do. These physiologic drains in female athletes could be offset by an iron-rich diet.

But insufficient iron can plague female athletes who are dieting, have eating disorders, or are vegetarian. The recommended dietary allowance for iron for women is 15 mg/day. Many competitive female athletes, however, notably "low-weight" athletes (e.g., ballet dancers, gymnasts, ice skaters, divers, distance runners) consume no more than 2000 kilocalories per day, which translates to only 12 mg of iron a day. In other words, they consume too little iron for their needs.

Contrary to popular belief, no good evidence exists for impaired iron absorption in athletes. But the iron in vegetarian diets (in grains and vegetables) is not highly bioavailable, and several studies agree that female athletes who shun red meat are prone to iron deficiency.

Finally, in any athlete with iron-deficiency anemia, one must consider incidental or sports-related GI bleeding (8). Diverse causes of GI bleeding, including ischemic colitis, are tied to sports. These are covered in another chapter.

Diagnosis of iron-deficiency anemia hinges on finding microcytic, hypochromic red blood cells in an anemic patient with a serum ferritin under 12 ng/dL. The best treatment is ferrous sulfate, 325 mg two or three times a day, with meals. Ideally, after a delay of a week or so, the hemoglobin should rise at the rate of about 1 g/dL a week. In about 3 weeks the athlete's hemoglobin level should be halfway back to normal, and in about 2 months it should be normal.

Dietary prevention of iron-deficiency anemia is covered in detail elsewhere (5). Briefly, practical tips include the following:

1. Eat more lean red meat.
2. To boost iron absorption from iron-fortified bread and cereals, avoid coffee or tea with meals and consume a source of vitamin C, such as orange juice.
3. Cook eggs and acidic foods (e.g., tomato sauce, vegetable soup) in cast-iron cookware to leach iron into the food.
4. Eat poultry or seafood (which contain little iron) with dried beans, peas, or other legumes so that the animal protein will enhance absorption of iron from the legumes.

When a female athlete repeatedly develops iron-deficiency anemia despite dietary tips, consider supplementing with ferrous sulfate, 325 mg two or three times a week. Oral contraceptives, if otherwise indicated, can regulate menses and curb menstrual blood loss.

FOOTSTRIKE HEMOLYSIS

Footstrike hemolysis is the bursting of red blood cells in circulation (intravascular hemolysis) from the impact of footfalls. Because intravascular hemolysis occurs in other sports, such as aerobic dancing, rowing, weight lifting, even swimming, it is better termed *exertional hemolysis* (9).

Exertional hemolysis is usually mild and rarely exhausts haptoglobin. This means the iron released from hemolyzed red cells is recycled, not lost in urine. So exertional hemolysis rarely if ever drains iron stores. And the mild hemolysis can easily be offset by mild reticulocytosis, so exertional hemolysis rarely if ever causes anemia.

Diagnosis hinges on the triad of (1) high red cell mean cell volume, (2) reticulocytosis, and (3) low serum haptoglobin level. All three of these abnormalities are mild. The blood smear usually is normal or shows a rare crenated red cell. Hemoglobinuria is rare because serum haptoglobin is rarely exhausted.

Treatment of footstrike hemolysis involves the following measures to lessen impact:

1. Wear better-cushioned running shoes.
2. Lose weight.
3. Avoid a "stomping" gait; instead, learn to run light on the feet.
4. Run on soft surfaces such as grass or dirt roads.

Unclear is how to reduce the exertional hemolysis of other sports. Except among world-class distance runners, any exertional hemolysis is so mild as to need no treatment.

SICKLE-CELL TRAIT

Sickle-cell trait (SCT), present in about 8% of American blacks and in about one in 10,000 American whites, is generally covert and benign throughout life. Athletes with SCT have no anemia, no blood smear abnormalities, and few or no clinical consequences. Indeed, SCT is consistent with top athletic performance. Surveys find the expected number of athletes with SCT in the National Football League, in high school football, and in young elite athletes and runners in Africa. One recent study, however, does suggest that SCT runners in Africa are slower than peers without SCT when they race at high altitude (10).

For practical purposes, only three clinical complications are linked to SCT: (1) hematuria and hyposthenuria; (2) splenic infarction at moderate altitude; and (3) a rare and too often fatal syndrome of exertional sickling, fulminant rhabdomyolysis, and sudden collapse (11). All three of these complications are relevant to athletes.

The hematuria, which is due to sickling and papillary necrosis deep in the renal medulla, is not necessarily caused by sports play, but calls for rest until it clears. The hyposthenuria, also due to sickling in the medulla, may foster dehydration in athletes. Splenic infarction occurs because of splenic sickling from the hypoxia of altitude. It can occur at rest (at altitude), but some case reports suggest that exercise (at altitude) may increase the risk of splenic infarction. Examples are skiers and, in theory, black football players who are training hard when new at altitude. Physicians should suspect splenic infarction when any athlete who is new at altitude suffers acute abdominal pain or distress or a left-sided "side-stitch." Early diagnosis may obviate splenectomy; bed rest, oxygen, and hydration may suffice. The grave threat for athletes with SCT is the rare syndrome of heroic exercise and fatal collapse (11).

Emerging evidence shows that in some military recruits and athletes with SCT, all-out exercise, especially when new at altitude or to a hot, humid climate, can evoke an acute, life-threatening syndrome of sickling in the working limbs, fulminant rhabdomyolysis, lactic acidosis, collapse, acute renal failure, and hyperkalemia. The early symptoms or warning signs, often after running less than a mile, include undue fatigue and dyspnea and especially severe muscular cramping in the legs, buttocks, and low back. Over the past 25 years, more than 30 such cases, many fatal, have been reported. Milder cases, nonfatal, are also on record (12). Unfortunately, fatal cases are still being reported (13,14), and surely other cases have not been reported.

Physicians and trainers must know that this sickling syndrome can mimic other causes of sudden collapse and that prompt diagnosis and emergent therapy can save lives. To avoid this grave syndrome, all athletes—with or without SCT—should stay fit and train wisely, acclimatize themselves to any new environment before exercising all-out, stay hydrated at all times, rest when sick, heed unexpected environmental stress, be aware of the early symptoms; and never charge recklessly into heroic exercise.

BLEEDING AND CLOTTING PROBLEMS

Nosebleeds in athletes are usually local problems and will not be covered here. The three most common systemic bleeding disorders in young athletes are (1) immune thrombocytopenic purpura (ITP), which usually is either autoimmune or drug-induced; (2) hemophilia, an inherited deficiency of factor VIII or IX; and (3) von Willebrand's disease (VWD), an inherited disorder of platelet function (reflected by a prolonged bleeding time) and a partial deficiency of functional factor VIII. VWD, which occurs in about one in 100–1000 people, is more common than hemophilia, which occurs in about one in 5000 males. Essential thrombocythemia, a rare disorder that can pose a bleeding risk, has also been seen in young athletes.

Clues to underlying hemophilia in contact athletes are large, deep, slowly resolving hematomas, as in the thigh in football players. Hemarthroses, as in the knee, are also common. In any athlete crops of petechiae and purpura suggest thrombocytopenia; they often first appear in dependent areas, as about the ankles in a runner. The abnormal bleeding in VWD is often mucosal (epistaxes, GI bleeding) and in women includes menorrhagia; hemarthroses are rare. Any of these bleeding disorders can be worsened by the use of aspirin, which inhibits platelet function. Other nonsteroidal anti-inflammatory drugs (NSAIDs) also inhibit platelet function but not as much as aspirin does.

Diagnosing bleeding disorders is best done in concert with a hematologist. Routine starting tests are the complete blood count (CBC) to document thrombocytopenia and the prothrombin time and partial thromboplastin time (PT and PTT). A prolonged PTT can be the first clue to the diagnosis of hemophilia or VWD, both of which have been seen in young football players.

Therapy varies by case. In children most cases of ITP are self-limited. Other cases remit when the offending drug is stopped, as in a professional football player who developed ITP after taking quinine sulfate for muscle cramps (15). In adolescent and young adult athletes, however, most cases of ITP are autoimmune related and need therapy with corticosteroids and/or other measures, such as splenectomy. In mild ITP, if the platelet count stays above 100,000/mm^3, contact sports may be allowed. Hemophilia and VWD are lifelong problems that need close follow-up and judicious clotting-factor replacement; these disorders often preclude contact sports, certainly collision sports (16).

The main clotting problem for athletes is deep venous thrombosis (DVT), which can present as acute calf pain. DVT in the lower extremity—with or without pulmonary embolism—has been reported in football players, wrestlers, marathoners, triathletes, skiers, other recreational athletes, and even in umpires (17–19).

Predisposing factors to DVT of the lower limb in athletes may include dehydration, prolonged standing or squatting, constricting garments or braces, recent minor surgery, long plane or car rides after competition, elevated hemoglobin level from blood boosting, and trauma to the involved vein.

Regarding trauma to the vein, the analogy is to effort thrombosis, the syndrome of thrombosis of the axillary-subclavian vein that presents as acute or subacute painless or mildly painful arm swelling in weight lifters, wrestlers, baseball or tennis players, or runners who run with hand weights. The risk of major pulmonary embolism seems to be less from upper-limb DVT than from lower-limb DVT (20).

The athlete with DVT will usually present with fairly localized pain in the calf, popliteal area, groin, or axilla. Palpable cords and/or local inflammation may be present. Distal swelling, especially after effort, is usually present. Pulses are intact. Homan's sign, or calf pain upon ankle dorsiflexion, is unreliable as the sole diagnostic criterion. Acute calf pain in an athlete can be from DVT but also from muscle strain, calf hematoma, acute or chronic exertional compartment syndrome, cellulitis, or ruptured or dissecting Baker's cyst. In fact, cases of DVT in athletes have been first diagnosed as muscle strains. Sure diagnosis of DVT on physical examination is notoriously difficult; the team physician would be wise to maintain a high index of suspicion for DVT. Definitive testing should be done early rather than later. Early diagnosis and therapy minimizes the risk of pulmonary emboli and venous value damage that can lead to chronic venous insufficiency.

Diagnosis of DVT is usually made by clinical suspicion, positive physical findings, and imaging. The gold standard of imaging is still the venogram, but noninvasive diagnostic methods are gaining sway, especially compression ultrasonography or impedance plethysmography.

Standard therapy of DVT includes heparin for about 5 days (with warfarin) and then warfarin for several months. Optimal duration of warfarin is debated; cases should be individualized. Return to play decisions also vary by case. One report suggests that for a triathlete recovering from DVT, a graded return to full training can take place over 6 weeks (19). Athletes taking warfarin should not play contact sports and should avoid aspirin and other NSAIDs, which increase the risk of bleeding.

Hypercoagulability is increasing being suspected or documented in individual athletes, as it is in the general population. For example, hypercoagulability was suspected in an older male recreational skier who developed DVT (18). Also, likely hypercoagulability (resistance to activated protein C) was recently documented in a young, elite, female mogul skier who had a family history—but no personal history—of DVT. This athlete was warned about other predisposing factors for DVT, such as long plane rides and the dehydration and erythrocytosis of high-altitude training (21).

BLOOD BOOSTING

Altitude training is in vogue as a legal and ethical way to "blood boost": to increase hemoglobin concentration. Field research suggests that a practice known as "living high and training low"—living at moderate altitude and training at least in part at lower elevations—offers runners a competitive edge over those who live and train at sea level or those who live and train at altitude. That is, living high and training low can shave vital seconds off the 5-km running time, a racing improvement that is in direct proportion to the increase in maximal oxygen capacity (22).

Altitude training is legal, but using recombinant human erythropoietin (rhEPO) is not. Yet athletes have used and are using rhEPO to blood boost. Beginning in 1987, when rhEPO first appeared in Europe, and continuing into 1990, at least 18 competitive European cyclists died, most of them suddenly and unexpectedly. Suspected of playing a role in some of the deaths was rhEPO. Cycling officials denied it at the time, but several former European cyclists have recently admitted that they used rhEPO and have said that many racing cyclists still use it. Evidence also suggests that rhEPO is in use among endurance skiers and triathletes.

The problem for athletes is that if rhEPO drives the hemoglobin level too high, it increases the work of the heart and poses a risk of thrombosis. It also seems that rhEPO can increase exercising blood pressure (23). Methods to detect the use of rhEPO are being developed (24,25); perhaps soon its use in sports can be curbed. In the meantime, skiing and cycling federations are drawing blood samples before races and barring from the race any athlete with a hematocrit over 50%.

Now altitude houses are used to blood boost athletes. Finnish sports scientists built the first one in 1993. Skiers, rowers, biathletes, and runners in four European countries use them. The idea is to live high and train low without moving to the mountains. The athletes live and train at sea level, where oxygen is plentiful to support hard training. But for about 12 hours a day, they live and sleep in airtight houses or chambers with nitrogen mixed into the air supply to drop the normal oxygen content from 21% to 15%. This "thin air" leads to an increase in endogenous erythropoitin level and so an increase in hemoglobin level.

Altitude houses are legal, and many people think they are also ethical–just another technological advance, like clap skates. But are they safe? And are they fair? What price glory?

REFERENCES

1. Eichner ER, Scott WA. Exercise as disease detector. *Phys Sportsmed* 1998;26(3):41–52.
2. Yang RC, Mack GW, Wolfe RR, Nadel ER. Albumin synthesis after intense intermittent exercise in human subjects. *J Appl Physiol* 1998;84:584–592.
3. Gillen CM, Lee R, Mack GW, et al. Plasma volume expansion in humans after a single intense exercise protocol. *J Appl Physiol* 1991;71:1914–1920.
4. Eichner ER. Sports anemia, iron supplements, and blood doping. *Med Sci Sports Exerc* 1992;24:S315–S318.
5. Eichner ER. Minerals: Iron. In: Maughan RJ, ed. *Nutrition in sport*, Vol. VII, International Olympic Committee, ed. *Encyclopaedia of sports medicine.* Oxford, England: Blackwell Science Ltd, 1998:Chapter 24.
6. Waller MF, Haymes EM. The effects of heat and exercise on sweat iron loss. *Med Sci Sports Exerc* 1996;28:197–203.
7. Eichner ER. Hematuria: a diagnostic challenge. *Phys Sportsmed* 1990;18(11):53–63.
8. Eichner ER. Gastrointestinal bleeding in athletes. *Phys Sportsmed* 1989;17(5):128–140.
9. Selby GB, Eichner ER. Endurance swimming, intravascular hemolysis, anemia and iron depletion: a new perspective on athlete's anemia. *Am J Med* 1986;81:791–794.
10. Thiriet P, Le Hesran JY, Wouassi D, et al. Sickle cell trait performance in a prolonged race at high altitude. *Med Sci Sports Exerc* 1994;26:914–918.
11. Eichner ER. Sickle cell trait, heroic exercise, and fatal collapse. *Phys Sportsmed* 1993;21(7):51–64.
12. Browne RJ, Gillespie CA. Sickle cell trait: a risk factor for life-threatening rhabdomyolysis? *Phys Sportsmed* 1993;21(6):80–88.

13. Murray MJ, Evans P. Sudden exertional death in a soldier with sickle cell trait. *Military Med* 1996;161:303–305.
14. Kerle KK, Nishimura KD. Exertional collapse and sudden death associated with sickle cell trait. *Military Med* 1996;161:766–767.
15. Powell SE, O'Brien SJ, Barnes R, et al. Quinine-induced thrombocytopenia. *J Bone Joint Surg* 1988;70:1097–1099.
16. McLain LG, Heldrich FT. Hemophilia and sports: guidelines for participation. *Phys Sportsmed* 1990;18(1):73–80.
17. Johnson PR, Krafcik J, Greene JW. Massive pulmonary embolism in a varsity athlete. *Phys Sportsmed* 1984;12(12):61–63.
18. Williams JS Jr, Williams JS. Deep vein thrombosis in a skier's leg: did exertion contribute to clotting? *Phys Sportsmed* 1994;22(1):79–84.
19. Roberts WO, Christie DM Jr. Return to training and competition after deep venous calf thrombosis. *Med Sci Sports Exerc* 1992;24:2–5.
20. Martinnelli I, Cattaneo M, Panzeri D, et al. Risk factors for deep venous thrombosis of the upper extremities. *Ann Intern Med* 1997;126:707–711.
21. Hilberg T, Moessmer G, Hartard M, Jeschke D. APC resistance in an elite female athlete. *Med Sci Sports Exerc* 1998;30:183–184.
22. Levine BD, Stray-Gundersen J. "Living high-training low": effect of moderate-altitude acclimatization with low-altitude training on performance. *J Appl Physiol* 1997;83:102–112.
23. Ekblom B, Berglund B. Effect of erythropoietin administration on maximal aerobic power. *Scand J Med Sci Sports* 1991;1:88–93.
24. Wide L, Bengtsson C, Berglund B, Ekblom B. Detection in blood and urine of recombinant erythropoietin administered to healthy men. *Med Sci Sports Exerc* 1995;27:1569–1576.
25. Gareau R, Audran M, Baynes RD, et al. Erythropoietin abuse in athletes. *Nature* 1996;380:113.

CHAPTER 27

Renal Problems in the Athlete

Thomas H. Trojian and Douglas B. McKeag

INTRODUCTION

During exercise many changes occur in the kidneys. The renal blood flow decreases with the onset of exercise. Alterations occur at both the glomerulus and renal tubules that cause changes in urine content and output. Many of the metabolites and hormones that are produced during exercise have an effect on the glomeruli and tubules. The decrease in renal blood flow and the effects of metabolic products can lead to proteinuria and hematuria. When an athlete with urinary findings presents to the sports medicine physician for evaluation, the normal variants as well as the pathologic states need to be considered. The physician needs to avoid subjecting the athlete to expensive and potentially harmful invasive tests. We will discuss the physiologic changes in the kidneys during exercise and review proteinuria, hematuria, acute renal failure, and renal trauma.

PHYSIOLOGY

Ultrafiltration of the blood occurs at the glomerulus complex. The renal blood flow (RBF) to the glomerulus is controlled by afferent and efferent arterioles. The renal tubules then reabsorb components of ultrafiltrate to form the urine. During exercise there are changes in the ultrafiltration and reabsorption of components.

As exercise is initiated, renal blood flow (RBF) decreases. The renal plasma flow (RPF) is measured by *p*-aminohippuric acid (PAH) clearance. See Table 27–1 for details of the technique.

There is a linear correlation between exertion and the changes in RBF (1). The exertional changes in RBF are not altered with age during moderate exercise (2).

T. H. Trojian: Department of Family Medicine, Saint Francis Hospital and Medical Center, University of Connecticut Health Center, Hartford, Connecticut 06105.
D. B. McKeag: Department of Family Medicine, Indiana University School of Medicine, Indianapolis, Indiana 46202–5263.

Castenfors (3) and Grimby (4) showed that as the percentage of V_{O_2}max increases the RBF decreases. Poortmans (1) reported that moderate exercise results in a RBF reduction of nearly 30% and that strenuous exercise may cause a decrease up to 75%. Castenfors (3) showed no significant change in the reduction of RBF with hyperhydration. The work of Smith and colleagues (5) showed greater decrease in RBF, with a hypohydration of 4-8% reduction of body weight.

The cause of the RBF decrease has been investigated, and two mechanisms are probably involved. Tidgren and colleagues (6) showed both direct and indirect (through angiotensin II) effect of the sympathetic nervous system (SNS) on RBF. The SNS acts to cause constriction of the afferent and efferent arterioles of the glomeruli. This is mediated by increased levels of adrenaline and noradrenaline during exercise (1). Diabetics have lower noradrenaline levels during exercise and correspondingly have higher RBFs (7). Walker and colleagues (8) suggested that prostaglandins might modulate RBF, as prostaglandin reduction by indomethacin administration causes further decrease in RBF.

The glomerular filtration rate (GFR) does not respond to exercise as the RBF does. During light exercise (25% V_{O_2}max) GFR increases (3,9). Once exercise reaches greater than 50% V_{O_2}max, GFR decreases to a maximal 60% of resting GFR during heavy exercise (10). Mohan and colleagues (11) demonstrated that 1 hour of cycling at 40% V_{O_2}max caused no change in GFR. The GFR is affected by hyperhydration, which significantly diminishes the decrease seen during heavy exercise (3), while hypohydration increases the drop in GFR during exercise (12). The changes in GFR are not the same at higher altitudes as shown by Olsen and colleagues (13). The high-altitude GFR decreased only during heavy exercise, while the RBF changes were similar to those at sea level.

GFR and RBF affect the filtration fraction (FF): FF = GFR/ RBF. With an increase in workload during exercise, FF also increases (10). The rise in FF causes

TABLE 27-1. *PAH renal clearance calculation (input = output)*

Input	Output
Pa(PAH) · RPF	O + U(PAH) · uV
Pa(PAH) = Arterial PAH conc.	U(PAH) = Urine PAH conc.
RPF = Renal plasma flow	uV = Urine flow rate

capillary oncotic pressure to increase, thereby enhancing the uptake of sodium and water. The increase in FF preserves transfer of metabolites through the glomerulus.

The renal tubules function during exercise is altered compared to the resting state. The changes in levels of angiotensin, renin, aldosterone, vasopressin, atrial natrietic protein, and prostaglandins have been studied (3,6,9,14–17). The effect of these hormones at rest on the renal tubules is shown in Table 27-2. All of the hormones increase in relationship to the intensity of the exercise. This change causes a decrease in urine flow, sodium, and chloride excretion.

Vasopressin is the hormone responsible for the decrease in urinary volume during exercise (1). Castenfors (3) and Poortmans (1) separately demonstrated that the decrease in urine output is related to vasopressin. The decrease occurs in both men and women (17). By contrast, Zappe and colleagues (2) did not see a decrease in urinary volume in six men over 65 years of age. The magnitude, duration, and rate of decrease are not accurately predictable (18). This is most likely because vasopressin is not the sole controlling agent in urine output reduction. This was demonstrated by Kramer and colleagues (19) when they showed that prostaglandins potentiate the effect of vasopressin. Walker and colleagues (8) reconfirmed this by demonstrating an accentuation of the decrease of urinary volume postexercise with indomethacin compared to placebo.

The total urine output is altered by the hydration status of the athlete before exercise. Vasopressin levels are inversely related to the hydration level of the athlete before exercise (20,21). Dehydrated males have a decreased urine output correlated to intensity of exercise (22). Wade and Claybaugh (23) showed a linear correlation between exercise intensity and vasopressin. The increased vasopressin was hypothesized to be due to decreased renal and hepatic clearance during exercise. Poortmans (1) found no change in the urine output percent reduction due to hyperhydration. Vasopressin is elevated before exercise in dehydration and can cause a large decrease in urine output with exercise.

Urinary sodium is decreased during exercise. The decrease continues for up to 4 hours postexercise. Women have a faster return to normal sodium excretion than men and a quicker return to normal levels of aldosterone postexercise (17). As demonstrated by Tankersley and colleagues (24), the sensitivity of the renal tubules to aldosterone is altered by estrogen. The urinary sodium decrease has been associated with increased aldosterone. The rise in plasma aldosterone seems to be related to intensity of exercise. The renin-angiotensin-aldosterone axis causes an increase in aldosterone with the rise in renin during exercise. This was shown by Castenfors (3) using ganglionic blockers in rats, which nearly eliminated the change in renin with exercise and decreased aldosterone. As well, Maher and colleagues (25) showed that beta-receptor blockage prevented the rise of renin and the subsequent rise in aldosterone. Suzuki and colleagues (14) commented that the decrease in urinary sodium may not solely be the effect of aldosterone. Further work will need to be done to determine this.

Atrial natriuretic protein (ANP) is elevated with exercise. ANP acts directly and indirectly to excrete sodium and water (26). Its release is stimulated by the stretch of the atrium (1). ANP levels have been shown by Hodsman and colleagues (27) to increase dramatically during exercise; contrary to ANP's function, fractional excretion of sodium and urine output decreases, though during low-intensity exercise the urine output and osmotic clearance are elevated. This is due to an increase in ANP before the significant increase in vasopressin, aldosterone, and renin, causing increased sodium and water excretion (9). As exercise intensity increases, the urine volume and urinary sodium decrease, although ANP continues to increase. This is most likely due to the counterregulatory hormones: aldosterone and vasopressin.

TABLE 27-2. *Hormone effects on renal tubules*

Segment	Hormone	Effects
Proximal tubule	Angiotensin	Increases NaCl and water reabsorption
Thick ascending limb	Aldosterone	Increases NaCl reabsorption
	Vasopressin	Increases NaCl reabsorption
Distal tubules and collecting ducts	Vasopressin	Increases NaCl and water reabsorption
	Aldosterone	Increases NaCl and water reabsorption
	ANP	Decreases NaCl and water reabsorption
	Prostaglandins	Decreases NaCl and water reabsorption

HYDRATION

Body fluid is regulated by the water balance hormones AVP, aldosterone, and vasopressin. Cade and colleagues (28) and Davidson and colleagues (29) have reported that plasma volume (PV) decreases immediately after a marathon race. Maron and colleagues (30) observed no change in PV immediately. However, there is general agreement that a marathon, like other strenuous exercise, results in the expansion of PV 2-3 days after exercise.

Competitive marathon running can cause a decrease of up to 5 kg in body mass (31). Most of the loss is due to sweating and is really a deficit of body water. Pastene and colleagues (32) reported that the lack of a noted decrease in PV during exercise may be due to the production of metabolic water and the release of water stored in glycogen complexes in muscle and liver. Therefore the loss of body water from sweating may be partially replaced by the energy requirements of running.

An increase in PV days after exercise has been reported by numerous sources (28,32–34). The mechanism of maintaining an increased PV is reported by Pastene and colleagues as a protein shift from the intravascular space and by renal sodium retention. Irving and colleagues (35) noted the influx of albumin into the intravascular space with an associated increase in plasma sodium. The sodium retention was confirmed by Gillen and colleagues (36), but they noted that baroreflex function participates in the induction of PV expansion by intense exercise. Most likely, multiple factors control PV postexercise.

The postexercise hormones influence thirst and increase water intake postexercise (37). In the elderly, conversely, postexercise thirst is diminished (2,37). Normal PV expansion is not seen in the elderly to the same degree as it is in younger athletes (2). Decreased total circulating proteins compared to the 20–30 age group is one cause. Zappe and colleagues reported that the inability of the older subjects to increase PV after repeated days of exercise is not related to an impaired renal fluid and sodium conservation ability.

Most studies describing fluid balance during recovery have been conducted on men (17). Women have been noted to have a decreased sweat rate at similar core temperatures. Francesconi and colleagues (38) and Stachenfeld and colleagues (17) did not find a difference between men and women with respect to PV in response to exercise. Stachenfeld and colleagues stated that despite small differences in sodium retention and water reabsorption after dehydration, it appears that recovery from dehydrating exercise in well-trained men and women is remarkably similar.

Maintenance of intravascular fluid is similar between men and women, but it is altered with the aging process. This is probably due to loss of total plasma proteins and decreased thirst with age. Further studies are needed to determine whether the loss of PV occurs in elderly women and whether the effects of age on PV can be altered.

DRUGS AND THE KIDNEY

A number of different drugs are used by athletes either therapeutically or as ergogenic aids. Some have specific effects on the kidneys and will be addressed here (Table 27–3). Some drugs (e.g., diuretics) can fall into both categories. It is important to ask about these drugs when getting a history from athletes with renal problems.

Diuretics are used to treat many hypertensives and are used by athletes to reduce weight. The dehydrating effects of diuretics can lead to acute renal failure (ARF). The diuretics, such as hydrochlorothiazide, can lead to the production of renal stones by forming hyperuricemia. Combining diuretics and NSAIDs can lead to ARF, owing to their combined effects on the kidney.

Allopurinol is used in prophylactic treatment of gout. Older athletes may be using this medication and exercising. ARF can occur from allopurinol treatment (39) or from gout, even though, treatment is in process (40). Caution should be used when strenuous exercise is combined with this drug.

NSAIDs vary in their effect on the kidney. Most of the NSAIDs cause reduced RBF owing to inhibition of prostaglandins. The reduced renal blood flow may lead to ARF, hematuria, or proteinuria. Sulindac was shown not to reduce RBF as indomethacin does (41). Further discussions of NSAIDs are in each section.

Athletes use growth hormone to increase muscle mass. It affects the kidney indirectly by IGF-1 (42). IGF-1 has been used in renal failure patients to maintain renal blood flow. Studies have not been done to determine whether RBF is maintained during exercise. If RBF is maintained, then FF would remain low, and IGF-1 would decrease hematuria and proteinuria and prevent ARF. Growth hormone excess, like acromegaly, causes deleterious effects elsewhere in the body (43) if not in the kidney.

Anabolic steroids are associated with athletes and may be very commonly used. The renal effects have not been well studied, but ARF with steroid use has been

TABLE 27–3. *Drugs that can alter kidney function*

1. NSAIDs and aspirin	1. Reduce RBF by inhibiting prostaglandins.
2. Diuretics	2. Decrease total plasma volume.
3. Allopurinol	3. Toxic effect on kidney.
4. Growth hormone	4. May maintain RBF during exercise.
5. Anabolic steroids	5. ARF due to decreased RBF.

reported (44). It is important to be aware of the possible relationship in athletes, as many drugs can affect kidney function.

POSTEXERCISE PROTEINURIA

Proteinuria in healthy athletes after exercise has been reported since von Leube in 1878 (18). In 1956 Gardner coined the phrase *athletic pseudonephritis* in an attempt to differentiate the condition from nephrotic syndrome (45). The excess protein in the urine postexercise has been noted in many sports: rowing, bicycling, cross-country skiing, running, swimming, and football (1). The amount depends on intensity of activity.

Normal healthy athletes will excrete less than 50 mg of plasma proteins per day (1). A much larger volume of high-molecular-weight (HMW) proteins (such as albumin) and low-molecular-weight (LMW) proteins (such as retinol-binding protein, beta-2-microalbumin) from the plasma are filtered and reabsorbed (46). The reabsorption occurs in the proximal tubules. Foulkes (47) identified that the increase in excretion of HMW proteins reflects a change in the glomerulus and that the increase in the more readily filtered LMW proteins is due to an interference of the renal tubule reabsorption. Therefore changes in the HMW proteins would reflect changes at the glomeruli and increases of LMW proteins reflect changes at the renal tubules.

The postexercise protein found in the urine was identified as being from the plasma (48). Poortmans (1) and others (49,50) have shown a rise in the plasma proteins in urine postexercise. Measuring serial urines postexercise, Poortmans and colleagues (51) showed that the half-life is 54 minutes and the peak is 20–30 minutes postexercise.

The amount of protein in the urine postexercise seems to be exercise related. Kachadorian and colleagues (22) demonstrated that the postexercise proteinuria (PEP) is exertion related. Poortmans and colleagues (51) showed that the PEP changes with type of exertion. The 100-meter sprint (anaerobic) caused increase in albumin but not in beta-2-microalbumin. The longer events (aerobic) caused an increase in both proteins. They later showed that PEP was correlated to the lactate level ($r = 0.87$). In rats an angiotensin II infusion has been shown to increase albuminuria, which is secondary to an increase in FF (52,53). The same mechanism would explain the PEP changes seen in humans.

The effects of age and gender have been addressed in studies. Poortmans and colleagues (54) studied the effects of exercise on proteinuria in children. They found that PEP is present at maximal exercise from childhood to adolescence. The magnitude of protein excretion is strictly related to the absolute intensity of exercise (55). Peggs and colleagues (56) found proteinuria to be a very common occurrence in adolescents and recommended for preparticipation physical to discontinue the practice of screening urinalysis. Robertshaw and colleagues (57) did not find a difference in PEP between men and women. This was also seen in earlier work in adolescents by Houser (55). The effect of exertion on PEP is not altered by age or gender.

The changes in proteinuria can be altered by fitness, temperature, and drugs. Taylor (58) showed that there was a decrease in PEP with training. This is probably due to a decrease in lactate levels because of increased fitness. Neviackas and Bauer studied marathon runners and found a difference in the RBF and GFR between cold and warm weather (59). The runners had more proteinuria in the warmer dehydrating weather with an increase in FF.

There is a question of whether the renin-angiotensin system (RAS) or prostaglandins play a role in PEP. Numerous studies have shown ACE inhibitors decrease PEP (60). This would support the role of the RAS. Renal prostaglandins are inhibited by indomethacin but not by sulindac. Indomethacin has been shown to decrease RBF and FF (8) and, through this mechanism, increase proteinuria (41). In Mittleman and Zambraski's study (61) they did not find a change in placebo or ACE inhibitor but found that indomethacin attenuated the PEP. It is uncertain whether RAS, prostaglandins, or both are responsible for PEP at this time.

The classification of benign exercise-related urinary changes is described as the onset of the abnormal values after exercise and the clearing of these findings after rest. To test for proteinuria, the urine dipstick is a helpful test. The values for PEP are typically 2+ or 3+. The value should decrease to normal levels over the next 24–48 hours. Thereby, a repeat urinalysis with microscopy at 24–48 hours postexercise should be negative. As always, a good history and physical are needed to assess the possibility of other causes of proteinuria. If the value does not return to normal, then further workup is needed.

When investigating proteinuria that does not resolve, other forms of benign and common causes need to be considered. The most common kind of proteinuria in adolescents is benign positional proteinuria. This disorder, like PEP or fever-associated proteinuria, is transient. The renal function is normal, and no hematuria is found. The diagnosis is made by measuring a recumbent urine sample and then an upright sample and looking at the difference between the two samples. Constant or recurrent proteinuria needs further evaluation. See Figure 27–1 for a recommended workup. Electrophoresis may help to identify the location of the proteinuria; increased albumin is from damage to the glomeruli, and beta-2-microalbumin is from damage to the renal tubules.

When the proteinuria is due to exercise alone, it carries a benign prognosis with no long-term sequelae (62).

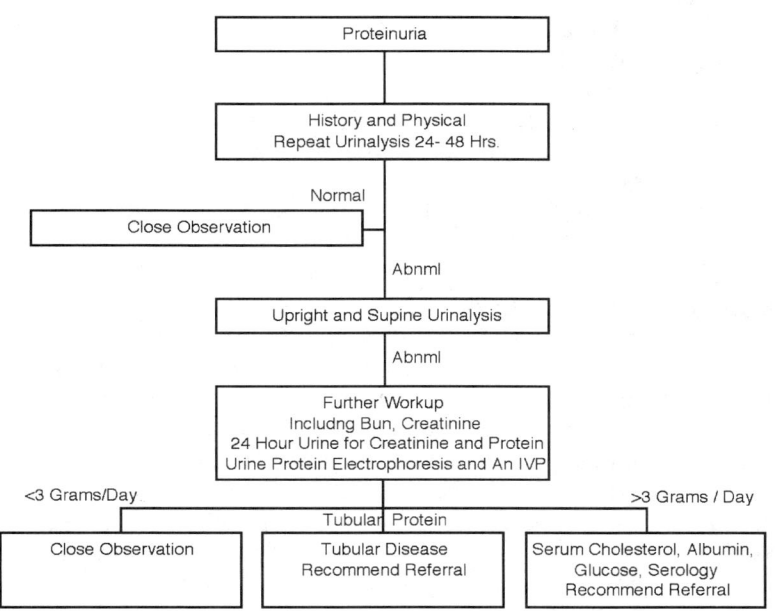

FIG. 27-1. Proteinuria workup. (Adapted from Goldszer RC, Siegel AJ. Renal abnormalities during exercise. In: Strauss, RH, ed. *Sports medicine,* 2nd ed. Philadelphia: WB Saunders, 1991.)

Bergamaschi and colleagues found in rats with chronic renal failure that physical training provoked a vasodilatation of the efferent arterioles, which induced the normalization of glomerular hypertension (63). The effect did not worsen or slow the decline in renal function. Further studies in humans are needed to prove that exercise has no long-term detrimental effects.

HEMATURIA

Hematuria can be a sign of serious disease. The athlete with red-colored urine needs to be carefully evaluated to determine whether the cause is hematuria. Most athletes under 40 years of age will have a benign cause. The heme-positive dipstick can be due to hemoglobinuria (whole red blood cells or hemoglobin) or a false-positive result. A false positive dipstick result can be caused by vegetable peroxide, bacterial enzymes, or other heme groups (myoglobinuria). Not all red urine is hematuria; pseudohematuria can be caused by certain drugs (pyridium, rifampin, nitrofurantoin, quinine, and phenytoin), vegetable dyes, and myoglobin. The use of microscopy will aid in determining whether a heme positive dipstick is from red blood cells (RBC). A positive result is considered >3 RBC per high-powered field averaged over 21 fields.

Microhematuria is prevalent in the general population with even greater percentage in athletes. In a Mayo Clinic study, 13% of adult men and women (≥55 years of age) had asymptomatic microhematuria (64). Mariani and colleagues (65) found that 15% of 1346 medical students had asymptomatic hematuria. In children a Finnish study found a rate of 4% (66). The rates in athletes are even higher and vary greatly from marathons (20%) to football (55%) to swimming (80%) (18,67).

Hematuria in athletes has been ascribed to a number of causes: bladder trauma, footstrike hemolysis, hypoxic damage to the nephrons, infection (pyelonephritis and STDs), medications, or cancer. Benign causes of hematuria—bladder traumas, footstrike hemolysis, and hypoxic damage to the nephrons—have been correlated to intensity of exertion. Eichner (68) states that the further the distance run, the more hematuria occurs. Kachadorian and colleagues showed that the faster the running speed, the more hematuria is found (22).

The exercise-related hematuria has been divided into different types (Table 27-4): duration-related, intensity-related, direct contact, and indirect contact. Direct contact hematuria will be discussed in the section on renal trauma. Indirect trauma is a part of the duration-related injuries in which the bladder or kidney is jarred during activity. Intensity-related injuries are due to changes in renal perfusion during exercise.

Intensity-related injuries are ischemic, hypoxic,

TABLE 27-4. *Causes of hematuria*

Categories	Type
Duration related	Footstrike hemolysis
	Bladder/kidney trauma
	Dehydration-induced hematuria
	Hyperexia hematuria
Intensity related	Ischemic insults
	Hypoxic insults
	Acidic insults
	Toxic insults
	Splenic lysis

acidic, or toxic insults. The insults allow whole RBC to enter the urine by crossing the glomeruli or from injury to the nephrons. The amount of exercise intensity correlates with increased findings of hematuria (22,69). The mechanism can be a combination of the above factors.

Hypoxic injury is due to decreased RBF during exercise. The damage is thought to be secondary to the spiral arteries to the renal papilla having diminished flow and being starved of oxygen. This leads to fragility of the arterioles and bleeding on reperfusion postexercise. During childhood the spiral vessels are less tortuous, which would explain the decreased rate of hematuria in children (70,71).

In ischemic injury, RBCs cross the glomeruli due to the increased FF (72). It has been noted that 54% of athletes taking NSAIDs have idiopathic hematuria (73). The use of NSAIDs, particularly indomethacin, has been shown to decrease RBF and increase FF. As was mentioned previously, both of these changes will cause hematuria. With acidic insult (increased lactate) or with myoglobinuria (toxic insult) the permeability of the glomeruli to proteins is increased (10). Both situations will allow RBCs through the membrane (72).

Intense exercise may cause the production of factors that destroys RBCs. Sjodin and colleagues (74) described free radical production during maximal exertion that can cause destruction of RBC and hematuria. Damage due to free radicals was also described by Szygula (75). Another reason for RBC destruction is the hemolytic factor in the spleen (lysolecithin). Shiraki and colleagues demonstrated that during severe exercise there is an increased destruction of erythrocytes due to the liberation of lysolecithin (72a). The adrenaline-mediated contracture of the spleen may mediate release of the lysolecithin. Hemolysis could be an adaptive measure, as reported by Yoshimura (76), to reutilize the proteins for muscle growth as seen in rats.

Hematuria has been described by Eichner (68) as a duration-dependent event. This is different from proteinuria, which does not occur if the intensity of exercise is below 50% VO_2max, as described earlier. The causes of the duration-related hematuria are footstrike hematuria, bladder or kidney trauma, dehydration, and/or hyperexia. The mechanism for hematuria is not unifactorial; multiple causes may occur simultaneously.

Footstrike hemolysis is probably the most recognizable cause of exercise hematuria. Hematuria was first described by an Italian physician, Ramazziani; in 1793 he wrote that runners would pass bloody urine (77). He attributed the hematuria to breaks in small veins in the kidney. Falsetti and colleagues (78) described foot impact as a cause of hematuria. Miller and colleagues (79) noted that running up hill, which has less heelstrike than running down hill, had less hematuria. Falsetti and colleagues (78) reported on the decrease in hematuria due to soft-soled running shoes. Poortmans and Henrist supported these results in their work on proteinuria (80). The rupture of RBCs in the heel due to impact causes the release of hemoglobin. If the repeated trauma is excessive, then haptoglobin binding of free Hgb is overwhelmed, and hemoglobin is excreted in the urine. This theory is supported by the finding of decreased plasma haptoglobin with hematuria (77,78,81).

Blacklock (82) coined the term *10,000 metres hematuria*. He found that eight runners had bladder contusions postexercise on cystoscopic examination. The contusions are found on the interureteric bar, on the posterior half of the rim of the internal meatus, and on the posterior bladder wall, in which position there is mirroring of the trigonal lesions (82). The contusions resolved, and so did the hematuria. Blacklock theorized that the amount of bladder urine volume would account for the variation in occurrence in the same athlete (83). Eichner (68) theorizes that emptying the bladder before running may cause the contusions. The time to last void has not been studied prospectively to determine whether this affects hematuria.

Hyperexia can cause lysis of RBCs, causing hemoglobinemia. The cause may be due to an increase in membrane fragility (84). This resulting hemolysis may lead to acute renal failure (18). Care should be taken while exercising in the heat. Proper hydration is important in maintaining plasma volume and preventing hemolysis.

Kidney trauma has been described as a cause of hematuria, either by a direct blow (football, boxing) or by jarring of the kidney (jumping, soccer, and basketball). In certain sports, such as soccer, a combination of direct blows and jarring can be the mechanism of hematuria. The effect of trauma on hematuria was shown by De Meersman and Wilkerson in a study of judo (85). Judo practices with falls and without falls did show differences in hematuria. Contrarily, the amount or type of proteinuria was not altered. We will further address trauma hematuria in the renal trauma section.

During continuous exercise the athlete will lose a large amount of fluid from sweating. Intravascular volume will not decrease significantly (32). If the athlete is dehydrated before exercise, then there will be a decrease in plasma volume and an increase in hematuria as exertion progresses. The cause is the decrease in RBF and the corresponding rise in FF.

The athlete with hematuria needs a thorough history and physical to evaluate whether the cause is exercise related. If there are no other ominous signs, then a repeat urinalysis at 24–72 hours can be done. The same rates of hematuria are seen in comparing men and women (86). Clean-catch urine needs to be obtained to differentiate menstruation from hematuria. Sexually transmitted diseases can present with microhematuria; therefore infection needs to be considered in sexually active athletes. If repeat urinalysis is negative, the athlete may return to exercise with no known long-term

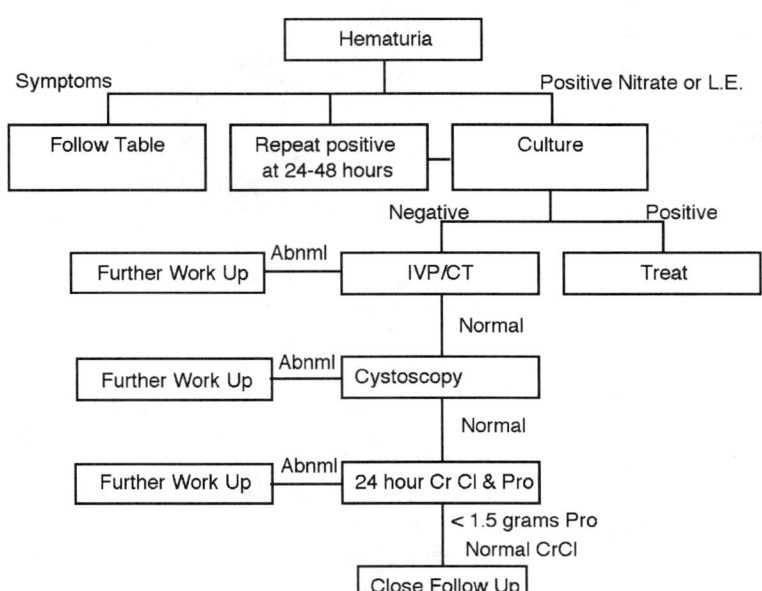

FIG. 27-2. Hematuria workup. (Adapted from Jones GR, Newhouse I. Sport-related hematuria: a review. *Clin J Sport Med* 1997;7:119–125.)

detriment to renal function (87). The athlete should be well hydrated before exercise to prevent the decrease in RBF.

Certain athletes need further attention when presenting with hematuria. Athletes with known metabolic diseases, such as sickle-cell trait, need further workup to eliminate the possibility of hemolysis. An athlete over age 40 needs further consideration, since the likelihood for renal or bladder tumors with painless hematuria is greatly increased. Chronic cases of repeated exercise-related hematuria can cause macrocytic anemia and further evaluation is warranted (88).

The workup for hematuria (Fig. 27–2) should involve microscopy to evaluate for whole or fragmented RBCs. If no RBCs are seen, then myoglobinuria should be considered. Bailey and colleagues (89) found myoglobinuria in 1.6% of athletes from various sports. It is more common in untrained individuals. Myoglobinuria will have a positive urinalysis dipstick for heme but a negative microscopic examination. For myoglobinuria, plasma CPKs should be measured, and the athlete should have aggressive fluid replacement.

An athlete with a positive urinalysis or urinary symptoms needs further workup (Table 27–5). A urine culture will help to evaluate whether the hematuria is secondary to infection. The dipstick test for leukocyte esterase and nitrate are usually positive with infection. Blood work for evaluation of renal function and sickle prep for sickle-cell trait can be helpful in diagnosis. An intravenous pyelogram (IVP) for renal functioning and evaluation for renal stones are important. The use of cystoscopy allows visualization of the bladder for tumors, contusions, or stones. A normal creatinine clearance or a negative workup needs close follow-up. The athlete may return to play after notification about the lack of long-term data concerning possible permanent renal damage.

The athlete with exercise-related hematuria needs to prevent chronic recurrence. This can be accomplished by maintaining hydration before and during exercise. Cycling training techniques can diminish hematuria, as

TABLE 27-5. *Hematuria: further workup*

Finding	Reason for workup	Important test to perform
Continuation of hematuria >24–72 hours	Renal contusion or renal cancer	CT scan of kidneys
Flank pain	Kidney stones, trauma, or pyelonephritis	Urine culture, IVP, CT
Urinary casts	Glomerular disease	Serum screen for compliment
Recurrent episodes	Bladder tumor	Cystoscopy
Mild, short-duration exercise	Another cause of hematuria	More thorough history
Age over 40 years	Renal tumor	CT scan with contrast

Adapted from Mariani AJ, Mariani MC, Macchioni C, et al. The significance of adult hematuria: 1,000 hematuria evaluations including a risk-benefit and cost-effectiveness analysis. *J Urol* 1989;141:350–355.

can the wearing of appropriate footwear with padded soles. Any athlete with repeated hematuria should have a further workup to rule out bladder or renal transitional cell tumors presenting as repeat exercise hematuria (90,91).

ACUTE RENAL FAILURE

Exercise-induced acute renal failure (EIARF) is uncommon, but it is the one of the most serious renal problems associated with exercise. RBF during exercise decreases owing to the increased demand of the muscles. Poortmans (1) estimates that 900 mL blood/min is shunted to the muscles during strenuous exercise. At a critical point, RBF becomes too low and causes renal ischemia and renal failure.

Another mechanism of EIARF is nephrotoxins such as myoglobin or hemoglobin. Myoglobin precipitates in the renal tubules, causing obstruction and renal tubule ischemia (92). Hemoglobinuria has been implicated in ARF (93), usually secondary to a hemolysis due to hyperexia. Both hemoglobin and myoglobin are released during severe exercise.

A third mechanism concerns metabolic diseases, such as renal hypouricemia or sickle-cell disease, that can cause acute renal failure with exercise. Renal hypouricemia is common in Japan at a rate of 0.2%. It can precipitate EIARF by increased uric acid excretion postexercise (94). The disease is found mostly in people of Asian descent. With sickle-cell anemia and sickle-cell trait, hemolysis can occur (95). Trait hemolysis occurs only during strenuous exercise and extenuating situations, such as severe dehydration, rapid altitude changes, or severe hypoxia (96). Strenuous exercise can cause hemolysis, which leads to EIARF.

Reduction of RBF during exercise needs to be augmented to cause EIARF (e.g., exercise and heat stroke, dehydration, or NSAIDs). ARF was increased in the military recruits after prolonged, strenuous exercise in the heat (97,98). Unacclimatized recruits developed hemoglobin and myoglobin in the plasma. Strenuous exercise decreases their RBF and, in combination with the nephrotoxic effects of myoglobin and hemoglobin, causes EIARF.

EIARF has been described as "raver's hematuria" (99) and "white collar rhabdomyolysis" (100); the two are similar conditions. The former results from strenuous, long-duration dancing and amphetamines; the latter is associated with strenuous exercise and alcohol use. Both situations augment the decrease in the RBF and cause production of myoglobin (from rhabdomyolysis), leading to potential renal failure.

NSAIDs such as indomethacin have been discussed as causing a decrease in RBF because of inhibition of prostaglandins. The prostaglandins cause renal vasodilation. The combination of severe exercise and NSAIDs

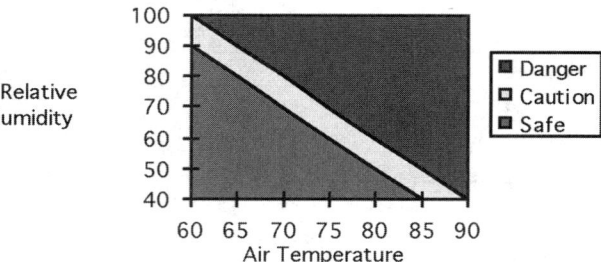

FIG. 27–3. Exercise heat risk chart.

on RBF can decrease perfusion to a critical level that precipitates renal failure. Sulindac does not appear to cause inhibition of renal prostaglandins. It may be a better choice if NSAIDs are needed to accompany strenuous exercise. Caution should be taken in using any NSAIDs before strenuous exercise.

Dehydration will cause a reduction in RBF. The combination of severe exercise and dehydration can cause EIARF. Dehydration is common practice in sports requiring a weigh-in procedure (wrestling, boxing, lightweight football). Careful attention to hydration should be used in these sports to prevent renal failure. A 2–5% body fluid loss will alter RBF; therefore a judicious guideline to follow would be to allow only 2% weight reduction before weigh-ins (101,102).

Prevention is the best treatment for EIARF. The athlete's environment needs to be monitored; maintaining a safe training wet bulb temperature (Fig. 27–3). There should be available fluids and encouragement to drink the fluids. Athletes should be cautioned about the use of NSAIDs before strenuous exercise and continue to drink fluids postexercise to produce urine flow within 1–2 hours. These measures will help to prevent EIARF.

The athlete with acute renal failure will usually do well with careful monitoring and intravenous fluids. Izumi and colleagues recently described the use of ultrasound Doppler technique to detect EIARF (103). If the oliguria persists despite fluid resuscitation, then further evaluation for life-threatening renal failure is needed. Insulinlike growth factor I has been safely used in people who are at risk of having acute renal failure and in patients with end-stage chronic renal failure to increase the glomerular filtration rate (104). Research to determine the role of IGF-I as a therapeutic agent for EIARF has not been done.

RENAL TRAUMA

The exact incidence of renal trauma is unknown. Many sports have been identified as generating renal trauma (e.g., football, soccer, rugby, horseback riding, diving, ice skating, hockey, and lacrosse) (18,105). Thirty percent of renal injuries in children occur during sports (106).

The kidney is well protected in the body. It is relatively mobile, so the kidney may be injured by contusion, fractured rib, or a sudden decelerating force. Renal injuries are classified by anatomic location and severity (renal contusions, caliceal lacerations, and renal fracture and vascular pedicle injuries).

The athlete will present with a range of symptoms, from mild flank pain to hematuria to shock. The symptoms are usually mild to moderate. The presence of hematuria is variable; up to 25% of renal injuries and 60% of renal pedicle injuries are without hematuria (107). CT scan is the recommended evaluation of renal trauma (108). An IVP may be used if CT is not available. Plain radiographs are of limited value; a loss of the psoas shadow may be helpful, though.

Renal contusions will present with microscopic hematuria or mild gross hematuria (109). Most often they are secondary to trauma, but these injuries can occur due to jarring. The athlete with renal contusion does well postinjury. Participation should be withheld until the hematuria resolves (usually 2–3 weeks); for contact sports 6 weeks is recommended (18). The CT scan can be used to document healing before return to play, if earlier return is needed.

Cortical or caliceal lacerations usually present with more hematuria than a contusion. The treatment is observation until hematuria resolves. CT scan is helpful in identifying the extent of injury. These lacerations usually do well with non-operative treatment (bed rest and observation for 7–8 days) (110). Follow-up with CT scan or IVP at 3 months is essential to document healing (111). Return to play occurs only after resolution of hematuria and documented healing of the laceration.

Renal fracture and vascular pedicle injuries are rare in sports. These injuries present with shock. Hematuria is not a reliable sign, since it is absent in up to 40% of cases (107). If an IVP is performed, it will not demonstrate the kidney with the vascular pedicle injury. In renal fracture there is intrarenal and extravasation of the dye during an IVP. Both injuries require surgical repair. The kidney can be salvaged in vascular pedicle injuries if it is treated urgently. Return-to-play guidelines require a minimum of 6 months to 1 year, if ever.

Renal trauma can be difficult to diagnosis, since hematuria may or may not be present. History of direct trauma is sometimes difficult to obtain in high-contact sports such as football. Not all people with hematuria need CT scans. In adults radiographic evaluation of the urinary tract is recommended only for patients with blunt trauma if associated with gross hematuria (4+), microscopic hematuria and hypotension, or microscopic hematuria and significant associated injuries (rib fracture, penetrating injury, etc.) (112). Stein and colleagues (113) studied children and renal trauma. They agreed with the adult recommendations but suggested that any child with a history of blunt abdominal trauma and any evidence of hematuria undergo abdominal and pelvic CT scanning for proper confirmation of diagnosis and staging of renal and other associated intraabdominal injuries. The kidney is less protected in children, and the amount of hematuria does not always correlate with extent of injury. Therefore further workup is required. Close observation and follow-up are needed to detect progression of renal damage. Renal contusion is more common than is recognized in collision sports (especially football).

SOLITARY KIDNEY AND PREPARTICIPATION

The issue of solitary kidney and participation is an interesting one. Anderson (114) surveyed members of the American Medical Society of Sports Medicine and found that a majority (54.1%) would allow athletes with solitary kidney to participate in contact and collision sports. This same group of physicians had mixed views when the question concerned their own children (41.6%). The type of kidney matters as well, since a horseshoe kidney has a better prognosis in injury owing to the dual blood supply. The rate of kidney loss from sports is extremely small, with no reported cases of blunt trauma causing kidney loss in over 25 years. In recommending participation, there should be a thorough discussion of the dangers of participation and guidance in the choice of activities.

CONCLUSION

The kidney adapts to exercise to prevent loss of fluids during exercise. The adaptation may cause proteinuria and hematuria. When hydration, drugs, or disease are present before exercise, changes in the kidney may cause renal failure or worsening of proteinuria or hematuria. Renal trauma is often minor and heals with rest. Changes in renal function due to severe exercise do not appear to have long-term detrimental effects.

REFERENCES

1. Poortmans JR. Exercise and renal function. *Sports Med* 1984; 1:125–153.
2. Zappe DH, Bell GW, Swartzentruber H, et al. Age and regulation of fluid and electrolyte balance during repeated exercise sessions. *Am J Physiol* 1996;270:R71–R79.
3. Castenfors J. Renal function during exercise. *Acta Physiol Scand* 1967;70:1–44.
4. Grimby G. Renal clearance during prolonged supine exercise, heat and dehydration. *J Appl Physiol* 1965;4:1294–1298.
5. Smith JH, Robinson S, Pearcy M. Renal response to exercise, heat and dehydration. *J Appl Physiol* 1952;4:659–665.
6. Tidgren B, Hjemdahl P, Theodorsson E, Nussberger J. Renal neurohormonal and vascular responses to dynamic exercise in humans. *J Appl Physiol* 1991;70:2279–2286.
7. Johansson BL, Berg U, Bohlin AB, et al. Exercise-induced changes in renal function and their relation to plasma noradrenaline in insulin-dependent diabetic children and adolescents. *Clin Sci* 1987;72:611–620.

8. Walker RJ, Fawcett JP, Flannery EM, Gerrard DF. Indomethacin potentiates exercise-induced reduction in renal hemodynamics in athletes. Med Sci Sports Exerc 1994;26:1302–1306.
9. Freund BJ, Shizuru EM, Hashiro GM, Claybaugh JR. Hormonal, electrolyte, and renal responses to exercise are intensity dependent. J Appl Physiol 1991;70:900–906.
10. Poortmans JR, Vanderstraten J. Kidney function during exercise in healthy and diseased humans: an update. Sports Med 1994;18:419–437.
11. Mohan BD, Sellens MH, McVicar AJ. Effects of moderate exercise on renal function in man. J Physiol 1993;467:64.
12. Dann EJ, Gillis S, Burstein R. Effect of fluid intake on renal function during exercise in the cold. Eur J Appl Physiol 1990;61:133–137.
13. Olsen NV, Kanstrup IL, Richalet JP, et al. Effects of acute hypoxia on renal and endocrine function at rest and during graded exercise in hydrated subjects. J Appl Physiol 1992;73:2036–2043.
14. Suzuki M, Sudoh M, Matsubara S, et al. Changes in renal blood flow measured by radionuclide angiography following exhausting exercise in humans. Eur J Appl Physiol 1996;74:1–7.
15. Wade CE, Hill LC, Hunt MM, Dressendorfer RH. Plasma aldosterone and renal function in runners during a 20-day road race. Eur J Appl Physiol 1985;54:456–460.
16. Wade CE, Dressendorfer RH, O'Brien JC, Claybaugh JR. Renal function, aldosterone, and vasopressin excretion following repeated long-distance running. J Appl Physiol 1981;50:709–712.
17. Stachenfeld NS, Gleim GW, Zabetakis PM, Nicholas JA. Fluid balance and renal response following dehydrating exercise in well-trained men and women. Eur J Appl Physiol 1996;72:468–477.
18. Cianflocco AJ. Renal complications of exercise. Clin Sports Med 1992;11:437–451.
19. Kramer HJ, Glanzer K, Dusing R. Role of prostaglandins in the regulation of renal water excretion. Kidney Int 1981;19:851–859.
20. Francesconi RP, Sawka MN, Pandolf KB. Hypohydration and heat acclimation: plasma renin and aldosterone during exercise. J Appl Physiol 1983;55:1790–1794.
21. Wade CE. Response, regulation, and actions of vasopressin during exercise: a review. Med Sci Sports Exerc 1984;16:506–511.
22. Kachadorian WA, Johnson RE, Buffington RE, et al. The regularity of "athletic pseudonephritis" after heavy exercise. Med Sci Sport Exerc 1970;2:142–145.
23. Wade CE, Claybaugh JR. Plasma renin activity, vasopressin concentration and urinary excretory responses to exercise in men. J Appl Physiol 1980;49:930–936.
24. Tankersley CG, Nicholas WC, Deaver DR, et al. Estrogen replacement in middle-aged women: thermoregulatory responses to exercise in the heat. J Appl Physiol 1992;73:1238–1245.
25. Maher JT, Jones LG, Hartley LH, et al. Aldosterone dynamics during graded exercise at sea level and high altitude. J Appl Physiol 1975;39:18–22.
26. Freund BJ, Wade CE, Claybaugh JR. Effects of exercise on atrial natriuretic factor release mechanisms and implications for fluid homeostasis. Sports Med 1988;6:364–377.
27. Hodsman GP, Phillips PA, Ogawa K, Johnston CI. Atrial natriuretic factor in normal man: effects of tilt, posture, exercise and haemorrhage. J Hypertens 1986;4:S503–505.
28. Cade R, Packer D, Zauner C, et al. Marathon running: physiological and chemical changes accompanying late-race functional deterioration. Eur J Appl Physiol 1992;65:485–491.
29. Davidson RJ, Robertson JD, Galea G, Maughan RJ. Hematological changes associated with marathon running. Int J Sports Med 1987;8:19–25.
30. Maron MB, Horvath SM, Wilkerson JE. Acute blood biochemical alterations in response to marathon running. Eur J Appl Physiol 1975;34:173–181.
31. Pugh LG, Corbett JL, Johnson RH. Rectal temperatures, weight losses, and sweat rates in marathon running. J Appl Physiol 1967;23:347–352.
32. Pastene J, Germain M, Allevard AM, et al. Water balance during and after marathon running. Eur J Appl Physiol 1996;73:49–55.
33. Green HJ, Thomson JA, Ball ME, et al. Alterations in blood volume following short-term supramaximal exercise. J Appl Physiol 1984;56:145–149.
34. Gillen CM, Lee R, Mack GW, et al. Plasma volume expansion in humans after a single intense exercise protocol. J Appl Physiol. 1991;71:1914–1920.
35. Irving RA, Noakes TD, Burger SC, et al. Plasma volume and renal function during and after ultramarathon running Med Sci Sports Exerc 1990;22:581–587.
36. Gillen CM, Nishiyasu T, Langhans G, et al. Cardiovascular and renal function during exercise-induced blood volume expansion in men. J Appl Physiol 1994;76:2602–2610.
37. Phillips PA, Rolls BJ, Ledingham JG, et al. Reduced thirst after water deprivation in healthy elderly men. N Engl J Med 1984;311:753–759.
38. Francesconi RP, Sawka MN, Pandolf KB, et al. Plasma hormonal responses at graded hypohydration levels during exercise-heat stress. J Appl Physiol 1985;59:1855–1860.
39. Handa SP. Drug-induced acute interstitial nephritis: report of 10 cases. Can Med Assoc J 1986;135:1278–1281.
40. Conger JD. Acute uric acid nephropathy. Med Clin North Am 1990;74:859–871.
41. Zambraski EJ, Dodelson R, Guidotti SM, Harnett CA. Renal prostaglandin E2 and F2a synthesis during exercise: effects of indomethacin and sulindac. Med Sci Sports Exerc 1986;18:678–684.
42. Ogle GD, Rosenberg AR, Kainer G. Renal effects of growth hormone: II. Electrolyte homeostasis and body composition. Pediatr Nephrol 1992;6:483–489.
43. O'Shea MH, Layish DT. Growth hormone and the kidney: a case presentation and review of the literature. J Am Soc Nephrol 1992;3:157–161.
44. Yoshida EM, Karim MA, Shaikh JF, et al. At what price, glory? severe cholestasis and acute renal failure in an athlete abusing stanozolol. Can Med Assoc J 1994;151:791–793.
45. Gardner KD. Athletic pseudonephritis: alteration of the urine sediment by athletic competition. JAMA 1956;151:1613–1617.
46. Voiculescu M. Advances in the study of proteinurias: I. The pathogenetic mechanisms. Med Interne 1990;28:265–277.
47. Foulkes EC. Tubular reabsorption of low molecular weight proteins. Physiologist 1982;25:56–59.
48. Poortmans JR. Postexercise proteinuria in humans: facts and mechanisms. JAMA 1985;253:236–240.
49. Miyai T, Ogata M. Changes in the concentrations of urinary proteins after physical exercise. Acta Med Okayama 1990;44:263–266.
50. Edes TE, Shah JH, Thornton WH Jr. Spontaneous decline in exercise–induced proteinuria during a 100–mile triathlon. South Med J 1990;83:1044–1046,1052.
51. Poortmans JR, Rampaer L, Wolfs JC. Renal protein excretion after exercise in man. Eur J Appl Physiol 1989;58:476–480.
52. Bohrer MP, Deen WM, Robertson CR, Brenner BM. Mechanism of angiotensin II-induced proteinuria in the rat. Am J Physiol 1977;233:F13–F21.
53. Myers BD, Deen WM, Brenner BM. Effects of norepinephrine and angiotensin II on the determinants of glomerular ultrafiltration and proximal tubule fluid reabsorption in the rat. Circ Res 1975;37:101–110.
54. Poortmans JR, Geudvert C, Schorokoff K, De Plaen P. Postexercise proteinuria in childhood and adolescence. Int J Sports Med 1996;17:448–451. [Published erratum appears in Int J Sports Med 1996;17:625.]
55. Houser MT. Characterization of recumbent, ambulatory, and postexercise proteinuria in the adolescent. Pediatr Res 1987;21:442–446.
56. Peggs JF, Reinhardt RW, O'Brien JM. Proteinuria in adolescent sports physical examinations. Journal Fam Pract 1986;22:80–81.
57. Robertshaw M, Cheung CK, Fairly I, Swaminathan R. Protein excretion after prolonged exercise. Ann Clinical Biochem 1993;30:34–37.
58. Taylor A. Some characteristics of exercise proteinuria. Clin Sci 1960;19:209.
59. Neviackus JA, Bauer JH. Renal function abnormalities induced by marathon running. South Med J 1981;74:1457–1460.
60. Esnault VL, Potiron-Josse M, Testa A, et al. Captopril but not

acebutolol, prazosin or indomethacin decreases postexercise proteinuria. *Nephron* 1991;58:437–442.
61. Mittleman KD, Zambraski EJ. Exercise-induced proteinuria is attenuated by indomethacin. *Med Sci Sports Exerc* 1992;24:1069–1074.
62. Goldszer RC, Siegel AJ. Renal abnormalities during exercise. In: Strauss RH, ed. *Sports Medicine,* 2nd ed. Philadelphia: WB Saunders, 1991.
63. Bergamaschi CT, Boim MA, Moura LA, et al. Effects of long-term training on the progression of chronic renal failure in rats. *Med Sci Sports Exerc* 1997;29:169–174.
64. Mohr DN, Offord KP, Owen RA, Melton LJ 3d. Asymptomatic microhematuria and urologic disease. A population-based study. *JAMA* 1986;256:224–229.
65. Mariani AJ, Mariani MC, Macchioni C, et al. The significance of adult hematuria: 1,000 hematuria evaluations including a risk-benefit and cost-effectiveness analysis. *J Urol* 1989;141:350–355.
66. Vehaskari VM, Rapola J, Koskimies O, et al. Microscopic hematuria in school children: epidemiology and clinicopathologic evaluation. *J Pediatr* 1979;95:676–684.
67. Siegel AJ, Hennekens CH, Solomon HS, Van Boeckel B. Exercise-related hematuria. Findings in a group of marathon runners. *JAMA* 1979;241:391–392.
68. Eichner ER. Hematuria: a diagnostic challenge. *Phys Sportsmed* 1990;18:53–63.
69. Helzer-Julin M, Latin RW, Mellion MB, et al. The effect of exercise intensity and hydration on athletic pseudonephritis. *J Sports Med Phys Fitness* 1988;28:324–329.
70. Lieu TA, Grasmeder HM 3d, Kaplan BS. An approach to the evaluation and treatment of microscopic hematuria. *Pediatr Clin North Am* 1991;38:579–592.
71. Hoover DL, Cromie WJ. Theory and management of exercise-related hematuria. *Phys Sportsmed* 1981;9:90–95.
72. Jones GR, Newhouse I. Sport-related hematuria: a review. *Clin J Sport Med* 1997;7:119–125.
72a. Yoshimura H, Inoue T, Yamada T, Shiraki K. Anemia during hard physical training (sports anemia) and its causal mechanism with special reference to protein nutrition. *World Rev Nutr Diet* 1980;35:1–86.
73. Kraus SE, Siroky MB, Babayan RK, Krane RJ. Hematuria and the use of nonsteroidal anti-inflammatory drugs. *J Urol* 1984;132:288–290.
74. Sjodin B, Westing YH, Apple FS. Biochemical mechanisms for oxygen free radical formation during exercise. *Sports Med* 1990;10:236–254.
75. Szygula Z. Erythrocytic system under the influence of physical exercise and training. *Sports Med* 1990;10:181–197.
76. Yoshimura H. Anemia during physical training (sports anemia). *Nutr Rev* 1970;28:251.
77. Brieger GH. The diseases of runners: a view from the eighteenth century—a commentary. *Pharos* 1980;43:29–32.
78. Falsetti HL, Burke ER, Feld RD, et al. Hematological variations after endurance running with hard and soft-soled running shoes. *Physician Sportsmed* 1983;11:118–120,122–124.
79. Miller BJ, Pate RR, Burgess W. Foot impact force and intravascular hemolysis during distance running. *Int J Sports Med* 1988;9:56–60.
80. Poortmans JR, Henrist A. The influence of air-cushion shoes on post-exercise proteinuria. *J Sports Med Phys Fitness* 1989;29:213–217.
81. Eichner ER. Runner's macrocytosis: a clue to footstrike hemolysis. Runner's anemia as a benefit versus runner's hemolysis as a detriment. *Am J Med* 1985;78:321–325.
82. Blacklock NJ. Bladder trauma in the long-distance runner: "10,000 metres haematuria." *Br J Urol* 1977;49:129–132.
83. Blacklock NJ. Bladder trauma in the long-distance runner *Am J Sports Med* 1979;7:239–241.
84. Shibolet S, Call R, Gilat T. Heat stroke: its clinical picture and mechanism in 36 cases. *QJM* 1967;36:535.
85. De Meersman RE, Wilkerson JE. Judo nephropathy: trauma versus non-trauma. *J Trauma* 1982;22:150–152.
86. Boileau M, Fuchs E, Barry JM, Hodges CV. Stress hematuria: athletic pseudonephritis in marathoners *Urology* 1980;15:471–474.
87. Abarbanel J, Benet AE, Lask D, Kimche D. Sports hematuria. *J Urol* 1990;143:887–890.
88. Balaban E. Sports anemia. *Clin Sports Med* 1992;11:313–326.
89. Bailey RR, Dann E, Gillies AH, et al. What the urine contains following athletic competition. *NZ Med J* 1976;83:309–313.
90. Mueller EJ. Thompson IM. Bladder carcinoma presenting as exercise-induced hematuria. *Postgrad Med* 1988;84:173–176.
91. Elliot DL, Goldberg L, Eichner ER Hematuria in a young recreational runner. *Med Sci Sports Exerc* 1991;23:892–894.
92. Grossman RA, Hamilton RW, Morse BM, Penn AS, Goldberg M. Nontraumatic rhabdomyolysis and acute renal failure. *N Engl J Med* 1974;291:807–811.
93. Stahl WC: March hemoglobinuria: report of five cases in students at Ohio State University. *JAMA* 1957;164:1458.
94. Yeun JY, Hasbargen JA. Renal hypouricemia: prevention of exercise-induced acute renal failure and a review of the literature. *Am J Kidney Dis* 1995;25:937–946.
95. Kark JA, Posey DM, Schumacher HR, et al. Sickle cell trait as a risk factor for sudden death in physical training. *N Engl J Med* 1987;317:781–787.
96. Gardner JW. Fatal rhabdomyolysis presenting as mild heat illness in military training. *Mil Med* 1994;159:160–163.
97. Vertel RM, Knochel JP. Acute renal failure due to heat injury: an analysis of ten cases associated with a high incidence of myoglobinuria. *Am J Med* 1967;43:435–451.
98. Schrier RW, Henderson HS, Tisher CC, Tannen RL. Nephropathy associated with heat stress and exercise. *Ann Intern Med* 1967;67:356–376.
99. Sultana SR, Byrne DJ. 'Raver's' haematuria. *J R Coll Surg Edinb* 1996;41:419–20.
100. Knochel JP. Catastrophic medical events with exhaustive exercise: "white collar rhabdomyolysis." *Kidney Int* 1990;38:709–719.
101. Zambraski EJ, Tipton CM, Jordon HR, et al. Iowa wrestling study: urinary profiles of state finalists prior to competition. *Med Sci Sport Exerc* 1974;6:129–132.
102. Zambraski EJ, Tipton CM, Tcheng TK, et al. Iowa wrestling study: changes in the urinary profiles of wrestlers prior to and after competition. *Med Sci Sport Exerc* 1975;7:217–220.
103. Izumi M, Yokoyama K, Yamauchi A, Horio M, Imai E. A young man with acute renal failure and severe loin pain. *Nephron* 1997;76:215–217.
104. Hammerman MR, Miller SB. Effects of growth hormone and insulin-like growth factor I on renal growth and function. *J Pediatr* 1997;131:S17–S19.
105. Lavard P, Holmich P. Renal laceration secondary to blunt trauma in soccer: case report. *Scand J Med Sci Sports* 1993;3:292–293.
106. Emmanuel B, Weiss H, Gollin P. Renal trauma in children. *J Trauma* 1977;17:275.
107. Amaral JF. Thoracoabdominal injuries in the athlete. *Clin Sports Med* 1997;16:739–753.
108. Leppaniemi A, Lamminen A, Tervahartiala P, et al. MRI and CT in blunt renal trauma: an update. *Semin Ultrasound CT MR* 1997;18:129–135.
109. Bergqvist D, Grenabo L, Hedelin H, Lindblad B, Maetzsch T. Blunt renal trauma: analysis of 417 patients. *Eur Urol* 1983;9:1–5.
110. Matthews LA, Smith EM, Spirnak JP. Nonoperative treatment of major blunt renal lacerations with urinary extravasation. *Urology* 1997;157:2056–2058.
111. Abdalati H, Bulas DI, Sivit CJ, et al. Blunt renal trauma in children: healing of renal injuries and recommendations for imaging follow-up. *Pediatr Radiol* 1994;24:573–576.
112. McAndrew JD, Corriere JN Jr. Radiographic evaluation of renal trauma: evaluation of 1103 consecutive patients. *Br J Urol* 1994;73:352–354.
113. Stein JP, Kaji DM, Eastham J, et al. Blunt renal trauma in the pediatric population: indications for radiographic evaluation. *Urology* 1994;44:406–410.
114. Anderson CR. Solitary kidney and sports participation. *Arch Fam Med* 1995;4:885–888.

CHAPTER 28

Cold-Related Injury in Athletes and Active People

William O. Roberts

INTRODUCTION

The human system operates in a narrow range of core body temperature. Athletic activity in cold conditions can overwhelm the normal balance of thermal regulation, resulting in lowered core or regional body temperatures. The body is functionally divided with regard to heat distribution into a core and a shell with a dynamically shifting boundary for thermal balance. The primary function of thermoregulation is to preserve the normal range of core temperature. The "normal" body temperature is 37°C (98.6°F) with a 1°C diurnal variation. The "physiologic range" of body temperature is from 36°C to 40°C (97–104°F) with higher temperatures occurring during exertion, heat exposure, and illness and lower temperatures occurring during exposure to cold environments with inadequate intrinsic heat production or excessive heat loss.

Acute thermal disorders below the normal range of body temperature include frostbite and hypothermia and can occur during exercise. Hypothermia is defined as a core temperature less than 36°C (97°F). Low cell temperatures require less cell metabolism and, to a degree, may lend to cell preservation. Very low tissue temperatures can lead to frostbite, which will destroy tissue and can result in marked tissue loss. Recognition is paramount to successful outcome, and hypothermia should be considered in all exertional settings when athletes collapse or develop changes in mental status in cold environments, especially in extremely cold conditions. Rapid onset of a cold-induced injury with rapid correction of core and tissue temperature results in a better outcome with both frostbite and hypothermia. Both problems should be considered preventable in the athletic setting. It is the responsibility of all who are involved in athletic activities to promote the prevention of cold injury.

HEAT BALANCE IN COLD CONDITIONS

Maintaining the normal core body temperature is a balance of heat gain and loss. The biologic system is not energy efficient; only 25% of the energy produced is converted to mechanical uses. In cold conditions athletes utilize this excess heat energy to maintain normal core temperature and, when working hard, can also increase core temperature and induce sweating. The paradox of activity in the cold lies in the "warmth" of activity balanced with the risk of cold injury during and after activity. Even in frigid environments sweating occurs in an effort to remove excess heat. In cold environments sweat becomes an enemy as wet clothing increases convective and conductive heat losses. As the Eskimos so succinctly phrased it, "Sweat kills."

THERMODYNAMICS IN THE COLD

Heat exchange occurs through conduction, convection, radiation, and evaporation. Conduction occurs during direct contact with a gas, fluid, or solid, as heat energy transfers from higher- to lower-temperature objects or surroundings. Water conducts heat approximately 32 times faster than air, and cold water is a dangerous heat sink for the human system.

Convection is the transfer of heat through contact with a flowing fluid. Moving water exchanges heat faster than still water does. Windchill is the common example of convective heat loss in which air is the fluid and reflects a rate of heat loss rather than an actual ambient air temperature.

Radiation is the electromagnetic energy transfer between two objects from warmer, higher-energy objects to cooler, lower-energy objects. The sun is the radiant

---

W. O. Roberts: MinnHealth Family Physicians, White Bear Lake, Minnesota 55115; and Department of Family Practice and Community Health, University of Minnesota Medical School, Minneapolis, Minnesota 55454.

heat source for our planet and is both friend and foe in athletic activity. In cold conditions radiant heat loss from the body can be substantial.

Evaporation is the most potent means of heat loss during exertion and can remove up to 1 kcal of heat energy per milliliter of sweat vaporized. Evaporation also accounts for respiratory heat loss, which can be considerable in cold, dry conditions. When an athlete sweats heavily during exertion in cold conditions, the combination of evaporative, conductive, and convective heat loss can result in hypothermia.

BODY TEMPERATURE REGULATION

The physiologic thermoregulatory system is under primary central control in the preoptic hypothalamus and secondary peripheral control in temperature-sensitive receptors in the skin. Heat is moved from the working muscles and metabolically active cells of the core to the shell via the circulatory system or is conducted directly to the shell from heat-producing centers. At the shell, heat is removed from the body by conduction, convection, and radiation of heat energy and by the evaporation of sweat. Heat dissipation acts in concert with other regulatory functions to maintain the overall integrity of the biologic system, and the regulatory functions are rank ordered in importance. Hypohydration will decrease blood pressure and produce several responses adverse to heat dissipation: intravascular volume for transport of heat is decreased, the peripheral vasodilatation required for heat dissipation is reversed to preserve adequate blood volume, and blood pressure; and sweating is decreased.

In cold conditions the body is faced with balancing heat dissipation and heat conservation. The system fares well when the heat produced is equal to or greater than the energy needed to preserve core temperature. The vasoconstriction resulting from cold stimulus to peripheral receptors increases the intravascular volume, but the vasoconstriction can be reversed by the need to remove heat. Sweating occurs in the face of extreme cold conditions with moderate to intense work. In athletic activity heat loss is generally not a problem unless the activity is stopped without adequate shelter, the clothing is inadequate to preserve intrinsic heat, or the system runs out of the fuel necessary to produce the heat that maintains core temperature.

COLD TOLERANCE

There is no known limit to cold stress in an adequately dressed athlete. Cold tolerance is mainly a function of environmental adaptation, and humans in arctic conditions still function in a "tropical microenvironment." The most common problem in the cold is removal of sweat from the skin layer to decrease the conductive heat losses.

In cold stress, the human system has a limited capacity for physiologic adaptation (1). The physiologic changes that have been demonstrated include increased peripheral vasoconstriction in Australian aborigines, increased fat layers with measurable increased skin fold thickness in men in Antarctica, and increased metabolic heat production in female Japanese pearl divers. Environmental and behavioral adaptations are the primary means of survival in cold conditions, including increasing layers of clothing, seeking shelter, and developing extrinsic heat sources. There may also be a degree of psychological adaptation with a mental toughness developing after exposure to extreme cold, making cold stress seem more tolerable.

BODY TEMPERATURE MEASUREMENT

Body temperature measurements in cold conditions are confounded by core-shell differences produced by the temperature gradient from the core to the environmentally cooled shell. A core temperature measurement is necessary to make an accurate assessment of cold illness. The core volume contains the organs that are vital to survival. At its minimum, in hypothermic conditions, the core includes the brain, heart, lungs, kidneys, liver, and central large vessels. The shell volume is the remaining muscle mass, skin, subcutaneous tissue, and other tissues that might be considered less critical for survival. The boundary between the core and shell has no definite tissue demarcation and varies with temperature and activity. Natural openings, such as the mouth, nasopharynx, and aural canal, are influenced by the shell temperature, which can spuriously decrease the measured temperature and lead to incorrect clinical assessment of the core temperature, especially in cold conditions (2). In the field and on the sidelines the rectal temperature is the basis of the diagnostic and treatment criteria for hypothermia. It is reliable in field measurement of body temperature, though it may lag behind rapid core temperature changes (3). The aural canal temperature is an analogue of tympanic membrane temperature clinically measured by an infrared temperature scanner. The infrared temperature scanner measures temperature precisely, but the core temperature is not accurately reflected in the aural canal during cool and sweating conditions because the aural canal becomes a part of the shell in these circumstances (2–5). In cold conditions this difference is accentuated (5). Oral temperatures are cooled by rapid respiratory rates and cool saliva. It takes 10 minutes for oral temperature to equilibrate in laboratory conditions, and it is unreliable in athletic settings. Axillary temperatures are cooled by evaporating sweat and also require several minutes for accurate measurements. Skin temperatures directly re-

TABLE 28-1. *Temperature cascades for cold injury and illness*

Temperature (°C/°F)	Cold injury and illness risks	MSHSL* cold weather guide
<−40/−40	Essential activity only	
<−29/−20	Severe frostbite and hypothermia risk	Recommended lower limit for practice for Nordic and downhill ski teams
<−20/−4	Increased frostbite and hypothermia risk	Cancel Nordic races and events > 1 min duration
<0/31	Frostbite risk	Increase protection during rest breaks and in windy conditions
<10/50	Increased hypothermia risk	Hypothermia risk with sweating or inadequate clothing
<18/65	Hypothermia can occur	

*Minnesota State High School League
Adapted from American College of Sports Medicine. Position statement on heat and cold illnesses during distance running. *Med Sci Sports Exerc* 28(12):i–vii, 1996.

flect shell temperature and are known to vary widely from core temperature. Urine temperatures are supply dependent, and although they tend to follow rectal temperature, the urine temperature is difficult to use in collapsed athletes, who are often dehydrated and unable to produce a urine specimen. Rectal temperature is the only reliable estimate of core temperature in field conditions (2–5).

COLD-RELATED DISORDERS

Exposure to cool or cold conditions increases the risk of cold-related disorders. In athletes the concerns are not as great during activity as after activity ceases or if injury forces cessation of activity, unless participating in extreme cold conditions (Table 28-1). Cold injury can be both life and limb threatening. The vasoconstriction response to cold exposure decreases blood and heat flow to the affected body area while increasing the insulating layer to protect the core temperature. Although cooling tissue does not damage individual cells as severely as overheating tissue does, actual freezing of cells destroys the cell membrane integrity and results in tissue loss.

SPECIFIC DISORDERS RELATED TO ACTIVITY IN THE COLD

Chilblains

Chilblains are vasculitis of the dermis caused by chronic exposure to cold conditions above freezing temperature levels. The most commonly affected areas are the face, the anterior tibia, and the dorsum of the hands and feet. Chilblains are most frequently found in laborers and military personnel.

Frostbite

Frostbite is the freezing of tissue, including intracellular contents, that occurs at −0.6°C to −2°C and is classified as superficial or deep on the basis of the depth of the freeze and tissue injury (6). Tissue injury can occur before actual freezing and is induced by severe vasoconstriction. Trench foot is a chronic form of prefreezing injury. Frost nip occurs when ice crystals form on the surface of the skin without actual freezing of the skin tissue. Frost nip is readily reversible and is often associated with numbness and blanching of the skin. The greatest risk of frostbite is in the appendages and watershed areas of the body, including the digits, feet, hands, ears, nose, cheeks, and genitalia. Frostbite of the male genitalia, referred to as *testicular nip,* is an intensely painful injury. Exposure to ambient temperatures in −29°C (−20°F) windchill for 1 hour will lead to frostbite of normal tissue (6). At −48°C (−55°F) windchill, flesh will freeze in 10 minutes (6).

A frostbite victim will often experience itching as the first sign of freezing tissue. Symptoms progress to pain, paresthesia, numbness, and loss of function. The clinical appearance of frostbite is red, swollen tissue progressing to white, waxy, cold, firm or hard tissue. There is obvious loss of blood flow when the tissue is frozen. Frostbite can be graded on the basis of the clinical appearance at the initial exam as superficial, with mobile subcutaneous tissue, or deep, with hard tissue extending deep to bone and insensitive tissue postthawing. Classification by frostbite severity rating can be assessed after several days with the following scheme (7):

First-degree
  Numbness
  Erythema
  Edema
Second-degree
  Clear, fluid-filled blisters
  Erythema
  Edema
Third-degree
  Hemorrhagic blisters

Fourth-degree
  Injury to bone and muscle
  Tissue mottled and lifeless

The risk factors for frostbite include outdoor sports and occupation exposures, tobacco use, black race, altered mental status, homeless living, exposure to spilled petroleum products, and previous frostbite. Previous frostbite also induces a twofold increased risk of frostbite in future exposures. At high altitudes the low O_2 tensions decrease mental sharpness and increase the risk of frostbite and other cold injuries (8).

The treatment of frostbite is rapid rewarming in a water bath at 40–42°C (104–108°F) (9). Rewarming frozen tissue should not be started until there is no risk of refreezing, as a second freeze-thaw cycle will markedly increase tissue destruction. Vascular changes and inflammation occur with rewarming, releasing free radicals, which produce oxidative stress and increased tissue damage. Oxidative stress also activates the clotting cascade, inducing capillary thrombosis, which compounds the physical tissue damage. Some studies have shown improved outcomes with the use of topical aloe vera (70% aqueous extract) and systemic ibuprofen at a dose of 400 mg twice daily beginning immediately after rewarming (10). Prophylactic antibiotic use is controversial. After thawing, there must be prolonged observation for demarcation of viable tissue before there is any amputation of affected tissue.

Prevention of frostbite is best accomplished through education. In severe cold conditions, especially if the windchill, either real or apparent, will be lower than −40°C, elective activities and races should be postponed or canceled as outlined in Table 28–1. The Federation Internationale de Ski rules require cancellation of Nordic ski races below −20°C because of the windchill generated by the speed of the skiers during the races. Strict attention to equipment and clothing needs is imperative in cold outdoor activities. Tight or restrictive clothing or boots that restrict blood flow to the extremities will increase the risk of frostbite and are a particular risk for downhill skiers with "race-fit" boots, as shown in Figure 28–1. Eye protection from the cold is critical in fast-moving activities, such as Nordic ski racing, in which the apparent windchill can produce frostbite of the cornea, resulting in blindness. Individuals whose activities will bring them away from immediate shelter must anticipate the conditions and carry the necessary equipment for their safety. A buddy system is helpful for preventing frostbite.

Hypothermia

Hypothermia is a multisystem disease that can ensue insidiously or rapidly. Hypothermia is defined as a core body temperature less than 36°C (97°F). Hypothermia can be classified as mild, 34–36°C (93–97°F); moderate, 30–34°C (86–93°F); or severe, <30°C (<86°F). Prompt recognition and treatment will decrease morbidity and mortality. Few medical centers, other than some remote medical stations in the popular mountain-climbing areas, have the casualty incidence to launch prospective studies of hypothermia. Hypothermia onset can be accidental or medical. Accidental hypothermia onset is rapid in cold-water immersion or severe cold exposure and slow in less severe exposure. Medical hypothermia is secondary to disease processes that do not provide the fuel or circulation for thermoregulation or may be induced for medical purposes. The lowest surviving accidental hypothermia victim had a core temperature of 15.2°C, and the surgically induced low is 6°C. Below 30°C core temperature the body is poikilothermic and assumes the temperature of the surrounding environment. The prevailing medical wisdom is that a hypothermia casualty is "not dead, until warm and dead," where warm equals 32–35°C core temperature.

The morbidity and mortality of hypothermia vary with the degree of severity. Mild hypothermic casualties have an excellent prognosis with general recovery through endogenous heat production. Moderate levels of hypothermia generally have a good recovery but often require active rewarming. Severe hypothermia will require active internal rewarming for the best chance of survival. Twenty years ago the mortality rates varied from 55% to 100% for accidental hypothermia (11). The most recent treatment protocols have lowered the mortality rate to 30%. A palpable pulse at initial exam correlates with better survival rates.

The environment, age, alcohol use, illicit and prescribed drugs, hypoglycemia, and medical conditions can predispose to hypothermia. Environmental factors include ambient temperatures less than 18°C (64°F); extreme cold, wet conditions; and cold-water immersion (12,13). Hypothermia occurs frequently in cool, wet conditions when hikers and slow long distance runners do not generate the necessary metabolic heat to keep the core temperature in the normal range. The thermal con-

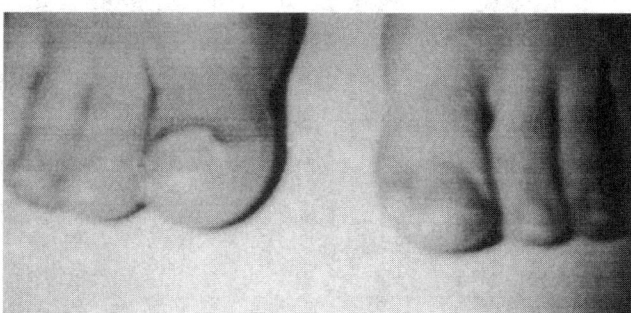

FIG. 28–1. Second-degree frostbite of the toes from "race-fit" ski boots. (Photo © W. O. Roberts, M.D.)

ductivity of water is 32 times greater than that of air, so heat loss is very rapid in cold-water immersion, especially if the neck, axilla, and groin are exposed (14). Older individuals have decreased metabolic rate and are more susceptible to exposure, and young children have a larger body surface to mass ratio, producing more rapid heat loss in comparison to adults in similar conditions. The risk of alcohol use in cold conditions is mainly due to altered, and often risky, behavior. Alcohol may also depress the myocardium, decreasing the ability of the heart to respond to cooling (5). Although the vasodilatation of alcohol use may contribute to mild hypothermia, truly significant vasodilatation does not occur until sublethal blood levels of alcohol are present. The pharmacologic agents from the barbiturate, halothane, phenothiazine, and ether classes have a direct effect on the temperature regulation center. They can reduce thermogenic shivering, induce cutaneous vasodilatation, and lower basal metabolic rate. Hypoglycemia can occur with diabetes mellitus treatment or depleted glycogen store from prolonged shivering or physical exertion. Hypoglycemia can set off thermogenic shivering through a centrally mediated mechanism. Administration of concentrated glucose or dextrose solutions can reverse the hypothermia associated with hypoglycemia and force a return of thermogenic shivering.

Other medical conditions can result in hypothermia and should be considered, especially in the elderly. The hypothermia of sepsis and head injury is the result of dysfunction of the central mechanism controlling core temperature. Hypothyroidism, with its decreased metabolic rate, hypopituitarism, and hypoadrenalism, is associated with low core temperature. Any condition with loss of shivering thermogenesis can result in hypothermia and will present most commonly with slow onset hypothermia.

The clinical presentation of hypothermia is not specific, and in exertional situations it can be identical to that of hyperthermic collapse (13). Impaired judgment, confusion, and apathy are early signs of hypothermia and can lead to worsening of the situation as critical decisions become unimportant to the individual at risk. This confusion is frequently demonstrated with paradoxical undressing in the moderate hypothermic range. Shivering decreases below 33°C core temperature but can continue to core temperatures of 24°C. Muscle stiffness is common with cooling tissues. As body temperature drops, the level of consciousness decreases; hypothermic casualties often become unconscious between 30°C and 32°C. Pulse and respiratory rate gradually slow in response to decreased metabolic rate and O_2 demands. Coma precedes death. Detection of hypothermia requires a high index of suspicion and a low-temperature thermometer that can register temperatures lower than 20°C.

The pathophysiology of hypothermia involves multiple systems. The initial response to cold stimulus and falling core temperature is peripheral vasoconstriction with progressive contraction of core volume to protect vital organs. Intense vasoconstriction can increase body insulation by a factor of 6. The Lewis Hunting reaction is a local vasodilatation due to paralysis of precapillary sphincter muscles in the peripheral vasculature, which allows local rewarming. The vasoconstriction response recurs as capillary sphincters become functional with local warming. The full reaction is the oscillation between threshold temperatures, causing alternate blanching and flushing of the skin. The Lewis Hunting reaction is most prominent in the digits, ears, and face and probably helps to prevent frostbite while conserving core temperature. Peripheral vasoconstriction also produces a relative increase in blood volume, which is sensed by the kidney as hypervolemia. Cold exposure alone augments urine flow as the kidney seeks to reestablish "normal" central volume. Hypothermic victims are usually hypohydrated because of the protective vasoconstriction response. In the hypothermic state, fluid will also extravagate into surrounding tissue, resulting in loss of intravascular volume (15). Dehydration is not as common in rapid onset hypothermia.

Hypothermia lowers the metabolic rate approximately 6% for each 1 C° decrease in core temperature. In many animals the diving reflex decreases cell metabolic rate in response to sudden immersion of the face in cold water. It may be present in children but is probably lost in adults.

Cardiac tissue cooling produces predictable changes, including progressive slowing of heart rate, which can be less than 3 beats per minute at 10°C core body temperature. Cardiac contractility will remain normal to profoundly cold temperatures. Atrial fibrillation is common below 30°C core temperature. Below 28°C core temperature the heart becomes irritable, and ventricular fibrillation often occurs, especially with rough handling during rescue and resuscitation. The risk of ventricular fibrillation is greatest between 20°C and 24°C core temperature and is difficult to treat below 28°C. Alcohol may lower the arrhythmia threshold by 2–5°C. Below 30°C core temperature there is poor response to defibrillation, antiarrhythmic drugs, cardioactive drugs, and pacemakers. Asystole is common below 20°C core temperature. The J-wave is an extra deflection at QRS-ST junction of the cardiac tracing. It once was considered pathognomonic of hypothermia. Although its presence is not obligatory, it is usually present in 80% of cases. The J-wave is also found in sepsis and central nervous system lesions. Cardiac catheterization may not be as risky as was once believed. CPR should be initiated for cardiac arrest but not for bradycardia and should be continued until the core is warmed and other resuscitation strategies become effective.

The chemistry changes associated with hypothermia

are of limited diagnostic value and generally reflect the elevated enzyme markers of cell injury. The acid-base balance usually demonstrates a combined respiratory and metabolic acidosis. Hyperglycemia occurs as a result of inhibited sympathetic insulin secretion and direct cooling of insulin secreting cells. This secondary increase of plasma glucose can contribute to the diuresis of hypothermia.

Rewarming is essential to the successful resuscitation of the hypothermic victim, but it can be a two-edged sword. Rewarming the periphery causes vasodilatation and can cause shock by overriding the compensation for hypothermia-induced hypovolemia. Rewarming also increases O_2 demand in warmed tissues. Afterdrop is a continued decrease in core temperature and occurs frequently as the cooling stimulus is removed and warming begins. The extended fall in core temperature can be 2–3°C in adults and 5°C in children. The mechanism of afterdrop was initially thought to be recirculation of cold blood from the extremities, but it is simply due to convective heat exchange cooling of blood circulating through cold peripheral tissues.

The basic treatment of hypothermia is either passive or active rewarming. Passive rewarming is accomplished through endogenous heat production. Victims usually warm at a rate of 1°C per hour and may increase the intrinsic heat production to 2°C per hour if shivering is present. Casualties should be warmed with exercise only if the core temperature is >35°C. Passive therapy begins with the first aid measures of removing the victim from the cold environment, removing wet clothing, drying the skin, and adding insulation layers (13,16).

Active rewarming implies the use of an exogenous energy supply to heat the cooled body core, either externally or internally. External methods are most convenient and accessible but are not as effective as internal methods for rapid rewarming. Internal methods are invasive, increasing the risk of therapy, but are necessary for successful treatment of severe hypothermia accompanied by cardiac instability.

External (surface) methods warm from the outside inward. Warm water immersion in a 40–45°C bath with the extremities out of water can raise the core temperature >5°C per hour and is the most effective of the external methods. It is difficult to do CPR in a tub if it is needed, and evaporative heat loss will occur when the victim is taken from the tub to initiate CPR. Heating blankets have also been used and have warming rates of 0.5–3°C per hour. There is an increased burn risk with heating blankets that are in direct contact with poorly perfused skin. Plumbed garments, heated objects or containers, and radiant heat sources have also been used in active external rewarming. In the field, one or two warm bodies in a sleeping bag with the casualty can be effective for rewarming mild- to moderate-level victims. Warmed water bags placed in the neck, axilla, and groin have been used to facilitate the warming of mild- to moderate-level hypothermia casualties in Nordic ski races.

Internal (core) rewarming heats from the inside out, a process that bypasses some of the problems of external techniques. Nearly every imaginable route of heat access has been tried. Warmed, humidified airway inhalation is used to augment field and hospital therapy, but better primary methods exist for use in the hospital. Warmed IV fluids are used whenever possible but probably do not contribute a significant heat load to the profoundly cold system. Gastric, rectal, and bladder irrigation can augment other methods but generally do not raise the temperature at the rates of more powerful methods. Gastric irrigation can raise the core temperature at a rate of 1–1.3°C per hour, similar to the rate for heating blankets.

Extracorporeal cardiopulmonary bypass is the most powerful means of rapidly increasing core temperature, with warming rates of up to 10°C per hour. Some centers have documented core temperature increases of 1–2°C every 3–5 minutes. The bleeding risk from heparin may be decreased with the introduction of new tubing, which may dramatically reduce or even eliminate the need for heparin. This is the method of choice in cardiac arrest, but its use is limited by availability of the apparatus. Continuous thoracostomy (pleural) lavage through two chest tubes is a relatively new method that is used mostly in Europe, with warming rates of 8°C per hour. Peritoneal irrigation or dialysis rewarms at rates of 4–6°C per hour. It is a relatively simple procedure done through two bladder catheters using 10–12 L/h of lactated Ringer's solution or saline at 40°C warmed in blood warmer. Mediastinal lavage rewarms at 2–3°C per hour. Extracorporeal hemodialysis has also been used.

The method of choice for treatment of hypothermia will vary with situation and location. The field protocol for casualties should be to handle gently; remove wet clothing; dry the skin; insulate the body from further heat loss; and, if available, ventilate with warmed, humidified air at 42–46°C; use O_2; and start EKG monitoring (16). The EKG electrodes often do not stick to cold skin, so it may be necessary to puncture the skin with a needle through the electrode pad to make electrical contact. The gain should be turned to maximum amplification if cardiac activity is not readily identified. In the field, CPR should be started only for pulseless and apneic casualties if it can be continued to the hospital. Rewarming for mild, conscious victims can be passive or active external treatment. Field rewarming for more severe victims should be passive with no active external rewarming initiated until the treatment facility is within reach.

Once the victim is in the medical facility, rapid internal rewarming should be instituted for severe hypothermia. The longer a victim is hypothermic, the greater the morbidity and mortality. Heated, humidified O_2, centrally administered warmed IV fluids at 43°C, and peritoneal dialysis or two-chest-tube irrigation should be used until extracorporeal cardiopulmonary bypass rewarming can be started. The endpoint for active internal rewarming is 32–34°C to avoid hyperthermia, which can increase cell metabolic demands and increase the overall damage to the system.

Fluid resuscitation will be needed to support the hypothermia-induced hypovolemia. Normal saline is the usual fluid of choice. Lactated Ringer's solution should not be administered because the cold liver cannot metabolize lactate. Other system support should include administration of 50 mL IV $D_{50}W$, 100 mg IV thiamine, and 0.8 mg IV naloxone for altered mental status; O_2 administration; glucose, electrolyte, and chemistry monitoring; and cardiac monitoring for arrhythmia. Ventricular fibrillation prophylaxis with bretylium (5 mg/kg) for temperatures lower than 28°C is recommended by some centers. Defibrillation is seldom successful in a cold heart, but a defibrillation trial of up to three shocks should be attempted for temperatures lower than 30°C. CPR is used when necessary. Prophylactic antibiotics are recommended to prevent secondary infection.

The complications of severe hypothermia include pneumonia, pulmonary edema, cardiac arrhythmia, myoglobinuria, disseminated intravascular coagulation, seizures, and compartment syndromes. Any complication will prolong hospitalization and can lead to the victim's demise.

In the athletic setting, hypothermia is a preventable illness. As with frostbite and hyperthermia, prevention is a function of environmental awareness and respect, preparation, and education.

SUMMARY

Cold-related illness and injury are preventable and can be treated with excellent outcomes if the problems are considered early in the presentation of collapsed athletes. Within the sports medicine community every effort should be made to educate all who are involved in the administration and training of athletes to prevent the onset and occurrence of cold illness. Prevention of cold injuries is easily accomplished by moving the event starting time to the safest available for the timing of the event and allowing the modification or cancellation of events that occur during unexpectedly severe environmental conditions. With the current knowledge of cold injury, an adverse outcome due to cold illness or injury sustained during extreme environmental conditions may be considered to result from negligence.

REFERENCES

1. Bittel J. The different types of general cold adaptation in man. *Int J Sports Med* 13[Suppl 1]:172–175, 1992.
2. Brengelman GL. The dilemma of body temperature measurement. In: Shiraki K, Yousef MK, eds. *Man in stressful environments: thermal and work physiology.* Springfield, IL: Thomas, 1987:Chapter 1.
3. Armstrong LE, Maresh CM, Crago AE, et al. Interpretation of aural temperatures during exercise, hyperthermia, and cooling therapy. *Med Exerc Nutr Health* 1994;3(1):9–16.
4. Deschamps A, Levy RD, Cosio MG, et al. Tympanic temperature should not be used to assess exercise induced hyperthermia. *Clin J Sports Med* 1992;2(1):27–32.
5. Roberts WO. Assessing core temperature in collapsed athletes. *Phys Sportsmed* 1994;22(8):49–55.
6. Siple PA, Passel CF. Measurements of dry atmosphere cooling in subfreezing temperatures. *Proc AM Philies Soc* 1975;89(1):177–199.
7. Stine RJ. *A practical approach to emergency medicine.* New York: Little, 1994:369–371.
8. Foray J. Mountain frostbite. *Int J Sports Med* 1992;13[Suppl 1]:195–196.
9. McCauley RL, Heggers JP, Robson MC. Frostbite: methods to minimize tissue loss. *Postgrad Med* 1990;88(8):67–77.
10. Heggers JP, Robson MC, et al. Experimental and clinical observations on frostbite. *Ann Emerg Med* 1987;16(9):1056–1062.
11. Lønning PE, Skulberg A, Åbyholm F. Accidental hypothermia. *Acta Anaesthesiol Scand* 30(8):601–613, 1986.
12. Crouse B, Beattie K. Marathon medical services: strategies to reduce runner morbidity. *Med Sci Sports Exerc* 1996;28(9):1093–1096.
13. Roberts WO. Exercise associated collapse in endurance events: a classification system. *Phys Sportsmed* 17(5):49–55, 1989.
14. Hayward JS, Collis M, Eckerson JD. Thermographic evaluation of relative heat loss areas of man during cold water immersion. *Aerospace Med* 1973;44(7):708–711.
15. Lauri T. Cardiovascular responses to an acute volume load in deep hypothermia. *Eur Heart J* 1996;17(4):606–611.
16. Mills WJ. Field care of the hypothermic patient. *Int J Sports Med* 1992;13[Supp 1]:199–202.
17. American College of Sports Medicine. Position statement on heat and cold illnesses during distance running. *Med Sci Sports Exerc* 1996;28(12):i–vii.

PART V
Overuse and Trauma

CHAPTER 29

Catastrophic Injuries in High School and College Sports

Frederick O. Mueller

INTRODUCTION

In 1931 the American Football Coaches Association initiated the First Annual Survey of Football Fatalities, and this research has been conducted at the University of North Carolina at Chapel Hill since 1965. In 1977 the National Collegiate Athletic Association initiated a national survey of catastrophic football injuries, which is also conducted at the University of North Carolina. As a result of these research projects important contributions to the sport of football have been made. Most notable have been the 1976 rule changes, the football helmet standard, improved medical care for the participants, and better coaching techniques.

Because of the success of these two football projects, the research was expanded to all sports for both men and women, and a National Center for Catastrophic Sports Injury Research was established. The decision to expand the research was based on the following factors:

1. Research based on reliable data is essential if progress is to be made in sports safety.
2. The paucity of information on injuries in all sports.
3. The rapid expansion and lack of injury information in women's sports.

For the purpose of this research the term catastrophic is defined as any severe injury incurred during participation in a school- or college-sponsored sport. Catastrophic will be divided into the following three definitions:

1. Fatal
2. Nonfatal: permanent severe functional disability

3. Serious: no permanent functional disability but severe injury. An example would be a fractured cervical vertebra with no paralysis.

Sports injuries are also considered direct or indirect. *Direct injuries* are injuries that result directly from participation in the skills of the sport. *Indirect injuries* are injuries that are caused by systemic failure as a result of exertion while participating in a sport activity or by a complication that was secondary to a nonfatal injury.

DATA COLLECTION

Data were complied with the assistance of coaches, athletic directors, executive officers of state and national athletic organizations, a national newspaper clipping service, and professional associates of the researchers. Data collection would not have been possible without the support of the National Collegiate Athletic Association, the National Federation of State High School Associations, and the American Football Coaches Association. On receiving information about a possible catastrophic sports injury, contact by telephone, personal letter, and questionnaire was made with the injured player's coach or athletic director. Data collected included background information on the athlete (age, height, weight, experience, previous injury, etc.), accident information, immediate and postaccident medical care, type of injury, and equipment involved. Autopsy reports are used when available.

In 1987 a joint endeavor was initiated with the Section on Sports Medicine of the American Association of Neurological Surgeons to enhance the collection of medical data. Dr. Robert C. Cantu, Chairman of the Department of Surgery and Chief of Neurosurgery Ser-

---

F. O. Mueller: Department of Exercise and Sport Science, University of North Carolina at Chapel Hill, Chapel Hill, North Carolina 27599–8605.

vice at Emerson Hospital in Concord, Massachusetts, has been responsible for contacting the physician involved in each case and for collecting the medical data.

SUMMARY

Fall Sports

Football is associated with the greatest number of catastrophic injuries. For the 1995 high school football season there was a total of 22 direct catastrophic injuries, which is a slight increase from 1994 (16 injuries) but a dramatic decrease when compared to the 1993 season (34 injuries) and one of the lowest numbers since 1982. College football was associated with four direct catastrophic injuries in 1995, which is a decrease from the eight in 1994. Rates per 100,000 participants for the years 1982–1983 through 1995–1996 are shown in Tables 29–1 through 29–4.

In 1990 there were no fatalities directly related to football. The 1990 football report is historic in that it is the first year since the beginning of the research (1931) that there was not a direct fatality in football at any level of play. The 1994 data shows zero fatalities at the high school level and one at the college level, with a slight rise in 1995 to four and zero. These numbers are very low when one considers that there were 36 direct fatalities associated with football in 1968.

In addition to the direct fatalities in 1995, there were eight indirect fatalities. Seven of the indirect fatalities were at the high school level, and one was at the college level. Five of the high school indirect fatalities were heat related, one was related to asthma, and one was heart related. The cause of the one indirect fatality at the college level was unknown.

In addition to the fatalities there were seven permanent paralysis cervical spine injuries in 1995. This number is also low when compared to the 25–30 cases every year in the early 1970s but was an increase from 1994. Six injuries were at the high school level, and one was

TABLE 29–1. High school fall sports: direct catastrophic injuries per 100,000 participants, 1982–1983 through 1995–1996

Sport	Fatalities	Nonfatal injuries	Serious injuries
Male			
Cross-country	0.00		0.00
Football	0.28	0.69	0.80
Soccer	0.13	0.06	0.16
Female			
Cross-country	0.00	0.00	0.00
Football	0.00	0.00	0.00
Soccer	0.00	0.00	0.00

TABLE 29–2. High school fall sports: indirect catastrophic injuries per 100,000 participants, 1982–1983 through 1995–1996

Sport	Fatalities	Nonfatal injuries	Serious injuries
Male			
Cross-country	0.41	0.00	0.00
Football	0.39	0.00	0.01
Soccer	0.45	0.00	0.00
Water polo (1992–1994)	4.83	0.00	0.00
Female			
Cross-country	0.07	0.00	0.00
Football	0.00	0.00	0.00
Soccer	0.06	0.00	0.00
Water polo	0.00	0.00	0.00

TABLE 29–3. College fall sports: direct catastrophic injuries per 100,000 participants, 1982–1983 through 1995–1996

Sport	Fatalities	Nonfatal injuries	Serious injuries
Male			
Cross-country	0.00	0.00	0.00
Football	0.48	1.71	5.81
Soccer	0.00	0.00	0.48
Field hockey	0.00	0.00	0.00
Female			
Cross-country	0.00	0.00	0.00
Football	0.00	0.00	0.00
Soccer	0.00	0.00	0.00
Field hockey	0.00	0.00	1.39

TABLE 29–4. College fall sports: indirect catastrophic injuries per 100,000 participants, 1982–1983 through 1995–1996

Sport	Fatalities	Nonfatal injuries	Serious injuries
Male			
Cross-country	0.74	0.00	0.00
Football	2.19	0.00	0.00
Soccer	0.97	0.00	0.00
Water polo	6.81	0.00	0.00
Female			
Cross-country	0.00	0.00	0.00
Football	0.00	0.00	0.00
Soccer	0.00	0.00	0.00
Water polo	0.00	0.00	0.00

at the college level. Football in 1995 was also associated with two subdural hematoma injuries that resulted in permanent disability. Both injuries were at the high school level.

Serious football injuries with no permanent disability accounted for 13 injuries in 1995: ten in high school and three in college. High school athletes were associated with two cervical spine fractures, four transient spinal cord injuries, and four subdural hematoma injuries with full recovery. College athletes were associated with two transient spinal cord injuries and one cervical spine fracture.

This decrease in catastrophic football injuries illustrates the importance of data collection, analysis of cause of injury, and the dissemination of that information to those responsible for conducting football programs. A return to the injury levels of the 1960s and 1970s would be detrimental to the game and its participants.

Cross-country was not associated with any direct injuries but was associated with one indirect fatality at the high school level in 1995. The indirect death was associated with sudden death and involved a male athlete. For the 14 years indicated, cross-country was associated with one direct nonfatal injury and 10 indirect fatalities at the high school level and one indirect fatality at the college level. All 11 of the indirect injuries were heart-related fatalities. Autopsy reports revealed congenital heart disease in three of these cases.

High school soccer had one direct nonfatal injury in 1995 and a total of 11 catastrophic injuries for the 14 seasons. The three direct catastrophic injuries in 1992 represented the highest number in the past 14 years. The one direct injury in 1995 occurred in a practice. The athlete was doing pull-ups on an unanchored goal, which fell over and hit the athlete's head. He was in a coma for 2 weeks. There was also one high school soccer indirect fatality in 1995, and the cause of death was heart related. In 1995 college soccer was associated with one indirect fatality, which was heart related.

In 1988 field hockey was associated with its first catastrophic injury since the study began in 1982. It was listed as a serious injury at the college level. The athlete was struck by the ball after a free hit. She suffered a fractured skull, had surgery, and recovered from the injury. The 1995 data show no field hockey direct or indirect injuries at either the high school or college level.

In 1992–1993 high school water polo was associated with its first indirect fatality, and in 1988–1989 college water polo had its first indirect fatality. The 1995 data show one indirect fatality at the high school level; it was heart related.

In summary, high school fall sports in 1995 were associated with 23 direct catastrophic injuries. Twenty-two were associated with football and one with soccer. There were four fatalities, nine injuries involved permanent disability, and 10 injuries were considered serious. For the 14-year period 1982–1995, high school fall sports had 363 direct catastrophic injuries, and 351, or 96.7%, were related to football participants. In 1995 high school fall sports were also associated with seven football indirect fatalities, one in cross-country, one in soccer, and one in water polo, for a total of 10 indirect fatalities. For the period from 1982 to 1995 there was a total of 106 indirect catastrophic injuries. Of the indirect injuries, 105 were fatalities, and 78 were related to football. Two of the indirect fatalities involved females: a soccer player in 1986 and a cross-country runner in 1992.

During the 1995 college fall sports season there was a total of four direct catastrophic injuries; all were in football. For the 14 years 1982–1995 there was a total of 86 college direct fall sport catastrophic injuries; 84 were associated with football. There were two indirect fatalities during the fall of 1995. One was associated with football and one with soccer. From 1982 through the 1995 season there was a total of 27 college fall sport indirect catastrophic fatalities. Twenty-three were associated with football.

High school football accounted for the greatest number of direct catastrophic injuries for the fall sports, but high school football was also associated with the greatest number of participants. Approximately 1,500,000 high school and junior high school football players participated each year. As is illustrated in Table 29–1, the 14-year rate of direct injuries per 100,000 high school and junior high school football participants was 0.28 fatalities, 0.69 nonfatal injuries, and 0.80 serious injuries. These catastrophic injury rates for football are higher than those for both cross-country and soccer, but all three classifications of catastrophic football injuries have an injury rate of less than 1 per 100,000 participants. Table 29–2 shows that the indirect fatality rates for high school football, soccer, and cross-country are similar and are also less than 1 per 100,000 participants. Water polo rates are high but are based on only 4 years of data, and water polo had only approximately 12,000 participants each year.

College football had approximately 75,000 participants each year, and the direct injury rate per 100,000 participants was higher than the rates for college cross-country, soccer, and field hockey. The rate of college football fatalities for the 14-year period indicated in Table 29–3 was less than 1 per 100,000 participants, but the rate increased to 1.71 per 100,000 for nonfatal injuries and 5.81 per 100,000 participants for serious injuries.

Indirect fatality rates were similar in college cross-country and soccer and increased in football, water polo being associated with the highest indirect fatality rate (Table 29–4). Water polo had approximately 1000 participants each year. Only one college female athlete received a direct or indirect catastrophic injury in a fall

TABLE 29-5. Participation figures, 1982-1983 through 1995-1996

	High school		College	
	Men	Women	Men	Women
Football	19,800,000	1,693	1,050,000	0
Cross-country	2,213,003	1,511,977	135,878	104,728
Soccer	3,075,836	1,664,024	206,086	93,534
Basketball	7,250,689	5,590,942	183,908	154,996
Gymnastics	67,790	394,464	10,932	21,900
Ice hockey	322,568	3,011	54,640	2,040
Swimming	1,094,920	1,243,852	109,599	108,552
Wrestling	3,323,523	3,892	102,174	0
Baseball	5,826,631	7,328	295,024	0
Softball	10,107	3,666,962	0	138,062
Lacrosse	264,659	133,076	68,738	42,694
Track	6,596,538	5,140,529	469,862	302,421
Tennis	1,864,069	1,800,639	108,278	102,625
Field hockey	174	705,822	0	71,817
Skiing	19,683 (1994-1996)	16,159 (1994-1996)	10,538	7,075
Water polo	41,384	10,178	14,688	0
Volleyball	60,269 (1994-1996)	697,752 (1994-1996)	1743 (1994-1996)	22,990 (1994-1996)
Total	51,831,843	22,592,300	2,822,088	1,173,434

sport for this 14-year period of time; it was a serious injury in field hockey.

Incidence rates are based on 14-year participation figures received from the National Federation of State High School Associations and the National Collegiate Athletic Association. (Table 29-5).

Winter Sports

High school winter sports were associated with three direct catastrophic injuries in 1995-1996. Two injuries were related to gymnastics, and one was related to wrestling. The disability injury in gymnastics was to a female, and the serious injury involved a male. The wrestling injury was also a serious injury.

High school winter sports were also associated with four indirect injuries during the 1995-1996 school year. Three of the injuries were fatalities, two being associated with wrestling and one with swimming. The fourth injury was a serious injury in swimming. Both of the swimming injuries involved females. All three of the fatalities were heart related; the cause of the one serious injury in swimming was unknown.

College winter sports were associated with two direct catastrophic injuries during the 1995-1996 season. Both injuries were disability injuries to ice hockey players. College sports were also associated with one indirect fatality in swimming during the 1995-1996 school year.

A summary of high school winter sports from 1982 to 1996 shows a total of 69 direct catastrophic injuries (five fatalities, 37 nonfatal injuries, and 27 serious injuries) and 73 indirect injuries. Wrestling was associated with 32, or 46.4%, of the direct injuries. Gymnastics was associated with 12, or 17.4%, of the direct injuries. Ice hockey was associated with 11 direct injuries, swimming with seven, volleyball with one, and basketball with six. Basketball accounted for the greatest number of indirect fatalities, with 51, or 69.9%, of the winter total.

College winter sports from 1982 to 1996 were associated with a total of 18 direct catastrophic injuries. Gymnastics was associated with six, ice hockey with six, basketball with three, swimming with one, skiing with one, and wrestling with one. There were also 18 indirect injuries during this time. Twelve, or 66.7%, were associated with basketball, two with ice hockey, three with swimming, and one with skiing.

High school wrestling accounted for the greatest number of winter sport direct injuries, but the injury rate per 100,000 participants was less than 1 for all three injury categories (Table 29-6). High school wrestling had approximately 238,000 participants each year. High school basketball and swimming were also associated with low direct injury rates. As is shown in Table 29-6, ice hockey and gymnastics were associated with the highest injury rates for the winter sports. Gymnastics had averaged approximately 5,000 male and 28,000 female participants during the 14-year period. Ice hockey averaged 23,000 participants each year. A high percentage of the ice hockey injuries involved a player being hit by an opposing player, usually from behind, and striking the skate rink boards with the top of his or her head.

Indirect high school catastrophic injury rates were all below 1 per 100,000 participants, as is indicated in Table 29-7.

Catastrophic direct injury rates for college winter sports were higher when compared to high school figures. Gymnastics had five nonfatal injuries and one seri-

TABLE 29-6. *High school winter sports: direct catastrophic injuries per 100,000 participants, 1982-1983 through 1995-1996*

Sport	Fatalities	Nonfatal injuries	Serious injuries
Male			
Basketball	0.00	0.01	0.05
Gymnastics	1.47	1.47	1.47
Ice hockey	0.62	1.24	1.55
Swimming	0.00	0.18	0.27
Wrestling	0.06	0.57	0.33
Female			
Basketball	0.00	0.02	0.00
Gymnastics	0.00	1.52	0.76
Ice hockey	0.00	0.00	0.00
Swimming	0.00	0.16	0.00
Wrestling	0.00	0.00	0.00
Volleyball	0.00	0.14	0.00

TABLE 29-8. *College winter sports: direct catastrophic injuries per 100,000 participants, 1982-1983 through 1995-1996*

Sport	Fatalities	Nonfatal injuries	Serious injuries
Male			
Basketball	0.00	0.54	1.09
Gymnastics	0.00	27.44	9.14
Ice hockey	0.00	5.49	5.49
Swimming	0.00	0.91	0.00
Wrestling	0.00	0.98	0.00
Skiing	0.00	0.00	0.00
Female			
Basketball	0.00	0.00	0.00
Gymnastics	0.00	9.13	0.00
Ice hockey	0.00	0.00	0.00
Swimming	0.00	0.00	0.00
Wrestling	0.00	0.00	0.00
Skiing	14.13	0.00	0.00

ous injury for the 14-year period, but the injury rate was 36.58 per 100,000 participants for nonfatal and serious male injuries and 9.13 per 100,000 for female nonfatal injuries (Table 29-8). Participation figures show approximately 780 male and 1564 female gymnastic participants each year during the 14-year period.

College ice hockey was associated with three serious injuries and three nonfatal injuries in the 14-year period, but the injury rate was 5.49 per 100,000 participants for both nonfatal and serious injuries. There were approximately 4000 ice hockey participants each year. Swimming nonfatal incidence rates were not as high as the rates for gymnastics or ice hockey but could be totally eliminated if swimmers would not use the racing dive into the shallow end of pools during practice or meets.

In fact, there has not been a direct injury in college swimming since one nonfatal injury in 1982-1983.

College wrestling had only one catastrophic injury from the fall of 1982 to the spring of 1996. For this period of time there were 102,174 participants in college wrestling, for an average of approximately 7298 per year. The injury rate for this 14-year period was 0.98 per 100,000 participants. College skiing had approximately 505 female participants each year, and one fatality in 1989-1990 produced a 14-year injury rate of 14.13 per 100,000 participants. This was the only skiing direct fatality since the study was initiated.

Injury rates for college indirect fatalities were high when compared with the high school rates. Basketball had an injury rate of 5.98 fatalities per 100,000 male participants, skiing had a rate of 9.49, ice hockey had a rate of 1.83, and swimming had a rate of 2.74 (Table 29-9). The female indirect injury rate for basketball was 0.64 per 100,000 participants.

Spring Sports

High school spring sports were not associated with any direct catastrophic injuries in 1996.

There was one indirect fatality in high school spring sports during the 1995-1996 school year; it was associated with lacrosse. The cause of death is unknown at this time.

College spring sports were not associated with any direct or indirect catastrophic injuries in 1996.

From 1983 through 1996, high school spring sports were associated with 58 direct catastrophic injuries. Seventeen were listed as fatalities, 20 as catastrophic nonfatal injuries, and 21 as serious injuries. Baseball accounted for 23, track for 32, lacrosse for one, and softball

TABLE 29-7. *High school winter sports: indirect catastrophic injuries per 100,000 participants, 1982-1983 through 1995-1996*

Sport	Fatalities	Nonfatal injuries	Serious injuries
Male			
Basketball	0.61	0.00	0.00
Gymnastics	0.00	0.00	0.00
Ice hockey	0.62	0.00	0.00
Swimming	0.00	0.00	0.00
Wrestling	0.39	0.00	0.00
Female			
Basketball	0.12	0.00	0.02
Gymnastics	0.00	0.00	0.00
Ice hockey	0.00	0.00	0.00
Swimming	0.32	0.00	0.08
Volleyball	0.14	0.00	0.00
Wrestling	0.00	0.00	0.00

TABLE 29-9. College winter sports: indirect catastrophic injuries per 100,000 participants, 1982–1983 through 1995–1996

Sport	Fatalities	Nonfatal injuries	Serious injuries
Male			
Basketball	5.98	0.00	0.00
Gymnastics	0.00	0.00	0.00
Ice hockey	1.83	1.83	0.00
Swimming	2.74	0.00	0.00
Wrestling	0.00	0.00	0.00
Skiing	9.49	0.00	0.00
Female			
Basketball	0.64	0.00	0.00
Gymnastics	0.00	0.00	0.00
Ice hockey	0.00	0.00	0.00
Swimming	0.00	0.00	0.00
Wrestling	0.00	0.00	0.00
Skiing	0.00	0.00	0.00

for two. Injury rates were less than 1 per 100,000 participants for each sport. There were two direct injuries to females in track and two in softball. There were also 26 indirect fatalities in high school spring sports during this time span. Seventeen were related to track, six to baseball, two to lacrosse, and one to tennis. Three of the indirect fatalities involved female track athletes.

College spring sports were associated with 14 direct catastrophic injuries from 1983 to 1996. Four of these injuries resulted in fatalities, four were listed as nonfatal injuries, and six were listed as serious injuries. Baseball accounted for three injuries, lacrosse for four, and track for seven. There were also six indirect fatalities in college spring sports during this time. Two indirect fatalities were associated with tennis, one with track, two with baseball, and one with lacrosse.

Injury rates for high school spring sports direct injuries were low, as is shown in Table 29–10. Baseball partic-

TABLE 29-10. High school spring sports: direct catastrophic injuries per 100,000 participants, 1982–1983 through 1995–1996

Sport	Fatalities	Nonfatal injuries	Serious injuries
Male			
Baseball	0.07	0.15	0.17
Lacrosse	0.38	0.00	0.00
Track	0.17	0.14	0.15
Tennis	0.00	0.00	0.00
Female			
Baseball	0.00	0.00	0.00
Softball	0.00	0.05	0.00
Lacrosse	0.00	0.00	0.00
Track	0.02	0.00	0.02
Tennis	0.00	0.00	0.00

TABLE 29-11. High school spring sports: indirect catastrophic injuries per 100,000 participants, 1982–1983 through 1995–1996

Sport	Fatalities	Nonfatal injuries	Serious injuries
Male			
Baseball	0.10	0.00	0.00
Lacrosse	0.76	0.00	0.00
Track	0.21	0.00	0.00
Tennis	0.05	0.00	0.00
Female			
Baseball	0.00	0.00	0.00
Softball	0.00	0.00	0.00
Lacrosse	0.00	0.00	0.00
Track	0.06	0.00	0.00
Tennis	0.00	0.00	0.00

ipation was approximately 416,000 players each year, track participation was 838,000, and tennis participation was 261,000. The baseball figures do not include the 261,000 softball participants each year. Lacrosse had approximately 28,000 participants each year. Injury rates for high school indirect injuries were also low, as is shown in Table 29–11.

College spring sports had low injury rates for direct injuries (Table 29–12). Men's lacrosse had two nonfatal injuries and two serious injuries, and the injury rates were slightly higher than those of the other sports. Participation figures reveal that approximately 4900 men and 3000 women played lacrosse each year. The 1991 injury was to a female lacrosse player.

Rates for indirect college fatalities in baseball and track were low, lacrosse and tennis having slightly higher rates (Table 29–13). There were two indirect tennis fatalities, one male and one female, but participation figures were low. Men averaged approximately 7700 participants, and women averaged 7300 participants each year.

TABLE 29-12. College spring sports: direct catastrophic injuries per 100,000 participants, 1982–1983 through 1995–1996

Sport	Fatalities	Nonfatal injuries	Serious injuries
Male			
Baseball	0.68	0.00	0.34
Lacrosse	0.00	1.45	2.91
Track	0.43	0.43	0.64
Tennis	0.00	0.00	0.00
Female			
Softball	0.00	0.00	0.00
Lacrosse	0.00	2.34	0.00
Track	0.00	0.00	0.00
Tennis	0.00	0.00	0.00

TABLE 29-13. *College spring sports: indirect catastrophic injuries per 100,000 participants, 1982–1983 through 1995–1996*

Sport	Fatalities	Nonfatal injuries	Serious injuries
Male			
Baseball	0.68	0.00	0.00
Lacrosse	1.45	0.00	0.00
Track	0.21	0.00	0.00
Tennis	0.92	0.00	0.00
Female			
Softball	0.00	0.00	0.00
Lacrosse	0.00	0.00	0.00
Track	0.00	0.00	0.00
Tennis	0.97	0.00	0.00

DISCUSSION

Football was associated with the greatest number of catastrophic injuries for all sports, but the incidence of injury per 100,000 participants was higher in both gymnastics and ice hockey. There have been dramatic reductions in the number of football fatalities and nonfatal catastrophic injuries since 1976, and the 1990 data illustrated an historic decrease in football fatalities to zero. This is a great accomplishment when compared to the 36 fatalities in 1968. This dramatic reduction can be directly related to data collected by the American Football Coaches Association Committee on Football Injuries (1931–1996) and the recommendations that were based on those data. Nonfatal football injuries involving permanent disability decreased to one for college football in 1995. There was a dramatic reduction in high school football from 13 in 1990 to four in 1991. There was an increase to seven in 1992 and 13 in 1993 but a reduction to five in 1994. The 1995 data show a slight increase to eight. Permanent disability injuries in football have shown dramatic reductions when compared with the data from the late 1960s and early 1970s, but a continued effort must be made to eliminate these injuries. In addition, there were 13 serious injuries in football in 1995: 10 in high school and three in college. All of the serious cases involved head or neck injuries; in a number of these cases excellent medical care saved the athlete from permanent disability or death.

Football catastrophic injuries may never be totally eliminated, but progress has been made. Emphasis should again be focused on the preventive measures that received credit for the initial reduction of injuries:

1. The 1976 rule change that prohibited initial contact with the head in blocking and tackling. There must be continued emphasis in this area by coaches and officials.
2. The National Operating Committee for Standards in Athletic Equipment (NOCSAE) football helmet standard that went into effect at the college level in 1978 and at the high school level in 1980. There should be continued research in helmet safety.
3. Improved medical care of the injured athlete with an emphasis on placing athletic trainers in all high schools and colleges. There should be a written emergency plan for catastrophic injuries at both the high school and college levels.
4. Improved coaching technique when teaching the fundamental skills of blocking and tackling, including *keeping the head out of football!*

It should be noted that since 1979, according to the Consumer Product Safety Commission, there have been 18 deaths and 14 serious injuries to children when movable soccer goals have fallen on them. The most recent case involved a 15-year-old high school male in September 1995. A soccer goal frame fell on his head while he was doing chin-ups on the crossbar of an unanchored goal. He was in a coma but has since recovered. According to the Consumer Product Safety Commission, climbing and hanging on the goals, as well as high winds, can cause the goals to tip. The Commission suggests that goals be anchored and that participants be warned not to climb on the goals. There has been one related fatality in this study, which involved a college athlete hanging on a soccer goal and the goal falling and striking the victim's head. A Loss Control Bulletin from K & K Insurance Group, Inc., Fort Wayne, IN, suggests the following safeguards:

1. Keep soccer goals supervised and anchored.
2. Never permit hanging or climbing on a soccer goal.
3. Always stand to the rear or side of the goal when moving it, *never* to the front.
4. Stabilize the goal as best suits the playing surface but in a manner that does not create other hazards to players.
5. Develop and follow a plan for periodic inspection and maintenance (e.g., dry rot, joints, hooks).
6. Advise all field maintenance persons to reanchor the goal if it is moved for mowing the grass or other purposes.
7. Remove goals from fields that are no longer in use for the soccer program as the season progresses.
8. Secure goals well from unauthorized access when stored.
9. Educate and remind all players and adult supervisors about the past tragedies of soccer goal fatalities.

A list of guidelines is available for movable soccer goal safety and warning labels. To obtain a copy, contact the following:

The Coalition to Promote Soccer Goal Safety
C/O Soccer Industry Council of America
200 Castlewood Drive
North Palm Beach, FL 33408

High school wrestling, gymnastics, ice hockey, baseball, and track should receive close attention. Wrestling was associated with 32 direct catastrophic injuries during the 14 years of the survey, but the injury rate per 100,000 participants was lower than the rates in both gymnastics and ice hockey. Because college wrestling was associated with only one catastrophic injury during this same time period, continued research should be focused on the high school level. High school wrestling coaches should be experienced in the teaching of the proper skills of wrestling and should attend coaching clinics to keep up to date on new teaching techniques and safety measures. They should also have experience and training in the proper conditioning of their athletes. These measures are important in all sports, but there are a number of contact sports, such as wrestling, in which the experience and training of the coach are of the utmost importance. Full-speed wrestling in physical education classes is a questionable practice unless there is proper time for conditioning and the teaching of skills. The physical education teacher should also have expertise in the teaching of wrestling skills.

Men's and women's gymnastics were associated with high injury rates at both the high school and college levels. Gymnastics needs additional study at both levels of competition. Both levels have seen a dramatic participation reduction, and this trend may continue, the major emphasis being in private clubs.

Ice hockey injuries were low in numbers, but the injury rate per 100,000 participants was high when compared to rates for other sports. Ice hockey catastrophic injuries usually occur when an athlete is struck from behind by an opponent and makes contact with the crown of his or her head and the boards surrounding the rink. The results are usually fractured cervical vertebrae with paralysis. Research in Canada has revealed high catastrophic injury rates with similar results. After an in-depth study of ice hockey catastrophic injuries in Canada from 1976 to 1983 (1), Dr. Charles Tator made the following recommendations concerning prevention:

1. Enforce current rules and consider new rules against pushing or checking from behind.
2. Improve the strength of neck muscles.
3. Educate players about risk of neck injuries.
4. Continue epidemiologic research.

Catastrophic injuries in swimming were all directly related to the racing dive in the shallow ends of pools. There has been a major effort by both schools and colleges to make the racing dive safer, and the catastrophic injury data support that effort. There has not been a high school swimming direct catastrophic injury in the last 6 years or a college injury for the past 13 years. The competitive racing start has changed and now involves the swimmer getting more depth when entering the water. Practicing or starting competition in the deep end of the pool could eliminate catastrophic injuries caused by the swimmer striking his or her head on the bottom of the pool. The National Federation of State High School Associations Swimming and Diving Rules Committee voted that in pools with a water depth less than 3.5 feet at the starting end, swimmers have to start the race in the water. This rule change is a refinement of a 1991–1992 rule change and took effect in the 1992–1993 season. The new rules read that in 4 feet or more of water, swimmers may use a starting platform up to a maximum of 30 inches above the water. Between 3.5 feet and 4 feet, swimmers may start no higher than 18 inches above the water. In April 1995 the National Federation revised rule 2-7-2, which now states that starting platforms shall be securely attached to the deck or wall. If they are not, they shall not be used, and deck or in-water starts will be required. These new rules point out the importance of constant data collection and analysis. Rules and equipment changes for safety reasons must be based on reliable injury data.

High school spring sports were associated with low incidence rates during the 14 years of the survey, but baseball was associated with 23 direct catastrophic injuries, and track was associated with 32. A majority of the baseball injuries were caused by the head-first slide or by being struck with a thrown or batted ball. If the head-first slide is going to be used, proper instruction should be involved. Proper protection for batting practice should be provided for the batting practice pitcher, and he or she should always wear a helmet, as should the batting practice coach. There are always a number of nonschool baseball injuries, and the cause of injury is usually the same. In 1994 information was received about a recreational player who had fractured his neck and died after sliding head first. Another case involved a college fraternity player sliding head first into home plate and fracturing a cervical vertebra, resulting in paralysis.

The pole vault was associated with a majority of the fatal track injuries. There were 10 high school fatal pole vaulting injuries from 1983 to 1996. In addition to the fatalities there were six permanent disability injuries and five serious injuries. All 21 of these accidents involved the vaulter bouncing out of or landing out of the pit area. The three pole vaulting deaths in 1983 were a major concern, and the National Federation of State High School Associations took immediate measures. Beginning with the 1987 season all individual units in the pole vault landing area had to include a common cover or pad extending over all sections of the pit.

These additional recommendations are in the 1991 rule book: Stabilize the pole vault standards so that athletes cannot fall into the pit, pad the standards, remove all hazards from around the pit area, and control traffic along the approach. Obvious hazards such as concrete or other hard materials around the pit should be eliminated.

There were also eight accidents in high school track involving participants being struck by a thrown discus, shot put, or javelin. In 1992 a female athlete was struck by a thrown discus in practice and died. In 1993 a track manager was struck in the neck by a javelin but recovered completely from the accident. In 1994 a female track athlete was struck in the face by a javelin and recovered. In 1995 a male athlete was struck in the head by a shot put during warm-ups and had a fractured skull. There was also a spectator struck in the head by a discus during a high school meet. Safety precautions must be stressed for these events in both practice and competitive meets to eliminate this type of accident. The National Federation of State High School Associations put a new rule in for the 1993 track season that the back and sides of the discus circle must be fenced off to help eliminate this type of accident. These types of injuries are not acceptable and should never happen.

The one fatality in high school lacrosse during the 1987 season was associated with a player using his head to strike the opponent. He struck the opponent with the top or crown of his helmet. This technique is prohibited by the lacrosse rules and should be strictly enforced. Lacrosse has been a safe sport, considering that high school lacrosse was involved with only one catastrophic injury in 14 years.

College spring sports were also associated with a low injury incidence. Injury rates were slightly higher in lacrosse, but the participation figures were so low that even one injury would increase the incidence rate dramatically. It is important to point out that there were only two college lacrosse catastrophic injuries during the survey years, and one injury was the first in women's lacrosse.

For the 14-year period from the fall of 1982 through the spring of 1996 there were 608 direct catastrophic injuries in high school and college sports. High school sports were associated with 82 fatalities, 196 nonfatal injuries, and 212 serious injuries for a total of 490. College sports accounted for 10 fatalities, 33 nonfatal injuries, and 75 serious injuries for a total of 118. During this same 14-year period there were a total of 256 indirect injuries, and all but three resulted in death. Of the indirect injuries, 205 were at the high school level, and 51 were at the college level. It should be noted that high school annual athletic participation for 1995–1996 included approximately 6,001,988 athletes (3,634,052 males and 2,367,936 females). National Collegiate Athletic Association participation for 1995–1996 included 323,388 athletes (199,556 males and 123,832 females).

During the 14-year period from the fall of 1982 through the spring of 1996, 74,424,143 high school athletes participated in the sports covered by this report. Using these participation numbers would give a high school direct catastrophic injury rate of 0.66 per 100,000 participants. The indirect injury rate is 0.27 per 100,000 participants. If both direct and indirect injuries were combined, the injury rate would be 0.93 per 100,000. This means that approximately one high school athlete out of every 100,000 participating would receive some type of catastrophic injury. The combined fatality rate would be 0.38 per 100,000, the nonfatal rate would be 0.26, and the serious rate would be 0.29.

During this same time period there were a total of 3,995,522 college participants with a total direct catastrophic injury rate of 2.95 per 100,000 participants. The indirect injury rate was 1.28 per 100,000 participants. If both indirect and direct injuries were combined, the injury rate would be 4.23. The combined fatality rate would be 1.50, the nonfatal rate would be 0.85, and the serious rate would be 1.88.

FEMALE CATASTROPHIC INJURIES

There were a total of 49 direct and 21 indirect catastrophic injuries to high school and college female athletes from 1982–1983 through 1995–1996, including cheerleading injuries. Thirty-three of these were direct injuries at the high school level, and 16 were at the college level. The 33 high school direct injuries included nine in gymnastics, 16 in cheerleading, two in swimming, one in basketball, two in track, two in softball, and one in volleyball. The 19 high school indirect fatalities included seven in basketball, five in swimming, three in track, one in soccer, one in cross-country, one in volleyball, and one in cheerleading. The 16 college direct injuries were associated with cheerleading (11), gymnastics (2), field hockey (1), skiing (1), and lacrosse (1). The two college indirect fatalities included one in tennis and one in basketball. Catastrophic injuries to female athletes have increased over the years. As an example, in 1982–1983 there was one female catastrophic injury, and during the past 13 years there has been an average of 5.4 per year. A major factor in this increase has been the change in cheerleading activity, which now involves gymnastic-type stunts. If these cheerleading activities keep increasing in difficulty and are not taught by a competent coach, catastrophic injuries are going to be a part of cheerleading. High school cheerleading accounted for 48% of all high school direct catastrophic injuries to female athletes and 68% at the college level. Of the 49 direct catastrophic injuries to female athletes from 1982–1983 through 1995–1996, cheerleading was related to 27, or 55%.

Athletic catastrophic injuries may never be totally eliminated, but with reliable injury data collection systems and constant analysis of the data, these injuries can be dramatically reduced. Athletic administrators and coaches should place equal emphasis on injury prevention in both female and male athletics. Injury prevention recommendations are made for both male and female athletes.

RECOMMENDATIONS FOR PREVENTION

1. Medical examinations should be mandatory, and a medical history should be taken before an athlete is allowed to participate.
2. All personnel concerned with training athletes should emphasize proper, gradual, and complete physical conditioning to provide the athlete with optimal readiness for the rigors of the sport.
3. Every school should strive to have a team trainer who is a regular member of the faculty and is adequately prepared and qualified. There should be a written emergency procedure plan to deal with the possibility of catastrophic injuries.
4. There should be an emphasis on employing well-trained athletic personnel, providing excellent facilities, and securing the safest and best equipment available.
5. There should be strict enforcement of game rules, and administrative regulations should be enforced to protect the health of the athlete. Coaches and school officials must support the game officials in their conduct of the athletic contests.
6. Coaches should know and have the ability to teach the proper fundamental skills of the sport. This recommendation includes all sports, not only football. The proper fundamentals of blocking and tackling should be emphasized to help reduce head and neck injuries in football. *Keep the head out of football.*
7. There should be continued safety research in athletics (rules, facilities, and equipment).
8. Strict enforcement of the rules of the game by both coaches and game officials will help to reduce serious injuries.
9. When an athlete has experienced or shown signs of head trauma (loss of consciousness, visual disturbance, headache, inability to walk correctly, obvious disorientation, memory loss), he or she should receive immediate medical attention and should not be allowed to return to practice or game without permission from the proper medical authorities. It is important for a physician to observe the head-injured athlete for several days following the injury.
10. Athletes and their parents should be warned of the risks of injuries.
11. Coaches should not be hired if they do not have the training and experience needed to teach the skills of the sport and to properly train and develop the athletes for competition.

ACKNOWLEDGMENT

Research funded by a grant from the National Collegiate Athletic Association.

REFERENCE

1. Tator CH, Edmonds VE. National survey of spinal injuries in hockey players. *CMAJ* 1984;130:875–880.

CHAPTER 30

Head Injuries

Margot Putukian

Head injuries occur commonly in sports participation and can have significant short- and long-term consequences. It is essential that health care providers be aware of the importance of detecting these injuries early on, treating them properly, and avoiding return to activity before the resolution of symptoms such that dangerous sequelae are prevented. The goal of this chapter will be to discuss the spectrum of head injuries that occur commonly in sport, as well as the evaluation and treatment of these injuries. Finally, a discussion of some of the new methods for evaluating and making decisions about return to play will be presented. The ultimate goal is that with an understanding of the complexity of head injuries as they occur in sport, as well as the importance of careful and close follow-up of these injuries, health care providers will be able to take care of head-injured athletes and avoid sequelae.

INTRODUCTION

The spectrum of head injuries is broad, yet in the realm of the athletic field, these injuries generally tend to be mild. Despite this, it is important to remember that severe injuries can occur in sport and that these as well as repetitive injuries can have long-standing and serious complications. Rapidly increasing vascular injuries can occur, often associated with skull fractures, and must be recognized early. Many head injuries occur in association with cervical spine injuries, which can be serious if not looked for and treated appropriately. In addition, the second impact syndrome (1), in which an athlete sustains a second head injury before completely recovering from a first one, can result in brain edema and death. Finally, postconcussive symptoms can occur that have a significant impact on an individual's activities outside of sport as well as long-term morbidity.

There has been some concern that an athlete who sustains repetitive head injuries may be at risk for long-term sequelae. This is most apparent in the sport of boxing, in which the main goal is to render the opponent unconscious by striking blows to the head. The cumulative injury to the brain that occurs because of the repetitive blows sustained has been referred to as the punch-drunk syndrome or posttraumatic encephalopathy, and many believe that this may increase an individual's risk for the developing dementia or Alzheimer's disease (2,3,4). There has also been concern that soccer may impose a similar risk from the repetitive heading of the ball that is part of the sport. The data for cumulative damage in the sport of soccer remain sparse and controversial.

The significance and natural history of head injuries are still unclear, and many head injuries continue to go undetected. Many younger athletes may not have access to a medical support staff that is trained to detect and treat these injuries. In many sports, head injuries are taken lightly, such that it is normal for a coach to say, "He was in a fog out there for most of the game, but that's football." A study of rugby players in Great Britain found that of 544 athletes, 56% had sustained at least one injury associated with amnesia after the event. In 58 players their posttraumatic amnesia lasted more than an hour, and only 38 of these athletes were admitted to the hospital for treatment (5). It is an intention of this chapter to impart a better understanding of the information that is known about head injuries and the importance of treating them with respect and concern.

INJURY EPIDEMIOLOGY

The exact incidence of head injuries is unknown, especially for the younger athlete, because many go unre-

---

M. Putukian: Primary Care Sports Medicine, Penn State University, and Department of Orthopedics and Rehabilitation, Hershey Medical Center, University Park, Pennsylvania 16803.

ported. Many athletes will sustain an injury and not mention it to anyone either because their symptoms resolve or because they believe that it is part of the game. In addition, many are fearful that if they admit injury, they will be taken out of play. Many athletes are evaluated but not sent to an emergency room, and therefore data from insurance agencies is likely to be an underestimation of the true incidence of injury, especially mild injury.

From the National Head Injury Foundation the causes of minor head injury include motor vehicle accidents (46%), falls (23%), sports (18%), and assaults (10%). In the United States in 1984, traumatic brain injuries accounted for approximately 500,000 hospital admissions or deaths, 3–10% of these having been caused by sports or recreational activity (6). Head injury accounts for 19% of all nonfatal injuries in football (7) and 4.5% of all high school sports injuries (8). It has been estimated that at the high school level, there is a risk of 15–20% for sustaining a minor head injury in one season, with 200,000 of these injuries occurring each year (9,10). An average of eight deaths per year occur as a result of head injury in football (11). For children at the elementary, junior, and high school level, football accounts for the highest incidence of injuries per player of any sport (12), and the incidence of concussion in young football players ranges from 4% to 5% (13). In a recent study, mild traumatic brain injury (MTBI) accounted for 5.5% of all injuries at the high school level, with football accounting for 63% of these injuries (14). The injury rates per 100 players for specific sports were 3.66 for football, 1.58 for wrestling, 1.14 for girls soccer, 1.04 for girls basketball, 0.92 for boys soccer, 0.75 for boys basketball, 0.46 for softball and field hockey, 0.23 for baseball, and 0.14 for volleyball.

National Collegiate Athletic Association (NCAA) data from 1984 to 1991 demonstrate that head concussions account for 1.8–4.5% of all injuries, with an injury rate of 0.11–0.27 injuries per 1000 athlete exposures. The NCAA data from 1995–1996 reveal higher numbers, with concussions accounting for 1.6–6.4% of all injuries and an injury rate of 0.06–0.55 injuries per 1000 athlete exposures.

The NCAA Injury Surveillance System (ISS) was developed in 1982 and has been instrumental in guiding the Committee on Competitive Safeguards and Medical Aspects of Sports within the NCAA. The data are reviewed and have resulted in implementations of new rules such that injuries can be prevented and/or decreased if possible. The definition of injury that the NCAA uses is one of time lost from play, and importantly, the data include an injury rate that is defined as the number of injuries per athlete exposure. The data for head injuries and concussion for 1995–1996 as well as some of the data from 1984–1991 are shown in Tables 30–1 and 30–2.

From the 1984–1991 data, ice hockey had the highest percentage of head injuries of the sports that were moni-

TABLE 30-1. NCAA injury surveillance system: head injury and concussion rate and severity in various sports: 1995–1996

Sport	Head injury Rate[a]	Head injury % Total injuries	Concussion rate Rate	Concussion rate % Total injuries	Concussion severity: Grade[b] I	II	III
Sports with no head protection							
Men's soccer	0.49	6.1	0.37	4.7	88.0	12.0	0.0
Women's soccer	0.48	6.9	0.41	5.8	95.0	5.0	0.0
Women's volleyball	0.08	1.8	0.06	1.6	100.0	0.0	0.0
Field hockey	0.53	8.0	0.28	4.1	100.0	0.0	0.0
Men's basketball	0.39	5.7	0.30	4.4	76.1	19.6	0.4
Women's basketball	0.23	3.4	0.20	3.0	100.0	0.0	0.0
Wrestling	0.55	5.6	0.30	3.1	76.0	24.0	0.0
Men's gymnastics	0.18	4.2	0.09	2.1	0.0	100.0	0.0
Women's gymnastics	0.30	2.0	0.34	3.5	85.7	14.3	0.0
Women's lacrosse	0.18	4.4	0.10	2.4	100.0	0.0	0.0
Sports with head protection							
Fall football	0.39	6.0	0.38	5.9	84.9	14.8	0.3
Ice hockey	0.45	6.9	0.42	6.4	87.8	12.2	0.0
Spring football	0.55	5.1	0.55	5.1	90.7	7.0	2.3
Men's lacrosse	0.19	3.5	0.17	3.2	84.6	15.4	0.0
Baseball	0.11	3.4	0.08	2.4	72.2	27.8	0.0
Softball	0.15	3.6	0.13	3.1	83.3	16.7	0.0

[a] Rate = number of injuries per 1000 athlete exposures.
[b] Grade I = no loss of consciousness (LOC), posttraumatic amnesia <1–2 min.
Grade II = LOC for <5 minutes, posttraumatic amnesia for up to 30 seconds.
Grade III = LOC for >5 minutes, extended amnesia.

TABLE 30–2. *NCAA head injury, concussion, and neck injury rate 1984–1991*

Sport	Head		Concussion[c]		Neck	
	IR[a]	%[b]	IR	%	IR	%
Sports with no head protection						
Field hockey	0.23	4.5	0.20	3.8	0.05	1.0
Women's lacrosse	0.17	4.1	0.16	3.9	0.03	0.7
Men's soccer	0.31	4.0	0.25	3.2	0.03	0.4
Women's soccer	0.29	3.7	0.24	2.8	0.08	1.0
Women's basketball	0.16	3.1	0.15	3.0	0.05	0.9
Men's basketball	0.14	2.5	0.12	2.1	0.04	0.8
Wrestling	0.28	2.9	0.20	1.8	0.51	5.4
Sports with head protection						
Ice hockey	0.30	5.4	0.25	4.5	0.09	1.7
Football	0.29	4.5	0.27	4.1	0.28	4.2
Men's lacrosse	0.22	3.2	0.19	3.0	0.12	1.7
Women's softball	0.11	2.9	0.11	2.9	0.06	1.6
Baseball	0.09	2.8	0.07	2.1	0.01	0.3

[a] Injuries expressed as IR = injuries per 1000 athlete exposures.
[b] Injuries expressed as % = percentage of all reported injuries.
[c] Concussions are a subset of all head injuries.

tored, followed by football and field hockey, women's lacrosse, and men's soccer. Injury rates in sports with no head protection such as men's soccer, women's soccer, and field hockey were comparable to rates in the helmeted sports of ice hockey, football, and men's lacrosse, respectively. In looking at concussion rates, the data reveal that football has the highest concussion rate, with ice hockey, men's and women's soccer, field hockey, and men's lacrosse falling slightly lower. These results are interesting in that the rates are similar despite a perceived difference in how much contact is involved in these sports; football and ice hockey have the reputation of involving much more contact than soccer, field hockey, and lacrosse.

Player contact was the primary injury mechanism for all but four of the sports in the 1984–1991 data given. For field hockey, contact with the stick was the primary mechanism of injury, whereas in women's lacrosse, softball, and baseball, contact with the ball created the most injuries. These data are useful in determining which sports pose a risk for head injury, as well as the extent to which head injuries are seen in particular sports. For example, head injuries occur commonly in football yet account for only between 4.5% and 6% of the injuries that occur in that sport.

When we look at the 1995–1996 data, the concussion rates are different in that spring football has the highest concussion injury rate, followed closely by ice hockey, women's soccer, fall football, and men's soccer. (The NCAA has only recently included spring football as a separate entity.) There is then a drop-off to other sports such as men's basketball, women's gymnastics, wrestling, and field hockey, and the remainder of the sports have even lower concussion rates. There has been much controversy over the high incidence of injury in spring football, and additional caution must be taken in comparing one year of data to data that span more than 7 years. At the same time the increase in concussions that is seen in spring football remains a concern. The increase in concussions in other sports has also raised some concern.

The 1995–1996 data are useful in and of themselves, as well as in comparison to the earlier data. Given that the injury surveillance system instituted by the NCAA is the same, the difference in head injury data between and within sports is very useful. They show that for many sports, head injuries and concussion injuries are on the increase. They also reiterate the point that though certain sports use head protection, this does not necessarily decrease the incidence of concussion and head injuries that occur. The increase in head injuries demonstrated within a sport may be due to a heightened awareness of these injuries and therefore an increased ability to detect these injuries when they have occurred. It may also be the result of an increase in supervision and medical care given to all athletes, such that mild injuries that were once ignored are picked up by an attentive athletic training and medical staff. This may be especially true for head concussions, for which symptomatology is often minimal.

The NCAA ISS injury data presented are also unique in that they represent university-level athletes participating in intercollegiate athletics. This feature in and of itself is a selection bias and might not represent the true incidence of injury at different levels of competition or age groups. As will be discussed later, how injuries are graded and when athletes are returned to play may differ depending on the athlete, the athletic trainers and physicians with whom they are in contact, and the level of competitive play. It may be that a collegiate athlete is taken care of differently than a high school or professional athlete. It is certainly true that the number of athletes who have direct interaction with a trainer or physician differs at different levels and may also differ depending on the gender of the athlete. This differential access to medical personnel may mean that minor injuries might not reach medical attention as easily and could go unnoticed.

The increase in head injuries and concussions seen in the NCAA data may also be due to an increased aggressiveness seen in various sports and an increase in the amount of contact seen in various sports. For example, basketball, which was characterized in the past as a noncontact/noncollision sport, appears to be much more aggressive, such that it is now a contact sport. The NCAA ISS data are very useful in looking at trends in injury data over time within and between sports and may help to answer some of these questions.

It is important in looking at injury data that one takes into account the biases that occur naturally as part of the group being studied. It is also important to use the information provided by injury data to make recommendations to improve the safety for that sport. For example, many have proposed that head injuries could be decreased in sports such as women's lacrosse and field hockey if these athletes were to wear helmets. If one looks at the injury data for these sports, however, head concussions are fairly uncommon. It may be useful to use helmets with shields to prevent facial lacerations, nasal fractures, and other facial and dental injuries, but given that the concussion rate is low already, will helmets make a significant difference in concussion rates? And will the addition of helmets create any new problems, such as an increase in aggressiveness and feelings of invulnerability in these athletes, that will actually increase in the incidence of head and neck injuries? It is essential that the existing data be used effectively to create rule and equipment changes that will truly increase safety and benefit the sport without unduly changing the nature of the sport.

The use of helmets has decreased the frequency of head injury in ice hockey and football (15,16). For football the number of fatal head injuries decreased substantially between 1975 and 1984 when compared to 1965–1974 (17). There has been a 50% decrease since 1976 (18), and this has been credited to rule changes implemented at that time forbidding spearing, along with improvements in helmet design and fit. In ice hockey there has been significant debate over whether helmets have changed the game. One study demonstrated that of 246 head injuries in ice hockey players, 75% were due to violence that was outside of the game, such as high sticking, deliberate pushing, and fistfights (19). From this study, it appears that better control of the game with enforcement of existing rules may be more important than protective equipment.

In baseball and softball the use of helmets is an easy and important means to protect these athletes from balls impacting their heads when they are batting. The use of helmets in this situation will not change the athletes' aggressiveness or the sport in any way other than to provide additional protection. That helmets are effective is well proven (20), and given that most of the head injuries that occur in these sports is due to contact with the ball (21), this intervention is well worth making.

The use of helmets is most clearly associated with a decrease in morbidity and mortality in recreational bicycling. Because of the surface on which bicyclists ride and the environment of the activity, including speed and motor vehicles, this activity poses an especially increased risk. It has been estimated that there is a 50% rate of head injury incurred from a fall from a bicycle and that if a bicyclist is traveling 20 miles per hour, the trauma can be fatal (22). In the United States 1300 deaths occur annually from bicycling accidents, most of these due to head injuries (23). It has also been demonstrated that the risk of brain injury is reduced by 88% with the use of an approved bicycle helmet (23). The use of helmets for all bicyclists is obviously essential in that the data clearly show a decrease in fatal injury with their use and virtually no ill effects.

From the injury data provided by the NCAA it is clear that head injuries and concussions are an important injury in both helmeted and nonhelmeted athletes. Given that these injuries may be associated with other injuries as well as long-term sequelae, it is important that health care professionals taking care of athletes understand the spectrum of head injuries that occur and the way in which these injuries can present in the athletic field or court. It is also important that the health care team have a well-thought-out plan of care for the head-injured athlete.

DEFINITIONS

Head injuries can be divided in practice into two general types: diffuse brain injury and focal brain injury. Focal injuries can be further subdivided into subdural hematoma, epidural hematoma, cerebral contusions, and intracranial hemorrhages, including subarachnoid hemorrhage and intracerebral hemorrhage. These focal injuries are often associated with loss of consciousness (LOC) and focal deficits and occur as a result of blunt trauma. Focal head injuries can occur in various sports and, though they generally are not missed, can sometimes be occult if LOC does not occur. The early detection and treatment of these injuries are essential and can at times be life saving.

FOCAL INJURIES

Subdural hematomas are often associated with loss of consciousness that may or may not occur with a history of slow deterioration in mental status and focal deficits. The accumulation of blood is secondary to a low pressure disruption of venous blood. Subdural hematomas are three times more common than epidural hematomas, described below. Subdural hematomas are further divided into simple or complex, depending on whether they are seen in association with underlying cerebral contusion or edema. Simple subdural hematomas are not associated with these complications and have a mortality rate of roughly 20%. Complex subdural hematomas involve a collection of blood in the subdural space associated with an underlying cerebral contusion or brain edema and swelling. (Figs. 30–1, 30–2). The mortality rate for complex subdural hematomas is greater than 50%.

Subdural hematomas in an older patient may not be associated with significant brain injury because the potential space in older individuals is larger, owing to the age-related atrophy that occurs (24). However, in the young athlete this potential space is much smaller, and the symptoms that occur with subdural blood accumulation are often due to compression of normal brain substance underlying, as opposed to symptoms related to a mass effect (25). Therefore the speed at which this subdural blood is removed may theoretically be more important in the young athlete.

Epidural hematomas are often associated with disruption of the middle or other meningeal arteries. These injuries, because of the high pressure vascular system, are generally associated with a very brisk accumulation of blood. In their classic form, epidural hematomas present with loss of consciousness at the time of injury, followed by recovery and a lucid interval. The patient often then develops a headache and subsequent deterioration of mental status with eventual loss of consciousness, pupillary abnormalities (unilaterally dilated pupil, usually ipsilateral to the clot), and decerebrate posturing with contralateral weakness (26). However, it is important to recognize that only one third of patients will actually present in this classic manner (25). (Fig. 30–3).

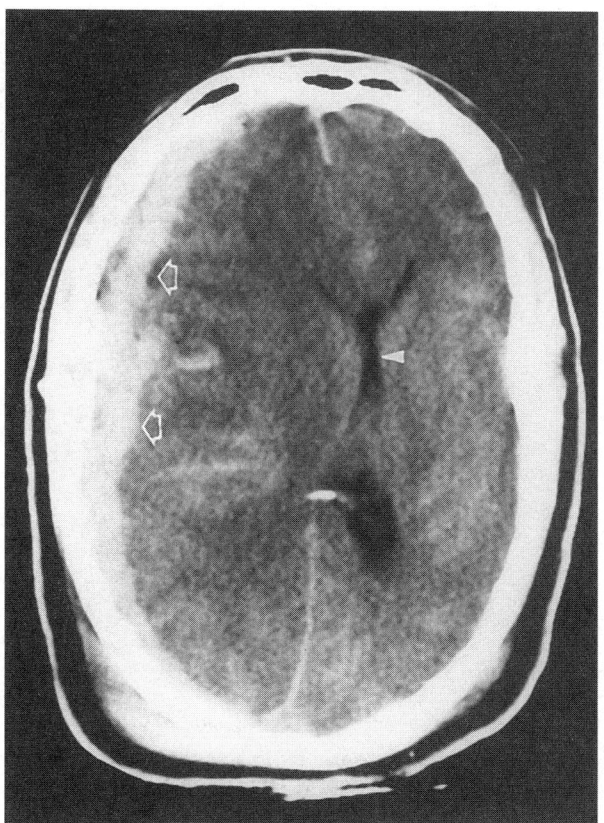

FIG. 30–2. Typical appearance of an acute subdural hematoma (*open arrows*) on an axial CT image. The degree of shift of the midline structures (*arrowhead*) is greater than the thickness of the subdural hematoma, suggesting significant parenchymal injury to the hemisphere in addition to the hematoma. (Reprinted with permission from Fu FH, Stone DA, eds. *Sports injuries: mechanisms, prevention, treatment.* Baltimore: Williams & Wilkins, 1994.)

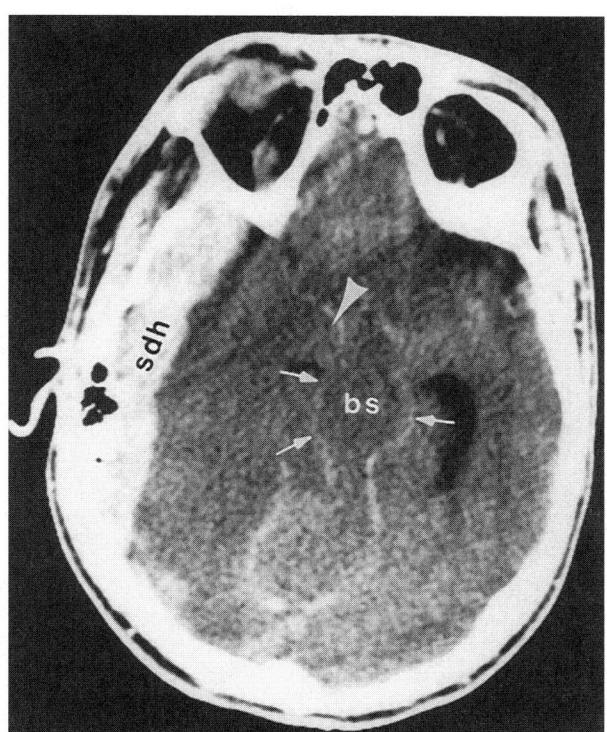

FIG. 30–1. Axial CT image demonstrating an acute subdural hematoma (sdh) on the right side, with herniation of the medial temporal lobe into the tentorial notch (*arrowhead*). The midbrain is outlined by subarachnoid hemorrhage in the perimesencephalic cistern (*arrows*). (Reprinted with permission from Fu FH, Stone DA, eds. *Sports injuries: mechanisms, prevention, treatment.* Baltimore: Williams & Wilkins, 1994.)

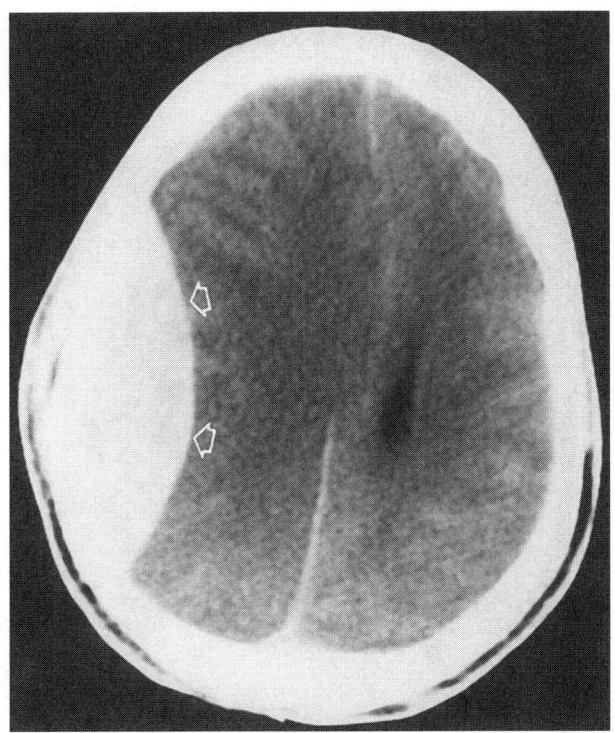

FIG. 30–3. Typical appearance of an epidural hematoma on an axial CT image. (Reprinted with permission from Fu FH, Stone DA, eds. *Sports injuries: mechanisms, prevention, treatment.* Baltimore: Williams & Wilkins, 1994.)

Cerebral contusions and hemorrhage are the other types of focal injury that can occur in athletic head injury. Cerebral contusion, intracerebral hematoma, and hemorrhage often present without loss of consciousness, with headache and periods of confusion and post-traumatic amnesia being the more common presenting complaints. Hemorrhages can be either on the surface of the brain (subarachnoid) or located within the substance of the brain itself (intracerebral). Hydrocephalus and changes related to a mass effect can occur as complications of cerebral contusions or hemorrhages. (Figs. 30–4, 30–5).

Computerized tomography (CT) scanning, magnetic resonance imaging (MRI), and electroencephalography (EEG) may reveal abnormalities with head injury (27–32). In one study of severe closed head injuries in which loss of consciousness was persistent and patients were admitted to an intensive care unit, the degree and duration of brain injury related to the depth of the brain lesion on MRI, lesions being present in 88% of patients (33).

Epidural and subdural hematomas can be diagnosed by both CT scanning or MRI, though CT is often favored initially because it is better in detecting blood as well as bony abnormalities in acute injury. MRI may be more useful in detecting subtle injuries, especially when the study is obtained more than 48 hours after the injury (34–36). Though a MRI study may show greater volume of injury than CT scanning, lesions that require surgical intervention are detected by CT (37). When hematomas are diagnosed, emergent neurosurgical consultation is

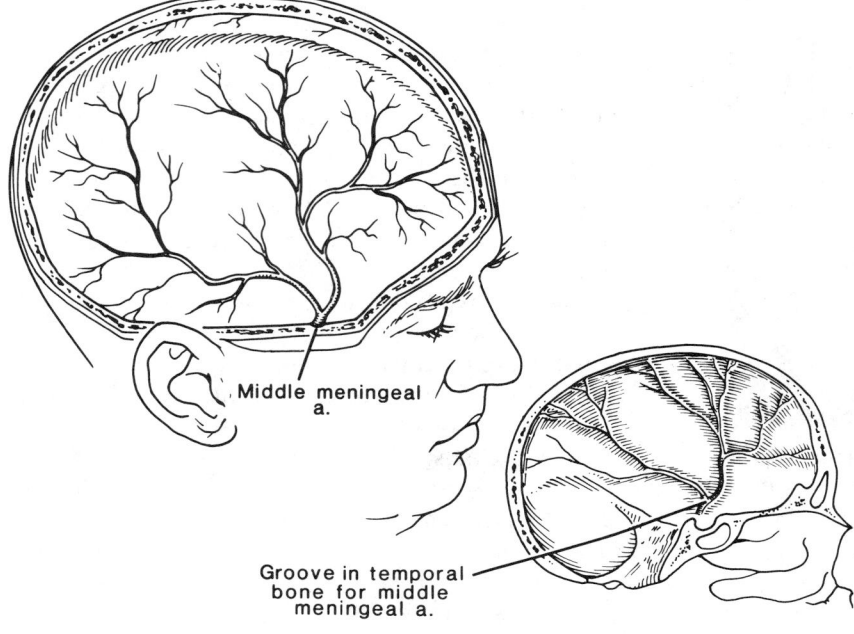

FIG. 30–4. The middle meningeal artery is tethered in a groove in the temporal bone and is easily lacerated by fractures through this bone. Hemorrhage from the middle meningeal artery causes an epidural hematoma. (Reprinted with permission from Fu FH, Stone DA, eds. *Sports injuries: mechanisms, prevention, treatment.* Baltimore: Williams & Wilkins, 1994.)

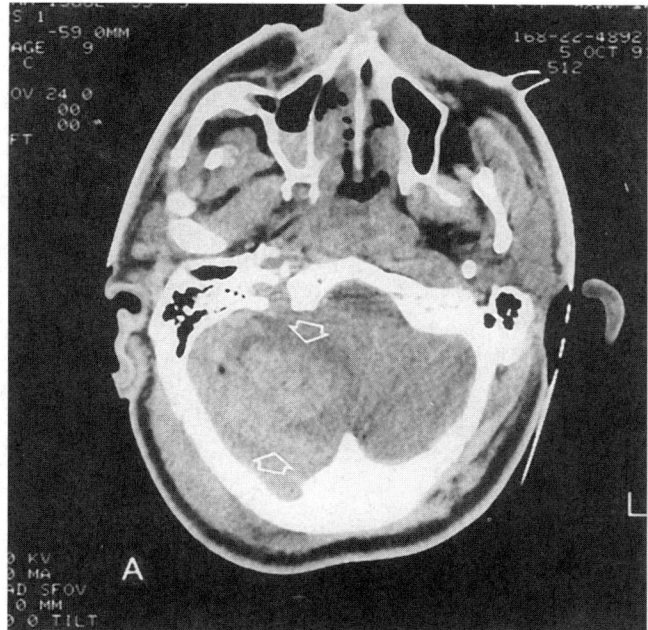 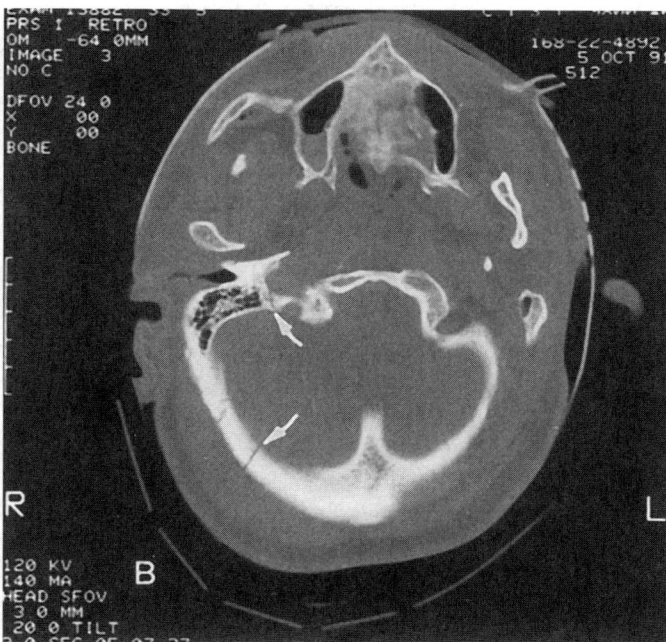

FIG. 30-5. Axial CT images demonstrate a hemorrhagic contusion of the right cerebellar hemisphere (**A**) associated with a fracture through the floor of the posterior fossa on the right side (**B**). (Reprinted with permission from Fu FH, Stone DA, eds. *Sports injuries: mechanisms, prevention, treatment.* Baltimore: Williams & Wilkins, 1994.)

warranted. Surgical intervention may be indicated, and the time between injury and treatment is crucial in terms of recovery of function.

NONFOCAL INJURIES

At the other end of the spectrum of head injuries are diffuse brain injuries, which are those not associated with focal intracranial injuries. Diffuse brain injury also represent a continuum of progressively more severe brain dysfunction depending on the amount of structural or anatomic disruption that occurs. At the least severe are nonstructural brain injuries, which are less severe because anatomic integrity appears to be maintained. Cerebral concussion is generally considered in this category, though as will be discussed below, concussion can be associated with structural abnormalities.

At the most severe are structural diffuse brain injuries, which, as their name indicates, are injuries associated with anatomic disruption. Diffuse axonal injury is generally associated with prolonged brain injury and coma, with loss of consciousness often persisting longer than 6 hours. Diffuse axonal injury is associated with residual neurologic, psychological, and personality deficits because of the axonal disruption that occurs in the white matter of the cerebral hemispheres and the brain stem.

Cerebral concussion was defined in 1966 as "a clinical syndrome characterized by immediate and transient impairment of neurologic function secondary to mechanical forces" (38). Cerebral concussions may or may not be associated with loss of consciousness and/or memory dysfunction. The hallmarks of concussion include confusion and amnesia. Various other symptoms may be present, as listed in Table 30-3, and the severity of injury

TABLE 30-3. *Signs and symptoms of cerebral concussion*

Loss of consciousness (LOC)	Slurred/incoherent speech
Confusion	Excessive drowsiness
Posttraumatic amnesia (PTA)	**Symptoms consistent with postconcussive syndrome**
Retrograde amnesia (RGA)	
Disorientation	Loss of intellectual capacity
Delayed verbal and motor responses	Poor recent memory
	Personality changes
Inability to focus	Headaches
Headache	Dizziness
Nausea/vomiting	Lack of concentration
Visual disturbances (photophobia, blurry vision, double vision)	Poor attention
	Fatigue
	Irritability
Disequilibrium	Phonophobia/photophobia
Feeling "in a fog," "zoned out"	Sleep disturbances
	Depressed mood
Vacant stare	Anxiety
Emotional lability	
Dizziness	

relies on the presence and persistence of these symptoms as well as other measures of cognitive functioning.

The most common head injury in the realm of athletics is head concussion, which, when compared to the spectrum of injuries seen in motor vehicle accidents and other high-velocity injuries, tends to be mild. This implies that on the spectrum presented above, head injuries that occur in sport will tend to be mild, with only a small extent of anatomic disruption. However, one message of this chapter is that *there is no such thing as a minor head injury*. Mild cerebral concussions can occur in association with the focal injuries discussed above and can also be associated with significant morbidity and mortality in and of themselves if they are not detected and treated appropriately. These injuries will be the focus of the remainder of this chapter.

MECHANISMS AND PATHOPHYSIOLOGY

Several mechanisms can occur in head injuries that may be useful in predicting outcome (39–41). Understanding these mechanisms and the pathophysiology that occurs as a result of head trauma in sport may also help to guide further interventions that may decrease injury or prevent them. The research behind the mechanisms and pathophysiology is well established, though new research is expanding this knowledge dramatically.

Diffuse brain injuries are associated with anatomic disruption, and these have been well demonstrated in research models. These changes can include axonal and myelin sheath disruption throughout the white matter of the hemispheres and brainstem, petechial hemorrhages in periventricular regions, and chromatolysis and cell loss throughout the cortical gray matter and brain stem nuclei (42–45). With repetitive injury these changes can evolve into gross atrophy (46). In the athletic setting, the acceleration and impact forces tend to be equal and can be thought of similarly (47). It appears that rotational forces and subsequent shearing stress account for more severe structural injuries (41,47,48). The neuropathology of head injuries has been recently reviewed (24) with much research ongoing.

There are basically three different mechanisms that occur in athletic head injuries: A stationary head is struck with a forceful blow (impact or compressive force), a moving head strikes a nonmoving object (acceleration or tensile force), or the head is struck parallel to its surface (shearing or rotational force). Impact forces, such as occur when a football lineman is struck in the head, are often considered coup injuries, the maximal area injury being the area of the brain lying underneath the area struck. Acceleration injuries, such as occur when a basketball player dives to the ground and strikes his or her head, are often considered contracoup injuries because the area of the brain opposite the area struck is injured. Shearing injuries can occur whenever there is a rotational force applied to the head, such as when a boxer is struck by a left hook. These mechanisms can occur together and can be useful in predicting injury severity. A combined mechanism can also occur, in which rotation and acceleration occur together; these injuries may have more severe consequences (49).

If one considers that the brain tissue itself is floating in a protective container (the skull) with fluid (cerebrospinal fluid (CSF)) surrounding it, these mechanisms are understandable. As the head accelerates, the brain lags behind and moves toward the back of the skull, thinning out the layer of protective CSF. On striking the ground or object, the brain is least protected at the site opposite to where the head hits. There are several sites within the skull that present significant perils; these are the bony ridges and the dura mater–brain attachments (falx cerebri, tentorium cerebelli) (50). These structural limitations are important and can help to predict what part of the brain will be injured.

It is also important to consider the neck musculature in considering the biomechanic forces that may affect injury severity. In applying Newton's second law (force = mass × acceleration or acceleration = force/mass), it makes sense that the forces imparted to the brain also depend on whether or not the head and neck muscles are rigid. If the neck muscles are rigid, as when one sees the blow coming or when striking a soccer ball with the head, the mass of the head takes on an approximation of the mass of the body. This means that if the mass is higher, it takes more force to create the same acceleration (since acceleration = force/mass). If the neck muscle are not rigid, then the forces that strike the head act on the mass of the head alone, a much smaller number, imparting much more acceleration. This would imply that proper technique in sport-specific skills (heading in soccer, tackling in football) as well as strengthening and conditioning of the neck muscle can potentially reduce injury.

There has been a great deal of exciting research into the neurochemical and neurometabolic changes that occur with concussive brain injury. Animal research suggests that when brain injury occurs, ionic fluxes, in part owing to the release of excitatory amino acids such as glutamate, occur that disrupt the way in which cells utilize oxygen (51,52). During a concussive injury cells that are mechanically normal, and thus not irreversibly damaged, are then exposed to these ionic fluxes in the setting of an increased need for glycolysis. The increase in glucose metabolism following brain injury has been demonstrated in animals by using [^{14}C]2-deoxy-D-glucose autoradiography (53,54). At the same time, the cerebral blood flow is decreased (55). In the setting of reduced blood flow, this leads to a mismatch between glucose demand and cerebral blood supply, which can lead to cell dysfunction and may also put the cell at risk for a second insult (56).

The research in humans appears to be consistent in that there is an increase in cerebral glucose metabolism in brain-injured patients that occurs as a result of ionic shifts (57). The changes include alterations in glutamate, potassium, and calcium and cerebral blood flow, and oxidative metabolism is reduced. These changes have been demonstrated in severely head-injured patients by [^{18}F]fluorodeoxyglucose-positron emission tomography scanning studies (57,58).

EVALUATING THE HEAD-INJURED ATHLETE

Initial management and evaluation of an athlete who sustains a head injury are important and involve a well-prepared protocol and qualified medical personnel. Evaluation includes a complete physical examination with particular attention to the neurologic examination and level of cognitive functioning. The close follow-up of an athlete with a head injury is crucial in management issues and return-to-play issues. The return-to-play issues are difficult and require an individualized approach that takes into account several factors, as well as neuropsychological data if available. Watching for postconcussive sequelae is also important.

When an athlete is initially evaluated, a high suspicion for associated injuries such as cervical spine and skull fractures should be maintained. It is helpful to ask the athlete whether he or she is experiencing any head or neck pain and, if so, to describe it. If the athlete describes neck pain or if the injury occurred in a mechanism that puts the cervical spine at risk, it is better to err on the side of safety and stabilize the cervical spine immediately. Spine boards and cervical collars may be necessary. If the athlete has a helmet in place, it should be left on unless an airway needs to be secured and the face mask cannot be cut away (59). If the athlete has no neck pain and the cervical spine is not tender, further history from the patient should be obtained.

Asking the athlete what he or she remembers of the injury and how it occurred, as well as what he or she remembers before the injury and directly afterward, can be very useful. If the athlete is being examined at the site of the athletic event, it is also useful to ask what the score of the contest is, what part of the game the athlete is in, and what the name of the opponent is. These questions can help to determine the athlete's orientation as well as whether the athlete is having difficulty with retrograde memory. If the athlete is being evaluated in the office setting, these questions can also be useful, and an attempt should be made to determine whether there was witnessed LOC as well as other pieces of information that the athlete may not recall. Having teammates or family members present can be useful, though an attempt to have the athletes answer the questions themselves should be made whenever possible.

Other questions that are very useful at the site of the injury include more sophisticated questions pertaining to anterograde memory, such as specific plays. Asking a teammate or coach to ask the athlete, "What do you do on the head-tap or basic play" can help to determine whether the athlete has memory for information learned in previous practices. Asking the athlete to remember five objects shortly after being presented to them and asking what happened directly after the injury are examples of tests which look at anterograde memory. This information can help to determine the severity of injury as well as being useful in demonstrating to the coach that the athlete has a significant injury and therefore cannot return to the athletic contest.

Head injuries can present with a variety of symptoms, and besides retrograde and anterograde amnesia and loss of consciousness, other symptoms such as headache, nausea, dizziness, tinnitus, imbalance, and "feeling in a fog" should be addressed. Symptoms that correlate to a focal deficit, such as visual disturbances, motor or sensory deficits, and problems with gait should be addressed. It is very important to ask about any previous head or neck injuries in terms of when they occurred, how severe they were, and what, if any, additional tests were obtained. This past history is very important in making return-to-play decisions.

In evaluating the head-injured athlete, the first task is to assess for difficulties in airway, breathing, and circulation, followed by any associated cervical and skull injuries. If the athlete is alert and can answer questions, a thorough history can be obtained. The Glasgow Coma Scale (GCS) is very useful in that it is well known and established (Table 30–4). It also is a good prognosticator in that if the GCS is less than 5, 80% of patients will die or remain in a vegetative state. If the GCS is greater than 11, then more than 90% will have complete recovery (50). The prognosis improves as the GCS score improves and therefore should be assessed serially.

Once an assessment of orientation is undertaken, the pupils should be assessed for symmetry as well as direct and indirect pupillary constriction in response to light. An assessment of the cranial nerves should be performed, followed by an assessment of upper and lower

TABLE 30-4. Glasgow coma scale

Item	Score
Eye opening	
Eyes open spontaneously	4
Eyes open to verbal command	3
Eyes open only with painful stimuli	2
No eye opening	1
Verbal response	
Oriented and converses	5
Disoriented and converses	4
Inappropriate words	3
Incomprehensible sounds	2
No verbal response	1
Motor response	
Obeys verbal commands	6
Response to painful stimuli (upper extremities)	
Localizes pain	5
Withdraws from pain	4
Flexor posturing	3
Extensor posturing	2
No motor response	1
Total score = eye opening + verbal response + motor response	

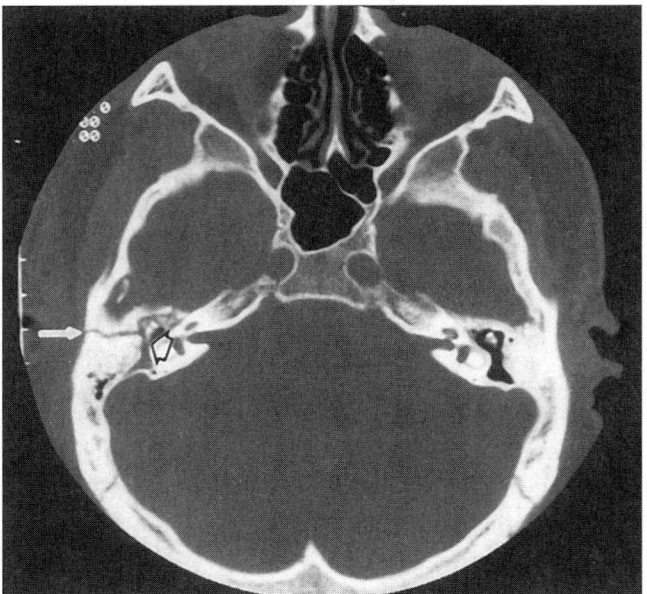

FIG. 30-6. A basilar skull fracture involving the petrous bone is seen on this axial CT image (*solid arrow*). The fracture extends into the middle ear (*open arrow*) and can cause a conducive hearing loss by disrupting the tympanic membrane or the ossicles of the middle ear. The fracture also can cause hemorrhage into the middle ear cavity, which will result in hearing loss. (Reprinted with permission from Fu FH, Stone DA, eds. *Sports injuries: mechanisms, prevention, treatment.* Baltimore: Williams & Wilkins, 1994.)

motor and sensory function, reflexes, and cerebellar examination. Any deficits in a complete neurologic examination should be noted, and serial examinations are needed.

Evidence for an associated basilar skull fracture should be assessed for in the evaluation of the head-injured athlete. A skull fracture should be considered if one sees any of the abnormalities listed in Table 30-5. If these are present, a CT scan should be obtained immediately (Figs. 30-6, 30-7). In addition, extreme precautions should be taken to avoid infection, and the athlete should be transferred to an emergency medical center as soon as possible with neurosurgical consultation available.

If there has been sustained loss of consciousness or any evidence of focal deficits, then imaging of the brain should be performed; CT scanning often provides the best initial study. If the athlete gives a history of a lucid interval with progressive decline or presents with worsening symptoms, imaging is also indicated. In a setting in which an athlete cannot be watched closely or when an athlete is getting worse instead of better, obtaining some type of imaging as well as a safe place for observation may be indicated. This will often ease much discomfort in the acute setting and may prevent a catastrophic event from occurring.

An athlete should have monitoring of the neurologic examination, and care should be taken to note any new or resolving symptoms. If an athlete is first assessed on the field and has only minor symptoms of headache and nausea, she or he should also be closely followed. No athlete should be allowed to return to the event if there are any symptoms whatsoever, including a mild headache. Once the athlete is completely asymptomatic, care should be taken to make note of when this occurs, and further management can be undertaken. This may include allowing the athlete to return to the activity or keeping the athlete out of activity until he or she remains symptom free for a specific time interval. For a mild injury when no loss of consciousness and no memory deficits occur, an observation period of at least 20 minutes symptom free is often used, followed by an exertional challenge before returning the athlete to competition. However, these recommendations must be

TABLE 30-5. *Signs of skull fracture*

Battle's sign: Postauricular hematoma
Rhinorrhea: CSF leaking from the nose
Otorrhea: CSF leaking from the ear canal
Raccoon eyes: Periorbital ecchymosis due to leakage of blood from anterior fossa into periorbital tissues
Hemotympanum: Blood behind the eardrum
Cranial nerve injuries: Especially involving the facial nerve
Palpable malalignment of calvarium

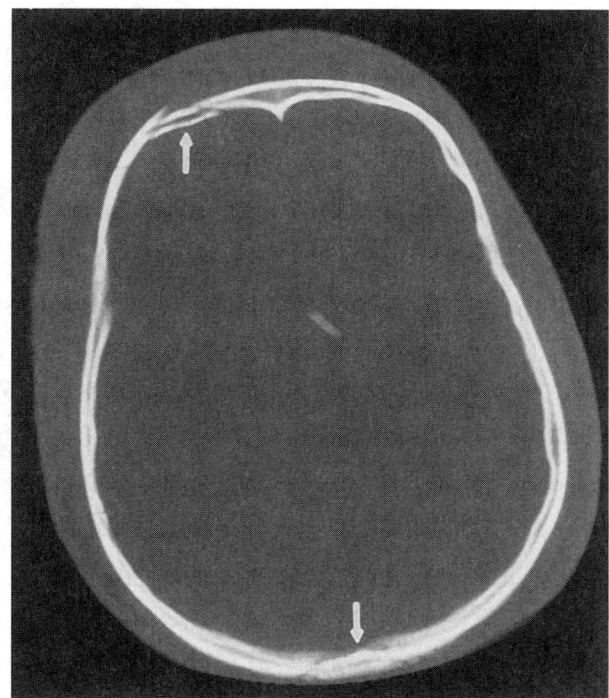

FIG. 30–7. Axial CT image of right frontal and occipital comminuted skull fractures. The occipital fracture is particularly ominous because it lies over the superior saggital sinus and may have lacerated it, causing an intracranial hematoma. (Reprinted with permission from Fu FH, Stone DA, eds. *Sports injuries: mechanisms, prevention, treatment.* Baltimore: Williams & Wilkins, 1994.)

individualized and will be discussed in further detail below.

COMPLICATIONS AND SEQUELAE OF HEAD INJURY

Certain sequelae and complications can occur after head injury that should be considered and watched for. These include cervical and skull fractures, posttraumatic seizures, second impact syndrome, and postconcussive syndrome. Of major importance is educating the head-injured athlete, coach, and parents to the seriousness of head injury, such that the probability that complications will occur will be decreased and, if they do occur, they are detected and treated promptly.

Skull fractures may occur in association with head injuries and should be assessed for. They are often associated with underlying injury to the brain surface or structure, as well as focal neurologic deficits or seizure activity. The risk for underlying intracranial hemorrhage has been estimated to be 20 times higher when a skull fracture is present compared to that seen in head injury without a skull fracture (60). There is also a concurrent risk for infection, given that these fractures will allow for an open transmission of organisms to the structures inside the calvarium. This is obviously of significant concern and consequence.

Cervical spine injuries also occur in association with head injuries and should be assessed for at the initial evaluation as well as in follow-up. In severe head injury, cervical spine injuries are present in 5–10% of patients (61). If an athlete initially complains of neck pain or there is palpable cervical spine tenderness, the neck should be stabilized until diagnostic testing is complete. Often, this includes a lateral and anteroposterior and open-mouth odontoid views. The lateral should include the occiput and the upper margin of the first thoracic vertebral body. If these are normal, flexion and extension lateral films should also be obtained to ensure that the cervical spine is stable. If radiographs are normal but the athlete complains of neck pain or demonstrates focal neurologic symptoms related to the cervical spine, MRI should be obtained to ensure that a soft tissue compression from a herniated disc or vascular lesion is not present.

Seizures may occur after head injury and generally occur in association with a skull fracture or intracranial hemorrhage. Seizure disorders may complicate head injury in roughly 5% of cases and generally occur within 1 week of trauma. Children younger than age 16 are less likely to develop seizures after depressed skull fractures than are adults. Head-injured individuals are at increased risk for developing posttraumatic epilepsy if they have seizures within 1 week of injury, posttraumatic amnesia greater than 12 hours, intracranial hemorrhage, or any neurologic deficit after injury. A normal EEG does not help to predict the risk for developing posttraumatic seizure disorders (62). Whether individuals with epilepsy should participate in contact sports with a risk of head injury is discussed elsewhere (63).

Postconcussive syndrome can occur after significant or recurrent head injury and is characterized by persistent headache, inability to concentrate, irritability, fatigue, vertigo, gait unsteadiness, sleep disturbances, visual disturbances, and emotional lability (Table 30–6). It may take several weeks for these symptoms to occur, and their presence and persistence are variable. CT or MRI scanning should be obtained to rule out intracranial lesions. There is some controversy over whether the duration of loss of consciousness or posttraumatic amnesia has any clear relationship to whether postconcussive syndrome will occur (64). In addition, it is also difficult to separate postconcussive syndrome from persistent symptoms after head injury. Finally, many individuals will also experience trauma-induced migraine, which may be also particularly difficult to treat in the athletic setting.

Criteria for postconcussive disorder were presented in preliminary form in the *1994 Diagnostic Statistical Manual* (DSM-IV) of the American Psychiatric Association. These were based on recommendations from

TABLE 30-6. *Proposed criteria for postconcussive syndrome*

A. History of head injury that includes at least two of the following:
   1. Loss of consciousness for 5 minutes or more
   2. Posttraumatic amnesia of 12 hours or more
   3. Onset of seizures (posttraumatic epilepsy) within 6 months of head injury
B. Current symptoms (either new symptoms or substantially worsening preexisting symptoms) to include
   1. At least the following two cognitive difficulties:
      a. Learning or memory (recall)
      b. Concentration
   2. At least three of the following affective or vegetative symptoms:
      a. Easy fatigability
      b. Insomnia or sleep/wake cycle disturbances
      c. Headache (substantially worse than before injury)
      d. Vertigo/dizziness
      e. Irritability and/or aggression on little or no provocation
      f. Anxiety, depression, or lability of affect
      g. Personality change (e.g., social or sexual inappropriateness, childlike behavior)
      h. Aspontaneity/apathy
C. Symptoms associated with a significant difficulty in maintaining premorbid occupational or academic performance or with a decline in social, occupational, or academic performance

From Brown SJ, Fann JR, Grant I. Postconcussional disorder: time to acknowledge a common source of neurobehavioral morbidity. *J Neuropsychiatry Clin Neurosci* 1994;6:15–22, with permission.

Brown and colleagues (65), and include criteria that must be met to carry that diagnosis. The initial criteria include posttraumatic amnesia for more than 12 hours, head injury with loss of consciousness, and seizure activity within 6 months of head injury. The individual must have two of these three criteria to have the diagnosis. The other proposed criteria are presented in Table 30-6. Many clinicians believe that these criteria are too strict and generally use the diagnosis of postconcussive syndrome for any head-injured individual who presents with typical symptoms after sustaining any head injury, no matter how seemingly mild.

Postconcussive syndrome can be very difficult to treat and generally includes a multidisciplinary approach using medications, psychotherapy, behavior modifications, biofeedback, and physical therapy. It appears that the same biochemical changes that occur with acute head injury may also explain the pathogenesis of posttraumatic headache and migraine. In both situations there may be evidence for changes in electrolytes (potassium, sodium, calcium, and chloride), excitatory amino acids, serotonin, catecholamines and endogenous opioids, impaired glucose utilization, and neuropeptides (66). The beta-adrenergic blockers and tricyclic antidepressants are the medications that have provided the best response clinically. The management of postconcussive syndrome and postconcussive headaches is discussed in recent reviews (67–69).

Of utmost concern in terms of complications of head injury is the second impact syndrome (SIS), described by Saunders and Harbaugh (1) and Schneider (70). In SIS an individual who is still recovering from a prior concussion sustains a second, even mild, head injury. This second impact can lead to fatal brain swelling. The symptoms from the first injury may include dizziness or vertigo, visual motor or sensory changes, or memory difficulty but may also be as mild as a persistent headache. The second impact may also be minor, including a blow to the chest that jerks the athlete's head (50). After the second impact occurs, the athlete collapses, generally within seconds to minutes, and quickly becomes semicomatose with rapidly dilating and fixed pupils and respiratory failure followed by death. It has been reported in both children as well as adults (71,72) and is obviously of major concern.

The pathophysiology of SIS is believed to be due to an increased sensitivity in the cerebral vasculature that occurs after the first head injury occurs. The second impact then causes a dysfunction in the autoregulation of the cerebral blood supply leading to vascular congestion and significant increases in intracranial pressure. The increase in intracranial pressure is associated with herniation of the brain and brainstem compromise with resultant coma and respiratory failure (73). The SIS exemplifies the need to follow head-injured athletes closely, look for symptomatology, and educate athletes as to the necessity and importance of reporting symptoms.

Another area of significant concern is that of recurrent head trauma and chronic traumatic encephalopathy (CTE). CTE is thought to be the premature loss of normal central nervous system function. This is believed to occur in the realm of athletics because of the cumulative effect of multiple blows to the head that results in pathologic changes in brain substance. It can occur in boxers who have had no episodes of loss of consciousness, and it may be difficult to predict the point at which CTE is likely to occur. It is likely impossible to determine the number of head impacts that can be sustained before brain dysfunction and CTE will occur (74). Recurrent head injury is discussed in further detail later in this chapter.

CLASSIFICATION SYSTEMS

It is helpful to understand some of the classification systems that have been presented in that they provide a historical look at head injury in sport. In the realm of head injury, most of those that occur in sport are considered mild unless they involve focal brain injuries or associated cervical spine or skull fractures. Yet within the realm of sports medicine differentiating a minor head injury from a more severe one and making decisions regarding return to play are among the most important roles that the medical team has in care of the athlete. If an error is made in this regard, it puts the athlete at risk for consequences that may be life threatening. At this time these decisions must be made on an individual basis with an understanding of the athlete's previous history, the nature of their injury, and the sport in which the athlete participates. With all of these parameters taken into account, an individualized plan can be undertaken to ensure the athlete's well-being and safe return to sport.

Several classification systems exist for head injury, and most include return-to-play guidelines (74–79). It is probably more important that the physician, trainer, and other health care professionals taking care of the same athletes understand the grading system being used than which classification system they feel best correlates with their own practice patterns. The existing guidelines are not based on long-term prospective data on athletes, yet there is some merit in understanding some of these as they relate to the athlete. All of the classification systems use loss of consciousness, retrograde and anterograde memory deficits, and symptoms or physical findings to differentiate different severity of injury. Examples of several classification systems are given in Table 30–7.

The need for a standard classification system is apparent. Based on the presentation and symptoms of a particular athlete, different grades of concussion exist. For example, in an athlete with significant retrograde and posttraumatic amnesia but no loss of consciousness (49), classifications include a Torg grade IV, a Nelson III, a Cantu II, or Colorado Medical Society III. It is probably more useful to include descriptive nomenclature such as loss of consciousness, retrograde or posttraumatic amnesia, and specific symptoms or physical findings as well. While these classification systems are different and each has its own merit, the consistency with which one is used is more important than the specific classification that is chosen.

RETURN-TO-PLAY GUIDELINES

Once an athlete sustains a head injury and is adequately treated, the next controversy is deciding when it is safe for the athlete to return to activities. This is especially true when the athlete participates in sports or activities that have a high risk for head injury. Examples of sports with a high risk include football, ice hockey, gymnastics, wrestling, martial arts, boxing, rugby, and soccer. Several other activities put the head at risk for injury, including equestrian sports; motorcycle, automobile, and boat racing; and sky diving. Return-to-play decisions include those for focal head injuries and structural abnormalities, as well as mild head injury.

Recent data have questioned the assumption that the presence of LOC correlates with more severe injuries. Lovell (80) used neuropsychologic data to demonstrate that cognitive deficits after head injury did not correlate with the presence or absence of LOC. Thus the athlete with brief LOC and no other symptoms may not necessarily have a more severe injury when compared to an athlete without LOC who experiences significant difficulties with memory or persistent symptoms. These data may challenge several of the current classifications systems. The presence of LOC, however, still raises significant concern for the possibility of intracranial vascular emergencies and should be treated accordingly.

Many of the classification systems discussed earlier also include guidelines for return to play (74–78). These again are not based on prospective studies and remain as guidelines. It is important to treat each head-injured athlete individually, on the basis of the specific injury, past history, complications, clinical course, and readiness to return. Though there may be some fault in being too conservative in returning an athlete to competition, most would agree that this is certainly better than allowing an athlete to return to play early and possibly contributing to a severe consequence. The most important points are that careful assessment and close follow-up are essential and that individualization of treatment remains ideal until further research is completed.

The return-to-play guidelines for focal and structural diffuse brain injuries are not based on prospective studies, and the decision to return these athletes to play is based on judgment and experience. The lesions that are generally considered include all types of intracranial hemorrhage (epidural hematoma, subdural hematoma, intracerebral hematoma, and subarachnoid hemorrhage), as well as SIS and diffuse axonal injury. Cantu has suggested that an athlete who sustains any of these injuries can return to play as long as she or he does not have any of the following five contraindications: persistent postconcussive symptoms, permanent central neurologic sequelae (organic dementia, hemiplegia, homonymous hemianopsia), hydrocephalus, spontaneous subarachnoid hemorrhage from any cause, or symptomatic neurologic or pain-producing abnormalities about the foramen magnum (50). In addition, an athlete who has been treated surgically for any of the intracranial hematomas should be seriously discouraged from participating in contact sports. This is because the surgical procedure itself may cause scarring within the subdural space and resultant tethering of the brain and abnormalities in CSF cushioning. The only exception is the epidural hematoma with no underlying brain injury. In these injuries, or other injuries in which surgery is not required and none of the contraindications exist, return to play can be allowed after at least one full

TABLE 30-7. *Classification systems and return to play guidelines*

Torg: Grades of cerebral concussion, 1982

I. Short-term confusion, no LOC, no amnesia
II. Confusion + amnesia, no LOC, + posttraumatic amnesia (PTA)
III. Confusion + amnesia, no LOC, + PTA, + (RGA)
IV. +LOC (immediate transient), + amnesia (PTA, RGA)
V. +LOC (paralytic coma)→ coma vigil, respiratory arrest
VI. +LOC (paralytic coma)→ death

Nelson: Classification of concussion, 1984

0. No complaints initially, + subsequent complaints of headache, difficulty with sensorium
I. + stunned or dazed, no LOC or amnesia, clears quick (<1 min)
II. Headache, cloudy sensorium (>1 min), no LOC, + amnesia
III. + LOC (<1 min), not comatose, Grade II symptoms during recovery
IV. + LOC (>1 min), not comatose, Grade II symptoms during recovery

Cantu: Grading system for concussion, 1986

I. Mild: no LOC, PTA < 30 min
II. Moderate: + LOC < 5 min, or PTA > 30 min but < 24 hr
III. Severe: + LOC > 5 min, or PTA > 24 hr

Colorado Medical Society: Guidelines for the Management of Concussion in Sport, 1991

I. Confusion without amnesia, no LOC
   Remove from contest.
   Examine immediately and every 5 min for the development of amnesia or postconcussive symptoms at rest and with exertion.
   Permit return to contest if amnesia does not appear and no symptoms appear for ≥20 min.
II. Confusion with amnesia, no LOC
   Remove from contest and disallow return.
   Examine frequently for signs of evolving intracranial pathology.
   Reexamine the next day.
   Permit return to practice after 1 full week without symptoms.
III. +LOC
   Transport from field to nearest hospital by ambulance (with cerebral spine immobilization if indicated).
   Perform thorough neurologic evaluation emergently.
   Admit to hospital if signs of pathology are detected.
   If findings are normal, instruct family for overnight observation.
   Permit return to practice only after 2 full weeks without symptoms.

American Academy of Neurology, 1997

I. Transient confusion, no LOC, concussion symptoms or mental status abnormalities on exam resolve in <15 min.
   Remove from contest.
   Examine immediately and at 5-min intervals for development of mental status abnormalities or postconcussive symptoms at rest and with exertion.
   May return if abnormalities/symptoms clear within 15 min.
   Second grade I concussion in same contest eliminates player from contest, returning only if asymptomatic for 1 week at rest and exertion.
II. Transient confusion, no LOC, concussion symptoms or mental status abnormalities last >15 min.
   Remove from contest, no return that day.
   Examine on site frequently for signs of evolving intracranial pathology.
   Reexamine athlete following day.
   Neurologic exam by M.D. one week after asymptomatic before return.
   CT or MRI if headache or other symptoms worsen or persist >2 weeks.
   Following second Grade II, return to play deferred until at least 2 weeks symptom free at rest and with exertion.
   Terminating season mandated by any abnormality on CT or MRI consistent with brain swelling, contusion, or other intracranial pathology.
III. Any LOC, either brief (seconds) or prolonged (minutes)
   Transport from field to ER by ambulance if unconscious or worrisome signs. Consider cervical spine immobilization.
   Thorough neurologic exam emergently, including appropriate neuroimaging procedures.
   Admit if any signs of pathology or mental status abnormalities.
   If normal evaluation, may send athlete home.
   Neurologic status should be assessed daily thereafter until all symptoms have stabilized or resolved
   Prolonged LOC, persistent mental status alterations, worsening symptoms, or abnormalities on neurologic exam require urgent neurosurgical evaluation or transfer to trauma center.

TABLE 30-7. Continued.

After brief (sec) Grade III concussion the athlete should be held out until asymptomatic for 1 week at rest or with exertion.
After prolonged (min) Grade III concussion athlete should be withheld from play for 2 weeks at rest and with exertion.
Following second Grade III concussion athlete should be withheld from play for min of 1 asymptomatic month. M.D. may elect to extend that period beyond 1 month, depending on clinical evaluation and other circumstances
CT or MRI reecommended for athletes whose headache or other associated symptoms worsen or persist >1 week.
Any abnormality on CT or MRI consistent with brain swelling, contusion, or other intracranial pathology should result in termination of the season for that athlete, and return to play in the future should be seriously discouraged in discussions with the athlete.

Return to Play Decisions

Cantu guidelines: return to play after concussion

Grade I: *First concussion*: May return to play if asymptomatic (no headache, dizziness, or impaired orientation, concentration, or memory during rest/exertion) for 1 week.
Second concussion: Return to play in 2 weeks if asymptomatic at that time for 1 week.
Third concussion: Terminate season, may return to play next season if asymptomatic.
Grade II: *First concussion*: May return to play after asymptomatic for 1 week.
Second concussion: minimum of 1 month; may return to play then if asymptomatic for 1 week, consider terminating season.
Third concussion: Terminate season, may return to play next season if asymptomatic.
Grade III: *First concussion*: Minimum of one month; may then return to play if asymptomatic for 1 week.
Second concussion: Terminate season; may return to play next season if asymptomatic.

Colorado Medical Society guidelines: return to play

Grade I: *First concussion*: Remove from contest. Examine immediately and every 5 minutes for the development of amnesia or postconcussive symptoms at rest and with exertion. May return to contest if amnesia does not appear and no symptoms appear for at least 20 minutes.
Second concussion: If in same contest, eliminate from competition that day. Otherwise, treat as grade I.
Third concussion: Terminate season. No contact sports for at least 3 months, and then only if asymptomatic at rest and exertion.
Grade II: *First concussion*: Remove from contest and disallow return. Examine frequently for signs of evolving intracranial pathology. Reexamine the next day. May return to practice after 1 full wk without symptoms.
Second concussion: Defer return to play for one month. Termination of season considered.
Third concussion: Termination of season mandated. (Also terminate season if any abnormality on CT/MRI.)
Grade III: *First concussion*: Transport from field by ambulance (with cervical spine immobilization if indicated) to nearest hospital. Thorough neurologic evaluation emergently. Hospital confinement if signs of pathology are detected. If findings are normal, instructions to family for overnight observation. May return to practice (no contact) only after 2 full weeks without symptoms. Return to full contact activity at one month only if athlete has been asymptomatic at rest and exertion for at least 2 weeks.
Second concussion: Terminate season. (Also terminate if any abnormality on CT/MRI.) Return to contact sports should be seriously discouraged.

---

year after the injury or neurologic recovery is complete (50).

As was already discussed, CT, MRI, and EEG may not always detect deficits in the mildly head-injured, particularly the mild head injuries that are sustained in athletic competition. It can be particularly frustrating to the athlete, parents, and health care professional to witness significant disruption in cognitive function yet have normal findings on EEG, MRI, and CT scanning. The athlete has difficulty answering questions, remembering events, and performing simple tasks, yet every sophisticated medical test reveals no abnormalities. When is the athlete truly back to normal? Do we know whether the athlete's ability to make decisions, recognize situations, and concentrate such that he or she is not at an increased risk for further injury is where it should be? Most health care professionals will agree that head injuries are different from ankle sprains; one might allow an athlete to get taped or braced and play on an ankle injury that is 80%, but allowing that to occur in a head-injured athlete is inappropriate.

No matter what the individual's particular situation is, it is imperative that the athlete not return to activity if he or she has any symptoms and that some form of exercise challenge be performed before the athlete is allowed to return. This ensures that exertion alone will not bring on any symptoms and gives the athlete confidence that he or she can expect to run and exercise without symptoms. It also ensures that if an athlete is not ready to return to activity, that athlete is not put at the additional risk of significant contact if exertion alone brings on symptoms.

Depending on the situation, an athlete can gradually be returned to activity once she or he is symptom free in a manner that allows the athlete to return to some of the rigors of the sport without the risk of further head injury. In other words, if an athlete sustains a more serious head injury with retrograde and/or anterograde amnesia, the decision might be made to keep the athlete out of activity for a specific time period. At that point she or he may perform an exercise challenge such as exercising on a bicycle to see whether exertion alone will provoke any symptoms. An athlete who remains asymptomatic might be then allowed to participate in sport-specific activities. For a soccer player this might include passing a ball back and forth or dribbling with the ball. For a basketball player this might mean shooting baskets or working on footwork. For different sports there are many examples of sport-specific activity that will allow the athlete to return to practices yet not be put at risk. The athlete is present at practice and is still part of the team but is kept out of contact drills and full competition if the sport involves contact or collision. Obviously, for some sports such as tennis or golf, little if any risk for contact exists, and getting the athlete back into full activity is a much simpler process.

It is important to discuss with the athlete, as well as the athlete's parents and coaches, the rationale for holding the athlete out of play until the symptoms resolve, as well as the importance of reporting any symptoms. Explaining the SIS (1) and explaining the risks of recurrent head injury can sometimes make the athlete understand how important these symptoms can be. An athlete who has had a concussion is at a 4–6 times greater risk of incurring a second concussion than a nonconcussed athlete (7,81). This risk for recurrent head injury is difficult to predict, though it is safe to say that as more time passes, the risk diminishes. Return-to-play guidelines attempt to diminish these risks by taking into account the severity of injury and not allowing an athlete to return to competition if she or he has symptoms. In addition, if symptoms are reproduced with a cardiovascular challenge alone without contact, return to contact play should not be seriously contemplated. Finally, it is also important to get an idea of whether the athlete is at all apprehensive about returning to play. These fears should be discussed, and no assumptions should be made about how the athlete feels about returning to activity.

Neuropsychological testing has been shown to be very useful in the assessment and recovery phases of head injury (82–84). It has been used specifically in the setting of head injury in athletes with particular success (33,49,85,86). Neuropsychological testing is now gaining attention, and though it has not been included in grading systems in the past, it may change how head injuries in the athlete are treated in the future. In addition, other tools that measure objectively the subtle deficits that occur in the head-injured athletes are being assessed, and these too may change the evaluation of the head-injured athlete. Research is currently underway to determine which of these tools can provide sensitive and specific information that relates to the deficits seen in head-injured athletes.

As we define the assessment tools that objectively measure deficits seen in the head-injured athlete, the next step is deciding at what point is it safe to return these athletes to their sport. If the tests are extremely sensitive and we insist that an athlete must be at 100% before returning to competition, one might argue that we might prevent an athlete from participating who could have done so without significant risk. At the other extreme, if we allow an athlete to return to competition when testing reveals deficits in reaction time or information processing, then one might argue that we are knowingly putting the athlete at a significant risk. Making these decisions will always be difficult. Having objective measurements will require some form of baseline testing against which to compare and certainly will increase the time spent during the preparticipation examination as well as time spent after head injury has occurred. However, it will also likely improve the level of care that is provided to the athlete.

NEW WAYS TO EVALUATE HEAD INJURY IN ATHLETES

Exciting research is currently underway in assessing mild head injury in athletes, and this research may change the way in which athletes are evaluated and the manner in which return-to-play decisions are made. It may also change the preparticipation examination to include some form of baseline testing that assesses the areas of cognitive function that are most affected by head injury such that if an injury occurs, any deficits can be detected. What this measure is and how difficult it is to perform remain unclear. What seems clear is that this measure is probably a battery of tests rather than a single test and that a baseline test will be necessary.

Though much of the research in the use of neuropsychological testing as part of the evaluation of head-injured athletes is underway, there is already good evidence that this form of testing will enhance our knowledge of brain injury as well as recovery for the future. Neuropsychological testing provides a reliable assessment and quantification of brain functioning by examining brain–behavior relationships. These instruments are used to measure the broad range of cognitive function: speed of information processing, attention and concentration, reaction time, scanning and visual tracking ability, memory recall, and problem-solving abilities. They have been useful in detecting mild head injuries (37,82–84,86–88). Neuropsychological testing can be used to detect acute and chronic head injury and may be more sensitive in assessing cognitive function (49,85) than classic medical testing.

Neuropsychological testing has been investigated in relationship with MRI and CT scanning in head-injured patients. Levin and colleagues assessed 20 patients with minor or moderated closed head injury with neuropsychological testing, MRI, and CT scanning (37). They found that MRI demonstrated more intracranial lesions than CT scanning, though none that required surgical evacuation. Neuropsychological testing during the initial hospitalization revealed deficits that correlated to the size and location of lesions defined by MRI. Follow up testing at 1 and 3 months after injury revealed a decrease in lesion size, which correlated with an improvement in memory and cognition.

Alves and colleagues tested U.S. college football players and found that, though there were no deficits after one head injury, if another injury occurred soon after, there were detrimental effects in cognitive function (85). This highlights the second impact syndrome discussed earlier. In other preliminary research, neuropsychological testing has detected deficits compared to baseline testing when CT scan and MRI tests have been normal in college athletes with cerebral concussions (89). These data also suggest that a higher percentage of tests are abnormal, and that they stay below baseline for a longer time, if the concussion sustained is more severe. Because an individual will generally have different strengths and weaknesses in these functions, individuals will often score differently from each other. This again underscores the need for baseline testing with a battery of tests instead of a single measure.

The head-injured individual has been shown to demonstrate deficits in neuropsychological tests that resolve with time. The use of neuropsychological testing in athletes with head injury is not new and is now entering an exciting time in that the research being performed is assessing changes in athletes at the high school, college, and professional levels. Importantly, much of the research is utilizing baseline testing, which is paramount given the complexity of the tests and the individuality explained above.

There has also been recent interest in assessing postural sway as a sensitive tool to assess for deficits in head-injured athletes. A recent study looked at both cognitive tests (Trail Making Test, Digit Span Test, Stroop Test, and Hopkins Verbal Learning Test) and a postural stability tests (NeuroCom Smart Balance Master) (90). Tests were performed on athletes with and without head injury, and despite a small study, the results found that postural testing revealed deficits in the injured athletes at 1 day after injury, whereas the cognitive tests did not show any difference. In addition, the postural tests remained below controls 3–5 days later, though the differences were no longer statistically significant.

These studies raises some important questions. Are the small deficits seen in postural sway or neuropsychological testing important in terms of putting the athlete at risk for further injury? In other words, when we evaluate ankle injuries, most would agree that despite there still being some swelling present, with functional testing and prophylactic strapping, one might allow an athlete to participate with minimal risk. Thus, despite the fact that the injury is still apparent on some form of assessment, the athlete may be capable of protecting himself or herself and be at minimal risk of recurrent injury. In the case of a head-injured athlete we are willing to take fewer risks; however, just because there is a slight aberration from normal, does that mean that the athlete is at any risk, or does it mean that the tests we are using are overly sensitive? One might argue that these are the most important questions that remain to be answered.

There are other new imaging studies that may be useful in the future of head injury assessment. These include near-infrared spectroscopy (91,92), single photon emission computed tomography (SPECT) (93,94), and magnetic resonance angiography (95) and diffusion weighted magnetic resonance imaging (96). How these studies can apply to the brain injuries that occur in sport will be elucidated in the years ahead. These noninvasive tests may offer additional information that correlates with the metabolic and neurochemical changes that occur and may also detect injury at a more minor level than that detected with tests such as MRI and CT, which appear to be superior at assessing focal brain lesions. As these new technologies advance and the natural history of head injuries in the athlete accumulates, the manner in which head injuries are taken care of in the athlete may change significantly. The additional information can only expand and improve the manner in which we deliver care to the head-injured athlete.

SPECIFIC SPORTS: IMPLICATIONS AND DEBATES

For many sports the evaluation and treatment of head injuries are very similar. The return-to-play guidelines will also be similar, taking into account sport-specific differences in skill, protective equipment, and risk for subsequent injury. It is important for the health care professional to consider the sport in which the head-injured athlete is involved and be familiar with what the sport-specific demands may be. This familiarity can be very useful in determining when it is safe to return these athletes to activity. There are a few sports, however, that deserve special consideration because of the nature of the sports. Soccer and boxing are two sports that will be briefly discussed below.

Boxing

The sport of boxing is unique in considering head injuries, and a full discussion of this issue is not possible. Recent reviews have assessed the chronic effects of boxing on brain function (97). The consensus from the available data is that boxing is associated with chronic brain injury, first termed the punch-drunk syndrome in 1928 (98) and later described as dementia pugilistica (99) or chronic progressive traumatic encephalopathy (100). This syndrome occurs in professional boxers with an incidence of between 9% and 25% and appears to correlate with the length of a boxer's career and the number of fights the boxer was in (101). The symptoms include cerebellar, pyramidal, extrapyramidal, and occasionally cognitive and personality impairments. These chronic changes tend to occur on average 16 years (with a range of 7–35 years) after a career in boxing is initiated, and they progress slowly over time through stages of increasing dysfunction and disability (97).

Boxing has been studied by MRI, CT scanning, and EEG, and there have been data to suggest that boxers show abnormalities on these types of testing compared with controls (102,103). Cerebral atrophy has been identified in boxers (103,104). In one large study of 338 active professionals, cerebral atrophy was noted on CT scanning, with 7% abnormal CT scans and 22% borderline scans. In this study a history of knockout or technical knockout correlated with a tendency for an abnormal CT scan finding (103). However, a retrospective study of boxers and soccer players and track and field athletes did not show any differences when assessed by EEG, CT, MRI, or neuropsychological testing (97). Further prospective data are necessary to accurately define the impact of head injury on cognitive function and chronic brain injury.

There have been attempts to prevent catastrophic outcome in the sport, and certain states have set up specific guidelines for return to competition after head injury has occurred. A mandatory 45-day suspension for mild concussions, 60-day suspension for moderate concussions, and 90-day suspension along with normal CT and EEG testing results for severe concussions are the guidelines set forth by the New York State Boxing Commission (105). These guidelines were put in place to protect the athlete from incurring bad sequelae in a sport that obviously has a high risk for head injury by its very nature.

Soccer

A recent debate has begun in the sport of soccer, a contact sport in which head injuries occur frequently and striking the ball with the head, a complex activity that is unique to soccer, occurs as part of the game. "Heading" the ball is used offensively in an attempt to strike it into the goal or redirect it to a teammate, as well as defensively in an attempt to clear it away. Different heading techniques exist for these skills, and there has been some speculation that this repetitive striking of the ball may put these athletes at risk for cumulative head injury, such as that seen in boxers.

The technique of heading has been compared to a catapult in which both the upper body and lower body go into extension before impact, then contract forcefully such that the head strikes through the ball as the trunk goes into flexion. In skilled players the neck becomes rigid as the head impacts the ball (106), which decreases the angular acceleration of the head and ultimately the risk of injury to the head and neck (107). There has been speculation that younger players, who are still learning the skill of heading, may be at the largest risk, with poor technique a culprit for putting the head and neck at risk.

It has been estimated that in a typical male soccer player's career, approximately 300 games are played and 2000 blows to the head are sustained (32). The kicked ball travels at an average speed of 114.4 km/h and, from 10 meters away, has an average impact speed of 116 kpm, though it can reach 200 kpm at full force (108,109). The ball is in contact with the head from 1/63 to 1/128 second, and the longer that the ball is in contact with the head, the smaller the impact force. These forces occurring repetitively throughout a soccer player's career are what has raised concern for head and neck injury.

In 1982 Sortland and colleagues reported that in 40-year-old soccer players, degenerative changes in the cervical spine were noted equivalent to those seen in 50- to 60-year-old nonplayers (110), and this was thought to be secondary to the cumulative effect of repetitive heading. Similarly, in a study of Norwegian professional players, central cerebral atrophy was noted on CT scanning, and these changes were more likely to be present if the player was a "typical header" (likely to head the ball) (32). In another study, EEG changes were seen in soccer players with acute or protracted complaints secondary to heading, some symptoms persisting for months or years (110). These studies have not gained recognition because they have significant flaws in methodology, including lack of proper control groups, no control for acute head injuries, and lack of screening for other problems (motor vehicle accidents) and alcohol use.

Neuropsychological testing, as well as MRI, CT scanning, and EEG, were used in a study on boxers in which soccer players as well as track and field athletes were used as controls. This study failed to demonstrate abnormalities in any of these measures between these groups (97). A recent well-controlled study of U.S. national team soccer players found no statistical difference between soccer players and track athletes on MRI evaluation (111). More prospective studies are necessary to determine whether there are chronic changes as a result of heading the ball and to separate this mechanism from the collision and contact mechanisms that also occur in the sport of soccer.

There are important differences in the biomechanics of heading a soccer ball and those that occur in boxing, in which the punch-drunk syndrome has been described. First, the acceleration forces in heading are severalfold less in soccer than in boxing: 20 gs versus 100 gs, respectively (112). Second, the forces in soccer generally occur in a linear direction, with muscular support from the muscles of the cervical spine, hip, and trunk. The forces that occur in boxing are often rotational, and these are thought to be more harmful because of the shearing of bridging veins that can occur (31) (Figs. 30–8, 30–9). In addition, the action of heading is generally occurring as a skill performed by the athlete with contraction of the paraspinal muscles such that the neck is rigid. This is different from a situation in which the neck is not rigid and the head is subsequently without support. As was discussed earlier, this means that the forces are significantly less in soccer heading if the proper technique is used.

In 1998, Boden performed a prospective study of Division I collegiate mens and womens soccer players and found injury rates of 0.6 and 0.4 per 1000 athlete exposures for men and women, respectively (113). The mechanism of injury was contact with another player's head in 28%; contact with the ground in 14%; and contact with the opponent's elbow, knee, or foot or a combination of these with the ground in 16%. In 24% the mechanism

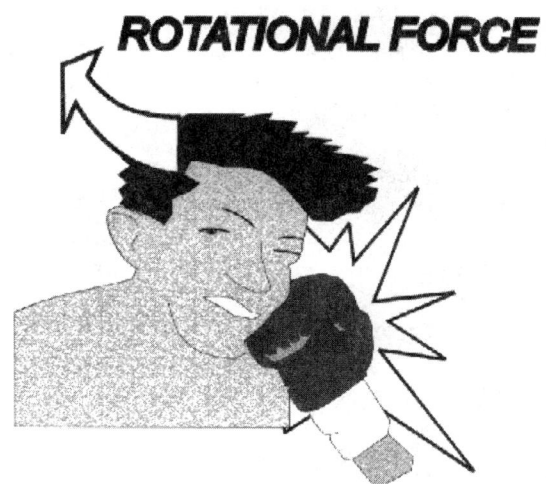

FIG. 30–9. Punching impact in boxing often produces rotational force.

was contact with a ball, but in none of these was the concussion due to purposeful heading.

In two studies Matser and colleagues (114,115) has shown a decrease in neuropsychological tests of soccer players compared to track athletes and swimmers. In one of these studies, however, researchers demonstrated an inverse relationship between poor NP performance and number of concussions, and in neither study did they partial out the effect of concussions from heading.

In a prospective pilot study of collegiate soccer players, no acute changes due to heading were noted by neuropsychological tests performed before and after a practice session (116).

There has been concern about head injuries in soccer, and the NCAA data do include soccer as one of the sports with the highest injury incidence of concussion. However, when one looks at the data, almost all of these injuries again occur as a result of impact of the head with another player, the ground, or the goalposts. The head injuries that occur are often concussions, and these are generally mild injuries. More long-term prospective studies that can differentiate the effects of multiple and severe concussions from the effects of heading are needed.

CONCLUSIONS

Head injury in sport is common and can be extremely incapacitating. It varies from mild injury after which an individual can return to competition 20 minutes later to severe injury with significant and even fatal complications. The health care team taking care of athletes must maintain a high index of suspicion for injury, especially in sports in which head injury is common. A careful and systematic approach should be followed with all head injuries, even seemingly mild ones. Additional diagnos-

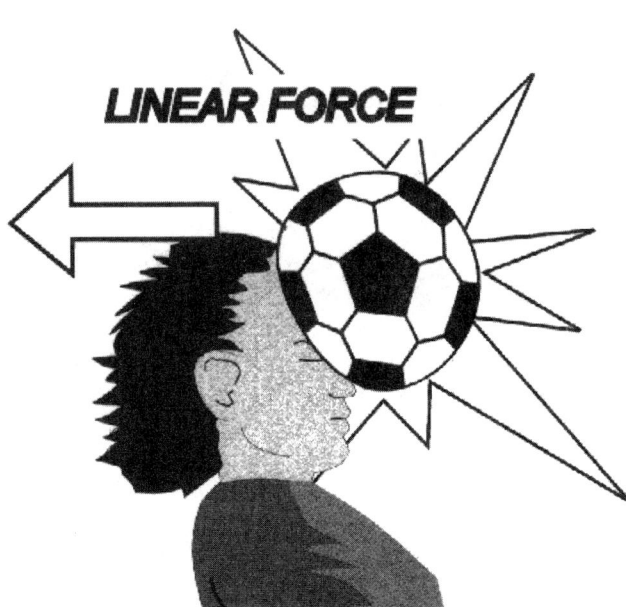

FIG. 30–8. Soccer heading typically produces linear force to the head.

tic testing may be necessary to exclude focal intracranial injuries or other associated injuries, and close follow-up and additional monitoring are essential. With a systematic approach, head injuries can generally be handled appropriately without consequence.

Several new techniques for assessing head concussion are evolving that may change the way in which these head injuries are assessed. These techniques may be more sensitive to the cognitive dysfunction that occurs in concussion. These techniques may also change the preparticipation examination and return-to-play guidelines that currently exist. More long-term prospective studies in an athletic population are needed before any conclusions can be made. As more information is obtained about these complex injuries, the health care provided to the athlete will certainly improve.

REFERENCES

1. Saunders RL, Harbaugh RE. The second impact in catastrophic contact-sports head trauma. *JAMA* 1984;252:538–539.
2. Spear J. Are footballers at risk for developing dementia? *Int J Geriatr Psychiatry* 1995;10:1011–1014.
3. Mayeux R, et al. Genetic susceptibility and head injury as risk factors for Alzheimer's disease among community-dwelling elderly persons and their first degree relatives. *Ann Neurol* 1993;33:494–501.
4. Mortimer JA, French LR, Hutton JT, et al. Head injury as a risk factor for Alzheimer's disease. *Neurology* 1985;35:264–266.
5. McLatchie G, Jennett B. ABC of sports medicine: head injury in sport. *Brit Med J* 1994;308:1620–1624.
6. Kraus JF. Epidemiology of head injury. In: Cooper PR, ed. *Head injury*, 2nd ed. Baltimore: Williams & Wilkins 1987:1–197.
7. Gerberich SG, Priest JD, Boen JR, et al. Concussion incidence and severity in secondary school varsity football players. *Am J Public Health* 1983;73:1370–1375.
8. Garrick JG, Requa RK. Medical care and injury surveillance in the high school setting. *Phys Sportsmed* 1981;9:115.
9. Buckley WE. Concussions in college football. *Am J Sports Med* 1988;16:1.
10. Wilberger JE. Minor head injuries in American football. *Sports Med* 1993;15:5.
11. Torg JS, et al. The National Football Head and Neck Injury Registry: 14 year report on cervical quadriplegia, 1971–1984. *JAMA* 1985;254:3439.
12. Bruce DA, Schut L, Sutton LN. Brain and cervical spine injuries in children and adolescents. *Prim Care* 1984;11(1):175–194.
13. Zariczny B, Shattuck LJ, Mast TA, et al. Sports related injuries in school age children. *Am J Sports Med* 1980;8:318–324.
14. Powell JW, Parber-Fass KD. Traumatic brain injury in high school athletes. *JAMA* 1999;282:958–963.
15. Hodgson VR. National operating committee on standards for athletic equipment: football helmet certification program. *Med Sci Sports* 1975;7:225–232.
16. Bishop PJ. Impact performance of ice hockey helmets. *Safety Res* 1978;10:123–129.
17. Mueller FO, Blyth CS. Fatalities from head and cervical spine injuries occurring in tackle football: 40 years' experience. *Clin Sports Med* 1987;6:185–196.
18. Cantu RC, Mueller F. Catastrophic spine injury in football 1977–1989. *J Spinal Dis* 1990;3:227.
19. Pforringer W, Smasal V. Aspects of traumatology in ice hockey. *J Sports Sci* 1987;5:327–336.
20. Goldsmith W. Performance of baseball headgear. *Am J Sports Med* 1982;10(1):31–37.
21. Dick, Randy. National Collegiate Athletic Administration. *Injury surveillance 1983–91*. Overland Park, KS.
22. Greensher J. Non-automotive vehicle injuries in adolescents. *Pediatr Ann* 1988;17:114–121.
23. Thompson RS, Rivara FP, Thompson DC. A case-control study of the effectiveness of bicycle safety helmets. *N Engl J Med* 1989;320:1361–1367.
24. Graham DI. Neuropathology of head injury. In: Narayan RK, Wilberger JE Jr, Povlishock JT, eds. *Neurotrauma*. New York: McGraw-Hill, 1996:46–47.
25. Bruno LA, Gennarelli TA, Torg JS. Management guidelines for head injuries in athletics. *Clin Sports Med* 1987;6:1.
26. Warren WL, Bailes JE. On the field evaluation of athletic head injuries. *Clin Sports Med* 1998;17(1):13–26.
27. Borczuk P. Predictors of intracranial injury in patients with mild head injury. *Ann Emerg Med* 1995;25:731–736.
28. Davis RL, Mullen N, Makela M, et al. Cranial computed tomography scans in children after minimal head injury with loss of consciousness. *Ann Emerg Med* 1994;24:640–645.
29. Hoffman JR. CT for head trauma in children. *Ann Emerg Med* 1995;24:713–715.
30. Jordan BD. Head injury in sports. In: Jordan BD, Tsairis, WR, eds. *Sports neurology*. Gaithersburg, MD: Aspen Publishers, 1990.
31. Lampert PW, Hardman JM. Morphological changes in brains of boxers. *JAMA* 1884;251(20):2676–2679.
32. Tysvaer AT, Storli OV, Bachen NI. Soccer injuries to the brain: a neurologic and electroencephalographic study of former players. *Acta Neurol Scand* 1989;80:151–156.
33. Levin HS, Williams D, Crofford MJ, et al. Relationship of depth of brain lesions to consciousness and outcome after closed head injury. *J Neurosurg* 1988;69(6):861–866.
34. Mittl RL, Grossman RI, Heihle JF, et al. Prevalence of MR evidence of diffuse axonal injury in patients with mild head injury and normal CT findings. *Am J Neuroradiol* 1994;15:1583–1589.
35. Gentry LR, Godersky JC, Thompson B, et al. Prospective comparative study of intermediate field MR and CT in the evaluation of closed head trauma. *Am J Neuroradiol* 1988;150:673.
36. Jenkins A, Teasdale G, Hadley DM, et al. Brain lesions detected by magnetic resonance imaging in mild and severe head injuries. *Lancet* 1986;iii:445.
37. Levin HS, Amparo E, Eisenberg JM, et al. Magnetic resonance imaging and computerized tomography in relation to the neurobehavioral sequelae of mild and moderate head injuries. *J Neurosurg* 1987;66:706–713.
38. Report of the Ad Hoc Committee to Study Head Injury Nomenclature. Proceedings of the Congress of Neurological Surgeons in 1964. *Clin Neurosurg* 1966;12:386–394.
39. Ryan AJ. Protecting the Sportsman's Brain. *Br J Sports Med* 1991;25(2):81–86.
40. Macciocchi SN, Barth JT, Littlefield LM. Outcome after mild head injury. *Clin Sports Med* 1998;17(1):27–36.
41. Elson LM, Ward CC. Mechanisms and pathophysiology of mild head injury. *Semin Neurol* 1994;14:8–18.
42. Adams H, Mitchell DE, Graham DI, et al. Diffuse brain damage of immediate impact type: its relationship to "primary" brain stem damage. *Brain* 1977;100:489–502.
43. Nevin NC. Neuropathological changes in the white matter following head injury. *J Neuropath Exp Neurol* 1967;26:77–84.
44. Peerless SJ, Rencastle NB. Shear injuries of the brain. *Can Med Assoc J* 1967;96:577–582.
45. Chason JL, Hardy WG, Webster JE, et al. Alterations in cell structure of the brain associated with experimental concussion. *J Neurosurg* 1958;15:135–139.
46. Hugenholtz H, Richard MT. Return to athletic competition following concussion. *Can Med Assoc J* 1982;127:827–829.
47. Ommaya AK. Head injury mechanisms and the concept of preventative management: a review and critical synthesis. *J Neurotrauma* 1996;12:527–546.
48. Ommaya AK, Gennarelli TA. Cerebral concussion and traumatic unconsciousness: correlation of experimental and clinical observations in blunt head injuries. *Brain* 1974;97:633–654.
49. Putukian M, Echemendia RJ. Managing successive minor head injuries: which tests guide return to play? *Physician Sportsmed* 1996;24(11):25–38.
50. Cantu RC, Micheli J, eds. *American College of Sports Medicine's*

guidelines for the team physician. Philadelphia: Lea & Febiger, 1991.
51. Katayama Y, Becker DP, Tamura T, et al. Massive increases in extracellular potassium and the indiscriminate release of glutamate following concussive brain injury. *J Neurosurg* 1990;73: 889–900.
52. Katayama Y, Cheung MK, Alves A, et al. Ion fluxes and cell swelling in experimental traumatic brain injury: the role of excitatory amino acids. In: Hoff JT, Betz AL, eds. *Intracranial pressure,* vol. 7. Berlin: Springer, 1989:584–588.
53. Yoshino A, Hovda DA, Katayama Y, et al. Hippocampal CA3 lesion prevents the post-concussive metabolic derangement in CA1. *J Cereb Blood Flow Metab* 1991;11[Suppl 2]:S343.
54. Yoshino A, Hovda DA, Kawamata T, et al. Dynamic changes in local cerebral glucose utilization following cerebral concussion in rats: Evidence of a hyper- and subsequent hypometabolic state. *Brain Res* 1991;561:106–119.
55. Yamakami I, McIntosh TK. Alterations in regional cerebral blood flow following brain injury in the rat. *J Cereb Blood Flow Metab* 1991;11:655–660.
56. Jenkins LW, Moszynski, Lyeth BG, et al. Increased vulnerability of the mildly traumatized rat brain to cerebral ischemia: the use of controlled secondary ischemia as a research tool to identify common or different mechanisms contributing to mechanical and ischemic brain injury. *Brain Res* 1989;477:211–224.
57. Hovda DA, Lee SM, Smith ML, et al. The Neurochemical and metabolic cascade following brain injury: moving from animal models to man. *J Neurotrauma* 1995;12(5):143–146.
58. Bergsneider M, Hovda DA, Shalmon E, et al. Cerebral hyperglycolysis following severe traumatic brain injury in humans: a positron emission tomography study. *J Neurosurg* 1997;86:241–251.
59. Kleiner DM, Cantu RC. Football helmet removal. American College of Sports Medicine, Current Comment, Indianapolis, IN, 1996.
60. Edna TH. Acute traumatic intracranial hematoma and skull fracture. *Acta Chir Scand* 1983;149:449–451.
61. Marion DW. Head injuries. In: Fu FH, Stone DA, eds. *Sports injuries: mechanisms, prevention, treatment.* Baltimore: Williams & Wilkins, 1994:813–831.
62. Henderson JM, Browning DG. Head trauma in young athletes. *Med Clin North Am* 1994;78(2):289–303.
63. Cantu RC. Epilepsy and athletics. *Clin Sports Med* 1998; 17(1):61–69.
64. Bornstein RA, Miller HB, van Schoor JT. Neuropsychological deficit and emotional disturbance in head-injured patients. *J Neurosurg* 1989;70:509–513.
65. Brown SJ, Fann JR, Grant I. Postconcussional disorder: time to acknowledge a common source of neurobehavioral morbidity. *J Neuropsychiatry Clin Neurosci* 1994;6:15–22.
66. Packard RC, Ham LP. Pathogenesis of post traumatic headache and migraine: a common headache pathway? *Headache* 1997; 37(3):142–152.
67. Rizzo M. Overview of head injury and postconcussive syndrome. In: Rizzo M, Tranel D, eds. *Head injury and postconcussive syndrome.* New York: Churchill Livingstone, 1996:1–18.
68. Troncosco JC, Gordon B. Neuropathology of closed head injury. In: Rizzo M, Tranel D, eds. *Head injury and postconcussive syndrome.* New York: Churchill Livingstone, 1996:47–56.
69. Barcellos S, Rizzo M. Post-traumatic headaches. In: Rizzo M, Tranel D, eds. *Head injury and postconcussive syndrome.* New York: Churchill Livingstone 1996:139–175.
70. Schneider RC. *Head and neck injuries in football.* Baltimore: Williams & Wilkins, 1973.
71. McQuillen JB, McQuillen EN, Morrow P. Trauma, sports, and malignant cerebral edema. *Am J Forensic Med Path* 1988; 9:12–15.
72. Bruce DA, Alavi A, Bilaniuk L, et al. Diffuse cerebral swelling following head injuries in children: the syndrome of "malignant brain edema." *J Neurosurg* 1981;54:170–178.
73. Cantu RC. Second-impact syndrome. *Clin Sports Med* 1998; 17(1):37–44.
74. Quality Standards Subcommittee, American Academy of Neurology, Practice Parameter. The management of concussion in sports (summary statement). *Neurology* 1997;48:581–585.
75. Cantu RC. Return to play guidelines after a head injury. *Clin Sports Med* 1998;17(1):45–60.
76. Colorado Medical Society. *Guidelines for the management of concussion in sports.* Colorado Medical Society, Sports Medicine Committee, May 1990 (revised May 1991).
77. Nelson WE, Jane JA, Gieck JH. Minor head injury in sports: a new classification and management. *Phys Sportsmed* 1984; 12(3):103–107.
78. Torg JS. *Athletic injuries to the head, neck, and face.* St. Louis: Mosby-Year Book, 1991.
79. Kelly JP, Rosenburg JH. Diagnosis and management of concussion in sport. *Neurology* 1997;48:575–580.
80. Lovell MR, Iverson GL, Collins MW, et al. Does loss of consciousness predict neuropsychological decrements after concussion? *Clin J Sports Med* 1999;9:193–198.
81. Zemper E. Analysis of cerebral concussion frequency with the most commonly used models of football helmets. *J Athletic Training* 1994;29(1):44–50.
82. Abreau F, Templer DI, Schuyler BA, et al. Neuropsychological assessment of soccer players. *Neuropsychology* 1990;4:175–181.
83. Rimel RW, Giordani B, Barth JT, et al. Disability caused by minor head injury. *Neurosurgery* 1981;9(3):221–228.
84. Rimel RW, Giordani B, Barth JT, et al. Moderate head injury: completing the clinical spectrum of brain trauma. *Neurosurgery* 1982;11(3):344–351.
85. Alves WM, Rimel RW, Nelson WE. University of Virginia prospective study of football-induced minor head injury: status report. *Clin Sports Med* 1987;6(1):211–218.
86. Tysvaer AT, Lochen EA. Soccer injuries to the brain: a neuropsychologic study of former soccer players. *Am J Sports Med* 1991;19(1):56–60.
87. McLatchie G, Brooks N, Galbraith S, et al. Clinical neurological examination, neuropsychology, electroencephalography and computed tomography head scanning in active amateur boxers. *J Neurol Neurosurg Psychiatry* 1987;50:96–99.
88. Porter MD, Fricker PA. Controlled prospective neuropsychological assessment of active experienced amateur boxers. *Clin J Sports Med* 1996;6:90–96.
89. Putukian M, Echemendia RJ, Phillips TG. Neuropsychological baseline testing in the management of head injured college athletes: the Penn State Concussion Program. Presented at American Medical Society for Sports Medicine Annual Meeting, Colorado Springs Colorado, April 6, 1997.
90. Guskiewicz KM, Riemann BL, Perrin DH, et al. Alternative approaches to the assessment of mild head injury in athletes. *Med Sci Sports Exerc* 1997;27(7):213–221.
91. Kirkpatrick PJ. Use of near-infrared spectroscopy in the adult. *Philos Trans R Soc Lond B Biol Sci* 1997;352(1354):701–705.
92. Robertson CS, Gopinath SP, Chance B. A new application for near-infrared spectroscopy: detection of delayed intracranial hematomas after head injury. *J Neurotrauma* 1995;12(4):591–600.
93. Masdeu JC, Abdel-Dayem H, Van Heertum RL. Head trauma: use of SPECT. *J Neuroimaging* 1995;5[Suppl 1]:S53–S57.
94. Lewis DH. Functional brain imaging with cerebral perfusion SPECT in cerebrovascular disease, epilepsy, and trauma. *Neurosurg Clin North Am* 1997;8(3):337–344.
95. James CA. Magnetic resonance angiography in trauma. *Clin Neurosci* 1997;4(3):137–145.
96. Ono J, Harada K, Takahashi J, et al. Differentiation between dysmyelination and demyelination using magnetic resonance diffusional anisotropy. *Brain Res* 1995;671(1):141–148.
97. Haglund Y, Eriksson E. Does amateur boxing lead to chronic brain damage? a review of some recent investigations. *Am J Sports Med* 1993;21:97–109.
98. Martland HS. Punch drunk. *JAMA* 1928;91:1103–1107.
99. Millspaugh JA. Dementia pugilistica. *US Naval Med Bull* 1937; 35:297.
100. Critchley M. Medical aspects of boxing, particularly from a neurological standpoint. *Br Med J* 1957;1:357–362.
101. Mortimer JA. Epidemiology of post-traumatic encephalopathy in boxers. *Minn Med* 1985;68:299–300.
102. Jordan B, Zimmerman R. Computed tomography and magnetic resonance imaging comparisons in boxers. *JAMA* 1990;263: 1670–1674.

103. Jordan B, Jahre C, Hauser A, et al. CT of 338 active professional boxers. *Radiology* 1992;185:509–512.
104. Bogdanoff B, Natter H. Incidence of cavum septum pellucidum in athletes: a sign of boxer's encephalopathy. *Neurology* 1989; 39:991–992.
105. Wilberger JE Jr, and Maroon JC. Head injuries in athletes. *Clin Sports Med* 1989;8:1.
106. Burslem I, Lees A. Quantification of impact accelerations of the head during the heading of a football. In: Reilly T, Lees A, Davids K, et al., eds. *Science and football: proceedings of the First World Congress of Science and Football.* London: E&FN Spon Ltd, 1987:243–248.
107. Tysvaer AT. Head and neck injuries in soccer: impact of minor trauma. *Sports Med* 1992;14(3):200–213.
108. Schneider PG, Lichte H. Untersuchungen zur groesse der krafteinwirkung beim kopfballspiel des fussballers. *Sportarzut und sportmedizin* 1975;26:10.
109. Smodlaka VN. Medical aspects of heading the ball in soccer. *Phys Sportsmed* 1984;12(2):127–131.
110. Sortland O, Tysvaer AT, Storli OV. Changes in the cervical spine in association football players. *Br J Sports Med* 1982;16: 80–84.
111. Jordan SH, Green GA, Galanty HL, et al. Acute and chronic brain injury in United States national team soccer players. *Am J Sports Med* 1996;24(2):205–210.
112. Green GA, Jordan SE. Chronic head and neck injuries. In: Garrett WE, Kirkendall DT, Contiguglia SR, eds. *The US soccer sports medicine book.* Baltimore: Williams & Wilkins, 1994: 191–204.
113. Boden BP, Kirkendall DT, Garrett WE. Concussion incidence in elite college soccer players. *Am J Sports Med* 1998;26:238–241.
114. Matser EJT, Kessels AG, Lezak MD, et al. Neuropsychological impairment in amateur soccer players. *JAMA* 1999;282:971–973.
115. Matser EJT, Kessels AG, Jordan BD, et al. Chronic traumatic brain injury in professional soccer players. *Neurology* 1998;51: 791–796.
116. Putukian M, Echemendia RJ, Macken S. The acute neuropsycholgical effects of heading in soccer: A pilot study. *Clin J Sports Med* 2000;10:104–109.

CHAPTER 31

Abdominal Injuries

Cindy J. Chang, Howard C. Lin, and Julie A. Pryde

INTRODUCTION

Injuries to the abdomen can occur with any sport but are more often seen in those involving sudden deceleration and impact, such as football, ice hockey, skiing, or mountain biking. Although these injuries do not occur as frequently as injuries to the extremities, it is imperative that they be immediately recognized and appropriately managed. Unfortunately, the situation can often be life threatening when involving the internal organs, and the hallmarks of an accurate evaluation include repeated assessments and a high index of suspicion. Once a severe abdominal injury has been recognized, standard protocol, including stabilization and transfer to the nearest emergency facility, should be followed.

Less minor in severity, but with an obviously important impact on an athlete's ability to participate in his or her sport, are the traumatic and overuse types of injuries involving the abdominal musculature. Essential elements to full recovery of these injuries are the length of relative rest and the type of rehabilitation prescribed. These are dependent on the type of injury sustained, as well as the type of surgery that may have been performed.

SPLENIC INJURIES

The spleen is the most commonly injured organ in the abdomen. Contributing to its high incidence of injury are its anatomic location and its ligamentous attachments, which fix the organ in the peritoneal cavity (Fig. 31–1). Decelerating forces lead the stomach and transverse colon to produce shearing motions on the splenic capsule and vessels. The incidence of splenic injuries ranges from 11.2% to 30% in studies of patients with traumatic abdominal injuries [1,2]. The risk of splenic rupture increases with the presence of infectious illnesses such as infectious mononucleosis, malaria, and typhoid fever, as well as certain pathologic disease processes such as sarcoidosis, lymphoma, and hemolytic anemias, which cause enlargement of the spleen. In the athletic population the mechanism of injury relates to a blunt traumatic force to the left upper abdomen and lower chest.

Initial symptoms include left upper quadrant pain radiating to the left flank or left shoulder (Kehr's sign), which can progress to diffuse abdominal tenderness and distension. The pain can be exacerbated by inspiration. There may also be the presence of fixed dullness in the left flank (Ballance's sign) as well as neck pain referred from phrenic nerve pressure (Seagasser's sign) [3]. Significant blood loss causing hemodynamic compromise can occur fairly early, although nonspecific symptoms such as nausea, vomiting, and tachycardia may be the only initial symptoms. There may be associated left-sided tenth to twelfth rib fractures and abdominal contusions. Lab values may be variable depending on the severity and timing of the injury. The hemoglobin and hematocrit may not be significantly lowered for 6–8 hours postinjury if the spleen is bleeding slowly. There also may be an elevated white blood cell count from a demargination effect seen in acute stress.

Decision for nonoperative management versus surgical intervention may be aided by the use of diagnostic peritoneal lavage (DPL) and/or computed tomography (CT) scan of the abdomen. DPL is the preferred method of assessing an unstable patient, given its high sensitivity for identifying intraabdominal bleeding. The presence of 5 mL of free blood or greater than 100,000 red blood

---

C. J. Chang: Intercollegiate Athletics and University Health Services, University of California–Berkeley, Berkeley, California 94720; Departments of Family and Community Medicine, University of California–San Francisco and University of California–Davis, San Francisco, California 94110 and Sacramento, California 95817.

H. C. Lin: Intercollegiate Athletics and University Health Services, University of California–Berkeley, Berkeley, California 94720; Departments of Internal Medicine and Sports Medicine, Kaiser Permanente Medical Center, Santa Clara, California 95051.

J. A. Pryde: Department of Physical Therapy, Samuel Merritt College, Oakland, California 94609.

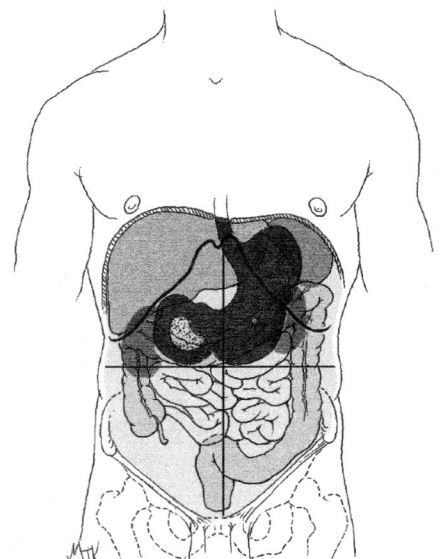

FIG. 31-1. Abdominal anatomy with quadrant separation.

cells/mm³ in the lavaged fluid is noted as a positive test. Contraindications to the DPL are indication for immediate laparotomy, pregnancy, pelvic fracture, significant obesity, and coagulopathy.

CT is more useful in stable patients because of the ability for selective management of solid organ injuries, though bowel, pancreas, and diaphragmatic injuries have a lower detection rate. This may be improved by the use of oral and rectal contrasts. The CT studies allow classification of the splenic injury into the American Association for Surgical Trauma Spleen Injury Scale (4) (Table 31-1). Success in splenic salvaging courses occur in the grade I to II injuries, though early detection of grade II to III injuries may improve the outcome of nonoperative course or even splenic repair (splenorrhaphy) (5).

More recently, ultrasound has been evaluated in its role as an emergent trauma screening tool for intraabdominal fluid and for organ injuries. The sensitivity for detecting free intraperitoneal fluid ranges from 81% to 100.0%, and the specificity ranges from 92.0% to 100% (6). However, sensitivity for organ lesion detection is much poorer, as low as 43.6% in one study, though specificity was much better at 99.6% in the same study (6). It is thought that the ultrasound is much better at rapid assessment of intraperitoneal fluid than at screening for solid organ injuries. Table 31-2 offers a comparison of these screening modalities.

Though sepsis in postsplenectomy patients has decreased in the era of vaccination and improved health care delivery, it remains important to spare the patient from unnecessary surgical risks, the risk of postsplenectomy infectious sequelae, and asplenic thrombocytosis when reasonably feasible. When conservative therapy is chosen, admission into an intensive care unit with aggressive delivery of crystalloid and blood products to replace hypovolemia is initiated with close monitoring of hemodynamics. Stable patients who do not require blood transfusions can be monitored on the surgical ward. Strict bed rest is enforced for 2–3 days, and mobilization thereafter is recommended on the basis of the clinical progress of the patients. The total hospital stay usually ranges from 7 to 14 days (7). However, if blood transfusions exceed 4 units over 48 hours, exploratory laparotomy should be considered for control of bleeding and splenorrhaphy. Because of their increased susceptibility to sepsis from encapsulated organisms, splenectomy patients should be considered for vaccination against encapsulated organisms such as *Streptococcus pneumoniae*, *Haemophilus influenzae*, and *Neisseria meningitidis*. In the nonsplenectomy cases, follow-up CT scan or ultrasound can be performed at 1- to 2-month intervals after discharge from the hospital until documentation of healing (7) (Fig. 31-2A-D).

A recent study attempts to predict follow-up time for ultrasonography (8). Using Buntain's classification of splenic injuries, ultrasound images are obtained at specified time periods correlating to severity of splenic injury on the initial CT scan, then subsequently followed at 4-week intervals until ultrasonographic documentation of healing is achieved. However, CT confirmation may still be needed in the follow-up evaluation of a fractured but healed spleen. Return to contact sports

TABLE 31-1. *Spleen injury classification*

Grade	Injury type	Injury description
I	Hematoma	Subcapsular, <10% surface area
	Laceration	Capsular tear, <1 cm parenchymal depth
II	Hematoma	Subcapsular, 10–50% surface area; intraparenchymal, <5 cm in diameter
	Laceration	1–3 cm parenchymal depth which does not involve a trabecular vessel
III	Hematoma	Subcapsular, >50% surface area or expanding; ruptured subcapsular or parenchymal hematoma Intraparenchymal hematoma >5 cm or expanding
	Laceration	>3 cm parenchymal depth or involving trabecular vessels
IV	Laceration	Laceration involving segmental or hilar vessels producing major devascularization (>25% of spleen)
V	Laceration	Completely shattered spleen
	Vascular	Hilar vascular injury that devascularizes spleen

From Moore EE, Cogbill TH, Jurkovich GJ, et al. Organ injury scaling: spleen and liver (1994 revision). *J Trauma* 1995;38(3):323–324.

TABLE 31–2. *Comparison of screening modalities in abdominal trauma*

Method	Advantages	Disadvantages
Ultrasound	Bedside availability Rapid use Noninvasive Widespread availability Easy to repeat Assess retroperitoneum	Operator dependent Obscured by obesity and subcutaneous emphysema Composition of fluid not assessed
Diagnostic peritoneal lavage	Widespread availability Detection of bowel contents Detection of abdominal fluid and composition	Invasive Possible complications Multiple contraindications Possibly time consuming Does not assess retroperitoneum
Computed tomography	Noninvasive Reproducibility Assess retroperitoneum	May not be easily accessible Need for contrast Radiation Time consuming Dependent on stable and cooperative patient

Rothlin MA, Naf R, Amgwerd M, et al. Ultrasound in blunt abdominal and thoracic trauma. *J Trauma* 1993;34(4):488–495.

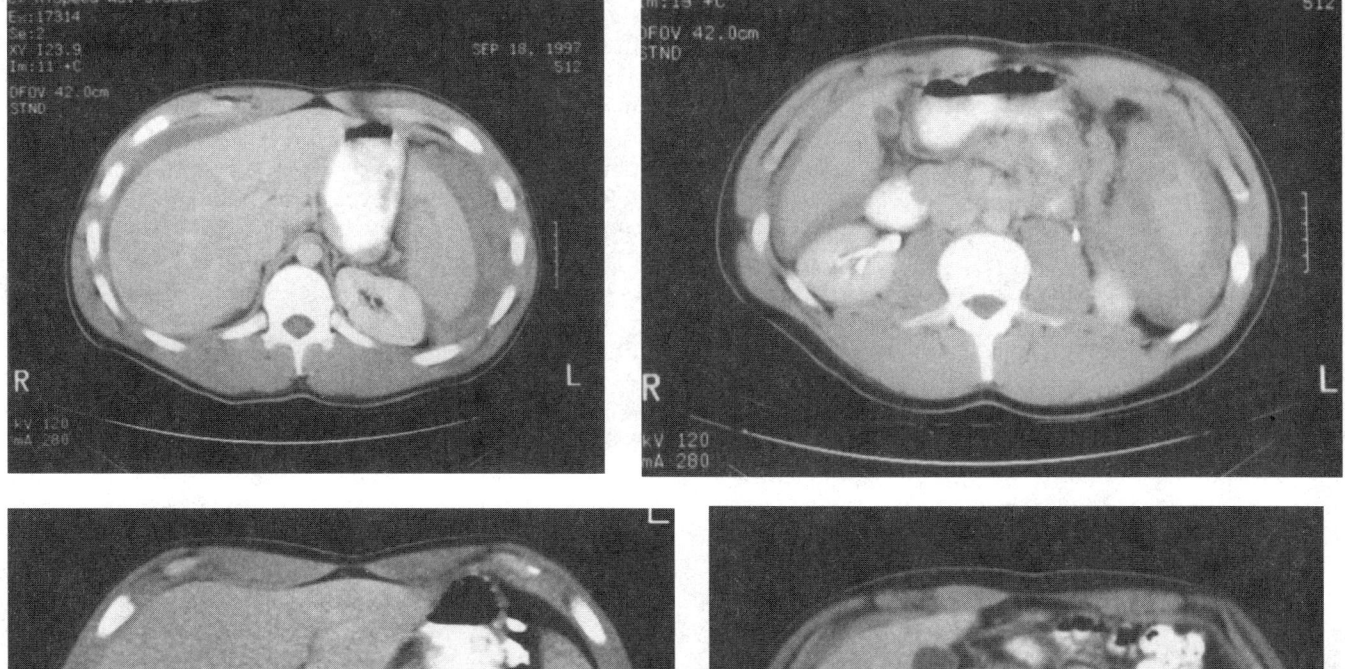

FIG. 31–2. **A** and **B:** CT scans of ruptured spleen in a 19-year-old baseball player on the day of injury. Note also the hemoperitoneum surrounding both the spleen and liver. **C** and **D:** CT scans at same approximate levels 3 months later (taken at a different facility). The spleen is now normal in size with homogeneous density.

TABLE 31-3. *Buntain's splenic injury classification with recommended period for follow-up ultrasound*

Grade	Description of inury	Initial follow-up ultrasound
I	Localized capsular disruption or subcapsular hematoma without significant parenchymal injury	4 weeks
II	Single or multiple capsular and parenchymal disruptions that do not extend into hilum or involve major blood vessels	8 weeks
III	Major blood vessels	12 weeks
IV	Completely shattered or fragmented spleen or separated from its normal blood supply at the pedicle	20 weeks

From Lynch JM, Meza MP, Newman B, et al. Computed tomography grade of splenic injury is predictive of the time required for radiographic healing. *J Pediatr Surg* 1997; 32(7):1093–1096.

is generally discouraged for a minimum of 3 months (Table 31-3).

A subset of splenic ruptures mentioned above may occur during infectious mononucleosis in the active person. Caused by the Epstein-Barr virus, splenomegaly is seen in 50–75% of cases by week 2, occasionally accompanied by hepatomegaly (9) (Fig. 31-3). Most patients recover within 4–6 weeks though some patients require 4–6 months before returning to full function. Delayed ruptures typically occur between 2–4 weeks of onset of illness. Most cases occur with simple Valsalva maneuvers such as sneezing, lifting objects, straining to defecate, or coughing. A full discussion of this infection is included in Chapter 18 on infectious mononucleosis in the athlete.

LIVER INJURIES

The liver is probably the second most commonly injured organ in the abdomen, owing to its large size and anatomic location. The incidence of liver injuries has ranged from 4.4% to 4.9% of pediatric abdominal injuries (10,11). It should be considered in blunt trauma to the right upper abdomen or lower chest and from the front, back, or right side. Associated findings include rib fractures, typically the tenth to twelfth ribs, and right upper quadrant pain with or without radiating pain to the right shoulder. Hypovolemic shock is not uncommon in significant liver injuries, though abdominal discomfort, nausea, vomiting may be the only initial symptoms. Diagnostic peritoneal lavage and abdominal CT scan may confirm suspected liver lacerations (Fig. 31-4).

In the initial triage, multiple large-bore (16 gauge) intravenous catheters should be started with large amounts of crystalloid and blood available for replacement. As in many blunt injuries to the solid organs in the abdomen, there has been considerable advancement in the conservative nonoperative care of liver injuries. To meet criteria for conservative care, a patient must maintain hemodynamic stability after initial resuscitation, have no preexisting liver disease that would complicate the bleeding, and be able to be monitored in an intensive care unit. Success in nonoperative management is seen primarily in the grade I to III injuries (Table 31-4).

Once the injury is identified, the patient is admitted to the intensive care unit for strict bed rest and observation. Blood transfusions are given as needed, though some have argued for a limitation of 2 units of packed red blood cells in 24 hours to maintain a conservative course (12). Patients who maintain hemodynamic stability after 48–72 hours can be transferred to the ward, with gradual progression of activity level over the next

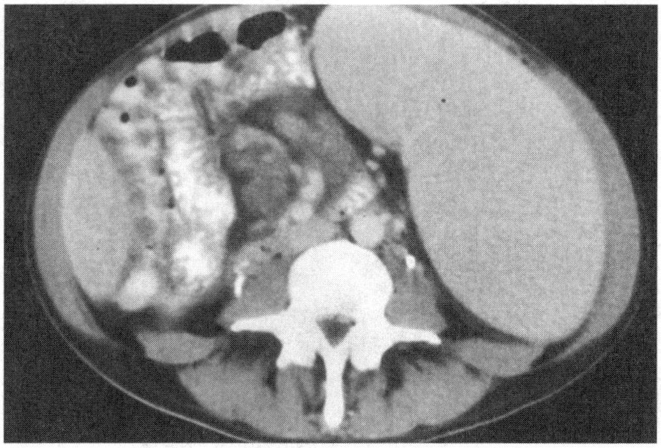

FIG. 31-3. CT scan of splenomegaly from infectious mononucleosis.

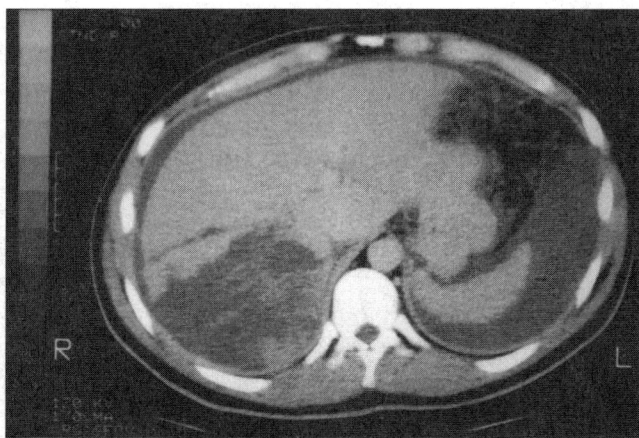

FIG. 31-4. CT scan of liver laceration with huge hemoperitoneum in a 28-year-old male who was involved in motorcycle trauma.

TABLE 31-4. *Liver injury classification*

Grade	Injury type	Injury description
I	Hematoma	Subcapsular, <10 % surface area
	Laceration	Capsular tear, <1 cm parenchymal depth
II	Hematoma	Subcapsular, 10–50% surface area: intraparenchymal, <10 cm in diameter
	Laceration	1–3 cm parenchymal depth, <10 cm in length
III	Hematoma	Subcapsular, >50% surface area or expanding; ruptured subcapsular or parenchymal hematoma Intraparenchymal hematoma, >10 cm or expanding
	Laceration	>3 cm parenchymal depth
IV	Laceration	Parenchymal disruption involving 25–75% of hepatic lobe or 1–3 Coulnaud's segments within a single lobe
V	Laceration	Parenchymal disruption involving >75% of hepatic lobe or >3 Coulnaud's segments within a single lobe
	Vascular	Juxtahepatic venous injuries; i.e., retrohepatic vena cava/central major hepatic veins
VI	Vascular	Hepatic avulsion

From Moore EE, Cogbill TH, Jurkovich GJ, et al. Organ injury scaling: spleen and liver (1994 revision). *J Trauma* 1995;38(3):323–324.

14 days. If there is any deterioration of hemodynamic stability, surgical intervention should be initiated without delay with consideration for celiotomy and exploration for concomitant abdominal injuries. A repeat CT scan or ultrasound should be repeated at 10–14 days and should be followed up in 2–4 weeks and at 2- to 6-month intervals until complete healing is noted (13). At this time most physicians would agree that full activity may be resumed with a normal CT scan or ultrasound. Common complications of liver injuries include delayed rupture of hematomas, hemobilia, bile leak, and infection.

HOLLOW VISCOUS INJURIES

Blunt injuries to the stomach, small bowel, and intestine remain rare, but typical mechanisms of injury include a fall onto bicycle handlebars, direct blows to the abdomen from a helmet or hockey stick, and diving decompression accidents. The mechanisms that have been proposed include a sudden increase in the intraluminal pressure, compression of the small bowel against the vertebrae, and deceleration at or near a point of fixation. Previous abdominal surgeries with adhesion formations have also been postulated as a possible risk factor for intestinal injury.

Deceleration injuries can lead to mesentery avulsion and devascularization of the small bowel, avulsion of the stomach near the pylorus where it is anchored by the retroperitoneal duodenum, and intramural hematomas. Sixty to seventy-five percent of intestinal injuries are associated with other abdominal injuries (14). A transverse fracture through the lower thoracic or lumbar vertebra (Chance fracture) should be suspicious for associated bowel injuries.

Initial presenting signs and symptoms may include abdominal contusion with diffuse abdominal and back pain, progressing to nausea, vomiting, absent bowel sounds, abdominal distension, bloody stool, and peritoneal signs. Physical examination findings may also reveal flank percussion dullness and tenderness. Hypotension and tachycardia may appear with concomitant vascular or solid organ injuries or portend a progression to intraperitoneal sepsis. Digital rectal examination for blood is indicated in all suspected rectal trauma.

DPL may detect early intraabdominal injuries, though sensitivity may decrease in the case of the duodenum and colon because of the retroperitoneal position of the organs. Free air under the diaphragm or along the iliopsoas muscle may be seen on plain upright or decubitus radiographs, though sensitivity is less than 50% in patients with intestinal perforation from blunt trauma (14). Bowel edema, air fluid levels, and ileus may be detected on plain radiographs. CT scan with water-soluble oral and rectal contrast may help to define intramural edema or air in the duodenum, jejunum, and colorectal regions as well as reveal pneumoperitoneum and extravasation of contrast (Fig. 31–5). Nasogastric tube placement to check for gastric blood is neither

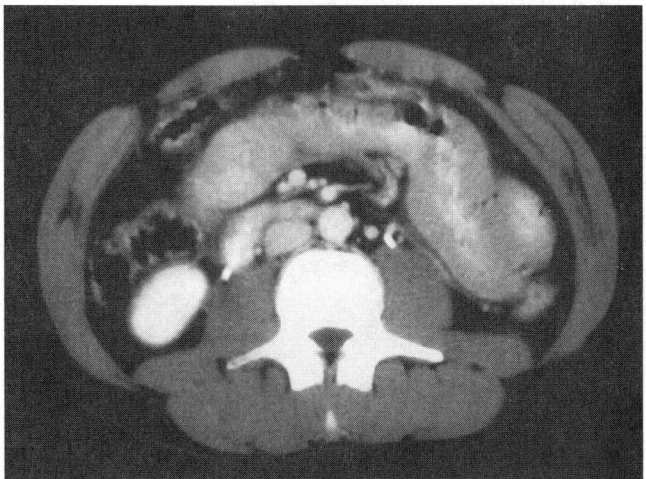

FIG. 31-5. CT scan of rupture of the proximal jejunum with small hemoperitoneum. Note the edema and free air in the bowel wall.

sensitive nor specific for other sites of injury. Morbidity and mortality are related to the relative speed of diagnosis and development of intraperitoneal sepsis before intervention. Urgent intraoperative exploration and repair are indicated in suspected hollow viscous injuries.

Interestingly, there have been case reports of delayed intestinal obstructions. These may occur from 10 days to 6 weeks after the abdominal trauma (15). Therefore the clinician should maintain vigilance for evidence of bowel obstructions in follow-up evaluations even with negative initial assessments at the time of injury.

PANCREATIC INJURIES

Though not frequently injured in sports, the pancreas can be at risk for life-threatening injury because of late recognition of associated intraabdominal injuries such as liver lacerations, bowel injuries, and major vessel lacerations, leading to development of systemic sepsis and hemodynamic instability. Overall, mortality in such patients with delayed diagnosis is estimated at 20%, with nearly all deaths occurring in the first 48 hours (16,17).

If suspected, serum amylase level can be obtained, along with an abdominal CT with water-soluble oral contrast. Hyperamylasemia may be seen in significant pancreatic injuries, but a direct correlation between elevated serum amylase levels and the degree of pancreatic injury is questionable. CT scan is helpful in assessing for hematoma or transection of the pancreas, in addition to screening for concomitant abdominal injuries (Fig. 31-6). A positive DPL is helpful, but a negative one does not exclude retroperitoneal injury. In addition, the testing of amylase level in the peritoneal lavage fluid may be misleading, given that elevation of the amylase level in the peritoneal fluid often is not evident for 24-48 hours.

Injuries are distributed fairly evenly among the head, body, and tail of the pancreas. The typical mechanism is a direct blow to the midabdomen from football helmets, bicycle handlebars, or karate kicks. Clinical symptoms include diffuse abdominal pain with possible peritoneal signs and hypovolemia. Hemorrhagic signs include bruising noted in periumbilical or left flank regions (Cullen and Turner-Grey signs).

Localized resection and/or percutaneous drainage can manage most injuries. Late complications include infection and development of pseudocysts, which can cause persistent abdominal pain, nausea, and vomiting. Antibiotic and percutaneous drainage are indicated in those situations, though a partial pancreatectomy may occasionally be needed for persistent pancreatic edema or hemorrhage. CT scan follow-ups can sometimes demonstrate cleaved pancreas posthealing, without further sequelae.

DIAPHRAGMATIC RUPTURE

Traumatic injuries to the diaphragm occur due to a high intraperitoneal force, usually resulting from severe blunt trauma. There is a high incidence of associated injuries to other abdominal organs such as splenic ruptures (25-50%), liver lacerations (10-50%), pelvic fractures (30-50%), and thoracic aorta tears (3-10%) (18). Left-sided injuries are 4-5 times more common than right-sided ruptures (possibly because of the presence of the large fixed liver) with the possible migration of stomach, spleen, or colon into the left hemithorax (18,19).

Presenting symptoms may be chest pain, shortness of breath, and nausea or vomiting, with physical examination revealing decreased breath sounds or even bowel sounds in the left lung field. Clinical examination is typically poor for diagnosis, however, and only 31% of diaphragmatic injuries are diagnosed before surgery (18).

Although diaphragmatic injuries may be suspected on chest radiographs, only 25-30% are actually diagnostic for diaphragmatic rupture (20-22). Typical features on the radiograph include an elevated or indistinct hemidiaphragm, blunted costophrenic angle, and hemopneumoperitoneum. A nasogastric tube may be seen on radiograph to curl back into the left hemithorax. CT scan and ultrasound have not proven to be useful tools for routine initial screening diaphragmatic hernias, though they are performed for evaluation of concomitant abdominal organ injuries (Fig. 31-7). Laparoscopy and thoracoscopy may be useful, though exploratory laparotomy remains the standard, as other abdominal injuries may be evaluated at the same time.

Treatment of the rupture is usually a primary repair. Complications include subdiaphragmatic abscess, pneumonia, empyema, and sequelae of associated injuries. The overall mortality rate falls in the 20-25% range (18).

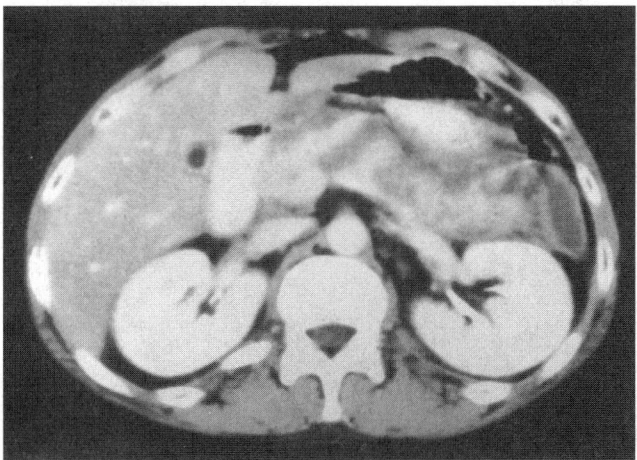

FIG. 31-6. CT scan of a pancreatic fracture.

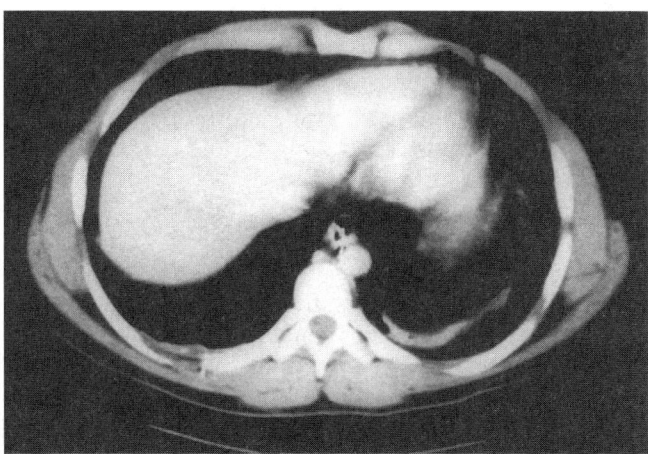

FIG. 31–7. CT scan of a diaphragmatic rupture. Note the presence of fatty tissue in the left hemithorax.

shearing forces that are distributed across a bony prominence of the pelvis or lower rib cage (23).

Most often, there is a preexisting condition with a potential for development of a hernia, such as a predisposing weakness of abdominal muscle or fascia or a partly obliterated processus vaginalis. In the latter case a strong impact to the lower abdomen can cause an expansion of the small bowel loops inside the tunica vaginalis (24), producing acute pain and swelling of only the scrotum.

Most of the time, hernias produce no symptoms until either the athlete notices a lump in the groin or sudden pain and swelling appear during some strenuous activity such as weight lifting. Some may complain of an aching sensation or radiation of pain into the scrotum.

A hernia can be diagnosed in a standing position, in a relaxed position when supine, or during maneuvers that increase intraabdominal pressure, such as a Valsalva maneuver or cough. Often the only symptom with which the athlete will present is an aching sensation and occasionally tender swelling in the area of the hernia.

In the case of an incisional hernia (or ventral hernia) a bulge along the operative scar is present, especially during abdominal contraction (Fig. 31–8A). About 10% of all abdominal operations result in incisional hernias. The etiologic factors are many, including postoperative wound infection, poor surgical technique, and obesity. A controversial factor is the type of incision used; some argue that transverse and oblique wounds heal better than vertical ones, while paramedian incisions heal better than midline ones (25). Incisional hernias should be repaired early to avoid bowel obstruction or at least should be controlled with a corset until definitive therapy is considered. Recurrence rates range from 2–5% to as high as 25%, depending on the size of the hernia, and these rates increase with each subsequent repair.

HERNIAS

The protrusion of any structure through a weak point in the abdominal wall is a hernia. The hernia can be congenital or acquired. In a majority of cases a hernia will involve only an empty peritoneal sac. However, if the contents of a hernia include bowel, for example, there is increased potential for an incarceration (irreducible hernia) or strangulation (twisting of the hernia), which may lead to interruption of blood supply, bowel obstruction, and toxicity. A Richter hernia, which occurs when only a part of the circumference of the bowel wall becomes incarcerated or strangulated, is uncommon but very dangerous. Although this type of hernia can spontaneously reduce (return to the abdomen), the compromised bowel section resulting in gangrene can be overlooked, and peritonitis from its perforation can result.

The three most common hernias in adults are indirect inguinal, direct inguinal, and femoral. Seventy-five percent of hernias occur in the groin; other abdominal wall hernias include incisional or ventral hernias (10%), umbilical and paraumbilical hernias (3%), and epigastric or linea alba defects. Occasionally, an indirect hernia can enter the scrotum; these are then called scrotal hernias.

The most frequent mechanism of injury for hernias is repetitive lifting activities; activities that increase the intraabdominal pressure, such as tackling during football or rugby; or rowing. A lower abdominal blow can also cause a sudden increase in intraabdominal pressure, or the trauma can directly cause a hernia, such as the impact from a bicycle handlebar on the abdominal wall. The traumatic hernias may either involve a considerable blunt force that is distributed over a surface area large enough to prevent frank penetration but small enough to remain focal (e.g., a handlebar of a bicycle) or involve

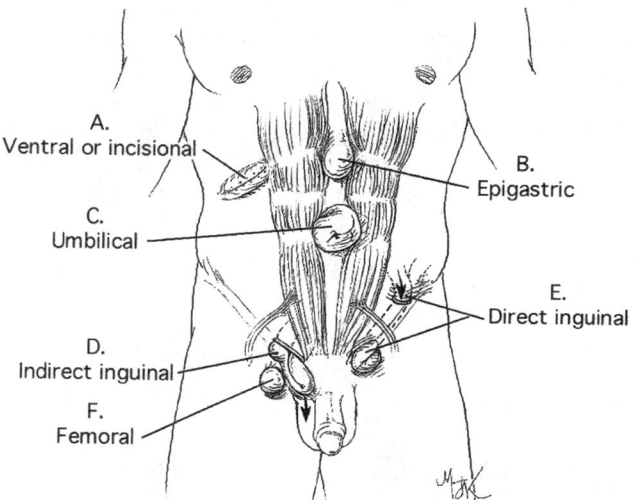

FIG. 31–8. The locations of various abdominal hernias.

An epigastric hernia, also known as fatty hernia of the linea alba, is more easily palpated than seen in the midline of the epigastric region (Fig. 31–8B). It usually consists of only a small bulge of fat protruding from an opening in the linea alba above the level of the umbilicus and can occasionally be reduced. Larger hernias can occasionally contain a loop of bowel. The athlete may present with symptoms similar to those of peptic ulcer disease with some relief in the supine position, but most epigastric hernias are painless. Three to five percent of the population are affected, with increased frequency in men and those between the ages of 20 and 50. Twenty percent of epigastric hernias are multiple in nature (25). Repair is recommended because of the risk of incarceration, especially in the smaller hernias. However, the recurrence rate is high at 10–20%, probably because of the failure to recognize and repair multiple small defects (25).

There are two types of umbilical hernias: congenital type and adult type (paraumbilical) (Fig. 31–8C). In either the navel may protrude during relaxation or when intraabdominal pressure is increased when standing. In the congenital type, palpation of the umbilical ring reveals a complete fibrous collar continuous with the linea alba. This is frequently found in newborns, especially premature infants. Forty to ninety percent of black newborns, compared to 10% of white newborns, are born with umbilical hernias (26). However, defects that are less than 1 cm in diameter will close by 6 years of age in 95% of cases. Although incarceration rarely occurs in this type of hernia, surgical repair is indicated if the defect is greater than 1 cm and in all children over 4 years of age (27).

In the adult type, the collar is not present; rather, the fascial ring is incomplete, and the superior portion of the hernia is covered only by skin. The adult type more frequently develops with long-standing increase in intraabdominal or intrathoracic pressure, such as with pregnancy, ascites, or chronic pulmonary disease. It is more common in women than men, and rather than resolving spontaneously like the congenital type, it increases steadily in size. Strangulation is also more common, as the neck of the hernia is quite narrow in comparison to the size of the herniated mass; therefore repair is recommended. Sharp pain can be experienced during coughing or straining, and the very large hernias produce a constant aching sensation.

In over 80% of newborn infants the processus vaginalis, the peritoneal extension whereby the testis descended into the scrotum, remains patent. However, by 2 years only 40–50% remain patent, and by adulthood 25% are still open (27). An indirect inguinal hernia occurs when the sac passes through the internal inguinal ring, the defect in the transversalis fascia halfway between the anterior iliac spine and the pubic tubercle (Fig. 31–8D). Although the hernia may have been "congenital," the clinical symptoms usually do not appear until years later when increased intraabdominal pressure and dilatation of the internal inguinal ring occur. Typically, if an inguinal hernia is found in infancy or childhood, it is repaired soon after diagnosis. Bilateral hernias are found in 15% of cases.

In the male the inguinal canal, which lies just above and parallel to the inguinal ligament, contains the spermatic cord; in females it contains the round ligament. In either gender the hernia can produce a bulge over the midpoint of the inguinal ligament, at the internal inguinal ring. On examination with the tip of the finger placed through the external inguinal ring into the canal, an impulse and/or an elliptical mass descending along the spermatic cord and felt at the tip of the finger with coughing or straining is diagnostic. Unfortunately, it is more difficult to palpate in a female, owing to the lack of slack tissue such that the scrotum offers.

The recurrence rate after repair is reported as <5% (25).

One type of indirect inguinal hernia is a sliding inguinal hernia, in which the wall of a viscus organ (typically the cecum or sigmoid colon but can also be the bladder or an ovary) is fixed to the posterior wall of the peritoneal sac. Diagnosis of this is essential so as not to inadvertently incise these lumens during repair of the hernia.

An acquired hernia through the posterior wall of the inguinal canal is a direct inguinal hernia (Fig. 31–8E). This bulge is close to the pubic tubercle just above the inguinal ligament and almost directly behind the external inguinal ring (thus medial to the bulge of an indirect hernia). There is usually no pain associated with a direct inguinal hernia. On physical examination the examiner's finger should be placed perpendicularly into the external ring so that the tip rests on the posterior wall of the canal; some find that it is easier to feel the impulse along the bottom of the finger close to the pubis if one simply places the volar aspect of the finger along the posterior wall of the canal. Direct hernias are less likely to incarcerate or strangulate, but repair is nonetheless advisable because of the frequent difficulty of differentiating them from indirect hernias. The repair is more extensive, however, and the recurrence rate has been reported to be as high as 28% (25).

Femoral hernias originate from the femoral canal, an empty space medial to the lacunar ligament (the lower end of the inguinal ligament) and lateral to the femoral vein (Fig. 31–8F). They are acquired and are found more commonly in women, making up one third of groin hernias in women, compared to 2% of groin hernias in men (25). However, inguinal hernias are still more common than femoral hernias in women. They are typically asymptomatic until incarceration or strangulation occurs, and even then the pain is typically localized in the abdomen rather than the femoral region. When a mass is present, it can appear in the upper medial thigh just below the inguinal ligament or even above the inguinal ligament if it becomes deflected upward in front of the ligament. Surgery is highly recommended, and the recurrence rate of 5–10% is similar to that of direct inguinal hernias (also involving a defect of the transversalis fascia).

Other rare types of abdominal hernias include a Littre hernia, which is a Meckel diverticulum in the hernia sac and can be found (in order of frequency) in the inguinal, femoral, and umbilical regions. When found in the groin, it is more common in men and on the right side. Its clinical presentation when strangulation occurs is pain, fever, and symptoms of bowel obstruction. The acquired Spigelian hernia occurs through the linea semilunaris (the line where the sheaths of the lateral abdominal muscles fuse to form the lateral rectus sheath). Diagnosis is often eluded because the mass is not easy to demonstrate, though there is usually localized pain at the hernia orifice. Because of its high incidence of incarceration, repair is necessary.

One last type of hernia that has recently been discussed extensively in the sports literature is the "sports hernia." It has been described as a syndrome caused by a distension of the posterior inguinal wall; effectively, it is an early direct inguinal hernia (28). Another term used is "groin insufficiency," a generalized weakness of the muscular fascial anatomy of the groin, an intrinsic weakness caused by the embryonic derivation of the inguinal canal that puts a male more at risk for injury.

A review of 189 athletes with chronic groin pain found that 50% of cases had an incipient hernia during surgery (29). Another study of elite hockey players with career-ending groin pain found that although there was no hernia on physical examination, during surgical exploration tears were found in the floor of the inguinal ring (30). After repair, all the athletes returned to hockey.

Meyers and associates (31) looked at the pathophysiologic processes of severe lower abdominal or inguinal pain in high-performance athletes and found a distinct syndrome of lower abdominal/adductor pain in male athletes that appeared correctable by a procedure designed to strengthen the anterior pelvic floor. In their study, 152 of the 175 athletes who underwent the pelvic floor repairs returned to their previous level of performance. Adductor releases were also later performed, as 88% of the athletes studied who had never undergone previous surgery in that area also had adductor pain as well as the lower abdominal or inguinal pain. The cause of "athletic pubalgia" appears to be a combination of abdominal hyperextension and thigh hyperabduction, with the pivot point being the pubic symphysis. Osteitis pubis, a very closely related entity, is discussed in greater detail later in this chapter. In fact, the surgery described above often completely resolves the pain at the symphysis pubis joint.

Another study of 11 professional ice hockey players discussed the concomitant involvement of the ilioinguinal nerve (32). All complained of lower abdominal pain with exertion without a specific traumatic event, and all underwent surgical exploration after failure of conservative therapies. In all cases extensive tearing of the external oblique aponeurosis in the direction of its fibers was seen, as well as a lateral tear of the superficial inguinal ring, but no hernia sac. The ilioinguinal nerve was also found trapped in scar tissue formed at the area of the torn aponeurosis and was fibrosed, which was confirmed by pathology. Surgical treatment included repair of the aponeurosis and a neurectomy proximal to the entrapment, and after 8 weeks all the athletes returned to hockey. Ilioinguinal nerve blocks near the anterior superior iliac spine, away from the abdominal wall defect, completely resolved the pain in the two athletes in whom it was attempted.

The diagnosis of some hernias is difficult to make despite careful physical examination, especially in the case of a traumatic hernia where there is an adjacent hematoma or wound infection or in larger, obese patients. There is also a high incidence of associated intra-abdominal injuries with traumatic hernias, and often a diagnostic peritoneal lavage will be done first in the emergency department.

Imaging studies can be helpful. Sonography is helpful in the evaluation of a traumatic acute incarcerated scrotal hernia, an intensely painful and swollen process, and can usually differentiate a mass containing fluid or gas from a solid lesion (24). Ultrasounds can also image tendons and identify true inguinal hernias, and attempts to make the test more dynamic by recreating movements that initiate pain have had some success. However, skilled musculoskeletal ultrasonographers are difficult to find in the United States. CT scans can help in the diagnosis of calcified tendinitis or bony abnormalities at tendon insertions, but MRI is far superior in detecting minor muscular injuries related to microruptures. Often these can appear as edema or inflammation with high signals on T2-weighted spin echo images or fat-suppressed images. The MRI appearance of an inguinal hernia is high signal fat in the inguinal canal on T1-weighted images.

The use of herniography is widely reported in the European literature for the diagnosis of the occult-type hernias or sports hernia. X-rays of the pelvis are obtained after intraperitoneal injection of a contrast medium through the abdominal wall to assess the integrity of the posterior inguinal wall and inguinal canal by demonstrating any filling defects. Herniography has been touted as an accurate means of identifying groin hernias when the clinical diagnosis is uncertain. Inguinal, femoral, and ventral hernias are well demonstrated on herniography, whereas the herniation of only fat and supine imaging may lead to misdiagnosis with CT or ultrasound. Spigelian hernias, however, are better depicted with cross-sectional imaging (33). In another study (34) there was an 84% incidence of inguinal hernia by herniography in soccer players with groin pain, and only 8% were detectable by physical examination. One study investigated over 1000 patients, of whom 78 male athletes had groin pain (35). Only 8% of hernias were palpable on physical examination, but at herniography 84% were found on the symptomatic groin sides. However, hernias were also found in 49% of asymptomatic groin sides.

A recent study of herniograms calculated false-positive and false-negative rates of 18.7% and 7.9%, respectively, thus casting doubt on its reliability in the diagnosis of occult hernias (36). One study found the predictive value of herniography to be 89% but the specificity to be only 64%, concluding that it should not be used as a screening tool but only to confirm an incipient hernia before surgical intervention (29). Another study reviewed 308 operations for unexplained, chronic groin pain that was suspected to be caused by an imminent but not demonstrable inguinal hernia (37). Herniography was used consistently in the diagnostic process in all the studies. However, in 49% of cases hernias were also demonstrated on the opposite, asymptomatic groin side.

The procedure, although used extensively in Europe, is not readily available in the United States. One reason may be its risks, which include hollow viscus perforation and allergic reactions to the contrast agents.

An incarcerated, painful, or tender hernia usually requires an emergency operation because of the possibility of strangulation. In general, one should never use force to reduce a hernia, as the result may be rupture of a strangulated bowel or a reduction of the entire mass such that the peritoneal sac accompanies the loop of bowel and the strangulation is not relieved, just pushed back into the abdominal cavity. However, when an operation is not possible or is risky, nonoperative reduction could be attempted by elevating the hips and sedating the athlete enough to relax the abdominal musculature before performing gentle manipulation. However, because of the possiblity of gangrenous tissue, operative repair should still be performed as soon as possible.

Recently, laparoscopic surgery has been touted as a way to repair hernias effectively with minimal time lost from work or athletic activity because of the smaller skin wounds and the lack of muscle or aponeurotic incision. However, a British study found that laparoscopic repair, though reducing postoperative muscular pain, was associated with a higher risk of complication than an open repair. Furthermore, costs were more than those of an open repair, operating time was longer, and return to normal activity was not significantly different (38). Entrapment of the lateral cutaneous nerve of the thigh is a recognized complication of laparoscopic hernia repair (39). Yet other studies have shown that laparoscopic inguinal herniorrhaphy is a safe and comparable alternative to standard open repairs (26,40). Unfortunately, there is little information about long-term recurrence rates with laparascopic surgery.

Nonsurgical management for athletes who refuse surgery or wish to complete their seasons may include a truss, which attempts to provide external compression over the defect in the abdominal wall. However, some claim that this may mask worsening symptoms and, in reality, provides little protection in this population. Most important are education of the athlete about potential complications if he or she were to continue participating and serial examinations to follow the development of any new symptoms. Although the decision to operate now or after the season should be made on an individual basis, depending on the type of athlete and sport, most would agree that if a hernia is symptomatic at all, it should be repaired immediately.

On the basis of studies evaluating the tensile strength of healing wounds, and with the knowledge that exercise increases intraabdominal pressure, which in turn leads to stress on surgical wounds, general guidelines have been developed concerning safe return to activity. Typical standards are return to noncontact sports by 6–8 weeks and to contact sports by 8–10 weeks for indirect hernia repairs in adults, with half that time for children. Umbilical hernias follow a similar and often shorter time frame. Progressive resistance exercises and conditioning can typically begin at 2–3 weeks. The more extensive repairs that are involved in direct inguinal hernias and femoral hernias take a longer recovery; two more weeks are advised before contact is allowed. For the ventral hernia repairs, because of the failed initial incision, a duration of 8 weeks before conditioning and 3–6 months before noncontact activities is recommended, and there is some question as to whether full contact activity is ever advisable for this group. For other uncomplicated abdominal surgeries, ranges vary from 4 to 12 weeks depending on the type of incision performed.

ABDOMINAL MUSCLE STRAINS AND HEMATOMAS

Abdominal muscle strains are extremely common athletic injuries. The most commonly injured muscle is the rectus abdominis. Certain forms of abdominal muscle strains, especially those that occur at the ribs, pubis, or iliac crest, may lead to chronic symptoms. Osteitis pubis will be discussed in greater detail following this section.

In general, there are two main categories of muscle injuries in athletes. The first results from direct trauma to muscle, or a contusion. The abdominal musculature often receives the initial force of a blow to the abdomen. The majority are mild and resolve spontaneously, but some can develop a hematoma or even myositis ossificans. The second main type of muscle injury is caused by excessive muscle stretching. This can be caused by a sudden violent muscular contraction or recurrent microtrauma from overuse (repetitive abdominal contractions). Muscles are most susceptible to this type of injury when performing an eccentric action, that is, being tense while being forced to stretch. Most muscle strains and tears occur at the myotendinous junction, the weakest point in the muscle–tendon unit.

Both external and internal mechanisms can precipitate a muscle strain. External mechanisms include activities that stretch a muscle beyond its limit, and internal mechanisms include a shortened or weakened muscle or imbalance. One should also evaluate for an anterior or posterior tilted pelvis or innominate bone.

Like other muscle strains, the severity of an abdominal strain is divided into three categories, and the degree of muscle strain is proportional to the degree of impairment in muscle function. In a first-degree strain, the athlete develops mild pain on active contraction and on passive lengthening but usually does not have too much difficulty with activities of daily living (ADL). There is no loss of strength of limitation of motion. In a second-degree strain, there is moderate pain on active contraction and passive lengthening with difficulty with ambulation and ADL. With third-degree strain, the athlete experiences intense pain and weakness on active contraction and intense pain with stretching. There is usually also an extremely decreased muscle length.

MRI can be helpful in determining the presence of a complete tear if an athlete shows loss of function after a muscle injury, which usually will require surgery to prevent long-term weakness. There may also be instances in which an MRI would be used to determine the severity of a muscle injury to better estimate an elite athlete's return to competition. On MRI a muscle strain presents as intramuscular high signal on T2-weighted images without disruption of the muscle. This can persist for weeks, peaking at 24 hours to 5 days after the injury (41). If the muscle is torn, either second degree or third degree, there is a discontinuity in the muscle, and it may be retraction. The edema and hemorrhage at the tear site are high signal on T2-weighted images. If the tear is chronic, fibrosis could have developed at the tear site, resulting in a muscle–tendon unit that can no longer contract fully, leading to weakness and an easily restrained muscle. This fibrous tissue is low signal on both T1- and T2-weighted sequences.

Muscle contusions are rare in noncontact sports. With a muscle contusion there is localized tenderness over the area of impact, with no referred pain. If the contusion occurred in the upper abdominal wall, the lower anterior floating ribs should be evaluated. It is essential to differentiate this injury from any intraabdominal injury. In a contusion the appearance is very similar to that of a first-degree muscle strain, with high signal on T2-weighted sequences within the traumatized area.

A rectus sheath hematoma (RSH) is a rare cause of abdominal pain. The rectus abdominis receives its blood supply from branches of the underlying inferior epigastric arteries. Sudden severe motions such as abrupt twisting of the trunk, sudden contraction of abdominal muscles, or sudden extension of the spine can tear the muscle, and the shearing force can rupture the supplying artery. This may result in an abdominal wall hematoma, which, depending on its location and size, can produce symptoms and clinical findings that are compatible with a variety of acute intraabdominal conditions. The incidence rate of RSH is estimated to be 3.5 per 100,000 per year, with a frequency of approximately 0.9% in patients admitted with "acute abdomen" (42).

Predisposing factors to the development of a hematoma are coagulation disorders, including people on coumadin (43), blood dyscrasias, or degenerative vascular diseases. The literature has also noted a predominance of pregnant patients among those affected with this ailment. Unfortunately, the clinical manifestations of rectus muscle hematoma are sometimes so dramatic that laparotomy is performed in the belief that intraabdominal pathology is present. An example is a suspected abruptio placenta misdiagnosed by clinical and ultrasound examination that was subsequently discovered to be a RSH at the time of surgery (44). Other cases have included an incorrect diagnosis of splenic enlargement (45) and appendicitis (46). Another unusual diagnosis was made in a bodybuilder who presented with acute abdominal pain 1 week after a vigorous workout. Only after a muscle biopsy was performed that showed muscle fiber necrosis was the diagnosis of rhabdomyolysis of the rectus abdominis muscle made (47). The single most important factor in the diagnosis of hematoma of the rectus abdominis is awareness of its existence; it should be included as a differential in all patients who present with an acute abdomen or abdominal pain.

There are few data on athletes with this injury. A study in the Netherlands involved 40 patients treated for hematoma of the rectus abdominis muscle (48). The mean age of the patients was 63 years (range 31–83), and just over half were women. Predisposing factors included the use of anticoagulant, the presence of scars on the abdominal wall, persistant coughing, and coexistent cardiovascular disease. The majority of the hematomas were in the right or left lower quadrant; only four were in the upper part of the rectus. Eight patients had bled severely enough to require blood transfusion, and 32 were successfully treated conservatively.

After blunt trauma the usual presenting sign of RSH is abdominal pain in the right lower abdomen, which can be sudden and severe in onset or slowly progressive. There can also be rapid swelling, muscle guarding, and nausea and vomiting. The athlete is most comfortable in a supported flexed position. Sometimes a bluish discoloration around the periumbilical region is present (Cullen sign), usually 72 hours after injury, and also the left flank (Grey-Turner's sign). A very tender fixed mass within the abdominal wall is palpable, and the pain and swelling are accentuated with abdominal muscle contraction (e.g., partial sit-up) or resisted hip flexion. Hyperextension of spine also causes pain in the anterior abdominal wall.

A cross-table lateral X-ray can often demonstrate the soft tissue swelling external to the abdominal cavity. If DPL is done on suspicion of intraabdominal injury, it should be done lateral to the rectus abdominis muscle. If the diagnosis remains in question, an ultrasound or CT scan can be used. In one small study, CT (9/9) appeared to be more accurate than ultrasonography (15/21) in facilitating the diagnosis of RSH (49). Sonographically, these hematomas may be confused with abdominal wall tumors. On CT scans, a hyperdense mass posterior to the rectus abdominis muscle with ipsilateral anterolateral muscular enlargement is characteristic of an acute RSH, though a chronic RSH may be isodense or hypodense relative to the surrounding muscle. An MRI can depict muscle strain and allow differentiation of moderate or severe injuries from mild lesions. However, whereas a CT scan can show a difference between hematoma and muscle tissue immediately after injury, an MRI may not. The appearance of a hematoma depends on the age of the lesion. If only days to a few weeks old, the RSH displays an intermediate to high signal on T1 and variable signal intensity on T2. If chronic and weeks to months old, the hemosiderin is low signal on both.

A method of classification for hematomas of the rectus abdominis has been proposed based on findings observed in CT in 13 cases of RSH (50). Type I hematomas are slight and do not require hospitalization. Type II and type III are moderate and severe hematomas, respectively, and do require hospitalization. The patients with type III hematomas in the study were all undergoing anticoagulant therapy and presented with a picture of acute abdomen, and in all five cases blood transfusion was carried out.

The treatment for all abdominal muscle injuries is to reduce pain, restore muscle function (regain length and strength), and prevent the likelihood of reinjury. The concepts of relative rest and protection of the injured muscle by limiting activity by pain are important to follow. Occasionally, a chronic muscle tear can remain symptomatic despite rehabilitation and rest, and surgery involving a tenotomy of an injured rectus abdominis can have good results with no loss of strength (51).

For a contusion or muscle strain, the immediate treatment is ice and compression. For a hematoma, immediate ice and pressure are also needed to keep the swelling localized, since the muscle is sectioned in fascia. Local heat can be applied after 48–72 hours. Activities to be avoided include rotation, stretching, and flexion of trunk or lower extremities. In a hematoma, operation is indicated if the pain is severe, with evacuation of the clot and control of the bleeding with surgical ligation of the affected epigastric artery. Typically, if the injury treated conservatively, the acute pain resolves within 72 hours, and the athlete can usually return to participation in 2 weeks, though the mass may remain fairly prominent for several weeks.

OSTEITIS PUBIS

Groin injuries are very common among athletes in sports that demand eccentric muscle contractions about the hip and lower abdominal muscles, such as soccer, hurdling, and ice hockey. Most of the time the injury involves the adductor longus, rectus femoris, rectus abdominis, or iliapsoas muscles. In the case of the rectus abdominis it is often strained at its insertion into the pelvis, and pain in that area can often also be confused with a hernia.

Osteitis pubis is an inflammatory process involving the symphysis pubis in athletes without an infectious etiology; it may also involve the adjoining pubic bones, the perichondrium, and the periosteum. The joint is a nonsynovial lined, amphiarthodial joint located between the two pubic bones. The innominate bones function as arches, thus transferring the weight of the upright trunk from the sacrum to the hips. The richly innervated symphysis acts to connect the two weight-bearing arches. The surrounding muscles including the pyramidalis, rectus abdominis, gracilis, and adductors.

The pathogenesis of this disease is controversial, despite a very consistent clinical presentation. It was first described by Beer in 1924 following a suprapubic operation; Beer further suggested that causes may be trauma to the periosteum of the pubis by retractors used during surgery, external closed trauma, or a prolonged vaginal delivery. In a study of 45 patients between 1935 and 1958, Coventry and Mitchell concluded that the underlying difficulty was venous congestion secondary to inflammation in the adjacent urinary tract (52). Infectious osteitis pubis is well recognized as a postoperative complication of gynecologic and urologic surgical procedures and is commonly reported in that literature.

The current etiology of noninfectious osteitis pubis is that overuse and microtrauma of the muscles associated with running and kicking occur, with degenerative changes at the site of bony origin of these muscles. Predisposing factors such as excessive frontal, up-and-down, or horizontal side-to-side pelvic motion or a limitation of hip joint movement have been implicated. This overuse also may result in a shearing stress at the symphysis, causing instability of the sacroiliac joint or unrecognized or subclinical subluxation of the symphysis with traumatic arthritis. Other sequelae may include avascular necrosis of part of the pubic bone (osteochondritis dissecans) or a fatigue fracture of the pubis at the symphysis. It has been reported in published literature in sports such as ice hockey, running, wrestling, rugby, tennis, football, and basketball. It is also prevalent in soccer and other one-legged activities.

The pattern of pain is perhaps most important in differentiating osteitis pubis from many other causes of groin pain (53). It usually emanates from the area of symphysis pubis and radiates into the lower rectus abdominis, the upper adductors, and the perineum and scrotum. The pain can be unilateral or bilateral, can involve one or more sites at variable times, and, though it can present acutely, is usually more by gradual onset. The majority complain of a gradual onset of groin or adductor pain that is associated with heavy impact loading, lateral side-to-side movements, or accelerating or decelerating while running. They also may have pain in the pubic symphysis and lower abdominal muscles that increases with sit-ups and other abdominal muscle-strengthening exercises. Rarely, there can be painful clicking at the pubic symphysis with movements such as rolling over in bed, reflecting potential instability of the pelvis.

Often the symptoms can be vague with nonspecific presenting complaints, leading to a prolonged diagnosis. The joint is innervated by both the genitofemoral (L1–2) and pudendal (S2–4) nerves. Thus symptoms can be referred to the various dermatomes and myotomes of these levels, which include the inguinal, greater trochanter, lower back, anterior thigh, hip flexors and adductors, perineum, medial thigh, lower sacrum, and buttocks, to name a few.

On physical examination, the most specific finding is point tenderness at the symphysis pubis. Also prevalent is loss of internal rotation of the hips, as well as decreased hip abduction and adductor pain and tightness. There may be a positive lateral compression test, in which the athlete is placed in the lateral decubitus position and pressure is applied to the iliac wing, with resulting discomfort over the pubis. If the athlete is febrile, check a complete blood count with differential and urinalysis.

Early in course of the disease, radiographs will be normal. It may take 6 months of symptoms before X-rays show a frayed appearance of the pubic periosteum, loss of cortex, symphyseal widening often greater than 7 mm, erosions and cyst formation, and sclerosis along the articular border, which can persist even after the symptoms resolve (Fig. 31–9A,B). These changes are usually bilateral and symmetric. However, the X-ray is not specific, as changes can be seen in normal athletes who have never had pelvic pain.

If the athlete allows himself or herself to rest and heal, gradual reossification will occur with complete restoration of bone but will take months. Usually, however, healing will result in residual sclerosis, spur formation, and even ankylosis of the symphysis. If instability is present, also evaluate the sacroiliac joints. A flamingo view can also be done with the athlete standing first on one leg then on the other during the X-ray to see whether any shift occurs across the symphysis. Significant pubic instability is movement across the joint of greater than 2 mm. However, even this can be asymptomatic.

A bone scan is positive on delayed views with increased uptake in the pubic bones on both sides of the symphysis (Fig. 31–10). This symmetry helps to rule out tumors and pelvic stress fractures, which are characteristically asymmetric. Yet there have been athletes with clinical findings of osteitis pubis with a negative bone scan.

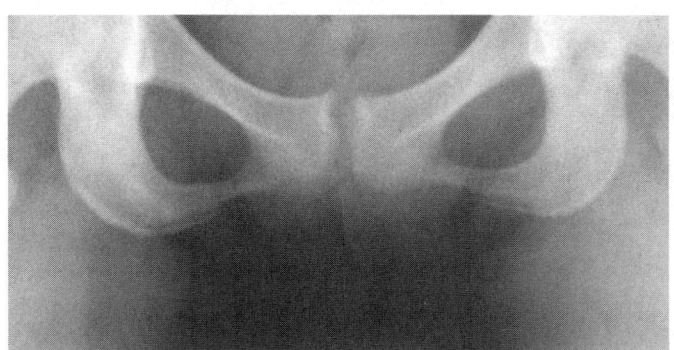 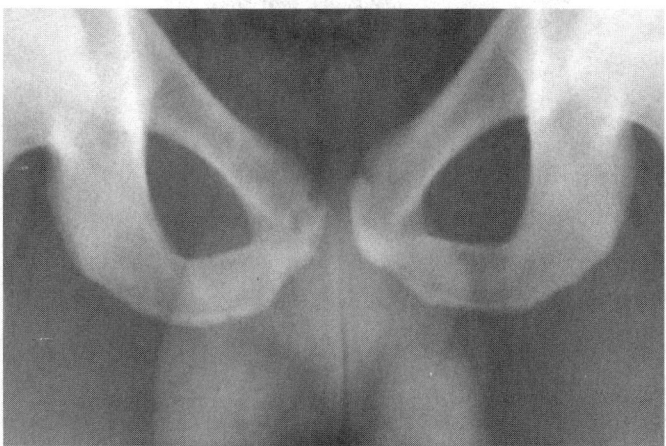

FIG. 31–9. A: Cortical irregularity and sclerosis of the pubic symphysis in a 21-year-old female gymnast with a 1-year history of osteitis pubis. **B:** Widening and subchondral cyst formation on the right in a 20-year-old male basketball player with a 2-year history of right groin and lower abdominal pain.

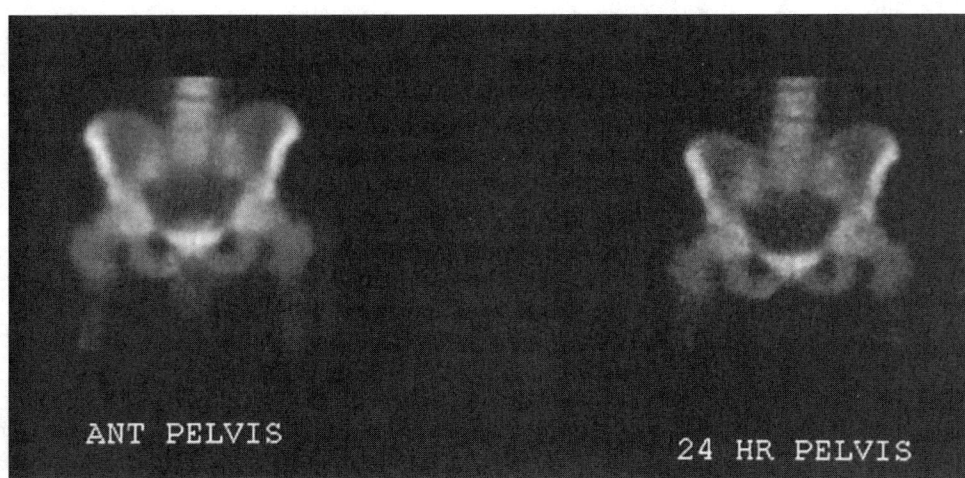

FIG. 31–10. Bone scan in an 18-year-old male rower with negative X-rays showing symmetrically increased uptake in the pubic symphysis.

An MRI can show disruption of cartilage, bone, or periosteum. Early on after development, a high-intensity signal within the pubic symphysis as well as marrow edema in the adjacent pubic bones is evident (Fig. 31–11A,B). Later in the disease, when fibrosis and adjacent bony sclerosis occur with minimal inflammation now at the eroded symphyseal cartilage and disc, there is a low signal on both T1- and T2-weighted MRIs (41). Pathology of the resected tissue has shown only scattered fibrosis and chronic inflammation.

The list of other causes of lower abdominal and groin pain can be exhaustive. The majority are types of muscle strains. Hernias, such as the incipient direct inguinal hernias, were mentioned earlier, as well as the ilioinguinal nerve entrapment. However, not to be missed are pelvic or femoral neck stress fractures or avulsion-type fractures.

Gracilis syndrome is an avulsion fracture at the origin of the gracilis muscle, at the lower half of the anterior edge of the symphysis pubis. Although symptoms are similar to those of osteitis pubis and the cause is also secondary to overuse such as kicking, an X-ray showing the fracture or an asymmetric bone scan can help to differentiate between the two. Treatment is typically conservative with rest, but in some cases only surgical removal of the bony fragment will resolve the symptoms (54). Another cause of chronic groin pain in athletes that can be misdiagnosed as osteitis pubis is obturator

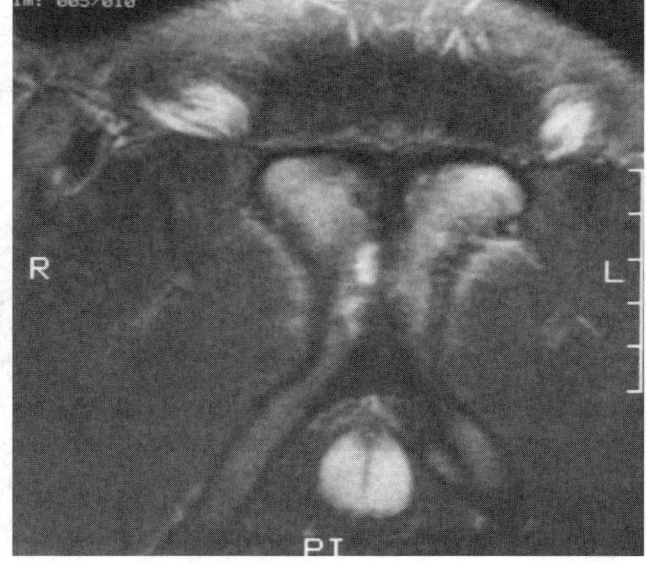 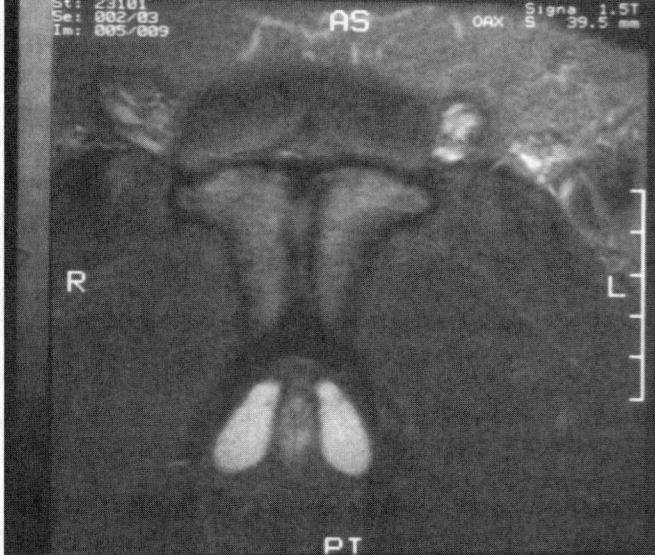

FIG. 31–11. A: MRI of a 20-year-old male hurdler showing bony erosions and subchondral edema (increased signal intensity) more prominent on the right. **B:** Normal MRI of pubic symphysis for comparison.

neuropathy, a fascial entrapment of the obturator nerve where it enters the thigh (55).

The treatment includes rest from physical activity and reassurance that the disease is self-limiting and that the athlete should expect to get better. Most are unsure whether continued activity delays recovery, but it is prudent to avoid activities that are painful and worsen the condition but to stay aerobically fit with swimming, cycling, and other activities that cause no pain. Initial rehabilitation involves improving flexibility of hips and any limitation of movement at the SI joints or even lumbosacral region, which may promote excess movement at the pubic symphysis.

Supportive shorts of neoprene for local warmth and some mechanical support, as well as antiinflammatory medications, can be helpful. Unfortunately, a study by Fricker and colleagues of 59 athletes reported that the average time to full recovery was 9.6 months (ranging from 3 weeks to 48 months); most other studies have reported resolution of symptoms after 3–6 months of rest (56).

Holt and fellow investigators have recommended an injection (1 cc 1% lidocaine, 1 cc 0.25% bupivacaine, and 4 mg dexamethasone) in the pubic symphysis if there is no decrease in symptoms after 7–10 days of rest, oral nonsteroidal antiinflammatory drugs, and hip-stretching exercises (57). In their study, three collegiate athletes all returned to full athletic competition within 2 weeks of injection. After the injection the athlete resumed stretching but did no impact-loading activities for a minimum of 3 days. Despite the apparent success of this treatment, others claim that the injections could be counterproductive and risk loosening the symphysis (53).

As a last resort, surgical fusion of the pubic symphysis or a wedge resection can be done, but results in athletes and return to previous level of activity have not been well documented. It remains debatable how much of a role the symphysis pubis has in pelvic stability.

GENERAL ABDOMINAL REHABILITATION AFTER INJURY

Patterns of pelvic and groin injuries have been observed in different sports; for example, in ice hockey, right groin injuries occur in left-sided shooters and vice versa, and in soccer the side of the dominant shooting leg is more commonly injured (32). Further exploration of the biomechanical aspects of these injuries will aid in their possible prevention and recurrence. Musculoskeletal fatigue at the end of long practices if athletes are not conditioned can lead to poor biomechanics and muscle imbalance. Poor training techniques also lead to weak abdominal musculature. Overtraining should be avoided by evaluation of the practice and game schedule. Poorly fitted equipment, such as a field hockey stick that is too short, could also be a culprit.

It is important to consider the nature of the injury as well as the sport, position, and body type of the athlete in designing a rehabilitation timeline after an abdominal injury. Whether the injury resulted in a surgical procedure or was solely musculoskeletal will play a major role in the development of a rehabilitation strategy. Surgical incisions to the abdominal area must be given sufficient time for adequate collagen strength to develop. The size and location of the incision, as well as the nature of the procedure and any resulting complications, must be considered. Protective equipment as well as padding of the area may be necessary if the athlete is to return to a contact sport.

The importance of the abdominal musculature cannot be overstressed, in its function in core stability and power as well as a protection of the abdominal viscera. Therefore, it is paramount to return the athlete to prior functional levels of strength and endurance before a progressive return to competition is allowed.

It is important to modulate the athlete's activity and progressively return him or her to competition. As was mentioned earlier, the time of relative rest before general progressive resistance exercise and conditioning activities can commence depends on the type of surgery that was performed. The athlete should then be gradually returned to controlled, noncontact drills and skills work for the next several weeks before finally returning to full activity and contact. In planning a strengthening program for the abdominals, it is important to tailor a program to the individual, taking into account body type, activity level, sport, and position. The clinician must first determine the relative strength of these muscles through proper testing, as the ability to perform a sit-up is not necessarily indicative of adequate abdominal strength. Abdominal strength is often broken up into upper and lower abdominals, including the obliques.

To determine upper abdominal strength, Kendall and colleagues advocate the use of the trunk curl (58). An athlete who is able to perform this maneuver with his or her arms straight out in front of the body is graded as having 60% of normal strength. If the athlete can complete the test with the arms crossed on the chest, the grade is 80%. A grade of 100% is attained if the movement is complete with the arms clasped behind the head. However, this test does not take into account muscular endurance.

According to Kendall and colleagues, weakness of the lower portion of the abdominals is the most common finding (58). To determine the strength of these muscles, a leg-lowering test is used. This test is performed by having the patient lie supine. The clinician raises both hips to 90° in relation to the trunk, keeping the knees straight. The athlete is asked to contract the abdominal muscles and maintain a posterior pelvic tilt while slowly

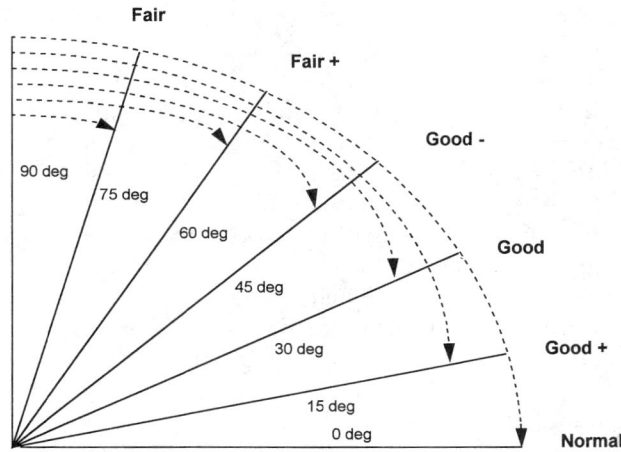

FIG. 31–12. Hip flexion angles and associated muscle strength grades of the lower abdominals. (Modified from Kendall FP, McCreary EK, Provance PG. *Muscle testing and function,* 4th ed. Baltimore: Williams & Wilkins, 1993.)

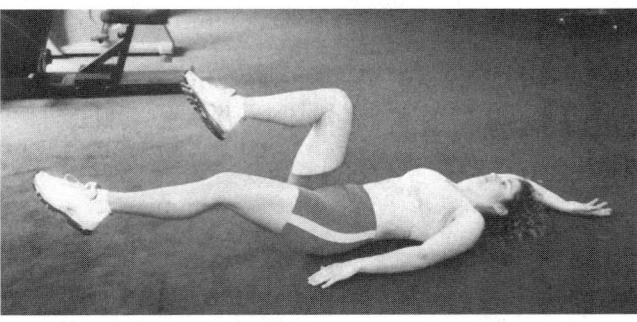

FIG. 31–14. The deadbug is a more advanced abdominal strengthening exercise in which the athlete is asked to maintain a posterior pelvic tilt while moving both the upper and lower extremities through the available ranges of flexion and extension.

lowering the legs to the table. The hip flexion angle at which the posterior pelvic tilt is lost is then measured and translated into a muscle strength grade or percentage (Fig. 31–12).

Once the relative strength of the abdominals is objectified, training can begin. If the athlete is severely deconditioned or recovering from an injury or surgery, abdominal bracing or posterior pelvic tilts may be the initial starting point. The abdominal curl can also be modified by placing a wedge-shaped pillow under the athlete's head and shoulders to allow him or her to begin strengthening in a shortened range.

Abdominal curls, both straight and diagonal, are commonly prescribed initial exercises for upper abdominal strength. Bent-knee fall-outs, deadbugs, and hip lifts are often used in the strengthening of the lower abdominals (Figs. 31–13, 31–14).

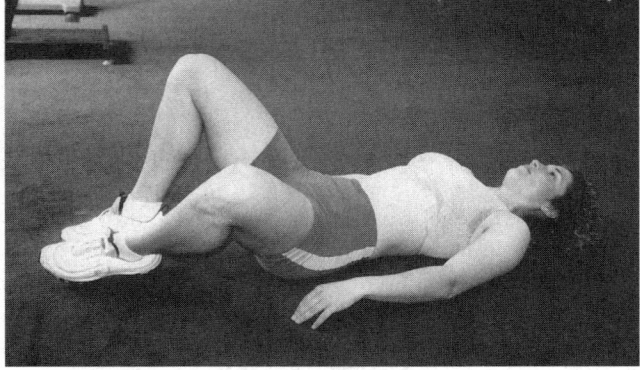

FIG. 31–13. The bent-knee fall-out exercise used to strengthen the lower abdominals. The athlete begins the exercise in a supine hooklying position and is asked to contract the lower abdominals while allowing one leg to "fall out" while avoiding movement in the opposite side of her pelvis.

Training can be progressed through the use of gymnastic balls to facilitate a greater range of motion or combination of stabilization with the other trunk musculature. Combinations of upper and lower extremity movements facilitate functional movements that often incorporate a rotatory component. The use of machines such as the Roman chair combine the strengthening of both the abdominals and the hip flexors and should be undertaken only if the athlete has a sufficient base of strength. External resistance to increase physical demands on these muscles can be added through the use of plate weights, cable columns, and plyoballs. The use of resistance should not be at the expense of limiting the high number of repetitions or proper form. Exercises that train the trunk muscles synergistically through functional movements can also be added to assist the athlete in the development of power. Many of these activities utilize a plyoball or medicine ball in functional or sport-specific positions. Such exercises are limited only by the imagination of the clinician.

To illustrate a rehabilitation progression, a specific program for the treatment of osteitis pubis is outlined (Table 31–5). Because of the critical role of both the abdominal and adductor muscles in performance and the inability to participate in athletic endeavors without using them, the treatment of osteitis pubis can be a slow and often frustrating task for both the athlete and the clinician.

In initiating treatment, it is important to consider whether the injury is caused by an overuse problem or is acute or chronic. This often dictates the speed through which one can progress the phases of rehabilitation. Identifying and correcting any underlying problem such as a sacral-iliac dysfunction are also imperative.

To achieve optimal results, the process of rehabilitation is broken up into five phases, each progression moving the athlete closer to the ultimate goal of returning to participation in his or her sport. The goal of the initial phase of rehabilitation (Phase I) is to decrease

TABLE 31-5. *Sample osteitis pubis rehabilitation program*

Phase I
    Ice
    Therapeutic modalities
    Active rest
    Abdominal bracing: various positions
    Pelvic tilt: various positions
Phase II
    Multiple angle adductor isometrics in supine
    Concentric/eccentric adductor contractions-painfree range
    Supine 90/90 position:
        Lower abdominal lift (to increase difficulty add manual resistance to knee, adductor isometric)
        Same as above with arms held straight up toward the ceiling (to increase difficulty, add manual resistance to upper extremities and/or diagonally to both the upper and lower extremities)
    Prone on elbows and toes (Fig. 31-17):
        Lower pelvis as close to the table until pain is noted (to increase difficulty add manual resistance)
Phase III
    Three-position isometric squats with body weight
    Controlled partial squats
    Positions: Slight trunk tilt with arms in 90° flexion
               Reaching back between legs as much as possible
    Closed hip to open hip squats
        Variations: Isometric holds
                Foot position
                Width of stance
                Step backward with each repetition
    Multihip flexion/abduction/adduction standing on the involved leg
    Abdominal crunches: straight and diagonal
    Manual resistance exercise:
        In the supine position, nonexercised knee bent:
            Hip flexion
            Hip abduction with knee bent
            Hip adduction with knee bent
            Lower abdominal
            Upper abdominal
        In the prone position:
            Hip internal rotation
            Hip external rotation
    Variations: Increase reps, sets, resistance (in that order of progression)
Phase IV
    Forward lunges
    Diagonal lunges with upper body in a forward flexed hip hinge
    Exercises perfomed with resistance utilizing elastic band or tubing
    Resistance from behind
    Step forward with high knee
    Resistance from the side
    Side steps in 1/4 squat position with 5 sec. isometric hold
    Resistance from the front
    Step to open hip position and perform a squat with a 5 sec. hold
Phase V
    Pool work:
        Running: conventional, high knees, butt kicks, backward
        Lateral: lunges, high knees, carioca, shuffle
        Standing hamstring curls
        Standing knee extensions
        Internal and external rotations
        Hip adduction and abduction, one leg at a time
        Hip circumduction: clockwise and counterclockwise
        Soccer kicks
        Running with flotation vests

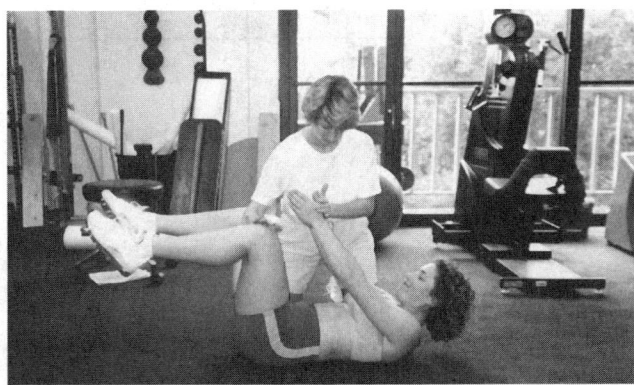

FIG. 31–15. In phase II, manual resistance can be applied to the athlete in the supine 90/90 position to increase the difficulty of the exercise.

the inflammation and pain. This is accomplished through the use of ice, electrotherapeutic modalities, and active rest. Active rest should include activities that do not cause pain to the injured area, as well as the introduction of pelvic tilts and abdominal bracing.

The remaining phases address the correction of soft tissue dysfunction through stretching and strengthening of the involved tissues, stabilization of the pubic symphysis, and ultimately returning the athlete to full participation in his or her sport.

During the remaining four phases of rehabilitation, the athlete needs to maintain pelvic neutral and abdominal bracing throughout the exercise regimen. The exercises, which are aimed at addressing both the adductors and abdominal muscles as well as the other stabilizers of the symphysis pubis, are ideally performed in a pain-free range of motion. Repetition and/or length of contraction should be increased before resistance is applied.

The exercises in phase II are designed to provide a strong base of strength and stabilization before progressing to the dynamic, functional movements in the latter phases. These exercises are performed with both a pelvic tilt and abdominal crunch, to fatigue. The first exercises in phase II are isometric, take place in one plane of movement, and involve the upper portion of the abdominal muscle more than the lower portion. They progress to controlled, limited range isotonics, adding multiple muscle groups, diagonal movement patterns, and including greater involvement of the lower abdominal musculature (Fig. 31–15).

Phase III places the athlete in a more functional squat position. The athlete starts with an isometric squat in various positions and progresses to a controlled repeated dynamic squat. Sufficient recovery time is imperative. Progression from closed to open hip squats follows with variations in isometric holds, foot position, width of stance, and dynamic movement such as stepping backward to increase the difficulty. Various stabilization exercises utilizing gymballs and foam roller can also be added to increase the variety of the program, which fosters improved motivation and compliance (Figs. 31–16, 31–17).

In phase IV, dynamic movement and resistance through elastic tubing are added. The first movement is the forward lunge, followed by a diagonal lunge, keeping the upper body in a forward lean to minimize the stress on the pubic symphysis. The next movement includes forward step-ups and side step-ups, adding resistance through the use of elastic tubing. Again, gymball or ethafoam stabilization activities of increasing complexity can be added to further challenge the athlete.

The final phase (phase V) before returning the athlete to sport-specific drills is an aquatic program that is designed to improve dynamic flexibility, strength, endurance, and function. Activities should include variations of forward, backward, and lateral running as well as isolated movements. Repetitions should be increased, followed by increased speed of movement. Ultimately, multiplanar functional movements such as soccer kicks, jumps, and cutting movements are added.

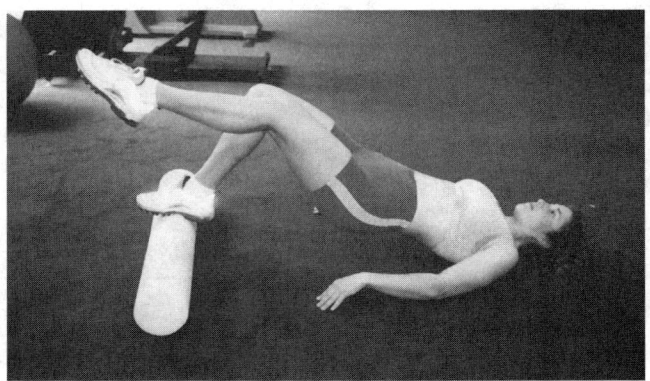
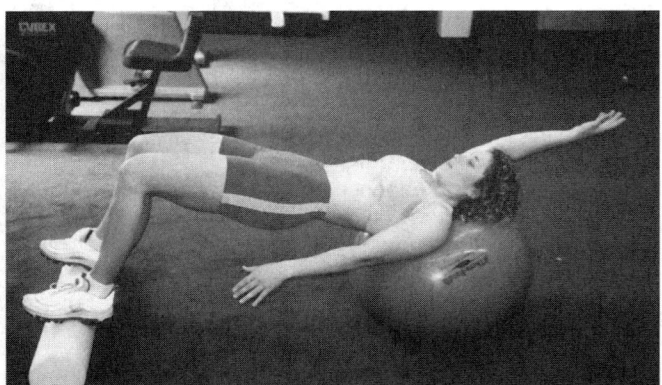

FIG. 31–16. Various stabilization exercises using foam rollers and/or gymnastic balls can be added to increase the complexity and difficulty of exercise.

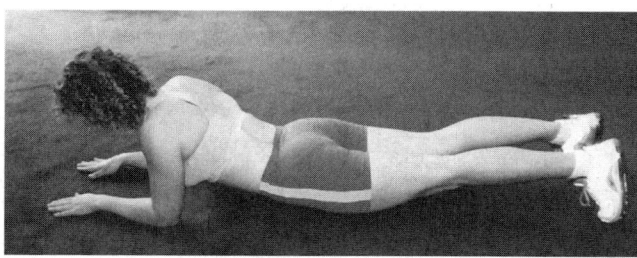

FIG. 31–17. An athlete demonstrating the end position in the prone on toes and elbow progression.

Finally, returning the athlete to running and functional sport specific drills on his or her sport-specific surface is the ultimate test before allowing the athlete back into actual competition.

REFERENCES

1. Berqvist D, Hedelin H, Karlsson G, et al. Abdominal injuries in children: an analysis of 348 cases. *Injury* 1985;16(4):217–220.
2. Lieberman ME, Levitt MA. Spontaneous rupture of the spleen: a case report and literature review. *Am J Emerg Med* 1989;7(1):28–31.
3. Eschelbach, MM. Splenic trauma in mountain biking. *Your Patient & Fitness* 1996;10(3):20–23.
4. Moore EE, Cogbill TH, Jurkovich GJ, et al. Organ injury scaling: spleen and liver (1994 revision). *J Trauma* 1995;38(3):323–324.
5. Buntain WL, Gould HR, Maull KI. Predictability of splenic salvage by computed tomography. *J Trauma* 1988;20(1):24–34.
6. Rothlin MA, Naf R, Amgwerd M, et al. Ultrasound in blunt abdominal and thoracic trauma. *J Trauma* 1993;34(4):488–495.
7. Pearl RH, Wesson DE, Spence LJ, et al. Splenic injury: a 5-year update with improved results and changing criteria for conservative management. *J Pediatr Surg* 1989;24(1):121–125.
8. Lynch JM, Meza MP, Newman B, et al. Computed tomography grade of splenic injury is predictive of the time required for radiographic healing. *J Pediatr Surg* 1997;32(7):1093–1096.
9. Eichner ER. Infectious mononucleosis: recognizing the condition, 'reactivating' the patient. *Phys Sportsmed* 1996;24(4):49–54.
10. Berqvist D, Hedelin H, Karlsson G, et al. Abdominal injury from sporting activities. *Br J Sports Med* 1982;16(2):76–79.
11. Berqvist D, Hedelin H, Karlsson G, et al. Abdominal trauma during thirty years: analysis of a large case series. *Injury* 1981;13(2):93–99.
12. Knudson MM, Lim RC Jr, Oakes DD, et al. Non-operative management of blunt liver injuries in adults: the need for continued surveillance. *J Trauma* 1990;30(12):1494–1500.
13. MacGillivray DC, Valentine RJ. Non-operative management of blunt pediatric liver injury-late complications: case report. *J Trauma* 1989;29(2):251–254.
14. Chiang W. Isolated jejunal perforation from nonpenetrating abdominal trauma. *Am J Emerg Med* 1993;11(5):473–475.
15. Kurkchubasche AG, Fendya DG, Tracy TF, et al. Blunt intestinal injury in children: diagnostic and therapeutic consideration. *Arch Surg* 1997;132:652–658.
16. Curreri WP. Management of the acutely injured person. In: Sabiston DC, ed. *Sabiston's essentials of surgery*. Philadelphia: WB Saunders Company, 1987:194.
17. Rizoli DB, Boulanger BR, McLellan BA, et al. Injuries missed during initial assessment of blunt trauma patients. *Accid Anal Prev* 1994;26(5):681–686.
18. Meyer BF, McCabe CJ. Traumatic diaphragmatic hernia: occult marker of serious injury. *Ann Surg* 1993;218(6):783–790.
19. Sukul DM, Kats E, Johannes EJ. Sixty-three cases of traumatic injury of the diaphragm. *Injury* 1991;22(4):303–306.
20. Aronoff RJ, Reynolds J, Thal E. Evaluation of diaphragmatic injuries. *Am J Surg* 1982; 144(6):671–675.
21. Johnson CD. Blunt injuries of the diaphragm. *Br J Surg* 1988;75(3):226–230.
22. Morgan AS, Flanebaum L, Esposito T, Cox EF. Blunt injury to the diaphragm: an analysis of 44 patients. *J Trauma* 1986;26(6):565–568.
23. Damschen DD, Landercasper J, Cogbill TH, Stolee RT. Acute traumatic abdominal hernia: case reports. *J Trauma* 1994;36(2):273–276.
24. Mucciolo RL, Godec CJ. Traumatic acute incarcerated scrotal hernia. *J Trauma* 1988;28:715–716.
25. Deveney KE. Hernias and other lesions of the abdominal wall. In: Way LW, ed. *Current surgical diagnosis and treatment*, 9th ed. Norwalk, CT: Appleton Lange, 1991;700–712.
26. Tetik C, Arregui ME, Dulucq JL, et al. Complications and recurrences associated with laparoscopic repair of groin hernias: a multi-institutional retrospective analysis. *Surg Endosc* 1994;8(11):1316–1322.
27. deLorimer AA, Harrison MR, Adzick NS. Pediatric surgery. In: Way LW, ed. *Current surgical diagnosis and treatment*, 9th ed. Norwalk, CT: Appleton Lange, 1991;1199–1201.
28. Hackney RG. The sports hernia: a cause of chronic groin pain. *Br J Sports Med* 1993;27(1):58–62.
29. Lovell G. The diagnosis of chronic groin pain in athletes: a review of 189 cases. *Aust J Sci Med Sport* 1995;27(3):76–79.
30. Simonet WT, Saylor HL III, Sim L. Abdominal wall muscle tears in hockey players. *Int J Sports Med* 1995;16(2):126–128.
31. Meyers WC, Foley DP, Garrett WE, Lohnes JH, Mandlebaum BR. Management of severe lower abdominal or inguinal pain in high-performance athletes. PAIN (Performing Athletes with Abdominal or Inguinal Neuromuscular Pain Study Group). *Am J Sports Med* 2000;28(1):2–8.
32. Lacroix VJ, Kinnear DG, Mulder DS, Brown RA. Lower abdominal pain syndrome in National Hockey League players: a report of 11 cases. *Clin J Sport Med* 1998;8(1):5–9.
33. Harrison LA, Keesling CA, Martin NL, et al. Abdominal wall hernias: review of herniography and correlation with cross-sectional imaging. *Radiographics* 1995;15(2):315–332.
34. Eames NW, Deans GT, Lawson JT, et al. Herniography of occult hernia and groin pain. *Br J Surg* 1994;81(10):1529–1530.
35. Smedberg SGG, Broome AEA, Gullmo A, et al. Herniography in athletes with groin pain. *Am J Surg* 1985;149(3):378–382.
36. Loftus IM, Ubhi SS, Rodgers PM, Watkin DF. A negative herniogram does not exclude the presence of a hernia. *Ann R Coll Surg Engl* 1997;79(5):372–375.
37. Fredberg U, Kissmeyer-Nielsen P. The sportsman's hernia: fact or fiction? *Scand J Med Sci Sports* 1996;6(4):201–204.
38. Lawrence K, McWhinnie D, Goodwin A, et al. Randomised controlled trial of laparoscopic versus open repair of inguinal hernia: early results. *BMJ* 1995;311(7011):981–985.
39. Broin EO, Horner C, Mealy K, et al. Meralgia paraesthetica following laparoscopic inguinal hernia repair: an anatomical analysis. *Surg Endosc* 1995;9(1):76–78.
40. Fallas MJ, Phillips EH. Laparoscopic inguinal herniorrhaphy. *Curr Opin Gen Surg* 1994:198–202.
41. Tuite MJ, DeSmet AA. MRI of selected sports injuries: muscle tears, groin pain, and osteochondritis dissecans. *Semin Ultrasound CT MR* 1994;5(5):318–340.
42. Andreassen KH, Olesen TE, Jacobsen PT. [Spontaneous rectal hematoma]. *Ugeskrift for Laeger* 1996;158(16):2254–2257.
43. Chi TW, Ma YC. Spontaneous rectus sheath hematoma during treatment of pulmonary embolism with warfarin: report of a case. *Kao-Hsiung i Hsueh Ko Hsueh Tsa Chih* [*Kaohsiung Journal of Medical Sciences*] 1996;12(10):601–604.
44. Ramirez MM, Burkhead JM III, Turrentine MA. Spontaneous rectus sheath hematoma during pregnancy mimicking abruptio placenta. *Am J Perinatol* 1997;14(6):321–323.
45. Buckingham R, Dwerryhouse S, Roe A. Rectus sheath haematoma mimicking splenic enlargement. *J R Soc Med* 1995;88(6):334–335.
46. Lohle PN, Puylaert JB, Coerkamp EG, Hermans ET. Nonpalpable rectus sheath hematoma clinically masquerading as appendicitis: US and CT diagnosis. *Abdom Imaging* 1995;20(2):152–154.

47. Schmitt HP, Bersh W, Feustel HP. Acute abdominal rhabdomyolysis after body building exercise: is there a 'rectus abdominis syndrome'? *Muscle Nerve* 1983;6:228–232.
48. Verhagen HJ, Tolenaar PL, Sybrandy R. Haematoma of the rectus abdominis muscle. *Eur J Surg* 1993;159(6–7):335–338.
49. Moreno Gallego A, Aguayo JL, Flores B, et al. Ultrasonography and computed tomography reduce unnecessary surgery in abdominal rectus sheath haematoma. *Br J Surg* 1997;84(9):1295–1297.
50. Berna JD, Garcia-Medina V, Guirao J, Garcia-Medina J. Rectus sheath hematoma: diagnostic classification by CT. *Abdom Imaging* 1996;21(1):62–64.
51. Martens MA, Hansen L, Mulier JC. Adductor tendinitis and musculus rectus abdominis tendopathy. *Am J Sports Med* 1987;15(4):353–356.
52. Coventry MB, Mitchell WC. Osteitis pubis: observations based on a study of 45 patients. *JAMA* 1961;178(9):130–137.
53. Fricker PA. Management of groin pain in athletes. *Br J Sports Med* 1997;31(2):97–101.
54. Wiley JJ. Traumatic osteitis pubis: the gracilis syndrome. *Am J Sports Med* 1983;11(5):360–363.
55. Bradshaw C, McCrory P, Bell S, Brukner P. Obturator nerve entrapment: a cause of groin pain in athletes. *Am J Sports Med* 1997;25(3):402–408.
56. Fricker PA, Taunton JE, Ammann W. Osteitis pubis in athletes: infection, inflammation, or injury? *Sports Med* 1991;12:266–279.
57. Holt MA, Keene JS, Graf BK, Helwig DC. Treatment of osteitis pubis in athletes. *Am J Sports Med* 1995;23:601–606.
58. Kendall FP, McCreary EK, Provance PG. *Muscle testing and function,* 4th ed. Baltimore: Williams & Wilkins, 1993.

CHAPTER 32

Genital Injuries in Sports

Andrew W. Nichols

Trauma of the genitalia is a common form of athletic injury. Male athletes are more susceptible to injury than females because of the greater anatomic exposure of the male external genitalia. The majority of athletic-related genital injuries are self-limited and not associated with serious consequences. The common mechanisms of genital injuries are blunt trauma, straddle fall injuries, and direct blows. Blunt trauma frequently occurs in sports such as football, soccer, rugby, and basketball; straddle fall injuries typically take place in gymnastics and bicycling; and direct blows usually transpire in sports that use hard implements, such as baseball, softball, hockey, and lacrosse.

The testes are the male anatomic structures that are most susceptible to injury, as they hang freely and lack the protection of the skeleton and abdominal wall. The use of athletic supporters and protective cups by male participants is highly effective in preventing such injuries. The penis, owing to its soft and pliable form, is only rarely injured. The most common female genital injuries are perineal contusions and hematomas. More severe gynecologic injuries, such as vaginal lacerations and vaginal water injection injuries, may produce severe complications if not promptly diagnosed and treated. The successful management of genital injuries requires early recognition and treatment. The clinician must also express a sympathetic concern for the potential psychological impact that a genital injury may have on an adolescent or teenage athlete who is undergoing sexual development.

INJURIES OF THE MALE GENITALIA

Testicular and Scrotal Injuries

The testes and scrotum are commonly injured in sports such as hockey, baseball, softball, and lacrosse. The free-hanging, extraabdominal scrotal location of the testes makes them susceptible to injury; though the thighs do provide some protection from injury. The right testis is more often injured than the left, owing to its lower-hanging position. Testicular injury is uncommon in young boys and infants because of the small size and mobility of the testes. Instinctive cremasteric muscle contraction recoil from a threatened blow to the groin serves an additionally protective function by elevating the testes to render the blow less severe. A properly fitting athletic supporter provides a significant defense against injury by holding the external male genitalia firmly against the body. The genital cup provides further protection.

It is often difficult to differentiate a mild scrotal injury from a severe injury because of similarities in their initial clinical presentations. Early signs and symptoms of all scrotal injuries usually include localized scrotal pain, swelling, and ecchymosis. It is crucial that the clinician maintain a high index of suspicion when evaluating scrotal injury to identify time-critical injuries, such as testicular rupture or torsion, in which a delay of diagnosis may lead to the loss of a testicle.

Scrotal Skin Injuries

A scrotal contusion typically results from blunt trauma. Signs and symptoms of a contusion include ecchymosis, hematoma formation, and concurrent intrascrotal injuries. Scrotal lacerations, though not commonly seen in sports, should be treated with debridement and primary wound closure. Avulsion of the scrotal skin is a rare but serious injury that is frequently associated with machinery-related trauma. Reflexive recoil of the testes at the time of scrotal skin avulsion injury helps to preserve the spermatic cord structures. The treatment of scrotal skin avulsion involves a surgical transfer of the testes and cord structures into the subcutaneous tissues of the upper thighs until skin grafting and scrotal reconstruc-

---

A. W. Nichols: John A. Burns School of Medicine, University of Hawaii at Manoa, Honolulu, Hawaii 96822.

tion can be performed, at which time the testes and cord structures are relocated to the scrotum.

Hematocele

A hematocele results from the accumulation of blood in the scrotum. The most common cause of a hematocele is blunt scrotal trauma that ruptures the spermatic cord's pampiniform plexus venous network. The presence of a hematocele should prompt the physician to determine the source of bleeding, so as to specifically rule out testicular rupture. The treatment of a simple hematocele involves bed rest, cool pack application, and scrotal elevation. If scrotal bleeding continues, despite these measures, the surgical ligation of bleeding vessels may be indicated. Individuals with varicoceles caused by chronic engorgement of the pampiniform plexus may be predisposed to developing hematoceles.

Testicular Rupture and Laceration

Testicular ruptures and lacerations are the most serious groin injuries. Most such injuries occur during participation in high-velocity sports such as in bicycling when a testis becomes trapped between the pubic symphysis and the hard bicycle seat. The impact causes rupture or laceration of the tunica vaginalis, the structure that covers the vascular and tubular components of the testis. Fortunately, ruptures and lacerations are rare because of the mobility of the testes. Clinical findings are scrotal pain, bleeding, swelling, and a failure of the scrotum to transilluminate. Prompt surgical treatment with hematocele evacuation, debridement of devitalized tissue, and primary testicular closure is essential for organ salvage. Ultrasonographic findings of rupture include hematocele, mixed parenchymal echogenicity, intraparenchymal hemorrhage, and disruption of the tunica albuginea or parenchymal interface. Despite the accuracy of ultrasonography, surgical exploration is the only certain way to establish a diagnosis of rupture or laceration. Equivocal ultrasonographic findings or a clinical picture consistent with testicular rupture, despite a negative ultrasound examination, should lead to surgical exploration of the scrotum. Immediate surgery has been shown to help salvage the testis, shorten recovery time, and reduce the risk of infection. Surgical delay of 3 or more days produces a significantly lower testicular salvage rate, and nonoperative treatment of rupture results in eventual orchiectomy in greater than 45% of cases (1,2).

Testicular Contusion

Testicular contusion, the most common groin injury, rarely results in long-term complications. Although the immediate pain experienced with a testicular contusion is often excruciating, recovery is generally rapid. An early physical examination is particularly useful in the evaluation of this injury, as the onset of scrotal swelling and hydrocele formation limits the diagnostic accuracy of the examination. The initial treatment of a testicular contusion includes supine position bed rest, scrotal elevation, cool pack application, and oral analgesics. Ambulation is permitted once pain has resolved and swelling has stabilized. A scrotal support should be worn for several days thereafter. Severe pain can be managed with an ilioinguinal nerve block, by injecting bupivacaine (without epinephrine) near the spermatic cord at the level of the external inguinal ring (3). An old athletic trainer's trick for relieving testicular contusion pain is to pull the injured player to a seated position on the field, grasp both axillae, lift him 10–12 inches off the ground, and drop him on his buttocks. The maneuver may reduce pain by overriding the pain from the testicles with new stimuli resulting from the drop (4).

Testicular Torsion

Torsion of the spermatic cord and testicle must be considered in any case of groin pain, scrotal swelling, and tenderness. Whether torsion occurs as a response to scrotal trauma is controversial, though it has been reported to take place spontaneously after a blow to the groin or as a result of a forceful cremasteric muscle contraction. Exercise or even cold exposure may provoke such a cremasteric contraction that pulls the testis superiorly over the pubis and twists the cord (Fig. 32–1). Williamson found 7% of torsion cases to be associated with antecedent trauma (5). Torsion has also been reported to afflict adolescent male bicyclists. The injury may result from the testis becoming twisted between

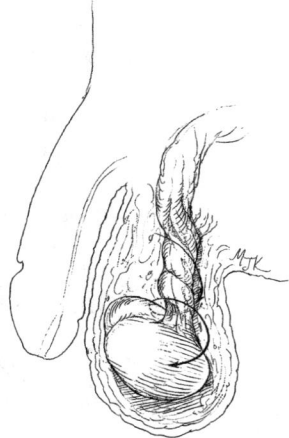

FIG. 32–1. Torsion of the testis is the result of twisting of the spermatic cord. (From Weinerth JL. The male genital system. In: Sabiston DC, ed. *Textbook of surgery*, 13th ed. Philadelphia: WB Saunders, 1986:1678.)

the thigh and bicycle seat as the legs pedal up and down (6).

Torsion must be diagnosed early, as ischemia occurs rapidly and treatment delays may result in the loss of a testis. Physical findings of torsion include testicular swelling, tenderness, and poor scrotal structure definition. Radionuclide scanning will show reduced uptake in the affected testicle, and Doppler probe evaluation reveals an absence of the spermatic artery pulse at the hilum of the injured testis. The initial treatment of torsion may be an attempt to externally reduce the testicle. If the testis cannot be reduced by using a closed technique, the torsion should be surgically reduced and the testicle fixed to the scrotum to prevent recurrence.

Highball Syndrome and Testicular Dislocation

A sudden blow to the groin may provoke a forceful contraction of the cremasteric muscle that draws the testes upward into the inguinal region, known as the highball syndrome. The testes generally reduce spontaneously into their proper anatomic positions as the cremasteric muscle relaxes. Japanese sumo wrestlers often experience highball syndrome, since they are taught to voluntarily contract their cremasteric muscles so as to protect the testes from human scrotal bites, a known sumo fighting technique. The treatment of recurrent highball syndrome, such as the case of a lacrosse player who experienced recurrent inguinal pain during exercise due to cremasteric muscle contraction–induced irritation of the testes at the external inguinal rings, is surgical orchiplexy (7).

Severe groin trauma may result in acute dislocation of one or both testicles into the inguinal, pubic, penile, perineal, or crural areas. Dislocated testicles can sometimes be reduced by external manipulation if edema and hematoma have not yet developed. Persistent dislocations are treated with surgical relocation and orchiplexy.

Other Scrotal or Testicular Conditions

Other conditions that must be considered in the evaluation of an athlete who presents with groin pain are epididymitis and neoplasms. Epididymitis typically manifests with a gradual onset of scrotal pain in young males. Early in the course of the disease, it may be possible to differentiate a soft, nontender testis from the adjacent, discretely tender and swollen epididymis by palpation. The presence of pyuria lends further support to the diagnosis. Most cases resolve with antibiotic treatment, though surgical drainage may also be necessary for severe infections.

The most common cause of a palpable testicular mass in a young man is the benign hydrocele. However, since testicular carcinomas are among the most frequently occurring neoplasms in this age group, this diagnosis must also be considered in the evaluation of any testicular mass. Testicular swelling—even that which appears to be clearly associated with trauma—must be followed for complete resolution to avoid overlooking a neoplasm. Some studies have suggested an association between testicular carcinoma and antecedent trauma; others have identified no such relationship (8). Apparent correlations may be due to heightened awareness and more thorough testicular self-examination in males who have sustained previous testicular trauma.

Recommendations regarding participation in competitive athletics by males with a single-functioning testicle are controversial, and an extensive discussion is beyond the scope of this chapter. Although the incidence of significant gonadal injury in sports that requires subsequent orchiectomy is quite small, general guidelines are that males who choose to participate in contact or collision sports should use protective cups.

Evaluation of the Acute Scrotal Injury

The most common causes of scrotal masses are illustrated in Figure 32–2. Medical evaluation of athletic scrotal trauma should begin with a thorough history and physical examination. The examination is best performed with the individual lying supine, to relieve discomfort and reduce the tug of gravity on the testicles. Each testis, epididymis, and spermatic cord should be systematically palpated. If scrotal swelling is detected, a light source should be used to determine whether the scrotum transilluminates. Hydroceles will transilluminate and consequently produce testicular shadows. On the other hand, hematoceles and testicular tumors do not transilluminate. Testicular torsion can be ruled out by the Doppler probe detection of a spermatic artery pulse at the testicular hilum. Ultrasonography, the most useful noninvasive imaging technique, helps to identify hematoceles, testicular masses, and epididymal swelling and to outline the integrity of the testicle. Diagnostic percutaneous needle aspiration of scrotal fluid should generally be avoided because of the risk of introducing infection. Scrotal aspiration is typically reserved for the therapeutic release of a tensely swollen scrotum (3). Testicular rupture is suggested by a history of recent groin trauma, the finding of a nonpalpable testicle, and failure of the scrotum to transilluminate. In such cases urgent urologic consultation should be obtained.

Injuries of the Penis

The penis is rarely injured during athletics due to its mobility and pliability. The use of an athletic supporter provides additional protection by holding the penis firmly against the body. Most significant penile injuries result from a blow to an erect penis that causes penile

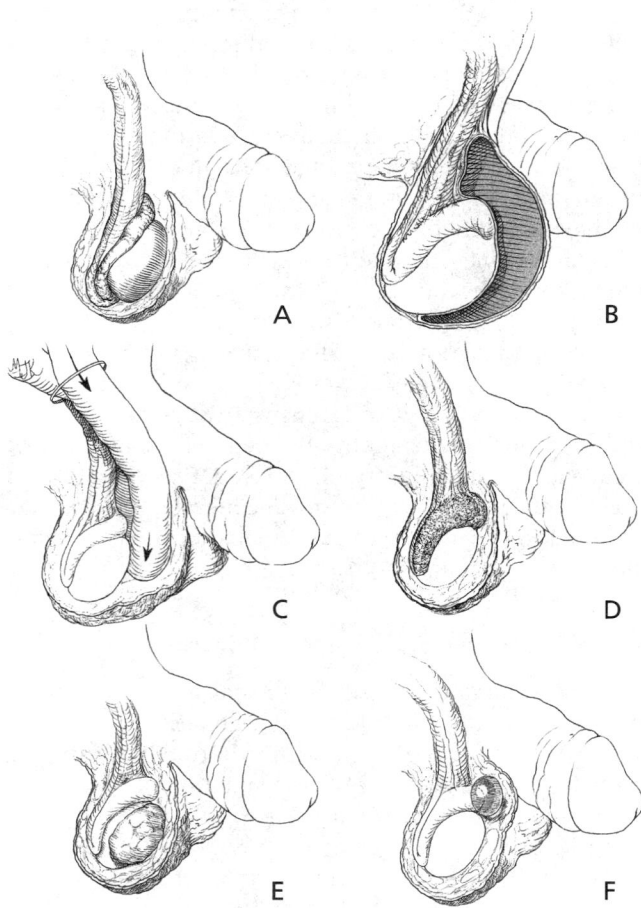

FIG. 32–2. Common scrotal masses. **A:** Normal anatomy. **B:** Hydrocele. **C:** Inguinal hernia entering scrotal compartment. **D:** Epididymitis causing induration and enlargement of epididymis but not testis. **E:** Testicular tumor intrinsic to testis. **F:** Epidermal cyst or spermatocele extrinsic to testis. (From Weinerth JL. The male genital system. In: Sabiston DC, ed. *Textbook of surgery,* 13th ed. Philadelphia: WB Saunders, 1986:1680.)

fracture or corpus cavernosum rupture. Severe penile injuries should be treated with primary repair and hematoma evacuation to help prevent the development of fibrosis and erectile dysfunction. Minor injuries generally require only hemorrhage control.

Bicyclists' Pudendal Neuropathy

Bicycle racers often experience traumatic irritations of the pudendal and genitofemoral nerves due to prolonged episodes of direct pressure against the hard bicycle saddle while riding. A survey found that 50% of male bicyclists who participated in day-long rides reported neuropathy symptoms; many experienced frequent recurrences, and 8% had to modify their riding styles to reduce the discomfort (6). Signs and symptoms of bicyclists' neuropathy include transient numbness of the penile shaft, hypothesia of the scrotum, and priapism. Acute impotence affected 13% of male participants in a 540-kilometer bicycle tour, half of whom continued to have symptoms after one week (9). Impotence may result from vascular compromise due to pressure of the penis against the nose of the bicycle or compression of the dorsal branch of the pudendal nerve, dorsal nerve of the penis, or cavernous (vasomotor) nerves of the penis against the bony pubic arch (10). Symptoms can usually be relieved by discontinuing bicycle riding, using a padded or furrowed saddle, tilting the seat farther forward, or standing frequently while riding.

Urethral Injuries

Urethral injuries are rare and most often affect males. The majority of urethral injuries occur as a result of straddle falls or pelvic fractures. Urethral trauma may affect the anterior urethra (bulbous and pendulous portions) or the posterior urethra (prostatic and membranous portions). Potential types of urethral injuries include lacerations, transections, contusions, and hematomas. The posterior urethra is relatively immobile in comparison to the anterior portion and is consequently more subject to trauma. The short female urethra, which is not fixed posteriorly, is only rarely traumatized.

Anterior Urethral Injuries

The male anterior urethra, referring to the portion distal to the urogenital diaphragm, is susceptible to lacerations and contusions during straddle falls. Urethral contusions and perineal hematomas from crush injuries usually resolve spontaneously. Severe straddle fall injuries may produce urethral wall lacerations with extravasation of urine into the scrotum, along the penile shaft, within Colles' fascia, and superiorly into the abdominal wall. Delays in the recognition of urethral lacerations may lead to sepsis (Fig. 32–3).

Anterior urethral injury is associated with urethral meatus bleeding, perineal pain and hemorrhage, urinary urgency, and sudden local swelling after voiding due to urinary extravasation. The physical examination shows tenderness and swelling of the perineum and a normal prostate gland. Massive urinary extravasation may predispose localized infections of the perineum, scrotum, and lower abdominal wall skin or sepsis. The presence of traumatic urethral meatus bleeding contraindicates the insertion of a urethral catheter until the integrity of the urethra has been assessed by urethrography. A urethrogram is performed by inserting 15–20 mL of water-soluble contrast into the urethra to demonstrate the presence and location of extravasation, corresponding to the site of urethral rupture or laceration. Urethral contusions fail to demonstrate extravasation of contrast.

Shock occurring secondary to urethral injuries is rare,

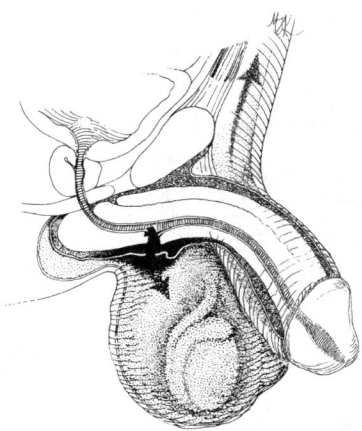

FIG. 32–3. Injury to the anterior urethra. The most common mechanism of injury is a perineal blow or straddle fall with crushing of urethra against inferior edge of pubic symphysis. (From McAninch JW. Injuries of the genitourinary tract. In: Tanagho EA, McAninch JW, eds. *Smith's general urology,* 14th ed. Norwalk, CT: Appleton & Lange, 1995:330.)

as the amount of blood loss is generally small. If heavy hemorrhage does occur, the application of direct local pressure will usually provide adequate bleeding control. No specific treatment is required for urethral contusions in which the patient is able to void without pain or bleeding. A urethral catheter should be inserted only in cases of persistent bleeding. Minor to moderate urethral lacerations are best treated with urinary flow diversion through a suprapubic cystostomy tube or percutaneous cystostomy while permitting the lacerations to heal. As was previously discussed, urethral instrumentation should be avoided in the presence of urethral lacerations. Minor extravasation injuries may be reevaluated to assess healing with a repeat voiding urethrogram approximately 7 days after placement of the suprapubic cystostomy. Follow-up urethrography should be delayed for 2–3 weeks in the reassessment of more severe injuries. Stricture formation at the site of healing is a frequent complication of urethral laceration, which is identifiable by determining urinary flow rates. Most strictures are mild and require no treatment. Severe urethral lacerations are generally treated with surgical urinary diversion and drainage of any urine that has extravasated into the scrotum, perineum, and lower abdomen. Some surgeons prefer to treat lacerations with primary surgical repair, although it is technically difficult and often results in stricture formation.

Posterior Urethral Injuries

Blunt pelvic trauma or fractures may cause the posterior urethra to be sheared off just proximal to the urogenital diaphragm (Fig. 32–4). The prostate may be forced into superior displacement by the resultant developing hematoma. Posterior urethral injuries are associated with lower abdominal pain, the inability to urinate, blood at the urethral meatus, suprapubic tenderness, the presence of a pelvic fracture on X-ray, perineal or suprapubic contusions, and a large developing pelvic hematoma. Rectal examination may reveal displacement of the prostate gland from its normal position, although a tense pelvic hematoma may resemble a prostate on digital examination. The presence of blood at the urethral meatus should prompt the physician to obtain a urethrogram before passing a urethral catheter, as blind insertion of the catheter could result in the introduction of infection into adjacent hematomas or the conversion of an incomplete laceration into a complete one. The treatment of posterior urethral injuries is suprapubic urinary diversion followed by immediate or delayed surgical urethral realignment and reconstruction. The delayed procedure is preferred by many surgeons as the incidence of stricture formation and impotence is lower.

Mechanical Urethritis

Direct chronic pressure applied by a bicycle seat may predispose some long-distance bicyclists to a mechanical urethritis. Resultant urethral inflammation potentially produces a susceptibility to bacterial urethritis. The workup of dysuria in a bicyclist should include mechanical urethritis in the differential diagnosis. Symptoms may be relieved by increasing the padding or altering

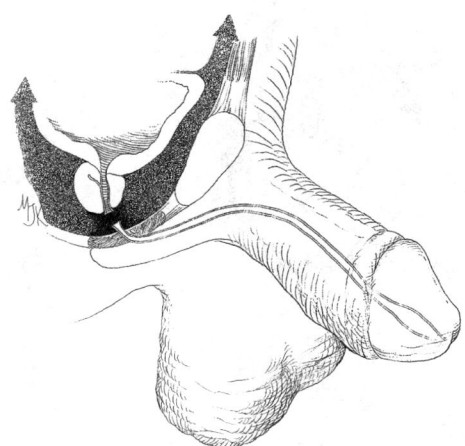

FIG. 32–4. Injury to the posterior urethra. The prostate has been avulsed from the posterior urethra secondary to pelvic fracture. Extravasation occurs above the triangular ligament and is periprostatic and perivesical. (From McAninch JW. Injuries of the genitourinary tract. In: Tanagho EA, McAninch JW, eds. *Smith's general urology,* 14th ed. Norwalk, CT: Appleton & Lange, 1995:328.)

the pitch of the bicycle saddle and by encouraging the bicyclist to stand periodically while riding.

Prostate Injuries

The prostate may become displaced superiorly owing to hematoma formation that results from severe pelvic trauma and rupture of the puboprostatic ligaments. Both recreational and elite long-distance bicyclists are predisposed to prostatitis owing to the chronic pressure applied on the prostate by the bicycle seat. Older men are more frequently affected with prostatitis, though it has been reported in men as young as 25 years of age. Avoidance of bicycle riding, good hydration, and adjustment of the seat height are effective techniques to prevent prostate irritation.

The administration of anabolic steroids presents another potential risk to the prostate gland by predisposing to prostatic enlargement and possibly malignancy. Anabolic steroids have been shown to increase prostatic volume, reduce urinary flow rates, and increase episodes of nocturia. The discontinuation of anabolic steroids led to a gradual return of these abnormalities to normal levels (11). Prostate specific antigen levels do not appear to be influenced by exogenous anabolic steroid administration (11). Metastatic adenocarcinoma of the prostate at a young age has been reported in a 38-year-old male bodybuilder who had taken anabolic steroids for 18 years (12).

Subcutaneous Perineal Nodules

Elite and professional bicyclists may form subcutaneous perineal nodules on one or both sides of the perineal midline, just posterior to the scrotum (6) (Fig. 32–5). Also known as "accessory testicles," or "third testes" when occurring unilaterally, the nodules develop only in males and have not been reported in recreational bicyclists. Fine needle aspirate histologic analysis of the nodules reveals pseudocysts that are relatively devoid of cellular material (13). The nodules represent areas of microtrauma-induced aseptic necrosis in the superficial perineal fascia due to prolonged pressure against the bicycle seat. The nodules have known effective treatment and may become a serious handicap to professional bicyclists.

INJURIES OF THE FEMALE GENITALIA

The female reproductive organs, despite being well protected behind the pubic bone, are occasionally injured during sports participation. The most common mechanism of injury is the straddle fall. Potential injuries of the female genitalia include labial and vulvar contusions; lacerations of the vulva, labia, periclitoral area, vagina, periurethral region, and anterior urethra; and vaginal water injection injuries to the deeper pelvic structures. Female genital injuries are often difficult to diagnose owing to the presence of profuse bleeding that may be out of proportion to the extent of injury and that may interfere with visualization of the injury. Sedation or general anesthesia may be required to obtain an adequate examination, particularly in an anxious, frightened, or uncooperative patient. The examiner must be especially sensitive to the injured patient so as to minimize any psychosocial trauma that may be associated with genital injuries (14).

Perineal Injuries

The most common injury of the female external genitalia is the labial or vulvar contusion. Contusions produce edema and hematomas, which are best treated with cool pack application and injury site protection. Lacerations of the perineum often bleed profusely, which may limit the physician's ability to evaluate the extent of injury and thus determine appropriate management. The degrees of perineal lacerations and appropriate treatments appear in Table 32–1. It is particularly important to identify and repair anal sphincter or rectal mucosa damage, as a failure to repair these structures may lead to chronic fecal incontinence. The pain from perineal laceration injury or repair may be reduced with anesthe-

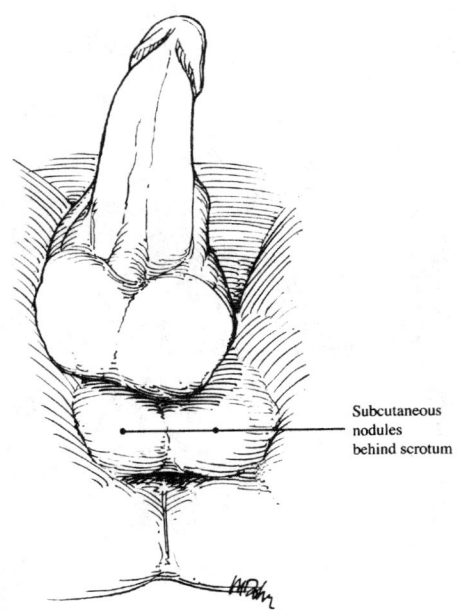

FIG. 32–5. Subcutaneous nodules in a long-distance cyclist. The photograph illustrates bilateral subcutaneous nodules located posterior to the scrotum in an elite-class bicyclist. (From Vuong PN, Camuzard P, Schnoonaat MF. Perineal nodular indurations "accessory testicles" in cyclists. *Acta Cytol* 1988;32:86–90.)

TABLE 32–1. Classification and treatment of perineal lacerations

Degree	Structures involved	Treatment
First	Skin only	Repair necessary only in cases of persistent bleeding
Second	Skin and subcutaneous tissues	Two-step episiotomy repair
Third	Into anal sphincter	Anal sphincter repair and two-step episiotomy repair
Fourth	Completely through anal sphincter and rectal mucosa	Anal sphincter repair and two-step episiotomy repair

tic sprays, heat lamps directed toward the perineum, or Sitz baths.

The astute clinician must be aware of the potential of sexual abuse injuries in the differential diagnosis of young girls and adolescents who present with genital trauma. An alleged athletic injury that fails to correspond with an athletic-related mechanism should raise suspicion. Types of genital injury that are specifically associated with sexual abuse include lacerations of the vagina and anal canal, anal fissures, and perineal trauma with coexisting higher visceral injuries.

Vaginal Water Injection Injuries

A forced sudden injection of water into the vagina may severely damage the vagina, uterus, and fallopian tubes. Such injuries have been reported to occur in women participating in water sports who fall perineum-first against the water surface with the legs in an adducted position. Vaginal water injection injuries have been reported in water skiers who fall backward while attempting to assume a squat position, in personal water craft (jet-ski) passengers who fall with their legs adducted in the line of the jet-ski's spray, and in surfers who land directly on the perineum during a fall (15–18). The injury affects only women who lack perineal protection, such as those wearing ordinary bathing suits, and may be prevented by wearing neoprene shorts or wetsuits.

TABLE 32–2. Female genital injuries associated with vaginal water injection trauma

Vulvar/labial hematomas	Tuboovarian abscesses
Vulvar/labial contusions	Partial avulsions of the cervix
Vaginal lacerations	Traumatic abortions
Broad ligament tears	Anal tears
Salpingitis	Shock
Peritonitis	

From Solomon S, Cappa KG. Impotence and bicycling. *Postgrad Med* 1987;81:99–101.

Vaginal lacerations are the most common of the various types of vaginal water injection injuries listed in Table 32–2. Vaginal lacerations average 3–5 cm in length and are located in the upper vagina in 75% of cases. The posterior upper vaginal wall and lateral fornices (right more frequently than left) are the most frequent sites of lacerations. The typical clinical presentation of vaginal lacerations is profuse, painless vaginal bleeding that progresses to hypovolemic shock in 15% of cases (17). Most vaginal lacerations require surgical repair, and treatment decisions are based on the depth and location of the laceration, concurrent injury to other intraabdominal organs, and the potential for infection. Since the injury extent may not be evident during the repair of the laceration, exploratory laparotomy or laparoscopy may be necessary to rule out intraabdominal involvement through broad ligament laceration extension or by vaginal perforation. Hypogastric artery ligation and intraarticular embolization may be required to control severe reproductive tract hemorrhage (17). Antibiotics are frequently used to treat or prevent infection. Minor vaginal lacerations or those located in the lower vagina may be successfully treated with vaginal packings to control hemorrhage. Salpingitis from bacterial contamination of the fallopian tubes after water injection may not appear clinically for several days after the injury has occurred. The patient may consequently not associate the vaginal water injection with the infection.

Hematomas of the Genital Tract

Blunt perineal trauma or vaginal water injection may produce hematomas of the vulva, vagina, or broad ligament. Hematoma bleeding that results from a ruptured artery in the perineal or paravaginal regions may extend downward to the vulva, laterally into the paravaginal area, or upward into the broad ligament. The clinical signs of genital tract hematomas include urinary and/or defecation urgency due to pressure applied by the hematoma on the bladder and/or rectum; bruising of the vulva and perineum; and a tender, large paravaginal mass on rectal examination. Treatment includes hemodynamic support, evacuation of the clot under anesthesia, and ligation of the bleeding vessel. Hematomas of the broad ligament are particularly worrisome, as they may extend into the peritoneal cavity and cause peritonitis.

REFERENCES

1. Schuster G. Traumatic rupture of the testicle and a review of the literature. *J Urol* 1982;127:1194.
2. McAleer IM, Kaplan GW. Pediatric genitourinary trauma. *Urol Clin N Am* 1995;22:177–188.
3. Hoover DL. How I manage testicular injury. *Phys Sportsmed* 1986;14:127–129.

4. O'Donoghue DH. *Treatment of injuries to athletes,* 4th ed. Philadelphia: WB Saunders, 1984:418.
5. Willliamson RCN. Torsion of the testis and allied conditions. *Br J Surg* 1976;63:465.
6. Weiss BD. Clinical syndromes associated with bicycle seats. *Clin Sports Med* 1994;13:175–186.
7. Mandell J, Cromie WJ, Caldamone AA, et al. Sports-related genitourinary injuries in children. *Clin Sports Med* 1982;1:483–493.
8. Swerdlow AJ, Huttly SRA, Smith PG. Is the incidence of testis cancer related to trauma or temperature. *Br J Urol* 1988;61:518–521.
9. Andersen KV, Bovium G. Impotence and nerve entrapment in long distance amateur cyclists. *Acta Neurol Scand* 1997;95:233–240.
10. Solomon S, Cappa KG. Impotence and bicycling. *Postgrad Med* 1987;81:99–101.
11. Wemyss-Holden SA, Hamby FC, Hastie KJ. Steroid abuse in athletes, prostatic enlargement and bladder outflow obstruction: is there a relationship? *Br J Urol* 1994;74:476–478.
12. Roberts JT, Essenhigh DM. Adenocarcinoma of prostate in a 40-year old body-builder [letter]. *Lancet* 1986;2:742.
13. Vuong PN, Camuzard P, Schnoonaat MF. Perineal nodular indurations "accessory testicles" in cyclists. *Acta Cytol* 1988;32:86–90.
14. Pokorny SF, Pokorny WJ, Kramer W. Acute genital injury in a prepubertal girl. *Am J Obstet Gynecol* 1992;166:1461–1466.
15. Kalaaichandran S. Vaginal laceration: a little-known hazard for women water-skiers [Letter]. *Can J Surg* 1991;34:107–108.
16. Rudoff JC. Vulvovaginal water-skiing injury [Letter]. *Ann Emerg Med* 1993;22:1072.
17. Haefner HK, Andersen F, Johnson MP. Vaginal laceration following a jet-ski accident. *Obstet Gynecol* 1991;78:986–988.
18. Wein P, Thompson DJ. Vaginal perforation due to a jet ski accident. *Aust NZ J Obstet Gynecol* 1990;30:384–385.

CHAPTER 33

Physeal Injuries

Manuel Leyes and Jack T. Andrish

EMBRYOLOGY

During the sixth week of embryonic development mesenchymal cells differentiate into chondrocytes to form a cartilaginous model of the future skeleton (1). In the midportion of this cartilaginous anlage, a primary diaphyseal center of ossification is gradually formed. The chondrocytes hypertrophy, their lacunae enlarge, and the matrix becomes calcified. At the same time the osteogenic cells of the perichondrium deposit a thin periosteal collar of bone (2). By the end of the eighth week, vascular invasion brings mesenchymal cells into the midportion of this cartilaginous anlage (3). These osteoprogenitor cells differentiate into osteoblasts and osteoclasts. The osteoblasts produce an osteoid matrix on the surfaces of the calcified cartilage to form the primary trabeculae, while the osteoclasts remove bone to form the medullary canal. This process of replacing the cartilage model by bone is called endochondral ossification, in contrast to intramembranous ossification in which bone is formed without a previous cartilaginous model. The flat bones of the skull, the sternum, and the scapula are examples of bones that develop by intramembranous ossification, while the long bones of the limbs and the ribs develop by endochondral ossification.

This primary diaphyseal center of ossification grows and expands centrifugally and eventually becomes confined to two platelike structures oriented toward each end of the bone. These platelike structures are the physes, or growth plates (4). At a rather definite time in the development of each long bone a secondary center of ossification appears within the cartilaginous epiphysis. Mechanical forces (5) and growth factors produced by the hypertrophic chondrocytes (6) stimulate the development of this center. The secondary center of ossification grows and expands centrifugally in all directions. The portion of the epiphysis that faces the growth plate eventually closes (Fig. 33–1) and becomes sealed with condensed bone, termed the bone plate (4).

ANATOMY

Knowledge of the normal anatomy of the physis is vital in understanding its injuries. The physis separates the epiphysis from the metaphysis in the immature skeleton. The bony surfaces of the epiphysis and the metaphysis are irregular, with small bony projections termed mammillary processes (7). The physis, which lies between those bony surfaces, is not a smooth plate, but rather is uneven with undulations. The cartilaginous component of the physis is encircled on the periphery by two fibrous structures: the perichondral ring of LaCroix and the ossification groove of Ranvier (Fig. 33–2). The cells in the ossification groove contribute to the horizontal growth of the physis. The fibrocartilaginous tissue of the perichondral ring is contiguous with the adjacent periosteum and serves to support the chondro-osseus junction (8).

Histologically, the physis consists of three zones (Fig. 33–2). The reserve zone is the part of the physis that is closest to the epiphyseal ossification center. It is broad in rapidly growing cartilage and decreases in width as the end of growth approaches. The chondrocytes in this zone are relatively few in comparison with other zones and exist singly or in pairs (4). They are active in protein synthesis (9), but they do not proliferate. Their intracellular calcium content is the lowest in the physis (10). The matrix contains type II collagen that inhibits calcification and acts as a barrier to the advancing front of the secondary center of ossification in the epiphysis

---

M. Leyes: Department of Orthopaedics, Cleveland Clinic Foundation, Cleveland, Ohio 44195.

J. T. Andrish: Section of Sports Medicine, Section of Pediatric Orthopaedics, Department of Orthopaedics, Cleveland Clinic Foundation, Cleveland, Ohio 44195.

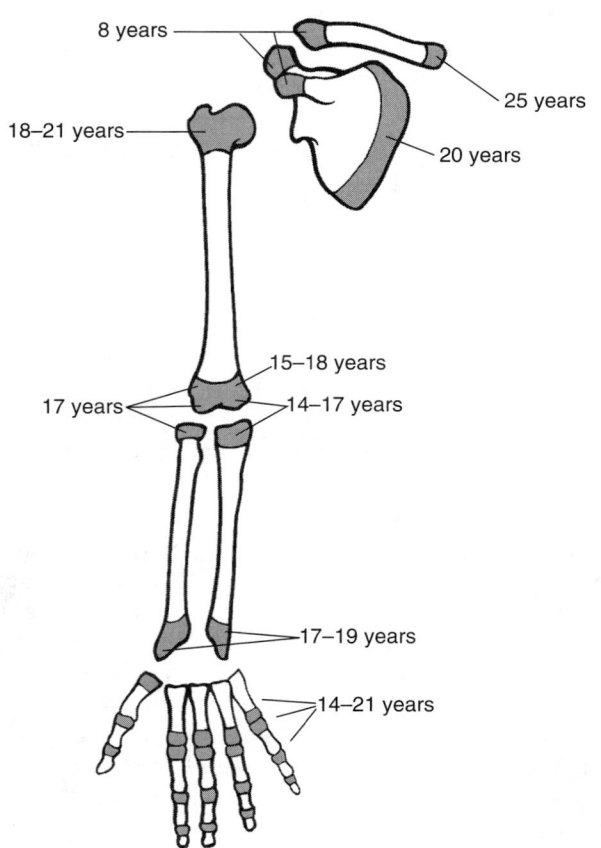

FIG. 33–1. The sequence of closure of the different physes is generally consistent. (Modified from Ogden JA. *Skeletal injury in the child.* Philadelphia: Lea & Febiger, 1982.)

(11). The collagen fibers exhibit random distribution and orientation. There are large numbers of vesicles in the matrix, but they do not participate in mineralization. Although vascular channels pass through this zone, they do not appear to supply it, and the oxygen tension is low (12). The function of the reserve zone is not clear. It does not actively participate in longitudinal growth.

In the proliferative zone the chondrocytes are bound in columns parallel to the axis of the bone. The uppermost cell in each column is the progenitor cell, which is not derived from the reserve zone cells. The total intracellular calcium content is similar to that in the reserve zone, but the ionized calcium concentration is significantly increased (10). The matrix contains randomly distributed collagen fibrils and matrix vesicles. The epiphyseal vessels that cross the resting zone terminate in this zone, yielding the highest oxygen tension in the physis (12). Aerobic metabolism occurs; glycogen is stored, and mitochondria form ATP. The proliferative zone is the major contributor to longitudinal growth achieved by cellular division and matrix production. The rate of chondrocyte replication is regulated by mechanical factors (2), systemic growth factors (growth hormone and parathormone), and local factors synthesized by the chondrocytes (somatomedin-C, insulinlike growth factor I, basic fibroblast growth factor, and transforming growth factor) (11). The receptors for systemic growth factors have been found primarily in this zone (13,14).

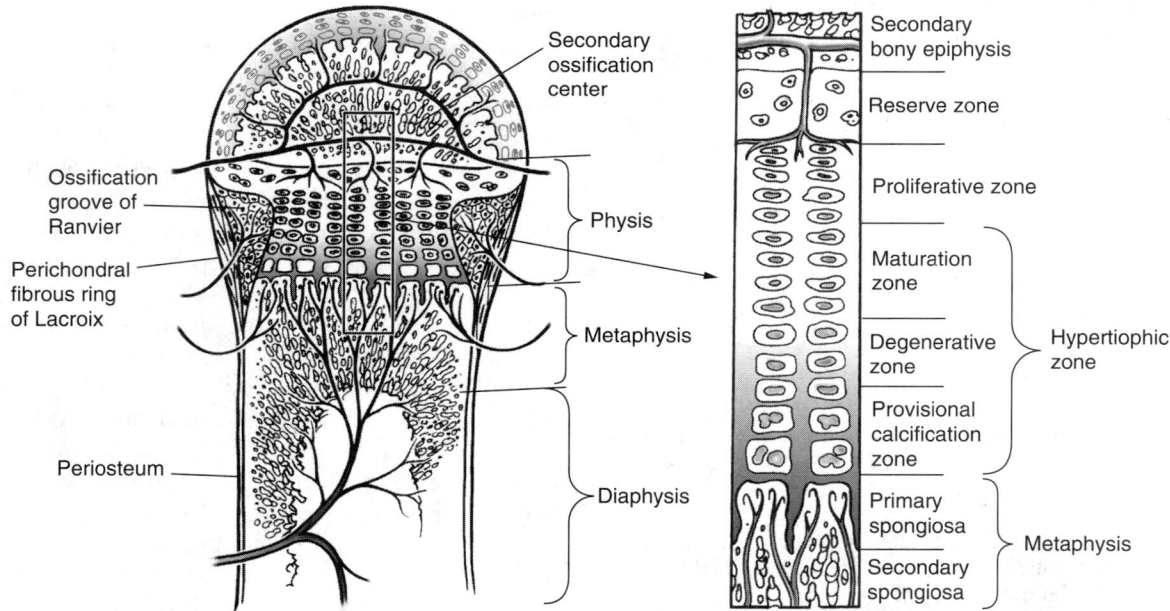

FIG. 33–2. Anatomy and histology of the growth plate. (Modified from Netter FH. *The CIBA Collection of Medical Illustrations.* Summit, N.J.: Ciba-Geigy Corporation, 1987.)

The hypertrophic zone is characterized by cellular enlargement from 5 to 10 times the size of the proliferative zone cell (9,15). It is subdivided into three zones: the maturation zone, the degenerative zone, and the zone of provisional calcification, which is adjacent to the metaphysis. The function of the cells of the maturation and degenerative zones is to prepare the matrix for calcification, which ultimately takes place in the provisional calcification zone. Biochemical analysis has shown that the hypertrophic zone chondrocytes are very active metabolically (2). There is no vascular supply to the chondrocytes, and anaerobic metabolism accounts for the synthesis of type X collagen and proteoglycans. Glycogen is consumed, and the mitochondria switch from forming ATP to accumulating calcium. In the zone of provisional calcification, glycogen supplies are depleted; the calcium concentration in the mitochondria can no longer be maintained, and calcium is released into the matrix. Calcification of the matrix further decreases diffusion of nutrients and oxygen to the chondrocytes. Anaerobic glycolysis occurs, and the mitochondria continue releasing calcium. This cycle ultimately results in the death of the hypertrophic chondrocyte.

The physis has three major vascular supplies. The terminal branches of the epiphyseal artery pass through canals in the reserve zone to terminate at the uppermost part of the proliferative zone. No vessels pass through the proliferative zone to supply the hypertrophic zone. Terminal branches of the nutrient artery supply the central region of the metaphysis, while metaphyseal arteries and a perichondrial artery to the perichondrial ring of LaCroix supply the periphery. Terminal branches from the nutrient and metaphyseal arteries pass vertically toward the bone-cartilage junction of the physis and end at the last cartilaginous transverse septum at the base of the cartilage portion of the physis. No vessels pass from the metaphysis into the hypertrophic zone. They turn back on themselves to form a venous return (16). Several perichondrial arteries supply the groove of Ranvier and the perichondrial ring of LaCroix.

BIOMECHANICAL PROPERTIES

Physeal injuries are typically due to shear and/or tension (80%) or compression and/or splitting forces (20%) (17). In adolescents the physis is 2–5 times weaker than the adjacent joint capsule and ligamentous structures (18). As a result, every adolescent who is suspected of having torn a major ligament should have a radiographic examination to study the epiphyses of the area (19).

The periosteum plays an important role in stabilizing the physis (20). Morscher and colleagues (21) showed that when the periosteum was removed, the load-to-failure values of the physis decreased to almost half of the values with intact periosteum. The periosteum is firmly attached to the epiphysis and to the physis at the perichondrial ring. The latter provides mechanical support, acting as a limiting membrane (4). The undulations of the physis are also thought to help resist displacement due to shear stress (22). Tendons and ligaments tend to insert at the area of the perichondrium, resulting in tensile forces transmitted to the physis. It has been long recognized that mechanical stimuli, compression, and tensile forces can influence bone growth in length, but the relationship between the specific character of the load and the physeal response is unknown (22).

The physis is most resistant to tension and least resistant to torsion (23). In the cartilaginous portion of the physis it is the intercellular substance and not the cells that provides the strength, particularly its resistance to shear (19). The collagen fibers of the epiphyseal plate are arranged longitudinally and play a role similar to that of the steel rods in reinforced concrete (19).

The different zones of the physis have different biomechanical properties. The weakest portion of the physis is the hypertrophic zone, in which the matrix volume is low and the cellular content is high (22). The orientation of the hypertrophic cell columns is an important microstructural feature that influences the tensile behavior (24). The proliferative layer is most susceptible to tensile forces, and the zone of calcification and the metaphyseal bone are most susceptible to compressive forces (25). Lee and colleagues (26) studied the mechanical properties of the mineralized bone around the physis and found that the primary spongiosa in the metaphysis had an elastic modulus and hardness that were significantly lower than those of the epiphyseal trabecular bone.

The age of the patient also influences the mechanical properties of the physes. The shear strength of the physis increases with age, and the pattern of physeal fracture also changes with age (22). For example, Type I fractures are more frequent in the very young, while in older bones Types II and IV fractures are more common.

CLASSIFICATION OF PHYSEAL INJURIES

Although other fracture classifications exist, the Salter-Harris classification (27) remains the most practical and widely used. In this classification system, five types of fracture patterns are described (Fig. 33-3).

Type I

In the Type I fracture, there is a complete separation of the epiphysis from the metaphysis. The line of cleavage is confined to the physis without extension into the

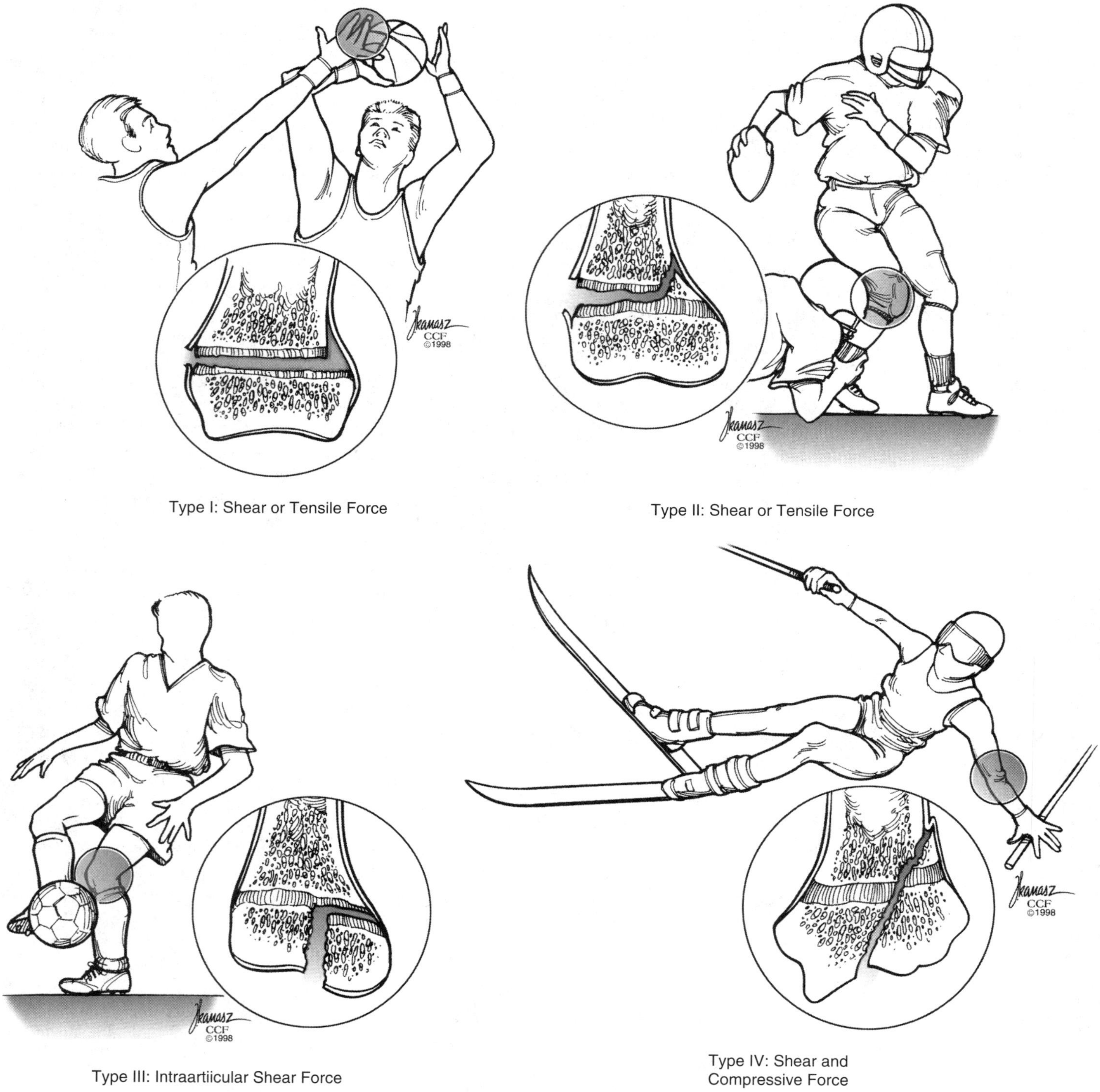

Type I: Shear or Tensile Force

Type II: Shear or Tensile Force

Type III: Intraarticular Shear Force

Type IV: Shear and Compressive Force

FIG. 33-3. Classification of Salter and Harris (27) with examples that illustrate the mechanism of injury.

epiphysis or metaphysis. The injury is caused by a shear or tensile force. The reserve zone of the physis remains attached to the epiphysis. Growth retardation is rare after this injury. It is more common in birth injuries and early childhood and may also be seen in pathologic separations of the epiphysis associated with rickets, scurvy, osteomyelitis, and endocrine imbalance (19). The diagnosis is often difficult because the periosteal attachment is usually intact and these fractures tend not to be displaced.

Type IV

In the Type IV fracture, the fracture line extends vertically through the epiphysis, the physis, and on through the metaphysis. The articular surface and the reserve zone are damaged, and there is a great potential for growth disruption. Most occur at the lateral humeral condyle and the distal tibia (17).

Type V

The Type V fracture is a pure compressive injury to the physis that is not associated with immediate clinical or radiographic findings of a fracture. It most commonly involves the distal femoral (Fig. 33–4) and proximal tibial physes (17). This injury is diagnosed in retrospect if premature physeal closure occurs and the radiographs at the time of injury were normal.

Other Types of Fractures

Some authors include a Rang-Salter-Harris Type VI injury (31), which represents an injury to the perichondrial ring with damage to the physis secondary to disruption of nutrient blood flow coming from the perichondrial ring. The perichondrial ring can be damaged by a

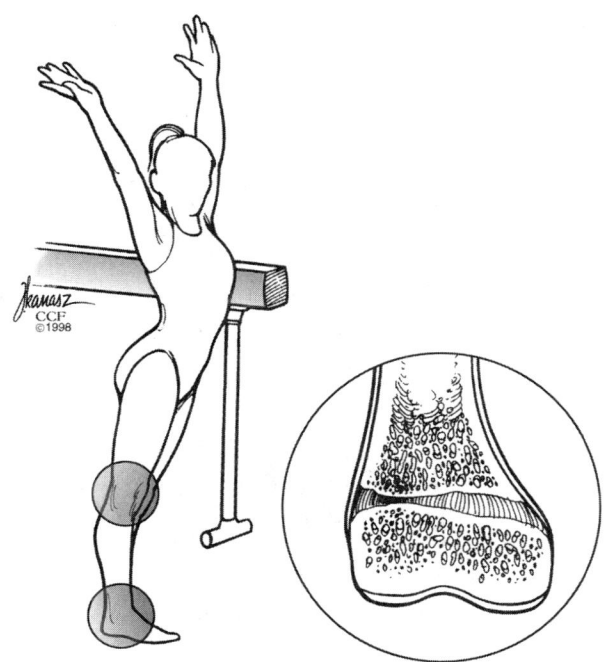

Type V: Compressive Force

FIG. 33–3. *Continued.*

Type II

Type II fractures are the most common type of physeal injury (28,29). The fracture line passes through the physis and extends into the metaphysis, separating a triangular metaphyseal fragment sometimes referred to as the Thurston Holland sign or corner sign. It is produced by shear or tensile forces. The periosteum is torn on the convex side of the angulation and intact on the side of the metaphyseal injury. The reserve zone is usually not disturbed, and growth arrest is rare except for the distal femur and proximal tibia (30), where any type of growth plate injury may cause growth arrest. Type II fractures frequently occur at the distal radius in children older than 10 years.

Type III

Type III is a fracture pattern that is produced by an intraarticular shear force. The line of fracture runs vertically through the epiphysis and then extends horizontally at the physis to its periphery. It is an uncommon injury that usually happens near the end of skeletal growth (19). The most frequent sites of involvement are the upper and lower tibial epiphyses, the distal femur, and the distal phalanges (17,19). The reserve zone and the articular cartilage are disrupted. The prognosis depends on the accuracy of reduction and the preservation of the blood supply.

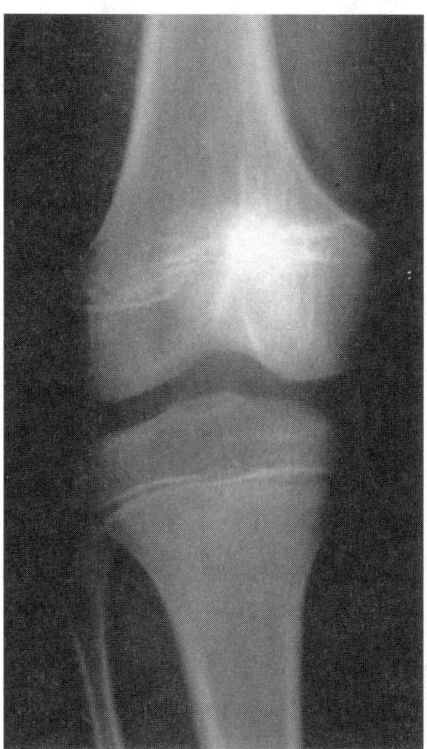

FIG. 33–4. This young patient sustained a Salter-Harris Type V fracture of the distal femur. The anteroposterior radiograph of the knee demonstrates varus angulation secondary to partial physeal arrest.

direct blow in a closed injury or by a sharp object in an open injury or avulsed by an injury to an attached ligament. The diagnosis may be challenging, since the initial radiographs are normal. In Type V and VI injuries, no structure is broken, and the term *injury* is more appropriate than *fracture* (30).

Peterson (32) has described two physeal fractures that were not previously classified. First is a transverse fracture of the metaphysis with the fracture line or lines extending to the physis but without propagation through the physis. Second is an open fracture in which a portion of the physis was missing. The former was a common fracture, occurring in 15.5% of patients in his study.

MICROSCOPIC ANALYSIS OF PHYSEAL FRACTURES

Salter and Harris based their classification on the belief that physeal fracture propagation was almost invariably through the layer of hypertrophic cells at approximately the junction of the calcified and uncalcified matrices (27). However, this is not always the case. Both experimental studies in animals (33–35) and human biopsy samples (36–38) have demonstrated an inconsistent cleavage plane in 50–85% of the cases. In these studies, the fracture line was often sinusoidal and could involve any zone of the cartilage. In some cases the fracture line extends to the zone of provisional calcification, and the radiograph shows fragments of bone on the metaphyseal side of the physeal injury (11). Experimental studies have shown that the extent of skeletal maturation and the direction and rate of application of the deforming force affect the physeal fracture patterns (25,33,39). When the shear force is dominant, there is a tendency toward production of a Type I injury with failure occurring between the upper zone of columnation and lower zone of hypertrophy (Fig. 33–5). If the compression component increases, particularly in the lower extremity, the likelihood of a Type II injury also increases (25,27,29). Torsional forces result in failure through all zones (25). Finally, the shape of the physeal plate and the obliquity of the forces also affect the level of the physeal fracture (40).

EPIDEMIOLOGY OF PHYSEAL INJURIES

Over recent decades there has been an increase in sports participation by young athletes (41). It has been estimated that more than 35 million children and adolescents in the United States participate in some kind of sport activity (42). Unfortunately, injury is an inherent risk in sports participation. Between 3% and 11% of school-aged children are injured each year in sport activities (43–45). Sports involving contact and jumping have the highest incidence of injuries (46).

In an epidemiologic study by Peterson and colleagues (28), the overall age- and sex-adjusted incidence of physeal fractures was 279.2 per 100,000 person-years. In Mann and Rajmaira's series (47), physeal injuries accounted for 30% of 2650 long-bone fractures in children, while Worlock and Stower (48) reported that 18.5% of fractures in children 12 years of age or younger involved the physis. This finding was similar to the 18% incidence of physeal injuries in 2000 fractures studied by Mizuta and colleagues (29). The variation in incidence between these different studies depends partly on whether injuries of the hands and feet are included. In fact, the actual incidence may be even higher than those reported, given that Type I injuries and some Type II injuries may be difficult to diagnose on routine radiographs.

Boys sustain twice as many physeal injuries as girls (28,29,49), probably because, in general, boys participate more in activities with increased physical risk.

Physeal injuries are also more common during periods of rapid skeletal growth. Girls with physeal fractures are, on average, 1.5 years younger than boys with the same type of fracture in the same location (47). In Peterson's series, incidence rates were found to be greatest among 11- to 12-year-old girls and 14-year-old boys (28). In contrast, physeal injuries are uncommon in children younger than 5 years of age (48). The increasing incidence of physeal injuries with age may be related to both the increased vigor of the activities and the relative weakening of the physis during puberty (50).

The physes of the upper extremities are involved

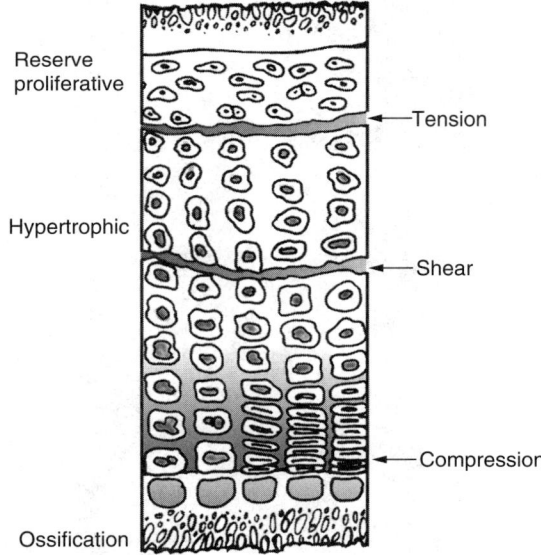

FIG. 33–5. The histologic failure pattern of the physis varies with the type of load. (Modified from Moen CT, Pelker RR. Biomechanical and histological correlations in growth plate failure. *J Pediatr Orthop* 1984;4(2):180–184.)

three times more often than those of the lower extremities (28,29). Distal physes are injured more frequently than proximal ones, except for the proximal humerus (28). The most common sites of physeal fractures are the phalanges of fingers and the distal radius (28,29,49).

EVALUATION OF PHYSEAL INJURIES

Although the accurate diagnosis of physeal injury depends on the radiographic examination, this lesion can be suspected on the basis of the history and clinical examination. The knowledge of the mechanism of injury may also help in the diagnosis, especially in crush injuries. The typical presentation of a physeal injury includes swelling, hyperemia, and tenderness over the physis. Deformity may or may not be apparent.

Most physeal fractures as well as the late complication of physeal bridges can be detected with plain radiographs. Anteroposterior and lateral radiographs are recommended as the initial imaging procedure. Additional oblique views are often required at the ankle (51) and the knee (52).

Radiographically, most physeal injuries are characterized by some combination of widening of the physis, displacement of the epiphysis, and blurring of the opposing margins of the metaphysis and epiphysis (17). In physeal fractures in which the cleavage line has extended to the zone of provisional calcification, small fragments of bone, the so-called lamellar fragments, may be seen within the physis (52).

Physeal injuries often result from an initial displacement of the epiphysis, followed by a reduction to the normal position, in which radiographs may be initially interpreted as normal. Comparative views of the opposite uninjured extremity and stress views (51) may be helpful in the diagnosis of nondisplaced physeal fractures. Stress views have been proven to be useful in the diagnosis of Type III injuries of the distal femoral epiphysis and Type I injuries of the distal fibula (52). However, some orthopedic surgeons believe that such maneuvers should be avoided because of the risk of producing further injury to the physis. (53). The delayed diagnosis of nondisplaced physeal fractures can be made by the demonstration of subperiosteal new bone formation in the metaphyseal region 10–14 days after the initial injury.

After a temporary slowdown or cessation of rapid longitudinal growth, plain radiographs may show transversely oriented lines parallel to the contours of the contiguous physis. These so-called Harris growth-arrest lines are located in the metaphyses or diaphyses, and when they converge with the physis, damage of growth is likely to be present (54). Plain radiographs are also used to assess the potential for remaining growth (55) and to measure limb length discrepancy and angulation.

Multiplanar tomography is a reliable method of evaluating the location, extent and contours of a physeal bar, but the radiation exposure is high (56). It is being replaced by computed tomography (CT) scan and magnetic resonance imaging.

With CT scan images the normal physis is visualized as a low-density layer of tissue between adjacent sclerotic margins of the epiphysis and the metaphysis (57). CT is most commonly used in the ankle and is particularly useful in triplane fractures (52). It has also been used to assess the alignment of the articular surfaces in Types III and IV physeal fractures (52) and to determine the extent and location of physeal bony bars (58,59). Two pitfalls of the CT scan, however, are that the entire physis cannot be captured on one cut in the transverse plane and that the normal juxtaphyseal bone sclerosis may mimic a bony bridge (30).

Magnetic resonance imaging (MRI) has facilitated the study of physeal injuries by demonstrating the extra-osseous and cartilaginous component of these lesions (60). This is particularly useful in epiphyseal separations about the knee where MRI depicts associated ligament injuries, which occur in half of these patients (52). Yet another advantage of MRI is its multiplane imaging capability without the use of ionizing radiation.

The MRI pattern of epiphyseal vessels and the degree of enhancement of the physis change with maturity (61). In the young patient the physis is uniformly hyperintense in gradient echo images and contrasts with the surrounding hypointense signal of bone (62). As the patient approaches maturity, the physis narrows and becomes less clear on MR images. Different physes show different patterns of physeal closure (63). After closure the physis is seen as a single hypointense band, which often persists into adult life. Some coronal and sagittal images of the normal knee show discontinuity of the physeal cartilage (drop-out sign), which should not be mistaken for premature closure (64).

Although it is very useful, MRI is not required in the diagnosis of most physeal injuries. Petit and colleagues (65) performed a study to assess the benefit of MR imaging compared with plain film radiography in the diagnosis and immediate treatment of acute fractures of the distal tibial physis. Only 1 of 29 fractures (3%) was misclassified by plain film radiography. MR imaging never caused the treatment plan to be modified. However, the position of fracture fragments in Salter-Harris IV and triplane fractures was always better appreciated on MR images, facilitating more accurate surgical treatment.

In any case, MRI has become the method of choice for the detection of fibrous or bone bridging of the physis (Fig. 33–6), the assessment of growth arrest, and the detection of avascular necrosis of the epiphyses and infarction of the metaphyses following epiphyseal injury (52). Its efficacy exceeds that of multiplanar tomography, specifically when the physis cannot be properly

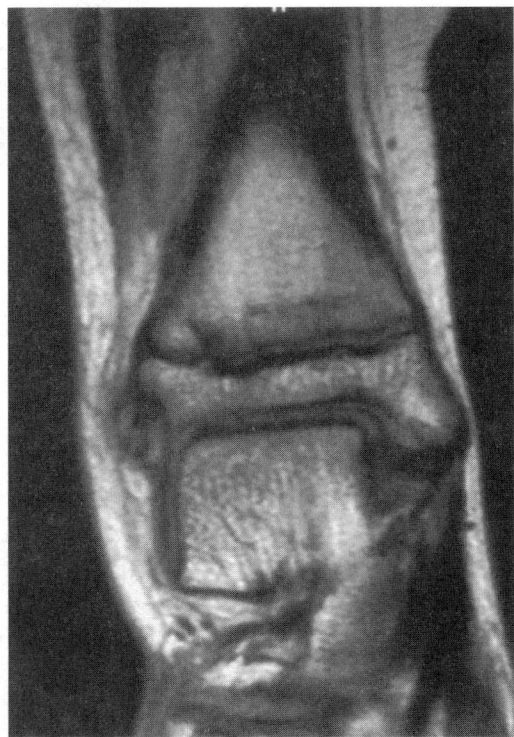 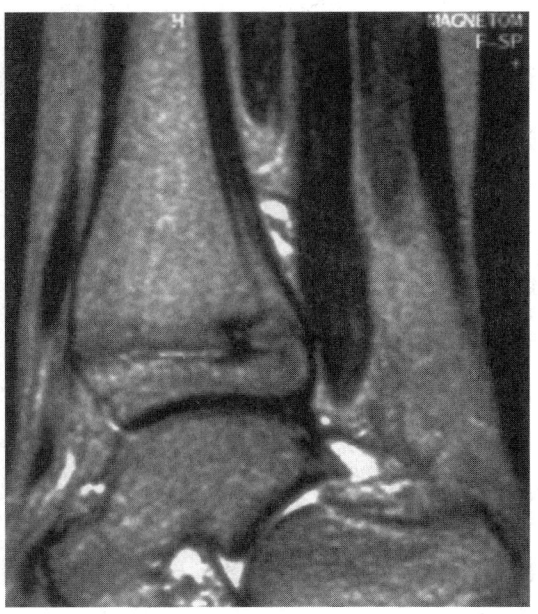

FIG. 33–6. Coronal T1–weighted (**A**) and sagittal T2–weighted (**B**) magnetic resonance images of the ankle depicting a physeal bony bridge.

oriented for tomographic evaluation, when more planes are desired, and when radiation exposure is thought to be excessive (56). Physeal bridging is shown as a hypointense line or bar disrupting the hyperintense physis (17). Physeal cartilage changes are best visualized on the gradient echo images (62). If bony bridges occur, fatty marrow may be seen on T1-weighted images (66). Furthermore, imaging data can be processed to yield both 3D rendered and projection physeal maps that are particularly useful in preoperative planning (66,67).

MR imaging also detects abnormalities in the cartilage that are significant predictors of subsequent growth disturbance (66). Examples are physeal widening of focal tongue morphology, central location of the lesion in the metaphysis, and coexistent epiphyseal signal after a single-event insult (68). Finally, MRI may also be used in the follow-up of patients after epiphysiodesis, since it provides excellent visualization of the anatomical changes that lead to closure of the physis (69).

Unlike other diagnostic studies, which basically provide anatomic information, radionuclide bone scanning reflects the physiologic status of the physis and is valuable in defining its viability (70,71). Technetium-99m diphosphonate is taken up at the zone of provisional calcification (72) and in the primary spongiosa adjacent to the physis (54). In the scintigraphic assessment of a physis, it is very important to compare it with the contralateral normal physis, symmetrically positioned on the same large view (73).

A physeal fracture results in uniformly increased physeal activity. Walter and colleagues (74) have successfully used bone scintigraphy to diagnose Type I and V Salter-Harris fractures of the physis at an early stage. Decreased radiopharmaceutical uptake is noted at the time of skeletal maturity and at both physiologic and surgical closure of the physis (54). In fact, bone scintigraphy may be used to document the success of the procedure (73).

Although visual interpretation is usually adequate, computer-assisted quantitative methods of assessing bone scan activity permit a more objective measurement and may detect asymmetric activity at the physis in angular deformities (75,76). The half of the physis with the greater mechanical loading becomes more active than the other half (73).

Bone single-photon emission computed tomography (SPECT) is capable of creating maps of the distribution of osteoblastic activity in the physis and may be useful in patients who are suffering from growth arrests. In a study performed by Wioland and Bonnerot (77) in patients with partial epiphysiodeses, the SPECT indicated the percentage of the remaining normal physis, located the bony bridge within the physis and showed the slowdown of the growth of the remaining normal physis induced by the bony bridge.

TREATMENT PRINCIPLES

A comprehensive discussion on the specific treatment for each physeal injury is beyond the scope of this chapter. Therefore we shall focus on the general principles of physeal injury management.

The goal of treatment of physeal fractures is not only the restoration of articular congruity and physeal anatomy, but also the restoration of physeal function (30,78). To prevent damage of the physis, manipulation of a physeal fracture should be gentle. It is better to accept an imperfect reduction and perform a corrective osteotomy later, if necessary, than to persist with forceful, repeated manipulations (19). In young children general anesthesia allows for the gentlest manipulation (78).

The best time to reduce a physeal fracture is the day of the injury (19). Delay makes reduction more difficult, particularly in the young child with a very rapid presence of healing callus. In experimental studies, onset of union by endochondral ossification was observed within 2 days of injury in immature rabbits with Salter-Harris Type I or Type II physeal fractures (79). When a child presents with a Type I or Type II fracture a week after the injury, it is better to accept malunion than to damage the physis by forceful manipulation. Osteotomy may be performed later if remodeling fails (80). On the other hand, because of the high incidence of growth disturbance with displaced Type III and IV injuries, it is preferable to perform delayed reduction rather than to accept the malunion (80).

When open reduction is required, the extent of soft tissue stripping should be limited to prevent avascular necrosis of the epiphysis (19). Care should be taken not to apply direct pressure on the physis with the surgical instruments (30). Inserting screws or threaded wires across the physeal plate should be avoided (19). Instead, fine smooth Kirschner wires that cross the physes at right angles and spare the perichondrial ring may be used, but these must be removed as soon as the injury is healed.

Absorbable pins have been successfully used in internal fixation of physeal fractures of the distal humerus (81,82) and distal femur (83). The main advantage of this method is that hardware removal procedures are not required (84). Although clinical (81–85) and experimental studies (86–88) have shown promising results, further experience with these materials is necessary before this method can be safely recommended (89).

The clinical criteria for an acceptable reduction will vary according to the location and type of fracture. The criteria are less rigid in the region of a multiplane joint, such as the shoulder, than in the region of a single plane joint such as the knee. Criteria are also less rigid in Type I and II fractures. For example, in Type I and II fractures, perfect reduction is desirable but not mandatory, since bone remodeling will correct moderate residual deformities, especially deformities that are in the same plane of motion as the nearest joint (80). Type III and IV fractures must be perfectly reduced to prevent articular degeneration (19).

As a rule, the younger the patient, the shorter the time to healing (90). Type I, II, and III injuries unite in approximately half the time that is required for union of a fracture through the metaphysis of the same bone in the same age group. Type IV injuries require the same period of immobilization as metaphyseal fractures. In physeal fractures about the knee, obese patients typically require more extensive immobilization (78). During healing of the fracture, weight bearing should be discouraged to prevent further damage to the physis (78).

Evaluation of growth arrest after physeal injuries requires radiographs of both extremities at 3- to 6-month intervals (17). Ideally, a child who sustained a physeal fracture must be followed until skeletal maturity (91). Since growth disturbance can be delayed for up to 1 year, this period of observation is considered to be the minimum follow-up required. More recently, MRI has been shown to be a sensitive indicator of impending physeal growth arrest as well as providing an early depiction of bone bridging (52,66).

Most Type I injuries are readily reduced by closed means, and the reduction is easily maintained. Cast immobilization for 3–4 weeks is usually sufficient (30). Displaced distal femoral physeal fractures are the exception. Published reports (92,93) have shown that the best results occur when fractures are anatomically reduced and fixed with pins.

In Type II injuries as well, closed reduction can usually be accomplished. The metaphyseal fragment prevents overreduction (30), and the intact periosteum on the metaphyseal side adds stability to the fracture (90). After reduction, protection is maintained until healing occurs, usually at 4–6 weeks. The prognosis depends on the amount of physis involved, the degree of displacement, the patient's age, and the particular physis involved. A flat physis, such as the distal radius, is less prone to develop growth arrest than undulating physes such as the distal femur or proximal tibia (30).

The Type III fracture is an intraarticular fracture and requires accurate reduction to restore a smooth joint surface. In Type IV injuries perfect reduction is also essential. Not only the articular surface but also the physeal plate should be accurately realigned to prevent bony union across the plate and eventual growth arrest (19). Unless the fracture is nondisplaced, open reduction is necessary.

In Type V injuries displacement of the epiphysis is unusual, and the treatment consists of protection and avoidance of weight bearing for approximately 6 weeks (90).

PROGNOSIS OF PHYSEAL INJURIES

The clinical outcome of a physeal injury depends on many factors. Parameters include the severity of the injury, the patient's age at the time of injury, the particular physis injured, the presence of damage to the blood supply of the epiphysis, the method and accuracy of reduction, and the type of physeal injury (30,40,94). Of these, the most important factor is the severity of the injury. Significant initial displacement, comminution, crush injury, and open fractures are all associated with a worse prognosis (19,30,40). In Lombardo and Harvey's series (40), initial metaphyseal displacement greater than one half the diameter was associated with a higher incidence of subsequent growth arrest after distal femoral physeal fractures. In open injuries portions of the physis may be missing (32) with the added factor of contamination and infection, which can destroy the physeal plate (19).

Age is the second most important factor in determining the prognosis. The younger the patient at the time of injury, the greater the amount of expected growth remaining and the more potential for serious growth disturbance outcome, should the complication of premature closure occur (19).

The prognosis also depends on the site of the physeal injury. In the upper extremity the prognosis for growth is good after Type I, II, and III injuries but is guarded in Type IV and poor in Type V (17). The likelihood of growth arrest is higher in the weight-bearing lower extremity, particularly at the distal femur (30,78,95), distal tibia (96-100), and proximal tibia (95,101–103). The high frequency of growth arrest after distal femoral and proximal tibial physeal injuries is related to the fact that they are the largest and fastest-growing physes (40,104) and that their irregular shape predisposes to fracture through more than one zone (104). Significant shortening occurs in 30–50% of adolescent distal femoral physeal fractures and more than 50% of juvenile fractures (40,104,105).

Disruption of the epiphyseal circulation, which commonly occurs with proximal femoral and radial head physeal fractures (19), is an important factor in the premature closure of the physis (38). Trabecular bone forms along the damaged vessels, and over time a bony bar bridges between epiphysis and metaphysis. Furthermore, if epiphyseal circulation is interrupted, the zones of cellular growth associated with these particular vessels cannot undergo appropriate cell division (38). On the other hand, damage of the metaphyseal circulation has minimal if any effect on physeal development (91).

With regards to the type of injury, in general, Type I, II, and III injuries have a good prognosis for growth if the blood supply is intact and the injury has not been severe (19). The prognosis for Type IV injuries is poor unless the fracture is completely reduced. Type V injuries carry the worst prognosis (19). However, it should be remembered that prognosis made on the basis of the Salter-Harris classification alone has been shown to be unreliable (29,40,95).

Reports of the percentage of physeal fractures that are associated with growth disturbance range between 1% and 14% (28,29,49). A partial physeal arrest is more common than a complete cessation of growth. The partial physeal arrest may present in three patterns (106). The most common pattern is a peripheral bar that causes angular deformity. The second most common pattern is a central bar that causes longitudinal growth disturbance and eventual articular surface distortion. The third pattern, also referred to as a linear bar, is a combined one that involves some areas of the peripheral and central physis. The resultant deformity includes intraarticular incongruity and progressive angular growth disturbance (106).

If the entire physeal plate ceases to grow, the result is significant progressive shortening without angulation. Complete growth arrest may be seen after a crush injury to the growth plate.

Cessation of growth does not necessarily occur immediately after injury to the physis. Usually, partial growth arrest is first recognized 3–6 months after the injury, but some bony bars may not become clinically evident until years after the initial injury. Early radiographic signs of growth disturbance after physeal injury include blurring and narrowing of the physis, areas of reactive bone condensation, and development of asymmetric Harris lines (107,108). Once the diagnosis of physeal arrest has been made, it is very important to accurately determine the extent and location of the bar. The role of diagnostic imaging methods in the evaluation of the physeal bars has already been discussed.

TREATMENT OF PHYSEAL ARREST

The treatment of partial physeal damage depends on the location of the bone bridge, the size of the bar, and the age of the patient. Physeal bar resection is indicated in patients with more than 2 years or 2 cm of growth remaining and less than 50% of the cross-sectional area of the physis involved (106). In the very young child resection of bars larger than 50% of the physis is occasionally successful (30). Resection of central bars is technically more difficult. A direct approach is not possible, and it may be difficult to locate the bar through the metaphyseal window. Nevertheless, the best results of physeal bar resection are obtained with central bars because the periphery of the physis maintains the longitudinal growth (106).

Various interpositional materials have been used to

prevent reformation of the transphyseal bone bridge after resection. The most popular materials are fat, bone wax, silastic, and methylmethacrylate (30). Fat has the advantage of being autogenous, but a second incision may be needed. Clinical, radiographic, and histologic studies in a rabbit model (109,110) have shown that a physeal graft, harvested from the iliac apophysis, is superior to silastic and fat in terms of correction of angular deformity as well as contributing to longitudinal growth after resection of a large peripherally situated bone bridge. Unfortunately, interposition of physeal allografts has not achieved comparable results (111).

In a more recent experimental study in rabbits (112), transfer of cultured chondrocytes prevented growth arrest and angular deformation after excision of the medial half of the proximal growth plate of the tibia, as well as after excision of an established bone bridge.

When more than 50% of the physis is involved, the partial arrest can be surgically converted into a complete arrest to prevent further angulation. If the resultant limb length inequality is less than 2 cm, it is usually managed conservatively with a shoe-lift. Larger discrepancies require contralateral epiphysiodesis or, rarely, an ipsilateral limb-lengthening procedure (30,106). Percutaneous epiphyseodesis has proven to be successful. The advantages of this technique include a cosmetic scar, short hospital stay, low incidence of complications, and reliable physeal arrest (113,114).

In children who are near skeletal maturity it is also possible to simultaneously correct angular deformities and bone shortening secondary to bony bridges by physeal distraction (115,116).

The treatment of a complete physeal arrest depends on the age of the patient and the involved physis. In children who are close to skeletal maturity, with little growth remaining, no treatment is required. In younger children the options include shoe-lift, epiphysiodesis of the contralateral bone, ipsilateral bone lengthening, contralateral bone shortening, or a combination of procedures.

STRESS-RELATED INJURIES AND APOPHYSEAL INJURIES

Several authors have described physeal stress-related injuries of the skeletally immature shoulder (117–122), wrist (123–130), and elbow (131,132).

The entity referred to as "Little League shoulder" is characterized by pain occurring in the dominant shoulder of a skeletally immature throwing athlete. Radiographs demonstrate widening of the proximal humeral physis. Cystic changes in the metaphysis may also be present. This condition is considered to be either a stress-related physeal widening or a subacute Type I growth plate fracture. The treatment consists of abstinence from throwing for 4–6 weeks. Complete healing occurs uniformly, and no adverse sequelae result.

Distal radial stress injuries are common in skeletally immature gymnasts. The mechanism of injury includes repetitive hyperextension, compression, and rotation, which occur in activities such as handsprings, vaulting, and maneuvers on the bar apparatus (126). The dowel grip, used by gymnasts to increase their hook-grip strength, has also been associated with stress-related changes of the distal radial and ulnar physes (133). Such repetitive injury of the wrist may lead to a premature closure of the distal radial physis, resulting in secondary ulnar overgrowth (125,127,134). The risk of growth disturbance is higher with increasing levels of competition and years of participation (125). Radiographic changes in stress-related wrist injuries include widening, irregularity, and haziness of the physis; cystic changes in the metaphysis; and displacement of the epiphysis (135). The treatment consists of avoiding weight bearing of the affected limb until the wrist is completely asymptomatic and nontender and has a full free range of motion (135).

In skeletally immature athletes repetitive microtrauma caused by the traction of the muscles or tendons may cause avulsion of apophyses or traction apophysistis. The most common locations are the tibial tubercle (Osgood-Schlatter disease), the distal pole of the patella (Sinding-Larsen-Johansson syndrome), the calcaneus (Sever's disease), the medial epicondyle of the humerus, (Little League elbow), the pelvic apophyses, and the vertebra (atypical Scheuermann's disease). These entities are described in the chapters on traction apophysitis and stress reaction-stress fractures.

ANTERIOR CRUCIATE LIGAMENT INJURY IN THE SKELETALLY IMMATURE ATHLETE

The basic principles of diagnosis and conservative treatment of anterior cruciate ligament injuries (ACL) are the same for the skeletally immature and for the adult patient (136). However, in the truly immature patient, with wide open physes, the surgical options may be restricted. Most techniques for anterior cruciate ligament (ACL) reconstruction involve drilling holes through the tibia and the lateral femoral condyle. In skeletally immature patients standard holes would cross the physes of the proximal tibia and distal femur. Because of the fear of physeal damage during the surgical reconstruction of the ACL, nonoperative management has traditionally been advised for isolated ACL tears in children. Operative intervention is delayed until skeletal maturity has been achieved. Unfortunately, the functional results of the nonsurgical treatment of ACL injuries are poor, and during this waiting period the risks of reinjury and further meniscus and cartilage damage are significant (137–143).

Encouraged by the recognized increased healing potential of young patients, some authors (143–146) have performed primary repair of the torn ACL in skeletally immature knees. However, the results were poor, and good clinical outcomes were achieved only with osseous avulsion-type injuries. In an effort to spare the open physes, Parker and colleagues (147) advocated operative reconstruction using hamstring tendons. A groove is placed over the front of the tibia and another groove over the top of the femur without violating the physes. A disadvantage of this technique is the predisposition for intercondylar notch impingement of the ACL graft that may adversely affect postoperative motion as well as leading to graft failure. Nakhostine and colleagues (148) reported good results in five adolescents with open physes who underwent extraarticular reconstruction of ACL using a strip of iliotibial band. However, there is concern with extraarticular reconstructions that they do not follow the principles of isometry (149).

The demand for an optimal level of knee function after ACL injury has prompted many authors (137,142, 150–154) to perform intraarticular reconstructions of the ACL in young patients. The risk of physeal damage with ACL reconstruction is related to the immaturity of the distal femoral and proximal tibial physes (155). Therefore assessment of maturity on the basis physiologic criteria (Tanner stage (156), menarche, axillary hair development), radiologic criteria (skeletal age as determined by the Greulich and Pyle atlas (55), Risser sign), and family height is critical before the formulation of a specific treatment regimen.

In the adolescent patient who is close to skeletal maturity, an intraarticular reconstruction with transphyseal bone patellar tendon bone grafts can be performed. McCarroll and colleagues (142) reported no growth disturbance using this technique in 60 patients whose age ranged between 13 and 17 years.

The use of bone patellar tendon bone grafts in the very skeletally immature knee has been discouraged because of the presumed high risk of physeal closure and subsequent deformity. In a recent experimental study, successful ACL reconstruction in young animals with an open physis, using bone patellar tendon bone autografts and iliotibial band, resulted in angulation and shortening of the leg (157). Valgus deformities and shortening of the tibia in rabbits have also been described after intraarticular ACL reconstruction with semitendinous grafts passed through open physes (158).

On the other hand, other experimental studies (159,160) have shown that soft tissue grafts placed in drill holes across open physes can prevent bone bridge formation. This contradictory finding may be related to the size of the physeal injuries. In rabbits the relative size of physeal drill injury necessary to cause growth disturbance has been found to be 7–9% of the total cross-sectional area of the physis (160). In humans the maximum diameter of graft tunnel that will not cause physeal closure has not been determined. However, intraarticular ACL reconstruction in truly skeletally immature patients using a soft tissue graft through a transphyseal tibial tunnel of 6–7 mm and the over-the-top position on the femur has been shown not to cause early physeal closure, leg length discrepancy, or angular deformity (150,151,154). Nevertheless, care should be taken to place the tibial tunnel through the center of the physis, avoiding damage to the periphery (150). Lipscomb and Anderson (137) reported a patient with a significant growth abnormality after ACL reconstruction, but it was attributed to the fixation of the graft with staples on both the femoral and tibial side.

On the basis of the data reported in the literature and our own experience, we recommend the following treatment algorithm: activity modification, bracing, and rehabilitation in patients with Tanner stage I and II; isometric reconstruction with hamstring tendons passed through tibial and femoral transphyseal tunnels in Tanner stage III patients; and isometric transtibial and transfemoral reconstruction with the surgeon's autograft technique of choice in Tanner stage IV and V patients. In Tanner stage I and II patients with very unstable knees, if reconstruction is deemed necessary, a physeal sparing procedure should be performed.

WHEN TO REFER

For the primary care physician, clarification regarding which physeal injuries are best managed by referral to an orthopedist is needed. Since virtually all physeal injuries are vulnerable to complication arising from premature closure, the ultimate "safe" action is to refer all documented physeal injuries regardless of type and location. However, some tempering of this attitude is warranted. Often, the initial radiograph does not confirm the clinical suspicion of physeal injury. Nondisplaced physeal fractures may not become apparent on the radiograph until 7–14 days after the injury when features of periosteal reaction and/or bone resorption about the fracture make the diagnosis possible. Because of this, a child presenting with a clinical suspicion of physeal fracture but with a normal radiograph may be managed with protection for 10–14 days before confirmation of the presence or absence of physeal fracture with a repeat radiograph. Protection may be defined as a cast or splint for an upper extremity injury and as crutches and a splint for a lower extremity injury.

Physeal injuries of the lower extremities carry an increased risk of late complication of partial or complete premature closure. This is particularly true for physeal fractures involving the distal femur or distal tibia, regardless of the fracture type. Furthermore, the complication of angular deformity or length inequality of a weight-bearing limb can lead to significant morbidity and disability, though there can also be morbidity from similar complication of upper extremity injuries as well. Because of this, it is probably best to refer any documented physeal injury of a lower extremity to an orthopedic surgeon.

Physeal injuries of the upper extremity may also be problematic but are more often related to fracture type and initial displacement. Because of this, nondisplaced and nonangulated physeal fractures involving bones of the upper extremity may be managed by the primary care physician who is knowledgeable and experienced with the principles of appropriate immobilization and radiographic follow-up. The exception to this is injury and fracture to any aspect of the elbow, where complications can be devastating. Immediate referral of even suspected physeal injuries of the elbow is therefore warranted.

ACKNOWLEDGMENTS

The authors thank Joseph Kannasz for his illustrations.

REFERENCES

1. Streeter GL. Developmental horizons in human embryos: a review of the histogenesis of cartilage and bone. *Contrib Embryol* 1949;33:149.
2. Iannotti JP. Growth plate physiology and pathology. *Orthop Clin North Am* 1990;21(1):1–17.
3. Gardner E. Osteogenesis in the human embryo and fetus. In: Bourne GH, ed. *The biochemistry and physiology of bone*, 2nd ed. New York: Academic Press, 1971.
4. Brighton CT. The growth plate. *Orthop Clin North Am* 1984;15(4):571–595.
5. Carter DR, Wong M. Mechanical stresses and endochondral ossification in the chondroepiphysis. *J Orthop Res* 1988;6(1):148–154.
6. Floyd WE III, Zaleske DJ, Schiller AL, et al. Vascular events associated with the appearance of the secondary center of ossification in the murine distal femoral epiphysis. *J Bone Joint Surg Am* 1987;69(2):185–190.
7. Shapiro F. Epiphyseal growth plate fracture-separations: a pathophysiologic approach. *Orthopedics* 1982;5:720–736.
8. Oestreich AE, Ahmad BS. The periphysis and its effect on the metaphysis: I. Definition and normal radiographic pattern. *Skeletal Radiol* 1992;21(5):283–286.
9. Brighton CT, Sugioka Y, Hunt RM. Cytoplasmic structures of epiphyseal plate chondrocytes: quantitative evaluation using electron micrographs of rat costochondral junctions with special reference to the fate of hypertrophic cells. *J Bone Joint Surg Am* 1973;55(4):771–784.
10. Iannotti JP, Brighton CT. Cytosolic ionized calcium concentration in isolated chondrocytes from each zone of the growth plate. *J Orthop Res* 1989;7(4):511–518.
11. Robertson WW Jr. Newest knowledge of the growth plate. *Clin Orthop* 1990;253:270–278.
12. Brighton CT, Heppenstall RB. Oxygen tension in zones of the epiphyseal plate, the metaphysis and diaphysis: an in vitro and in vivo study in rats and rabbits. *J Bone Joint Surg Am* 1971;53(4):719–728.
13. Crabb ID, O'Keefe RJ, Puzas JE, Rosier RN. PTH effects on chondrocytes from the different maturational stages of the growth plate. *ORS Trans* 1989;14:84.
14. Trippel SB, Doctrow S, Whelan MC, Mankin HJ. Modulation of growth plate chondrocyte response to Sm-C/IGF-I and basic FGF by growth factor interaction. *ORS Trans* 1989;14:256.
15. Hunziker EB, Schenk RK, Cruz-Orive LM. Quantitation of chondrocyte performance in growth-plate cartilage during longitudinal bone growth. *J Bone Joint Surg Am* 1987;69(2):162–173.
16. Anderson CE, Parker J. Invasion and resorption in enchondral ossification: an electron microscopic study. *J Bone Joint Surg Am* 1966;48(5):899–914.
17. Kao SC, Smith WL. Skeletal injuries in the pediatric patient. *Radiol Clin North Am* 1997;35(3):727–746.
18. Schwab SA. Epiphyseal injuries in the growing athlete. *Can Med Assoc J* 1977;117(6):626–630.
19. Salter RB. Injuries of the epiphyseal plate. *Instr Course Lect* 1992;41:351–359.
20. Ogden JA. Skeletal growth mechanism injury patterns. In: Uhthoff HK, Wiley JJ, eds. *Behavior of the growth plate*. New York: Raven Press, 1988.
21. Morscher E, Desaulles PA, Schenk R. Experimental studies on tensile strength and morphology of the epiphyseal cartilage at puberty. *Ann Paediatr Int Rev Pediatr* 1965;205(2):112–130.
22. Iannotti JP, Goldstein S, Kuhn J, et al. Growth plate and bone development. In: Simon SR, ed. *Orthopaedic basic science*. Rosemont, IL: American Academy of Orthopaedic Surgeons, 1994.
23. Ogden JA. *Skeletal injury in the child*. Philadelphia: Lea & Febiger, 1982.
24. Cohen B, Chorney GS, Phillips DP, et al. The microstructural tensile properties and biochemical composition of the bovine distal femoral growth plate. *J Orthop Res* 1992;10(2):263–275.
25. Moen CT, Pelker RR. Biomechanical and histological correlations in growth plate failure. *J Pediatr Orthop* 1984;4(2):180–184.
26. Lee FY, Rho JY, Harten R Jr, et al. Micromechanical properties of epiphyseal trabecular bone and primary spongiosa around the physis: an in situ nanoindentation study. *J Pediatr Orthop* 1998;18(5):582–585.
27. Salter RB, Harris WR. Injuries involving the epiphyseal plate. *J Bone Joint Surg Am* 1963;45:587–622.
28. Peterson HA, Madhok R, Benson JT, et al. Physeal fractures: 1. Epidemiology in Olmsted County, Minnesota, 1979–1988. *J Pediatr Orthop* 1994;14(4):423–430.
29. Mizuta T, Benson WM, Foster BK, et al. Statistical analysis of the incidence of physeal injuries. *J Pediatr Orthop* 1987;7(5):518–523.
30. Peterson HA. Physeal and apophyseal injuries. In: Rockwood CA, Wilkins KE, Baety JH, eds. *Fractures in children.*, 4th ed. Philadelphia: Lippincott-Raven, 1996.
31. Rang M. *The growth plate and its disorders*. Baltimore: Williams & Wilkins, 1969.
32. Peterson HA. Physeal fractures: 2. Two previously unclassified types. *J Pediatr Orthop* 1994;14(4):431–438.
33. Lee KE, Pelker RR, Rudicel SA, et al. Histologic patterns of capital femoral growth plate fracture in the rabbit: the effect of shear direction. *J Pediatr Orthop* 1985;5(1):32–39.
34. Gomes LS, Volpon JB, Goncalves RP. Traumatic separation of epiphyses: an experimental study in rats. *Clin Orthop* 1988;236:286–295.
35. Makela EA, Vainionpaa S, Vihtonen K, et al. The effect of trauma to the lower femoral epiphyseal plate: an experimental study in rabbits. *J Bone Joint Surg Br* 1988;70(2):187–191.
36. Johnston RM, Jones WW. Fractures through human growth plates. *Orthop Trans* 1980;4:295.
37. Smith DG, Geist RW, Cooperman DR. Microscopic examination of a naturally occurring epiphyseal plate fracture. *J Pediatr Orthop* 1985;5(3):306–308.
38. Ogden JA, Ganey T, Light TR, Southwick WO. The pathology of acute chondro-osseous injury in the child. *Yale J Biol Med* 1993;66(3):219–233.
39. Rudicel S, Pelker RR, Lee KE, et al. Shear fractures through the capital femoral physis of the skeletally immature rabbit. *J Pediatr Orthop* 1985;5(1):27–31.
40. Lombardo SJ, Harvey JP Jr. Fractures of the distal femoral epiphyses: factors influencing prognosis: a review of thirty-four cases. *J Bone Joint Surg Am* 1977;59(6):742–751.
41. Maffulli N, Baxter-Jones AD. Common skeletal injuries in young athletes. *Sports Med* 1995;19(2):137–149.
42. Landry GL. Sports injuries in childhood. *Pediatr Ann* 1992;21(3):165–168.
43. Gallagher SS, Finison K, Guyer B, Goodenough S. The incidence

44. Zaricznyj B, Shattuck LJ, Mast TA, et al. Sports-related injuries in school-aged children. *Am J Sports Med* 1980;8(5):318–324.
45. Tursz A, Crost M. Sports-related injuries in children: a study of their characteristics, frequency, and severity, with comparison to other types of accidental injuries. *Am J Sports Med* 1986;14(4):294–299.
46. Backx FJ, Beijer HJ, Bol E, Erich WB. Injuries in high-risk persons and high-risk sports: a longitudinal study of 1818 school children. *Am J Sports Med* 1991;19(2):124–130.
47. Mann DC, Rajmaira S. Distribution of physeal and nonphyseal fractures in 2,650 long-bone fractures in children aged 0–16 years. *J Pediatr Orthop* 1990;10(6):713–716.
48. Worlock P, Stower M. Fracture patterns in Nottingham children. *J Pediatr Orthop* 1986;6:656–660.
49. Krueger-Franke M, Siebert CH, Pfoerringer W. Sports-related epiphyseal injuries of the lower extremity: an epidemiologic study. *J Sports Med Phys Fitness* 1992;32(1):106–111.
50. Morscher E. Strength and morphology of growth cartilage under hormonal influence of puberty: animal experiments and clinical study on the etiology of local growth disorders during puberty. *Reconstr Surg Traumatol* 1968;10:3–104.
51. Heim M, Blankstein A, Israeli A, Horoszowski H. Which X-ray views are required in juvenile ankle trauma? *Arch Orthop Trauma Surg* 1990;109(3):175–176.
52. Rogers LF, Poznanski AK. Imaging of epiphyseal injuries. *Radiology* 1994;191(2):297–308.
53. Rogers LF. *Radiology of skeletal trauma*, 2nd ed. New York: Churchill Livingstone, 1992.
54. Guille JT, Yamazaki A, Bowen JR. Physeal surgery: indications and operative treatment. *Am J Orthop* 1997;26(5):323–332.
55. Greulich WW, Pyle SI. *Radiographic atlas of the skeletal development of the hand and wrist*. Stanford, CA: Stanford University Press, 1959.
56. Gabel GT, Peterson HA, Berquist TH. Premature partial physeal arrest: diagnosis by magnetic resonance imaging in two cases. *Clin Orthop* 1991;272:242–247.
57. De Campo JF, Boldt DW. Computed tomography of partial growth plate arrest: initial experience. *Skeletal Radiol* 1986;15(7):526–529.
58. Loder RT, Swinford AE, Kuhns LR. The use of helical computed tomographic scan to assess bony physeal bridges. *J Pediatr Orthop* 1997;17(3):356–359.
59. Young JW, Bright RW, Whitley NO. Computed tomography in the evaluation of partial growth plate arrest in children. *Skeletal Radiol* 1986;15(7):530–535.
60. Jaramillo D, Shapiro F. Musculoskeletal trauma in children. *Magn Reson Imaging Clin N Am* 1998;6(3):521–536.
61. Barnewolt CE, Shapiro F, Jaramillo D. Normal gadolinium-enhanced MR images of the developing appendicular skeleton: I. Cartilaginous epiphysis and physis. *Am J Roentgenol* 1997;169(1):183–189.
62. Jaramillo D, Hoffer FA. Cartilaginous epiphysis and growth plate: normal and abnormal MR imaging findings. *Am J Roentgenol* 1992;158(5):1105–1110.
63. Chung T, Jaramillo D. Normal maturing distal tibia and fibula: changes with age at MR imaging. *Radiology* 1995;194(1):227–232.
64. Harcke HT, Synder M, Caro PA, Bowen JR. Growth plate of the normal knee: evaluation with MR imaging. *Radiology* 1992;183(1):119–123.
65. Petit P, Panuel M, Faure F, et al. Acute fracture of the distal tibial physis: role of gradient-echo MR imaging versus plain film examination. *Am J Roentgenol* 1996;166(5):1203–1206.
66. Jaramillo D, Hoffer FA, Shapiro F, Rand F. MR imaging of fractures of the growth plate. *Am J Roentgenol* 1990;155(6):1261–1265.
67. Borsa JJ, Peterson HA, Ehman RL. MR imaging of physeal bars. *Radiology* 1996;199(3):683–687.
68. Laor T, Hartman AL, Jaramillo D. Local physeal widening on MR imaging: an incidental finding suggesting prior metaphyseal insult. *Pediatr Radiol* 1997;27(8):654–662.
69. Synder M, Harcke HT, Bowen JR, Caro PA. Evaluation of physeal behavior in response to epiphyseodesis with the use of serial magnetic resonance imaging. *J Bone Joint Surg Am* 1994;76(2):224–229.
70. Murray IP. Bone scanning in the child and young adult: part I. *Skeletal Radiol* 1980;5(1):1–14.
71. Harcke HT, Zapf SE, Mandell GA, et al. Angular deformity of the lower extremity: evaluation with quantitative bone scintigraphy. Work in progress. *Radiology* 1987;164(2):437–440.
72. Christensen SB, Krogsgaard OW. Localization of Tc-99m MDP in epiphyseal growth plates of rats. *J Nucl Med* 1981;22(3):237–245.
73. Harcke HT, Mandell GA. Scintigraphic evaluation of the growth plate. *Semin Nucl Med* 1993;23(4):266–273.
74. Walter E, Feine U, Anger K, et al. The scintigraphic diagnosis and follow-up of injuries to the epiphyseal plates. *ROFO Fortschr Geb Rontgenstr Nuklearmed* 1980;132(3):309–315.
75. Keret D, Harcke HT, Bowen JR. Tibia valga after fracture: documentation of mechanism. *Arch Orthop Trauma Surg* 1991;110(4):216–219.
76. Zionts LE, Harcke HT, Brooks KM, MacEwen GD. Posttraumatic tibia valga: a case demonstrating asymmetric activity at the proximal growth plate on technetium bone scan. *J Pediatr Orthop* 1987;7(4):458–462.
77. Wioland M, Bonnerot V. Diagnosis of partial and total physeal arrest by bone single-photon emission computed tomography. *J Nucl Med* 1993;34(9):1410–1415.
78. Edwards PH, Grana WA. Physeal fractures about the knee. *J Am Acad Orthop Surg* 1995;3(2):63–69.
79. Iwabu S, Sasaki T, Kameyama M, et al. Primary healing of physeal separation under rigid fixation. *J Bone Joint Surg Br* 1998;80(4):726–730.
80. Rang M. *Children's fractures*. Philadelphia: JB Lippincott, 1975.
81. Makela EA, Bostman O, Kekomaki M, et al. Biodegradable fixation of distal humeral physeal fractures. *Clin Orthop* 1992;283:237–243.
82. Hope PG, Williamson DM, Coates CJ, Cole WG. Biodegradable pin fixation of elbow fractures in children: a randomised trial. *J Bone Joint Surg Br* 1991;73(6):965–968.
83. Partio EK, Tuompo P, Hirvensalo E, et al. Totally absorbable fixation in the treatment of fractures of the distal femoral epiphyses: a prospective clinical study. *Arch Orthop Trauma Surg* 1997;116(4):213–216.
84. Bostman O, Makela EA, Tormala P, Rokkanen P. Transphyseal fracture fixation using biodegradablepins. *J Bone Joint Surg Br* 1989;71(4):706–707.
85. Bostman O, Makela EA, Sodergard J, et al. Absorbable polyglycolide pins in internal fixation of fractures in children. *J Pediatr Orthop* 1993;13(2):242–245.
86. Gil-Albarova J, Fini M, Gil-Albarova R, et al. Absorbable screws through the greater trochanter do not disturb physeal growth: rabbit experiments. *Acta Orthop Scand* 1998;69(3):273–276.
87. Donigian AM, Plaga BR, Caskey PM. Biodegradable fixation of physeal fractures in goat distal femur. *J Pediatr Orthop* 1993;13(3):349–354.
88. Nordstrom P, Pihlajamaki H, Toivonen T, et al. Tissue response to polyglycolide and polylactide pins in cancellous bone. *Arch Orthop Trauma Surg* 1998;117(4–5):197–204.
89. Svensson PJ, Janarv PM, Hirsch G. Internal fixation with biodegradable rods in pediatric fractures: one-year follow-up of fifty patients. *J Pediatr Orthop* 1994;14(2):220–224.
90. Kaeding CC, Whitehead R. Musculoskeletal injuries in adolescents. *Prim Care* 1998;25(1):211–223.
91. Ogden JA, Ganey TM, Ogden DA. The biological aspects of children's fractures. In: Rockwood CA, Wilkins KE, Baety JH, eds. *Fractures in children*, 4th ed. Philadelphia: Lippincott-Raven, 1996.
92. Thomson JD, Stricker SJ, Williams MM. Fractures of the distal femoral epiphyseal plate. *J Pediatr Orthop* 1995;15(4):474–478.
93. Graham JM, Gross RH. Distal femoral physeal problem fractures. *Clin Orthop* 1990;(255):51–53.

94. Chadwick CJ, Bentley G. The classification and prognosis of epiphyseal injuries. *Injury* 1987;18(3):157–168.
95. Bylander B, Aronson S, Egund N, et al. Growth disturbance after physeal injury of distal femur and proximal tibia studied by roentgen stereophotogrammetry. *Arch Orthop Trauma Surg* 1981;98(3):225–235.
96. Moon MS, Kim I, Rhee SK, et al. Varus and internal rotational deformity of the ankle secondary to distal tibial physeal injury. *Bull Hosp Jt Dis* 1997;56(3):145–148.
97. Peterson HA Premature physeal arrest of the distal tibia associated with temporary arterial insufficiency. *J Pediatr Orthop* 1993;13(5):672–675.
98. Kling TF Jr, Bright RW, Hensinger RN. Distal tibial physeal fractures in children that may require open reduction. *J Bone Joint Surg Am* 1984;66(5):647–657.
99. Karrholm J, Hansson LI, Selvik G. Changes in tibiofibular relationships due to growth disturbances after ankle fractures in children. *J Bone Joint Surg Am* 1984;66(8):1198–1210.
100. Cass JR, Peterson HA. Salter-Harris Type-IV injuries of the distal tibial epiphyseal growth plate, with emphasis on those involving the medial malleolus. *J Bone Joint Surg Am* 1983;65(8):1059–1070.
101. Gautier E, Ziran BH, Egger B, et al. Growth disturbances after injuries of the proximal tibial epiphysis. *Arch Orthop Trauma Surg* 1998;118:37–41.
102. Takai R, Grant AD, Atar D, Lehman WB. Minor knee trauma as a possible cause of asymmetrical proximal tibial physis closure: case report. *Clin Orthop* 1994;307:142–145.
103. Pappas AM, Anas P, Toczylowski HM Jr. Asymmetrical arrest of the proximal tibial physis and genu recurvatum deformity. *J Bone Joint Surg Am* 1984;66(4):575–581.
104. Riseborough EJ, Barrett IR, Shapiro F. Growth disturbances following distal femoral physeal fracture-separations. *J Bone Joint Surg Am* 1983;65(7):885–893.
105. Stephens DC, Louis E, Louis DS. Traumatic separation of the distal femoral epiphyseal cartilage plate. *J Bone Joint Surg Am* 1974;56(7):1383–1390.
106. Devito DP. Management of fractures and their complications. In: Morrisy RT, Weinstein SL, eds. *Lovell and Winter's pediatric orthopaedics*. Philadelphia: Lippincott-Raven, 1996.
107. Hynes D, O'Brien T. Growth disturbance lines after injury of the distal tibial physis: their significance in prognosis. *J Bone Joint Surg Br* 1988;70(2):231–233.
108. Ogden JA. Growth slowdown and arrest lines. *J Pediatr Orthop* 1984;4(4):409–415.
109. Lee EH, Gao GX, Bose K. Management of partial growth arrest: physis, fat, or silastic? *J Pediatr Orthop* 1993;13(3):368–372.
110. Olin A, Creasman C, Shapiro F. Free physeal transplantation in the rabbit. an experimental approach to focal lesions. *J Bone Joint Surg Am* 1984;66(1):7–20.
111. Martiana K, Low CK, Tan SK, Pang MW. Comparison of various interpositional materials in the prevention of transphyseal bone bridge formation. *Clin Orthop* 1996;325:218–224.
112. Lee EH, Chen F, Chan J, Bose K. Treatment of growth arrest by transfer of cultured chondrocytes into physeal defects. *J Pediatr Orthop* 1998;18(2):155–160.
113. Gabriel KR, Crawford AH, Roy DR, et al. Percutaneous epiphyseodesis. *J Pediatr Orthop* 1994;14(3):358–362.
114. Horton GA, Olney BW. Epiphysiodesis of the lower extremity: results of the percutaneous technique. *J Pediatr Orthop* 1996;16(2):180–182.
115. Cañadell J, de Pablos J. Breaking bony bridges by physeal distraction: a new approach. *Int Orthop* 1985;9(4):223–229.
116. Hamanishi C, Tanaka S, Tamura K, Fujio K. Correction of asymmetric physeal closure: rotatory distraction in 3 cases. *Acta Orthop Scand* 1990;61(1):58–61.
117. Adams JE. Little league shoulder: osteochondrosis of the proximal humeral epiphysis in boy baseball pitchers. *Calif Med* 1966;105(1):22–25.
118. Torg JS. The little league pitcher. *Am Fam Physician* 1972;6(2):71–76.
119. Tullos HS, Fain RH. Little league shoulder: rotational stress fracture of proximal epiphysis. *J Sports Med* 1974;2(3):152–153.
120. Cahill BR, Tullos HS, Fain RH. Little league shoulder: lesions of the proximal humeral epiphyseal plate. *J Sports Med* 1974;2(3):150–152.
121. Barnett LS. Little League shoulder syndrome: proximal humeral epiphyseolysis in adolescent baseball pitchers: a case report. *J Bone Joint Surg Am* 1985;67(3):495–496.
122. Albert MJ, Drvaric DM. Little League shoulder: case report. *Orthopedics* 1990;13(7):779–781.
123. Auberge T, Zenny JC, Duvallet A, et al. Etude de la maturation osseuse et des lesions osteoarticulaires des sportifs de haut niveau. *J Radiol* 1984;65(8-9):555–561.
124. Carter SR, Aldridge MJ. Stress injury of the distal radial growth plate. *J Bone Joint Surg Br* 1988;70(5):834–836.
125. Mandelbaum BR, Bartolozzi AR, Davis CA, et al. Wrist pain syndrome in the gymnast: pathogenetic, diagnostic, and therapeutic considerations. *Am J Sports Med* 1989;17(3):305–317.
126. Caine D, Roy S, Singer KM, Broekhoff J. Stress changes of the distal radial growth plate: a radiographic survey and review of the literature. *Am J Sports Med* 1992;20(3):290–298.
127. De Smet L, Claessens A, Lefevre J, Beunen G. Gymnast wrist: an epidemiologic survey of ulnar variance and stress changes of the radial physis in elite female gymnasts. *Am J Sports Med* 1994;22(6):846–850.
128. Chang CY, Shih C, Penn IW, et al. Wrist injuries in adolescent gymnasts of a Chinese opera school: radiographic survey. *Radiology* 1995;195(3):861–864.
129. Bak K, Boeckstyns M. Epiphysiodesis for bilateral irregular closure of the distal radial physis in a gymnast. *Scand J Med Sci Sports* 1997;7(6):363–366.
130. DiFiori JP, Puffer JC, Mandelbaum BR, Dorey F. Distal radial growth plate injury and positive ulnar variance in nonelite gymnasts. *Am J Sports Med* 1997;25(6):763–768.
131. Maffulli N, Chan D, Aldridge MJ. Overuse injuries of the olecranon in young gymnasts. *J Bone Joint Surg Br* 1992;74(2):305–308.
132. Chan D, Aldridge MJ, Maffulli N, Davies AM. Chronic stress injuries of the elbow in young gymnasts. *Br J Radiol* 1991;64(768):1113–1118.
133. Yong-Hing K, Wedge JH, Bowen CV. Chronic injury to the distal ulnar and radial growth plates in an adolescent gymnast: a case report. *J Bone Joint Surg Am* 1988;70(7):1087–1089.
134. Albanese SA, Palmer AK, Kerr DR, et al. Wrist pain and distal growth plate closure of the radius in gymnasts. *J Pediatr Orthop* 1989;9(1):23–28.
135. Roy S, Caine D, Singer KM. Stress changes of the distal radial epiphysis in young gymnasts: a report of twenty-one cases and a review of the literature. *Am J Sports Med* 1985;13(5):301–308.
136. Stanitski CL. Anterior cruciate ligament injury in the skeletally immature patient: diagnosis and treatment. *J Am Acad Orthop Surg* 1995;3:146–158.
137. Lipscomb AB, Anderson AF. Tears of the anterior cruciate ligament in adolescents. *J Bone Joint Surg Am* 1986;68(1):19–28.
138. Kannus P, Jarvinen M. Long-term prognosis of nonoperatively treated acute knee distortions having primary hemarthrosis without clinical instability. *Am J Sports Med* 1987;15(2):138–143.
139. Angel KR, Hall DJ. Anterior cruciate ligament injury in children and adolescents. *Arthroscopy* 1989;5(3):197–200.
140. Brief LP. Anterior cruciate ligament reconstruction without drill holes. *Arthroscopy* 1991;7(4):350–357.
141. Graf BK, Lange RH, Fujisaki CK, et al. Anterior cruciate ligament tears in skeletally immature patients: meniscal pathology at presentation and after attempted conservative treatment. *Arthroscopy* 1992;8(2):229–233.
142. McCarroll JR, Shelbourne KD, Porter DA, et al. Patellar tendon graft reconstruction for midsubstance anterior cruciate ligament rupture in junior high school athletes. An algorithm for management. *Am J Sports Med* 1994;22(4):478–484.
143. Bradley GW, Shives TC, Samuelson KM. Ligament injuries in the knees of children. *J Bone Joint Surg Am* 1979;61(4):588–591.
144. Clanton TO, DeLee JC, Sanders B, Neidre A. Knee ligament injuries in children. *J Bone Joint Surg Am* 1979;61(8):1195–1201.
145. DeLee JC, Curtis R. Anterior cruciate ligament insufficiency in children. *Clin Orthop* 1983;172:112–118.
146. Engebretsen L, Svenningsen S, Benum P. Poor results of anterior cruciate ligament repair in adolescence. *Acta Orthop Scand* 1988;59(6):684–686.

147. Parker AW, Drez D Jr, Cooper JL. Anterior cruciate ligament injuries in patients with open physes. *Am J Sports Med* 1994; 22(1):44–47.
148. Nakhostine M, Bollen SR, Cross MJ. Reconstruction of midsubstance anterior cruciate rupture in adolescents with open physes. *J Pediatr Orthop* 1995;15(3):286–287.
149. Kurosawa H, Yasuda K, Yamakoshi K, et al. An experimental evaluation of isometric placement for extra-articular reconstructions of the anterior cruciate ligament. *Am J Sports Med* 1991; 19(4):384–388.
150. Andrews M, Noyes FR, Barber-Westin SD. Anterior cruciate ligament allograft reconstruction in the skeletally immature athlete. *Am J Sports Med* 1994;22(1):48–54.
151. Lo IK, Kirkley A, Fowler PJ, Miniaci A. The outcome of operatively treated anterior cruciate ligament disruptions in the skeletally immature child. *Arthroscopy* 1997;13(5):627–634.
152. Matava MJ, Siegel MG. Arthroscopic reconstruction of the ACL with semitendinosus-gracilis autograft in skeletally immature adolescent patients. *Am J Knee Surg* 1997;10(2):60–69.
153. Pressman AE, Letts RM, Jarvis JG. Anterior cruciate ligament tears in children: an analysis of operative versus nonoperative treatment. *J Pediatr Orthop* 1997;17(4):505–511.
154. Bisson LJ, Wickiewicz T, Levinson M, Warren R. ACL reconstruction in children with open physes. *Orthopedics* 1998;21(6): 659–663.
155. Lo IK, Bell DM, Fowler PJ. Anterior cruciate ligament injuries in the skeletally immature patient. *Instr Course Lect* 1998;47: 351–359.
156. Tanner JM, Whitehouse RH, Marshall WA. *Assessment of skeletal maturity and prediction of adult height (TW2 Methods)*. London: Academic Press, 1975.
157. Ono T, Wada Y, Takahashi K, et al. Tibial deformities and failures of anterior cruciate ligament reconstruction in immature rabbits. *J Orthop Sci* 1998;3(3):150–155.
158. Guzzanti V, Falciglia F, Gigante A, Fabbriciani C. The effect of intra-articular ACL reconstruction on the growth plates of rabbits. *J Bone Joint Surg Br* 1994;76(6):960–963.
159. Stadelmaier DM, Arnoczky SP, Dodds J, Ross H. The effect of drilling and soft tissue grafting across open growth plates: a histologic study. *Am J Sports Med* 1995;23(4):431–435.
160. Janarv PM, Wikstrom B, Hirsch G. The influence of transphyseal drilling and tendon grafting on bone growth: an experimental study in the rabbit. *J Pediatr Orthop* 1998;18(2):149–154.

CHAPTER 34

Traction Apophysitis

Douglas F. Hoffman and Robert J. Johnson

INTRODUCTION

Growth cartilage in the skeletally immature athlete is located at three sites: the epiphyseal plate, the joint surface, and the apophyseal insertions of major muscle–tendon units. The apophyses are defined as physes that are subjected to traction forces, as opposed to the usual compressive forces of the epiphyseal plates of long bones. The growth plates may be injured from either acute macrotrauma or repetitive microtrauma. The apophyses are particularly susceptible to the latter, since they are the weak link in the muscle–tendon units that are subjected to repetitive stresses during common motions in sports such as throwing, jumping, and running.

Varied terminology has been used to describe overuse injuries to the apophyses. Older names such as *epiphysitis* and *osteochondritis* have been abandoned, since they denote a primary inflammatory cause rather than an overuse etiology. Similarly, the term *nonarticular osteochondrosis*, defined as disordered endochondral ossification of the normal developing apophysis (1), has given way to the favored nomenclature of *traction apophysitis*, since this term emphasizes the repetitive tensile forces that predominate as the primary etiology. Many of these disorders are more commonly identified by their eponyms, such as Osgood-Schlatter disease or Sever's disease, though the word *disease* is misleading and should be replaced by terms such as *disorder* or *syndrome*.

EPIDEMIOLOGY

In referring to the increasing incidence of overuse injuries in children, George Sheehan said that no horse ever ran itself to death until there was a rider on its back (2). With the growing participation of both preadolescents and adolescents in organized sports, particularly the young female athlete, the incidence of overuse disorders to the apophysis would be expected to experience a parallel rise. The epidemiology of the traction apophysitises as an entity has not been well studied. Micheli and Fehlandt (3) retrospectively reviewed 724 cases of overuse tendinitis or apophysitis in 445 athletes ages 8–19 years. Twenty-five percent of all injuries were diagnosed as an apophysitis, the majority of which occurred in the lower extremity. Overuse apophyseal injuries occurred more commonly in males (60%) than in females (40%). Calcaneal apophysitis was the most common, in both females and males, followed by iliac and tibial tubercle apophysitis.

PREDISPOSING FACTORS

Repetitive submaximal tensile forces are thought to be the common pathway that result in microtrauma to the apophyses and its clinical manifestation as pain and edema (3–7). Both extrinsic and intrinsic factors can potentiate or modify the stresses that are placed on the apophyses (Table 34–1). Excessive training is one of the most important predisposing factors to injury (2,5). The emphasis that is often placed on winning in organized sports at the youth level translates into increased practice time, more intense training, and a greater number of games per season. In addition, it is not uncommon for young athletes to participate on several teams in the same or a different sport during a season. The increasing frequency of tournaments, which may result in multiple games during a several-day period, also places excessive stresses on the apophysis.

Footwear is another factor to consider. Shoes that fit poorly or provide little arch support, as occurs with soccer cleats, may increase the stresses placed on the apophyses of the lower extremity.

D. F. Hoffman: Department of Orthopedics and Sports Medicine, St. Mary's Duluth Clinic, Duluth, Minnesota 55805.
R. J. Johnson: Division of Primary Care Sports Medicine, Department of Family Practice, Hennepin County Medical Center, Minneapolis, Minnesota 55408.

TABLE 34-1. *Predisposing factors to overuse injury of the apophysis*

Extrinsic factors	Intrinsic factors
Training	Growth
Footwear	Biomechanics
Playing conditions	Malalignment
Protective equipment	Inherent joint laxity
Weather	Strength imbalances
Supervision	Inflexibility
	Deconditioning
	Chronic disease

Biomechanics play an important role in the distribution of stresses during athletic activity. The forces transmitted to the medial epicondylar or olecranon apophysis, for example, are directly related to throwing mechanics. Similarly, biomechanical factors in weight-bearing sports influence the stresses to the apophyses of the lower extremity.

Growth in children is not linear and typically occurs in phases of accelerated growth or growth spurts (8). The pubertal growth spurt for females begins at approximately 10 years of age, reaches a peak velocity at age 12, and decelerates toward zero as epiphyseal fusions occur at age 15. For males this pattern begins around age 12, reaches peak velocity at age 14, and culminates in epiphyseal closure at approximately 17 years of age. Animal studies have shown a decrease in tensile strength of the physis during pubescence (9,10). This phenomenon can be extrapolated to humans by the fact that the peak incidence of all types of physeal injuries occurs during the same period of maturation (11–13). Additionally, during growth spurts, longitudinal bone growth occurs at a faster rate than muscle or tendon elongation (4,14,15). As a result, there is an increase in muscle–tendon tightness, which in turn may transmit greater tensile forces to their apophyseal attachments.

UPPER EXTREMITY APOPHYSEAL INJURIES

Upper extremity apophyseal injuries are primarily related to throwing sports, implicating too much throwing and throwing with poor biomechanics (16–22). Typical differences in throwing biomechanics between youth and adult throwers that increase the stresses placed on the upper extremity include poor balance, a short throwing stride that does not permit normal force transfer from the trunk to the arm, and a posture that is too upright (23). Children also tend to generate less velocity during internal rotation of the shoulder and have lower shoulder compression forces (23). It has also been noted that young throwers who perform using a sidearm motion are three times more likely to develop problems than are overhand throwers (24). The improperly thrown curveball further compounds the abnormal stresses on the upper extremity.

Efforts at primary prevention of these throwing injuries should be initiated in "at-risk" sports. Proper throwing techniques must be taught to youth baseball and softball coaches as well as to the athletes who are involved in these sports. Limiting the number of pitches thrown in each game or week may reduce the risk. Organizations tend to limit the number of innings pitched in a given week. Our preference would be to limit pitching on the basis of pitch counts. The exact number of pitches permitted to protect the young thrower at a given age is unknown. We recognize that major league pitchers are allowed approximately 100 pitches early in the season before they are relieved. Some fraction of this number is probably appropriate for adolescents.

Medial Epicondylar Apophysitis

Medial epicondylar apophysitis is the classic upper extremity overuse apophyseal injury, seen predominantly in the young throwing athlete. The term *Little League elbow* denotes a group of pathologic entities in and about the elbow joint that result from excessive and abnormal forces created by the throwing motion; medial epicondylar apophysitis is the most common of these entities (16). The stresses placed on the elbow during throwing depend on both the technique and the phase of the throwing motion (23). The phases of throwing are commonly broken down into windup, cocking, acceleration, release and deceleration, and follow-through. Both a valgus (traction) force on the medial side of the elbow and a varus (compressive) force on the lateral side are generated with throwing. Repetitive valgus strain at the elbow resulting in excessive tensile forces and consequent microtrauma at the medial epicondylar apophysis has been reported to occur in both the late cocking phase and the early acceleration phases of throwing (16,25–29). These tensile forces on the medial side of the elbow are further magnified by throwing curve balls (23).

Medial epicondylar apophysitis most commonly occurs in baseball players between the ages of 9 and 12 years of age (29). Since the medial epicondylar apophysis is the last to close (at age 17–19 years), this may occur in older adolescents as well (4). Medial elbow pain aggravated by throwing is the predominant complaint by the athlete, although a reduction in throwing velocity and diminished control is also common (30). Physical examination findings include palpable tenderness and edema over the medial epicondyle and pain elicited by wrist flexion and forearm pronation. A flexion contracture may also be present, though this may be a common finding in the asymptomatic throwing athlete (30,31).

Elbow radiographs are important to obtain and may show irregularity and widening of the medial epicondylar apophysis (29,32). Comparison views are often helpful. Acute avulsions may occur in response to violent valgus and terminal flexion forces in the presence of chronic symptoms (23). These avulsions may be confirmed by X-ray, though not all avulsions will be significantly displaced (33).

Treatment of the athlete who has experienced persistent symptoms requires an accurate diagnosis followed by modification or complete cessation of throwing activities. In those less symptomatic cases, switching the athlete from pitcher or catcher to a position that requires fewer throws frequently permits recovery without discontinuing sport participation. As symptoms improve, strengthening of the forearm, as well as the shoulder girdle musculature, should be instituted. Ideally, a throwing analysis and instruction in proper throwing mechanics should precede a graduated throwing program and return to competition.

Treatment of acute avulsions that are minimally displaced is controversial. Several authors advocate a nonoperative approach with complete cessation of throwing activities for 4–6 weeks (23,34–37). Complete immobilization must be limited and used cautiously for fear of a permanent flexion contracture. Others, however, believe that in the throwing athlete internal fixation is necessary to restore medial elbow stability against valgus stresses (38–40). In situations in which the apophysis is separated from the humerus by more than 2 mm, surgical reduction and fixation may be necessary. Since surgical indications are relative and vary from region to region, an orthopedic consultation is warranted.

Long-term sequelae of chronic medial epicondylar apophysitis may be bony overgrowth and joint stiffness. Those who try to pitch "through the pain" may be at greater risk of disability and intra-articular disturbance.

Olecranon Apophysitis

Olecranon apophysitis also predominates in the throwing athlete but is much less common than medial epicondylar apophysitis (21). This injury is not uncommon in gymnasts (41,42) and in those who weight-train. In the throwing athlete rapid elbow extension occurs from its flexed position during the late acceleration and follow-through phases, placing tensile stresses on the olecranon apophysis. Posterior elbow pain may also occur during the late cocking or early acceleration phases from valgus overload resulting in abutment of the medial aspect of the olecranon process against the olecranon fossa (43).

This entity is distinguished from an apophysitis by the phase of throwing at which pain occurs, pain to palpation over the posteriomedial joint line, and absence of a posteriomedial osteophyte on a lateral or axial radiograph.

The athlete with an olecranon apophysitis will experience pain with palpation over the olecranon apophysis and the tip of the olecranon at the insertion of the triceps muscle. Pain is exacerbated by resisted elbow extension. Radiographs may be normal or show irregular patterns of ossification at the secondary ossification center of the olecranon (21). Pappas notes that this injury pattern can progress to avulsion fragments or lack of fusion between the ossified secondary center and the olecranon (21).

Treatment of the overuse apophysitis involves reducing or stopping the throwing activities until symptoms resolve, with institution of the usual local measures and analgesics as necessary. A rehabilitation program addressing strength deficits of the shoulder girdle and forearm and a gradual return to a throwing program stressing proper mechanics are important to prevent recurrence once the athlete returns to competition.

Avulsions of the olecranon apophysis have also been reported in the setting of a particularly forceful throw, though this is a rare injury (44–46). A displaced avulsion usually requires surgical reduction.

Long-term overuse may result in significant sequelae to the patient. Hypertrophy and spurring of the olecranon may cause impingement in the olecranon fossa during elbow extension. This impingement, as well as avulsion fragments from the apophysis, can form loose bodies in the joint requiring surgical intervention (44–46). A nonunion between the olecranon and its secondary ossification center has also been reported (47,48).

Little League Shoulder

Though not a true apophyseal injury, Little League shoulder can be grouped with upper extremity injuries because of its similarity in cause and its relationship to throwing. First described in 1953 (49), Little League shoulder is a stress reaction of the proximal humeral epiphyseal plate that results from repetitive traction forces and improper mechanics during the throwing motion. This injury most often occurs in male pitchers 11–13 years of age. It has also been reported in an elite junior badminton player (50). The usual clinical symptom is proximal shoulder pain while throwing. Physical examination may elicit tenderness over the proximal humerus. Radiographs reveal widening of the humeral epiphysis with metaphyseal cystic changes or

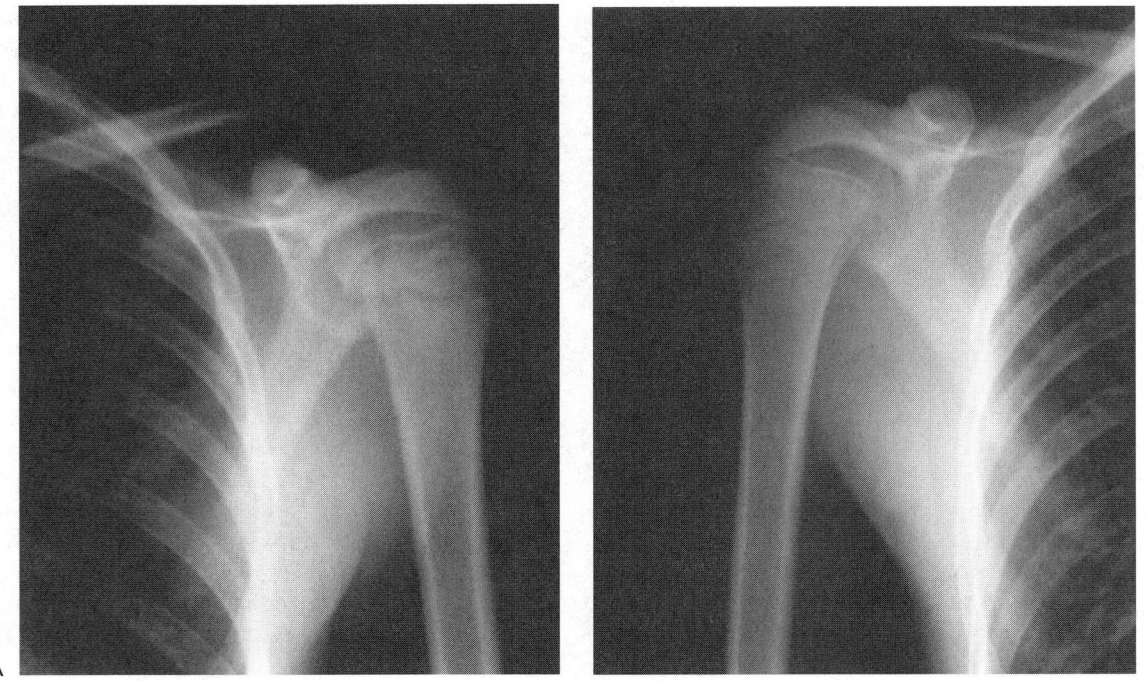

FIG. 34–1. A: Radiograph of a 14-year-old baseball pitcher with right shoulder pain during and after throwing for 8 weeks. The proximal humeral physis shows epiphyseal widening and metaphyseal cystic and sclerotic changes indicative of Little League shoulder. **B:** Comparison view of a normal left shoulder in the same patient.

sclerosis (51,52) (Fig. 34–1). The treatment is to restrict throwing until symptoms subside. When symptoms improve, resume throwing with a graduated program under proper tutelage to eliminate the mechanical errors. Long-term complications are rare.

Acromial Apophysitis

A rare upper extremity apophysitis is acromial apophysitis. Morisawa and colleagues reported in a small series of two male and one female athlete ages 12–14 that all three experienced pain at the top of the shoulder during and after sporting activities (53). Daily activities were pain free. Examination of the shoulder demonstrated tenderness at the acromion accompanied by a feeling of warmth. X-rays confirmed the diagnosis with sclerosis and irregularity of the secondary ossification center of the acromion. Conservative treatment involving cessation of aggravating activities resulted in improvement.

APOPHYSEAL INJURIES OF THE HIP AND PELVIS

Apophyseal injuries about the hip and pelvis are classified as acute avulsion fractures, or the less common overuse traction apophysitis. Once thought of as rare fractures (54), acute apophyseal avulsions comprise a significant portion of pediatric pelvic fractures in several reported series (55,56). These fractures occur predominantly in young athletes who participate in strenuous sports, especially those requiring sprinting, rapid acceleration or deceleration, or jumping (56–65). The usual mechanism for acute avulsion injuries is a sudden forceful concentric or eccentric contraction of a large muscle in an attempt to accelerate or decelerate the body mass (56,62). Direct trauma is an uncommon cause of these injuries (57,58,66). The appearance and fusion of the secondary ossification centers of the hip and pelvis occur in a predictable sequence (Fig. 34–2). Several studies have shown that the ability of the apophysis to resist tension is weakest around the time of its appearance (67,68). Case series have also supported this finding revealing that most acute apophyseal avulsions occur between the ages of 13 and 17 (55,56,58,62). The majority of apophyseal avulsions of the pelvis are treated nonoperatively (54,56–58,60–62,65,69–73). A comprehensive rehabilitation program is essential for optimizing return to sport as well as minimizing the risk of recurrence. Table 34–2 shows a modified rehabilitation program, outlined by Metzmaker and Pappas (62), that can serve as a guideline for return to sport after an apophyseal avulsion frac-

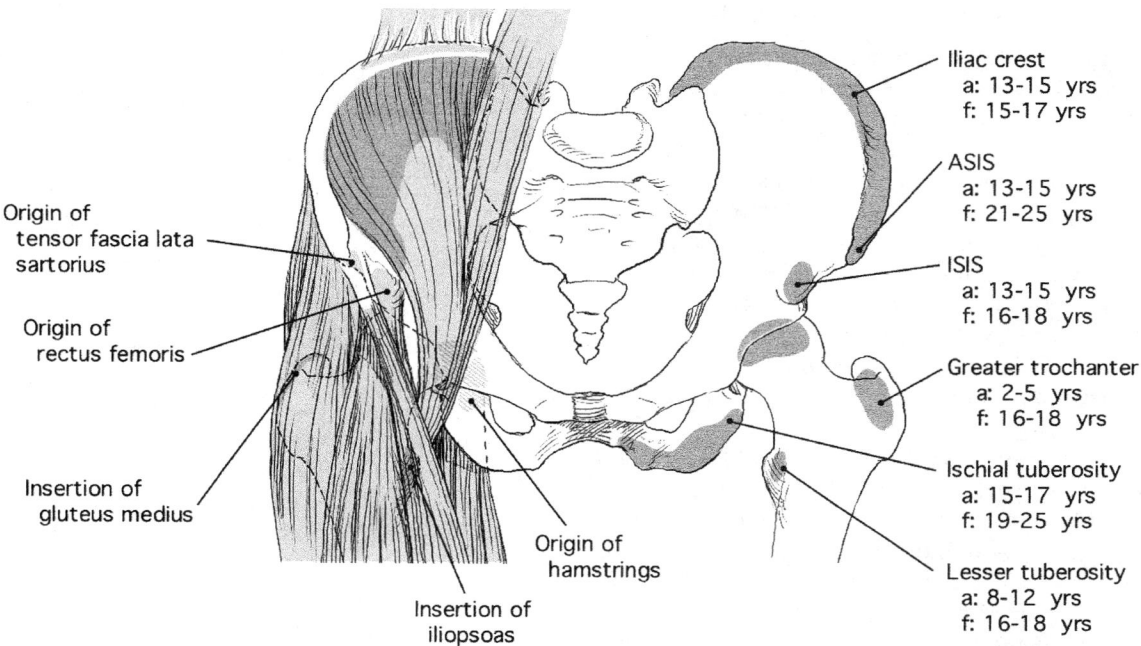

FIG. 34–2. The pelvic apophyses. On the right side the muscular attachments are shown. On the left are the average age of appearance (a) and the average age of fusion (f) of the apophyses.

ture of the pelvis. Important components of a rehabilitation program include a thorough assessment of the kinetic chain with correction of deficits and functional exercises that are specific to the athlete's sport before return to full activity. Avulsion fractures involving a greater displacement of the fragment, particularly those involving the ischial tuberosity, may warrant surgical reduction (54,63,64,66). There are wide variations in treatment recommendations, which are influenced by variables such as the athlete's age, the site of the injury, the sport of participation, and regional practice patterns.

TABLE 34–2. Phases of rehabilitation for apophyseal avulsion injuries of the hip and pelvis

Treatment phase	Days after injury	Subjective pain	Palpation	Range of motion	Muscle strength	Rehabilitation	X-ray appearance
I	0–10	Moderate to severe	Moderate to severe	Very limited	Poor	None, protected gait	Osseous separation
II	7–21	Minimal to moderate	Moderate	Improving with guided exercise	Fair	Protected gait, WBAT, aerobic conditioning with UBE, early trunk stabilization, static proprioception	Osseous separation
III	14–28	Minimal with stress	Minimal to moderate	Normal	Good	Trunk stabilization, dynamic proprioception, strengthening	Early callus formation
IV	21–35	None	Minimal	Normal	Good to normal	Sports-specific strengthening, progressive functional rehabilitation	Maturing callus
V	35–return	None	None	Normal	Normal	Normal	Maturing callus

WBAT, weight-bearing as tolerated; UBE, upper body ergometer
Modified from Metzmaker JN, Pappas AM. Avulsion fractures of the pelvis. *Am J Sports Med* 1985;13:349–358.

Avulsion of the Anterior Superior Iliac Spine

The avulsion of the anterior superior iliac spine (ASIS) is at the origin of the sartorius muscle. Some fibers of the tensor fascia lata also originate from this site. Avulsion of the ASIS most commonly occurs from sudden and forceful contraction of the sartorius muscle with the hip in extension and knee in flexion. Running, particularly sprinting, is reported to be the most common activity at the time of injury (54,58,62,65,69). This injury may also occur from the kicking motion (65,69). The athlete will often experience a pop or tearing sensation followed by intense pain over the region of the anterior superior iliac spine. Carp reported that immediate disability occurred in 76% of the patients in his series (69).

Physical examination demonstrates localized edema and palpable tenderness over the ASIS. In some cases a displaced fragment may be palpable (69). Pain is elicited with passive hip extension or active flexion. X-rays will confirm the diagnosis and most often show an inferiorly and laterally displaced fragment (58,69). Since the displaced fragment is inferior, care must be taken to avoid confusing this with an anterior inferior iliac spine avulsion.

The majority of ASIS avulsions can be treated nonoperatively with excellent results (54,55,58,62,65,69,70). The initial treatment period consists of rest, ice, analgesia, and crutch ambulation with early initiation of a rehabilitation program as outline in Table 34–2. Several authors have advocated surgical reduction in cases of severe displacement or rotation of a large fragment, though others maintain that there are good results in these cases with a nonoperative approach (54,74,75). Veselko and Smrkolj (64) reported two cases of open reduction in competitive athletes that allowed return to active training in 3–4 weeks. On the basis of their experience they advocate open reduction in situations in which return to competition is a priority.

A traction apophysitis of the ASIS resulting from repetitive traction forces of the sartorius muscle is much less common than the acute avulsion. Examination will reveal mild edema and tenderness directly over the ASIS. Resistance to active hip flexion elicits pain. Radiographs are often normal, though, rarely, mild displacement of the apophysis and exostosis may be present in cases of chronic and prolonged injury (76). Treatment is directed at relative rest and a progressive rehabilitation program.

Avulsion of the Anterior Inferior Iliac Spine

The avulsion of the anterior inferior iliac spine (AIIS) is the origin of the straight head of the rectus femoris whose functions include assisting the iliopsoas muscle in hip flexion and acting in concert with the quadriceps muscles in knee extension (54). Acute avulsion fractures of the AIIS appear to occur less commonly than fractures of the ASIS (55,62,65). The secondary ossification center, which appears at age 13 or 14, typically fuses at age 16–18, which has been implicated as the reason these injuries are less likely to occur in older adolescents than ASIS injuries (60). Similar to ASIS avulsions, running (especially sprinting) appears to be the most common mechanism of injury (54,60,77,78). Kicking (54,65) and slipping (78) are also reported as causes of AIIS injuries. Gomez (60) reported a bilateral AIIS avulsion injury in a 14-year-old sprinter.

The athlete usually reports an acute onset of groin pain that tends to be less localized than that of an ASIS avulsion, since the AIIS lies deep to the sartorius and iliopsoas (60). Fernbach and Wilkinson noted that AIIS avulsions seem to be less painful than those involving the ASIS (58). Examination reveals pain with palpation over the AIIS that is intensified with passive hip hyperextension and active hip flexion. Pain with active knee extension is also common and helps to distinguish this injury from an ASIS avulsion (60). Radiographs will often show minimal inferior displacement of the fragment (55,58,65,78). Wider displacements are uncommon, owing to the stabilizing effects of the conjoined tendon and reflected head of the rectus femoris (55,62). Surgical intervention for this injury is rare, and nonoperative treatment is similar to that of injuries of the ASIS (54,55,58,60,62,65,70). Irving (79) reported two cases of formation of an exostosis at the AIIS as a rare complication of an avulsion injury. The exostosis resulted in persistent functional disability that was alleviated with excision.

Avulsion of the Ischial Tuberosity

The ischial tuberosity is the origin of the hamstring muscles. The apophysis appears and fuses later than other hip and pelvic secondary ossification centers (Fig. 34–2); therefore this injury may occur in athletes into their third decade. The ischial tuberosity has been reported to be the most common site of avulsion fracture of the hip in the skeletally immature athlete (55,56,58,70).

Explosive or sudden eccentric contraction of the hamstring muscles while the hip is in flexion and the knee is extended (such as during hurdling or doing the splits) is the most common mechanism of injury (63,66). The athlete usually experiences the sudden onset of lower buttock pain, which may radiate along the posterior thigh (54,70). The examiner will find tenderness to palpation at the ischium with pain reproduced by passively stretching the hamstrings and during resisted hip extension. Patients may find it difficult to sit during the acute phase of this injury. Radiographs reveal a crescent-shaped fragment that, when displaced, occurs distally and laterally (54,63,70).

For injuries involving minimal or no displacement, bony union is likely, and most authors recommend a nonoperative approach (54,55,58,62,63,66,70,71,80). For avulsed fragments with wider separation, controversy exists as to the best approach to treatment. Good clinical outcomes have been reported for cases in which the fragment healed by fibrous union (66). Additionally, several authors demonstrated good results from late excision of a persistently painful fibrous nonunion (63,66). However, injuries that heal by fibrous union or nonunion may have an increase risk of developing significant prolonged disability, including buttock pain, difficulty in sitting, weakness, and diminished athletic performance (54,63,66,81). Consequently, numerous authors have advocated surgical reduction for displaced fragments, particularly if the fracture fragment is displaced greater than 2 cm (54,56,63,66,80,82,83). Healing by exuberant bony overgrowth resulting in persistent symptoms and disability is another potential complication of an ischial tuberosity apophyseal fracture, though relief of symptoms can be expected from surgical excision (54,66,81).

Apophysitis of the ischial tuberosity from repetitive stress can also occur in athletes (71). Radiographs are often normal, though differences in the ossification centers may be demonstrated between the two sides. Bone scan or MRI will confirm the diagnosis but is rarely necessary. Treatment consists of relative rest, a progressive rehabilitation program, and gradual resumption of athletic activity.

Avulsion of the Greater Trochanter

Avulsion of the greater trochanteric apophysis is a rare injury (73). The appearance of the secondary ossification center occurs between ages 2 and 5 and fuses at 16–18 years of age. It is the attachment site of the gluteus medius and minimus muscles as well as the external rotators of the hip. Avulsion fractures may occur in the athlete who performs abrupt cutting motions or side-to-side movements (70). The athlete may be unable to ambulate after the injury and will often hold the injured leg in slight flexion and abduction (54). On examination the greater trochanter is tender to palpation with pain elicited with resisted abduction and external rotation. A positive Trendelenburg test is usually present. Radiographs are diagnostic with displacement occurring proximally, posteriorly, and medially (73). Occasionally, the presence of an accessory ossification center may confuse the diagnosis (54). The clinical history, examination, and comparison views with the contralateral side should clarify the diagnosis.

Several authors advocate nonoperative treatment (Table 34–2) for minimally displaced fragments and surgical reduction and internal fixation for those that have displaced greater than one centimeter (54,70,84).

Avulsion of the Lesser Trochanter

The lesser trochanter is the insertion site of the iliopsoas muscle. Appearance of the secondary ossification center occurs between 8 and 12 years of age with fusion occurring at 16–18 years of age. An uncommon injury, avulsion of the lesser trochanter usually results from sprinting or kicking (57,70). The athlete typically presents with the acute onset of groin or anterior hip pain followed by immediate disability. Examination reveals an antalgic gait, tenderness over the lesser trochanter, and the inability to flex the hip while in the supine position (57). Pain accompanied by an inability to actively flex the hip when in the seated position is referred to as the Ludolph sign (54). An AP pelvic radiograph will demonstrate the avulsed fragment in most cases, since the hips normally resume a position of slight external rotation exposing the lesser trochanters (57). A film with the hip in external rotation may be necessary to adequately visualize the avulsed fragment. Treatment of this injury is nonoperative (Table 34–2), with excellent results uniformly reported (57,58,62,70,72). The degree of displacement of the avulsed fragment appears to have no relationship to symptomatology of the prognosis (57).

Injuries of the Iliac Apophysis

The iliac crest is the site of attachment of several muscles including the internal and external oblique abdominal muscles, the transverse abdominus muscles, the gluteus medius, and the tensor fascia lata. The appearance of the apophysis occurs in a progression from anterior to posterior beginning at age 12–15 years (54). Closure may be delayed until the midtwenties. Injuries of the iliac crest can result from either acute trauma or repetitive microtrauma. Acute avulsion of the iliac apophysis occurs predominantly in runners, particularly sprinters, though a sudden twisting movement, such as swinging a baseball bat, can also result in injury (61,62,76). It is unclear which specific muscles are involved in the avulsion, though the abdominals have been implicated (61,85). At the time of injury, athletes will often experience a pop followed by intense pain over the anterior portion of the iliac crest. Most patients will be unable to ambulate in the acute stage of this injury. Physical examination reveals tenderness over the anterior portion of the iliac crest, limited hip range of motion, and pain with contraction of the abdominal muscles. Radiographs of the pelvis will show an avulsion of the anterior portion of the iliac crest with varying degrees of displacement. Treatment is nonoperative as outlined in Table 34–2. Trunk stabilization is emphasized in the latter stages of rehabilitation.

Iliac apophysitis from repetitive microtrauma is not uncommon in the adolescent runner. Lombardo and colleagues (86) reported this overuse injury in a small series of adolescents who were diagnosed with "hip pointers." These diagnoses were actually made by radiographs that demonstrated discontinuity of the anterior aspect of the iliac apophysis. In this series, eight of nine improved with conservative treatment. The length of time to recovery ranged from 1 to 8 months. Bilateral symptoms were uncommon. There was no evidence of stress fractures, since serial X-rays failed to show any healing. Furthermore, all radiographic abnormalities disappeared at skeletal maturity. In our experience, virtually all runners recover after a period of relative rest and a trunk stabilization program.

LOWER EXTREMITY APOPHYSEAL INJURIES

Apophyseal injuries of the lower extremity are relatively common and account for the majority of growth plate injuries resulting from overuse (3). Although the traction apophysitises may result in significant short-term morbidity for the skeletally immature athlete, the majority of these injuries are self-limited as the secondary growth center begins to fuse. Addressing both the extrinsic and intrinsic predisposing factors may enhance recovery and minimize morbidity.

Tibial Tubercle Apophysitis (Osgood-Schlatter's Lesion)

Tibial tubercle apophysitis, commonly known as Osgood-Schlatter's lesion (OSL), is an overuse injury to the apophysis at the tibial tubercle as a result of repetitive submaximal tensile stresses. Osgood (87) and Schlatter (88) independently described, in 1903, injury to the tibial tubercle apophysis, distinguishing this overuse injury from an acute tibial avulsion fracture.

The prevalence of OSL is unknown. Previous retrospective studies (89–91) have shown that this condition is more common in boys than in girls. However, the number of preadolescent and adolescent females who are engaged in organized sports has steadily increased over the last 10 years, and the current epidemiology of OSL would be expected to include a higher proportion of females than previously reported. Participation in sports, particularly those involving repetitive impact, such as football, hockey, soccer, basketball, running, and gymnastics, is associated with an increased incidence of this condition (4,5,90).

Females generally develop symptoms at a younger age than males do because of females' earlier onset of skeletal development. The peak incidence of OSL for females occurs between ages 11 and 13, and that for males occurs between ages 12 and 14, corresponding to the periods of rapid skeletal growth (89,90,92).

Previous theories have attributed OSL to aseptic necrosis, infection, endocrine abnormalities, ectopic calcification, and partial or complete avulsion of the patellar tendon from the tibial tuberosity (93,94). However, it is generally accepted that OSL results from repetitive tensile forces of the patellar tendon onto its apophyseal insertion on the proximal tibia (4,91–99). Ogden and Southwick (93) described the lesion of OSL as an avulsion of segments (ossicles) of the anterior portion of the developing secondary ossification center and overlying hyaline cartilage of the tibial tuberosity, with formation of callus in the intervening area. In their model, the tuberosity of the growth plate remains intact (Fig. 34–3). However, several authors have questioned whether these presumed avulsions of the tibial tuberosity are the sole cause of symptoms. Lanning and Heikkinen (100) used ultrasound to compare the knees of those with and without OSL. While patients with OSL showed soft tissue swelling and elevation of the anterior portion of the apophysis and edema anterior to the tibial tubercle, which is in support of Ogden and Southwick's model, distal patellar tendon thickening and edema was uniformly demonstrated, a finding suggesting that involvement of the patellar tendon was an important feature of OSL.

Rosenberg and colleagues (94) addressed whether symptoms of OSL are due to a patellar tendinitis versus avulsion fractures by comparing three-phase bone scintigraphy, computed tomography (CT), and magnetic resonance (MR) in patients with OSL during and after the disappearance of symptoms. Soft tissue changes indicative of an insertional patellar tendinitis were present

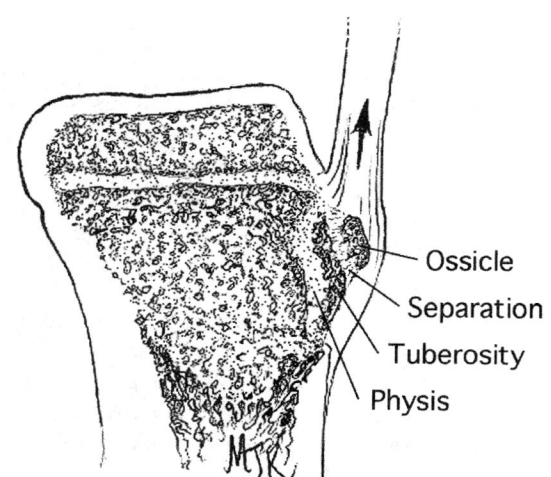

FIG. 34–3. Schematic of the secondary ossification center of the tibial tuberosity. **A:** Normal. **B:** Osgood-Schlatter's condition with fragmentation of the ossification center. **C:** Enlargement showing avulsion of the ossicle from the anterior portion of the developing ossification center. The region of separation fills in with fibrous and fibrocartilaginous tissue which eventually ossifies. (Reprinted with permission from Ogden JA, Southwick WO. Osgood-Schlatter's disease and tibial tuberosity development. *Clin Orthop* 1976:116.)

in all patients symptomatic with OSL. Additionally, deep and infrapatellar bursae were commonly noted among symptomatic patients. Both of these findings showed partial or complete resolution on follow-up scans. Bone abnormalities, mainly ossicles anterior to the ossification center of the tibial tuberosity, were an inconsistent finding. However, in several of these cases a defect in the ossification center of the tibial tubercle, similar in shape to the ossicle, was demonstrated on CT scans and MR images, suggesting that a bone detachment off the tibial tubercle had occurred. On several follow-up CT scans of these patients, fusion of the ossicle to the tubercle was demonstrated, though abatement of symptoms also occurred in patients in whom the ossicle did not fuse. In several patients MR images reveal marrow edema of the tibial tubercle and tibial epiphysis. In some of these cases the MR findings partially returned to normal on repeat studies. Three-phase bone scans on all but one symptomatic patient were negative. These findings suggest that, while avulsion fractures from the ossification center of the tibial tubercle do occur, the symptoms of OSL are probably more directly related to an insertional patellar tendinitis, surrounding bursitis, and, in a few cases, marrow edema of the tubercle and tibial epiphysis.

The most common symptom of OSL is pain at the tibial tubercle that is often aggravated by running or activities that require eccentric quadricep contraction such as jumping and squatting. Direct trauma to the tibial tubercle is extremely painful, and most patients find it difficult to kneel. Physical examination reveals a characteristic prominence of the tibial tubercle (Fig. 34-4) and marked pain to direct palpation over the tubercle. The distal patellar tendon and peripatellar soft tissue structures may be tender as well. Slipped capital femoral epiphysis may coexist with OSL (101). A hip examination should be part of the evaluation of any child with symptoms of knee pain.

The importance of obtaining radiographs of the knee in patients with clinically apparent OSL has been stressed by several authors, who cite the rare occurrence of entities that can mimic OSL, including osteomyelitis, arteriovenous malformation, and bone tumor (4,101–103). Also, radiographs are essential in distinguishing OSL from a true acute fracture of the proximal tibial epiphysis in patients with more acute onset of symptoms. Common findings on a lateral radiograph in patients with OSL include soft tissue swelling anterior to the tibial tubercle, prominence of the bony portion of the tubercle, fragmentation of the epiphysis, and bony fragments or a separated ossicle anterior to the tibial tubercle (Fig. 34-5).

Several authors have noted a relationship between patellar alta, as determined by a lateral radiograph of the knee, and OSL, though this association remains controversial (104–106). Aparicio and colleagues (104)

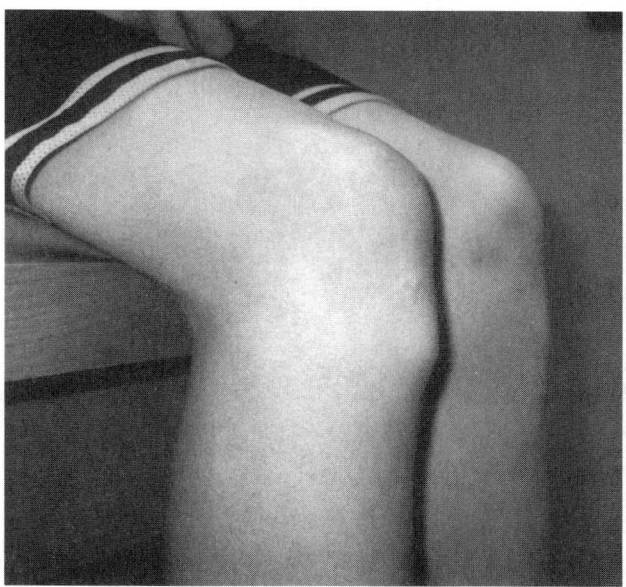

FIG. 34-4. A 13-year-old male with Osgood-Schlatter's condition of the right knee that developed during football season.

recently compared patellar height in patients with OSL to controls by using a radiographic method that is not influenced by skeletal maturation or inprecisions in determining the insertion of the patellar tendon. They found a strong association between patella alta and

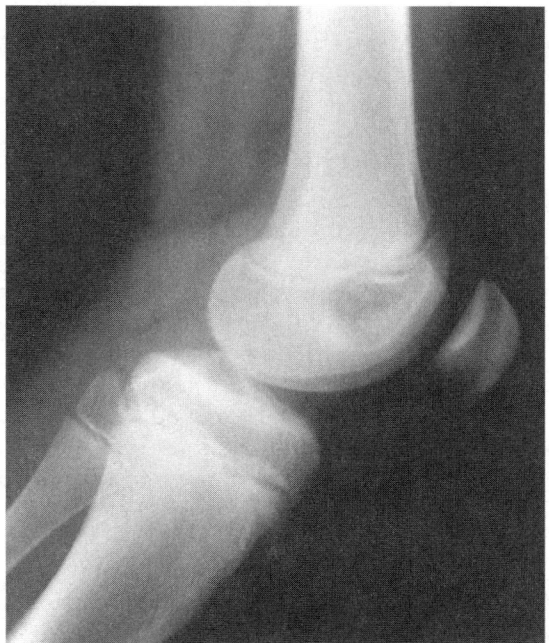

FIG. 34-5. Radiograph of the right knee of a 13-year-old male with symptomatic Osgood-Schlatter's condition showing a separated ossicle anterior to the tibial tubercle.

OSL, though their study design does not allow a cause-and-effect conclusion.

The natural history of OSL was retrospectively studied by Krause and colleagues (89) and revealed that the majority of patients experienced limitation in activities and inability to kneel without pain during the symptomatic phase of their condition. At follow-up (average 9 years, range 3–30 years), 60% were still unable to kneel without pain, and 18% had tenderness over the tibial tubercle. Additionally, the outline of the tibial tubercle remained abnormal in 70% of the knees. However, only 18% of the patients experienced limitations in activity due to tenderness of the tibial tubercle. These findings support the view that the pain associated with OSL most often spontaneously resolves with skeletal maturation.

The treatment of OSL is primarily nonoperative (4,91,97,102). Education of both the athlete and parents regarding the relationship to growth, natural history, and treatment is paramount for a successful outcome. Regular icing, limited use of anti-inflammatory medication, and occasionally modalities are helpful in controlling symptoms and maintaining physical activity. Modification of sports activity depends on pain tolerance and severity of symptoms. Relative rest with activities that have less eccentric loading to the quadriceps muscles is often necessary to overcome persistently severe symptoms or flare-ups. Occasionally, a young athlete will need to modify or change sports for a season. Avoiding excess kneeling or squatting is also important. An appropriately contoured knee pad may reduce symptoms in patients who are engaged in contact sports. With the above approach, it has been our experience that only a limited number of athletes have had to resort to complete cessation of physical activity.

The severity and duration of symptoms, however, depend on the presence and modification of both intrinsic and extrinsic predisposing factors. Improvements in lower extremity flexibility, particularly the hamstrings and quadriceps muscles, may help to decrease the tensile forces transmitted by the patellar tendon onto the tibial tubercle (4). The forces that are generated by the extensor mechanism of the knee are affected by weak links along the kinetic chain of the lower extremity; therefore all parts of the kinetic chain need to be assessed. Frequently, enhancing stability of the trunk and gluteal muscles has helped to unload the quadricep mechanism during squatting or jumping motions. Finally, patients who demonstrate marked pronation may benefit from full-length arch supports, in the form of either an over-the-counter or custom orthosis.

Several other treatment approaches have been described in the literature that warrant discussion. Previously, the pain associated with OSL was assumed to arise predominantly from small avulsion fractures; therefore immobilization was a viable treatment option (87,93,95,99). Currently, the pain associated with OSL is known to result from insult to both tendon and surrounding soft tissue, and routine immobilization is discouraged except in the most extreme cases.

Steroid injections into or around the tibial tubercle is contraindicated. Rosenberg and colleagues (94), however, reported immediate and long-lasting relief from one or two lidocaine injections into the soft tissues around the tibial tubercle in patients with OSL. Further studies validating this treatment approach have not been performed.

Currently, the role of surgery is reserved for the rare patient who exhibits persistent symptoms that interfere with sports or activity of daily living past the age of skeletal maturity (4,98,107,108). Mital and colleagues (98) reported excellent results in patients with persistent symptoms (average age: 16) after surgical removal of a separate ossicle that was attached to the distal part of the undersurface of the patellar tendon.

In summary, OSL is a common traction apophysitis resulting from repetitive tensile forces at the insertion of the patellar tendon onto the maturing tibial tubercle. While small avulsion fractures occur at the anterior portion of the tubercle, both an insertional tendinitis and surrounding bursitis are part of the syndrome and correlate with patient's symptomatology. Treatment is aimed at symptom reduction with rest, ice, compression, and elevation (RICE); activity modification; and correction of underlying extrinsic or intrinsic predisposing factors. Surgery is rarely required and is reserved for the persistently symptomatic individual who has reached skeletal maturity.

Sinding-Larsen-Johansson Syndrome

Sinding-Larsen and Johansson independently described, in 1921 and 1922, respectively, a syndrome of pain accompanied by radiographic changes at the inferior pole of the patella in the skeletally immature athlete (109,110). Analogous to the Osgood-Schlatter's lesion, Sinding-Larsen-Johansson syndrome (SLJS) is thought to result from repetitive tensile stresses of the patellar tendon at its origin on the inferior pole of the patella (109–112).

The etiology of the pain that is characteristic of SLJS is not fully understood. Whether SLJS is due to small avulsion fractures of the ossification center at the inferior pole of the patella, from soft tissue changes of the patellar tendon, or from a combination is unclear. Radiographic changes of SLJS have been reported as an incidental finding in an asymptomatic basketball player (113). Medlar and Lyne (112) noted that several patients in their series had no initial radiographic abnormalities but developed calcification at the inferior pole of the patella as they were followed over time. Whether pain over the inferior pole of the patella is accompanied by X-ray abnormalities and is therefore termed SLJS or does not result in radiographic abnormalities and is called patellar tendinitis becomes an academic discussion, since treatment is directed at the symptomatology rather than at radiographic findings.

SLJS occurs predominantly in preadolescents and adolescents aged 10–14 who are involved in sports that require running, jumping, or kicking (112–114). The pain is often accentuated by squatting, kneeling, or climbing stairs. Several authors have noted the simultaneous occurrence of SLJS with other traction apophysitises, mainly Osgood-Schlatter's lesion (112–114). However, these studies have not addressed whether individuals with a traction apophysitis are predisposed to another one.

The diagnosis of SLJS is made by the presence of pain at the inferior pole of the patella accompanied by radiographic abnormalities in a young athlete (Fig. 34–6). Radiographic findings have been classified into four stages based on the observations of Medlar and Lyne (112).

Stage I: normal patella on a lateral X-ray.
Stage II: irregular calcifications at the inferior pole of the patella.
Stage III: coalescence of the calcification.
Stage IVa: incorporation of the calcification into the patella
Stage IVb: coalesced calcification mass separate from the patella

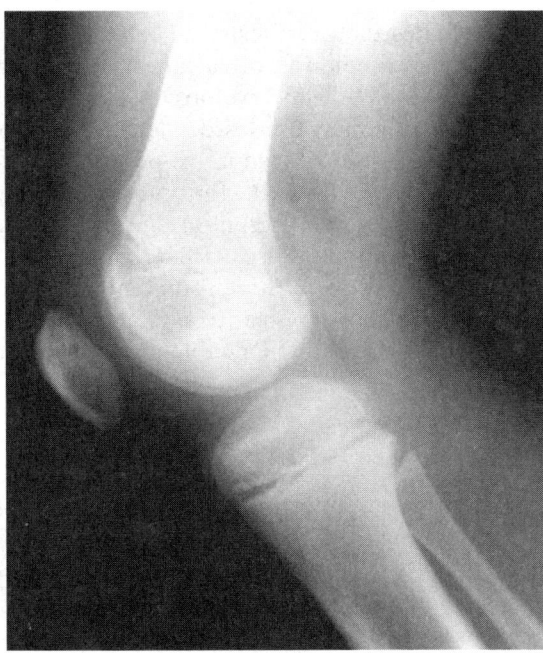

FIG. 34–6. Radiograph of a 10-year-old male with pain at the inferior pole of the patella showing calcification at the inferior pole consistent with Sinding-Larsen-Johansson syndrome (Medlar and Lyne stage III).

Fragmentation of the proximal pole of the patella has also been described in patients with the clinical features of SLJS or OSL. In their case description of six patients, Batten and Menelaus (115) noted that none of the patients in whom X-rays revealed fragmentation of the proximal pole of the patella had signs or symptoms at that site. Follow-up radiographs 8 months to 2 years later varied from complete healing, often with a more pointed contour of the superior pole, to persistent fragmentation. It appears that fragmentation at either pole of the patella may be an incidental finding in some patients and that treatment decisions are determined by the patient's clinical manifestations.

In patients who present with a more acute onset of pain at the inferior pole of the patella, a patellar stress fracture or sleeve fracture should be considered. Patellar sleeve fracture may be overlooked on initial evaluation, since X-rays may be normal or show only subtle abnormalities (116,117). Patients who present with a sleeve fracture are usually between ages 9 and 12 and experience a more acute onset of pain and marked disability than those with SLJS. The usual mechanism of injury is a forceful eccentric contraction of the quadricep muscles against a slightly flexed knee, resulting in an avulsion of the patellar tendon complex at the inferior pole of the patella (111,116). The patient describes a sudden, painful giving way of the knee followed by an inability to bear weight. Physical examination reveals a hemarthrosis, patella alta, and point tenderness with a palpable defect at the inferior pole of the patella. Radiographs reveal an effusion and patella alta. The avulsed segment of bone from the inferior pole of the patella may not be evident on initial X-rays, obligating the clinician to make the diagnosis on clinical grounds (111). Sleeve fractures require open reduction and internal fixation to restore intra-articular alignment and quadriceps mechanism congruency.

Treatment of SLJS is nonoperative and is similar to that of OSL (102,111–113). Ice, anti-inflammatory medication, and activity modification are the mainstay of controlling symptoms, while a rehabilitation program that is designed to correct intrinsic and extrinsic predispositions, especially lower extremity flexibility, is undertaken. As we noted above, rehabilitation decisions as well as sports participation are based solely on symptomatology; X-ray findings have no clinical significance. Like most traction apophysitises, symptoms are often self-limited as skeletal maturity ensues. Persistent symptoms that occur beyond skeletal maturation are uncommon, though the risk of developing future patellar tendinitis in patients with SLJS is unknown.

Medial Malleolus Apophysitis

Ishii and colleagues (118) described three cases of traction apophysitis of the medial malleolus, an uncommon injury, in young athletes ranging from age 8 to age 11. In this age group an accessory ossification center separate from the secondary ossification center of the distal tibial epiphysis is often present and is subject to traction forces from the attachment of the deltoid ligament. Diagnosis is based on the presence of swelling over the medial malleolus and pain elicited by palpation over the anterior portion of the medial malleolus as well as valgus movement of the foot. X-rays may reveal a more separated ossification center or fragmentation. MR imaging of the patients in the above study showed varied degrees of avulsion of the apophyseal cartilage from the distal tibial epiphyseal center.

Treatment of this apophysitis includes relative rest until asymptomatic, which ranged from 1 to 6 months in Ishii and colleagues' study. Resolution of symptoms appeared to correlate with healing or fusion of the accessory ossification center as indicated by follow-up radiographs or MR images.

Calcaneal Apophysitis

Calcaneal apophysitis, or Sever's disease, is the most common cause of heel pain in the preadolescent or adolescent athlete (119). In a retrospective review of young athletes presenting to a sports medicine clinic over a 10-year period, Micheli and Fehlandt revealed that calcaneal apophysitis was the most common traction apophysitis among both males and females (3). Soccer and running were the most common sports associated with heel pain in males, while soccer and gymnastics were the most common among the female athletes. Micheli and Ireland (119) noted in their retrospective review of 85 children with calcaneal apophysitis that soccer leads the list as the cause of symptoms in males, while gymnastics was most common among females. In our experience, soccer is by far the most common sport associated with this disorder.

The etiology of calcaneal apophysitis has been controversial, ranging from macrotrauma or microtrauma to tensile, compressive, or shear forces (120). Unlike other traction apophysitises, in which repetitive tensile stresses are the predominant forces resulting in tissue microtrauma, calcaneal apophysitis appears to result from a combination of repetitive stresses of both traction and impact. This concept was proposed by Liberson and colleagues (120) after comparing the radiographs of 35 children with calcaneal apophysitis to 52 asymptomatic control patients and evaluating those with heel pain with computed tomography (CT). They also performed a histologic study postmortem on six heels that showed radiographic features of calcaneal apophysitis. Comparison of lateral radiographs of the heel revealed that children with calcaneal apophysitis all showed fragmentation lines, compared to 27% of the control group. In three children with severe symptoms, radiographs revealed slight displacement of the apophyseal fragments along the lucent lines or appearance of bony callus. CT studies further showed that the location of the fragmentation lines were not haphazard, occurring in the inner two quarters of the apophysis. Histologic study of the sites corresponding to these fragmentation lines revealed fibrous tissue plates, oriented perpendicularly to the apophyseal bone, abruptly interrupting the normal architecture of the bone. Further histologic examination within these fibrous plates showed changes indicative of a reparative or remodeling process. On the basis of these observations the authors hypothesized that the calcaneal apophysis is growing under the influence of both repetitive tensile stresses from the insertion of the Achilles tendon and repetitive impact forces that occur during the gait cycle (Fig. 34–7). These forces, particularly in the young athlete, can exceed a given threshold and result in the breakdown of bone along the fibrous plates that manifests as heel pain.

The clinical presentation of calcaneal apophysitis is one of a young athlete who develops the insidious onset of posterior heel pain, often associated with a growth spurt (119). The onset of symptoms occurs most commonly between ages 10 and 12 for both boys and girls, though this disorder can present at age 7 or 8, earlier than most other apophysitises. Bilateral involvement has been reported to occur more commonly than unilateral symptoms (119). Physical examination rarely reveals erythema or swelling. Palpable tenderness is elic-

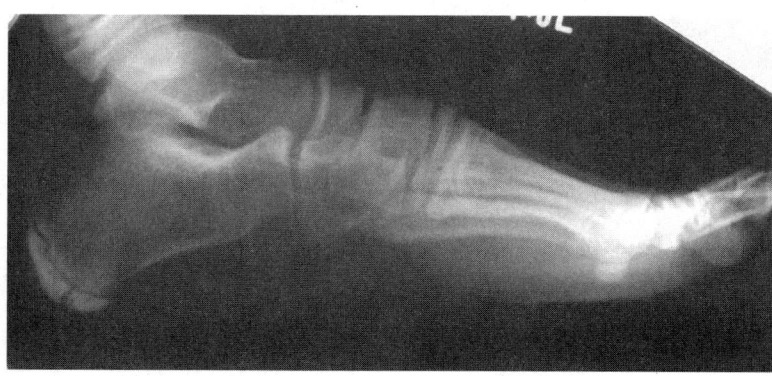

FIG. 34–7. Lateral radiograph of the foot of a 12-year-old female with clinically apparent calcaneal apophysitis. The increase in density of the calcaneal apophysis and fragmentation line are not specific to patients with calcaneal apophysitis. The apophysis is growing under the influence of repetitive tensile forces from the insertions of the Achilles tendon and plantar fascia and intrinsic muscles (longer arrows) and repetitive impact forces from the gait cycle (short arrow). (Adapted from Liberson A, Lieberson S, Mendes DG, et al. Remodeling of the calcaneus apophysis in the growing child. *J Pediatr Orthop* 1995;4:77.)

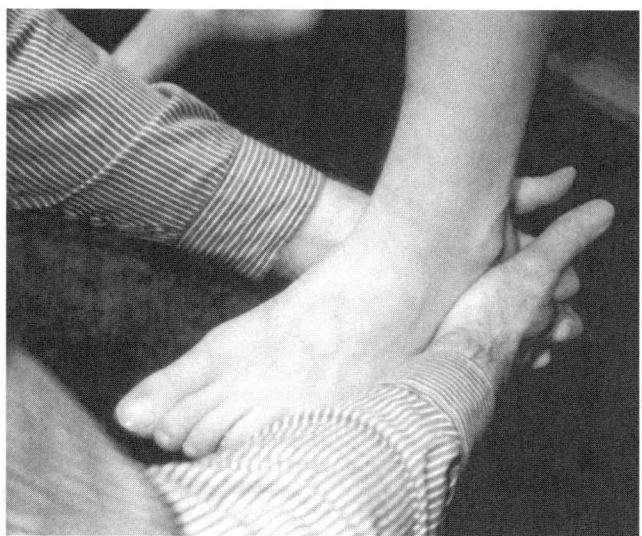

FIG. 34-8. The calcaneal compression test. Gentle medial and lateral compression of the calcaneus elicits pain in the patient with calcaneal apophysitis.

ited with medial and lateral heel compression over the course of the apophyseal plate (Fig. 34-8). Other associated findings in patients with calcaneal apophysitis include deficits in dorsiflexion and malalignments that may result in an increase pronation during the gait cycle.

Radiographs of the heel are not specific for the diagnosis of calcaneal apophysitis. As we noted above, fragmentation lines can been seen in radiographs of asymptomatic children. Similarly, an increase in the density of the calcaneal apophysis is not specific to patients with calcaneal apophysitis and is observed in the majority of children without pain (see Fig. 34-7) (120). However, routine radiographs, including lateral and axial views, are recommended to exclude the rare presence of an os calcis stress fracture, infection, or neoplasm.

The approach to treatment for calcaneal apophysitis is similar to that of the other traction apophysitises. Micheli and Ireland (119) demonstrated that a regimen of relative rest, gastrocnemius–soleus stretching, dorsiflexion strengthening, and orthotics for those with foot malalignments resulted in symptomatic relief and return to desired athletic activity in an average of 2 months (with a range of 1–6 months). The temporary use of heel cups, which are thought to reduce the impact to the posterior heel, or heel lifts, which lessen the pull of the gastrocnemius-soleus complex on the apophyses, may benefit those with no obvious foot malalignments. For the rare patient who experiences more persistent and severe heel pain accompanied by radiographic evidence of apophyseal displacement along the fragmentation line or the appearance of a bony callus, a short period of immobilization or more prolonged rest may be warranted. Persistent symptoms beyond the age of closure of the calcaneal apophysis are rare. After skeletal maturation the physiologic stresses no longer concentrate at the apophysis but become distributed among a larger portion of the calcaneus.

Traction Apophysitis at the Base of the Fifth Metatarsal (Iselin's Disease)

Described by Iselin in 1912 (121), traction apophysitis that occurs at the base of the fifth metatarsal is not uncommon in young athletes who are engaged in sports requiring running, jumping, cutting, or inversion stresses. The secondary ossification center at the base of the fifth metatarsal is a thin, shell-shaped bone onto which the tendon of the peroneus brevis inserts. This apophysis generally appears in females at age 10 and in males at age 12, with fusion occurring several years later. The apophysis is usually visible only on an oblique radiograph of the foot (Fig. 34-9).

Clinically, the patient presents with pain at the base of the fifth metatarsal exacerbated by running, cutting, or jumping (122). Occasionally, symptoms begin after

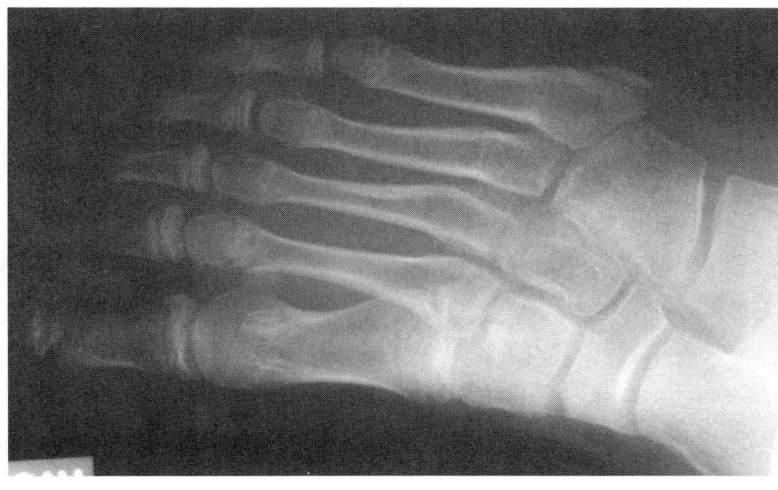

FIG. 34-9. Oblique radiograph of the foot of a 13-year-old male showing a normal apophysis at the base of the fifth metatarsal.

the athlete receives a direct blow to the area, such as during a soccer tackle. Examination reveals a prominent tuberosity from the associated edema as compared to the uninvolved side. Tenderness is elicited by direct palpation at the base of the fifth metatarsal as well as by having the patient resist both eversion and plantar flexion. An oblique radiograph may show an enlarged apophysis with fragmentation (123).

Treatment consists of relative rest, ice application, and exercises emphasizing stretching of the evertors and plantar flexors and strengthening of the invertors and dorsiflexors. Since the peroneus brevis has an eccentric role in controlling pronation during the gait cycle, orthotics may be useful in patients who exhibit excessive pronation. For severe symptoms that are unresponsive to the above measures, a short course in a walking cast boot, coming out daily for range-of-motion and gentle stretching exercise, may be warranted.

REFERENCES

1. Katz JF. Nonarticular osteochondrosis. *Clin Orthop* 1981;158:70–76.
2. Sports in childhood: a round table. *Phys Sports Med* 10(8), 1982.
3. Micheli LJ, Fehlandt AL. Overuse injuries to tendons and apophyses in children and adolescents. *Clin Sports Med* 1992;11(4):713–727.
4. Micheli LJ. The traction apophysitises. *Clin Sports Med* 1987;6(2):389–405.
5. Outerbridge AR, Micheli LJ. Overuse injuries in the young athlete. *Clin Sports Med* 1995;14(3):503–516.
6. Stanitski CL. Pediatric and adolescent sports injuries. *Clin Sports Med* 1997;16(4):613–633.
7. Steinish UD. Overuse injuries in athletes: a perspective. *Med Sci Sports Exerc* 1984;16(1):1–7.
8. Roemmich JN, Rogol AD. Physiology of growth and development: its relationship to performance in the young athlete. *Clin Sports Med* 1995;14(3):483–502.
9. Bright RW, Burstein AH, Elmore S. Epiphyseal-plate cartilage. *J Bone Joint Surg Am* 1974;56:688–703.
10. Morscher E. Strength and morphology of growth cartilage under hormonal influence of puberty. *Reconstr Surg Traumatol* 1968;10:3–104.
11. Mann DC, Rajmaira S. Distribution of physeal and non-physeal fractures in 2,650 long-bone fractures in children aged 0–16 years. *J Pediatr Orthop* 1990;10:713–716.
12. Mizuta T, Benson WM, Foster BK. Statistical analysis of the incidence of physeal injuries. *J Pediatr Orthop* 1987;7:518–523.
13. Peterson CA, Peterson HA. Analysis of the incidence of injuries to the epiphyseal growth plate. *J Trauma* 1972;12:275–281.
14. Kirchner G, Glines D. Comparative analysis of Eugene, Oregon, Elementary school children using the Kraus-Weber test of minimum muscular fitness. *Res Q Exerc Sport* 1957;28:16–25.
15. Phillips M, Bookwalter C, Denman C, et al. Analysis of results from the Kraus-Weber test of minimum muscular fitness in children. *Res Q Exerc Sport* 1955;26:314–323.
16. Adams JE. Injury of the throwing arm: a study of traumatic changes in the elbow joints of boy baseball players. *Calif Med* 1965;102:127.
17. Barnes DA, Tullos HS. An analysis of 100 symptomatic baseball players. *Am J Sports Med* 1978;6(2):62–67.
18. Gugenheim JJ, Stanley RF, Woods GW, et al. Little League survey: the Houston study. *Am J Sports Med* 1976;4(5):189–200.
19. Larson RL, Singer KM, Bergstrom R, et al. Little League survey: the Eugene study. *Am J Sports Med* 1976;4(5):201–209.
20. Lipscomb AB. Baseball pitching in growing athletes. *Am J Sports Med* 1975;3:25–34.
21. Pappas AM. Elbow problems associated with baseball during childhood and adolescence. *Clin Orthop* 1982;164:30–41.
22. Stanitski CL. Combating overuse injuries: a focus on children and adolescents. *Phys Sports Med* 1993;21:87.
23. Ireland ML, Hutchinson MR. Upper extremity injuries in young athletes. *Clin Sports Med* 1995;14(3):533–569.
24. Albright JA, Jokl P, Shaw R, Albright JP. Clinical study of baseball pitchers: correlation of injury to the throwing arm with method of deliver. *Am J Sports Med* 1978;6:15–21.
25. Indelicato PA, Jobe FW, Kerlin RK, et al. Correctable elbow lesions in professional baseball players. *Am J Sports Med* 1979;7:72.
26. King JW, Brelsford JH, Tullos HS. Analysis of the pitching arm of the professional baseball pitcher. *Clin Orthop* 1969;67:116.
27. Tullos HS, King JW. Lesions of pitching arm in adolescents. *JAMA* 1972;220:264.
28. Wilson FD, Andrews JR, Blackburn TA, McCluskey G. Valgus extension overload in the pitching elbow. *Am J Sports Med* 1983;11:83–87.
29. Gill TJ, Micheli LJ. The immature athlete: common injuries and overuse syndromes of the elbow and wrist. *Clin Sports Med* 1996;15(2):401–423.
30. Morrey BF, Regan WD. Throwing injuries. In: DeLee JC, Drez DD, eds. *Orthopaedic sports medicine,* vol 2, 1st ed. Philadelphia: WB Saunders, 1994:882–889.
31. Morrey BF, An KN. Stability of the elbow joint: a biomechanical assessment. *Am J Sports Med* 1984;12:315–319.
32. Grana WA, Rashin A. Pitcher's elbow in adolescents. *Am J Sports Med* 1980;8(5):333–336.
33. Wilson FD, Andrews JR, Blackburn TA, McCluskey G. Valgus extension overload in the pitching elbow. *Am J Sports Med* 1983;11:83–87.
34. Bede WB, Lefebure AR, Rosmon MA. Fractures of the medial humeral epicondyle in children. *Can J Surg* 1975;18:137–142.
35. Bernstein SM, King JD, Sanderson RA. Fractures of the medial epicondyle of the humerus. *Contemp Orthop* 1981:637–641.
36. Smith FM. Medial epicondyle injuries. *JAMA* 1950;142:396–402.
37. Wilson NIL, Ingran R, Rymaszewski L, Miller JH. Treatment of fractures of the medial epicondyle of the humerus. *Injury* 1988;19:342–344.
38. Ireland ML, Andrews JR. Shoulder and elbow injuries in the young athlete. *Clin Sports Med* 1988;7(3):473–494.
39. Micheli LJ. Elbow pain in a Little League pitcher. In: Smith NJ, ed. *Common problems in pediatric sports medicine.* Chicago: Yearbook Publishers, 1989:223.
40. Wilkins KE. Fractures and dislocations of the elbow region. In: Rockwood CA, Wilkins KE, King RE, eds. *Fractures in children,* 3rd ed. New York: JB Lippincott, 1991.
41. Aronem JG. Problems of the upper extremity in gymnasts. *Clin Sports Med* 1985;4:61–70.
42. Goldberg MJ. Gymnastic injuries. *Orthop Clin North Am* 1980;11:717–732.
43. Wilson FD, Andrews JR, Blackburn TA, McCluskey G. Valgus extension overload in the pitching elbow. *Am J Sports Med* 1983;11:83–87.
44. DeHaven HE, Evarts CM. Throwing injuries of the elbow in athletes. *Orthop Clin North Am* 1973;4:801–808.
45. Gore RM, et al. Osseous manifestations of elbow stress associated with sports activities. *Am J Roentgenol* 1980;134:971.
46. Morrey BF. *The elbow and its disorders,* 2nd ed. Philadelphia: WB Saunders, 1993.
47. Torg JS, Moyer RA. Non-union of a stress fracture through the olecranon epiphyseal plate observed in an adolescent baseball pitcher: a case report. *J Bone Joint Surg* 1997;59A:264.
48. Pavlov H, Torg JS, Jacobs B, et al. Non-union of olecranon epiphysis: two cases in adolescent baseball pitchers. *Am J Roentgenol* 1981;136(4):216–222.
49. Dotter WE. Little Leaguer's shoulder: a fracture of the proximal epiphyseal cartilage of the humerus due to baseball pitching. *Guthrie Clinic Bull* 1953;23:68.
50. Boyd KT, Batt ME. Stress fracture of the proximal humeral

epiphysis in an elite junior badminton player. *Br J Sports Med* 1997;31(3):252–253.
51. Barnett LS. Little league shoulder syndrome: proximal humeral epiphyseolysis in adolescent baseball pitchers. *J Bone Joint Surg* 1985;67A(3):495–496.
52. Wilkins KE. Shoulder injuries. In: DeLee JC, Drez DD, eds. *Orthopaedic sports medicine,* vol 3, 1st ed. Philadelphia: WB Saunders, 1994:175–182.
53. Morisawa K, Umemura A, Kitamura T, et al. Apophysitis of the acromion. *J Shoulder Elbow Surg* 1996;5(2, pt 1):153–156.
54. Paletta GA, Andrish JT. Injuries about the hip and pelvis in the young athlete. *Clin Sports Med* 1995;14(3):591–628.
55. Canale ST, King EK. Pelvic and hip fractures. In: Rockwood CA, Wilkins KE, King R, eds. *Fractures in children,* 3rd ed. Philadelphia: JB Lippincott, 1991:991–1120.
56. Sundar M, Carty H. Avulsion fractures of the pelvis in children: a report of 32 fractures and their outcome. *Skeletal Radiol* 1994;23:85–90.
57. Dimon JH III. Isolated fractures of the lesser trochanter of the femur. *Clin Orthop* 1972;82:144–148.
58. Fernbach SK, Wilkinson RH. Avulsion injuries of the pelvis and proximal femur. *Am J Roentgenol* 1981;137:581–584.
59. Goodshall RW, Hansen CA. Incomplete avulsion of a portion of the iliac epiphysis: an injury of young athletes. *J Bone Joint Surg* 1973;55A:1301–1302.
60. Gomez JE. Bilateral anterior inferior iliac spine avulsion fractures. *Med Sci Sports Exerc* 1996;28(2):161–164.
61. Lambert MJ, Fligner DJ. Avulsion of the iliac crest apophysis: a rare fracture in adolescent athletes. *Ann Emerg Med* 1993; 22:1218–1220.
62. Metzmaker JN, Pappas AM. Avulsion fractures of the pelvis. *Am J Sports Med* 1985;13:349–358.
63. Rogge EA, Romano RL. Avulsion of the ischial apophysis. *Clin Orthop* 1957;9:239–243.
64. Veselko M, Smrkolj V. Avulsion of the anterior-superior iliac spine in athletes: case reports. *J Trauma* 1994;36:444–446.
65. Weitzner I. Fracture of the anterior superior spine of the ilium in one case and anterior inferior in another case. *Am J Roentgenol* 1935;33:39–40.
66. Martin TA, Pipkin G. Treatment of avulsion of the ischial tuberosity. *Clin Orthop* 1957;10:108–118.
67. Curry JD, Butler G. Mechanical properties of bone tissue in children. *J Bone Joint Surg* 1975;57A:810–814.
68. Morscher E, Desaulles PA, Schenk R. Experimental studies on tensile strength and morphology of the epiphyseal cartilage at puberty. *Ann Pediatr* 1965;205:112–130.
69. Carp L. Fracture of the anterior superior spine of the ilium by muscular violence. *Ann Surg* 1924;79:551–560.
70. Combs JA. Hip and pelvis avulsion fractures in adolescents. *Physician Sportsmed* 1994;22(7):41–49. Hamada G, Rida A. Ischial apophysiolysis: report of a case and review of the literature. *Clin Orthop* 1963;31:117–130.
71. Kujala UM, Orava S. Ischial apophysis injuries in athletes. *Sports Med* 1993;16(4):290–294.
72. Green JT, Gay FH. Avulsion of the lesser trochanter epiphysis. *South Med J* 1956;49:1308–1310.
73. Merlino AF, Nixon JE. Isolated fractures of the greater trochanter: report of twelve cases. *Int Surg* 1969;52:117–124.
74. Howard MF, Piha RJ. Fractures of the apophyses in adolescent athletes. *JAMA* 1965;192:842.
75. Watts HG. Fractures of the pelvis in children. *Orthop Clin North Am* 1976;33:39.
76. Winkler AR, Barnes JC, Ogden JA. Break dance hip: chronic avulsion of the anterior superior iliac spine. *Pediatr Radiol* 1987;17:501–502.
77. Gallagher JR. Fractures of the anterior inferior iliac spine of the ilium: sprinter's fracture. *Ann Surg* 1935;102:86–88.
78. Lagier R, Jarret G. Apophysiolysis of the anterior inferior iliac spine. *Arch Orthop* 1975;83:81–89.
79. Irving MH. Exostosis formation after traumatic avulsion of the anterior inferior iliac spine. *J Bone Joint Surg* 1964;463:720–722.
80. Schlonsky J, Olix ML. Functional disability following avulsion fracture of the ischial epiphysis: report of two cases. *J Bone Joint Surg* 1972;54A:641–644.
81. Barnes ST, Hinds RB. Pseudotumor of the ischium: a late manifestation of avulsion of the ischial epiphysis. *J Bone Joint Surg* 1972;54A:645–647.
82. Wootton JR, Cross MJ, Holt KW. Avulsion of the ischial apophysis: the case for open reduction and internal fixation. *J Bone Joint Surg* 1990;72B:625–627.
83. Howard FM, Phia RJ. Fractures of the apophyses in adolescent athletes. *JAMA* 1965;192:842–844.
84. DeLee JC. Fractures and dislocations of the hip. In: Rockwood CA, Green DP, Bucholz RW, eds. *Fractures in adults,* vol 2, 3rd ed. Philadelphia: JB Lippincott, 1991:1560–1562.
85. Godshall RW, Hansen CA. Incomplete avulsion of a portion of the iliac epiphysis: an injury of young athletes. *J Bone Joint Surg* 1973;55A:1301–1302.
86. Lombardo SJ, Retting AC, Kerlan RK. Radiographic abnormalities of the iliac apophysis in adolescent athletes. *J Bone Joint Surg* 1983;65A:444–446.
87. Osgood RB. Lesions of the tibial tubercle occurring during adolescence. *Boston Med Surg J* 1903;148:114–117.
88. Schlatter C. Verletzungen des schnabelfoemingen fortsatzes der oberen tibiaepiphyse. *Beitr Klin Chir* 1903;38:874.
89. Krause BL, Williams JPR, Catterall A. Natural history of Osgood-Schlatter disease. *J Pediatr Orthop* 1990;10(1):65–68.
90. Kujala UM, Kvist M, Heinonen O. Osgood-Schlatter's disease in adolescent athletes: retrospective study of incidence and duration. *Am J Sports Med* 1985;13(4):236–240.
91. Willner P. Osgood-Schlatter's disease: etiology and treatment. *Clin Orthop* 1969;62:178–179.
92. Yashar A, Loder RT, Hensinger RN. Determination of skeletal age in children with Osgood-Schlatter's disease by using radiographs of the knee. *J Pediatr Orthop* 1995;15:298–301.
93. Ogden JA, Southwick WO. Osgood-Schlatter's disease and tibial tuberosity development. *Clin Orthop* 1976;116:180–189.
94. Rosenberg ZS, Kawelblum M, Cheung YY, et al. Osgood-Schlatter's lesion: fracture or tendinitis? scintigraphic, CT, and MR imaging features. *Radiology* 1992;185:853–858.
95. Ehrenborg G. The Osgood-Schlatter lesion: a clinical study of 170 cases. *Acta Chir Scand* 1962;124:89–105.
96. Holstrin A, Lewis GB, Schulze R. Heterotopic ossification of the patellar tendon. *J Bone Joint Surg* 1968;45A:656.
97. Katz JF. Nonarticular osteochondroses. *Clin Orthop* 1981;158:70–76.
98. Mital MA, Matza RA, Cohen J. The so-called unresolved Osgood-Schlatter lesion. *J Bone Joint Surg* 1980;62A:732–739.
99. Ogden JA. *Skeletal injury in the child,* 2nd ed. Philadelphia: WB Saunders, 1990:812–815.
100. Lanning P, Heikkinen E. Ultrasonic features of the Osgood-Schlatter lesion. *J Pediatr Orthop* 1991;11:538–540.
101. Stanitski CL. Osgood-Schlatter disease. In: Stanitski CL, DeLee JC, Drez DD, eds. *Orthopaedic sports medicine,* vol 3, 1st ed. Philadelphia: WB Saunders, 1994:320–324.
102. Stanitski CL. Anterior knee pain syndromes in the adolescent. *J Bone Joint Surg* 1993;75A:1407–1416.
103. D'Ambrosia RD, NacDonald GL. Pitfalls in the diagnosis of Osgood-Schlatter disease. *Clin Orthop* 1975;110:206.
104. Aparicio G, Abril JC, Calvo E, et al. Radiologic study of the patellar height in Osgood-Schlatter disease. *J Pediatr Orthop* 1997;17:63–66.
105. Jakob RP, VonGumppenberg S, Engelhardt P. Does Osgood-Schlatter disease influence the position of the patella? *J Bone Joint Surg* 1981;63B:579–582.
106. Lancourt JE, Cristini JA. Patella alta and patella infera: their etiological role in patellar dislocation, chondromalacia, and apophysitis of the tibial tubercle. *J Bone Joint Surg* 1975;51A:1112–1115.
107. Glynn MK, Regan BF. Surgical treatment of Osgood-Schlatter's disease. *J Pediatr Orthop* 1983;3:216–219.
108. Robertsen K, Kristensen O, Sommer J. Pseudoarthrosis between a patellar tendon ossicle and the tibial tuberosity in Osgood-Schlatter's disease. *Scand J Med Sci Sports* 1996;6:57–59.
109. Sinding-Larsen MF. A hitherto unknown affection of the patella in children. *Acta Radiol* 1921;1:171–173.
110. Johansson S. En forut ecke beskriven sjukdom i patella. *Hygiea* 1922;84:161–166.

111. Gardiner JS, McInerney VK, Avella DG, et al. Injuries to the inferior pole of the patella in children. *Orthop Rev* 1990;19(7):643–649.
112. Medlar RC, Lyne ED. Sinding-Larsen Johansson disease: its etiology and natural history. *J Bone Joint Surg* 1978;60A:1113–1116.
113. Stanitski CL. Osgood-Schlatter disease. In: Stanitski CL, DeLee JC, Drez DD, eds. *Orthopaedic sports medicine,* vol 3, 1st ed. Philadelphia: WB Saunders, 1994:325–328.
114. Traverso A, Baldari A, Catalani F. The coexistence of Osgood-Schlatter's disease with Sinding-Larsen Johansson's disease: case report in an adolescent soccer player. *J Sports Med Phys Fitness* 1990;30(3):331–333.
115. Batten J, Menelaus MB. Fragmentation of the proximal pole of the patella: another manifestation of juvenile traction osteochondritis? *J Bone Joint Surg* 1985;67B:249–251.
116. Houghton GR, Ackroyd CE. Sleeve fractures of the patella in children: a report of three cases. *J Bone Joint Surg* 1979;61B:165–168.
117. Beaty JH, Roberts JM. Fractures and dislocations of the knee. In: Rockwood CA, Wilkins KE, King R, eds. *Fractures in children,* 3rd ed. Philadelphia: JB Lippincott, 1991:1222–1233.
118. Ishii T, Miyagawa S, Hayashi K. Traction apophysitis of the medial malleolus. *J Bone Joint Surg* 1994;76B:802–806.
119. Micheli LJ, Ireland ML. Prevention and management of calcaneal apophysitis in children: an overuse syndrome. *J Pediatr Orthop* 1987;7:34–38.
120. Liberson A, Lieberson S, Mendes DG, et al. Remodeling of the calcaneus apophysis in the growing child. *J Pediatr Orthop* 1995;4:74–79.
121. Iselin H. Wachtumsbeschwerden zur zeit dur knochernen entwicklung der tuberositas metatarsi quint. *Dtsch Z Chir* 1912;117:529–535.
122. Lehman RC, Gregg JR, Torg E. Iselin's disease. *Am J Sports Med* 1986;14:494–496.
123. Canale ST. Osteochondroses and related problems of the foot and ankle. In: Stanitski CL, DeLee JC, Drez DD, eds. *Orthopaedic sports medicine,* vol 3, 1st ed. Philadelphia: WB Saunders, 1994:351–352.

CHAPTER 35

Avulsion Injuries

Keith L. Stanley

INTRODUCTION

This chapter will attempt to define avulsion injuries for the sports medicine physician. Additionally, specific avulsion injuries as they occur to specific anatomic regions of the human anatomy will be identified. We will attempt to delineate the mechanisms of injuries, and we will discuss current treatment options for each of the injuries listed.

AVULSION INJURIES DEFINED

Avulsion comes from Latin *avulsio*: "a," meaning away, plus "velere," meaning to pull. Therefore the term *avulsion injury* means the tearing away of a part of structure (1).

Avulsion injuries can involve most anatomic structures, including skin, teeth, nerves, or ears, for example. For the purpose of this chapter our reference will be restricted to the musculoskeletal system. This discussion will also exclude avulsion injuries as they apply to amputation-type mechanisms.

Avulsion injuries of the musculoskeletal system usually occur around joints but may include bony processes without an articular relationship. Typically, the injury involves the pulling away of a tendinous or ligamentous attachment to an osseous structure.

In this chapter, discussion will be directed to specific anatomic regions and the common and uncommon avulsion injuries occurring there.

AVULSION INJURIES TO THE HAND

Avulsion Fractures of the Metacarpals

Avulsion fractures of the metacarpals involving the index metacarpal and the long metacarpal are rare (2,3).

K. L. Stanley: Eastern Oklahoma Orthopedic, Tulsa, Oklahoma 74136.

Avulsion fractures of the index metacarpal involve the tendon attachment of the extensor radials longus (3–5). Avulsion fractures of the long finger metacarpal involve the tendinous attachment of the extensor carpi radialis brevus.

These patients generally present with marked dorsal hand swelling and tenderness over the base of the carpal metacarpal articulation; wrist extension generally will cause pain. X-rays generally will show a displaced dorsal fracture fragment.

Since these fractures, if not properly reduced and treated, can lead to instability to axial load of the metacarpal, it is important to get anatomic reduction of the fracture (2). These fragments are usually fixed with a tension band wire (2,6). Cast immobilization is also part of the postsurgical treatment for up to 3–4 weeks after a progressive immobilization rehabilitation program is initiated to regain range of motion and strength.

Avulsion Fractures of the Thumb Metacarpophalangeal Joint

Avulsion fractures of the thumb metacarpophalangeal joint also require adequate treatment to prevent joint instability (7–10). Metacarpophalangeal joint instability may result if an avulsion fragment is displaced or rotated so that it compromises the ligamentous support of the joint. This type of injury is a common one during athletic activities. These skier's thumb injuries do not always involve a bony avulsion, and the treatment of ulnar collateral ligament sprains will be discussed elsewhere. For patients who do have an associated avulsion injury, the fractures have been classified by Jupiter and Shepherd (11) (Fig. 35–1).

These patients have a history of a fall, usually during athletic activities, such as skiing or from a grasping attempt such as a football player making a tackle. On

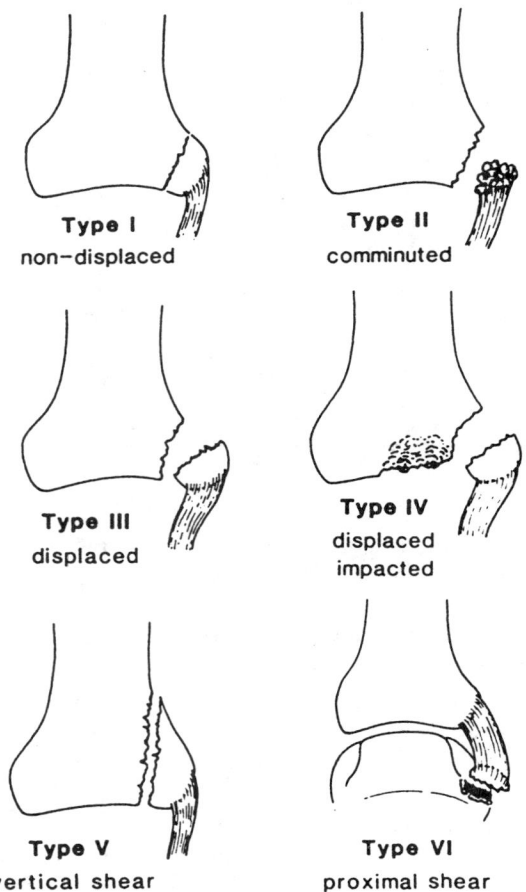

FIG. 35–1. Classification of collateral ligament avulsion fracture. (From Jupiter JB, Shepherd JE. Tension wire fixation of avulsion fractures in the hand. *Clin Orthop* 1987;214:113–120.)

physician examination they will have pain over the ulnar aspect of the first metacarpal phalangeal joint. They also may demonstrate instability by stress testing of the ligament. The X-rays may reveal an avulsion fracture. A variety of types of fractures may be found, as seen in Figure 35–1 (11).

Treatment for these injuries should attempt to restore the normal anatomy. If a fracture is present, surgical treatment is usually indicated. The Stener's lesion has been discussed extensively in the literature as an indication for surgery. But any of the fracture types described by Jupiter and Shepherd, including the Stener's lesion, should be considered for surgical treatment. Kozin and colleagues described the technique with tension wire fixation as an operative method for the treatment of these avulsion fractures of the first metacarpophalangeal joint (7). Bovard and colleagues described a technique using a mitek suture anchor as a method of achieving internal fixation of the fracture fragment (12).

Avulsion Fractures about the Proximal Interphalangeal Joint

Avulsion fractures around the proximal interphalangeal joint can involve either the ulnar collateral, radial collateral, volar plate, or dorsal central slip, which are stabilizers of the joint. Combined injuries may also be present (13).

These are common injuries in athletics. The athlete may present with pain and swelling of the proximal interphalangeal joint. If these avulsion injuries do not involve intraarticular fragments, as in the case of some collateral ligament avulsion injuries, conservative treatment may be adequate. Volar plate or dorsal-type avulsion injuries may require surgical treatment, especially if the injury involves a significant size fragment affecting 25% or greater of the articular surface. Conservative treatment may even be possible for dorsal central slip avulsions of the extensor tendon if there is minimal displacement. Splinting in extension is recommended to try to preserve the continuity of the extensor mechanism. Operative treatment needs to be considered for larger fragment sizes or for any that has significant displacement. Tension band wire fixation is usually recommended as an operative procedure.

Boutonniere Deformity Secondary to Central Slip Avulsion Injuries

These injuries may occur with or without an avulsion fracture. The extensor tendon may avulse from its insertion of the dorsal base of the middle phalanx without a bony fragment, while others may actually have a bony fragment of varying size. The deformity that results is one with flexion of the proximal interphalangeal and hyperextension of the DIP joint. As the lateral bands progressively tear or stretch after this injury, they actually act as flexors as they slip volar past the axis of the proximal interphalangeal joint (14).

Clinically, the athlete may present with pain over the dorsal aspect of the proximal interphalangeal joint and difficulty extending the PIP joint. The deformity may not be immediately apparent but may progress over several days.

Treatment many times is splinting, but one may opt for surgical repair if there is a large fracture fragment or if one has difficulty keeping the deformity reduced.

Mallet Finger Associated with Avulsion Fracture of the Distal Phalanx

Mallet finger deformities are a result of the avulsion of the extensor tendon from the dorsal aspect of the distal phalanx or avulsion fracture of its bony attachment. The mechanism of injury is usually one of a sudden blow to the tip of an extended finger (14).

The patient generally presents with an inability to extend the distal interphalangeal joint. They may be very painful to palpation over the dorsal aspect of the distal interphalangeal joint.

Treatment is generally one of splinting in an extended position with the exception being those that have a volar subluxation. It is typically recommended that those undergo open reduction and internal fixation (15,16). In those treated conservatively, the extension splinting may need to be as long as 6–8 weeks and the splinting should be continuous, including nighttime for at least 4–6 weeks.

Avulsion of the Flexor Digitorum Profundus

An injury that is sometimes referred to as "jersey finger" in football players is one of an avulsion of the flexor digitorum profundus from its insertion at the base of the distal phalanx on the flexor surface. The ring finger is the finger most often involved (17).

Three different types of flexor digitorum profundus avulsion injuries have been identified (18). In Type I the tendon retracts into the palm, severing the blood supply to the tendon. Type II injuries involve retraction of the tendon to the level of the proximal interphalangeal joint. In Type III a large bony fragment is involved by the tendon and is usually lodged at the distal pulley.

The athlete usually presents with a history of having grabbed a jersey trying to make a tackle in football or having caught a finger on the rim of a goal while slam-dunking a basketball (19). There may be associated pain at the sight of the avulsion injury, and one may actually even palpate the tendon to the point at which it is entrapped. The athlete will also have an inability to flex the distal interphalangeal joint. X-rays should be taken to determine whether an avulsed fracture fragment is involved. These can be very small or very large (19,20).

In general, early treatment is highly recommended for any of the three types of flexor digitorum profundus injuries. In Type I injuries repair should be done within 7–10 days or the retracted tendon deteriorates and makes the repair difficult and the prognosis less favorable (19). Type II lesions should also be treated early, but successful repair has been reported to have been done as late as 3 months after injury (19). Type III injuries should also be treated early, and an attempt to make a true reduction of this avulsed fragment is important. Return to athletic competition is usually not possible until the fracture is completely healed, which usually takes approximately 8 weeks (19).

AVULSION FRACTURES OF THE WRIST

Considering the multiple ligamentous attachments of the distal radial ulnar joint and the carpal bones, numerous injuries can occur. This discussion will focus primarily on the triangular fibral cartilage complex and some mention of other less common avulsion injuries.

AVULSION FRACTURES OF THE TRIQUETRUM

This injury may actually be a heralding signal of more significant injuries to the perilunate ligaments (21). The avulsion fractures of the triquetrum generally occur on the radial aspect of the volar triquetral bone. These injuries are best seen on lateral radiographs. Patients may present as being tender over the triquetrum. Treatment for the volar avulsion fractures is typically conservative with cast or splint immobilization.

AVULSION INJURIES OF THE ULNAR STYLOID

Avulsion fractures of the ulnar styloid can be an isolated injury or associated with other fracture injuries (for example, radius fracture + ulnar styloid fracture). The fracture fragment is usually attached to the ulnotriquetral ligament. These injuries should be considered serious until they have been more thoroughly evaluated. The reason for this is that there may be an associated avulsion injury to the triangular fibral cartilage complex, which is the primary stabilizer of the distal radioulnar joint (22).

These injuries are usually a result of a fall on an outstretched hand, which can occur in a sporting or athletic situation. Mikic and Sad (22) found that the injuries to the triangular fibral cartilage complex were isolated lesions in only 15% of the patients in their series. More frequently, they were associated with other fractures (22). Treatment revolved around treating the associated injury such as fractures of the distal radius; then the attention was directed toward stabilization of the distal radioulnar joint. Sennwald and colleagues describes a procedure for reattachment of the triangular fibral cartilage that included an articular shortening osteotomy of the radial head. The purpose was to give one an opportunity to have maximal reattachment of the triangular fibral cartilage complex to its anatomic mooring (23). This effort is made to try to restore the normal pronation and supination function of the distal radial ulnar joint, since it is largely controlled by the triangular fibral cartilage complex (23,24).

In the athlete who has an ulnar styloid fracture, one must consider the possibility that significant injury has occurred to the triangular fibral cartilage complex and subsequently, significant injury to the distal radioulnar joint. One needs to make sure that they have thoroughly evaluated this injury before deciding upon the appropriate treatment plan.

AVULSION FRACTURES ABOUT THE ELBOW

Avulsion Fractures of the Medial Epicondyle

Epicondyle avulsion fractures are primarily seen in the pediatric age group. In athletics these are seen predominantly in throwing athletes but can occur under other situations in which valgus stress applied through the elbow (25). Some patients may actually have a prelude to an avulsive injury by experiencing onset of pain before an acute traumatic event.

These patients may present with a history of an acute pain or even a "pop" that resulted from a throwing motion. On physical exam the patients are usually very point tender over the medial epicondyle and have an inability to fully extend the elbow. Displacement can be either minimal or significant. The separation occurs along the cartilaginous ephyseal growth plate, which is weaker than the actual tendinous attachment (26). Two types of medial epicondylar avulsion injuries have been described (27). Type I lesions are those that occur in younger children and produce a larger fragment. It often will be displaced and rotated. A Type II lesion occurs in older adolescents and produces only a small fracture fragment.

There is controversy concerning the treatment of these injuries. Most protocols revolve around millimeters of displacement of the fracture fragment. The difficulty is interpreting the literature as to what is a significant displacement. Surgical treatment would be recommended if the displacement were in excess of 3–8 mm (26,27). One can do a gravity-stressed radiograph to determine whether there is elbow instability. If instability is indicated by gravity stressed radiograph, surgical treatment is recommended (28). Others would not accept any degree of medial epicondylar displacement and recommend anatomic surgical reduction (29).

Avulsion Fractures of the Olecranon

Avulsion injuries to the olecranon are seen during adolescence. These occur around an ossification center. In some patients a delay in the fusion of the ossification center predisposes them to avulsion-type injuries (30). Avulsion injuries of young adults or older adults have also been reported. Any displacement of an olecranon avulsion injury should be considered for operative treatment. In adults one may have to consider other possible pathologies that may coexist, such as posterior osteophytes and posterior medial osteophytes. Avulsion fragments in adolescents may be treated by arthroscopic removal. An unfused apophysis may be responsive to conservative treatment, but in those that have persistent symptoms, operative treatment may be necessary (25).

Avulsion Fractures of the Coronoid Process

Ulnar coronoid process injuries are usually associated with posterior elbow dislocations (31). These fractures have been categorized into three types, which relate to the insertions of the medial colateral ligament the elbow joint capsule and the brachialis muscle and in the different regions of the coronoid process.

Type I fractures involve the coronoid tip, Type II fractures involve 50% or less than the coronoid height, and Type III fractures involve greater than 50% of the coronoid height. Of these three types it is thought that Type II and Type III are true avulsion-type injuries, whereas Type I is more of a shear injury (31). Type II fractures do include the attachment of the anterior capsule and may affect the instability of the elbow joint. Type III fractures include the insertions of the anterior bundle of the medial collateral ligament and the brachialis muscle and may cause marked instability of the elbow joint.

Treatment of these injuries is determined by whether instability of the elbow is significant; if so, the treatment should be directed toward stabilizing the elbow.

AVULSION FRACTURES OF THE SHOULDER

Distal Coronoid Process Avulsion Fractures

Avulsion fractures of the coronoid tip are usually a result of an indirect force applied through the conjoined tendon that is concentrated at its attachment to the coronoid process (32).

Displacement can be significant, but nonoperative treatment is usually recommended (33,34). Some have recommended open reduction and internal fixation in athletes in throwing or racquet sports. If the displaced fracture fragment causes soft tissue irritation, surgical excision may also be considered (34,35). In either conservative management or surgical management, return to activity is based on full rehabilitation of the shoulder.

There is an association of an avulsion fracture of the coronoid process with a Grade 3 disruption of the acromioclavicular joint (32,36–38). It appears that the injury that causes the Grade 3 separation of the acromioclavicular joint results in an avulsion fracture of the coronoid base or the attachment of the coracoiclavicular ligament to the angle of the coronoid process (39).

Weight-bearing X-rays of this injury on an AP projection may show the displacement of the clavicle above the acromion, but the coronoid clavicular interval remains normal.

Treatment basically follows the guidelines for Grade 3 acromioclavicular joint injuries.

Avulsion Fractures of the Base of the Coronoid Process

Base fractures of the coronoid process are probably most commonly due to a direct blow from the outside or from the dislocating head of the humerus during a shoulder dislocation injury. The avulsion fractures that involve the coronoid process are usually by strong traction forces (40).

Usually, displacement is minimal, and asymptomatic nonoperative care is adequate. Recovery is usually accomplished within 6 weeks (33,34).

Avulsion Fractures of the Acromial Process

An avulsion fracture of the origin of the deltoid muscle is a significant injury because of the function of the deltoid as it pertains to the glenohumeral joint (37). This fracture is likely to require surgical treatment to restore function of the deltoid about the glenohumeral joint.

Avulsion Fractures Through the Main Body of the Acromion

Two case reports have been described concerning this injury (41,42). These fractures are a result of muscular forces applied along the main body of the acromion. The deltoid muscle is one of the primary muscles involved in this phenomenon. Since this is a rare injury and only a few cases have been reported, there is not a clear advantage between nonoperative and operative treatment. The case reports have reported good results with both treatments.

Avulsion Fractures of the Scapula

Avulsion fractures of the scapula have been described as having three possible mechanisms of injury:

1. A severe uncontrolled muscular contraction, as seen for example in an epileptic seizure or in electric shock (37,43)
2. Trauma due to strong indirect forces applied to the scapula
3. Stress or fatigue fractures as a result of a repetitive traumatic event (44)

In diagnosing avulsion fractures of the scapula, plain radiographs such as AP and lateral projections are standard, but a true axillary view of the glenohumeral joint is also helpful. Computed tomography scans may also be necessary to evaluate fully the potential trauma to the scapula.

Treatment can largely be nonoperative except in cases of significant displacement. Table 35–1 is a listing of avulsion fractures of the scapula that have been reported and are categorized into those treated successfully nonoperatively and those that at least deserve operative consideration (32,37,39,43,45–48).

TABLE 35–1. *Treatment options for avulsion fractures of the scapula*

Scapular avulsion fractures successfully treated nonoperatively	Scapular avulsion fractures to consider operative treatment
Avulsion fracture of the superior angle of the scapula	Avulsion of the lateral margin of the acromial process
Avulsion fracture of the superior border of the scapula	Avulsion fracture of the distal tip of the coracoid process
Avulsion fractures to the body of the scapula	Avulsion fracture of the superior angle of the coracoid process
Avulsion fractures of the intraglenoidtubical	Avulsion fracture of the inferior angle of the scapula
Avulsion fractures of the lateral border of the scapula	Avulsion fracture of the supraglenoid tubercle

AVULSION FRACTURES OF THE LUMBAR SPINE

This discussion on avulsion fractures as they apply to the spine will be limited to those occurring to the lumbar spine, specifically transverse process avulsion fractures of the lumbar vertebral bodies. These fractures are largely considered benign fractures. They are usually related to direct trauma or an avulsion of the origin of the psoas muscle (49). In athletes the mechanism of injury could be from a direct hit, such as a football player being speared in the lumbar spine, or from resistance applied against a forceful contraction of the hip flexors.

These patients usually present with a severe low back pain that is localized by palpation along the paraspinal area of the side involved. Rotation, flexion, and extension of the spine, as well as resisted hip flexion, may elicit pain. Plain radiographs will many times easily identify these transverse process avulsion fractures. One must keep in mind that sometimes a transverse process avulsion fracture is accompanied to a much more severe injury to the spine. Krueger and colleagues found that 3 of 28 patients in their series, or 11%, had lumbar spine fractures that were not diagnosed from the plain radiographs but were identified by CT (49).

Treatment of transverse process avulsion fractures is conservative. Isolated transverse process avulsion fractures of the lumbar spine are considered benign fractures and usually require lumbar support, analgesia for the acute pain, and rest. Once the acute period of this injury is past, then a progressive rehabilitation program is followed until the patient is able to return to full activities. In cases in which more significant injuries are associated, the treatment of the more severe injury obviously takes precedence.

AVULSION FRACTURES OF THE PELVIS AND HIP

Pelvic bony injuries are uncommon in children except for avulsion fractures (50). Avulsion fractures of the hip and pelvis usually involve the adolescent age group. Hence the injury is usually to an open apophysis of the hip or pelvis.

The mechanism of injury in general terms will be discussed here, but specific mention will be made with each category. The injury mechanism is usually due to a sudden violent muscular contraction or an excessive amount of muscle stretch across an open apophysis (51). A pertinent consideration in athletics is that many times these injuries occur without an external trauma but are the result of the individual athlete's particular muscle function that he or she voluntarily directs (52,53). While these are more common injuries in the 14- to 17-year-old age group, one must remember that the apophyses of the hip may not close in some patients until well into their twenties. In this age group, one must always be aware that a complaint of a strain injury associated with muscles that attach to the pelvis should be evaluated thoroughly for a possible avulsion fracture.

While avulsion fractures can occur around the hip and pelvis from any of the apophyseal sites, Sundar and Carty found in their series of 32 avulsion fractures, the three sites that were most commonly involved were the anterior superior iliac spine, the anterior inferior iliac spine, and the ischial tuberosity. They also noted that they had seven cases for which there were multiple or bilateral sites of an avulsion injury (54).

The following will be a discussion on each individual apophyseal site.

Avulsion Fracture of the Anterior Superior Iliac Spine

An avulsion fracture of the anterior superior iliac spine (ASIS) occurs when an excessive force or stress is applied through the sartorius muscle, which attaches at the ASIS. In athletes this usually occurs during jumping or running. The hip is typically extended and the knee flexed when the avulsion occurs (55,56).

The athlete typically will present with local pain and local edema. Any attempt to flex or abduct the affected thigh actively will elicit pain. Plain radiographs will show a displacement of the ASIS. Displacement is usually minimal because the tensor fascia lata and the lateral portion of inguinal ligament prevent marked displacement (57).

Treatment is usually nonoperative, although there have been cases reported in which open reduction internal fixation was elected. Most authors concur that most of these fractures can be treated nonoperatively (51, 54, 55, 58). If pain is severe, these patients could be placed at bed rest; otherwise, weight bearing to tolerance may be allowed or partial weight bearing with use of crutches. An elastic wrap placed in a hip spica fashion may also give some comfort to this injury. A progressive rehabilitation program following the recovery from the acute phase of the injury is recommended; return to activity should be based on when the athlete has gained full strength, a painless range of motion, and integration of the muscle into the athletic activity in which he or she engages.

Avulsion Fracture of the Anterior Inferior Iliac Spine

Avulsion fractures of the anterior inferior iliac spine (AIIS) are reported to be less common than avulsion fractures in the ASIS. The reason suggested is the AIIS ossifies earlier and generally less tension is applied through the apophysis of the AIIS (59).

The mechanism of injury for an AIIS avulsion fracture is a vigorous contraction of the straight head of the rectus femorus muscle. The classic mechanism is kicking. Tension is generated both as the knee is extended and as the hip flexed with that motion (60).

These patients usually are tender at the sight by palpation and may have local edema. On X-rays there will be a displacement of the AIIS. Marked displacement is usually prevented by the intact reflected head of the rectus femorus and through the conjoin tendon (55). To rule out the possibility of an os acetabuli, contralateral radiographs should be obtained for comparison.

The treatment for AIIS injuries is usually conservative; there is no apparent advantage to doing anything operative, as is shown by the lack of case reports of operative treatment for this injury (58). Bed rest followed by protected weight bearing with progression to full weight bearing as tolerated is the recommended course of treatment. One can recommend progression to flexibility and strengthening exercises and on to functional activity as tolerated once a full range of motion and equal strength are attained (53).

Ischial Avulsion Fractures

Ischial avulsion fractures usually occur when increased tension is applied through the hamstring either by resistance of active flexion of the knee or by eccentric overload of the hamstring muscle. These injuries can be missed by assuming that a hamstring tear has occurred.

When the pain is more proximal, AP pelvis X-rays should be obtained to evaluate for a possible ischial avulsion injury.

The patient may present with pain with any attempt to flex the knee, actively or against resistance, or have exquisite pain in an attempt to stretch the hamstring. The patient may be point tender at the ischial tuberosity. Plain radiographs will show the avulsion injury (Fig. 35–2).

As compared to other avulsion injuries about the pelvis, this injury does generate some controversy concerning the appropriate treatment. Traditional treatment is nonoperative (53,60–63). Conservative care generally includes bed rest or protective hip motion with the hip in extension and in some external rotation followed by protective weight bearing with crutches. Up to 6 weeks may be required for healing to be completed (58). While some have recommended that operative treatment should be considered, others have reserved operative treatment for excision of exuberant callous after conservative treatment has been completed. There have been reports that functional disability has occurred after conservative treatment for ischial avulsion fractures (65). In view of the literature, both traditional and current, conservative treatment is likely the treatment of choice. Surgery may need to be considered in cases in which a complication is present or there is exuberant callous or disability following conservative treatment. The conservative treatment should involve a progressive rehabilitation program to restore normal flexibility and strength to the hamstring mechanism. Once the patients have progressed through a functional rehabilitation period, then return to sport is possible.

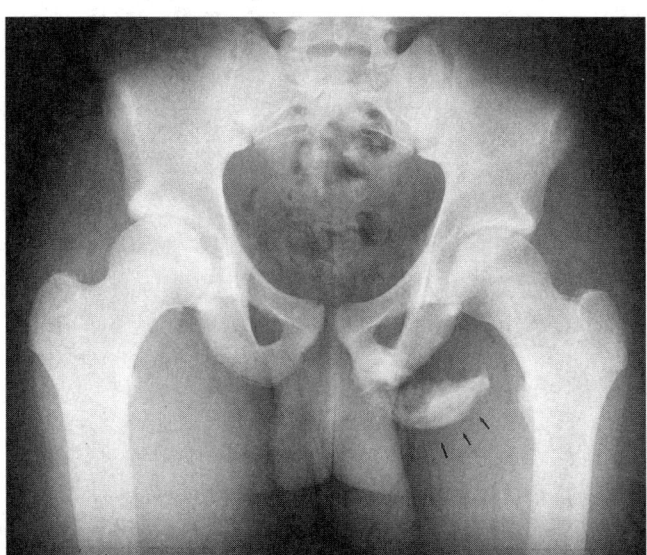

FIG. 35–2. X-ray of an ischial avulsion fracture.

Avulsion Fractures of the Iliac Crest

Avulsion fractures of the iliac crest are often confused with the terminology of hip pointers. While a direct blow or contusive-type injury could cause a fracture of the iliac crest with displacement of the apophysis, atypical avulsion fracture is due more to a pull of the abdominal musculature at the attachment site on the iliac crest. While the clinical presentation is very similar, these are probably distinctly different entities. Closure of the iliac crest apophysis typically occurs between 14 and 16 years of age (58).

The athlete's presentation is one of pain and tenderness over the iliac crest and pain with resisted abduction of the hip. Plain radiographs may not show significant separation in every injury to this area. Occasionally, oblique films of the injured with comparison views of the uninjured side may help one in defining a diagnosis of an iliac crest avulsion. This should be distinguished from iliac crest apophysitis, which can also occur. Treatment may be very similar for both entities.

The treatment for iliac crest avulsion fractures is conservative. Usually, a period of protected weight bearing or supportive weight bearing until the acute symptoms subside is followed by a progressive rehabilitation program. Most of these will resolve in 4–6 weeks, and return to sport is allowed as soon as the athlete can do functional integrated activities.

Avulsion Fractures of the Lesser Trochanter

Avulsion fractures of the lesser trochanter are due to a sudden contracture of the iliopsoas muscle. These usually occur while the athlete is running (58).

The patient generally presents with pain in the anterior medial aspect of the hip and is found to have pain with resisted hip flexion. Plain radiographs will reveal an avulsed fragment of the lesser trocanter. Treatment is usually conservative for this injury. This may include bed rest if necessary, protected weight bearing, and then a progressive rehabilitation program (66,67). Surgery for lesser trochanter avulsion fractures has been advocated if a wide separation is present (66,68). In one study, it was found that there was no prognostic difference in the degree of displacement (66). Therefore bed rest followed by progressive weight bearing and progressive rehabilitation until full strength returns is the recommended treatment. This is usually accomplished within 6–8 weeks.

Avulsion Fractures of the Greater Trochanter

Avulsion fractures of the greater trochanter are extremely rare (69). This occurs at the insertion of the abductor of the hip. This injury could occur in a broad spectrum of sports, but since it is a rare injury, general trends are difficult to establish (51). Pain is generally significant at the site of the greater trochanter. Patients will experience pain with abduction of the hip. Plain radiographs should easily confirm this diagnosis.

Treatment generally is conservative and follows the guidelines mentioned for the previous injuries above.

General Principles Concerning Avulsion Fractures of the Hip and Pelvis

As one might have determined from the previous discussions, conservative treatment is generally recommended for avulsions of the hip and pelvis (51,54,58). In the area of diagnosis, one particular concern is confusing these injuries with possible malignancies. It is very important to take a good history to determine whether trauma was associated with these presentations. As reported by Resnick and colleagues, in a case of an avulsion fracture of the anterior inferior iliac spine, the abundant reactive ossification cause some concern for this being a presentation of a possible neoplasm (70). In such cases an experienced pathologist should be asked to review any biopsies that are taken of this bone mass. Reactive bone formation of an apophyseal avulsion injury may mimic such concerning neoplasms as parosteal osteosarcoma, high-grade osteosarcoma, and periostial osteosarcoma. As was noted by Resnick and colleagues, this would be an unusual place for these to occur, but one has to consider these possibilities (70). There may be a place for magnetic resonance imaging, as suggested by Watanabe and colleagues, for trying to differentiate traumatic pathologies versus neoplastic pathologies (71).

Additionally, treatment for avulsion-type injuries can follow conservative guidelines in most cases. Metzmaker and Pappas outlined a five-stage progressive rehabilitation program in a series they published (53). The following is a summary of those stages:

1. Rest. The salient point with the rest stage is to position the involved muscle group in a state of being relaxed. Ice and analgesics are also initiated at this time.
2. Gradual increase in the excursion of the injured musculotendinous unit. This should be conducted after pain has subsided.
3. When the athlete has regained a full active range of motion, a resistive exercise program is instituted.
4. When approximately 50% of the strength has been recovered, an integrated functional rehabilitation program to incorporate the injured musculotendinous unit is initiated.
5. When full strength and functional integration have been achieved, then the specific athletic activity can then be reinstituted.

AVULSION FRACTURES OF THE KNEE

Avulsion fractures about the osseous structures of the knee are not uncommon. They can be the primary injury or indicative of a more severe insult.

Segond Fracture

Segond fracture was first described by Paul Segond in 1897 (72,73). The Segond fracture is a bony avulsion of the meniscotibial ligament. (73,74) (Fig. 35–3).

The mechanism of injury is usually internal tibial rotation with the knee in flexion (73,75). This usually occurs after damage to the anterior cruciate ligament (ACL). Therefore the Segond fracture is considered a continuation of an injury event. Once the anterior cruciate ligament, the primary stabilizer of knee, gives way, the tibia is allowed to internally rotate, resulting in this injury.

Hess and colleagues found in 151 patients with ACL tears, 9% had this fracture. In another large group of

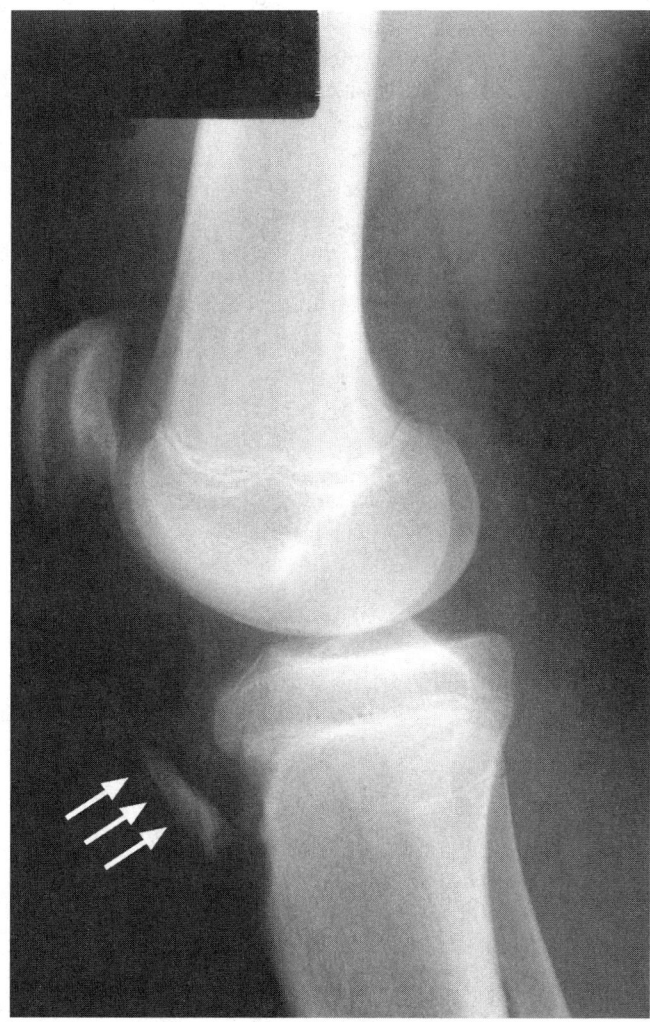

FIG. 35–3. X-ray of a Segond fracture.

patients without ACL damage, only one patient had a Segond fracture (73).

When one observes this finding on a plain X-ray, one should be concerned about an accompanying ACL injury. Several studies have supported this relationship of the Segond fracture and an anterior cruciate ligament tear (73,74,76–79).

Treatment should be directed to the primary pathology, which is usually a rupture of the anterior cruciate ligament. Correcting the instabilities in the knees is usually a primary concern. Attention to the meniscal pathology should also be given; otherwise, no direct treatment to the segond fracture is usually indicated.

Tibial Spine Avulsion Fractures

The tibial spine avulsion fracture is a rare but specific plain radiograph finding associated with anterior cruciate ligament injuries. It is most common in children (75,80). In children these tibial spine avulsions may be isolated injuries, but in adults they are usually associated with other ligament or meniscal pathology (75,81). The treatment of these injuries should be directed at the primary pathology, usually an anterior cruciate ligament injury. In children an isolated avulsion injury may be repaired by internal fixation of the avulsed fragment rather than reconstructive surgery of the anterior cruciate ligament. In adults with a tibial spine avulsion fracture, the primary pathology is usually an anterior cruciate ligament tear, and reconstruction is usually indicated, provided that other treatments are not deemed appropriate for that specific athlete (82).

Posterior Cruciate Avulsion Fractures

Three common mechanisms of injuries to the posterior cruciate ligament have been described by Trickey (83):

1. Anterior posterior force on the front of the flexed knee
2. Hyperextension of the joint
3. Posteriorly directed rotatory injury (83,84)

Any of these mechanisms could result in the avulsion of the posterior cruciate ligaments attachment. Posterior cruciate avulsion fractures have been associated with other, more significant injuries to the knee, such as medial tibial osteochondral fragments (84). Isolated avulsion fractures of the PCL attachment are rare but have been reported (85).

Treatment of isolated injuries should be based on recommendations for posterior cruciate ligament instabilities. This will be discussed in another portion of the text. Treatment for those avulsion injuries associated with other trauma would depend on definitive treatment of the other pathology (84).

Avulsion Fracture of the Tibial Tubercle

Avulsion fractures of the tibial tubercle are seen in the skeletally immature patient. Because of the physiologic process of growth, the skeletal system of the adolescent athlete is more vulnerable to this type of injury (86–88). Tibial tuberosity avulsion fractures in adolescent athletes is truly quite uncommon (89–92). The more extensive of these injuries are considered a Type III Salter-Harris fracture. These fractures make up 0.4–2.7% of all epiphyseal injuries. These injuries can occur in any sport but are most commonly seen in sports that require jumping (Fig. 35–4).

The mechanism of injury that is involved is one of forced flexion of the knee against a straining quadriceps contraction, or a violent quadriceps contraction against a fixed foot (93). The susceptibility to this injury by these mechanisms is thought to be related to the changes that occur during this time period in the adolescent. At this point, the proximal tibial epiphysis and the second-

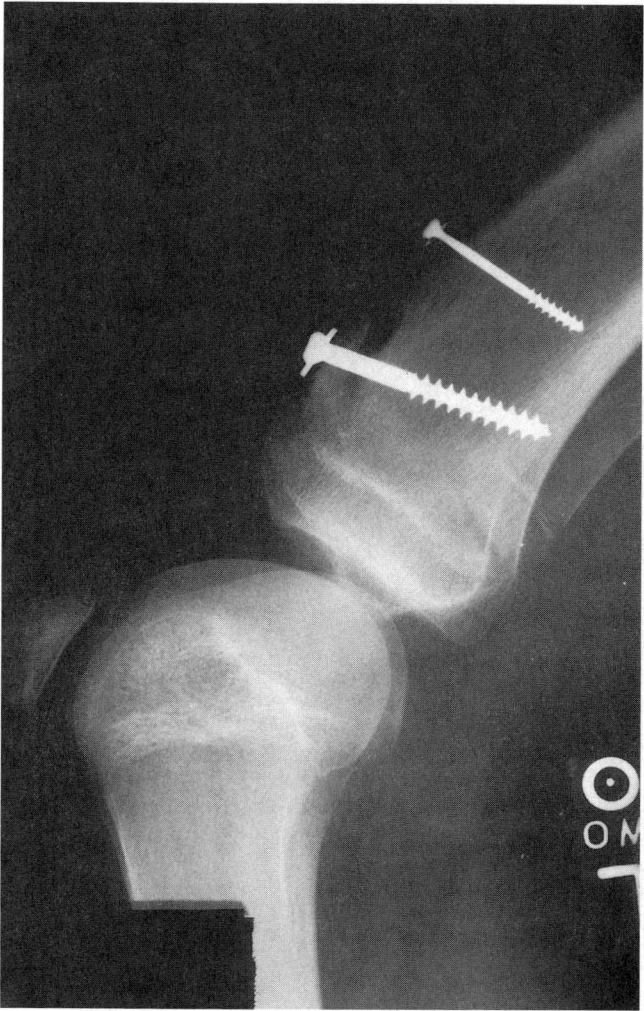

FIG. 35–4. X-ray of a tibial eminence avulsion fracture.

ary ossification center of the tubercle are undergoing change. It has been suggested that these areas are beginning to fuse and transit from a more fibrous to hyaline-type cartilage, thus being unable to resist tensile stress as well. There does not appear to be a causal relationship between this fracture and Osgood-Schlatter disease. The fracture generally occurs in a different area than the location of the typical tibial tuberosity aphophysitis (92).

There has been an attempt to classify the different types of tibial tuberosity injuries. Figure 35-5 is based on Ogden's classification (94). Type I fractures involve a small fragment of the tuberosity shown in Figures 35-5A and 35-5B. Type II fractures are shown in Figures 35-5C and 35-5D. In this type a large anterior portion of the proximal tibial ephysis is hinged forward. These are Type II fractures and occur when the secondary ossification center of the tuberosity has fused with the proximal tibial epiphysis. Type III fractures shown in Figures 35-5E and 35-5F are Salter-Harris Type III fractures that do extend intraarticularly. There have been case reports of bilateral avulsion fractures of the tibial tubercle (95,96).

Treatment of a Type I fracture may be conservative if it is a small nondisplaced fragment. Protection from stress should be considered, as by using a knee immobilizer to prevent any tensile load from being applied through this attachment. Type II and Type III fractures should be treated by open reduction and internal fixation. There have been reports of an arthroscopic procedure for Type III fractures (97). If a complication of an extension deficit would occur after conservative treatment of any of these fractures, a procedure for arthroscopic roof plasty has also been reported (98).

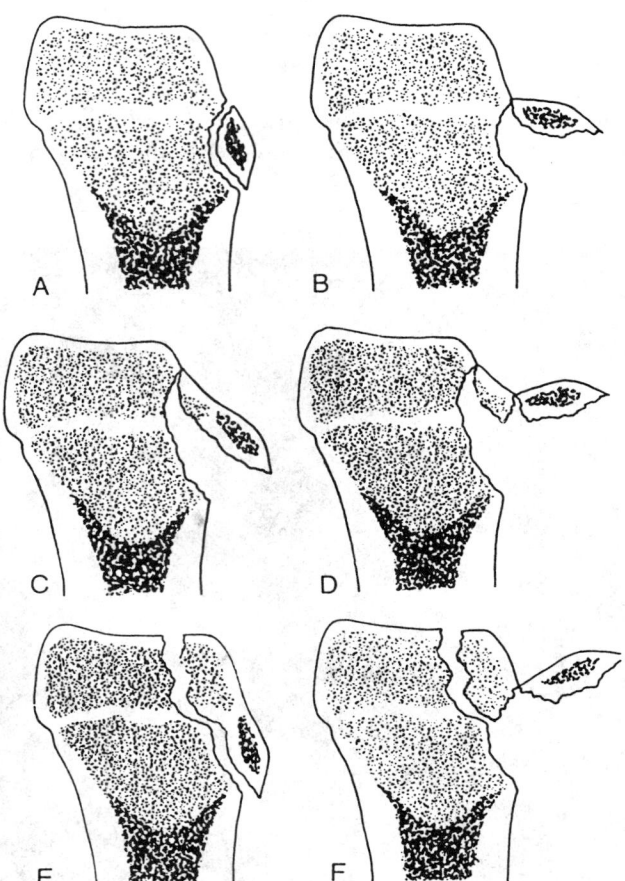

FIG. 35-5. A and **B**: Ogden classification scheme for tibial tuberosity fractures. Types IA and IB fractures are distal to the normal junction of the ossification centers of the proximal end of the tibia and tuberosity. Type IA fractures (**A**) are minimally displaced, while Type IB (**B**) are hinged anteriorly and proximally. **C** and **D**: Type IIA and IIB fractures are characterized by fracture lines at the junction of the ossification of the proximal end of the tibia and the tuberosity. **D**: Comminution of the tuberosity fragment characterizes Type IIB injuries. **E** and **F**: Fracture extension into the joint with resultant joint incongruity defines a Type IIIA or IIIB injury. **F**: In Type IIIB injuries the large joint/tuberosity fragment is comminuted. (From Polakoff DR, Bucholz RW, Ogden JA. Tension band wiring of displaced tibial tuberosity fractures in adolescents. *Clin Orthop* 1986;209:61.)

Avulsion Fractures of the Patella

Avulsions of the pole of the patella constitute approximately 5% of all patellar fractures. There is also a consideration for a distinct injury called a patellar sleeve fracture that occurs in the pediatric population. These typically occur in the 8- to 12-year-old athlete. In the sleeve fractures, a large avulsion of a small bony fragment is accompanied by a large piece of cartilage (99). Magnetic resonance imaging may be helpful in determining the significance of this injury, since the bony avulsion may be a very small component and could lead one to believe that there is a less serious injury (100).

The mechanism of injury for avulsion fractures of the patella and patellar sleeve fractures usually involves a lateral patellar dislocation or subluxation (101). Another potential mechanism would be a forceful contraction of a quadriceps muscle against a partially flexed knee (100).

These patients will present with a painful, swollen area in the area of the patella. Patients may have difficulty with active or resisted knee extension or with passive knee flexion in avulsion injuries to the patella. Radiographic evaluation usually will help to identify these lesions. One must be aware of the bipartite patella and be astute in clinical evaluation to determine whether this truly represents an avulsion injury or a true bipartite phenomenon. Treatment of avulsion fractures depends on the size, location, and displacement of the fragment. Nondisplaced avulsion fractures may do well with conservative management. One must give consideration with polar avulsions to excision of the fragment or reattachment of the extensor mechanism. If the fragment is large enough, open reduction and internal fixation may be considered (89). In sleeve fractures, anatomical reduction is absolutely necessary to preserve the extensor mechanism (99,102,103).

Badly comminuted avulsion fractures of the inferior polar patella have been reported and did require open reduction and internal fixation to give adequate anatomic restoration (104).

AVULSION FRACTURES OF THE ANKLE

Injuries about the ankle can have many different avulsion fractures associated. Many times the avulsion injury may accompany a much more severe derangement such as a fracture or dislocation. Other times it may be associated with more isolated injuries such as a ligament sprain.

The complex topic of ankle fractures and dislocations is not possible to cover in this chapter and likely will be discussed elsewhere. This discussion will be limited to the avulsion fractures of the malleoli of the ankle, that is, the lateral malleolus and the medial malleolus.

Lateral Malleolus Avulsion Fractures

Avulsion fractures of the lateral malleolus are usually associated with lateral ligament sprains of the ankle. The usual mechanism of the injury is one of inversion and plantar flexion. The athlete usually has pain and swelling localized to the area of the injury, that is, the lateral aspect of the ankle.

If an avulsion fracture of the lateral malleolus accompanies an inversion-type injury, most of these are treated conservatively, much as one would treat an ankle sprain. Larger fragments that are true avulsion injuries are probably rare. If a large fragment is displaced significantly, true avulsion injuries are probably rare. If a large fragment is displaced significantly, true anatomic reduction is necessary, by either closed reduction, percutaneous fixation, or open reduction and internal fixation. Since most of these lateral malleolar avulsion injuries are truly associated with a lateral ankle sprain, the treatment recommendation is usually either short-term casting or moving directly to a controlled motion brace and early mobility and rehabilitation of the injury (105). A more in-depth discussion of ankle sprain treatments is given in Chapters 45 and 50 of the companion book *Principles and Practice of Orthopaedic Sports Medicine*.

Medial Malleolar Avulsion Fractures

Medial malleolar avulsion fractures are typically related to injuries to the deltoid ligament. Most deltoid ligament injuries are associated with fractures and/or dislocations of the ankle (105).

The mechanism of injury for more isolated avulsion injuries and deltoid ligament sprains would typically be an eversion-type stress. But since avulsion injuries to the medial malleolus may be associated with more significant fracture and silocation events, they are many times characterized as pronation-abduction, pronation-external rotation, and supination-external rotation of the foot by the Lauge-Hansen classification of ankle fractures (106,107). Treatment of avulsion-type injuries to the medial malleolus depends on whether other, more serious injuries are present. If other fractures an/or a dislocation is involved, more serious injuries would need to be treated appropriately, followed by determination of whether the deltoid ligament injury needed to be addressed specifically (105).

There is some controversy concerning the treatment of deltoid ligament injuries (105). Most would agree that partial tears can be treated conservatively by casting or bracing.

Complete tears of the deltoid, with or without other significant injuries, may need consideration for surgery. With or without an avulsion fragment, complete tears may need operative repair for satisfactorily stabilization (108–110). Other studies have shown that conservative treatment of a deltoid injury has done well, provided that other associated fractures or instabilities were repaired (111–113).

If the sports medicine physician does identify an avulsion injury by plain radiograph, this should alert him or her to evaluate more closely the possibility of other associated injuries.

AVULSION FRACTURES OF THE FOOT

Avulsion Fractures of the Anterior Process of the Calcaneous

There is more than one mechanism of injury for anterior process fractures of the calcaneous. But one type, referred to as Type I, is truly an avulsive injury. These Type I injuries occur when the foot is forcibly plantar flexed and abducted. The bifurcate ligament, which attaches to the anterior process of the calcaneous, causes a bony avulsion (114,115) (Fig. 35–6).

Since the athlete may complain of an ankle-type injury and describe an inversion-type mechanism, avulsion fractures of the foot can be easily missed by someone who does not pay particular attention to the physical exam. These typically are more swollen distal to the lateral malleolus. An area of point tenderness inferior to that area is usually present. Adduction of the forefoot with the hindfoot stabilized will many times elicit exquisite pain. Supination of the forefoot with the hindfoot stabilized may also elicit pain.

There is not a consensus on the treatment of these injuries. Recommendations of treatment may vary from a very conservative approach with a soft wrap and early motion. What has been recommended most often is

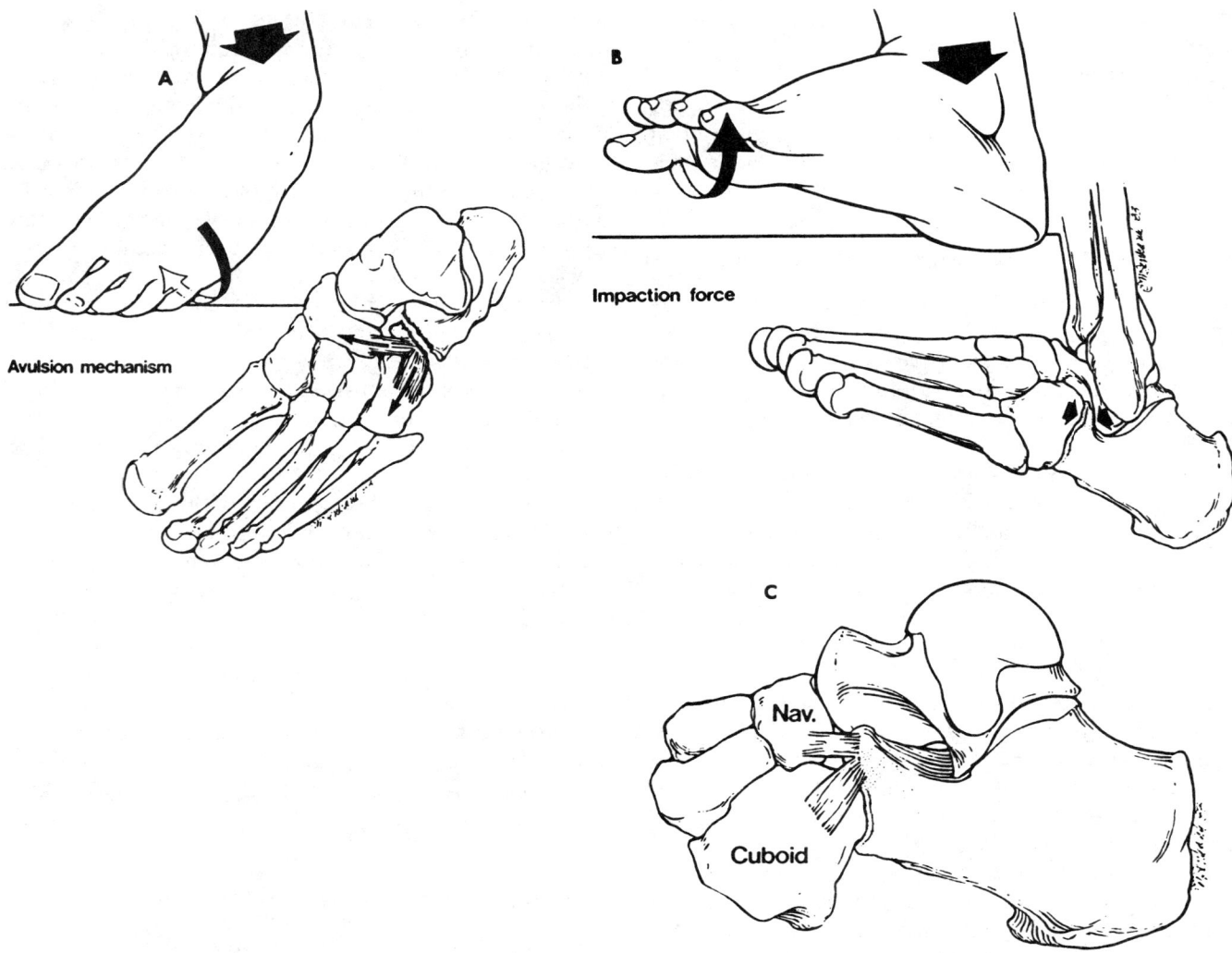

FIG. 35–6. A: Inversion and plantar flexion results in avulsion of the anterior process by the bifurcate ligament. This is the same mechanism that produces a sprain of the anterior talofibular ligament, hence the term sprain fracture. **B**: The anterior process is forced inward against the cuboid and produces an impaction force that fractures the anterior process. **C**: Abduction and supination of the forefoot force the cuboid against the inferior aspect of the calcaneus. This portion of the anterior process is compressed and posteriorly displaced. (From DeLee JC. Fractures and dislocations of the foot. In: Mann RA, Coughlin MJ, eds. *Surgery of the foot and ankle.* St. Louis: Mosby, 1993:1703.)

non-weight-bearing casting for 2–4 weeks. This may be followed by an additional time of weight-bearing casting if pain remains. Otherwise, the athlete may be placed into a brace and rehabilitation begun (114,115).

For persistent painful nonunions of these anterior process fractures, surgical treatment should be considered. The procedure may be excision for small fragments or intermedulary fixation for larger fragments (116).

Fractures of the Lateral Process of the Talus

These injuries many times occur with a history typical for a lateral ligamentous injury of the ankle or in an incident of violent trauma (117).

The lateral talocalcaneal ligament originates from the tip of this process. These injuries constitute approximately 1% of ankle injuries. A concerning statistic is that only 50% of these fractures are recognized early (118). These patients usually present with swelling and ecchymosis over the lateral aspects of the ankle, as is typically seen with the lateral inversion injury. The area of point tenderness may be just anterior and inferior to the distal portion of the lateral malleolus. Because of some variability in this injury, a classification scheme of the three types has been presented. Type I is a simple chip-type fracture located at the anterior surface of the lateral process. Type II may be displaced or nondisplaced but extends from the talofibular articulation of the lateral process to the anterior process of the posterior facet of the subtalar joint. A Type III avulsion fracture is comminuted fracture of the lateral process involving the talofibular joint and the posterior facet of the talocalcaneal articulation (119).

The recommended treatment for Type I injuries is short leg casting for 6 weeks. Some would recommend that the first 4 weeks be non-weight-bearing, while others would consider partial weight bearing as tolerated (117).

Type II fractures that are undisplaced or reducible can be treated with short leg casting. The recommendation is non-weight-bearing for 4 weeks followed by 2 weeks of additional casting while weight bearing. For displacement of greater than 2 mm, open reduction with internal fixation is recommended (114).

Primary excision is the usual recommendation for comminuted Type III fractures. A period of casting is usually suggested for up to 3 weeks, followed by a progressive return to full weight bearing.

Proximal Fifth Metatarsal Fractures

Proximal fifth metatarsal fractures are subdivided into two types. Type I fractures are referred to as Jones' fracture and involve the junction of the metatarsal shaft and the metatarsal base. These will not be discussed in this section, since they are not considered an avulsion-type injury. These definitely need to be differentiated from the Type II fractures, which are of the styloid process of the base of the fifth metatarsal. These are further divided into Types IIA and IIB, with IIA being extraarticular and IIB having extension into the intraarticular space (114).

The mechanism of injury usually is sudden inversion of the foot against the contracting perineous brevis muscle (120).

The athlete usually will present with tenderness, swelling, and pain with ambulation and exquisite pain with direct palpation at the base of the fifth metatarsal. There may also be exquisite pain with resisted eversion of the foot.

Avulsion fractures at the base of the fifth metatarsal can usually be treated conservatively. Clapper and colleagues showed that most of these avulsion fractures healed in an average of 4.7 weeks. There did not appear to be a significant difference in treatment with a cast versus treatment with a healing shoe (121). Wiener and colleagues had similar results. They actually found that the average time for healing was 33 days in patients treated with a soft Jones' dressing as compared to 46 days for those treated in a short leg cast (122). Other studies support these findings (123–127). Even in patients who have a fibrous union, most are asymptomatic. Excision of these may be indicated in the rare instance that a nonunion would remain painful (120,122). Some controversy arises with intraarticular styloid fracture, that is, Type 2B. Undisplaced intraarticular fractures should be treated by non-weight-bearing in a short leg cast and ultimately progress to weight-bearing cast treatment. Four to six weeks of cast protection may be required. Large displaced intraarticular fractures have been shown to have good results with conservative treatment (123). Open reduction with internal fixation is an alternative suggested by some, especially if it is a large, displaced intraarticular fragment (114).

Avulsion Fractures of the Calcaneal Tuberosity

Avulsion fractures of the calcaneal tuberosity involves a posterior superior aspect of the calcaneous. These are rare, constituting approximately 3% of all calcaneal fractures (127,128). These avulsion fractures of the calcaneal tuberosity are a result of the pull of the tendo Achillis. These can occur in adults (129) or in children, in whom the injury is through the calcaneal apophysis (130). Those involving the apophysis in children are extremely rare. The treatment that is chosen should accomplish complete anatomic reduction, since anything short of complete reduction would affect the function of the Achilles tendon. Conservative treatment would entail casting for 6 weeks in plantar flexion in nondisplaced fractures or in those anatomically positioned by closed reduction (115). Open reduction internal fixation by cancellous screws or by tension band technique may be used (129,130).

Avulsion Fractures of the Tarsonavicular

Avulsion fractures of the tarsonavicular must be differentiated from injuries associated with an accessory navicular ossicle. The mechanism of this injury can occur through acute eversion injuries of the foot. The increased tension of the tibialis posterior tendon results in an avulsion fracture of the navicular tuberosity (115,131).

Fractures of the navicular tuberosity have also been associated with other injuries to the foot or ankle. Hunter and Sangeorzan describes a fracture of the tuberosity associated with cuboid fracture, or the so-called nutcracker fracture (132).

Since the tibialis posterior tendon has other insertion sites, these fragments are not often significantly displaced. Treatment can usually be conservative, with cast immobilization or some type of support dressing or brace to relieve the tension off of the tuberosity fragment. This may be needed for up to 4 weeks or until the examination shows no significant pain to palpation at the navicular tuberosity (133,134). Treatment for symptomatic nonunions is usually surgical excision. Raw surfaces of the tendon are sutured in place, and casting is done for 3–4 weeks (115).

REFERENCES

1. *Dorland's illustrated medical dictionary,* 25th ed. Philadelphia: WB Saunders, 1974:173.
2. Cobbs KF, Owens WS, Berg EF. Extensor carpi radialis brevis avulsion fracture of the long finger metacarpal: a case report. *J Hand Surg [Am]* 1996;21A(4):684–686.
3. DeLee J. Avulsion fracture of the base of the second metacarpal by the extensor carpi radialis longus. *J Bone Joint Surg* 1979; 61A:445–446.
4. Crichlow T, Hoskinson J. Avulsion fracture of the metacarpal base: three case reports. *Hand Surgery* 1988;13B:212–214.
5. Treble N, Arif S. Avulsion fracture of the index metacarpal. *J Hand Surg [Am]* 1987;12B:38–39.
6. Bischoff R, Buechler V, De Roche R, Jupiter J. Clinical results of tension band fixation of avulsion fractures of the hand. *J Hand Surg [Am]* 1994;19A:1019–1026.
7. Kozin SH, Bishop AT. Tension wire fixation of avulsion fractures at the thumb metacarpophalangeal joint. *J Hand Surg [Am]* 1994;19A(6):1029–1031.
8. Bowens WA, Hurst LC. Gamekeeper's thumb: evaluation by arthrography and stress roentgenography. *J Bone Joint Surg* 1977;59A:519–524.
9. Frank WF, Dobyus JH. Surgical pathology of collateral ligament injuries of the thumb. *Clin Orthop* 1972;83:102–114.
10. Stener B. Displacement of the ruptured ulnar collateral ligament of the metacarpophalangeal joint of the thumb: a clinical and anatomical study. *J Bone Joint Surg* 1962;44B:869–879.
11. Jupiter JB, Shepherd JE. Tension wire fixation of avulsion fractures in the hand. *Clin Orthop* 1987;214:113–120.
12. Bovard RS, Derkash RS, Freeman JR. Guide III: avulsion fracture repair on the UCL of the proximal joint of the thumb. *Orthop Rev* 1994:167–169.
13. Lo I, Richards RS. Combined central slip and volar plate injuries at the PIP joint. *Br Soc Surg Hand* 1995;20B(3):390–391.
14. Idler RS. *The hand: examination and diagnosis,* 3rd ed. New York: Churchill Livingstone, 1990:1–127.
15. Culver JE. Sports-related fractures of the hand and wrist. *Clin Sports Med* 1990;9(1):85–109.
16. Eaton RG, Malerich MM. Volar plate arthroplasty of the proximal interphangeal joint: a review of ten years' experience. *J Hand Surg [Am]* 1980;5:260–268.
17. Bynum DK, Gilbert JA. Avulsion of the flexor digitorum profundus: anatomic and biomechanical considerations. *J Hand Surg [Am]* 1988;13:222–227.
18. Leddy JP, Packer JW. Avulsion of the profundus tendon insertion in athletes. *J Hand Surg [Am]* 1977;2:66–69.
19. Green DP, Strickland JW. The hand. In: DeLee J, Drez D, eds. *Orthopedic sports medicine principles and practice.* Philadelphia: WB Saunders, 1994;945–1017.
20. Kevu JE, Calder SJ, Cleary JE. Complete avulsion of the palmar cortex of the distal phalanx. *J Hand Surg [Br]* 1996;21B:758–759.
21. Smith DK, Murray PM. Avulsion fractures of the volar aspect of the triquetral bone of the wrist: a subtle sign of carpal ligament injury. *Am J Roentgenol* 1996;166:609–614.
22. Mikic ZD, Sad N. Treatment of acute injuries of the triangular fibrocartilage complex associated with distal radioulnar joint instability. *J Hand Surg [Am]* 1995;20A:319–323.
23. Sennwald GR, Lautenburg M, Zdravkovic. A new technique of reattachment after traumatic avulsion of the TFCC at its ulnar insertion. *J Hand Surg [Am]* 1995;20B:178–184.
24. Acosta, HNAT W, Scheker LR. Distal radio-ulnar ligament rotation during supination and pronation. *J Hand Surg [Am]* 1993;18B:502–505.
25. Bradley JP. Upper extremity: elbow injuries in children and adolescents. In: Stanitski CL, DeLee JC, Drez D, eds. *Pediatric and adolescent sports medicine.* Philadelphia: WB Saunders, 1994: 242–261.
26. Bennett JB, Tullos HS. Ligamentous and articular injuries in the athlete. In: Morrey BF, ed. *The elbow and its disorders.* Philadelphia: WB Saunders, 1985:502–522.
27. Woods GW, Tullos HS. Elbow instability and medial epicondyle fractures. *Am J Sports Med* 1977;5:23–30.
28. Hunter SC. Little League elbow. In: Zarins B, Andrews JR, Carson WG, eds. *Injuries to the throwing arm.* Philadelphia: WB Saunders 1985.
29. Ireland ML, Andrews JR. Shoulder and elbow injuries in the young athlete. *Clin Sports Med* 1988;7:473–493.
30. Pappas AM. Elbow problems associated with baseball during childhood and adolescents. *Clin Orthop* 1982;164:30.
31. Cage DJN, Abnaus RA, Callahan JJ, Bottle MJ. Soft tissue attachments of the ulnar coronoid process. *Clin Orthop* 1995;320:154–158.
32. Goss TP. The scapula: coronoid acromial and avulsion fractures. *Am J Orthop* 1996;2:106–115.
33. Wong-Pack WK, Bobechko PE, Becker EJ. Fractured coronoid with anterior shoulder dislocation. *J Can Assoc Radiol* 1980; 31:228.
34. Zilberman Z, Rejovitzky R. Fracture of the coronoid process of the scapula. *Injury* 1982;13:203–206.
35. Garcia-Elias M, Salo JM. Non-union of a fractured process after dislocation of the shoulder. *J Bone Joint Surg* 1985;67B:722–723.
36. DeRosa GP, Kettelkamp DB. Fracture of the coronoid process of the scapula case report. *J Bone Joint Surg* 1977;59A:696–697.
37. Heyse-Moore GH, Stoken DJ. Avulsion fractures of the scapula. *Skeletal Radiol* 1982;9:27–32.
38. Smith DM. Coronoid fracture associated with acromioclavicular dislocation: a case report. *Clin Orthop* 1975;108:165–167.
39. Mongomery SP, Loyd RD. Avulsion fracture of the coronoid epiphysis with acromioclavicular separation. *J Bone Joint Surg* 1977;59:963.
40. Mariani PP. Isolated fracture of the coronoid process in an athlete. *Am J Sports Med* 1980;8:129–130.
41. Mugikura S, Hirayama T, Tada H, Takemits Y. Avulsion fracture of the scapular spine: a case report: *J Shoulder Elbow Surg* 1993;3(1):3.
42. Rask MR, Steinberg LH. Fracture of the acromion caused by muscle forces. *J Bone Joint Surg* 1978;60A:1146–1147.
43. Tarquinio T, Weinstein ME, Vingilio RW. Bilateral scapular fractures from accidental electric shock. *Trauma* 1979;19: 132–133.
44. Warner J, Port J. Stress fracture of the acromion. *J Shoulder Elbow Surg* 1994;3(4):262–265.
45. Ishizuki M, Yamaura I, Isobe Y. Avulsion fracture of the superior border of the scapula: a case report of five cases. *J Bone Joint Surg* 1981;63A:820–822.
46. Wolfe AW, Shojitt, Chuinard RG. Unusual fracture of the coronoid process: case report and review of the literature. *J Bone Joint Surg* 1976;58A:423–424.
47. Hayes J, Zehr D. Traumatic muscle avulsion causing winging of the scapula. *J Bone Joint Surg* 1981;68A:495.
48. Iannotti JP, Wang ED. Avulsion fracture of the supraglenoid tubercle: a variation of the SLAP lesion. *J Shoulder Elbow Surg* 1992;1(1):26–30.
49. Krueger MA, Green DA, Hoyt D, Garfin SR. Overlooked spine injuries associated with lumbar transverse process fractures. *Clin Orthop* 1996;327:191–195.
50. Rieger H, Brug E. Fractures of the pelvis in children. *Clin Orthop* 1996;336:226–239.
51. Waters PM, Millis MG. Hip and pelvic injuries in the young athlete. *Clin Sports Med* 1998;7:513.
52. Fernbach SK, Wilkinson RH. Avulsion fractures of the pelvis and proximal femur. *Am J Roentgenol* 1981;137:581–584.
53. Metzmaker JN, Pappas AM. Avulsion fractures of the pelvis. *Am J Sports Med* 1985;13:349–358.
54. Sundar M, Carty H. Avulsion fractures of the pelvis in children: a report of thirty two fractures and their outcome. *Skeletal Radiol* 1994;23:85–90.
55. Canale ST, King RE. Pelvic and hip fractures. In: Rockwood CA, Wilkins KE, King RE, eds. *Fractures in children.* Philadelphia: JB Lippincott, 1984.
56. Kane WJ. Fractures of the pelvis. In: Rockwood CA, Green DP, eds. *Fractures in adults.* Philadelphia: JB Lippincott, 1984.
57. Robertson RC. Fracture of the anterior superior spine of the ilium. *J Bone Joint Surg* 1935;17:1045.
58. Gross ML, Nasser S, Finerman GA. Hip and pelvis. In: DeLee JC,

Drez D, eds. *Orthopedic sports medicine principles and practice.* Philadelphia: WB Saunders, 1994:1063–1085.
59. Weitzner I. Fracture of the anterior superior spine of the ilium in one case and anterior inferior in another case. *Am J Roentgenol* 1935;33–39.
60. Watson-Jones R. Dislocations and fracture dislocations of the pelvis. *Br J Surg* 1938;25:773.
61. Watson-Jones R. *Fractures and joint injuries.* Baltimores: Williams & Wilkins, 1957.
62. Kelly J. Ischial epiphysitis. *J Bone Joint Surg* 1963;45A:435.
63. Watts HG. Fractures of the pelvis in children. *Orthop Clin N Am* 1976;7:615.
64. Rogge EA, Romano RL. Avulsion of the ischial apophysis. *J Bone Joint Surg* 1956;38A:442.
65. Schlonsky J, Olix ML. Functional disability following avulsion fracture of the ischial apophysis. *J Bone Joint Surg* 1972;54A:641.
66. DeLee JC. Fractures and dislocations of the hip. In: Rockwood CA, Green DP, eds. *Fractures in adults.* Philadelphia: JB Lippincott, 1984.
67. Dimon JH. Isolated fractures of the lesser trochanter of the femur. *Clin Orthop* 1972;82:144.
68. Poston H. Traction fracture of the lesser trochanter of the femur. *Br J Surg* 1921;9:256.
69. Ogdon JA, Trauma, Hip development and vascularity. In: Tronzo RG, ed. *Surgery of the hip joint.* New York: Springer-Verlag, 1984.
70. Resnick JM, Carrasco CH, Edeiken J, et al. Avulsion fracture of the anterior inferior iliac spine with abundant reactive ossification in the soft tissues. *Skeletal Radiol* 1996;25:580–584.
71. Watanabe H, Shinozaki T, Arita S, Chigira M. Irregularity of apophysis of the ischial tuberosity evaluated by magnetic resonance imaging. *Can Assoc Radiol J* 1995;46:380–385.
72. Segond P. Recherches cliniques et experimentales sur les epanchements sanguins du genou par entorse. *Prog Med* 1879;7:297.
73. Hess T, Rupp S, Hopf T, Gleitz M, Liebler J. Lateral tibial avulsion fractures and disruptions to the anterior cruciate ligament: a clinical study of their incidence and corrilation. *Clin Orthop* 1994;303:193–197.
74. Davis DS, Post WR. Segond fracture: lateral capsular ligament avulsion. *J Orthop Sports Phys Ther* 1997;23:2:103–106.
75. Kezdi-Rogus PC, Lomasney LM. Plain film manifestations of ACL injury. *Orthopedics* 1994;17:967–973.
76. Dietz GW, Wilcox DM, Mongomery JB. Segond tibial condyle fracture: lateral capsular ligament avulsion. *Radiology* 1986;159:467–469.
77. Woods GW, Stanley RJ, Tullos HS. Lateral capsular sign: X-ray clue to significant knee instability. *Am J Sports Med* 1979;7:27–33.
78. Kerr HD. Segond fracture: hemarthrosis and anterior cruciate ligament disruption. *J Emerg Med* 1990;8:29–33.
79. Scharf W, Schabus R, Wagoner M. Das laterale kapselzeichen. *Unfallheikunde* 1991;84:518.
80. Mink JH, Reicker MA, Crues JV, Deutsch AL. *Magnetic resonance imaging of the knee.* New York: Raven Press 1993:141–162.
81. Rogers LF. *Radiology of skeletal trauma.* New York: Churchill Livingstone, 1992:1245–1248.
82. Veselko M, Senekovic V, Tonin M. Simple and safe arthroscopic placement and removal of canulated screw and washer for fixation of tibial avulsion fracture of the anterior cruciate ligament. *Arthroscopy* 1996;12;2:259–262.
83. Trickey EL. Injuries to the posterior cruciate ligament. *Clin Orthop* 1980;147:176.
84. Ho TK, Fang D. Posterior cruciate avulsion fractures associated with a large inverted medial tibial osteochondral fragment. *Trauma* 1995;38:4;653–657.
85. Torisu T, City K. Isolated avulsion fractures of the tibial attachment of the posterior cruciate ligament. *J Bone Joint Surg* 1977;59A:68.
86. Maffulli N, Grewal R. Avulsion of the tibial tuberosity: muscles too strong for growth plate. *Clin J Sports Med* 1997;7:129–133.
87. Maffulli N. Intensive training in young athletes: the orthopedic surgeons viewpoint. *Sports Med* 1990;9:229–243.
88. Maffulli N, Pintore E. Intensive training in young athletes. *Br J Sports Med* 1990;24:237–239.
89. Cohn SL, Sotta RB, Bergfeld JA. Fractures about the knee in sports. *Clin Sports Med* 1990;9(1):121–139.
90. Christie MJ, Dvonch VM. Tibial tuberosity fracture in adolescents. *J Pediatr Orthop* 1991;1:391–394.
91. Mirbey J, Besancenot J, Chambers RT, et al. Avulsion fractures of the tibial tuberosity in the adolescent athlete: risk factors, mechanism of injury and treatment. *Am J Sports Med* 1988;16:336–340.
92. Ogden JA, Trass RB, Murphy MJ. Fractures of the tibial tuberosity in adolescents. *J Bone Joint Surg* 1980;62A:205.
93. Levi JH, Coleman CR. Fractures of the tibial tubercle. *Am J Sports Med* 1976;4:254.
94. Polakoff DR, Bucholz RW, Ogden JA. Tension band wiring of displaced tibial tuberosity fractures in adolescents. *Clin Orthop* 1986;209:61.
95. Henard DC, Boho RT. Avulsion fractures of the tibial tubercle in adolescents. *Clin Orthop* 1983;177:182.
96. Mirly HL, Olix ML. Bilarteral simultaneous avulsion fractures of the tibial tubercle. *Orthopedics* 1996;19:1:66–68.
97. Prince AR, Moyer RA. Arthroscopic treatment of an avulsion fracture of the intracondular intercondylar eminence of the tibia. *Am J Knee Surg* 1995;8:3:114–116.
98. Freedman KB, Glasgow SG. Arthroscopic roof plasty: correction of the extension deficit following conservative treatment of a Type III tibial avulsion fracture. *Arthroscopy* 1995;11:2:231–234.
99. Roberts JM. Fractures and dislocations of the knee. In: Rockwood CA, Wilkins KE, King RE, eds. *Fractures in children.* Philadelphia: JB Lippincott, 1984:919.
100. Bates DG, Hresko MT, Jaramillo D. Patellar sleeve fracture: demonstration with MR imaging. *Radiology* 1994;193:3:825–827.
101. Heckman JD, Alkire CC. Distal patellar fractures. *Am J Sports Med* 1984;12:424.
102. Shands PA, McQueen DA. Demonstration of avulsion fracture of the inferior polar patella by magnetic resonance imaging. *J Bone Joint Surg* 1995;77A(11):1721–1723.
103. Houghton GR, Ackroyd CE. Sleeve fractures of the patella in children: a report of three cases. *J Bone Joint Surg* 1979;61(B2):165–168.
104. Veselko M, Smrolj V, Tonin M. Comminuted avulsion fractures of the inferior polar patella. *Unfalchirurg* 1996;99:71–72.
105. Renstrom P, Kannus T. *Injuries of the foot and ankle.* Philadelphia: WB Saunders, 1994:1705–1767.
106. Lauge-Hansen N. Fractures of the ankle: II. Combined experiemental surgical experimental roetgenologic investion. *Arch Surg* 1950;60:957–985.
107. Yde J, Lauge-Hansen N. Classification of malleolar fractures. *Acta Orthop Scand* 1980;51:181–192.
108. Canale ST, Beaty JH. Injuries of the talus. In: Hamilton WG, ed. *Traumatic disorders of the ankle.* New York: Springer-Verlag, 1984:244–250.
109. Hamilton WG, ed. *Traumatic disorders of the ankle.* New York: Springer-Verlag, 1984:1–293.
110. Yablon IG, Segal B. Ankle fractures. In: Evarts MC, ed. *Surgery of the musculoskeletal system.* New York: Churchill Livingstone, 1983:97–100.
111. Mast JW, Teipner WA. A reducable approach to the internal fixation of adult ankle fractures: rationale, technique, and early results. *Orthop Clin N Am* 1980;11:6661–6669.
112. Harper MC. The deltoid ligament: an evaluation of need for surgical repair. *Clin Orthop* 1988;226:156–168.
113. DeSouza LJ, Gustilo RB, Meyer TJ. Results of operative treatment of displaced external rotation-abduction fractures of the ankle. *J Bone Joint Surg* 1985;67A:1066.
114. Davis AW, Alexander IJ. Problematic fractures and dislocations in the foot and ankle of athletes. *Clin Sports Med.* 1990;9(1):163–181.
115. DeLee JC. Fractures and dislocations of the foot. In: Mann RA, Coughlin MJ, eds. *Surgery of the foot and ankle.* St. Louis: Mosby, 1993:1703.
116. Degan TJ, Moorey MD, Braun DP. Surgical excision for anterior process fractures of the calcaneous. *J Bone Joint Surg* 1982;64A:519–524.
117. Heckman JD, McLean MR. Fractures of the lateral process of the talus. *Clin Orthop* 1985;199:108–113.

118. Mukherjee SK, Pringle RM, Baxter AD. Fracture of the lateral process of the talus: a report of thirteen cases. *J Bone Joint Surg* 1974;56B:263–273.
119. Hawkins LG. Fracture of the lateral process of the talus. *J Bone Joint Surg* 1965;47A:1170–1175.
120. Sammarco GJ. Perineal tendon injuries. *Orthop Clin N Am* 1994;25:1:135–145.
121. Clapper MF, O'Brien TJ, Lyons PM. Fractures of the fifth metatarsal: analysis of a fracture registry. *Clin Orthop* 1995;315:238–241.
122. Wiener BD, Linder JF, Giattini FG. Treatment of fractures of the fifth metatarsal: a prospective study. *Foot Ankle Int* 1997;267–269.
123. Dameron TB. Fractures and anatomical variations of the proximal portion of the fifth metatarsal. *J Bone Joint Surg* 1985;57A:788–792.
124. Kavanaugh JH, Brewer TD, Mann RV. The Jones' fracture revisited. *J Bone Joint Surg* 1978;60A:776–782.
125. Heckman JD. Fractures and dislocations of the foot. In: Rockwood CA, Green DP, eds. *Fractures*. Philadelphia: JB Lippincott, 1981:2155–2159.
126. Richili WR, Rosenthal DI. Avulsion fracture of the fifth metatarsal: experimental study of patho-mechanics. *Am J Roentgenol* 1994;143:889–891.
127. Rowe CR, Sakellarides HT, Freeman PA, Sworbie C. Fracture of the oscalcus. *JAMA* 1963;184:920–923.
128. Lyngstadaas S. Treatment of avulsion fractures of the tuber calcanei. *Acta Chir Scand* 1971;137:579–581.
129. Levi N, Garde L, Kofed H. Avulsion fracture of the calcaneous: a report of a case using a new tension band technique. *J Orthop Trauma* 1997;1:61–62.
130. Birtwristle SJ, Jacobs L. An avulsion fracture of the calcaneal apophysis in a young gymnast. *Injury* 1995;26;6:409–410.
131. Heckman JD. Fractures in athletes. In: Rockwood CA, Green DP, eds. *Fractures,* vol 2. Philadelphia: JB Lippincott, 1975:1703–1832.
132. Hunter JC, Sangeorzan BJ. A nutcracker fracture: cuboid fracture with an associated avulsion fracture of the tarsal navicular. *Am J Roentgenol* 1996;166:878.
133. Garcia A, Parkes JC. Fractures of the foot. In: Giannesteras NJ, ed. *Foot disorders: medical and surgical management,* 2nd ed. Philadelphia: Lea & Febiger, 1973.
134. Coker TP, Arnold JA. Sports injuries to the foot and ankle. In: Jahss MH, ed. *Disorders of the foot,* vol 2. Philadelphia: WB Saunders, 1982.

CHAPTER 36

Stress Fractures

Thomas P. Knapp and William E. Garrett, Jr.

INTRODUCTION

Aristotle (384–322 B.C.) correctly characterized "Olympic Victors" by stating that they are "those who do not squander their powers by early and overtraining." Stress fractures have received various names when diagnosed in the tibia, including exertional posterior compartment syndrome, fatigue fractures, shin splints, anterior tibial periostitis, and medial tibial stress syndrome. What, then, is a stress fracture? Pentecost (1) describes an insufficiency fracture as that produced by normal or physiologic stress applied to bone with deficient elastic resistance. In contrast, a fatigue (stress) fracture occurs when abnormal stress is applied to a bone with normal elastic resistance.

Stress fractures in amateur and professional athletes are becoming very common worldwide. For example, 9 of the 24 members of the 1994 U.S. National World Cup Soccer team were diagnosed with stress fractures. In the United States today an ever-increasing number of people participate in sporting activities. Those who are competing and training including elite, recreational, youth, and female athletes. It is important to consider each of these groups separately, as each has special potential problems that must be addressed. If not properly diagnosed early, these injuries can cause significant lost time from participation or even early retirement. With greater numbers of people participating, engaging in longer hours and higher intensity, the medical professional must understand the proper diagnosis, treatment, and prevention of these injuries.

This article will serve as an overview to the general concepts of stress fractures, including history, epidemiology, and etiology. The proper diagnosis, confirmatory studies, and treatment regimens will be presented. Finally, the timing of the athlete's return to sports and stress fracture prevention will be reviewed.

HISTORY

The original description of stress fractures was by Briethaupt, a Prussian military physician, in 1855. He described the clinical signs and symptoms and the time course in the development of a stress fracture of the metatarsal. This was commonly known as a march fracture or Deutschlander's fracture. It took an additional 40 years before the advent of radiographs allowed visual confirmation of his theory.

Devas, in 1958, was the first to describe this injury in athletes. Since then there have been numerous reports of stress fractures in athletes including runners (2,3) and dancers (4).

EPIDEMIOLOGY

Stress fractures have been described in relation to age, race, sex, specific sport, and bone location patterns. The earliest report of a stress fracture was in an 18-month-old child (5). More typical is a nonexperienced, nonconditioned runner who tends more to jog than to participate in either competitive or competitive-recreational running. These individuals usually run fewer than 20 miles a week and develop discomfort with the sudden initiation of an intensive training program (6).

The common dictum is that stress injuries are rare in the dark-skinned and black races. However, Markey (5) found that in a racially mixed population undergoing the same military training, the incidence of stress fracture was similar for all races.

There appears to be a lower incidence of stress fractures in men, for whom lean body mass is greater and

---

T. P. Knapp: Santa Monica Orthopaedic and Sports Medicine Group, Santa Monica, California 90404.
W. E. Garrett, Jr.: Department of Orthopaedics, University of North Carolina, Chapel Hill, North Carolina 27599.

overall bone structure is larger; the converse is true for women. According to Markey (5), the relative higher incidence of female-related stress injuries in running sports may reflect the fact that the shorter women, in comparison to the men, are being overstressed. Several authors have shown that women develop up to 10 times as many stress fractures as men on the same training course (7,8). This was documented by Jones and colleagues (9), who prospectively measured 310 army trainees during 8 weeks of basic training. They found that women had a significantly higher incidence of time-loss injuries than men: 44.6% compared to 29.0%. Similarly, Orava and colleagues (10) discovered that adolescents younger than 16 years of age had nearly equal numbers of stress fractures in boys and girls. This is important, since fewer girls participate in running and jumping activities.

Most studies generally reveal the tibia as the most frequent site of stress fractures. McBryde (4) in a literature review, reported on the most common bones involved by sporting activity. These are listed in Table 36–1.

Matheson and colleagues (11) reported on 320 cases of bone scan-positive stress fractures. Their study included 145 males and 175 females. In their series the tibia was the most frequent site of injury (49.1%), the tarsals being the second most common (25.3%). The remaining stress fractures were to the metatarsals (8.8%), femur (7.2%), fibula (6.6%), pelvis (1.6%), sesamoids (0.9%), and back (0.6%); 16.6% of the cases were bilateral. Femoral and tarsal stress fractures were more common in older athletes, and fibular and tibial stress fractures were more common in younger athletes. In a retrospective review of radiographic case of stress fractures, Wilson and Katz (12) reported metatarsals as the most common (35.2%), followed by the calcaneus (28.0%), tibia (24.0%), ribs (5.6%), femur (3.2%), fibula (3.2%), spine (0.4%), and pubic ramus (0.4%).

CAUSE

Why are sports-related stress fractures so common? Possible answers include playing fields that are too hard, poor shoe design, training errors, and overtraining. To fully comprehend how these extrinsic factors affect the athlete, one must first understand basic connective tissue physiology.

Knapp and Mandelbaum (13) have developed a hypothesis to account for adaptation of connective tissue to stresses. Wolff's Law of Transformation states that connective tissue will respond to external forces. Consequently, every change in form and function of bone results in a change in internal architecture. Figure 36–1 is the dose-response curve in relation to bone adaptation to stress. The y-axis represents the dose of a given activity, including duration, intensity, and frequency. The x-axis is the response to adaptation. A stress fracture is a maladaptation response to abnormal doses of stress. By modulation of the application of stress in a judicial manner, the injury is preventable. Adequate adaptive response requires that stress be applied in a cyclic fashion, alternating with periods of rest. The amount of rest and stress allowable is determined by the biologic status

TABLE 36–1. *Fractures by sporting activity*

Sport/Athletic activity	Bone commonly involved
Running	
Sprint (rare)	
Middle-distance	Fibula-tibia
Long-distance	
Hiking	Metatarsal (rare)
	Pelvis
Jumping	Pelvis, femur
Tennis	Ulna, metacarpal
Baseball	
Pitching	Humerus, scapula
Batting	Rib
Catching	Patella
Basketball	Patella, tibia, os calcis
Javelin	Ulna
Soccer	Tibia
Swimming	Tibia, metatarsal
Skating	Fibula
Curling	Ulna
Aerobics	Fibula, tibia
Ballet dancing	Tibia
Cricket	Humerus
Fencing	Pubis
Handball	Metacarpal
(Water skiing)	(Pars)

From McBryde AM. Stress fractures in athletes. *J Sports Med* 1975;3:212–217.

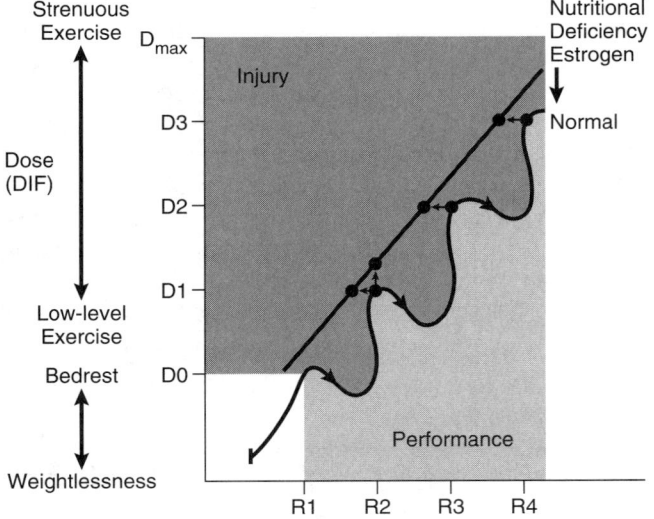

FIG. 36–1. Response of adaptation

of the host. This modulation is affected by intrinsic factors, including nutritional and endocrine variables. Inspection reveals that given the points on the curve between weightlessness and bed rest, performance adapts negatively and results in decreased bone mineral density, decreased tensile strength, and decreased new periosteal bone formation. This is because both of these "activities" lack ground reactive forces. The exercise portion of the curve demonstrates that it is essential that bone adapt in a cyclically progressive fashion. All points below the cyclical curve allow a positive adaptation, minimizing the probability of injury. Increasing the activity dose in a way that is inconsistent with the athlete's pattern and quality of response to adaptation, such as those practiced in a progressive training program, results in a maladaptive response and injury. In addition, in the moderate and high doses of exercises (as in any specific training program) dose response is key to understanding and integrating details of the adaptive response. This includes not only quality and quantity but also temporal relationships of the progress. Negative modulation, such as hormonal deficiency, nutritional deficiency, or increase in the duration, intensity, and frequency outside of the temporal response, will also cause this negative response to adaptation. When the maximal dose (D_{max}) is exceeded, there will also be a negative response with resultant maladaptation and the consequent stress fracture. This hypothesis provides the sports medicine professional with a conceptual and practical mechanism of interpreting stress maladaptation.

In general, there are varied theories that try to explain stress fracture etiology. The currently most widely held concept is that of repetitive stress causing a periosteal resorption that outstrips the rate of bone remodeling, weakening the cortex and resulting in a stress fracture (1). The previous concept of stress fractures stated that fatigue failure within the bone is preceded by fatigue in the surrounding muscles, which then allows excessive forces to be transmitted to the underlying bone. However, Stanitski and colleagues (14) believe that the reverse of this mechanism is true. They proposed that highly concentrated muscle forces acting across a specific bone from particular repetitive tasks enhance the loading that occurs. The rhythmic, repetitive muscle action causes subthreshold mechanical insults that sum up beyond the stress-bearing capacity of the bone, resulting in a stress fracture. This persistent overuse of bone that is unaccustomed to stress causes a rapid, focal, circumferential, periosteal resorption of bone formation of a small cortical cavity. At a lower rate, more dense, stronger lamellar bone is laid down along the lines of stress to the tibia. As the periosteal resorption outstrips the stronger lamellar bone formation, the net effect is transient weakening of the cortex, which may eventually rupture with continued stress and overuse. While multiple biologic and mechanical factors are involved in creating a stress injury to bone, the fracture process appears to be the same, whether it is in trabecular bone or cortical bone. This process is altered by various factors in addition to altered healing responses. These factors include disorders of collagen formation or nutrition that may prolong fracture healing or produce nonunion in a stress fracture of bone otherwise expected to heal (5).

Simple mechanical evaluation of bone, however, does not explain the biologic process involved in the development of a stress response and ultimate fracture. There are predilections for certain bones and certain sites on bones, depending on the type of stress, the age of the patient, and biologic fitness. For instance, in runners the tibia is the most frequent site of stress fractures because it bears five to six times the body weight (running magnifies the ground reactive forces by three times as compared to walking) (4). Additional examples are seen in athletes with tarsal navicular fractures. Typically, they all sustain repetitive high doses of stress. Intrinsic variables include foot abnormalities, including a short first metatarsal and metatarsus adductus, as well as limited dorsiflexion of the ankle and/or limited subtalar motion are sometimes present (15). Interestingly, microangiographic studies of the blood supply to the tarsal navicular by Torg and colleagues (16) demonstrated relative avascularity of the middle third of the bone. All of these findings suggest that repetitive cyclic loading, associated with some as-yet unidentified intrinsic variations in foot structure, may result in fatigue failure through the relatively avascular central portion of the tarsal navicular.

Stress fractures therefore must be considered as an injury spectrum (from stress response to stress fracture) because not all progress to the point of actual disruption of bony cortices and intramedullary changes that are detectable on radiographs. For example, simple cortical hypertrophy along the posterior medial cortex of the tibia may be the only radiographic sign. In 5 years, Jackson (6) saw more than 100 young athletes who had pain associated with this process, that is, benign cortical hypertrophy secondary to continued stress and overuse.

Training errors are the most frequently encountered cause of stress fractures. Orava and colleagues (10) discovered that athletes develop stress fractures mostly during a period of sequential stair-step increase/increase dose progression. Matheson and colleagues (11), in their survey of athletes, found training errors to be responsible for 22.4% of stress fractures. Pronated feet were most commonly found in tibial stress fractures and tarsal bone fractures and were least common in metatarsal fractures. Cavus feet were found most commonly in metatarsal and femoral stress fractures. At presentation 4.1% had positive radiographs (11).

In 1987 Jones and James (17) found, in their study of lower extremity injuries, that 2.4% of the men had stress fractures versus 12.3% of the women. In female athletes menstrual irregularities have been found to be a predisposing cause of stress fractures (3). Marcus and colleagues have shown that running-related fractures are more frequent in amenorrheic women (3). It appears that extreme weight-bearing exercise partially overcomes the adverse skeletal effects of estrogen deprivation; however, amenorrheic runners remain at high risk for exercise-related fractures (3). Frisch and colleagues (18) and Warren (19) have also proposed that prepubescent girls who initiate serious training and competition before menarche may have delayed menarche and be at increased subsequent risk for secondary amenorrhea and therefore stress fractures. Drinkwater and colleagues discovered that amenorrhea in female athletes is accompanied by a decrease in mineral density of the lumbar vertebrae, which is primarily trabecular bone (20). There was no such changes in the radius, which is primarily cortical bone. The amount of physical activity reported by amenorrheic athletes did not protect them from an apparent loss of vertebral bone. Marcus and colleagues (3) similarly found that mineral density of the lumbar spine in amenorrheic runners was lower than that in cyclic women and age-matched controls but higher than that in runners with secondary amenorrhea who were less physically active. Mineral density of the radius was normal in both groups. Myburgh and colleagues reported that in athletes with similar training habits, those with stress fractures are more likely to have lower bone density, lower dietary calcium intake, current menstrual irregularity, and lower oral contraceptive use (21). Bone mineral density measured by dual-energy X-ray absorptiometry was significantly lower in the spine, femoral neck, Ward's triangle, and greater trochanter (21).

Therefore the etiology of stress fractures has its basis in various intrinsic and extrinsic responses to periods of stair-step increase/increase activity doses rather than the proper adaptive cyclical progression. Breakdown due to stress is expected, as is the adaptation to breakdown. Repair simply cannot keep up with increased breakdown.

MAKING THE DIAGNOSIS

It is imperative that the stress fracture is diagnosed early, since delay may increase the athlete's morbidity. Johansson and colleagues (22) reported on 23 patients with stress fractures of the femoral neck (average of 6.5 years); 16 were recreational athletes, and 7 were elite athletes. An important finding of this study was that the diagnosis was confirmed an average of 14 weeks after onset of symptoms. Johansson believed that all of the elite athletes were forced to end their careers because of the delay in diagnosis. Therefore prevention is the ultimate objective of the sports medicine professional.

Athletes with stress fractures have a predictable, stereotypic historic course. In almost every instance there is a change in the dose of activity. This change may be over a period of time, or it may be a single event. Nonetheless, symptoms are gradual in onset over a 2- to 3-week period and in some cases up to 5 weeks. According to Markey (5), a prodrome of less than 24 hours generally indicates cancellous bone involvement.

Devas (23), in 1958, described the crescendo process elegantly:

> The symptoms start insidiously: at first the athlete feels a dull gnawing pain in one or other shin, which occurs toward the end of a run. The intensity of the pain, at first mild, gradually increases over the days, and will ultimately become so severe that running or sprinting cannot be continued. At first the pain passes off with rest, but recurs with further running. Over the days shorter and shorter distances produce the pain, which persists for some hours after athletic activity has ceased. Finally the pain continues during the night, but does not prevent sleep, and any attempt at running causes severe pain at once and training has to be discontinued. With a few days' rest from sport the athlete feels better and tries to run again, only to find that the pain recurs; in this way a whole season of training is [spoiled].

In addition to the athlete's history, a physical examination is important in correctly diagnosing the injury. The examiner must determine the point of maximum tenderness. Additionally, intrinsic anatomic variations must be carefully evaluated (e.g., cavus or pronated feet, pes planus, bony nodules, hyperkeratosis). One must be mindful of other problems that may mimic stress fractures. The differential diagnosis must include tumor (e.g., osteoid osteoma), chronic compartment syndrome, medial tibial stress syndrome, and infection.

Each stress fracture type has specific history and physical issues that aid in the proper diagnosis. In the tibia it is important to differentiate shin splints from stress fractures (24,25). Shin splints, according to the AMA Subcommittee Report on Classification of Sports Injuries, are characterized by "pain and discomfort in the leg from repetitive running on hard surfaces, or forcible, excessive use of the foot dorsiflexors; diagnosis should be limited to the musculotendinous inflammations, excluding fracture and ischemic disorders"(17). Shin splint pain is present at beginning of the workout and for several hours afterward. It is most often a dull, aching discomfort with a broad spectrum of intensity. Usually, there is a 3- to 6-cm area of tenderness over the posteromedial distal third of the tibia. Stress fractures show greater induration, erythema, and warmth, with a more localized pisiform-shaped area of tenderness. Shin splint pain occasionally is aggravated by active plantar flexion and inversion of the foot against manual resistance. In addition to local tenderness and edema, percussion at distance to the fracture causes transmission pain to the stress fracture site (5).

Metatarsal stress fractures generally present with vague mid/forefoot pain. It is often difficult to localize a point of maximum tenderness. Toe-walking will often aggravate the pain. Occasionally, mild soft tissue swelling will be present.

Tarsal navicular stress fractures are an underdiagnosed source of prolonged disabling foot pain in young athletes. Symptoms of the tarsal navicular stress fracture include the insidious onset of vague pain over the dorsum of the medial midfoot or over the medial aspect of the longitudinal arch. The pain is an ill-defined soreness, or there is a well-localized tenderness over the tarsal navicular or along the medial longitudinal arch. There is little if any swelling and no discoloration or lumps. There may be an associated decrease in dorsiflexion or subtalar motion. Torg and colleagues (16) described the diagnosis, fracture patterns, complications, and possible etiology of 21 tarsal navicular stress fractures in 19 patients. They discovered that the interval between the onset of symptoms and the diagnosis ranged from less than 1 month to 38 months (mean interval: 7.2 months) because the fracture was not evident or it was overlooked on the routine foot radiographs.

CONFIRMATORY STUDIES

Although most stress fractures are diagnosed from the history and physical examination, it is important for the clinician to corroborate the diagnosis by confirmatory studies. The clinical and radiographic criteria for the diagnosis of a stress fracture include premorbid normal bone, no direct trauma but a definite inciting activity, and pain and tenderness before radiographic evidence of fracture. Follow-up films must show resolution or remodeling at the fracture site (4).

The multifaceted variables in the development of the stress response account for the variation in radiographic appearance. Since this is an injury continuum, the exact time in the course of a developing stress fracture when the X-ray is taken also determines the radiographic appearances. Stress fracture radiographic signs include no abnormalities, periosteal new bone formation, and sometimes a lucency. Periosteal new bone is at a maximum by 6 weeks (5). In actual practice only 50% of stress fractures will be seen on plain films.

The diagnostic gold standard is the technetium-99 diphosphonate three-phase or single-phase bone scan or spec scan. Table 36–2 compares the bone scan appearance of stress fractures versus shin splints (26). Because this isotope is incorporated by the osteoblast in new bone formation, the area of a fracture will be easily detected. This may be as early as 48–72 hours after clinical signs of injury (5).

Bone scans offer a highly sensitive technique for the early diagnosis of stress fractures (27). Abnormalities on

TABLE 36–2. *Bone scan appearance: stress fracture versus shin splints* (26)

Characteristic	Stress fracture	Shin splints
Bone scan	Any phase can be positive	Positive only on delays
Intensity	Can be 1+ to 4+	Usually 1+ or 2+
Shape	Round/fusiform	Linear/vertical
Location	Anywhere in lower leg	Midposterior tibia

From Martire JR. The role of nuclear medicine bone scans in evaluating pain in athletic injuries. *Clin Sports Med* 1987; 6:713–737.

scans can be identified long before radiographic changes are observed. While the bone scan is highly sensitive in detecting stress fracture, it does lack specificity. Prather and colleagues reported that the plain radiographic false negative rate for stress fractures was 71% and the false positive rate for scintigraphy was 24% (28). The sensitivity and accuracy of the bone scan can be enhanced with high-resolution views of the suspected areas and comparison scans of the uninvolved limb. A negative bone scan virtually excludes the diagnosis of stress fracture. Table 36–3 compares the sequential pattern of stress fractures in regards to the athlete's symptoms, bone scan, and plain film results (26).

Computed tomography (CT) may be of use when the clinician wants to confirm a fracture, but this is not an accepted test routinely. It may be of value in determining fracture location, morphology, and state of healing.

Early reports showed that magnetic resonance (MR) imaging is not superior to bone scanning in the assessment of stress fractures (26). The relative sensitivity of MR imaging as compared to scintigraphy for detection of stress fracture has not been the subject of a critical study. Deutsch, Mink, and Kerr (29) believe that MR imaging, by virtue of its enhanced soft tissue contrast resolution, may permit early (preradiographic) detection of stress injuries of bone. Prefracture stress responses are most readily demonstrated on MR imaging in areas in which bone marrow is overwhelmingly fatty.

TABLE 36–3. *Sequential pattern of stress fractures* (26)

Stage	Symptoms	Scan	X-Rays
Normal bone remodeling (uneventful)	–	–	–
Accelerated bone remodeling ("stress remodeling")	+/–	+	–
Bone fatigue ("stress fracture")	+	+	–
Bone exhaustion (cortical break)	+	+	+

From Martire JR. The role of nuclear medicine bone scans in evaluating pain in athletic injuries. *Clin Sports Med* 1987;6: 713–737.

This is a distinct advantage of MR imaging in the imaging of the foot and lower extremity, which are overwhelmingly composed of fatty marrow except in the youngest individuals.

On MR imaging, stress responses appear as globular foci of decreased signal on T1-weighted sequences that are graphically demonstrated against a background of fatty (bright) marrow. The signal variably increases in intensity on T2-weighted sequences. Stress responses are exceedingly well demonstrated on STIR (Short Tau [T1] Inversion Recovery) sequences, in which they are depicted as areas of high signal intensity against the suppressed background of fatty marrow. While the detection of stress responses in fatty marrow is relatively straightforward, demonstrating the abnormalities in hematopoietic marrow can be more difficult. STIR sequences can be of considerable value in this setting (29). Therefore, according to Deutsch and colleagues, MR imaging is more specific than bone scan (29).

TREATMENT

Once the diagnosis is made, how does the sports medicine specialist treat this injury? The treatment must be multifaceted and multidisciplinary. Categorically, these are divided into general, psychological, medical, physical (duration, intensity, frequency), and surgical issues.

In general, athletes must maintain adequate nutritional integrity to avoid injury. This is particularly true of the young female athlete. Proper nutrition includes a low-fat, high-carbohydrate diet with avoidance of phosphate-containing sodas (studies suggest that excess phosphate intake may be an important variable in stress maladaptation). Calcium balance must be achieved at all times, since a negative balance will result in maladaptation. Supplementation should be encouraged, as most female athletes require 1000–1500 milligrams of calcium per day. Vitamins and trace elements are used only to prevent deficiency (the use of high-dose vitamins or trace elements has not been shown to have any benefit).

Eating disorders must always be considered. This is especially true in the female athlete with multiple recurrent stress fractures. When an eating disorder is identified, the physician must involve the coach, trainer, parent, and athlete as well as a psychiatrist or psychologist in the treatment program.

Medically, the athlete must be evaluated to ascertain that no concurrent medical condition exists that may affect bone integrity. Abnormal menstrual patterns in the female athlete must be identified (30). If such patterns are present, the primary care physician should evaluate for possible estrogen supplementation. Once the above factors have been evaluated, the athlete is then treated according to the bone-specific treatment algorithm. The most common factor that is found to modulate this injury in the healthy individual has been the application of cyclic stress. The cessation of stress (i.e., rest) will allow repair to dominate over resorption. Six to eight weeks is necessary for most fractures. Pubic rami fractures heal in 2–5 months (19). Andrish and colleagues (31), in their study of midshipmen, treated 97 men in whom shin splints developed by dividing them into five treatment regimens. All the regimens were effective to varying degrees. Prohibition of running was common to all the treatments.

Bracing may be important in limiting motion that may aggravate the injury. However, it may also transfer stress to other areas that may become symptomatic (5). Whitelaw and colleagues (32) reported on 17 competitive athletes with tibial stress fractures who were fitted with a pneumatic leg brace. All were able to ambulate without pain and were allowed to resume light training in an average of 1 week. They resumed intensive training at an average of 3.7 weeks postinjury. They returned to competition at the preinjury level in an average of 5.3 weeks after application of the brace. Whitelaw and colleagues theorized that the effect is due to accelerated healing caused by a venous tourniquet.

Surgery should be considered only for bones in which a complete fracture would have serious complications. Examples of this are the tibia, tarsal navicular, fifth metatarsal, and femoral neck (33). Figure 36–2 represents the treatment algorithm for athletes with suspected tibial stress fractures (13). After the history is taken and the athlete is examined, a plain film X-ray should be obtained, even though in the majority of cases it will be grossly negative. This is done for the occasional positive study and documentation for future X-rays. If these films are negative, proceed with either a bone scan or MR imaging. Once the diagnosis is confirmed, the athlete begins 6 weeks of rest from the aggravating activity. Crutches are utilized if a limp or significant pain is present. An important component of this time period is that the athlete should be allowed to maintain cardiovascular tone by cross-training, including swimming or bicycling (5). The athlete is reevaluated after 6 weeks. If pain free, the athlete is allowed to return to sporting activities via cyclical progression. If pain persists and plain films are negative for fracture propagation, cyclical progression is instituted. If plain films are positive for propagation of the fracture, step 1 is repeated for an additional 6 weeks. On reexamination after an additional 6 weeks, pain will determine whether return to sport is allowed. When pain remains, a CT scan is done (if radiographs are equivocal). If a large lucency is present or if the CT scan is positive, then reamed intramedullary rodding of the tibia is considered. In any event the athlete is then able to return to sport by way of cyclical progression.

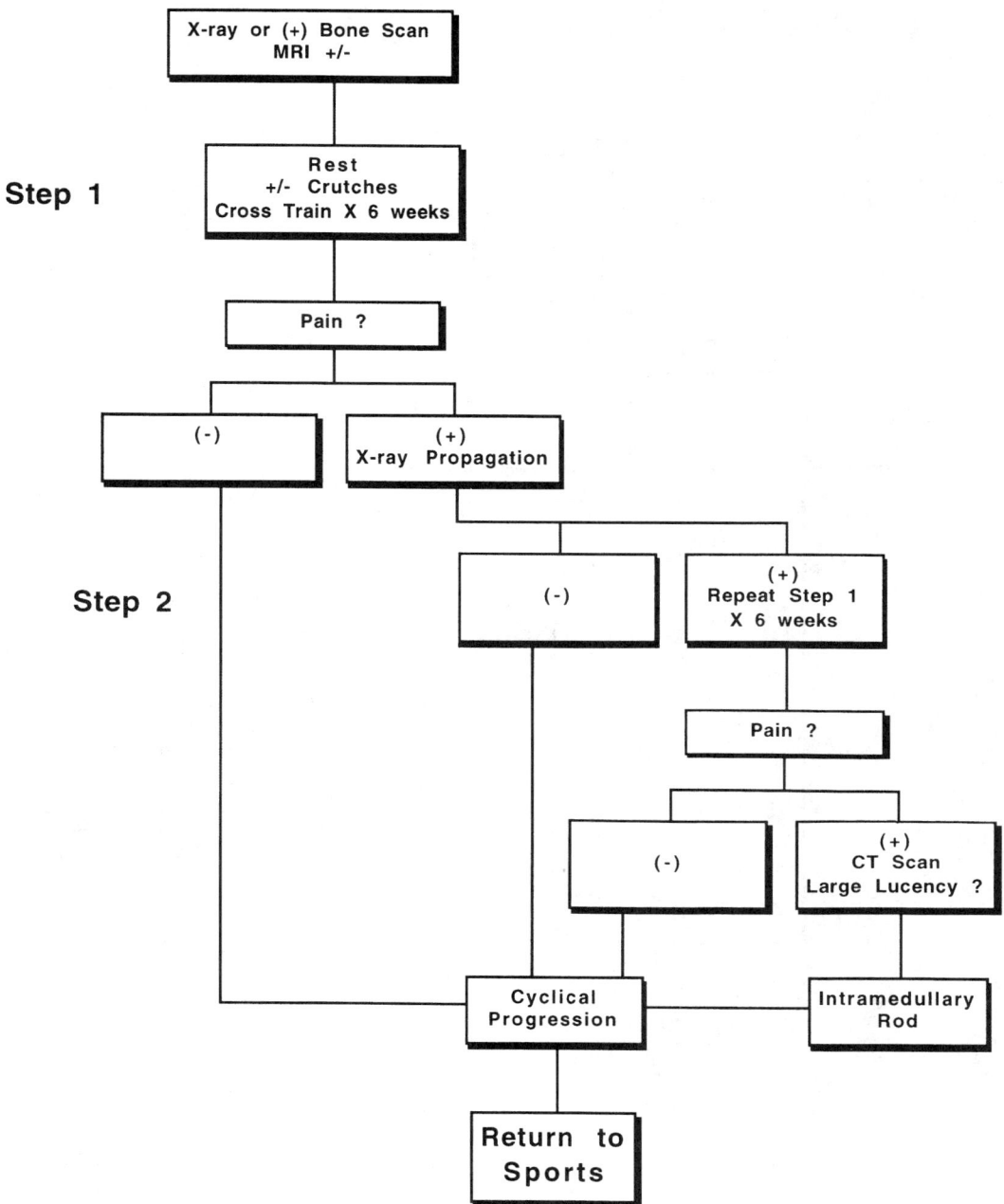

FIG. 36–2. Tibial stress fracture treatment algorithm

Figure 36–3 shows the treatment algorithm for the management of metatarsal stress fractures. The concepts are the same as for the tibia, with the exception that surgical intervention involves cancellous screw fixation +/− bone graft (13). Figure 36–4 is the treatment algorithm for tarsal navicular fractures developed by Torg and colleagues (15).

Uncomplicated partial fractures and nondisplaced complete fractures of the tarsal navicular should be treated by immobilization in a plaster cast with non weight bearing for 6–8 weeks. Return to weight bearing and activity should be guided by the patient's clinical picture as well as roentgenographic evidence of the union. Complete displaced fractures can be treated either with immobilization in a plaster cast with non weight bearing for 6–8 weeks or with open reduction and internal fixation, followed by immobilization and non weight bearing for 6 weeks. Fractures that are complicated by delayed union or nonunion should be treated with medullary curettage and inlaid bone grafting. In these situations a fibrous union may exist, and no attempt should be made to reduce the fragments. If the

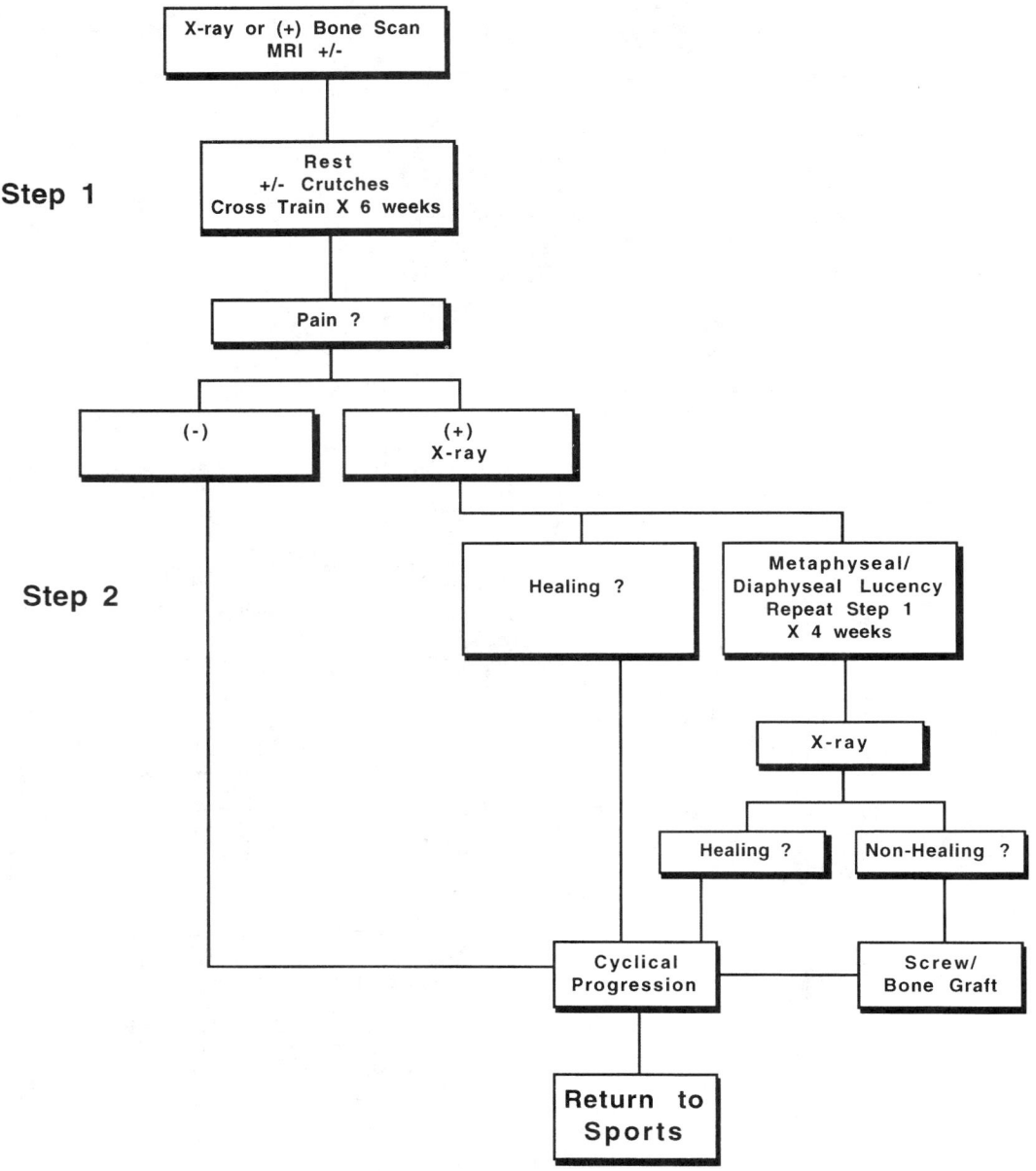

FIG. 36–3. Metatarsal stress fracture treatment algorithm

fragments are mobile, internal fixation should be effected by using a malleolar screw. After medullary curettage and inlaid bone grafting with or without internal fixation, the patient should be placed in a non-weight-bearing short-leg cast for 6–8 weeks. Again, mobilization and return to activity should depend on clinical and roentgenographic evidence of healing. It should be noted that in fractures treated by bone grafting, the healing course may be protracted, with firm bony union not occurring for 3–6 months. Partial fractures that are complicated by a small dorsal transverse fracture may require excision of the dorsal fragment. Complete fractures that are complicated by a large dorsal transverse fracture will go on to union with immobilization and do not require excision of the fragment. Associated dorsal talar beaks should be excised. Other than these and the small dorsal transverse fragments, sclerotic fragments associated with delayed union and nonunion should not be excised. These should be treated with medullary curettage and inlaid bone graft as indicated (15). Khan and colleagues (34) showed that non-weight-bearing cast immobilization is the treatment of choice for tarsal navicular stress fractures. The treatment compared favorably with surgical treatment for patients who presented after failed weight-bearing treatments. The CT scan appearance of healing fractures did not mirror clini-

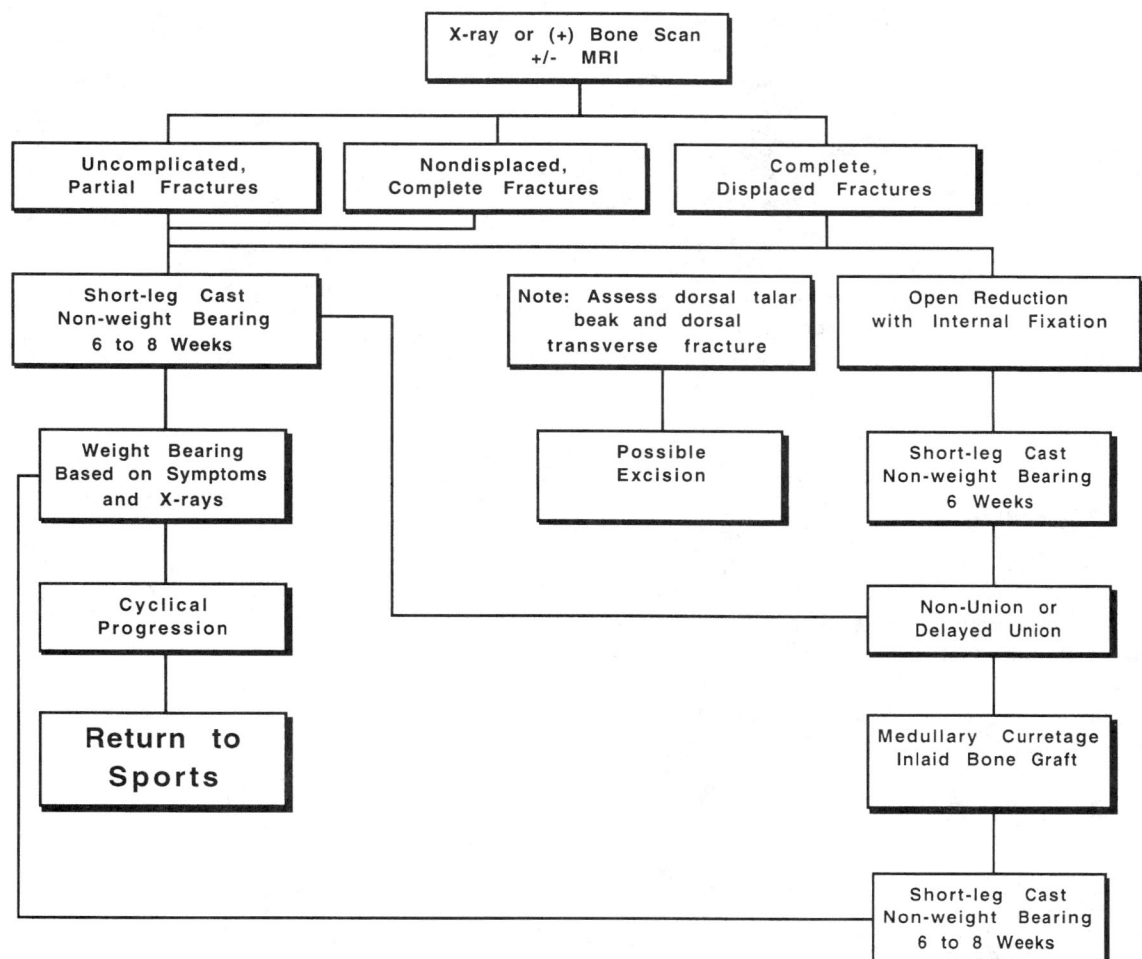

FIG. 36–4. Tarsal navicular stress fracture treatment algorithm

cal union. Authors suggest that postimmobilization management should be managed clinically. Twenty-eight of 35 (80%) healed with non-weight-bearing cast immobilization, compared with 12 of 40 (30%) with limitation of physical activity. Only one of five healed with continued sporting activity.

The only required medications are analgesics. As we stated, hormonal replacement in amenorrheic thin female athletes is often necessary. One should be on guard for rare metabolic abnormality in the otherwise healthy athlete. Altered magnesium and copper metabolism can result in a poor crystalline structure of bone. Additionally, osteomalacia rickets, whether primary or secondary, requires vitamin D supplementation as well as calcium to prevent insufficiency fractures (5).

Ultrasound is contraindicated because it aggravates the pain in the area of the fracture (although some studies suggest it may be of some diagnostic value). Application of ice and massage with gentle exercise relieves pain and increases the blood supply to the subcutaneous area (by reflex vasodilatation) (5).

RETURN TO SPORT

Most athletes will be able to return to sporting activities in 3–8 weeks. The athlete must be pain free and remain so during physical activity to begin rehabilitation.

PREVENTION

Andrish and colleagues (31) studied 2777 first-year midshipmen using four prophylactic programs for prevention of shin splints, including heel pads, tennis shoes, stretching exercises, and a graduated running program. None was effective.

The U.S. Soccer Federation has developed the following treatment guidelines in the prevention of stress fractures for their soccer players, but these easily apply to all athletes:

- Educate athletes, coaches, parents, trainers, and doctors.
- Training shoes and game shoes must be different.
- Training should be in a cyclical progression and in a

dose-responsive adaptation progression. Cross-train with bicycle, pool, or Stairmaster. Quality should take priority over quantity at all times. Monitor physical activity periods and rest periods carefully. Do not put all individuals in the same training program.
- Athletes in year-round programs must beware. The highest concentration of stress fractures are found in areas such as California and Florida.
- If the number of stress fractures seem to be inordinately high, consider changing the field if possible.
- Heed Aristotle's warning: "The child is not a small adult." Individualize programs by puberty stage, not by age.
- Be observant for eating disorders. Watch for multiple stress fractures.

FUTURE RESEARCH

Detailed studies must be undertaken on the prevalence and incidence of stress injuries. Biomechanical studies should be designed to look at shoe design and force concentration. Several trainers have raised the possibility of peroneal fatigue and its implications for stress fractures. Finally, nutritional concerns need to be addressed (e.g., vitamins, trace elements, and antioxidants).

REFERENCES

1. Pentecost RL, et al. Fatigue, insufficiency and pathologic fractures. *JAMA* 1964;187:1001–1004.
2. Lombardo SJ, Benson, DW. Stress fractures of the femur in runners. *Am J Sports Med* 1982;10:219–227.
3. Marcus R, et al. Menstrual function and bone mass in elite women distance runners. *Ann Intern Med* 1985;102:158–163.
4. McBryde AM. Stress fractures in athletes. *J Sports Med* 1975;3:212–217.
5. Markey KL. Stress fractures. *Clin Sports Med* 1987;6:405–425.
6. Jackson D. Shin splints: an update. *Phys Sports Med* 1978;6:51–61.
7. Greaney RB, Gerber FH, Laughlin RL, et al. Distribution and natural history of stress fractures in U.S. Marine recruits. *J Bone Joint Surg* 1983;146:339–346.
8. Protzman RR, Griffis CG. Stress fractures in men and women undergoing military training. *J Bone Joint Surg* 1977;59A:825.
9. Jones BH, Bovee MW, Harris JM, Cowan DN. Intrinsic risk factors for exercise-related injuries among male and female army trainees. *Am J Sports Med* 1993;21:705–710.
10. Orava S, Puranen J, Ala-Ketola L. Stress fractures caused by physical exercise. *Acta Orthop Scand* 1978;49:19–27.
11. Matheson GO, Clement DB, McKenzie DC, et al. Stress fracture in athletes. *Am J Sports Med* 1987;15:46–58.
12. Wilson ES, Katz FN. Stress fractures: an analysis of 250 consecutive cases, *Radiology* 1969;92:481–486.
13. Knapp TP, Mandelbaum BR. Stress fractures. In: Garrett WE, ed. *The U.S. soccer sports medicine book*. Baltimore: Williams & Wilkins, 1996.
14. Stanitski CL, McMaster JH, Scranton PE, et al. On the nature of stress fractures. *Am J Sports Med* 1978;6:391–395.
15. Torg JS, Pavlov H, Torg E. Overuse injuries in sport: the foot. *Clin Sports Med* 1987;6:291–320.
16. Torg JS, Pavlov H, Cooley LH, et al. Stress fractures of the tarsal navicular. *J Bone Joint Surg* 1982;63A:700–712.
17. Jones DC, James SL. Overuse injuries of the lower extremity: shin splints, iliotibial band friction syndrome, and exertional compartment syndromes. *Clin Sports Med* 1987;6:273–290.
18. Frisch RE, Gotz-Welbergen AV, McArthur JW, et al. Delayed menarche and amenorrhea of college athletes in relation to onset of training. *JAMA* 1981;246:1559–1563.
19. Warren M. The effects of exercise on pubertal progression and reproductive function in girls. *J Clin Endocrinol Metab* 1980;51:1150–1157.
20. Drinkwater BL, Nilson K, Chesnut CH, et al. Bone mineral content of amenorrheic and eumenorrheic athletes. *N Engl J Med* 1984;311:277–281.
21. Myburgh KH, Hutchins J, Fataar AB, et al. Low bone density is an etiologic factor for stress fractures in athletes. *Ann Intern Med* 1990;113:754–759.
22. Johansson C, Ekenman I, Tornkvist H, Eriksson E. Stress fractures of the femoral neck in athletes: the consequences of a delay in diagnosis. *Am J Sports Med* 1990;18:524–528.
23. Devas MB. Stress fractures of the tibia in athletes or "shin soreness." *J Bone Joint Surg* 1958;40B:227–238.
24. Clement DB. Tibial stress syndrome in athletes. *Am J Sports Med* 1974;2:81–85.
25. Detmer DE. Chronic shin splints: classification and management of medial tibial stress syndrome. *Sports Med* 1986;3:436–446.
26. Martire JR. The role of nuclear medicine bone scans in evaluating pain in athletic injuries. *Clin Sports Med* 1987;6:713–737.
27. Rosen PR, Micheli LJ, Treves S. Early scintigraphic diagnosis of bone stress and fractures in athletic adolescents. *Pediatrics* 1982;70:11–15.
28. Prather JL, Nusynowitz ML, Snowdy HA, et al. Scintigraphic findings in stress fractures. *J Bone Joint Surg* 1977;59A:869–873.
29. Deutsch AL, Mink JH, Kerr R. *MRI of the foot and ankle*. New York: Raven Press, 1992;79–84.
30. Wyshak G, Frisch RE, Albright TE, et al. Bone fractures among former college athletes compared with nonathletes in the menopausal and postmenopausal years. *Obstet Gynecol* 1987;69:121–126.
31. Andrish JT, Bergfeld JA, Walheim J. A prospective study on the management of shin splints. *J Bone Joint Surg* 1974;56A:1697–1700.
32. Whitelaw GP, Merrick MJ, Levy AS, et al. A pneumatic leg brace for the treatment of tibial stress fractures. *Clin Orthop* 1991;270:301–305.
33. Mendez AA, Eyster RL. Displaced nonunion stress fracture of the femoral neck treated with internal fixation and bone graft. *Am J Sports Med* 1992;20:230–233.
34. Khan KM, Fuller PJ, Brukner PD, et al. Outcome of conservative and surgical management of navicular stress fracture in athletes. *Am J Sports Med* 1992;20:657–666.

PART VI
Sports Epidemiology

CHAPTER 37

The Applied Physiology of Baseball

Kevin E. Wilk

Baseball is routinely described as America's pastime and has a large player and fan base world wide. The Sporting Goods Manufacturers Association estimates that in 1994 over 17 million Americans played baseball at least once and over 4 million Americans played frequently (52 times or more). Their data also show that an average of about 24% of boys between the ages of 6 and 17 years played baseball at least once in 1994. Add to this the 40 million people who play in recreational softball leagues, and there is an enormous player pool.

Baseball, and its companion sport, softball, are considered to be noncontact sports and thus a relatively safe activity. However, because of their huge player base, baseball and softball injuries lead to more emergency room visits than any other sport (1). It is surprising that little has been reported on the overall rate of injury for the games. Overall injury rates have been reported to be 1.6 injuries per 1000 practice/games (2) or 2–8% of participants per year (3). Acute injuries in the games typically occur during sliding, collisions, or falls (1), sliding-related injuries making up 71% of the total injuries during a university-based recreational softball league (4) or as many at one third of all lower extremity injuries (3).

Other traumatic injuries are due to collisions with players, bat, or ball. Softball and baseball appear to be the most common cause of eye injuries in sport (3), especially among 5- to 14-year-olds who are struck by a pitched ball. The rare catastrophic injury can occur when the player is struck in the head or chest with a bat or ball (3). In spite of this, the relative incidence of acute injury in baseball and softball appears to be quite low. The institution of equipment to minimize the effects of traumatic injury has lead to some drastic reductions in injury from predictable injury. For example, the use of batting helmets with face guards has helped to minimize bat and ball injuries to the head, face, and eyes. Breakaway bases have brought about significant reductions of sliding-related injuries. Chest protectors for catchers protect the chest from accidental ball contact. So rule changes, based on sound epidemiologic data, have been instituted, successfully reducing these predictable injuries.

A primary concern in baseball and softball is the development of overuse injuries from overhand throwing. Injuries to the shoulder and elbow can result in significant time loss from the game or even premature retirement from the game. Therefore this chapter will be directed toward a discussion of these complex injuries.

THE OVERHEAD ATHLETE

The overhead-throwing athlete is a highly skilled individual. To perform the overhead throwing motion successfully, the athlete must exhibit significant flexibility, muscular strength, coordination, synchronicity of muscle firing, and neuromuscular efficiency. In some instances the thrower may be throwing a baseball at velocities up to 97–100 mph. In other instances the thrower may be throwing a pitch, such as a curve ball or slider, that requires the same arm speed but creates much different, and in some instances higher, stresses at the elbow and shoulder joints.

The overhead throwing motion produces excessively high stresses because of the unnatural movements that are frequently performed by the overhead thrower. The thrower's shoulder must be flexible enough to allow the excessive external rotation required to throw a baseball. However, the thrower's shoulder must also be stable enough to prevent the shoulder joint from subluxation. Therefore a paradox appears to exist in describing the

K. E. Wilk: HealthSouth Rehabilitation Corporation, Birmingham, Alabama 35205.

thrower's shoulder: The thrower's shoulder must be loose enough to throw but stable enough to prevent humeral head subluxation. Hence the thrower's shoulder is in a delicate balance between mobility and stability.

The surrounding musculature of the thrower's shoulder must exhibit sufficient muscular strength, power, and neuromuscular control efficiency. The thrower's shoulder musculature must be strong enough to assist in arm acceleration but must also exhibit neuromuscular efficiency to enhance dynamic functional stability. The surrounding musculature work synergistically with the glenohumeral joint capsule to provide functional stability. The overhead throwing motion places tremendous demands on the shoulder and elbow joint complex musculature to produce functional stability, especially the shoulder joint. The musculature must function and react while the arm and shoulder joint are moving at incredibly high angular velocities. Furthermore, the shoulder musculature must function effectively throughout the entire range of motion, especially at end ranges, which are usually much greater than normal motions—all of which are occurring at tremendously fast speeds.

In this chapter the biomechanics of the overhead baseball throwing motion are briefly discussed, and key physiologic aspects are highlighted. Additionally, the physical requirements (such as range of motion, muscular strength, ligamentous stability, and neuromuscular control) are thoroughly described. Those physical requirements are then applied to a conditioning program to prevent injuries to the shoulder and elbow joint in the overhead thrower.

THE BIOMECHANICS OF THE OVERHEAD THROW

The overhead throwing motion is a highly skilled, extremely stressful, and violent activity. In general, the motion for throwing a baseball is similar to, but not exactly the same as, that of throwing a football or javelin. To understand the physical requirements for throwing a baseball and subsequent injuries from overhead throwing, one must understand the biomechanics of the overhead throwing motion.

The overhead pitching motion can be divided into five distinct phases (Fig. 37–1). These phases include the windup, early cocking, late cocking, acceleration, and deceleration follow-through (5). During the throw, the kinetic energy is generated from the legs and trunk and is transferred upward to the shoulder and arm (Fig. 37–2). At ball release and follow-through, the generated energy is transferred downward and back through the legs. It has been estimated that over 55% of the kinetic energy and momentum necessary to throw a ball is generated from the legs and lower trunk (6).

The Windup Phase

The windup begins when the pitcher initiates the first motion and ends with the ball being removed from the glove. During the pitching motion the athlete will pivot on the stance foot to a parallel position with the pitching rubber. The lead leg is then lifted concentrically by the hip flexors while the stance leg is slightly flexed to support the athlete's body weight. This position is referred to as the balanced position (Fig. 37–3). The pitcher must exhibit significant muscular strength not only in the stance leg but also in the pelvis and lower trunk to maintain this difficult balanced position. The quadriceps femoris of the stance leg performs an eccentric and isometric contraction to maintain the flexed knee posture, while the hip abductors and extensors cocontract to stabilize the pelvis. This balanced position is a very important position in the overhead pitching motion. The body must be vertical; therefore balance, proprioception, and kinesthesia are important attributes in maintaining this posture. The young thrower often mistakenly attempts to gain arm speed and ball velocity by propelling himself or herself toward the target too

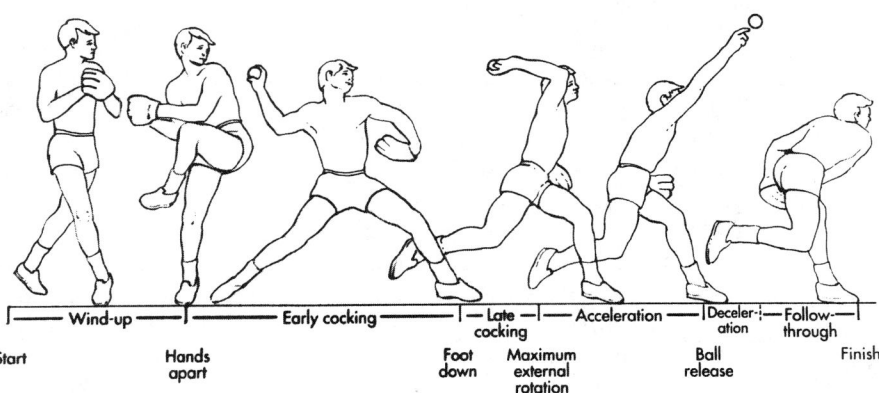

FIG. 37–1. The five phases of the overhead pitching motion. These phases include the windup, early cocking, late cocking, acceleration, and deceleration. (From DiGiovine NM, Jobe FW, Pink M, et al. An electromyographic analysis of the upper extremity in pitching. *J Shoulder Elbow Surg* 1992;1:15–24.)

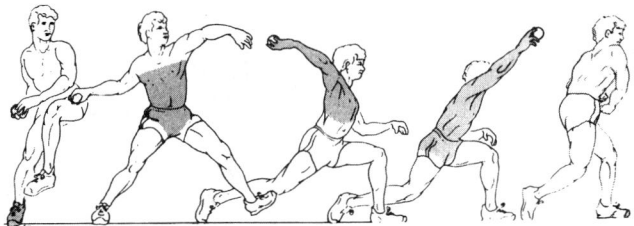

FIG. 37-2. During the pitch, the transfer of kinetic energy is generated from the legs and transferred upward. (From Jobe FW, Tibone JE, Jobe CM, et al. The shoulder in sports. In: Rockwood CA, Matsen FA, eds. *The shoulder.* Philadelphia: WB Saunders, 1990:961.)

soon and never accomplishes the balance position. This omission can lead to significant injuries to the shoulder from the shoulder's turning to the target too early. The main purpose of the windup phase is to place the thrower in an advantageous starting position to maximize the effort and perhaps act as a distraction to the batter.

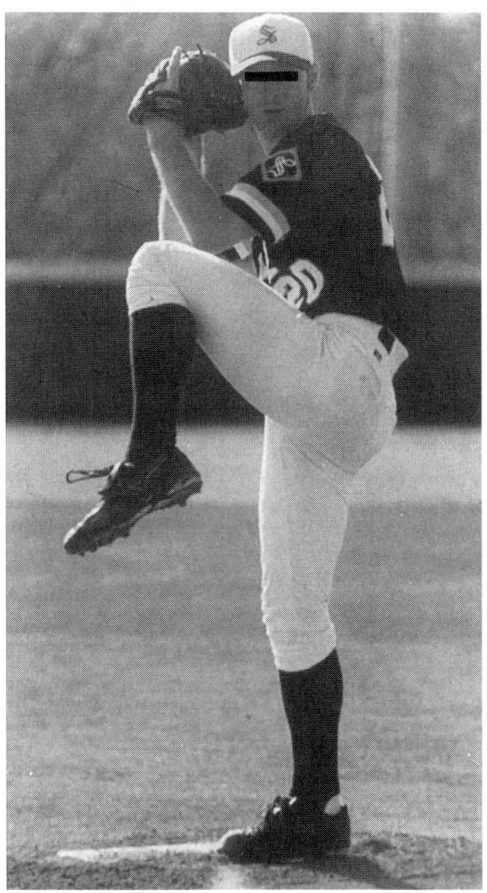

FIG. 37-3. The balanced position during the windup of the overhead pitch.

The Cocking Phase

The early cocking phase begins as the two arms separate (the ball being taken out of the glove). During this phase the pitcher pushes off the pitching rubber using a concentric contraction of the stance leg's hip extensors, hip abductors, knee extensors, and plantar flexors. The stride leg is lunged forward, with the lead foot pointed at the target. Usually, the lead foot is turned slightly inward (approximately 5–25°). The lead leg's knee is flexed to approximately 45–55° at foot contact. This position allows the body to rotate on this fixed and stable base of support. In addition, during this phase the shoulder is abducted externally and horizontally. During early cocking, the upper trapezius, supraspinatus, deltoid, and serratus anterior muscles exhibit moderately high to moderate levels of electromyographic (EMG) activity, respectively (Table 37-1) (7). The upper trapezius and serratus anterior musculature work synchronously to rotate the scapula upward while the deltoid muscle is elevating the arm and the rotator cuff muscles are cocontracting to stabilize the humeral head. The shoulder is abducted to approximately 80–100° (8). In addition, during this phase the elbow is flexed to approximately 80–100° while the arm is pronating. EMG analysis has shown that the wrist extensors (extensor carpi radialis, extensor carpi ulnaris, and extensor digitorum) exhibit moderately high levels of EMG activity (especially during late cocking).

During the late cocking phase the shoulder joint remains abducted approximately 80–100° while the arm externally rotates. Late cocking is characterized by the internal rotators acting eccentrically to control shoulder external rotation. The subscapularis exhibits high levels (99% MVIC) of EMG activity, while the pectoralis major and latissimus dorsi exhibit moderately high (56% and 50% MVIC, respectively) EMG activity (Table 37-1). Additionally, the serratus anterior exhibits extremely high muscular activity (106% MVIC), along with moderately high muscle activity of the levator scapula, middle trapezius, infraspinatus, and teres minor muscles. In addition, the internal rotators are elastically stretched to provide a stretch stimulus to the muscle spindle, provoking a powerful concentric contraction during the next phase of the throw, the acceleration phase. This type of stretch-shortening muscular contraction is referred to as a plyometric contraction. The throwing of a baseball is a classic example of a plyometric muscular contraction (9,10). It has been reported that during late cocking, the arm externally rotates to a maximum of approximately 165–180° (8). This excessive external rotation is the combination of scapular, thoracic, and lumbar spine motion. Nevertheless, for this motion to occur, the anterior glenohumeral joint capsule must exhibit significant laxity. During arm cocking, the shoulder joint angular velocity is approximately 1100° per second (8).

TABLE 37-1. EMG analysis of the overhead throw

	Number of pitchers	Windup	Early cocking	Late cocking	Acceleration	Deceleration	Follow-through
Scapular muscles							
Upper trapezius	11	18 ± 16	64 ± 53	37 ± 29	69 ± 31	53 ± 22	14 ± 12
Middle trapezius	11	7 ± 5	43 ± 22	51 ± 24	71 ± 32	35 ± 17	15 ± 14
Lower trapezius	13	13 ± 12	39 ± 30	38 ± 29	76 ± 55	78 ± 33	25 ± 15
Serratus anterior (sixth rib)	11	14 ± 13	44 ± 35	69 ± 32	60 ± 53	51 ± 30	32 ± 18
Serratus anterior (fourth rib)	10	20 ± 20	40 ± 22	106 ± 56	50 ± 46	34 ± 7	41 ± 24
Rhomboids	11	7 ± 8	35 ± 24	41 ± 26	71 ± 35	45 ± 28	14 ± 20
Levator scapula	11	6 ± 5	35 ± 14	72 ± 54	77 ± 28	33 ± 16	14 ± 13
Glenohumeral muscles							
Anterior deltoid	16	15 ± 12	40 ± 20	28 ± 30	27 ± 19	47 ± 34	21 ± 16
Middle deltoid	14	9 ± 8	44 ± 19	12 ± 17	36 ± 22	59 ± 19	16 ± 13
Posterior deltoid	18	6 ± 5	42 ± 26	28 ± 27	68 ± 66	60 ± 28	13 ± 11
Supraspinatus	16	13 ± 12	60 ± 31	49 ± 29	51 ± 46	39 ± 43	10 ± 9
Infraspinatus	16	11 ± 9	30 ± 18	74 ± 34	31 ± 28	37 ± 20	20 ± 16
Teres minor	12	5 ± 6	23 ± 15	71 ± 42	54 ± 50	84 ± 52	25 ± 21
Subscapularis (lower third)	11	7 ± 9	25 ± 22	62 ± 19	56 ± 31	41 ± 23	25 ± 18
Subscapularis (upper third)	11	7 ± 8	37 ± 26	99 ± 55	115 ± 82	60 ± 36	16 ± 15
Pectoralis major	14	6 ± 6	11 ± 13	56 ± 27	54 ± 24	29 ± 18	31 ± 21
Latissimus dorsi	13	12 ± 10	33 ± 33	50 ± 37	88 ± 53	59 ± 35	24 ± 18
Elbow and forearm muscles							
Triceps	13	4 ± 6	17 ± 17	37 ± 32	89 ± 40	54 ± 23	22 ± 18
Biceps	18	8 ± 9	22 ± 14	26 ± 20	20 ± 16	44 ± 32	16 ± 14
Brachialis	13	8 ± 5	17 ± 13	18 ± 26	20 ± 22	49 ± 29	13 ± 17
Brachioradialis	13	5 ± 5	35 ± 20	31 ± 24	16 ± 12	46 ± 24	22 ± 29
Pronator teres	14	14 ± 16	18 ± 15	39 ± 28	85 ± 39	51 ± 21	21 ± 21
Supinotor	13	9 ± 7	38 ± 20	54 ± 38	55 ± 31	59 ± 31	22 ± 19
Wrist and finger muscles							
Extensor carpi radialis longus	13	11 ± 8	53 ± 24	72 ± 37	30 ± 20	43 ± 24	22 ± 14
Extensor carpi radialis brevis	15	17 ± 17	47 ± 26	75 ± 41	55 ± 35	43 ± 28	24 ± 19
Extensor digitorum communis	14	21 ± 17	37 ± 25	59 ± 27	35 ± 35	47 ± 25	24 ± 18
Flexor carpi radialis	12	13 ± 9	24 ± 35	47 ± 33	120 ± 66	79 ± 36	35 ± 16
Flexor digitorum superficialis	11	16 ± 6	20 ± 23	47 ± 52	80 ± 66	71 ± 32	21 ± 11
Flexor carpi ulnaris	10	8 ± 5	27 ± 18	41 ± 25	112 ± 60	77 ± 42	24 ± 18

Means and standard deviations, expressed as a percentage of the maximal manual muscle test.

Additionally, maximum anterior shear force is approximately 380 ± 90 N, and compressive forces are 660 ± 110 N (8). Thus approximately 85 ± 36 lb of force are acting at the glenohumeral joint attempting to sublux the humeral head anteriorly while approximately 145 ± 28 lb of force are compressing the humeral head within the glenoid. A maximum elbow extensor torque of approximately 20–40 Nm has been noted during arm cocking phase (3). In addition, a significant varus torque of approximately 50–75 Nm that resists a valgus force occurs shortly before maximum shoulder external rotation (8,11).

The Acceleration Phase

Once the arm reaches maximal external rotation, the elbow joint begins to extend, and the shoulder joint rapidly internally rotates and adducts, initiating the acceleration phase of throwing. The acceleration phase of the overhead throw has been reported to be the fastest human motion recorded. During the acceleration phase the maximum internal rotation/adduction velocity exceeds 7000° per second (8). This phase of the throw takes approximately 0.03–0.04 second. Regardless of the type of pitch is thrown or the style of the pitcher (sidearm, overhead, three quarter, etc.), at ball release the shoulder joint is abducted between 90° and 100° (12). The difference between the overhead and the sidearm throw is not the amount of shoulder abduction, but rather the degree of lateral tilt of the trunk. During the acceleration the subscapularis, latissimus dorsi, and trapezius exhibit high levels of EMG activity (Table 37-1).

During arm acceleration the elbow begins to extend just before maximum shoulder external rotation; then shoulder internal rotation occurs. This sequence of integrated motions appears to enhance the velocity of internal rotation and thus arm speed and is an example of the synchronicity of joint motions exhibited during the overhead throwing motion. Maximum elbow angular velocity is approximately 2100–2400° per second. During this phase of pitching, a valgus stress is imparted onto the elbow joint. Shoulder internal rotation torque and elbow varus torque gradually decrease during the arm acceleration phase as the arm begins rotating forward, and near ball release low forces and torques are generated at the elbow and shoulder joints (11,13,14). The wrist flexors (flexor carpi radialis, flexor carpi ulnaris, and flexor digitorum superficialis) exhibit significantly high EMG activity during this phase. It should be noted that the muscle that exhibits the highest EMG activity of any muscle in the body is the flexor carpi radialis (120% MVIC). During this phase the elbow extends from approximately 85° elbow flexion to 20° elbow flexion (8). A maximum elbow compressive force of approximately 600–900 N is produced to prevent elbow joint distraction. The elbow flexors act eccentrically to control elbow extension and also act to compress the elbow joint contributing to joint stability.

Additionally, the trunk contributes greatly to arm speed. As the elbow extends and the shoulder internally rotates, the trunk forward flexes from an extended position. Forward flexion by the trunk occurs at an angular velocity of approximately 300–450° per second and is accomplished by the action of the hip flexors and abdominal muscles (rectus abdominals and obliques) (16). This rapid and forceful forward trunk flexion contributes to the vertical force generated through the upper body, which contributes to arm speed.

The Deceleration/Follow-through Phase

The arm deceleration/follow-through phase occurs from ball release to the termination of movement; this phase takes approximately 0.03–0.05 second to complete. After ball release the arm continues to adduct horizontally, extend, and to a lesser extent internally rotate as the kinetic energy is gradually dissipated through the lower extremity. During arm deceleration the forces at the glenohumeral joint reach relatively high levels. Maximum posterior shear force is approximately 400 ± 90 N, while the compressive force is approximately 1090 ± 110 N. This extremely high compressive force resists the distraction force generated at the glenohumeral joint. During deceleration large, eccentric muscle actions are needed at the shoulder and elbow joints. The teres minor exhibits significantly high EMG activity during this phase (84% MVIC); conversely, the infraspinatus exhibits relatively low musculature activity (37% MVIC). This discrepancy between the teres minor and infraspinatus during this phase would suggest that the teres minor plays a more significant role in arm deceleration than the infraspinatus muscle. Other muscles that exhibit significant EMG activity are the lower trapezius (78% MVIC), posterior deltoid (60% MVIC), and subscapularis (60% MVIC). At the elbow, wrist, and forearm the muscles that are most active are the flexor carpi radialis (79% MVIC), flexor carpi ulnaris (77% MVIC), supinator (59% MVIC), and brachialis (49% MVIC). The elbow extension motion terminates when the elbow is extended to approximately 15–25°. The follow-through phase of the pitch is the continuation of the deceleration phase, in which the joint forces and muscular torques are gradually diminished.

The tremendous energy generated during the acceleration phase of throwing must be gradually dissipated after ball release, during the deceleration and follow-through phases. This dissipation usually occurs by the action of the larger body segments and muscles. To reduce the distraction forces that were generated during the deceleration phase, the thrower should exhibit a complete follow-through path of motion, allowing the energy and momentum to be dissipated over a longer period of time. Decelerating too quickly or abruptly will result in excessively high forces, which may lead to injury.

Consequently, the throwing shoulder and elbow joint complexes are subjected to tremendous unnatural stresses. The thrower's shoulder joint must be loose enough to allow excessive motion, especially external rotation, yet maintain functional dynamic stability. Functional stability is provided by the integrated action of the joint capsule and surrounding musculature of the shoulder joint complex. There are muscles that appear to be primarily responsible for arm acceleration, such as latissimus dorsi, pectoralis major, triceps brachii, and wrist flexors. Conversely, there appear to be muscles that are primarily responsible for providing dynamic joint stability; these muscles include the supraspinatus, infraspinatus, subscapularis, serratus anterior, biceps brachii, and rhomboids. Dynamic stability is accomplished by coactivation of the stabilizing muscles. Because of the tremendous forces occurring at extremely high angular velocities and the repetitive nature of throwing, the thrower becomes susceptible to a variety of shoulder and elbow joint injuries. The most common shoulder joint complex injuries include overuse tendinitis, capsular hyperlaxity (subluxation), posterior rotator cuff impingement, undersurface tearing (fraying) of the rotator cuff, and glenoid labral lesions. The most common elbow joint injuries include flexor/pronator tendinitis, ulnar collateral ligament sprains, valgus extension overload syndromes, and posterior osteophyte formation. It is also important to note that there are significant differences in muscular activity and kinetics in the amateur and professional thrower, as well as in throwers with shoulder instability and those with a "normal" shoulder joint.

Gowan (17) compared the EMG activity of the shoulder musculature of amateur pitchers with that of professional pitchers. During arm cocking, the subscapularis muscle activity was approximately twice as great in the professional pitchers as that of the amateurs. Muscular activity of the biceps, serratus anterior, supraspinatus, and pectoralis major was approximately 50% greater in the amateur pitchers compared to that in the professional pitchers. During the acceleration phase muscle activity of the infraspinatus, teres minor, supraspinatus, and biceps brachii was two to three times greater in the amateur pitchers. Conversely, the muscle activity of the subscapularis, serratus anterior, and latissimus dorsi was significantly greater in professional throwers. These findings suggest that professional pitchers require less muscular activity of the stabilizing muscles because of improved throwing efficiency. During arm deceleration the amateur throwers had over twice the amount of muscle activity of the posterior deltoid and biceps brachii. This fact suggests that the less skilled thrower requires greater muscular activity to perform the same task owing to less efficient throwing biomechanics. This study may imply that the amateur pitcher may be more likely to sustain overuse tendinitis of the shoulder musculature than is the highly skilled pitcher. Several investigators have reported that the unskilled tennis player produces significantly greater EMG activity than the highly skilled player when performing the tennis service motion (18,19).

Gloussman and colleagues (20) examined and compared the EMG activity of the shoulder musculature in individuals with glenohumeral instability with that of individuals without instability during the overhead pitching motion. The investigators reported a marked increase in EMG of the supraspinatus, infraspinatus, and biceps brachii muscles during the cocking and acceleration phase in the individuals with instability. Additionally, the subscapularis, pectoralis major, latissimus dorsi, and serratus anterior muscles exhibited a significant decrease in muscular activity during the cocking and acceleration phases. These findings may suggest a conscious or subconscious compensatory mechanism for shoulder instability whereby the powerful accelerating muscles are inhibited and the stabilizing muscles act to a greater degree.

THE THROWER'S UPPER EXTREMITY

The Thrower's Shoulder

On physical examination of the thrower's shoulder and elbow joint, a characteristic pattern becomes obvious. The thrower's shoulder joint usually exhibits excessive external rotation (115–145°) and a significant reduction in internal rotation (35–55°) (Fig. 37–4). Additionally, the thrower's (particularly pitcher's) elbow joint usually exhibits a marked reduction in elbow extension; usually, in the pitcher a 5–20° flexion contracture is present.

Several investigators have examined the range of motion of the throwing shoulder in the pitcher as well as in the position players. Brown and colleagues (21) examined the range of motion of 41 professional players and compared 18 pitchers motion to 23 positional players. The investigators reported significant differences in range of motion of the dominant and nondominant arm for pitchers. Pitchers demonstrated 9° more external rotation, 15° less internal rotation, 11° less horizontal abduction, and 6° less elbow extension. Position players demonstrated 8° more external rotation, a 14° loss of horizontal abduction, and 8° loss of elbow extension. Additionally, pitchers exhibited 9° more external rotation in the dominant arm than did position players.

Johnson (22) reported the range of motion of 26 collegiate baseball players from two universities. The players included 17 infielders and outfielders and 9 pitchers. The author reported that the pitchers' dominant arm exhibited 136 ± 14° of external rotation; this was 8° greater than the nondominant shoulder, 15° greater than

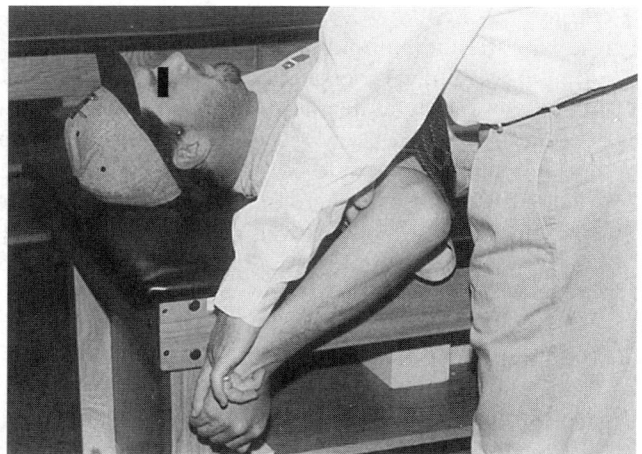
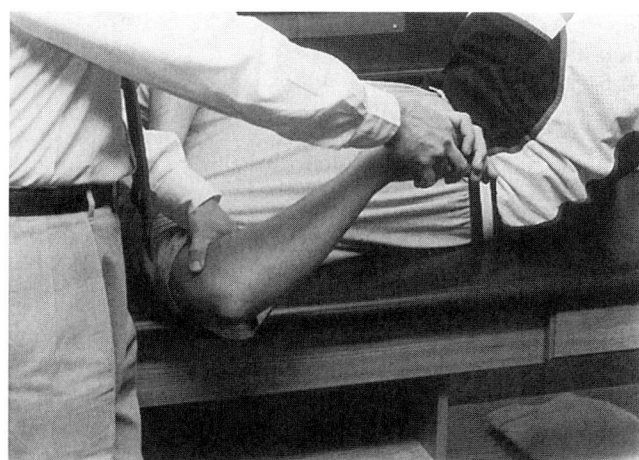

FIG. 37–4. The range of motion of the thrower's shoulder. **A:** External rotation to 138°. **B:** Internal rotation to 50°.

the outfielders' dominant shoulder, and 21° greater than the infielders' dominant shoulder. Also, the author reported that the pitcher's dominant shoulder exhibited greater internal rotation (111°) than that of the infielders' (110°) and outfielders' (106°) shoulders. This result is a little surprising to the author of this chapter. It has been the author's experience that the pitcher's shoulder usually exhibits significantly less internal rotation than reported by this study.

Recently, Bigliani and colleagues (23) examined the range of motion of 148 professional baseball players: 72 pitchers and 76 position players. The average external rotation with the arm positioned in 90° of abduction was statistically greater, and the average internal rotation was significantly less, in the dominant shoulders than in the nondominant shoulders, in both pitchers and position players. The authors reported that pitchers' external rotation with the arm abducted to 90° averaged 118° (range: 95–145°) in the dominant shoulder. Conversely, position players' dominant shoulder averaged 109° (range: 80–150°). In addition, the investigators noted that internal rotation was about the same for pitchers and position players.

The Thrower's Elbow

Several investigators have reported a significant decrease in elbow extension in pitchers as well as in position players (24–31). As was previously mentioned, Brown and colleagues (21) reported an elbow extension that was 6° less in pitchers and 8° less in position players when compared to the nondominant side. Other authors have noted a loss of elbow extension up to 15–20°. King and colleagues (27) examined the radiographic changes at the elbow in professional baseball pitchers and found consistent evidence correlating these changes with a decreased range of motion. Another possible cause of loss of elbow extension is soft tissue trauma during the ball release to deceleration phase of the throw. Additionally, as was stated previously, during arm acceleration through deceleration the elbow extends to an average of 20° flexion and does not fully extend (8). This may represent adaptive changes at the elbow joint due to throwing.

Shoulder Laxity

Shoulder laxity is defined as the ability to translate the humeral head on the glenoid. One would expect the thrower's shoulder to exhibit significant laxity because of motion requirements for throwing a ball and the range of motion exhibited on clinical examination. Although this assumption appears obvious, there are few studies that have documented shoulder laxity in the throwing athlete. Bigliani and colleagues (23) examined shoulder laxity in 72 professional baseball pitchers and 76 professional position players. The investigators noted a high degree of asymptomatic inferior glenohumeral joint laxity, with 61% of pitchers and 47% of position players exhibiting a sulcus sign on their dominant shoulders. Additionally, in the players who exhibited a positive sulcus sign on the dominant side, 54% of pitchers exhibited a sulcus sign on the nondominant shoulder; only 45% of position players exhibited a sulcus sign on the nondominant shoulder. The authors reported no correlation between laxity and players' age or length of professional baseball career in years.

Therefore it would appear from the findings of these studies and clinical observations that the following statements would be true:

1. The thrower's shoulder exhibits excessive external rotation.
2. The pitcher's shoulder exhibits greater external rotation than that of position players.
3. Shoulder laxity is greater on the throwing shoulder than non-throwing shoulder, but some throwers exhibit bilateral laxity.

Hence the question that remains is whether these differences in range of motion and laxity are adaptive (i.e., a physiologic response to repetitive microtrauma), selective (i.e., occurring in high-level athletes with inherent glenohumeral laxity), or a combination of the two. Some authors have stated that these differences are adaptive (21,32). Certainly, the presence of inferior laxity in the dominant shoulder of throwers can indicate an adaptive response to the repetitive throwing motion, particularly the higher degree of external rotation that is required during the late cocking and arm acceleration phases of throwing. However, Bigliani and colleagues (23) reported that a significant number of players exhibited a positive bilateral sulcus sign. Therefore the author of this chapter believes that while some shoulder laxity may be the result of an adaptive response to repetitive throwing, preexisting inherent glenohumeral laxity may play a role in the selection of athletes who are able to succeed at a high level of competition.

Because of the excessive glenohumeral joint motion exhibited by the throwing athlete, most frequently the anterior and inferior aspect of the shoulder joint capsule is lax. This excessive laxity allows the excessive range of motion that is necessary to perform the throwing motion fluently. The hypermobility of the shoulder joint capsule can be appreciated during the stability assessment of the glenohumeral joint, particularly during the anterior drawer, anterior fulcrum, and sulcus tests (33). On clinical examination the clinician will feel that the humeral head translates to a greater degree than a non-throwing shoulder. Additionally, the clinician should assess the end feel when performing these stability tests; this is an important variable to assess. The author of the chapter has referred to excessive laxity and increased motion as thrower's laxity (34).

TABLE 37-2. Unilateral muscle ratios (ER/IR)

		Angular velocity (deg/sec)						
		60	90	120	180	210	240	300
Alderink et al. (36)	D	—	66	68	—	71	—	70
	ND	—	70	72	—	76	—	76
Brown et al. (21)	D	—	—	—	67	—	61	65
	ND	—	—	—	71	—	66	65
Cook et al. (37)	D	—	—	—	70	—	—	70
	ND	—	—	—	81	—	—	81
Hinton (38)	D	—	69	—	—	—	71	—
	ND	—	76	—	—	—	80	—
Wilk et al. (39)	D	—	—	—	65	—	—	61
	ND	—	—	—	64	—	—	70

MUSCULAR STRENGTH AND PERFORMANCE

Several investigators have examined the muscular strength in the overhead throwing athlete (21,35–40), with varying results and conclusions. Alderink and colleagues (36) and Hinton (38) have reported the external rotator strength being greater on the nonthrowing side compared to the throwing shoulder. Conversely, Brown and colleagues (21) reported the throwing shoulder external rotators exhibited greater isokinetic strength. Cook and colleagues (37) reported that both shoulders were equal in strength. In the bilateral comparison of internal rotation strength, Alderink and colleagues (36) and Cook and colleagues (37) reported the throwing and nonthrowing shoulder as being equal, while Brown and colleagues (21) and Hinton (38) noted that the throwing shoulder's internal rotation was significantly stronger. Additionally, these investigators have published data regarding unilateral muscle ratios (ER/IR) of the shoulder (see Table 37-2).

Wilk and colleagues (40) reported the results of isokinetic muscular performance testing in 150 professional baseball pitchers. The results of external rotation strength testing indicated the dominant shoulder was weaker at 180° per second and bilaterally equal at 300° per second. The pitcher's internal rotation strength was slightly stronger on the dominant side at both test speeds (180° per second and 300° per second). The unilateral muscle ratios for the ER/IR muscles are represented in Table 37-3. Additionally, peak torque to body weight ratios are also illustrated in Table 37-3.

Wilk and colleagues (40) have also reported the abductor and adductor strength characteristics of professional baseball pitchers. The results indicated that shoulder abduction was approximately equal bilaterally; however, adduction was significantly stronger in the dominant shoulder. The abductor/adductor unilateral muscle ratios and peak torque to body weight ratios are represented in Table 37-3.

Often the question is raised, "Does a relationship between shoulder strength and the ability to throw exist?" Bartlett and colleagues (41) examined the relationship of shoulder strength and throwing speed in 11 professional pitchers and reported a positive statistical relationship between shoulder adductor strength and throwing speed. In comparison, Pedegona and colleagues (35), in a similar research design of eight professional baseball pitchers, found no direct relationship between adductor muscular strength and throwing speed.

Additionally, it is not uncommon for the pitcher to exhibit significant muscular weakness of the throwing shoulder. Often muscular weakness can be noted of the supraspinatus and external rotators when compared to the contralateral shoulder. Magnusson and colleagues (42) compared static muscular strength in professional pitchers to an age-matched nonthrowing control group. The pitcher's dominant shoulder was weaker in external rotation and "isolated" supraspinatus muscle testing than the nondominant side and significantly weaker than the control group. This is a common observation and is often reconfirmed when the strength of a professional pitcher is tested by a trainer or clinician.

TABLE 37-3. Data profile for the throwing athlete

Velocity (deg/sec)	Bilateral comparison			
	ER	IR	ABD	ADD
180	98–105	110–118	98–103	110–122
300	85–95	105–113	96–102	110–123

Velocity (deg/sec)	Unilateral muscle ratios	
	ER/IR	ABD/ADD
180	65–75	78–84
300	61–71	88–94

Velocity (deg/sec)	Torque to body weight ratios			
	ER	IR	ABD	ADD
180	18–23	27–33	26–32	32–38
300	15–20	25–30	19–25	28–34

Scapular muscular strength is also very important for the overhead thrower. To date, there have been no published studies that have documented the muscular strength of the scapular musculature in the overhead thrower. Scapular muscles of particular interest are the trapezius (upper, middle, and lower fibers), serratus anterior, rhomboids, and levator scapula. Scapular muscle strength is critical to the overhead athlete in establishing a stable base of support (foundation) from which the humerus and arm act (43–46). Trunk and leg musculature strength is also very important to the throwing athlete.

NEUROMUSCULAR CONTROL

Although muscular strength is an important physical attribute to the thrower's shoulder, perhaps as or more important is the neuromuscular control abilities exhibited by the athlete. As was previously mentioned, the thrower's shoulder must be lax enough to throw but stable enough not to sublux. The dynamic stability that is required to prevent glenohumeral subluxation is accomplished through the combined actions of the glenohumeral joint capsule and surrounding musculature. The glenohumeral joint musculature must work in a synchronized fashion to both accelerate the arm and dynamically stabilize the glenohumeral joint. The surrounding musculature of the glenohumeral joint must act to cocontract through coactivation to produce glenohumeral joint compression, thus creating dynamic stability. Dynamic stability occurs through the combined actions of the neurologic system through afferent sensory input and the muscular actions (efferent response) to the sensory input. This is referred to as neuromuscular control and is a critical aspect to sports performance and particularly the overhead throw.

Proprioception refers to the conscious and unconscious appreciation of joint position (47). Kinesthesia is the sensation of joint motion or acceleration. The efferent (motor) response to sensory information is referred to as neuromuscular control (48). All three components play a vital role in dynamic stabilization of the thrower's shoulder. Although proprioception and neuromuscular control are critical components for dynamic stability, there have been no published studies that have tested these areas in the overhead athlete. However, two studies have documented the effect of shoulder injury on proprioception (49,50).

Smith and Brunoli (49) were the first to investigate the effect of capsuloligamentous injury on proprioception in the shoulder. They reported that patients with unilateral, recurrent, traumatic anterior shoulder instability demonstrated proprioceptive sensory deficits. Lephart and colleagues' study (50) was the first performed comparing shoulder proprioception in groups of individuals with normal, unstable, and surgically repaired shoulders. The results revealed significant proprioceptive deficits in patients who have chronic, traumatic anterior shoulder instability and that surgical stabilization of such a shoulder normalizes proprioceptive sensibility. Voight and colleagues (51) examined the effects of muscular fatigue on shoulder joint proprioception in individuals without shoulder pathology. The investigators noted that shoulder proprioception was diminished in the presence of muscular fatigue, a result suggesting that various muscular receptors contribute to proprioception.

Therefore it would appear that proprioception and neuromuscular control abilities play a significant role in effective injury-free throwing. Although a standardized proprioceptive test has not been established for the throwing athlete, the author of the chapter has clinically utilized a test maneuver to assess proprioception and neuromuscular control. The patient lies supine with eyes closed; the clinician passively moves the patient's arm through a PNF D_2 flexion/extension path (52) of motion twice; then the patient is asked to replicate that path of motion as closely as possible with the eyes remaining closed (Fig. 37–5). The patients are evaluated as to how

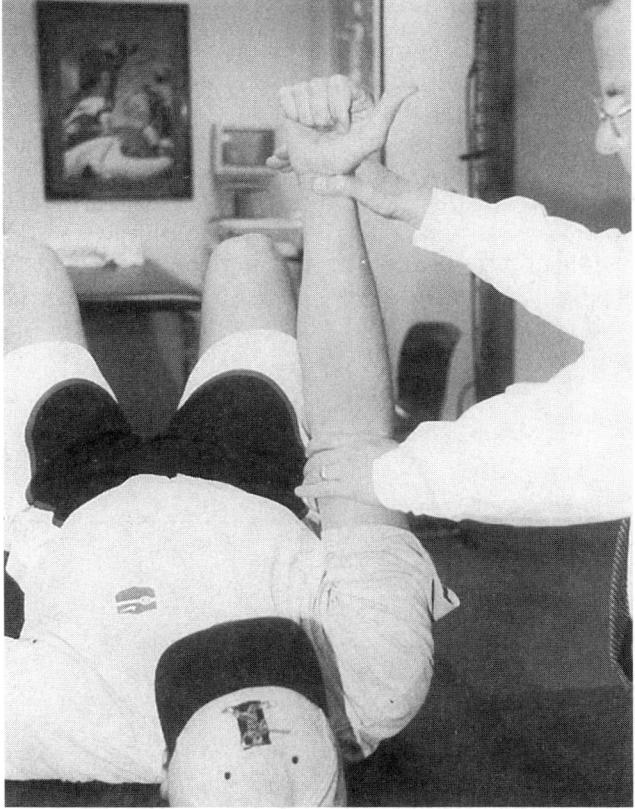

FIG. 37–5. Proprioceptive test for the overhead thrower. Initially, the patient's arm is passively taken though an arc of motion, tracking a D2 flexion/extension pattern; this is performed twice. Then the patient is asked to replicate the exact movement actively.

closely they can replicate the exact movement without deviating from the path of motion. A deviation in motion of more than 3 inches has been treated as significant by the author, and treatment would emphasize proprioceptive training to a greater extent than for the patient not exhibiting proprioception deficits.

Thus the physiologic requirements of the overhead thrower are numerous. The requirements to throw effectively centers on the paradox of the thrower's shoulder: The thrower's shoulder must be loose enough to be able to throw but exhibit enough stability to prevent glenohumeral joint subluxation. The thrower's shoulder appears to exhibit greater motion than the nondominant shoulder as a result of adaptive and inherent factors. Dynamic functional stability is accomplished through the combined efforts of the glenohumeral joint capsule and the neuromuscular systems. Muscular strength of the scapular region and the glenohumeral joint is an important component in training or rehabilitating an overhead athlete. Additionally, proprioception and neuromuscular control abilities are vital components and should also be included into the conditioning program.

REHABILITATION OF THE OVERHEAD ATHLETE

The majority of injuries to the shoulder and elbow joint can be successfully treated nonoperatively with a thorough and comprehensive rehabilitation program. For the nonoperative program to be effective, the clinician must identify the cause of the problem, establish a differential diagnosis, and identify all involved structures. The nonoperative rehabilitation program utilized for the overhead thrower involves a multiphase approach that is progressive and sequential. The specific goals of each of the four phases of the program are outlined in Table 37–4.

TABLE 37–4. *Conditioning program for the professional baseball player*

Phase I: Competition phase
In-season training
6 mo
April–September
Phase II: Postcompetition phase
Postseason (rest–recovery)
6–8 wk
October, November
Phase III: Preparation phase
Off-season conditioning
12 wk
Nov. 24–Feb. 15
Phase IV: Transitional phase
Spring training
6 wk
Feb. 16–Mar. 31

During the initial phase, one of the primary goals of the rehabilitation program is to normalize shoulder motion, particularly improving internal rotation and horizontal adduction. Therefore specific stretches to address posterior rotator cuff and capsular tightness should be performed. Another primary goal of the phase is to reestablish baseline dynamic stability as well as restoring proprioception and kinesthesia. Additionally, the patient's pain and inflammation are addressed and reduced through activity modifications, modalities, and gentle stretching.

In the second phase of the rehabilitation program, the primary goals are to enhance dynamic stability and to facilitate neuromuscular control. Additionally, the program should emphasize the restoration of muscular balance at the glenohumeral and scapulothoracic joints. During this phase the patient is placed on an isotonic strengthening program and a plyometric exercise program.

The primary goals of the third phase are to enhance dynamic stabilization, improve reactive neuromuscular control, and improve power and endurance. Also during this phase an interval throwing program can be initiated. The isotonic strengthening program and the thrower's ten program are continued, and manual resistance drills to enhance dynamic stability are also performed.

During the fourth phase the primary goals are a gradual return to throwing while maintaining the neuromuscular gains that have been established in the previous three phases. During this phase isotonic, plyometric, and manual resistance exercises are performed. Additionally, the interval throwing program is progressed. The interval throwing program is designed to gradually increase the number of throws and the distance, intensity, and types of throws to facilitate the restoration of normal biomechanics. The interval throwing program is organized into two phases: phase I is a long-toss program (from 45 to 180 ft), and phase II is an off-the-mound program for pitchers. The primary goal of the last phase is to enhance sport-specific techniques that reestablish proper biomechanics, thus reducing the chance of reinjury.

SUMMARY

Baseball and softball lead to more sports-related visits to the emergency room than any other sport, owing to its staggering number of participants. Acute injuries occur mostly during sliding, followed by collisions (with the bat, ball, or other player) and falls. Overall, the rate of injury is one of the lowest in team sports. Of particular interest is the risk of overuse injury from overhead throwing.

The thrower's shoulder and elbow joints are subjected to tremendous stresses and strains during the overhead throwing motion. Because of the excessive forces generated, significantly high muscular activity and tremendously high angular velocities at the shoulder and elbow joints are susceptible to injury. Additionally, the hypermobility of the anterior glenohumeral joint capsule contributes significantly to some of the common pathomechanics. Through proper conditioning and training, some of these injuries can be avoided.

Optimum sports performance requires skill and power. The conditioning program should address the development of both entities and should motivate the athlete to strive for a higher level of performance. In designing a conditioning program for the overhead athlete, specific elements should include flexibility, strengthening, proprioception, kinesthesia, neuromuscular control, endurance, power, core stability, and the concepts of periodization. The conditioning program should be manageable, measurable, and motivational. Additionally, the elements of a rehabilitation program were discussed in the chapter. The rehabilitation of the overhead has dramatically changed in the past decade. Currently, the goals of the rehabilitation are muscular balance, proprioception, neuromuscular control, scapular strengthening, dynamic stabilization, and a gradual return to throwing activities. By utilizing these principles and guidelines, athletes improve their chances to return to injury-free throwing.

REFERENCES

1. Janda DH, Wild DE, Hensinger RN. Softball injuries: aetiology and prevention. *Sports Med* 1992;13:285–291.
2. Harner CD, Bradley JP, McMahon PJ, Kocher MS. Baseball. In: Fu FH, Stone DA, eds. *Sports injuries: mechanisms, prevention, treatment.* Baltimore: Williams & Wilkins, 1994:191–207.
3. Committee on Sports Medicine and Fitness of the American Academy of Pediatrics. Risk of injury from baseball and softball in children 5–14 years of age. *Pediatrics* 1994;93:690–691.
4. Janda DH, Hankin FM, Wojtys EM. Softball injuries, cost, cause and prevention. *Am Fam Phys* 1986;33:143–144.
5. Jobe FW, Tibone JE, Jobe CM, et al. The shoulder in sports. In: Rockwood CA, Matsen FA, eds. *The shoulder.* Philadelphia: WB Saunders, 1990:961.
6. Toyoshima S, Hoshikawa T, Miyashita M, et al. Contribution of the body parts to throwing performance. In: Nelson RC, Morehouse CA, eds. *Biomechanics,* vol IV. Baltimore: University Park Press, 1974:169–174.
7. DiGiovine NM, Jobe FW, Pink M, et al. An electromyographic analysis of the upper extremity in pitching. *J Shoulder Elbow Surg* 1992;1:15–24.
8. Fleisig GS, Andrews JR, Dillman CJ, et al. Kinetics of baseball pitching with implications about injury mechanisms. *Am J Sports Med* 1995;23:233–239.
9. Verkhoshanski Y. Perspectives in the improvement of speed-strength preparation for jumpers. *Yessis Rev Soviet Phys Educ Sports* 1969;4:28–35.
10. Wilk KE, Voight ML, Keirns MA, Gambetta V. Stretch-shortening drills for the upper extremity: theory and clinical application. *J Orthop Sports Phys Ther* 1993;17:225–239.
11. Werner SL, Dillman CJ, Escamilla RF, et al. Biomechanics of the elbow during baseball pitching. *J Orthop Sports Phys Ther* 1993;17:274–278.
12. Dillman CJ. Proper mechanics of pitching. *Sports Med Update* 1990;5:15–21.
13. Fleisig GS, Dillman CJ, Andrews JR. Biomechanics of the shoulder during throwing. In: Andrews JR, Wilk KE, eds. *The athlete's shoulder.* New York: Churchill Livingstone 1994:355–368.
14. Fleisig GS, Dillman CJ, Andrews JR. Proper mechanics for baseball pitching. *Clin Sports Med* 1991;10:789–805.
15. Fleisig GS, Escamilla RF, Barrentine SW, et al. Kinematic and kinetic comparison between baseball pitching and football passing. *J Appl Biomech* 1996;12:207–224.
16. Moynes DR. Electromyography and motion analysis of the upper extremity in sports. *Phys Ther* 1986;66:1905–1911.
17. Gowan ID. Comparative electromyographic analysis of the shoulder during pitching. *J Sports Med* 1987;15:586–590.
18. Van Gheluwe B, Hebbelinck M. Muscle actions and ground reaction forces in tennis. *J Sport Biomech* 1986;2:88–93.
19. Miyashita M, Tsunoda T, Sakurai S, et al. Muscular activities in the tennis serve and overhead throwing. *Scand J Sports Sci* 1980;2:52–59.
20. Gloussman R, Jobe FW, Tibone JE, et al. Dynamic electromyographic analysis of the throwing shoulder with glenohumeral instability. *J Bone Joint Surg* 1988;70A:220–226.
21. Brown LP, Niehues SL, Harrah A, et al. Upper extremity range of motion and isokinetic strength of the internal and external shoulder rotators in major league baseball players. *Am J Sports Med* 1988;16:577–585.
22. Johnson L. Patterns of shoulder flexibility among college baseball players. *J Athl Trn* 1992;27:44–49.
23. Bigliani LU, Codd TP, Connor PM, et al. Shoulder motion and laxity in the professional baseball player. *Am J Sports Med* 1997;25:609–613.
24. Adams JE. Bone injuries in very young athletes. *Clin Orthop* 1968;58:129–140.
25. Albright JA, Jokl P, Shaw R, et al. Clinical study of baseball pitchers: correlation of injury to the throwing arm with method of delivery. *Am J Sports Med* 1978;6:15–21.
26. DeHaven KE, Evarts CM. Throwing injuries of the elbow in athletes. *Orthop Clin North Am* 1973;4:801–808.
27. King JW, Brelsford HJ, Tullos HS. Analysis of the pitching arm of the professional baseball pitcher. *Clin Orthop* 1969;67:116–123.
28. Slocum DB. Classification of elbow injuries from baseball pitching. *Texas Med* 1968;64:48–53.
29. Torg JS, Pollack H, Sweterlitsch P. The effects of competitive pitching on the shoulders and elbows of preadolescent baseball players. *Pediatrics* 1972;49:267–272.
30. Tullos HS, Erwin WD, Woods GW, et al. Unusual lesions of the pitching arm. *Clin Orthop* 1972;88:169–182.
31. Tullos HS, King JW. Lesions of the pitching arm in adolescents. *JAMA* 1972;220:264–271.
32. Tullos HS, King JW. Throwing mechanism in sports. *Orthop Clin North Am* 1973;4:709–720.
33. Wilk KE, Andrews JR, Arrigo CA. The physical examination of the glenohumeral joint: emphasis on the stabilizing structures. *J Orthop Sports Phys Ther* 1997;25:380–389.
34. Wilk KE. The thrower's shoulder: evaluation of common injuries. Presented at the 1997 Advances on the Knee & Shoulder. Cincinnati Sports Medicine Center, Hilton Head, SC, May 24, 1997.
35. Pedegona LR, Elsner RC, Roberts D, et al. The relationship of upper extremity strength to throwing speed. *Am J Sports Med* 1982;10:352–354.
36. Alderink GJ, Kuck DJ. Isokinetic shoulder strength of high school and college-aged pitchers. *J Orthop Sports Phys Ther* 1986;7:163–172.
37. Cook EE, Gray VL, Savinar-Nogue E, et al. Shoulder antagonistic strength rations: a comparison between college-level baseball pitchers and non-pitchers. *J Orthop Sports Phys Ther* 1987;8:451–461.
38. Hinton RY. Isokinetic evaluation of shoulder rotational strength in high school baseball pitchers. *Am J Sports Med* 1988;16:274–279.
39. Wilk KE, Andrews JR, Arrigo CA, et al. The strength characteristics of internal and external rotator muscles in professional baseball pitchers. *Am J Sports Med* 1993;21:61–66.
40. Wilk KE, Andrews JR, Arrigo CA. The abductor and adductor strength characteristics of professional baseball pitchers. *Am J Sports Med* 1995;23:307–311.
41. Bartlett LR, Storey MD, Simons DB. Measurement of upper

extremity torque production and its relationship to throwing speed in the competitive athlete. *Am J Sports Med* 1989;17:89–91.
42. Magnusson SP, Gleim GW, Nicholas JA. Shoulder weakness in professional baseball pitchers. *Med Sci Sports Exerc* 1994;26:5–9.
43. Kibler BW. The role of the scapula in the overhead throwing motion. *Contemp Orthop* 1991;22:525–531.
44. Paine RM. The role of the scapula in the shoulder. In: Andrews JR, Wilk KE, eds. *The athlete's shoulder.* New York: Churchill Livingstone, 1994:495–512.
45. Davies GJ, Dickoff-Hoffman SD. Neuromuscular testing and rehabilitation of the shoulder complex. *J Orthop Sports Phys Ther* 1993;18:449–456.
46. Moseley JB, Jobe FW, Pink M, et al. EMG analysis of the scapular muscles during a shoulder rehabilitation program. *Am J Sports Med* 1992;20:222–228.
47. Mooncastle VS. *Medical physiology,* 14th ed. St. Louis: Mosby, 1980.
48. Jonsson HJ, Karrholm J, Elmquist LG. Kinematics of active knee extensions after tear of the anterior cruciate ligament. *Am J Sports Med* 1989;17:796–802.
49. Smith RL, Brunoli J. Shoulder kinesthesia after anterior glenohumeral dislocation. *Phys Ther* 1989;69:106–112.
50. Lephart SM, Warner JJP, Borsa PA, Fu FH. Proprioception in the shoulder of healthy, unstable, and surgically repaired shoulders. *J Shoulder Elbow Surg* 1994;3:371–381.
51. Voight ML, Hardin JA, Blackburn TA, et al. The effects of muscle fatigue on and the relationship of arm dominance to shoulder proprioception. *J Sports Phys Ther* 1996;23:348–352.
52. Knott M, Voss D. *Proprioceptive neuromuscular facilitation.* New York: Hoeber Medical Division, Harper & Row, 1968:84–85.

CHAPTER 38

Cycling

Arnie Baker

BICYCLE SAFETY

Preventing accidents is the best strategy. Keep bicycle equipment safe, that is, well-maintained and in mechanically sound working order. Acquire the riding skills and techniques needed to operate a bicycle safely. Know how bicycle–car accidents commonly occur. Ride in a safe and defensive manner. Use specialized safety equipment.

Safe and Defensive Riding Style

Bicycle–car collisions account for only 10–20% of accidents, although they are what worry most cyclists and what cause the most serious accidents. Falls account for about 50% of accidents, and bicycle–bicycle collisions 10–20%. Bike–dog accidents and other causes split the remainder. Here are some rules for cyclists:

- Obey traffic codes. In most states bicycles are treated as vehicles. Learn the local bicycle laws and regulations.
- Be courteous as you share the road with others. Respect their rights and be tolerant if they trespass on yours.
- Assume that motorists will not see you. Motorists expect and look for other motorists but often have a blind eye for cyclists. Anticipate that a motorist will do something imprudent—for example, pull out in front of you.
- Look ahead of your current position; don't just look at the roadway beneath you. Anticipate possible problems down the road.
- Never have more people on a bicycle than there are seats. Never allow anyone to ride on your handlebars.

- Ride on the right side of the road (in the United States), not on the left and not on the sidewalk.
- Do not ride against traffic on one-way streets.
- Keep your hands on the handlebars. Do not ride no-hands.
- Use lights when riding at night.
- Obey stop signs or red lights.
- Do not hitch rides by holding onto other vehicles.
- Do not ride while under the influence of drugs or alcohol.
- Signal turns.
- Ride predictably in a straight line at a steady pace.
- When coming into a large road, yield to other vehicles.
- Look left, right, and left again (in the United States) before entering roads or intersections.
- Make eye contact with drivers. If you don't think they have seen you, shout politely and loudly, "Watch out!"
- Do not ride with headphones on.
- When riding alongside parked cars, check inside the car for a driver or passenger who may be preparing to open the car door.
- Even though you have the right of way, do not insist on it. Cars have much better protection against accidents than you do; you are more likely to be hurt than the motorist.

Safety Equipment

Protection Equipment

A helmet is an essential piece of safety equipment. Gloves protect against common hand scrapes that occur with most falls. They also provide comfort and prevent blistering, jarring, overuse, and hand nerve injuries.

Visibility Equipment

Lights are often required at night. Bright clothing is also useful. Vertical or horizontal flags are necessary for recumbent riders; they are also helpful to touring riders and used by commuters.

Other Equipment

Many riders consider mirrors essential. Bells alert other people to the cyclist's presence.

BICYCLE POSITION

Injuries in bicycling often result from either improper bicycling position or the lack of sufficient time for adaptation to a new position. Proper bicycle position and sufficient time for adaptation to a new position help prevent many injuries.

Certain general principles apply. There is a window of perfectly acceptable bike fit. The individual rider must make the final decision about position. Bicycle position is a compromise among many bicycling needs. The optimal position is different for maximizing muscle power, aerobic efficiency, and comfort and minimizing injury.

Too often riders are classically positioned without regard for their individual variations. Riders with anatomic variants—for example, upper or lower extremity discrepancy or turned-in or turned-out feet—should be fitted to allow for these differences.

Setup

The setup equipment includes the bicycle, a stationary trainer, bike tools, a plumb line, a level, a tape measure, calipers, and an assistant.

Level Bike

Set the bicycle on a trainer. Use blocks of wood to raise the front of the trainer to level the bicycle if necessary. Have the seat horizontal to start.

Warm-up

Pedal moderately for at least 10 minutes before adjusting. Pedal moderately for a few minutes between adjustments.

Where to Start

The order in which you perform adjustments is important. Some measurements depend on others. The order suggested works best for most riders.

Frame Sizing

When straddling a road bicycle, there should be an inch or two of clearance between the top tube and the crotch. For mountain bikes, there should be 2–3 inches of clearance. For road bikes, an alternative method is to measure the rider's inseam and multiply by 65%. This number is a starting point for the frame size you will need. Find the inseam by standing with back to the wall with a 1-inch book binding snug up against the crotch. Measure the distance from the floor to the top of the binding.

Pedal Fore-Aft

The cleat should be positioned so that the ball of the foot is over the pedal spindle. Sprint cyclists may prefer to back their feet out of the pedals a little more and be more on their toes.

Seat Height

Seat height is of paramount importance. Seat height selection is a compromise between aerobic efficiency, aerodynamics, power, and injury reduction. Cleat thickness, pedal type, and seat tube angle all influence this measurement. Formulas based on inseam measurements or other body dimensions can give only approximate results and can only provide starting points.

The higher the saddle, the more power can be generated and the less the aerobic cost. One must not be so far extended that the hips rock or that spin is restricted. Some riders determine position by raising the seat until their heels can just clear the pedals.

A seat height that results in 25–30° of knee flexion when the pedal is at the bottom of the stroke tends to result in the least injury but is not optimal for cycling power or for aerobic efficiency.

The higher the seat, the more likely the rider is to have pain in the back of the knee, Achilles tendon pain, or buttock ache. Low saddle positions are associated with anterior knee pain. Those with limited flexibility are the most likely to have problems.

Seat Position Fore-Aft

Some riders position the seat fore-aft by measuring the distance that a plumb line hanging from the nose of the saddle falls behind the bottom bracket. Road and mountain bike riders tend to have the seat an inch or more back. Sprinters and time trialists tend to have a more forward position.

Other riders determine their seat position by dropping a plumb line from the front of their knees when the cranks are horizontal. They look for the plumb to fall through the pedal axle.

After adjusting the fore-aft position, repeat the determination of seat height, since adjustment of saddle fore-aft may change the seat height.

Seat Angle

Most riders ride best when their seat is level. Sprinters, aero time trialists, and women may prefer to have the nose of the saddles pointing down slightly. Climbers may prefer to have the nose pointing upward slightly.

Pedal Rotation Angle

The cleat should be positioned so that the toes point nearly straight ahead. Some riders prefer their feet to be pointed slightly inward, while others prefer them slightly outward. Some may ride with cleats just slightly loose to determine the most comfortable position before the final tightening. Cleat position is not as critical with free-rotation systems.

In general, if the outside of the knee hurts, adjust the cleats to point the toes a little more outward. If the inside of the knee hurts, point the toes a little more inward.

Stem Height

The stem may be from 1–3 inches below the height of the saddle. The lower the stem, the more aerodynamic the rider. If the stem is too low, the rider may be uncomfortable, especially in the lower back, or lose power.

Stem Extension

Most bikes are sized so that most men end up needing stems 10–13 cm in length and most women require stems that are several centimeters shorter. When the handlebars are in the drop position, there should be scant clearance between the elbows and the knees, and the back should be flat. A rule of thumb is that the top of the bars should obscure the front axle when the rider looks down with his or her hands on the dropped handlebars.

Mountain bikers often prefer a combination of longer top tube and shorter stem for better handling on cross-country trails and downhill.

Handlebar Shape

The shape of the handlebar varies with the type of riding. For general road riding, a long top horizontal section is preferred for climbing comfort. The drop of handlebars is determined partially by the comfort level of the hands in the curve.

Handlebar Width

Handlebar width should be roughly the width of the shoulders.

Handlebar Angle

The handlebars should be angled so that the drops are perpendicular to the seat tube. This means that they are pointed downward about 15°.

Brake Levers

Brake levers are most comfortable when positioned such that their tips are in line with the bottom of the handlebar drops.

Leg-Length Discrepancy

Many riders have leg lengths that are different. This usually doesn't cause problems, especially if the difference is slight. But leg-length discrepancy can sometimes be a cause of knee, leg, or back discomfort. Shims, other devices, and cleat positioning can correct for leg-length discrepancy and can help alleviate these discomforts.

Although some theorize that correcting leg-length discrepancy results in a more effective stroke, no study has shown that correcting leg-length discrepancy improves power or aerobic economy.

Traditionally, differences less than $\frac{1}{4}$ inch (6 mm) are not considered significant. Some have claimed that differences of as little as $\frac{1}{8}$ inch (3 mm) are significant, especially for high-volume or high-intensity riders.

Measuring and Evaluating Leg Length

Leg-length differences can be in the upper leg (femoral) or in the lower leg (tibial). Leg length is traditionally determined by measuring the distance from the anterior superior iliac spine to medial malleolus. X-rays can be used to measure the length of the legs more accurately. It is easy to quickly eyeball and measure upper and lower leg-length differences:

Sit the rider with the back flat against a hard-backed chair, feet on the ground. Place a straightedge in front of the anterior (forward) protrusion of the kneecaps—point A in Figure 38-1. If an upper leg-length discrepancy is present, the straightedge will not be level against the knees. When the straightedge is level, the distance to the straightedge from the shorter leg is the upper leg-length discrepancy. Differences of a few millimeters are usually insignificant.

Place a straightedge on the superior (top) part of the knee—point B in Figure 38-1. If a lower leg-length discrepancy is present, the straightedge will not be level on the knees. When the straightedge is level, the distance to the straightedge from the shorter leg is the lower leg-length discrepancy. Differences of a few millimeters are usually insignificant.

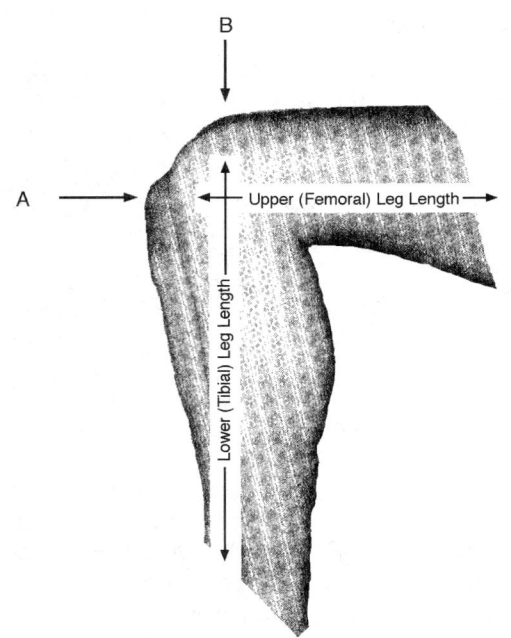

FIG. 38–1. Measuring upper and lower leg lengths.

Evaluating Leg Length by Knee Goniometry

Measuring leg length may not be the real issue. Some riders with no leg-length difference, for example, have an effective difference when riding because of arthritic changes in the hips or other factors. And some riders have accommodated to their differences with their pedaling styles.

Another approach is to measure the angles of the knees when pedaling. If they are equal, then the legs are effectively the same length. If they are different, the legs are effectively of different lengths, regardless of actual measurements.

The traditional method of measuring knee angles is to have the rider stop pedaling at the bottom of the stroke and measure knee angle with a goniometer.

Many riders change the angle of the knee when they stop pedaling by changing their ankle position. Measuring knee angles while the rider pedals using an electronic goniometer gives more accurate information.

How to Correct for Leg-Length Discrepancy

Set the seat height for the longer leg. Shim the exterior sole or cleat of the shoe of the shorter leg to equalize knee angles. In general, femoral (upper leg) differences require about one third correction, tibial (lower leg) differences about one half. So, for example, a femoral leg length discrepancy of 6 mm requires about a 2-mm shim. A tibial leg length discrepancy of 6 mm requires about a 3-mm shim.

Some femoral differences can also be partially accommodated by offsetting the cleat of the shorter leg forward (cycling more on the toes).

Small differences are sometimes shimmed with an insole. This often crowds the shoe interior and is not ideal. The insole of the shoe of the longer leg is sometimes removed as an easy fix for small differences. Again, a comfortable fit may now not be possible. Wearing different size shoes to accommodate different insole thickness is an unusual and rare alternative.

Some riders correct leg-length differences with eccentric chainrings, concentrically machined but off-center mounted chainrings, or different length cranks. These approaches are not recommended.

OVERUSE INJURIES

Overuse injuries are chronic, uncontrolled, overload, microtraumatic events.

Causes

Adaptation

Overuse injuries occur over a period of time when forces applied to a structure are increased faster than the structure can adapt or when the forces exceed the structure's limits of adaptation. Doing too much too soon often causes problems. In cycling, too many miles or mileage that is too intense, especially hills and big gears, often cause overuse injury. Less commonly, excessive spinning may cause problems.

Bicycle Fit

If a rider's fit or position is not optimal, it may contribute to overuse injuries.

Off-the-Bike Activities

Other athletic activities may help or hinder recovery. Weight lifting, running, jumping sports, and racquet sports may also cause or contribute to bicycle-related overuse problems. Weight training has many benefits, but it is taxing on the body. For example, many exercises that specifically strengthen the quadriceps—perhaps the most important bicycling muscle—also place big loads on the kneecap where it glides over the thigh bone. Full squats, leg extensions, and lunges are particularly grueling for knee structures. In the presence of knee pain, some weight training may need to be curtailed.

Running is also stressful on the knee. Running up and especially down hills places tremendous pressures on the knee. Running on inclines, such as along the beach or the side of a canted road, places stresses on the inside and outside of the knees. In the presence of knee pain, running may need to be stopped.

Anatomy and Overuse Injuries

A person's individual body type and construction may be a contributing factor. For example, some body types or anatomy predispose to certain overuse knee injuries:

- A wide pelvis places the knees farther apart and stresses the outside, or lateral, structures of the knee.
- The shinbone, or tibia, is twisted internally as a normal human variant in many people. This twist results in a tendency for the feet to turn inward. Trying to ride with toes pointed straight ahead may cause discomfort on the inside (medial) aspect of the knee.
- Unbalanced muscles or other anatomical variants may lead to the abnormal tracking of the kneecap.
- Leg-length discrepancy is not usually associated with problems in the general or recreational rider population unless the difference between the legs exceeds 6 mm ($\frac{1}{4}$ inch). However, long-distance riders or racers may experience leg-length discrepancy-related problems with as little as 3 mm ($\frac{1}{8}$ inch) difference.
- Excessive foot pronation is associated with medial (inside aspect of the) knee pain.

Riders with anatomic variants may require nonstandard configurations of their equipment—for example, asymmetrically positioned cleats in the case of leg-length discrepancy.

Specific Overuse Conditions and Injuries

This section will review specific cycling overuse injuries from the neck down. Bicycling-specific treatments will be emphasized; standard medical or surgical treatments will not. The lack of discussion of standard treatments is not meant to imply that these approaches are not important; rather, they are widely known, and space limitations prohibit their reiteration.

A considerable portion of this section will be devoted to the knee, since the knee is the most common site for overuse injury in cyclists, and bicycle-position adjustment for knee injury may be completely different depending on the type of knee injury.

Neck Pain

Consider a neurologic origin and consultation whenever neck pain is associated with upper extremity symptoms: pain, loss of sensation, or loss of power in the arms. Consider urgent or emergency medical consultation when pain in the front of the neck or pain in the jaw is associated with exercise: These symptoms may be of cardiac origin.

Etiology

Neck pain can follow strain or overuse. The pain may travel to the back of the head and become more generalized. If nerves are involved, it may travel to the arms. It is usually due to one or more of the following:

- Muscle strain and/or spasm
- Arthritis, usually degenerative osteoarthritis. Strain on the vertebral joints from misalignment, often secondary to disc degeneration, also causes pain.
- A bulge or herniation of an intervertebral disc. This may cause radicular pain.

In younger cyclists neck pain is usually due to muscle strain. In older cyclists a combination of muscle strain and degenerative changes is often responsible. Degenerative changes are usually aging-related, not cycling-related.

Cycling-related neck strain is often associated with long rides. Position on the bike can be important. Cyclists who lack flexibility may find the aerodynamic bent-over racing position uncomfortable. Anything that forces the rider to increase stretch in the neck may cause neck pain.

Women tend to ride bikes with top tubes that are too long. Most bikes are designed for men; women have relatively longer legs and relatively shorter reaches.

Jarring from rough mountain bike riding can be a factor. Road riders who keep their necks and shoulders locked and who forget to look around, are prone to neck pain.

Neck pain may be non-cycling-related, arising from muscle tension due to stress, anxiety, depression, or fatigue or from poor posture.

Treatment

If neck pain is due to long rides, allow for a gradual increase in endurance riding. Increase the length of endurance rides no more than 10% per week. Consciously relax the upper body—back, elbows, and neck—every few minutes. Change hand positions, which will change neck position and reduce strain. Stretch the neck on the bike. Look around: don't focus only on the pavement directly in front. A helmet is a must for safety, but make sure it is lightweight.

If pain is from craning the neck on the bike, ride with a more upright posture. Ride on the hoods or tops of the handlebars. Avoid the drops. Use a more upright bar. Reduce the distance needed to stretch. Raise or shorten the stem. Use narrower handlebars. Get a bike with a shorter top tube.

If pain is due to jarring, get a gel saddle. Use a suspension system. Ride a mountain bike on road rides. Consider a recumbent bike.

Scapula Syndrome

Physicians are concerned about pain in the upper back, around the shoulder blade. It may or may not be associ-

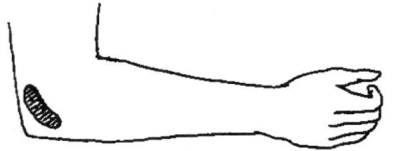 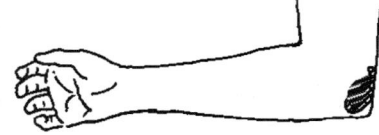

FIG. 38–2. Lateral (*left*) and medial (*right*) epicondylitis.

ated with neck, shoulder, or arm symptoms. It may or may not be related to cycling. The problem overlaps with those of neck ache, discussed above.

Cycling-Related Etiologies

Scapula syndrome may have the following causes:

- Extended saddle time. The longer one is in the saddle, the more other factors act to increase tension in this area.
- Rough terrain and jarring.
- Too much pressure. Weight distribution too far forward puts more pressure on the upper back and neck.
- Excessive use of upper back and neck muscles during sprinting, climbing, or other efforts.

Treatment

Reduce mileage and readapt slowly. Prevent jarring through the use of padded gloves and padded handlebar tape. Consider suspension. Reduce pressure: Sit more upright, vary position, raise stem height, and use a shorter stem. Check that the seat is not too far forward, and avoid tilting the saddle downward. Use a frame with a shorter top tube. Avoid strain: Reduce hard efforts involving the upper back muscles.

Epicondylitis

Physicians are concerned about pain at either the medial or lateral elbow that is unrelated to sudden injury. Injury, fracture, and swelling of the elbow are not discussed here (Fig. 38–2).

Etiology

Repetitive twisting usually causes the problem. The twisting irritates the forearm muscles as they rub over bony surfaces near the elbow. The irritation is often accompanied by microtears of the tendons. Pain at the outside of the elbow is lateral epicondylitis, or "tennis elbow." Pain at the inside is medial epicondylitis, or "reverse tennis elbow." Tennis is a frequent cause, but any repetitive twisting motion—whether it be polishing doorknobs, sorting items into slots, painting, or shaking hands—can cause the problem.

Cycling-related elbow pain is most frequent in mountain bikers who repetitively twist gear and brake levers. It may also occur in cyclists who ride tensed up with rigid outstretched arms.

Treatment

Be aware of twisting motions. Use a setup that reduces the need to twist or places shifters and brakes in a more ergonometric position.

Cyclist's Palsy: Ulnar Neuropathy

Practitioners should be concerned about pain, tingling, numbness, and weakness in the hand along the course of the ulnar nerve. Symptoms may be present in the fourth and fifth digits. Symptoms are worse during riding or for several hours afterward. Although this problem usually improves after riding stops, it can lead to permanent nerve injury if ignored (Fig. 38–3).

Etiology

The ulnar nerve is compressed in the heel of the hand—the fleshy part of the hand below the fifth digit. Cycling-related etiologies are as follows:

- Extended saddle time. The longer one is in the saddle, the more other factors act to press on the hand.
- Rough terrain, causing jarring of the hands while gripping the handlebars
- Improper hand position: too much time on the tops with the heel of the hand pressed against the bar
- Too much pressure. Weight distribution too far forward puts more pressure on the hands, wrists, and arms.

The affected hand is usually the one that stays on the handlebar—the one that doesn't reach for the water bottle.

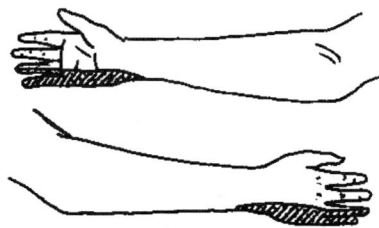

FIG. 38–3. Ulnar nerve pathway in the hand.

Treatment

Get pressure off the heel of hand when riding. Reduce mileage and readapt slowly. Prevent jarring by using padded or gel gloves; use padded, even double, handlebar tape; or try suspension. Improve hand position and reposition the hands frequently; relax the hands, wrists, and upper body. Reduce pressure and avoid placing pressure on the heel of the hand; vary position, raise stem height, check that the seat is not too far forward, use a shorter stem, avoid tilting the saddle downward, or use a shorter top tube.

Low Back Pain

Low backache makes riding uncomfortable. Low back pain is ubiquitous in noncyclists and cyclists alike.

Etiology

Acute low back pain can follow strain or overuse. The pain may travel to the buttock or thigh, but if nerves are not involved, it does not travel below the knee. It is usually due to one or more of the following:

- Muscle strain and/or spasm
- Arthritis—usually wear and tear/degenerative/osteoarthritis. Strain on the vertebral joints from misalignment, often secondary to disc degeneration, also causes pain.
- A bulge or herniation of an intervertebral disc

In younger cyclists, back pain is usually caused by muscle strain. In older cyclists, a combination of muscle strain and degenerative changes is usually responsible.

Cycling-related back strain is often related to long rides, big gears, or hill work. Big-gear riding and hill climbing—especially long grades—result in back pain because riders tighten their back muscles to get more power.

Position on the bike can be important. Cyclists who lack flexibility may find the aerodynamic bent-over racing position uncomfortable. Anything that forces the rider to increase stretch may cause back pain.

Jarring from rough riding can be a factor, and chronic low back pain may be due to non-cycling-related factors such as leg-length difference, lordosis, deconditioning and poor posture, and muscle tension due to stress, anxiety, depression, or fatigue.

Treatment

If back strain is due to excessive exercise load, allow for a gradual increase in endurance riding. Increase the length of endurance rides no more than 10% per week. If big gears are in the training program, allow time to adapt to them slowly.

If back strain is due to hills, reduce hill mileage, and then adapt to increased mileage slowly. Shift positions every so often from seating to standing. Consciously relax the back every few minutes when climbing. Take a rest break at the side of the road on long climbs and enjoy the view!

If back strain is related to an overly stretched out position on the bike, reduce stretch by assuming a more upright posture by a variety of methods: Ride on the hoods or tops of the handlebars, reduce the distance one needs to stretch, raise, or shorten the stem use narrower handlebars; or get a bike with a shorter top tube.

If buttock pain or sciatica is related to nerve pressure in the piriformis muscle, a gel-filled or more compliant saddle is sometimes effective.

If back strain is due to jarring, get a gel saddle; use a rear suspension system; ride a mountain bike on road rides; or consider a recumbent bike.

A heel lift, orthotic, or cleat shim may help if a leg-length difference exists.

Saddle Sores

Saddle sores may involve a number of separate problems involving the skin of the upper thigh, groin, and buttocks and are a common occupational hazard for the bicycle rider. Pressure, friction, and infection are the three main causes of saddle sores. Prevention is possible, and specific treatment is available.

Types of Saddle Sores

Furuncles and Folliculitis. Blocked and/or infected glands and lumps are a common cycling problem. These painful bumps are classic saddle sores.

Ischial Tuberosity Pain. Ischial tuberosity pain is pain in the area of the pelvic bones that bear the weight on the bicycle seat. Occasionally, pain in this area progresses to either a local bursitis or ulceration.

Chafing of the Thigh. Chafing of the inside of the upper leg is common in cyclists. It occurs because of friction caused by the repeated rubbing of the inside of the thigh during the up-and-down motion of the pedal stroke. Dampness of the cycling shorts related to sweat production and the lack of breathability of the shorts' material may make the problem worse.

Skin Ulceration. Skin ulceration is sometimes an extreme result of rubbing or pressure.

Relatively Rare Problems. Subcutaneous nodules are a specific type of lump found in elite male cyclists near the scrotum, sometimes called "extra testicles." A tailbone abscess is a genetic predisposition to a blocked pilonidal sinus that may be aggravated by cycling and become infected. Surgical treatment is often advised.

Etiology

There are two prevalent theories about the origin of classic saddle sores. The first has to do with infection and blocked glands: Bacteria get into glands and cause saddle sores. Therefore treatment is directed at reducing the level of skin bacteria and preventing pore blockage. The second theory has to do with pressure and friction. Saddle pressure creates local tissue ischemia. This causes a breakdown in the skin's defenses, pore irritation, and blockage. Trapped bacteria may proliferate. Treatment is directed at reducing tissue ischemia.

Riders who always get saddle sores on the same cheek may find that their leg on that side is shorter. The buttock of a shorter leg gets more bumping and bruising.

Prevention

Methods of prevention of saddle sores are as follows:

- Keep dry. Modern synthetics wick away moisture and are softer on the skin than traditional leather chamois. Don't wear wet, sweat-drenched shorts after riding. Change into loose shorts that allow air to circulate. After bathing, allow the crotch to dry completely before putting on tight-fitting shorts or cycling shorts. Powder in the shorts can prevent chafing that may lead to irritation and infected blocked glands (though powder may be linked to some cervical problems in women).
- Keep clean.
- Wear synthetic, padded cycling shorts.
- Wear clean cycling shorts. Soiled shorts not only have more bacteria, but also don't breathe as well as freshly laundered ones.
- Avoid cycling shorts that are pilled or have seams in areas that either rub the inside thigh or on which pressure is placed.
- Do not suddenly increase weekly mileage.
- Use seats that provide enough padding or support and spread the support over as wide an area as is compatible with the anatomy.
- Check the seat position.
- Avoid shaving above the short line to the groin.

Self-Treatment

Methods of self-treatment of saddle sores include the following:

- Apply the preventive measures described above.
- Modify training. The rider may need to reduce training or climb more out of the saddle.
- Soak in a comfortably hot bathtub three times a day for 15 minutes.
- For classic saddle sores or ischial tuberosity pain, pad the skin with padded tape or moleskin. A donut hole in the padding may help.
- Wear a second pair of shorts over the first; change to a padded seat or just a different seat.
- A padded seat cover may help.
- A different seat may help.
- Suspension may help. Rear-end suspension or beamed seat tubes reduce saddle pressure.
- A modification of seat position (nose up or down, forward or back) may help.
- Topical emollients, cortisone, or antifungal and antibacterial creams may help. A veterinary product, Bag Balm (8-hydoxyquinolone sulfate, petrolatum, lanolin), has a cultlike following.
- Shimming the shoe of the shorter leg may help if saddle sores are related to leg length discrepancy.

Medical and Surgical Treatment

If the area around the sore is infected, it may require surgical drainage or antibiotics. Uninfected saddle sores that remain painful, swollen, or lead to hard lumps can be treated with a cortisone injection. Occasionally, surgery may be required to remove chronic cysts.

Crotch Dermatitis

Crotch dermatitis is more common in women—specifically, irritation of the skin around the vagina, the clitoris, and the urethra. Crotch dermatitis is distinct from saddle sores.

Prevention

The best treatment is prevention. Some general measures will help almost all cases of crotch dermatitis. Some treatments may improve some cases but may make other cases worse. It is therefore important to determine the cause of crotch dermatitis.

Etiology

Many cases of crotch dermatitis are related to a combination of factors:

- Warmth and moisture
- Hygiene and irritants
- Friction
- Bicycle position and saddle
- Allergies
- Vaginal infections
- Medical problems, including dermatitis

Warmth and Moisture. Warmth and moisture aggravate most cases of crotch dermatitis. Avoid wearing bike shorts while traveling to races or rides; instead change into them on arrival. Use bike shorts with a breathable, moisture-wicking crotch. Change out of moist or wet bike shorts as soon as you can after riding. Wear loose-fitting shorts or a skirt, breathable fabrics, and cotton underwear. Avoid tight-fitting, nonbreathing underwear, or wear no underwear. Allow ventilation to cool and dry the area. Avoid sitting on nonbreathing surfaces such as plastic and leather. Use a car seat cover with air holes if the car has vinyl or leather seats.

Moisture and warmth cause yeast overgrowth—commonly called jock itch. Over-the-counter antifungal creams and powders may help to reduce yeast overgrowth. Occasionally irritated skin can also be helped by over-the-counter cortisone cream, though cortisone sometimes worsens yeast overgrowth.

Hygiene and Irritants. While stool is a powerful irritant, overzealous hygiene can be just as much of a problem as lack of hygiene. Excessive wiping and rubbing can cause chafing and irritation. Wipe from front to back, thus, in women, avoiding carrying bacteria toward the vagina and urethra. Such bacteria can aggravate crotch dermatitis as well as lead to urinary tract infections and vaginal infections. Avoid local irritants such as harsh soaps.

If crotch dermatitis extends to areas that one needs to wipe to keep clean, consider using facial tissue, medicated over-the-counter products such as Tucks, moistened toilet paper, or plain water. Clean, and then pat—not wipe—dry.

Friction. Using an emollient skin preparation, such as Vaseline, or an antiyeast cream can minimize friction. A seat pad or cover fitted over the saddle may allow slight movement and function similarly to a sock in the shoe.

Wearing two pairs of lightweight bicycling shorts or a lightweight bicycling liner may help to reduce friction-caused crotch dermatitis. But if crotch dermatitis is related to warmth and moisture, doubling up on shorts may make things worse.

Bicycle Position and Saddle. Most bicycles are sold for men; the top tube stem length results in too much reach for most women, leading to extra pressure on the crotch. Make sure the bicycle position is not too stretched out.

Saddle position and saddle type may be factors related to crotch dermatitis. Positioning the nose slightly downward may help, especially for time trial events or criterions in which one is in an aerodynamic position and putting a lot of pressure on the crotch. Some women prefer a nose-up position so that the saddle presses more on the pubic bone and less on the soft tissues around the vagina.

Move around frequently, and get off that saddle when possible. Stand up on the pedals to relieve crotch friction and pressure. Occasionally climb hills standing up. When descending, put weight on the pedals to relieve pressure on the crotch. This has the added benefit of allowing moving air to cool and dry the crotch. If riding tandem, be sure to take frequent breaks by getting out of the saddle at stop signs and stoplights and by standing at least every 15 minutes.

American-made Terry saddles have padding and are not as stiff as other saddles. Many women report that these saddles don't feel any different while riding, and at the end of a ride their crotches don't feel as much pressure. Recalcitrant cases of crotch dermatitis may require drastic measures; the rider may need to cut or pare the seat in order to keep riding.

Allergies. Many riders use a wide variety of products in the crotch area that may cause allergic reactions. To help with saddle sores near the crotch, riders may use tapes or pads, and they may have an allergic reaction to these. This can make the condition worse, turning saddle sores into saddle sores plus dermatitis. Some riders use perfumed or chemically treated products, including sprays, sanitary napkins, or lubricating oils, and they may be allergic to these.

Vaginal Infections. The extra moisture related to a vaginal infection may worsen crotch dermatitis, and treating the underlying vaginal discharge may help improve crotch dermatitis. Infected or otherwise blocked sweat or other glands may develop into crotch dermatitis if friction worsens these conditions.

Other Medical Problems

Riders with skin conditions such as herpes, psoriasis, or eczema may have flare-ups in this area related to friction and other general factors listed above. Prescription-strength cortisone creams are often the best help for this. Occasionally, other medical problems—such as lactose intolerance or pinworms—are the cause.

Knee and Lower Leg Problems

Overuse knee problems related to the repeated and constant stresses of riding over time are one of the most frequent reasons cyclists seek medical advice. Many bicyclists are former runners who have preexisting pathologies.

Some knee problems are sudden injuries related to trauma such as a bicycle crash or the sudden tearing of a cartilage or ligament. Sudden injuries, injuries with significant effusion, knee clicking, knee instability, and knee collapse are not discussed here. Torn ligaments, torn menisci, and fractures generally require standard, prompt orthopedic attention. Significant local redness or warmth may indicate an infection and requires prompt diagnosis. Those with a history of gout or other forms of arthritis are advised to seek medical attention. Mild problems may be self-treated, but any problem that does not respond within a couple of weeks is deserving of expert advice.

TABLE 38-1. Bicycle adjustment based on location of knee pain

Location	Etiology	Solutions
Anterior	Seat too low	Raise seat
	Seat too forward	Move seat back
	Climbing too much	Reduce climbing
	Big gears, low rpm	Spin more
	Cranks too long	Shorten cranks
Medial	Cleats—toes point out	Modify cleat position—toe in
		Consider floating pedals
	Floating pedals	Limit float to 5 degrees
	Exiting clipless pedals	Lower tension
	Feet too far apart	Modify cleat position—closer
		Shorten bottom bracket axle
		Use cranks with less offset
Lateral	Cleats—toes point in	Modify cleat—toe out
		Consider floating pedals
	Floating pedals	Limit float to 5 degrees
	Feet too close	Modify cleat position—apart
		Longer bottom bracket axle
		Use cranks with more offset
		Shim pedal on crank 2 mm
Posterior	Saddle too high	Lower saddle
	Saddle too far back	Move saddle forward
	Floating pedals	Limit float to 5 degrees

Bicycle Adjustment Based on Location of Knee Pain

Knee complaints can usually be identified as being anterior, medial, lateral, or posterior. Discussion of specific knee problems follows. Even without knowing the diagnosis, by knowing where the knee hurts, it is possible to make bicycle-position recommendations (Table 38–1 and Fig. 38–4).

Chondromalacia Patella

The patella glides over the proximal femur. Sometimes the undersurface of the patella is roughened or softened. Instead of gliding smoothly, it rubs roughly over the femur. This problem is also called patello-femoral dysfunction, or patello-femoral syndrome, because of the anatomic location of this problem.

A grating sensation at the front of the knee, pain going down stairs, and a general ache are frequent features. Stiffness after prolonged seating is common (Fig. 38–5).

Etiology. Excessive force pushing the patella onto the proximal femur creates excessive stress, which may result in patellar roughening. Some of the bicycling causes of excessive loading forces are hill climbing and big-gear time trialing. Weight training, running, squatting, kneeling, and climbing also place increased pressure on the patello-femoral surface.

A muscle or posture imbalance may cause the knee-

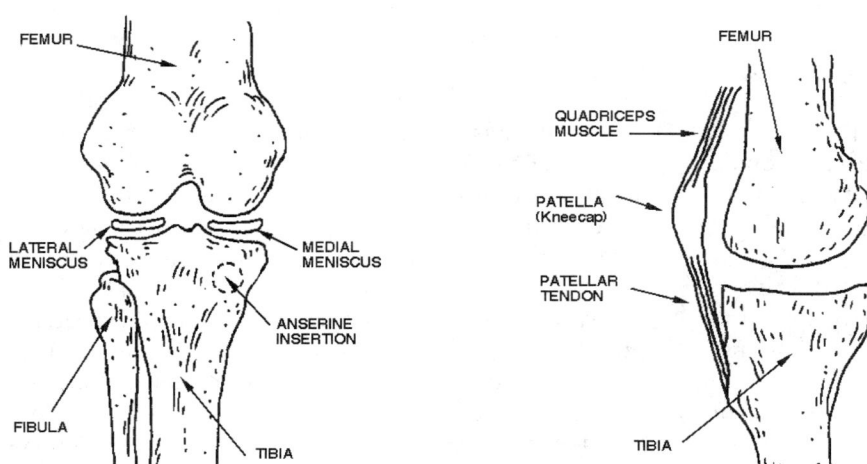

FIG. 38-4. Front (*left*) and side (*right*) view of the knee.

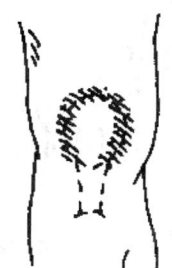

FIG. 38-5. Front-of-the-knee tenderness.

cap to stray from its ideal path over the surface of the femur. When not gliding over its ideal path, the patella is also subject to increased forces and becomes roughened. A relative weakness of the medial quadriceps muscle is often responsible. A wide pelvis and knock-knees may make the condition more likely.

Treatment. Bicycling correctly often helps this problem. Many runners suffer from chondromalacia, and bicycle riding is often suggested for therapy. A roughened kneecap may smooth out over time if the offending activities are stopped.

A position relatively high in the saddle helps—a knee that is not bent more than 25° from horizontal when the foot is at the bottom of the stroke. A position farther back in the saddle helps. Spinning rather than big gears—a cadence of 85 rpm or more—helps. Avoid hills, especially long climbs. Stand more when climbing and avoid long cranks.

If the problem is due to tracking rather than a load problem, pedals that allow some free rotation may help.

Off the bicycle, weight-lifting machines usually increase the load or shearing forces of the patella on the femur. Exercises in which the knee is bent more than 30° often worsen the problem. Squats, leg presses, and leg extensions all place increased loads on the patello-femoral surface. Avoid squatting or kneeling. Reduce walking down stairs or hills, and avoid running, especially down hills.

Look for exercises that involve only the last part of straightening the leg—terminal extension exercises that strengthen the quadriceps. Remember to be cautious about strength training when injured. Use strength training primarily to prevent reinjury.

Quadriceps stretching exercises are useful. If excessive foot pronation results in underneath-the-kneecap discomfort, orthotics may help. Surgery is the treatment of last resort. The underside of the roughed kneecap may have to be smoothed. If the gliding path of the kneecap is incorrect, repositioning the soft tissue may be tried, but this is a drastic step.

Patellar Tendinosis

The patellar tendon attaches the lower pole of the patella to the tibial tubercle. This type of tendinosis may take a relatively long time to resolve with continued riding.

Osgood-Schlatter disease, another form of patellar tendon problem found mostly in adolescent boys, results from growth-related traction. Pain is found where the patella tendon attaches to the tibia (Fig. 38-6), and there may be ossicles separated from the tibia.

Etiology. Tendinosis in this area from repetitive bicycling stress may follow a one-time injury to this area or may result from poor bike fit. Low saddle, forward position, big gears, and long hills all contribute to this problem. Tenderness at the kneecap's lower edge is occasionally due to a stress fracture.

In Osgood-Schlatter disease, growth of the bones during the growth spurt results in a pulling at the attachment of the patellar tendon at the tibial tubercle.

Treatment. On the bicycle, a position relatively high in the saddle helps—a knee that is not bent more than 25° from horizontal when the foot is at the bottom of the stroke. A position farther back in the saddle helps. Spinning rather than big gears—a cadence of 85 rpm or more—helps. Avoid hills, especially long climbs; avoid long cranks; and limit flotation to 5°.

Off the bicycle, the treatment is the same as that for chondromalacia. Jumping sports are particularly associated with patellar tendinosis.

Quadriceps Tendinosis

The quadriceps tendons attach the ends of the quadriceps muscles to either the upper pole of the patella. This type of tendinosis may take a relatively long time to resolve with continued riding.

Etiology. Tendinosis in this area from repetitive bicycling stress may follow a one-time injury to this area or may result from poor bike fit. A low saddle, a forward position, big gears, and long hills all contribute to this problem.

Treatment. Treatment is the same as that for patellar tendinosis and chondromalacia unless the medial quadriceps is involved, in which case terminal-extension strengthening exercises are to be avoided as well.

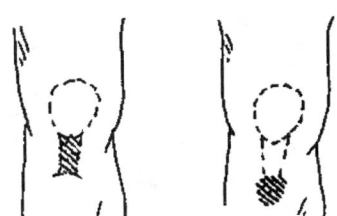

FIG. 38-6. Pain where the patellar tendon attaches to the shinbone.

Prepatellar Bursitis

Prepatellar bursitis is swelling and perhaps discomfort over the lower kneecap and patellar tendon caused by a swelling of the bursa. If this area is red, warm, or tender, it may be necessary to aspirate the bursa to make sure it is not infected.

Etiology. Continued irritation from an initial injury, such as a fall, may cause prepatellar bursitis. Overuse irritation from frequent prolonged kneeling, such as occurs in carpet laying or floor scrubbing ("housemaid's knee"), is also common.

Treatment. Treatment is the same as that for patellar tendinitis and chondromalacia above. Avoid kneeling, and use pads if kneeling must be continued. Nonsteroidal antiinflammatory drugs (NSAIDs), drainage and cortisone injection, and surgery are options, as for noncyclists.

Arthritis

The most common forms of arthritis—osteoarthritis, degenerative joint disease, or wear-and-tear arthritis—occur as we age. The additional knee stress of obesity, pushing big gears, or climbing may also contribute to this problem. Pain or aching is felt in the front of the knee or throughout the knee. Treatment is the same as that for chondromalacia. NSAIDs are a mainstay of treatment. Cortisone is occasionally used. Surgery—including total knee replacement—is used in the most severe cases.

Pes Anserine Tendinitis

The pes anserine tendon attaches at the proximal, medial aspect of the tibia (Fig. 38–7).

Etiology. Excessive forces may result from having the toes pointed outward or the knees too far apart when cycling. Exiting clipless pedals stresses the ligaments and tendons of the medial knee. Occasionally, improper saddle position is a factor. Some people's anatomy tends to predispose to this condition—those with tibial torsion, pronation, or bowed legs.

Treatment. If fixed cleats are used, adjust them so that the toes point a little more inward. If floating pedals are used, limit flotation to 5°. Reduce the tension of

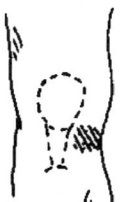

FIG. 38–7. Medial knee tenderness.

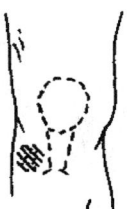

FIG. 38–8. Lateral knee tenderness.

clipless pedals to allow exit more easily. Reduce the distance between the feet by positioning the cleat so that the foot is closer to the crank, using a narrower bottom bracket axle, or using cranks with less offset. Use a proper saddle position and spin over 85 rpm and reduce mileage.

Off the bicycle, avoid running on inclines, especially when the affected leg is on the uphill side. Rollerblading and skiing may make this problem worse.

Plica or Patello-Femoral Ligament Inflammation

A plica is a fold or thickened band of tissue that arises within the knee, causing discomfort most frequently on the medial aspect of the knee. An inflamed medial patello-femoral ligament or torn medial meniscus causes similar symptoms. Often only surgery will distinguish the true diagnosis. Pain often occurs within a reproducible range of motion—once on the downstroke, once on the upstroke.

Etiology. Increased pressure on the inside of the knee is related to the problem. Extra force is caused by having the toes pointed outward or the knees too far apart when cycling. Occasionally, improper saddle position is a factor. Sometimes tibial torsion, pronation, or bowed legs tend to predispose selected cyclists to predispose to this condition.

Treatment. If fixed cleats are used, adjust them so that the toes point a little more inward. If floating pedals are used, limit flotation to 5°. Reduce the distance between the feet by positioning the cleat so that the foot is closer to the crank, using a narrower bottom bracket axle, or using cranks with less offset. Use a proper saddle position and spin over 85 rpm, and reduce mileage. Running, skiing, and rollerblading make the problem worse.

Iliotibial Band Syndrome

The iliotibial band is a fibrous band of tissue running along the lateral aspect of the knee. It rubs over the lateral surface of the knee, especially at the time when the knee is bent about 30°. It is commonly inflamed, causing pain in this area (Fig. 38–8).

Etiology. Excessive stretching in this area is the most

common cause. It results from too much pull on the lateral knee. Maladjusted cleat position, with the toes pointing inward, is the most frequent cause. A narrow bottom bracket or cranks with little offset may be associated with iliotibial band syndrome. Low saddle height and excessive forces due to big gears and hills are contributing factors. Sometimes iliotibial band syndrome develops after a fall and a bruise to this area. Those with a wide pelvis, tight gluteal muscles, or tight iliotibial band may be predisposed to this condition.

Treatment. Readjust the cleats to allow the toes to point outward a little more. Limit the flotation to 5°, and increase the distance between the feet by positioning the cleats so that the foot is farther from the crank by inserting a 2-mm spacer between the pedal and the crank, using a wider bottom bracket, or using cranks with more offset. Reduce hill work. Make sure the saddle height is neither too low nor too high and not too far back. Off the bicycle, avoid running, especially across inclines where the affected leg is uphill.

Tight Hamstrings

Tight hamstrings can be a cause of pain behind the knee.

Etiology. High seat position and sitting too far back in the saddle are contributing factors. Dropping the heel when climbing and pushing big gears worsen the problem. Lack of flexibility is usually present. Improper cleat position can be a factor in fixed-pedal systems. Sometimes excessive pedal float is related to this problem because the hamstrings help to stabilize the leg when pedaling. Relative weakness of the hamstrings, compared to the strength of the quads, can be a contributing factor.

Treatment. Sit farther forward in the saddle, and avoid a high saddle position. Avoid dropping the heels when pushing a big gear or climbing. Use pedals that limit float to less than 5°.

Baker's Cyst

A Baker's cyst is found behind the knee. It is a swelling of a sac that has its origins either within the knee or from a bursa associated with a muscle behind the knee. It is an occasional cause of posterior knee pain. If the cyst ruptures, it can cause calf pain, which may mimic the pain of thrombophlebitis.

Etiology. Baker's cyst is caused by a weakness in the tissues. When associated with a sac that has its origins within the knee, it often indicates a more serious problem within the knee.

Treatment. Sit farther forward in the saddle. Avoid a high saddle position. Avoid dropping the heels when pushing a big gear or climbing.

Tibialis Anterior Tendinosis

Etiology. This problem is caused by excessive tendon strain on the upstroke, especially when the foot is dorsiflexed.

Treatment. Avoid a forceful pull-up. Occasionally, a high saddle contributes to the problem. Lowering the saddle may help. This problem is more common in runners, so avoid running, especially on hills.

Achilles Tendinitis

Etiology. Excessive stretch from unaccustomed activity usually causes the problem. This most often results from a new shoe or cleat, especially when the net consequence is that the extension of the leg has been increased. Somewhat paradoxically, a seat that is too low can also cause Achilles tendinitis. In an attempt to get more power, the rider may drop the back of the foot, placing excessive and repeated stretch on the Achilles tendon.

With unequal leg lengths, the shorter leg is more likely to have an Achilles problem. A cleat that is too far forward or positioned so that the foot is toed-in occasionally causes this problem. Soft or flexible soles may contribute to the condition. Cold, wet weather riding, in which the back of the sock gets wet and cold, may also cause the problem.

Treatment. Ride if pain free and reduce hill mileage. To reduce stretch on the Achilles tendon, most riders lower the saddle a few millimeters. If the problem is associated with other activity, that activity may need to be modified. For example, if Achilles tendinitis is associated with new shoes with a lower heel used for walking or running, a heel pad or lift may help.

Achilles Bursitis

Achilles bursitis is also known as posterior calcaneal bursitis. The common term is pump bump.

Etiology. The heel counter of an offending shoe irritates the bursa, causing Achilles bursitis.

Treatment. Avoid wearing the offending shoe, or cut out the offending heel counter.

Foot Problems

Foot problems related to cycling include neuropathy and hot and cold feet.

Etiology. Pain, burning, or numbness is almost always caused by pressure around the foot. Old-style cleats with toe-straps that are too tight, shoes that are too tight, or shoe straps that are cinched too tightly are the usual causes. Occasionally, high mileage and an improperly positioned cleat contribute to the problem. Sometimes the cause is arthritis or a non-cycling-related medical condition.

In cool weather cold feet may result from compression of the foot and the resulting decrease in blood circulation.

Treatment. For pain, burning, or numbness the solution is to relieve the pressure. Loosen the toe-straps, loosen the shoes, or buy wider or larger shoes. When stopping for lunch or rest—even if only for a few minutes—take off the shoes and wiggle the toes.

Occasionally, the problem is due to cleat position. Usually, the cleat needs to be placed farther back, though solutions differ. Do whatever allows the foot more room in the shoe.

An irregularity of the sole of the shoe—occasionally a manufacturing defect—may press on the ball of the foot. Look carefully for cleat bolts that are pushing through the sole, causing it to be uneven.

Too much or too little cleat–shoe contact may contribute to the problem. Orthotics, which can spread the pressure, may help.

Occasionally, the problem relates to a Morton's neuroma. Local cortisone, orthotics, and surgical removal of the neuroma are options.

For cold feet, relieve the pressure, consider wider or larger shoes that allow room for thermal socks, or use shoe covers.

Male Problems

Pudendal Neuropathy

Men frequently experience penile paresthesia. Occasionally, priapism results. The problem is worse on long rides and worse after riding for prolonged periods bent over using dropped or aero bars.

Etiology. The pudendal nerve itself—or the small arteries that supply it—is compressed between the symphysis pubis and the bicycle seat.

Treatment. The best treatment is prevention. Since the usual cause is riding bent over for too long, remove the pressure from the genitals periodically by standing on the bike or otherwise changing position.

Adjust the seat position so the nose of the saddle is pointing downward a little more, or lower the height of the seat. A padded or different saddle—perhaps a differently shaped saddle with a different width—or padded bicycling shorts may help.

Long-Term Complications. Occasional nerve disturbance in this area usually resolves rapidly when pressure is relieved. Most riders have normal sensation return within minutes.

Sometimes as much as 24 hours is required for the nerve to return to apparently normal function. Rarely, more than a day is required. The longer it takes for the nerve to return to normal, the more damage is being done. Neuropathy should be avoided as much as possible because of the possibility of permanent nerve damage.

Impotence

It is not unusual for riders to have occasional difficulties in sexual relations because of riding. In some instances bicycling can cause permanent impotence.

Etiology. The nerve supply to the penis can be reduced from bicycle seat pressure. Decreased sensation in the penis can contribute to reduced sexual performance. This problem is usually a temporary one, although accident and injury can cause prolonged problems. There are reports of prolonged nerve damage from prolonged pressure.

Libido depends on many factors, including testosterone. Studies have shown that elite athletes have decreased levels of testosterone during their racing seasons. These factors, combined with the general exhaustion of training and racing, often result in decreased sexual activity.

Treatment. Avoid excessive compression of the genitals and nerve injury through proper bicycle position. Understand the physiologic effects of significant training on overall energy level and libido. Consider modifying the training schedule if training is interfering with the ability to maintain normal sexual activity.

Urinary Symptoms

Cycling-related pressure, leading to inflammation of the urethra, may cause frequent urination, dribbling, decreased urinary stream force, nighttime urination, or burning on urination. In addition, an infection can be a complication of this irritation.

Riders over the age of 40 may have difficulties that are related to the prostate. Hesitancy before urinating and dribbling after urinating are common problems with the prostate and are, for many men, a normal part of aging. Since other medical conditions may also cause these problems, a general physical examination that includes a prostate examination is advised. Cycling does not cause prostate pathology, but it is controversial whether it can worsen symptoms.

Pressure can be relieved by varying position, by using padded saddles, by using wider tires with lower air pressure, by using suspension, or by using less stiff bicycles or recumbent bikes.

Prostatitis

Although some believe that pressure on the prostate can cause or aggravate typical prostate symptoms, many physicians doubt this and find no scientific evidence to support the hypothesis. Most physicians doubt that infection of the prostate is related to cycling. Cancer of the prostate is not related to cycling.

Female Problems

While some problems specific to women have been discussed (e.g., crotch dermatitis), other conditions exist.

Nipple Friction and Pain

Riding can result in irritation of the nipples when clothing chafes at the skin and causes irritation. Once the nipples are irritated, repeated rubbing from clothing worsens the problem. Clothing that is wet is especially irritating.

A support or sport bra may help. A lightweight undershirt under the jersey will also reduce skin irritation. Sometimes an adhesive bandage covering helps a particularly irritated nipple, or an emollient, such as Vaseline, may protect the skin and reduce irritation. Riders should wear layers, dress appropriately for the weather, and change out of wet clothes as soon as possible.

Bicycle-Seat Discomfort

Whereas most men will find the same kinds of saddles comfortable, this is not the case for women whose pelvises have a number of anatomic variants. For this reason the shape of a saddle that will provide the most comfort is an individual affair. Riders must often try differently shaped saddles to determine the type that best matches their anatomy. Some saddles specifically marketed for women are likely to be more comfortable.

As stated earlier, most bicycles that are sold are designed for men. As a result, most bikes are sized with too long a top tube, and this stretched position can make the seat uncomfortable for women near the pubic bone. Traditionally seat position has been with the nose of the saddle pointed slightly upward or level. Some women find it more comfortable to position the nose of the seat slightly pointed downward; this will also help avoid irritation of the urethra.

The time trial position is often the worst for most women. Improved flexibility may allow pelvis rotation, reducing pressure on the pubic area, while at the same time allowing a more aerodynamic position.

Dyspareunia

For many women, riding places pressure on the vaginal and pubic areas. This pressure may result in local inflammation or irritation, including swelling and chafing. Since sexual activity often also places pressure on these areas and may cause similar soreness due to inflammation, some women have discomfort riding after sexual activities, and some women have difficulty with sexual activities soon after riding. Placing more pressure on the buttocks and away from pubic areas may be helpful. Riders should use the handlebar tops more than the drops. Make sure bike fit is correct—not too stretched out, with the nose of the saddle not too high. A different saddle may help.

Vulvar Swelling

Women who spend a lot of time on the saddle occasionally develop swelling of the vulva, often unilateral. Pain is not usually a problem. The etiology of the condition is uncertain. This problem is not considered dangerous, and riding is usually continued. Swelling due to Bartholin or other gland abscess requires standard treatment.

Tampon Hints

Tampon strings that are left outside the vagina may result in chafing. If flow is so heavy that one tampon is insufficient, using two tampons, placed side by side, may be more comfortable than using a tampon and a pad.

SPECIFIC TRAUMATIC INJURIES

Illustrative, specific traumatic injuries will be presented because of their frequency in cyclists or because of their cycling-specific treatment.

Serious head injury is not a common injury, and treatment for cyclists follows the same lines as treatment for other individuals. Because head injuries are potentially fatal, and often preventable with the use of helmets, this topic will also be discussed.

This section is not meant to be a comprehensive review of all traumatic injuries in cycling. Injuries that do occur in cyclists but with low frequency and injuries that are treated in the same way in noncyclists—such as splenic rupture or carpal bone fracture—will not be discussed.

Abrasions

Abrasions, also known as road rash, are the most common of bicycling injuries and can be treated in different ways.

Treatment Objectives

The objective of treatment is to heal the tissues as rapidly and effectively as possible. Goals of therapy include not allowing the depth of the rash to increase in severity, rapid healing, and minimizing pain.

Grading Road Rash

The severity of road rash is similar to that of burns:

- First-degree abrasion: Only the surface is reddened. This problem does not require active treatment.

- Second-degree abrasion: The surface layer of the skin is broken, but a deep layer remains that will allow the skin to replace itself and heal without significant scarring.
- Third-degree abrasion: The skin is entirely removed, perhaps with underlying layers of fat and other supporting tissue structures exposed. Such damage may require skin grafting.

Open Treatment

There are two general methods of treatment. The first is the traditional "let nature take its course" approach, also called the open method. This involves cleaning the wound with soap and water, hydrogen peroxide, an iodide, or something similar and then allowing the wound to dry out, form a scab, and heal on its own.

This method has drawbacks for all but the smallest and most superficial abrasions. Just because they have been cleaned once doesn't mean that abrasions will not get infected. Bacteria thrive on damaged skin. Infection can deepen the depth of the abrasion, making scarring and delayed healing more likely. Scabs can crack and become painful. Scabbed areas don't receive oxygen well from the surrounding air and therefore take much longer to heal.

Closed Treatment

The alternative is the closed approach: frequent cleansings and the application of topical antibiotics and dressings that keep the abrasion moist. The area is cleansed at least daily with wet compresses or bathing. Superficial debris is gently removed. An effort is made to remove soft-forming exudates with gentle scrubbing. These exudates usually form between the third and fifth days after injury. Pink, healthy, new-forming skin is what one wants to see. Second-degree abrasions usually take 2–3 weeks to heal.

Treatment Supplies

Silver sulfadiazine (Silvadene), mupirocin (Bactroban), or Polysporin is applied. A Vaseline gauze (e.g., Adaptic) is placed over this. This is a nonstick mesh that allows removal of the dressing without sticking. Padding in the form of gauze squares may be applied. Then a conforming gauze roll is wrapped around the area and taped in place. Finally, a tube stretch gauze (e.g., Tubigauze) is applied over this to keep everything in place and tidy. Alternatively, Tegaderm (3M) or Bioclusive (Johnson & Johnson) alone may be stretched over the antibiotic. The result is a dressing that allows maximum protection of the wound, minimum risk of infection, prevention of scabbing and its attendant cracking and pain, and healing as fast as possible.

Side Effects

People who are allergic to sulfa drugs should avoid sulfadiazine. As the skin nears complete healing, one may be tempted to become less attentive to treatment. Sun exposure may cause permanent pigmentary abnormality. Keep abrasions covered until they are completely healed or use adequate sunscreen (SPF > 15).

Clavicular Fracture

Fracture of the clavicle is the most common break in a fallen cyclist. A clavicular fracture is usually the result of falling on an outstretched hand, which causes indirect violence to the shoulder girdle.

Healing and Treatment

Most bones heal in about 6 weeks. The clavicle is no exception. About 80% of the time the clavicle breaks between the middle and distal third. This type of clavicular fracture, in which the bones are in good alignment, has an excellent prognosis. About 15% of the time the break is much closer to the acromioclavicular joint, in which case healing may be more difficult. Rarely, the break is near the sternum.

Most clavicular injuries will heal without much medical or surgical intervention. A figure-of-eight bandage, which pulls the shoulders back, is sometimes prescribed for a couple of weeks. This may help keep the ends of the bones in alignment and reduces discomfort. Additionally, the arm is often placed in a sling. Most patients discard the sling and bandage after a week or two.

Surgery may be required in the unusual case. Occasionally, the break compresses a nerve and surgery is required for decompression. Surgery may be advisable from the outset in some breaks close to the A-C joint associated with significant ligament damage.

Orthopedic surgeons rarely perform surgery on broken clavicles in the United States. Their European counterparts are more likely to consider a surgical option, especially for athletes, to provide a more rapid return to racing. New operative techniques for stabilization of displaced clavicular fractures may lead to more surgical management in the future.

Return to Riding

For aligned clavicle breaks in which normal healing is expected and the athlete is very motivated, training can resume almost immediately, usually in 48 hours. Since jarring of the road is uncomfortable, training is performed on a stationary trainer. A specific workout plan is invaluable; otherwise, most riders waste their time. Raising the front of the trainer a few inches (6 cm) will allow the rider to ride in a more upright position with less weight on the shoulder and less pain.

Active shoulder exercises may be begun when pain lessens, usually about a week after injury. Most riders with fractured clavicles can ride the road in about 2 weeks, especially on a hybrid or mountain bike with fat tires that absorb road shock. After an uncomplicated clavicle fracture, serious road riding and racing can resume in about 4–6 weeks. Mountain bike racing may be delayed another month.

The above are guidelines for motivated racers with "good" breaks. Some riders have won national or world championships within days of a clavicular fracture. Many others take several months to get back to competition.

Shoulder Separation

Shoulder separation, also known as A-C sprain, is a common bicycling injury. The clavicle is held to the shoulder blade at the A-C joint by a fibrous envelope or capsule. There are also two coracoclavicular ligaments—fibrous attachments between the clavicle and the coracoid part of the shoulder blade.

Severity of Injury

Shoulder separations are classified according to severity and X-ray appearance:

- First-degree separation: The capsule is stretched but not completely torn. Local pain at the A-C joint worsens with abduction of the arm. X-rays do not show any movement at the A-C joint.
- Second-degree separation: Capsule disruption is such that X-ray shows some movement of the acromion downward relative to the clavicle. This displacement is less than the width of the clavicle.
- Third-degree separation: The separation is as much as or more than the width of the clavicle. The coracoclavicular and A-C ligaments have been torn.

Treatment

First- and second-degree separations are treated with a sling. Range-of-motion exercises may begin when pain allows, usually within a week of the injury. Stationary trainer workouts may begin almost immediately. Road riding and racing can commence as discomfort allows. Third-degree separations may take as long as 6 weeks to heal on their own. Some orthopedic surgeons prefer operative treatment of third-degree separations.

Shoulder Dislocation

Anterior or posterior dislocations of the shoulder are usually reduced in emergency rooms, and neurovascular status is always checked before reduction. Although reduction can take place in the field, either the original injury or reduction can cause fracture. X-ray control before reduction properly identifies those fractures before reduction. A sling is often prescribed for discomfort. Although training on a stationary trainer may resume almost immediately, many physicians believe that keeping the arm in a sling for 3 weeks, together with physical therapy, helps to prevent recurrent dislocations.

Head Injury and Helmet Use

Head injury is the most common cause of cycling-related death:

- In the United States, about 1,000 bicycling deaths each year are caused by head injuries.
- About 80% of all cycling deaths result from head injuries.
- Sixty to seventy percent of all serious bicycle injuries involve head trauma.
- Fifty percent of head-injury deaths occur in adults, and 50% occur in children and adolescents.
- Head injury rates are reduced by as much as 85–95% by using a helmet.

To be effective, a helmet must be properly fitted. It needs to be the right size, it must be worn covering the top of the forehead, and straps must be snug. A number of helmet safety standards exist, including those of the American National Standards Institute (ANSI) and the Snell Memorial Foundation. Approved helmets carry a sticker.

Helmets lose much of their effectiveness after a crash and should be replaced. Helmet materials deteriorate with age, so helmets should be replaced at least every 5 years.

As in other professional sports, whenever new safety equipment is introduced, there is often resistance to the adoption of such equipment. For example, when hockey helmets were first introduced, complaints were loud and strong. After a few years, or even a generation of athletes, such safety requirements tend to be not only adopted, but also embraced by all.

Heat is not an issue. Although at rest wearing a helmet is hotter, while riding, modern well-ventilated helmets have no significant effect on overheating riders on hot days; some studies even show a cooling effect. Aerodynamics is improved in comparison with riding bare headed. Weight is of trifling significance since helmets weigh only about half a pound. Cost should not be an issue because the cost of a helmet is a fraction of the cost of a single emergency room visit and about the same as the cost of a routine doctor's office visit.

BIBLIOGRAPHY

Baker A. *Smart cycling: Successful training and racing for riders of all levels.* New York: Simon & Schuster, 1997.

Baker A. *Bicycling medicine.* New York: Simon & Schuster, 1998.

Birnbaum JS. *The musculoskeletal manual.* Orlando, FL: Grune & Stratton, 1986.

Garrick J, Webb D. *Sports injuries, diagnosis and management.* Philadelphia: WB Saunders, 1990.

Grisolfi CV, Rohlf DP, Navarude SN, et al. Effects of wearing a helmet on thermal balance while cycling in the heat. *Phys Sportsmed* 1988;16(1):139.

Lamb DR. *Physiology of exercise: Responses and adaptations.* New York: Macmillan, 1984.

McArdle W, Katch F, Katch V. *Exercise physiology.* Philadelphia: Lea & Febiger, 1994.

Mellion MB, Burke E. *Clinics in sports medicine: Bicycling injuries.* Philadelphia: WB Saunders, 1994.

Weiss BD. Bicycle-related head injuries. *Clin Sports Med* 1994;13(1):99–111.

Wilson JD, et al: *Harrison's textbook of internal medicine.* New York: McGraw-Hill, 1991.

CHAPTER 39

Dance

William T. Hardaker, Jr.

Theatrical dance is an art form and, as such, is to be distinguished from social and ballroom dance. It encompasses the disciplines of classical ballet, modern dance, ethnic dance, and various mixed forms, such as Broadway and jazz. The elite professional dancer is a combination of superior artist and high-performance athlete. Few would dispute the grace, elegance, and projection of the accomplished theatrical dancer. It has been only recently, particularly in the medical community, that many have come to recognize the strength, power, and coordination of these remarkable athletes. In essence, contemporary dancers must possess the agility and balance of the gymnast, the speed and strength of the football running back, the reaction time and hand-eye coordination of the baseball player, and the body control and jumping ability of the basketball player. Indeed, many exercise kinesiologists and physiologists consider the professional dancer to represent the ultimate athlete (1–4).

PATHOGENESIS

Dancers, as athletes, can become injured. Although acute injuries can occur in dance (5), the vast majority are chronic and relate to a single mechanism of injury: the repetitive impact loading of the lower extremities on a hard, unyielding surface of the dance floor. In this regard, dancers and long-distance runners share a common mechanism of injury with subtle yet significant differences. The runner is equipped with a specially constructed shoe utilizing high-technology materials with the major design emphasis directed toward maximum cushioning and stability. Blown and/or carbon rubber are components of a very durable outsole. Ethylene vinyl acetate and polyurethane, often encapsulating inert gas or silicone gels, provide cushioning and support within the midsole. Plastisote, Spenco, and other synthetic materials provide further support within the insole. The upper consists of lightweight nylon mesh.

In contrast, the classical ballet dancer wears nothing but a soft slipper or toe shoe, wherein the design emphasis rests on tradition and aesthetics. In further contrast, the materials that are used in the construction of ballet shoes include satin, leather, burlap, cardboard, and wheat paste. In modern dance the performers routinely wear no shoes at all. The majority of the forces of cyclic loading must therefore be dissipated in the lower extremities. It is the failure to effectively and efficiently dissipate these forces that can and does lead to the majority of chronic dance injuries (6).

The complex interplay of anatomic variation and improper technique often contributes to the production of dance injury. Anatomic variation within the foot and ankle can determine the effectiveness of energy absorption and dissipation within the lower extremity. Excessive femoral anteversion, genu varum, genu valgum, tibia vara, and leg length discrepancy all represent potential malalignments that can lead to ineffective shock absorption. The high cavus foot with its relatively rigid midtarsal joint, pronates incompletely, thereby absorbing energy poorly within the pronation cycle. The forces of cyclic loading may then be directed to structures that are poorly suited to absorb stress. Indeed, the cavus foot is especially vulnerable to midfoot strain, plantar fasciitis, and stress fractures about the foot, ankle, and lower leg (6).

The ability to externally rotate the hip, or "turn out," is fundamental to all forms of theatrical dance. Turnout is especially emphasized in classical ballet, in which each of the five basic positions have in common maximum external rotation of the leg (Fig. 39–1). Indeed, all ballet movements begin or end with one of the five basic positions.

Under optimum circumstances turnout would be achieved primarily at the hip, with smaller contributions

---

W. T. Hardaker: Division of Orthopaedic Surgery, Duke University Medical Center, Durham, North Carolina 27710.

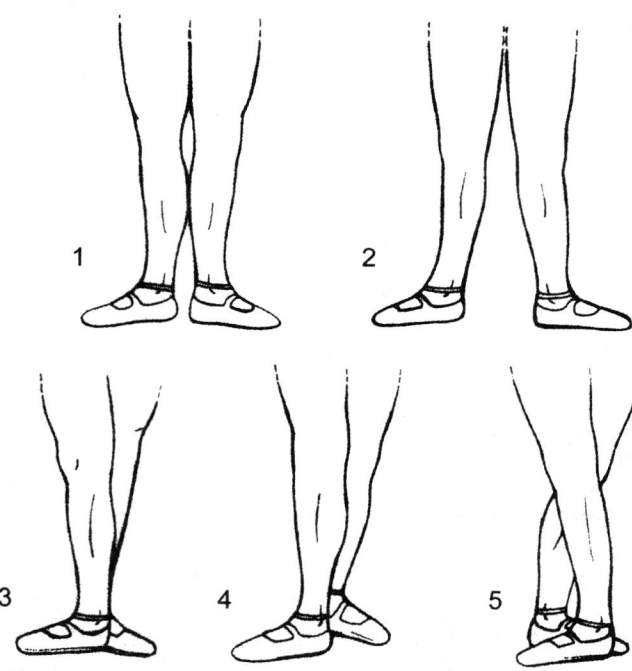

FIG. 39–1. The five basic positions of classical ballet have in common maximum external rotation of the leg.

coming from the foot, ankle, and knee joints (6,7). In the ideal sense, 60–70 degrees of turnout would occur at the hip, with the remaining 20–30 degrees occurring in combination from the foot, ankle, and knee (Fig. 39-2). Multiple factors determine the ability to externally rotate or turn out at the hip joint. These include the angle of femoral anteversion, the orientation of the acetabulum, the elasticity of the hip joint capsule, and, finally, the flexibility of the muscles that cross the hip joint (6). No alteration in the bony constraints of the acetabulum and femoral anteversion can be anticipated in the skeletally mature dancer. Dancers with inherent ligamentous laxity and those with flexible muscle units may increase their turnout at the hip joint with proper stretching protocols (8).

Dancers with poor "natural turnout" at the hip joint may force external rotation at the foot, ankle, or knee joints (Fig. 39-3). "Rolling-in" and "sickling" are dance terms that refer to excessive pronation/eversion at the foot and ankle joints and can represent techniques that some dancers use to compensate for inadequate external rotation of the hip. The consequence of either maneuver is to cause excessive strain on the medial structures of the foot and ankle joint and can lead to a variety of injuries to structures in this region (6,9–14).

Forced external rotation at the knee joint can lead to injury to both intraarticular and extraarticular structures. Chronic strain of the medial ligamentous complex can produce pain and abnormal laxity within the tibial collateral ligament and medial retinaculum. The medial meniscus can become trapped beneath the femoral condyle, leading to intersubstance degenerative change and eventual tears in this important structure. With retinacular laxity, the patella may sublux laterally, creating the environment for a variety of patellofemoral tracking disorders (6,7,10,15).

ANKLE SPRAINS

Ankle sprains represent the most common acute injury seen in theatrical dance (5,16). Inversion sprains are most frequently seen and involve injury to the lateral

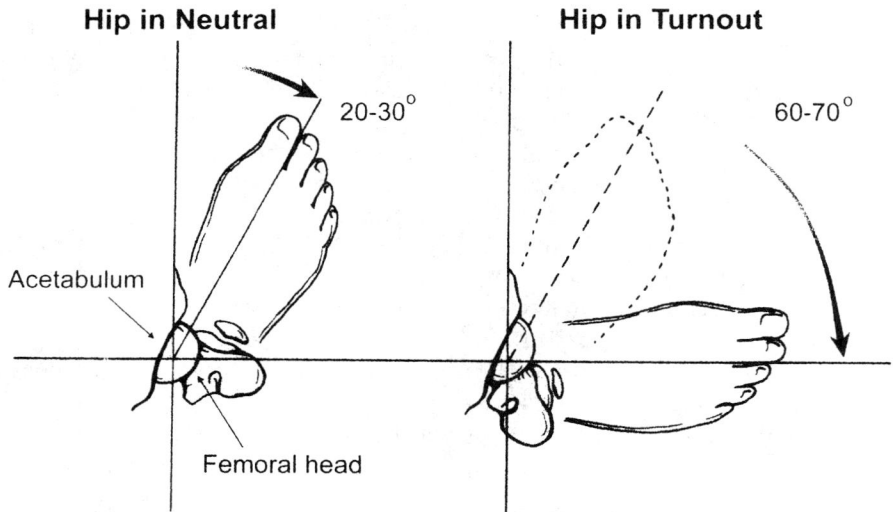

FIG. 39–2. The dancer's hip in turnout. Under ideal circumstances 90 degrees of turnout is achieved by a combination of external rotation at the hip, knee, and ankle joints. The greatest external rotation occurs at the hip joint (60–70 degrees), the remaining 20–30 degrees occurring in combination from the foot, ankle, and knee joints.

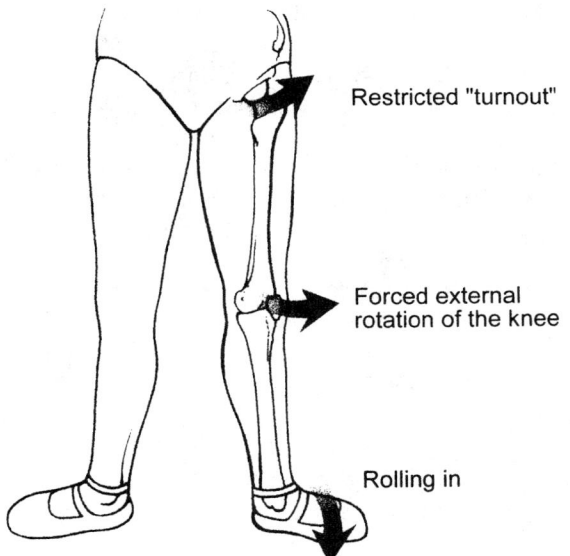

FIG. 39–3. Dancers with poor "natural turnout" may compensate for lack of external rotation at the hip by forcing external rotation at the knee and/or at the foot and ankle complex. "Rolling-in" refers to forced eversion in pronation at the foot and ankle complex and represents a maladaptive technique to increase external rotation of the leg.

ligamentous structures. Such sprains can result from forced inversion of the hindfoot while landing from a jump or from a misstep, particularly while partnering. The plantar-flexed foot renders the talus relatively unstable within the ankle mortise. The anterior talofibular ligament represents the primary static restraint to inversion stress. Forced inversion in the plantar-flexed position can lead to stretch or partial or complete tear of this important lateral structure. On examination tenderness may be isolated to the anterior talofibular ligament, suggesting injury to only that ligament. Tenderness and swelling over both the anterior talofibular and calcaneofibular ligaments indicate a more severe sprain involving both structures. Routine radiographic examination is recommended to rule out the possibility of fracture. If complete ligament rupture is suspected, stress X-rays performed under local anesthetic block are recommended. The anterior drawer test will determine the integrity of the anterior talofibular ligament. Anterior displacement of the talus beneath the ankle mortise indicates a positive test and complete tear of the anterior talofibular ligament. A positive talar tilt test (17) with inversion of the talus within the ankle mortise suggests tear of the calcaneofibular ligament.

Mild sprains are relatively stable injuries involving stretch or partial tear of the anterior talofibular ligament. Such sprains are stable on both clinical and radiographic examination and can be effectively treated with the time-honored principles of icing, elevation, and compression (18). The patient can be placed in an inflatable, semirigid orthosis. This device provides both medial and lateral support while restricting inversion and eversion of the ankle joint. Weight bearing is restricted until a normal heel-toe gait is possible.

Moderate sprains involve complete disruption of the anterior talofibular ligament concomitant with injury to the calcaneofibular ligament. The anterior drawer sign will be positive, and the talar tilt test will be negative. Serially applied soft tissue dressings and splinting may be required before effective application of the inflatable splint can be achieved.

Severe sprains involve disruption of not only the anterior talofibular ligament, but also the calcaneofibular ligament. Both the anterior drawer and talar tilt test will be positive, suggesting instability in both the coronal and sagittal planes. Although such injuries frequently can be managed successfully with immobilization, operative repair should be considered in the acute management of these injuries in dancers (5,16). Gymnasts, divers, and dancers all require uncompromising stability of the ankle in the plantar-flexed position. If the lateral ligamentous structures heal in a stretched position, this laxity can lead to chronic instability and diminished performance. Operative management provides functional restoration of the ligamentous complex and effectively decreases the possibility of long-term instability (19–22).

FRACTURES

The "dancer's fracture" results from an inversion injury of the forefoot with severe torsional forces transmitted to the metatarsal shaft. The injury represents a spiral fracture at the distal diaphyseal-metaphyseal junction of the fifth metatarsal. The fracture may be comminuted with the fragments frequently displaced. These fractures will usually heal within 6–8 weeks when immobilized in a conventional short leg cast. Severe displacement may require manipulative reduction and intramedullary fixation using heavy Kirshner wire(s) (12).

Stress fractures most commonly are found in the second and third metatarsals, the sesamoids, and the distal fibula. These injuries result directly from cyclic trauma and are more commonly seen in dancers who have rapidly increased their class or rehearsal schedules. The initial symptoms are rather insidious, but with time the pain will become localized to the precise area of fracture. Stress reaction of bone represents a continuum. Initial plain films may be negative, and only a bone scan will demonstrate the injury.

After a brief period of immobilization until the fracture is pain free, the dancer is placed in protective orthotics. A structured pool therapy program is recommended. Pool therapy allows restoration of range of motion, aerobic fitness, and functional exercise while taking advantage of the buoyant effect of water. The dancer is encouraged to perform barre exercises while

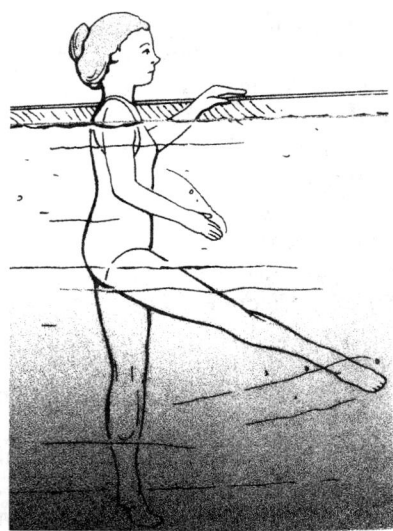

FIG. 39–4. Water barre exercises take advantage of the buoyant effect of water and represent an effective technique for rehabilitating dance injuries of the lower extremity.

in the pool (Fig. 39–4). The injured leg is used as the leg of support and the uninjured leg as the working leg. The dancer can return to dance when there is radiographic evidence of fracture healing.

IMPINGEMENT SYNDROMES

The extreme plantar flexion and dorsiflexion that certain dance positions require can lead to talar impingement syndromes involving the anterior and posterior aspect of the ankle joint. Demi-plié can lead to impingement of the anterior lip of the tibia on the talar neck (Fig. 39–5). The superior aspect of the talar neck contains a natural sulcus that accommodates the anterior tibial ridge in conventional dorsiflexion. The extreme dorsiflexion required by demi plié can lead to contact between the tibia and the talus. With time repeated impingement can lead to formation of exostoses on both the anterior lip of the tibia as well as the talar neck (9,11,23–25).

Initially, the dancer may complain of lack of satisfactory depth on plié. This may be interpreted as tightness within the gastroc soleus muscle groups, and the dancer may embark on an aggressive stretching program for those structures. This will only aggravate the condition and increase the pain of plié. With early impingement the pain is diffuse. With time the symptoms of impingement will become more localized to the anterior ankle joint. Mild swelling will be noted in this region.

On examination there will be tenderness along the anterior aspect of the ankle. The exostoses may be palpated about the anterior lip of the tibia as well as the talar neck. The symptoms of anterior impingement can be reproduced with dorsiflexion of the ankle and relieved by plantar flexion. Weight-bearing lateral X-rays with the ankle in hyperdorsiflexion often will demonstrate impingement of the anterior lip of the tibia on the talar neck. Symptomatic treatment can be achieved with a heel lift in street shoes, accompanied by antiinflammatories. Definitive treatment requires surgical excision of the exostoses. Such exostectomy can often extend the dancer's career. With time the impingement symptoms may recur, requiring repeat excision.

The relevé positions of demi-pointe and full pointe can produce symptoms of posterior talar impingement (Fig. 39–6). In contrast to anterior impingement, exostoses are not seen. Posterior impingement results from repetitive compression of the soft tissues in this region. Contributing factors include the presence of os trigonum, a large posterior tubercle, or a large dorsal process of the calcaneus. These structures can compress synovial and capsular tissues within the posterior ankle joint. With repeated compression the soft tissues become inflamed and, with time, thickened and fibrotic. The dancer will note decreased height in the demi-pointe and en-pointe positions with pain in the posterior aspect of the ankle joint (9,11,23,26,27).

On examination the pain of posterior impingement can be reproduced by hyper-plantar flexion. The symptoms can be relieved by dorsiflexion and confirmed with infiltration of xylocaine into the region. Tenderness, mild swelling, and crepitus are characteristic of this condition. Symptomatic treatment includes restriction of demi-pointe and full-pointe dance. In early presentation antiinflammatories and cortisone injections can be effective in reversing the inflammatory process. Refractory

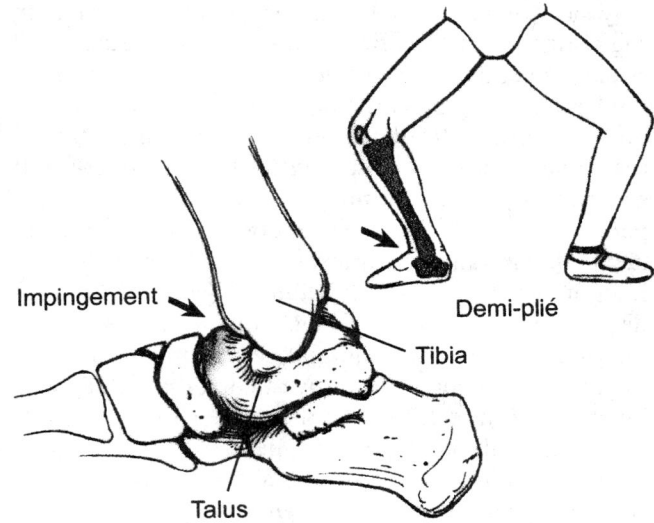

FIG. 39–5. Demi-plié is a position characterized by extreme dorsiflexion of the ankle joint and can lead to impingement of the anterior lip of the tibia on the talar neck.

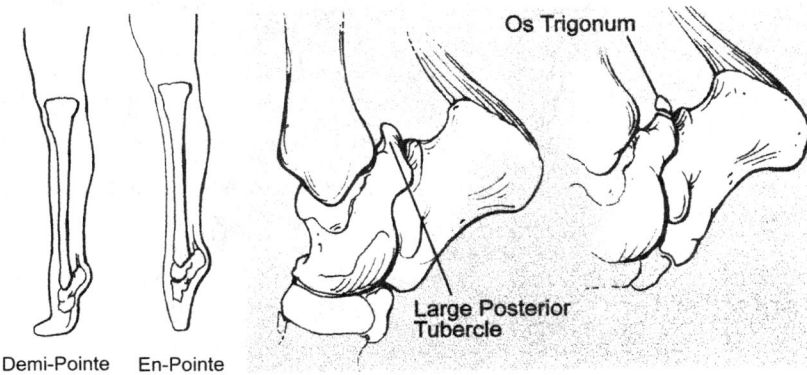

FIG. 39-6. The relevé positions of demi-pointe and full-pointe can lead to compression of posterior capsular and synovial structures from an enlarged os trigonum, posterior tubercle, or posterior process of the calcaneus.

cases require surgical excision of the offending structure(s).

FLEXOR HALLUCIS TENDINITIS

The flexor hallucis longus is the primary dynamic stabilizer of the plantar-flexed foot and ankle complex. Sickling and rolling-in are maladaptive techniques that can stress, stretch, and produce subsequent inflammation within the tendon (6,9–14). Chronic inflammation can lead to secondary degenerative changes within the tendon substance. Further degradation of tissue can lead to cyst and nodule formation. Thickening of the tendon occurs most commonly at the entrance of the fibroosseous canal. Nodules and cysts can impede the smooth sliding action of the tendon within the sheath, causing pain or, in some cases, triggering of the great toe. In advanced cases a partial rupture of the flexor hallucis longus tendon may occur (28).

On examination there will be tenderness, mild swelling, and crepitus along the posteromedial aspect of the ankle joint. Palpation may reproduce symptoms of pain and triggering of the inflamed tendon as it slides within the sheath.

Treatment consists of restriction of plié and pointe work. Emphasis should be placed on proper technique with prevention of sickling and rolling-in. Local heat, contrast baths, and pool therapy are recommended until resolution of symptoms. Tenolysis is reserved for cases in which conservative management is not successful.

INJURY PREVENTION

Prevention of dance injuries requires the concerted effort of all members of the dance medicine team, including the artistic director, the dance teacher, the dance therapist, and the company physician. The artistic director can assist in injury prevention by insisting on sufficient rest in the rehearsal and tour schedule, thus preventing fatigue among individual dancers and the company as a whole. One must insist on a proper floor surface and stage temperature for both rehearsal and performance. The artistic director must appreciate the physical limitations of each dancer in terms of choreographic demands. The dance teacher must create an awareness in each dancer of his or her physical limitations. The teacher is responsible for encouraging proper strengthening, conditioning, and technique. The teacher and therapist together must encourage dancers to adhere to principles of proper warm-up and stretching, emphasizing their role in injury prevention. Finally, physicians must be aware of the unique demands of dance. They must be cognizant of the mechanisms of dance injury, the role of contributing factors, the necessity of accurate diagnosis, and appropriate methods of treatment.

REFERENCES

1. Kirkendall D, Calabrese LH. Physiologic aspects of dance. *Clin Sports Med* 1983;2:525.
2. Micheli LJ, Gillespie WJ, Walaszek A. Physiologic profiles of female professional ballerinas. *Clin Sports Med* 1984;3:199–209.
3. Teitz C. Sports medicine concerns in dance and gymnastics. *Clin Sports Med* 1983;2:571–593.
4. Nicholas JA. Risk factors, sports medicine and the orthopedic system: an overview. *J Sports Med* 1975;3:243–259.
5. Hardaker WT Jr, Colosimo AJ, Malone TR, Myers, M. Ankle sprains in theatrical dancers. *Med Prob Perform Arts* 1988;3:146.
6. Hardaker WT Jr, Erickson L, Myers M. The pathogenesis of dance injury. In: Shell CG, ed. *The dancer as an athlete.* Champaign, IL: Human Kinetics Press, 1984:11–29.
7. Gelabert R. Turning-out. *Dance* 1977;Feb:86.
8. Clippinger K. Biomechanical considerations in turn-out. In: Solomon R, ed. *Preventing dance injuries: an interdisciplinary perspective.* Reston VA: National Dance Association, 1990.
9. Hardaker WT Jr, Morgello S, Goldner JL. Foot and ankle injuries in theatrical dancers. *Foot Ankle Int* 1985;6:59–69.
10. Miller EH, Schneider HJ, Bronson JL, McLain, DA. A new consideration in athletic injuries: the classical ballet dancer. *Clin Orthop* 1975;111:181–196.
11. Howse AJG. Orthopaedists aids ballet. *Clin Orthop* 1972;89:52.
12. Hamilton WG. Foot and ankle injuries in dancers. *Clin Sports Med* 1988;7:143.
13. Sammarco GJ, Miller EH. Forefoot conditions in dancers: parts I and II. *Foot Ankle Int* 1982;3:85–98.
14. Myers M. Talking technique: is the grand plié obsolete? *Dance* 1982;June.

15. Thomasen E. Diseases and injuries of ballet dancers. Universitetsforlaget 1. Arhus, Denmark, 1982.
16. Hamilton WG. Sprained ankles in ballet dancers. *Foot Ankle Int* 1982;3:99.
17. Almquist G. The pathomechanics and diagnosis of inversion injuries of the lateral ligaments of the ankle. *Am J Sports Med* 1974;2:109.
18. Garrick JG. A practical approach to rehabilitation illustrated by treatment of ankle injury. *Am J Sports Med* 1981;9:67–68.
19. Anderson KJ, LeCocq JF, LeCocq EA. Recurrent anterior subluxation of the ankle joint. *J Bone Joint Surg Am* 1952;34A:853–860.
20. Brostrom SL. Sprained ankles, treatment and prognosis in recent ligament ruptures. *Acta Chir Scand* 1966;132:537–550.
21. Cox JS. Surgical and non-surgical treatment of acute ankle sprains. *Clin Orthop* 1985;198:118–126.
22. Gould N, Seligson D, Gassman J. Early and late repair of lateral ligaments in the ankle. *Foot Ankle Int* 1980;1:84–89.
23. Hardaker WT Jr. Foot and ankle injuries in classical ballet dancers. *Orthop Clin North Am* 189;20:521–527.
24. Parks JC II, Hamilton WG, Patterson AH et al. The anterior impingement syndrome of the ankle. *J Trauma* 1980;20:895.
25. Kleiger B. Anterior tibial talar impingement syndrome in dancers. *Foot Ankle Int* 1982;3:69–73.
26. Hamilton WG. Tendinitis about the ankle joint in classical ballet dancers. *Am J Sports Med* 1977;2:84–88.
27. Howse AJG. Posterior block in the ankle joint in dancers. *Foot Ankle Int* 1982;3:81–84.
28. Sammarco GJ, Miller EH. Partial rupture of the flexor hallucis longus tendon in classical ballet dancers. *J Bone Joint Surg Am* 1979;61A:149.

CHAPTER 40

Football

John A. Bergfeld and Jonathan J. Paul

INTRODUCTION

Football is a violent sport and has led to the generation of a growing body of literature of football-related injuries. Some of this literature has been the impetus for rule changes in football. The elimination of the crackback block and penalties for grabbing the face mask have been implemented to help reduce the number and severity of injuries.

The player's position may predispose him or her to specific types of injuries (1) and is an important consideration in predicting return to participation. A fractured finger may not limit a lineman at all but may prevent a wide receiver from playing for up to 6 weeks. Football equipment has become lighter, less restrictive, and more effective at absorbing shock. In addition, football players have simply become stronger, bigger, and faster (2). These factors, combined with the advent of artificial turf, allow the game to be played at a faster pace.

Despite these changes in the game of football, Nicholas has reported that a 26-year analysis of regular season game injuries in a single National Football League (NFL) team revealed no increased incidence of injury. Nicholas attributes increased mass media attention to the perception that the incidence of football injuries is on the rise (3).

We have developed a grading system (Table 40–1) for football injuries that has proven valuable over the years in conversing with coaches, players, and others about the extent and prognosis of football-related injuries. Each of our coaches has a copy of this grading system, making communication about a player's injury more effective.

OVERVIEW

According to Powell, the most recent estimates are that over 1 million high school athletes and 75,000 college athletes play football in the United States each year (4). The number of injuries related to football has been estimated to be 600,000 per year (1,5). Wide variations of the injury rate (10–80%) have been reported (6–9). Prager and colleagues (10) have outlined the pitfalls of data collection related to sports. The adequacy of any injury surveillance program begins with the awareness of injuries. Currently, there is no universally accepted definition of what constitutes an injury or measurement of injury severity. This variation may be the result of differences in the definition of injury and severity, the identification of the population at risk, and exposure time. In DeLee and Famey's study (1) an injury was defined as any episode that caused the football player to miss time from a practice or game, any head injury, and any injury that required treatment by a physician and/or trainer. Their study population consisted of 100 randomly selected class 4A and class 5A high schools in Texas. The overall injury rate was 0.509 per football player per year. Over one season they documented 2228 injuries. Fifty-six percent of their injuries occurred during games. This relative increased frequency of injuries in games compared to practice is consistent with other studies (10–12). The risk of injury in a game has been reported to be 3–20 times higher than the risk during practice (13).

DeLee and Famey (1) defined a severe injury as one that required hospitalization and/or surgery. The injury rate for a severe injury was determined to be 0.031 per athlete per year. They calculated that a football player was almost twice as likely as the age-matched general population to sustain a severe injury. A football player was 5.8 times more likely to sustain a severe knee injury than the general population.

The most common types of injuries are sprains and strains, which account for 40% of all football injuries.

J. A. Bergfeld: Section of Sports Health, Cleveland Clinic Foundation, Cleveland, Ohio 44195.

J. J. Paul: Orthopaedic Group of Concord, Concord, North Carolina 28025.

TABLE 40–1. *Grading system for football injuries*

GRADE 0	Absolutely clean. No problems. Recommend drafting.
GRADE 1	Problem fully corrected. Cannot "go down" due to problem. Recommend drafting. Examples: 1. Meniscectomy, has played 2 or 3 seasons. 2. Minor hand and finger injuries. 3. Well-healed fracture
GRADE 2	Moderate problem. Could "go down" due to specific problem, but probably not. Has played 1 or more seasons after injury. Examples: 1. Chronic isolated PCL injury 2. ACL Surgery 3. Mild posttraumatic ankle X-ray changes 4. Asymptomatic spondylolysis 5. Third-degree AC sprain 6. Asymptomatic subluxating shoulder
GRADE 3	Major problem. Can play, but may "go down" any time. Examples: 1. ACL-deficient knee 2. Symptomatic subluxating shoulder 3. Rotator cuff problem in a thrower 4. Symptomatic cervical or lumbar HNP
GRADE 4	Significant risk for reinjury.
GRADE 5	Injured currently. Needs to be rechecked. Example: 1. Acute ACL injury with fracture

Second most common are contusions, which account for 25% of injuries. Fractures account for 10%. Concussions and dislocations each make up 5% of football injuries (13–16).

Approximately 50% of football injuries involve the lower extremity, and 30% involve the upper extremity. The knee is consistently the most common area injured (20–30%) followed by the ankle (15%) (1).

The highest percentage of injuries are sustained by running backs (43%), followed by tackles (18%), guards (12%), ends (10%), quarterbacks (6%), safeties (5%), and centers (5%) (10,17). Considering the relative risk for each position, again running backs have the highest risk for injuries (relative risk = 3.0), followed by quarterbacks (2.5), tackles (2.0), and centers (2.0). Guards (1.2) and ends (1.1) have the lowest relative risk for injury.

Most injuries occur during tackling (32%) or blocking (26%). The next most common activity at the time of injury is ball carrying (19%) and being blocked (10%). Less than 5% of injuries occur while passing, receiving, or running.

The peak injury rate occurs at midseason; fewer injuries occur in the final weeks of the season (16). A study by Moretz and colleagues suggested that preseason practices are 5.4 times more likely to produce injuries than are in-season practices (14).

RISK FACTORS

Numerous studies have attempted to identify football injury risk factors. Some of these studies have been the impetus for rule and equipment changes. The factors that were evaluated included playing surfaces, amount of contact during practice, tackling techniques, footwear, and various types of protective equipment.

Playing Surfaces

As we mentioned earlier, knee and ankle injuries are the most common football injuries. This has led to investigations of the significance of playing surface and footwear as potential contributing factors to these injures. Mueller and Blyth (6) resurfaced the fields of nine randomly selected high schools in North Carolina. The fields were maintained in good condition throughout the season. These authors then prospectively compared injury rates with those of schools that did not play on well-maintained fields. The athletes playing at schools that had fields resurfaced had a 31% reduction in knee and ankle injuries. Andresen and colleagues (16) demonstrated a lower injury rate on wet, slippery fields with normal grass cover. This reduction possibly is related to reduced speed of game and decreased friction between the shoe-playing surface interface (16). In contrast to Mueller and Blyth's prospective study, the highest injury rate was found with good field conditions in this retrospective study (defined as normal grass cover without recent or ongoing rain and without dry packed-down areas of bare dirt) (16).

Several studies have evaluated the effects of artificial turf on football injuries. The risk for injury on an artificial surface also may be reduced when the surface is wet (5). Powell and Schootman considered several risk factors simultaneously to arrive at the overall risk of knee injury while playing on Astroturf over eight seasons in the NFL (18). Over the study period (1980–1989), 46% of team games were played on natural surfaces, and 47% were played on Astroturf (Balsam, St. Louis, MO). The other 7% of games were played on Tartan-Turf (3M, St. Paul, MN) and Super Turf (Super Turf Inc., Dallas, TX) and were not included in the study. The average team incurred six game-related knee sprains per season. Overall, there was a tendency for increased knee sprains, medial collateral ligament (MCL) injuries, and anterior cruciate ligament (ACL) injuries under specific circumstances playing on Astroturf. For MCL injuries a higher rate for linemen was seen in playing on Astroturf. A higher incidence of ACL injuries and knee sprains was seen on Astroturf during punts and kickoffs. Unfortunately, in this study, no distinction was made between contact versus noncontact injury or type of shoe worn. Investigations on the risk of injury on artificial surface are incomplete; however, there is probably a relative increase in the risk of injuries to the lower extremity (19). More well-controlled studies are needed.

Footwear

Shoes have also been implicated as a source for injury. Two types of shoes are worn by football players: the football shoe with either long or short cleats and the soccer-style shoe. In the early 1970s a typical football shoe had seven cleats that were 0.5–0.75 inch long. In 1971 Torg and Quedenfeld (20) demonstrated a reduced incidence and severity of injuries when football shoes with long cleats were replaced with soccer-style shoes. This resulted in a change in the type of shoes worn by football players. The greater risk for injury with the long cleated shoes was thought to be that they rendered the shoe noncompliant to intrinsic and extrinsic forces. At present the standard football-style shoe has seven cleats that are 0.5 inch long and 0.375 inch in diameter. Mueller and Blyth, in the high school study mentioned previously, demonstrated a further reduction in injuries when shoes were changed to the soccer-style shoe (6). These shoes tend to be flexible and have led to an increased incidence of turf toe. Lambson and colleagues (21) performed a 3-year prospective study to evaluate the effect of the torsional resistance of modern football cleat design on the incidence of surgically documented ACL tears in high school football players wearing four different types of cleats. The cleat types were as follows:

1. Edge: long irregular cleats at the periphery of the shoe with smaller pointed cleats positioned interiorly
2. Flat: cleats on the forefoot that are the same height, shape, and diameter, such as are found on the soccer-style shoe
3. Screw-in: seven screw-in cleats of 0.5 inch height and 0.5 inch diameter
4. Pivot disk, a 10-cm circular edge on the sole of the forefoot with one 0.5-inch cleat in the center

The edge design produced significantly higher torsional resistance than the other designs. The edge design also was associated with a significantly higher ACL ligament injury rate (0.017%) than the other three designs combined (0.005%). Recently, Torg and colleagues investigated the effect of different temperature on the torsional resistance of different turf shoes. Increased turf temperature correlated with increased torsional resistance, potentially placing the athlete's knee and ankle at risk of injury. Only the flat-soled basketball-style turf shoe could be designated "safe" or "probably safe" at all five temperatures (20). Heidt and colleagues (23) evaluated the friction and torsional resistance differences of the shoe-surface interface of 15 football shoes made by three manufacturers. Shoes tested included traditional cleated football shoes, court shoes (basketball-style), molded-cleat shoes, and turf shoes. Shoes were tested on synthetic turf under wet and dry conditions and on natural stadium grass. Spatting, which is protective taping of the ankle and heel applied on the outside of the shoe, resulted in a reduction of forces generated in both translation and rotation. The only safe shoe-surface combination was court shoes on wet Astroturf. Molded-rubber cleats were unsafe on all surfaces, and cleated shoes were unsafe on all surfaces except wet Astroturf (probably unsafe). Significant difference between grass and Astroturf values were noted only for rotation in cleated shoes and in turf shoes.

Amount of Contact During Practice

Mueller and Blyth (6) were able to get six high schools in North Carolina to limit the amount of contact practices. The schools that had limited contact practices had a lower injury rate compared with schools that had regular contact practices. Similarly, Cahill and Griffith (24) in a study involving two football teams from the Big 10 demonstrated a 4.7 times greater risk of injury during contact practices compared to controlled practices.

Coaching Experience

Blyth and Mueller demonstrated an increased risk of injury for athletes who play for coaches with less experience and also for teams that have fewer assistant coaches (25).

Tackling Techniques

As a result of the work of the National Football Head and Neck Injury Registry, the National Collegiate Athletic Association (NCAA) Football Rules Committee in 1976 banned spearing, which is defined as intentionally striking an opponent with the crown of the helmet or otherwise using the helmet to butt or ram an opponent (26). A similar rule was adopted by the National Federation of State High School Associations. As a result of these rule changes, fractures, subluxations, and dislocations of the cervical spine have declined dramatically since 1976 (27). Football-related permanent cervical quadriplegia decreased from 34 cases in 1976 to five in 1984 (27). The yearly incidence of cervical spine fractures decreased from 110 to 42 over this same time period.

Head contact is inevitable in sports but should be minimized. To avoid head contact, players should be consistently reminded to initiate contact with their shoulders rather than their heads and to keep their heads up and "see what they hit". The rules instituted to ban spearing must be consistently and meticulously obeyed. Neck strengthening is an important (but often neglected) way to prevent neck injuries. While neck strengthening, according to Watkins, probably produces degenerative changes and developmental stenosis, it is imperative in preventing neck injuries in football players (28).

Protective Equipment

Protective equipment has become lighter, more comfortable, and more protective. The National Operating Committee on Standards for Athletic Equipment (NOCSAE) is responsible for establishing guidelines for equipment maintenance and reconditioning. NCAA rules state that players must wear a NOCSAE-approved helmet, soft neck pads that are at least 0.5 inch thick, shoulder pads, hip pads, thigh pads, and a mouthpiece.

The football helmet has evolved over the past century (27). Initially, no helmet was worn. In 1908 the first "helmet" was essentially a pair of heavy-duty leather earmuffs. By 1918 the helmet consisted of an outer leather piece and an inner felt piece. A more modern design was used by 1932 and included a primitive suspension webbing. Design and quality improved over the next 20 years, and in 1950 the plastic shell appeared, signifying a significant improvement in design and construction. Soon afterward, the kraycolite shell and web suspension system appeared. Early face protectors were improvisations to protect a fractured nose. By the early 1950s a single-bar mask and subsequently a double-bar mask was in widespread use to prevent injury. The current helmet-face mask unit is composed of a bird cage mask attached to a polycarbonate shell with a variety of pneumatic, hydraulic, and web suspension systems. Helmets are classified by the type of suspension system or padding within the shell. The types of suspension systems include air and fluid-filled cells, a combination of air and pads, pads alone, and suspension type (29). The outer shell of the helmet is made of polycarbonate that is an alloy polymer plastic called Kralite 11. This polymer is lightweight yet able to withstand high impact. All helmets that are used in high school, college, and professional football must have a NOCSAE seal of approval, indicating that the helmet has met the requirements established for safe use. Helmets also carry a warning sticker from NOCSAE that must be placed on the outer shell of the helmet (29).

Without proper fit and maintenance, equipment not only may fail to protect the athlete but may actually cause injury (29,30). An improperly fitted helmet may predispose the football player to injury to the head and neck. Shoulder pads are designed to absorb large forces and protect the athlete from injury to the shoulder and upper trunk. Serious injury may result from poorly fitted shoulder pads. The model and type of shoulder pads may need to be varied according to the player's position.

Other equipment worn by football players includes hip pads to protect the iliac crest and tailbone. Often these pads are inserted in a girdle. Thigh and knee pads are inserted in the pants. The pants should fit snugly to prevent slippage of these pads. All players should use a mouthpiece to reduce dental and head injuries. The mouthpiece should be form-fitted to the athlete's teeth. Players who are in particular positions may wear additional protective equipment. Quarterbacks may use a flak jacket to protect their ribs. Linemen typically use sparring gloves to protect their hands.

SHOULDER INJURIES

Shoulder injuries are common in football. Shields and Zommar reported that the frequency of shoulder injuries in football was second only to that of injuries of the knee (31). The shoulder is made up of four articulations (sternoclavicular, acromioclavicular, scapulothoracic, and glenohumeral), any of which may be injured. These injuries are not peculiar to football, but there are certain in injuries that occur more commonly in football players. These include acromioclavicular injuries, brachial plexus injuries, glenohumeral instability, rotator cuff injuries, contusions, and exostoses.

Rotator Cuff Injuries

Rotator cuff problems in athletes have typically been seen in overhead-throwing athletes, such as quarterbacks. In throwers, repetitive eccentric loading of the rotator cuff may lead to tendinitis or tendinosis and subsequent secondary impingement. This entity classically has been reported in throwers with multidirectional instability, a condition in which the rotator cuff is relied on more heavily to maintain the humeral head in the glenoid. Subsequently, it is thought, an overuse tendinitis develops in the rotator cuff. Athletes typically complain of pain with throwing and with overhead activities. Physical examination should include a careful evaluation for anterior instability. The natural history of partial thickness tears of the rotator cuff has not been clearly defined; therefore the role of arthroscopy for these lesions remains controversial and unclear.

Blevins and colleagues reported on rotator cuff surgery in ten football players, nine of whom played on the professional level (32). Only one of these patients was a quarterback. Each player had sustained a direct blow to the shoulder while playing football, either from a fall onto the shoulder or from direct contact with another player. One player had an anterior glenohumeral dislocation. The diagnoses for these patients were rotator cuff contusions in two, partial thickness tears in five, and complete rotator cuff tears in three. Their indications for surgery included physical examination consistent with rotator cuff injury and no improvement with nonoperative treatment consisting of rest, antiinflammatory medications, modalities, gentle range of motion, and progressive cuff-strengthening exercises. Time from injury to surgery averaged 9 weeks. Nine of the ten athletes returned to football at a very high level of play an average of 4 months after surgery. Seven of the ten judged that they had returned to the preinjury levels of play. These authors believe that arthroscopic evaluation should be considered for contact athletes with shoulder pain and weakness after a direct blow to the shoulder if they do not improve with a rotator cuff rehabilitation program. In their hands, surgical treatment of cuff and subacromial abnormalities lead to a high rate of return to football; however, strength may not be fully restored.

Acromioclavicular Injuries

Acromioclavicular joint injuries are a common football injury and are discussed in depth in the musculoskeletal injury volume of this series. In Cox's series, 41% of acromioclavicular injuries were football injuries (33). Acromioclavicular injuries in football are usually the result from a fall on the point of the shoulder. Management of these injuries has been described previously (34).

Sternoclavicular Dislocations

Anterior sternoclavicular dislocations are not uncommon in football. Reduction may be attempted, although these injuries are usually unstable after reduction.

Posterior sternoclavicular dislocations are potentially life-threatening injuries and fortunately are rare in football, though football injuries make up the majority of case reports for this injury (35). Physical examination and plain X-rays are unreliable in making the diagnosis, which usually necessitates CT scanning to differentiate anterior from posterior dislocation. Treatment is closed reduction. Return to football should be discouraged after a posterior dislocation

Contusions

Proximal humeral contusions are more common in defensive players. These contusions are usually a result of a direct blow, analogous to the iliac crest contusion, or hip pointer (36). Repetitive contusions to the subcutaneous part of the anterolateral humerus (a relatively unprotected area just distal to the edge of the shoulder pads) can result in "tacklers exostosis." In this condition the deltoid insertion or the brachialis origin are injured, resulting in periosteal injury and new bone formation. Radiographs may demonstrate a "dotted veil" in the region that later matures into an exostosis. A high index of suspicion is necessary to initiate early treatment, which includes compression wraps and icing as well as additional padding below the level of normal shoulder pads. Aspiration of a hematoma may be considered. Surgical excision may be necessary if a mature exostosis becomes symptomatic. This lesion can be differentiated from myositis ossificans, which has a radio-dense cleavage plane between the lesion and the humeral cortex.

Perlmutter and colleagues (37) performed long-term follow-up of 11 athletes (nine of whom were football players) who had sustained isolated injuries to their axillary nerves while tackling opposing players. There were no known shoulder dislocations. Electromyographs were taken of ten patients, and all patients had confirmation of clinically defined injuries that were confined to their axillary nerves. In seven athletes the mechanism of injury was a direct blow to the anterior lateral deltoid muscle. In four athletes there were simultaneous contralateral neck flexion and ipsilateral shoulder depression. At follow-up, all patients had residual deficits of axillary sensory and motor nerve function. There had been no deltoid muscle improvement in three patients, moderate improvement in two patients, and major improvement in six patients. However, shoulder function remained excellent, with all athletes maintaining full range of motion and good-to-excellent motor strength. Axillary nerve exploration and neurolysis in four patients did not significantly affect the outcomes. Although no patient had full recovery of axillary nerve function, ten of 11 athletes returned to their preinjury levels of sports activities, including professional football.

Glenohumeral Instability

Instability of the glenohumeral joint represents a spectrum from a sprain to a frank dislocation. Classification is based on the direction, degree, and chronology of the instability.

Anterior traumatic glenohumeral dislocation usually occurs when the shoulder is in the abducted and externally rotated position. A common improper tackling technique, in which the arm is completely abducted, predisposes the football player to this injury. Miller and colleagues (38) has pointed out that this vulnerable position may also lead to rupture of the pectoralis major in the football player. Management of acute dislocations consists of immediate reduction, immobilization for approximately 3 weeks, and rehabilitation. When full strength and motion are regained, the player is allowed to resume contact. The use of a Duke splint or other orthoses limiting abduction and external rotation may be helpful if the player tolerates it. For a dislocation that occurs in season, we think the approach of Speer's (39) is reasonable. The player is treated as above with the understanding that surgical stabilization will be planned after the season concludes. The role of arthroscopy in the management of acute shoulder dislocations is evolving. At the present time we believe that an open shoulder stabilization is the procedure of choice in the football player.

A posterior shoulder dislocation can result from a fall on an internally rotated adducted arm or a direct blow to the anterior aspect of the shoulder. This injury is rare in football, as it is in the general population. More common in football are recurrent posterior shoulder subluxations from repetitive trauma associated with blocking. This is commonly seen in offensive linemen, who are susceptible to this condition while blocking with their arms adducted and forward flexed. Because it is difficult for linemen to avoid this position and surgical treatment for this condition is not as successful as anterior stabilization, this can be a difficult problem to treat.

ELBOW INJURIES

Kenter and colleagues recently reported on the NFL experience of elbow injuries (40). In a survey of NFL physicians (25 of 30 responded, with an average of 8.2 years in NFL), 99 elbow injuries were reported over the period 1991–1995. Seventy-seven percent of these injuries were sprains, and 18% were dislocations. Fractures were very rare (4%). Of the sprains, 56% were from hyperextension, 20% were MCL injuries, and another 21% were nonspecific. Of the 14 dislocations, 13 were anterior. The only elbow dislocation that underwent surgery was in a quarterback. The most frequent activity at the time of dislocation was tackling. Forty-eight percent had returned to full participation by 4 weeks, and another 40% returned by 6 weeks. Only two of the physicians responding to the survey had a player with symptomatic posterolateral rotatory instability requiring reconstruction.

Medial elbow instability, though commonly thought of as occurring in baseball pitchers, is a condition that can exist in quarterbacks as well (29). D'Alessandro pointed out that it is unusual for a quarterback to demonstrate symptoms of MCL insufficiency because of different throwing biomechanics than a pitcher. Only one of the physicians in Kenter's survey has had a quarterback with symptomatic MCL insufficiency requiring reconstruction with a palmaris graft (40).

Forty-eight percent of NFL physicians have had an NFL player sustain a rupture of the distal biceps tendon. The most common activity during rupture is tackling (40). Fifty-six percent of these physicians have had a player sustain a triceps avulsion. Eleven of fourteen were in linemen (seven offensive, four defensive). All underwent surgical repair, and all returned to play.

INJURIES OF THE FOREARM

In football the forearm is prone to contusions, particularly when used for blocking. Forearm pads can be used to provide some protection. Repetitive forearm stresses in football may lead to periostitis (41). The athlete will typically have vague complaints of exercise-induced pain. The pain may worsen to the point at which it limits activities of daily living. Initial radiographs may appear normal. Repeat radiographs and a bone scan can be helpful in making the diagnosis. This condition is analogous to shin splints in the lower extremity and is treated in a similar manner (42). This condition is treated with relative rest, avoidance of painful activities, and then gradual return to full activities. Ward and colleagues have pointed out that this ossifying periostitis can masquerade as a malignancy (43). Forearm fractures are uncommon in football, but they can occur with direct blows, such as when arm tackling or from falling on the outstretched arm.

INJURIES OF THE WRIST AND HAND

Ellsasser and Stein (44) studied 38 players from one professional football team who had 46 major hand and wrist injuries during a 15-year period. Twenty-one of the injuries occurred in offensive players, and 25 occurred in defensive players. The injuries included fractures, dislocations, fracture dislocations, and soft tissue injuries. Twelve surgical procedures were performed over the 15-year observation period. Early aggressive surgery for intraarticular and certain metacarpal fractures achieved the best possible functional results.

Dorsal hand contusions are common in football. They usually occur as a result of a direct blow such as contact with a helmet or from being stepped on. Fractures of the metacarpals should be ruled out with an X-ray. Early return to play can be facilitated with padding to protect the hand from further injury.

Retig and colleagues (45) reviewed 29 metacarpal fractures in football.. The most common mechanism of injury was a direct blow or a fall on the outstretched hand. Most metacarpal fractures were undisplaced or minimally displaced and were considered to be stable. The fractures were evenly distributed among the fingers. Time lost from practice or play averaged 11 days for receivers but only 5.6 days for running backs. Most of metacarpal fractures in this series were successfully treated with the application of a cast and/or a splint. A hard cast was used during the week for practice. It was then replaced with a playing cast constructed of silicone rubber for games. At the completion of the game, the hard cast was reapplied. Cast use was maintained until there was radiographic evidence of healing. After healing, buddy taping was continued for the remainder of the season. Fractures that were displaced were treated with internal fixation. This allowed early motion and return to football with protective padding. Displacement of the fracture with return to football was not seen in their series.

Fractures of the scaphoid in football players have been studied by Riester and colleagues (46), who estimated an incidence of one scaphoid fracture per 100 college football players per year. The typical mechanism of injury is a fall on the outstretched arm with the wrist in the extended position. The athlete will present with pain and tenderness in the anatomic snuffbox. Pain can be increased with extension and radial deviation of the wrist. A high index of suspicion is needed to diagnose these injuries because radiographs may initially be negative. The fracture line may become evident with serial X-rays 10-14 days later. In the absence of a positive radiograph but with a history and physical examination consistent with scaphoid fracture, the athlete should be treated as if he or she has a fracture. A bone scan may be used to confirm this suspicion. Fractures that have a step-off or gap of less than 1 mm are considered to be nondisplaced. Since 1973 these authors (46) report they have been allowing athletes with stable scaphoid fractures to participate in contact sports with cast immobilization without limitation. They reviewed 14 such fractures studied over a 10-year period with an average follow-up of 4 years. Treatment consisted of a padded short arm thumb spica cast with the wrist in neutral for the week of practice. On game day the cast was replaced with a custom-made silastic short arm thumb spica. After the game a new thumb spica cast was applied. In their series, fractures of the middle third of the scaphoid that were detected and treated early (within 24 hours) healed; however, the average time of immobilization was 6 months. Two of three fractures of the proximal third did not heal. One of these players was operated on and subsequently refractured his scaphoid. The other player with a nonunion was asymptomatic and declined surgery. He played in the NFL for 8 years.

Raab and colleagues (47) reviewed the treatment and prognosis of lunate and perilunate carpal dislocations in the NFL over a 5-year period. There were seven lunate and three perilunate dislocations. The mechanism of injury was hyperextension in nine of ten players. Five players were treated by closed reduction and percutaneous pinning; the others were treated by open reduction and K-wire fixation. No player was treated by cast immobilization alone. A minimum of 4 weeks of playing time was lost. Their results demonstrated that lunate and perilunate dislocations do not mean the end of a career in professional football. Treatments varied with respect to open or closed reductions, placement of pins, casts, and of immobilization. None of the variations was clearly superior or detrimental, although four of the five players who returned to play in the same season were treated by closed reduction with percutaneous pinning.

Injury of the ulnar collateral ligament (UCL) of the first metacarpophalangeal joint ("gamekeepers thumb") is frequently seen in football. It may result from a fall on an outstretched hand or from tangling the thumb in a player's jersey. The injury usually results from forced abduction of the thumb. It can also occur as a combination of abduction and hyperextension and, less frequently, as a combination of abduction and flexion (48). The injury involves a partial or complete tear of the UCL. For unstable injuries (indicating a complete tear of the UCL), repair of the UCL to restore stability to the ulnar side of the thumb has been advocated by McCue and colleagues (48). The rationale for this is that in certain instances the adductor pollicis aponeurosis may become interposed between the UCL and its healing bed (Stenner's lesion), preventing proper healing. After partial or complete tear of the UCL, the player's thumb should be protected when he or she returns to activity. Protection may be provided by use of a splint or adhesive tape. For skilled players the tape should be applied in a figure of eight around the thumb. For nonskilled players who do not handle the ball, taping may be used to hold the thumb against the second finger or to anchor it to the index finger. Nonskilled players may return to activity during the period of immobilization, with a padded or silicone rubber-type cast. Football players who require use of their hands, such as quarterbacks and receivers, may not be able to return to football until the injury has healed. We believe that most poor results from nonoperative treatment of complete UCL tears have been from a lack of properly supervised controlled motion with adequate protection during contact. Our experience has been that complete tears of the UCL in football players heal satisfactorily with nonoperative, controlled motion to facilitate ligamentous healing, as outlined by Frank and Woo and colleagues (49,50). Protection with splinting during contact activities is critical if this approach is taken.

Fumich and colleagues (51) reported two cases involving dorsal dislocation of the metacarpophalangeal joint of the thumb in offensive linemen. This injury was caused by use of improper blocking technique in which the player dorsiflexed his wrist and drove his closed fist into the opponent's chest, using his thumb to push against the inferior border of the opposing player's shoulder pads. A dorsal dislocation of the phalanx occurred when the radial collateral ligament was torn when the thumb was flexed, driving the radial border of the thumb against the shoulder pads.

Weiland and Lister reported on volar fracture dislocation of the second and third metacarpal bases associated with acute carpal tunnel syndrome in a 17-year-old football player (52). This injury was treated with open reduction, via volar incision to decompress the carpal tunnel, and via a second dorsal incision for internal fixation of the fracture dislocations with Kirschner wire fixation and reinsertion of the avulsed extensor carpi radialis longus tendon.

Injuries to the interphalangeal joints of the finger are

common in football and are often the result of a player's fingers becoming entangled with the opposing player. These injuries need to be properly treated to avoid late deformity and loss of motion. After reduction of a dislocated IP joint, X-rays should be obtained to rule out an associated fracture. Treatment for most sprained fingers involves buddy taping and range-of-motion exercises. Complete tears of the ligament and certain fractures may require immobilization and/or internal fixation. Intraarticular fractures should be carefully reduced and internally fixated to ensure restoration of the normal geometry of the articular surface.

Jersey finger or avulsion of the flexor digitorum profundus most commonly occurs in the ring finger. These injuries all need to be surgically treated.

LUMBAR SPINE INJURIES

In football players mild injuries to the lumbar spine can be disabling. It has been reported that 30% of college football players will lose playing time because of a lumbar spine problem (53,54). A survey of injuries from 1980 to 1986 in the NFL reported a 12% incidence of spine injuries resulting in lost playing time (53).

Lumbar contusions or strains are the most common injuries (54). These are usually managed successfully by modification or restriction of participation, followed by conditioning and strengthening of the abdominal and lumbar muscles. The player is allowed to resume activity gradually when pain subsides. Most low back pain will respond to conservative care, including modalities and therapeutic exercise (29). If a player's symptoms persist, X-rays should be obtained.

A high incidence of spondylolysis has been reported in football players. The incidence of lumbar spondylolysis in the general population is approximately 6% (55–58). At Indiana University an X-ray was obtained on all 145 incoming freshmen football players over a 6-year period. A 15% incidence of lumbar spondylolysis was noted (59). This incidence did not significantly increase during their college careers (59). None of their players had a progression of spondylolisthesis, and none discontinued their careers because of their spondylolysis. Ferguson and colleagues (53) reported a 50% incidence of spondylolysis in symptomatic division 1 college interior linemen. Semon and Spengler (60) at the University of Washington reported that 27% (135 of 506) of football players had low back pain during their college careers, and of the 58 who had X-rays there was a 21% incidence of lumbar spondylolysis. They found that the players with spondylolysis did not have significantly greater time loss from games or practices than other players with low back pain. Spondylolysis is thought to be the result of repetitive loading of the posterior lumbar elements that occurs when the linemen come out of their stance into the blocking posture while excessively extending the lumbar spine. However, since other players besides linemen had spondylolysis in these studies, other sources of stress, such as weight lifting and other training techniques, may be additional causes. A wide spectrum of treatment plans has been used for this condition ranging from symptomatic treatment to surgical stabilization. We advocate rest, heat, and antiinflammatory medications and abdominal strengthening exercises. Return to play may be allowed once full range of painless motion is achieved.

Tewes and colleagues (61) reviewed 29 cases of lumbar transverse process fractures over a 9-year period in the NFL. Associated visceral injuries were rare, and the time lost from football was an average of 3.5 weeks.

Day and Friedman (63) reported on lumbar disc disease in 12 college football players at Florida over a 4-year period. The most common position affected was down-lineman. No players could recall the onset of symptoms relative to football activity, but weight lifting was associated with symptoms in three cases. In their experience, for failure of nonoperative treatment, discectomy was successful for disk herniations occurring at the L4-5 space or higher.

PELVIC AND HIP INJURIES

Pelvic and hip injuries are relatively rare in football and represent less than 3% of injuries(15,17).

The hip pointer is the most common of these injuries. This injury consists of a contusion of the iliac crest. Protective padding is the mainstay of prevention and treatment and may include the addition of a doughnut pad or custom-made thermoplastic pad to the area of injury. In the adolescent, complete avulsion of the iliac apophysis can occur. These avulsions are treated with activity limitation for 4–6 weeks (29).

Renstrom has written on the potentially serious consequences of contusions to the groin. These include phlebothrombosis, traumatic phlebitis, and femoral neuropathy (63). Common muscles that are strained around the groin include the illiopsoas and adductors. X-rays should be obtained to rule out avulsion of the lesser trochanter. The critical aspect of treatment of these injuries is stretching. Activity is protected to avoid reinjury during the healing phase.

While hip dislocation is very rare in football, hip subluxation has been reported (64–66). Moorman and colleagues have reported the largest series (eight players) of this injury to date in football players (66). Half of the players were running backs. The mechanism of injury in 75% of the injuries was a fall on a flexed, adducted knee. None of the players were able to continue playing acutely after the injury. Subsequently, avascular necrosis was noted in 25% of the players and necessitated total hip replacement. The other 75% of players returned to their previous level of play without limitation. This injury may lead to interruption of the blood supply and subsequent osteonecrosis. The resultant osteonecrosis of the femoral head can be devastating and can end an athlete's career. The natural history of osteonecrosis is unpredictable, and the athlete may actually be able to resume football (63) but should be advised against it. Early recognition of this disorder may help to avoid some of the disastrous sequela of this injury. If an athlete has a history of hip injury and subsequent limited range of motion and painful ambulation, then toe touch crutch walking should be initiated. Judet views should be obtained, as all eight of the patients in Moorman and colleagues' study had a posterior acetabular lip fracture that was not visualized on an AP pelvis view. An acute MRI may confirm the diagnosis but is an unreliable predictor of subsequent AVN. Delayed MRI at 6 weeks postinjury appears to be the best predictor of AVN. Patients with a full range of motion who are pain free and have no AVN by MRI at 6 weeks may return to play safely (66).

Osteitis pubis may be seen in the football player and may present with abdominal pain, groin pain, testicular pain, or hip pain (55). This multiplicity and lack of consistency of presenting complaints may lead to a delayed or misdiagnosis (55). The exact etiology is unknown but may be incited by a muscle strain around the pubic rami initiating an inflammatory reaction (55). Instability of the joint may ensue. Shear stress across the joint may lead to bony resorption. Early X-ray may be negative. The condition may be ruled out with a bone scan. Initial treatment includes rest, ice, and nonsteroidal antiinflammatory drugs. Once infection is ruled out, judicious use of corticosteroid injections may be of benefit. A stretching program is emphasized. Recurrence rates as high as 25% have been reported (55). Three to six months may be required to return to the preinjury level (55).

Karpos and colleagues have reported on osteomyelitis of the pubic symphysis in a college football player. This is a debilitating condition with an average return to sports at 5 months (67).

THIGH INJURIES

Quadriceps contusions result from a direct blow usually from an opposing player's helmet. Ryan and colleagues have pointed out that the quadriceps muscle lies in contact with the femur throughout the full length of the thigh and is particularly vulnerable to trauma (68). Blunt trauma causes transmission of force through the fluid compartment of the muscle, and damage occurs only in the layer next to the bone. This major muscle injury is associated with fiber disruption, capillary damage, and hemorrhage (69). This may lead to calcification of scar tissue, leading to the formation of myositis ossificans. In 1973, Jackson and Feagin (70), from their experience at West Point, described a classification scheme for quadriceps contusions. *Mild contusions* were characterized by localized tenderness in the quadriceps with more than 90 degrees of flexion without altered gait, *moderate contusions* had antalgic gait and less than 90 degrees of flexion, and *severe contusions* had a severe limp and less than 45 degrees of knee flexion. A second paper on quadriceps contusion from West Point was published in 1991 (68). Contrast of these two papers shows an evolution of treatment of these injuries to include resting the injured leg in flexion (as opposed to extension) and emphasis on achieving early knee flexion. The knee must be carefully evaluated with these injuries for ligamentous damage and effusion. Assistive devices are utilized until the athlete has at least 90 degrees of flexion, has good quadriceps control, and is able to walk normally. Quadriceps strength is then increased to prepare for return to football. To protect the area, additional padding should be added to a standard thigh pad. The thigh pad should be held in place with the use of an elastic bandage or tape to ensure that it does not slip (29). Ryan and colleagues (68) reported that the average period of disability for mild contusions was 13 days, that for moderate contusions was 19 days, and that for severe contusions was 21 days. Myositis ossificans developed in 4% of the mild contusions, 18% of the moderate contusions, and 13% of the severe contusions (68). There was an increased incidence of myositis ossificans in injuries occurring in football, previous quadriceps injury, delayed treatment greater than 3 days, and ipsilateral knee effusion. No cadet with knee flexion greater than 120 degrees at initial evaluation developed myositis ossificans. Irrgang and colleagues have noted that in their experience, myositis ossificans will develop if treatment in the early phase is too aggressive or if the athlete is reinjured (29).

Although rarely, a thigh contusion can result in development of a thigh compartment syndrome (71). A high index of suspicion is necessary to make this diagnosis. Thigh compartment syndrome should be considered when a player receives a direct blow to the anterior thigh with subsequent unrelenting pain, swelling, and loss of knee motion (71). The five classic signs of compartment syndrome are pain out of proportion to the injury, pain on passive motion of associated joints, pulselessness, paresthesia, and pallor (72). However, not all five need to be present for the diagnosis to be made. Confirmation of clinical suspicion can be achieved by monitoring intracompartment pressure. Treatment is emergent fasciotomy.

Football players, like other athletes, are susceptible to muscle strains. These injuries tend to occur in muscles that cross two joints, such as the rectis femoris, hamstrings, gastrocnemius, and wrist extensors. Most groin muscle strains involve the hip flexors. Hamstring strains are most commonly seen in speed players: running backs, wide receivers, and defensive backs. Rectus femoris strains are commonly seen in kickers and punters. Muscle strains occur with eccentric muscle contractions and usually occur through the muscle fibers near the musculotendinous junction. The cornerstone of treatment is controlled stretching to align the healing fibrous scar tissue with the muscle line of pull. Mild strains may disable the athlete for 1–2 weeks, while severe strains may disable the athlete for 6–8 weeks. Proper warm-up and conditioning as well as maintaining a normal hamstring-to-quadriceps strength ratio (approximately 0.6) may help to prevent muscle strains. One report demonstrated a reduction in the incidence of hamstring injuries with a stretching and year-round weight-training and running program.

KNEE INJURIES

Knee injuries account for 22–37% of all football injuries (1,5,13). The high demand in football for cutting, jumping, pivoting, and rapid starting and stopping, combined with contact, contributes to the predominance of knee injuries in football. The most common injuries in football in descending order are MCL injuries, meniscal injuries, and ACL injuries.

In diagnosing ligament injuries, the history of mechanism is important. The player who injures a knee by falling onto the ground, striking the flexed knee, may have torn the posterior cruciate ligament (PCL). The player who injures a knee while changing directions with no contact may have torn the ACL. Alternatively, the player who sustains a valgus contact injury likely has torn at least the MCL and perhaps the cruciate ligaments.

Prevention

Prevention of knee injuries in football is a controversial subject. We have previously outlined the literature on the risk of knee injury depending on the type of shoe worn and the playing surface. The most appropriate type of cleat is a low (less than 0.5 inch) and wide (0.375-inch diameter) cleat (29). Such a shoe can provide adequate traction for running, cutting, and turning but also tends to give way and slide with strong external forces. For artificial turf, Torg and colleagues (22) recommend a multicleat shoe with a polyurethane sole. A conditioning program focusing on strengthening of the quadriceps and hamstring muscles and stretching of the hamstrings and the iliotibial band should be maintained.

The use of a prophylactic knee brace in football remains controversial. Several articles (73–78) have attempted to address this issue, but most are nonrandomized studies with the usual problems that accompany this type of study. A review of these articles leaves confusion, as some report decreased injury (73–76) and others report increased injury (77,78) in wearing prophylactic knee braces. In a prospective randomized study at West Point, Sitler and colleagues (79) demonstrated that intramural tackle football players who wore a prophylactic knee brace while on defense had significantly fewer knee injuries. This benefit was not seen in offensive players. The severity of injuries to the MCL and ACL was not statistically significantly reduced. The most frequent mechanism of injury in that study was attributed to a direct lateral blow to the knee that produced a valgus force. There was no significant difference between the braced group and the control group in the frequency of ankle injuries. Footwear, playing surface, athlete exposure, and knee injury history were all controlled in this study. In Albright and colleagues' report in 1987 Big Ten players, for lineman, linebackers, and tight ends there was a consistent trend toward a lower injury rate in braced players (74). The braced players in the skill positions (backs, kickers) exhibited a higher injury rate. From these studies, it seems that the main advantage of prophylactic knee braces is to prevent MCL injuries that occur from a contact mechanism in offensive and defensive linemen and linebackers. The decision to use a prophylactic brace should be left to the player and not be recommended by the team physician. Further well-controlled studies are needed before definitive conclusions can be made.

Ligament Injuries

Medial Collateral Ligament

Injuries to the MCL are the most common ligament injuries around the knee in football. The injury is usually a contact-induced valgus stress to the knee with the foot fixed. In a grade 1 injury the knee is treated symptomatically, and the player is allowed to bear weight as tolerated. Once the athlete has full range of motion and strength, he or she may return to play. Isolated grade 2 and 3 injuries should be treated nonoperatively with a double upright knee brace and range-of-motion and rehabilitation exercises as soon as the athlete can tolerate them (80). In both grade 2 and grade 3 injuries, players may return to participation when swelling or tenderness subsides and a full range of motion and muscle function have been restored. Timing for return to play is athlete and position specific. In our experience taping has been a useful adjunct to bracing in returning players to competition (81). Return to play was 10.6 days for grade 1 injuries (81), 19.6 days for grade 2 injuries (81), and 29 days for grade 3 injuries (82). Grade 3 injuries may require up to 9–10 weeks before return to play (80).

Anterior Cruciate Ligament

Bradley (83) recently reported on the ACL injury rate in the NFL over the past 10 years. The yearly incidence has been fairly constant at 2% of total knee injuries. The ACL injury rate is approximately 1 per 20 games and 0.4 per 100 practices. There have been a total of 441 ACL injuries in the last 10 years in the NFL.

Decisions regarding treatment options for the football player with an isolated ACL-deficient injury need to consider several factors. Our experience has been that players at certain positions (offensive/defensive linemen) may be able to participate with an isolated ACL-deficient knee. Certainly, the risk of subsequent giving way episodes and risk of further meniscal damage needs to be discussed with the player and be considered when deciding on a treatment plan. Nonoperative treatment consists of an aggressive rehabilitation program, including hamstring strengthening and the use of a functional knee brace for return to football. Players who require the ability to accelerate, decelerate, and change direction quickly (running backs, linebackers, receivers, and defensive backs) may not be able to play with their ACL-deficient knee and likely will require reconstruction. Players with nonisolated ACL injuries should undergo ACL reconstruction. As with any knee exam, attention to detail to differentiate between isolated and nonisolated ACL injuries is crucial. The use of a functional knee brace after surgical reconstruction of the anterior cruciate ligament is generally recommended. While probably not providing any mechanical stability, a brace may provide proprioceptive feedback to the quadriceps-hamstring mechanism that may help to prevent recurrent injuries to the ACL.

Players with a partial tear of their ACL may also return to play with the understanding that they may sustain a subsequent injury completing the tear. Noyes and Barber-Westin's study of 32 partial ACL tears (one third were football players) showed that the amount of ligament tearing diagnosed arthroscopically was a significant predictor of subsequent tearing (84). Tears involving one fourth of the ACL rarely progressed, half tears progressed in 50%, and three quarter tears progressed in 86% of knees. The occurrence of a subsequent giving way episode was also a significant predictor of progression to a complete tear. Bracing and aggressive rehabilitation are recommended for players with a partial ACL tear.

Posterior Cruciate Ligament

Most PCL injuries in football occur as a result of a fall on a flexed knee with the foot in plantar flexion, leading to an isolated PCL injury. Other mechanisms include a direct blow to the anterior tibia, hyperextension and hyper flexion. Varus and valgus injuries can tear the PCL after the collaterals.

As in the ACL-deficient knee it is essential to differentiate between isolated PCL tears and a PCL tear with associated capsuloligamentous injuries.

As with the ACL-deficient knee the true natural history of a PCL-deficient knee is not known. Because the isolated posterior cruciate ligament injury syndrome may be relatively benign and has been unrecognized in the past, we believe that there is a large silent group of asymptomatic functionally stable knees with posterior laxity. Parolie and Bergfeld (85) have noted that at the NFL combine, approximately 2% of elite college players have a PCL-deficient knee. These authors retrospectively evaluated 25 isolated PCL injured knees in athletes with a mean follow-up of 6.2 years (2.2–16 years). Eighty percent were satisfied with their knees, and 84% had returned to their previous sport (68% at the same level). The mean quadriceps strength for the athletes who had fully returned to sports and were satisfied with their knees was greater than 100% of the uninvolved knee; conversely, those who were not satisfied with their knees all had values less than 100% of the uninvolved knee. Posterior drawer at follow-up ranged from 2.5 to 14.5 mm. Posterior drawer decreased in internal rotation in 76%. In 1990, Kaeding and Bergfeld prospectively evaluated 34 acute isolated PCL injuries at a mean follow-up of 7.5 years (86,87). KT-1000 measurements ranged from 4 mm to 10 mm, and all patients had decreased posterior drawer with internal rotation of the tibia. The average Lysholm knee score was 93. Seventeen had a negative bone scan, and three had positive bone scans. The results of PCL reconstruction are clearly inferior to ACL reconstruction. We advocate PCL reconstruction for nonisolated PCL injuries. An open technique may be superior to arthroscopic reconstruction in reducing residual laxity (87).

Meniscal Injuries

Meniscal injuries in football players usually result from rotation of the knee while the foot is planted. Arthroscopic meniscal excision is effective in returning players to competition expeditiously. Isolated repair of a meniscal tear in a football player without ligamentous reconstruction is debatable. Certainly, the increased stress on the articular cartilage and an increased chance of degenerative arthritis at a later date need to be considered in deciding on meniscal tear treatment. DeHaven (88) has pointed out that when viewed from the standpoint of the potential for normal knee function and absence of degenerative problems, participation in a particular season may be an inordinately high price to pay for undergoing partial meniscectomy rather than repair. Decisions such as these need to be made carefully between physician and player.

Patellofemoral Problems

A fairly unique condition that we have seen in football players has been a patellar chondral flap causing significant limitation of ability to play. Typically, this is seen in linemen who complain of giving way or weakness in pushing off from a stance. In our experience, arthroscopic debridement of the chondral flap has been effective in returning these players to play.

LEG INJURIES

A tibial stress fracture with the "dreaded black line" is a potentially disabling injury. Our experience and that of others (89) is that intramedulary nailing of the tibial is the treatment of choice in the athlete desiring to resume a football career.

Fibular shaft fractures are not as benign in the football player as they are in the general population. Slauterbeck and colleagues (90) at UCLA reported three such fractures, all appearing benign, treated nonoperatively. All three were what they considered delayed unions (average: 23 weeks), and each case was complicated by refracture.

FOOT AND ANKLE INJURIES

Ankle sprains are the most common ankle injury in football. As in other sports, lateral ligament sprains are most common. The most common mechanism is supination and external rotation. These injuries most commonly occur when the athlete is cutting and changing direction.

Particularly difficult to treat are deltoid and syndesmotic sprains because the time for recovery seems out of proportion to the injury. Syndesmotic injury typically results from pronation, external rotation injuries. Guise (91) presented 16 cases of pronation-external rotation sprains in professional football players that resulted in injury to the syndesmotic ligaments. There was a longer recovery time compared to the supination-internal rotation injury. Boytim reported a 6-year experience of ankle sprains of one NFL team (92). Fifteen syndesmotic sprains were compared with 28 significant lateral ankle sprains. The players with syndesmotic sprains missed significantly more games and received substantially more treatments than did players with lateral sprains. Taylor and colleagues (93), at Duke, reported a retrospective review of 44 syndesmotic sprains in football players. All players were treated nonoperatively with a regiment of ice, whirlpool therapy, taping, and activity restriction. Oral prednisone was prescribed in several cases. Return to full activity was allowed when the ankle tenderness resolved and the player had no functionally limiting pain. Players who were the slowest to return to full activity had the best long-term results. The average return time to full activity was 31 days. Pain with pushing off was a major factor preventing return to activity. At follow-up (average: 47 months) over one third complained of persistent mild to moderate stiffness of the ankle. Twenty-three percent had mild to moderate pain, usually with activity. Eighteen percent of the ankles had persistent mild to moderate swelling. Ankle function was treated as good to excellent in 86%. Twenty-two of the players had follow-up X-rays. Of these, one half had heterotopic ossification of the interosseous membrane, but no player had a frank synostosis. Functionally, there were no differences between these two groups. The group with heterotopic ossification had more recurrent lateral ankle sprains. Veltri and colleagues (94) reported two documented syndesmosis sprains in NFL players that went on to develop painful heterotopic ossification of the syndesmosis. Both players resumed play 5–6 weeks after initial injury. Both players then developed symptoms 8–12 months later, which were thought to be secondary to their heterotopic ossification. One lesion involved the anterior aspect of the posterior aspect of the syndesmosis. They underwent excision of the heterotopic ossification after their respective seasons and were asymptomatic at 1- to 2-year follow-up. Careful radiographic follow-up in the first 6 weeks of this injury is required to rule out subsequent ankle diastasis. Miller and colleagues reported on four football players with deltoid and syndesmotic ligament injury and diastasis of the ankle requiring syndesmotic screw. This diagnosis requires a high index of suspicion and may require stress radiographs (95).

Treatment of acute ankle sprains includes protection, rest, ice, compression, and elevation. Proprioception and strengthening exercises should be started as soon as possible to develop dynamic stability for the ankle. Typically, when a player returns to play ankle braces, taping, and/or high-top shoes are used for protection from reinjury. An ankle orthosis may be used to allow plantar flexion and dorsiflexion while preventing medial and lateral motion. Surgery for acute ankle sprains is rarely indicated. Surgery may be indicated to correct chronic ankle instability.

Turf toe is a sprain of the plantar capsular ligament of the first metatarsophalangeal joint (96). Rodeo and colleagues reported that forced dorsiflexion was the mechanism of injury in 85%, forced plantar flexion in 12%, and valgus stress in 4% of turf toe (96). These players typically complain of pain during pushing off. On X-ray, there may be diastasis of a bipartite sesamoid (96). As we noted previously, the soft-soled soccer style shoe has contributed to this entity. Physical therapy, taping, and use of a stiff-soled shoe are effective in treating this condition.

Ward and Bergfeld (97) have reported on acute disruption of the fifth metatarsophalangeal sesamoid with fracture of both sesamoids in a professional running back. They pointed out that fluoroscopic or stress radiographs may be useful in differentiating a fractured or disrupted partite sesamoid from intact partite sesamoids.

The NFL experience with stress fractures at the junction of the distal metaphysis and diaphysis of the fifth metatarsal (Jones fracture) has been reported by Browne (98). Of 3165 elite college football players evaluated at the NFL combine from 1980 to 1997, 42 fractures were identified in 39 athletes.

Losse reported his results of a survey of NFL physicians on Achilles tendon ruptures (99). These injuries average 1 injury per 5 years of NFL experience according to this survey. The average return to play was 5.5 months after surgical repair.

CONCUSSIONS

Concussions are the most common head injury in football (4,73,97). A concussion, as defined by the Committee on Head Injury Nomenclature of the Congress of Neurological Surgeons, is "a clinical syndrome characterized by immediate and transient post-traumatic impairment of neural function, such as alteration of consciousness, disturbance of vision, equilibrium, etc., due to brain stem involvement" (100). Concussions are graded as mild (no loss of consciousness), moderate (loss of consciousness with retrograde amnesia), and severe (unconsciousness greater than 5 minutes) (100).

It is estimated that for high school football players in the United States there is up to a 20% risk of minor head injury or concussion each season (101). The true incidence of concussions in football is unknown. It is believed that athletes grossly underreport concussions to their athletic trainers, coaches, and physicians for fear of being removed from the game or practice. In addition, an athlete does not always recognize that a concussion has occurred (101,102) The senior author (103) using confidential questionnaires, documented that over a single season for a single high school varsity football team, 203 "bell rung" episodes occurred. Only six of these episodes were reported to the athletic trainer (103).

An athlete who has sustained one concussion is at fourfold greater risk for sustaining another concussion (101,103). The available studies on the long-term consequences of these minor injuries in athletes shows definite, but probably reversible, neuropsychological impairment after a single minor head injury. Wilberger (101) performed neuropsychological testing on high school football players after concussions with a subset of 62 players who had suffered two concussions in a single season. Initial neuropsychological tests were abnormal in 47 of these 62 players (75%). At 1 month postinjury, 61% (29 of 47) of these players had abnormal neuropsychological testing; at 3 months postinjury, 34% (16 of 47) had continuing abnormalities. In these 16 players, subjective symptoms such as headache, dizziness, and difficulty concentrating also remained common.

The prevention of these minor head injuries, while a noble concept, is very difficult in practice, given the violent nature of the game of football. Certainly, proper tackling techniques (e.g., not initiating contact with the head) should be stressed. Alteration in the current football helmet has been investigated (103). The ProCap is a polyurethane pad that attaches to the outside of a standard football helmet that was designed to prevent recurrent concussions in a professional football player. A significant concern that has been raised about the ProCap is the theoretical risk of increasing cervical spine injuries because of increased friction between the surface of the ProCap and other helmets or objects during contact. A pilot study that was performed on a single varsity high school football team showed promising results in reducing minor head injuries. However, this study had a small study population, considered only a single season, and was not adequate to address the cervical spine injury concerns. There is no simple solution to the significant problem of concussions in football.

REFERENCES

1. DeLee JC, Farney WC. Incidence of injury in Texas high school football. *Am J Sports Med* 1992;20:575–580.
2. Williford HN, Kirkpatrick J, Scharff-Olson, et al. Physical and performance characteristics of successful high school football players. *Am J Sports Med* 1994;22(6):859–862.
3. Nicholas JA, Rosenthal PP, Gleim GW. A historical perspective of injuries in professional football: twenty-six years of game-related events. *JAMA* 1988;260(7):939–944.
4. Powell J. 636,000 injuries annually in high school football. *Athletic Training* 1987;22(1):19–22.
5. Adkison JW, Requa RK, Garrick JG. Injury rates in high school football: a comparison of synthetic surfaces and grass fields. *Clin Orthop* 1974;99:131–136.
6. Mueller FO, Blyth CS. North Carolina high school football injury study: equipment and prevention. *Am J Sports Med* 1974;2:1–10.
7. Backx FJG, Erich BM, Kemper ABA, et al. Sports injuries in school aged children. *Am J Sports Med* 1989;17:234–240.
8. Blyth CS, Mueller FO. Football injury survey: III. Injury rates vary with coaching. *Phys Sportsmed,* 1974;2(11):45–50.
9. Robey JM, Blyth CS, Mueller FO. Athletic injuries: application of epidemiologic methods. *Phys Sportsmed* 1984;12(9):79–84.
10. Prager BI, Fitton WL, Cahill BR, Olson GH. High school football injuries: a prospective study and pitfalls of data collection. *Am J Sports Med* 1989;17:681–682
11. McLain LG, Reynolds S. Sports injuries in a high school. *Pediatrics* 1989;84:446–450.
12. Lowe EB, Perkins ER, Herndon JH. Rhode Island high school athletic injuries 1985–1986. *R I Med J* 1987;70:265–270.
13. Olson OC. The Spokane study: high school football injuries. *Phys Sportsmed* 1979;7(12):75–82.
14. Moretz A, Rashkin A, Grana WA. Oklahoma high school football injury study: a preliminary report. *J Okla State Med Assoc* 1978;71:85–88.
15. Hal RW, Mitchell W. Football injuries in Hawaii in 1979. *Hawaii Med J* 1981;40:180–182.
16. Andresen BL, Hoffman MD, Barton LW. High school football injuries: field conditions and other factors. *Wisconsin Med J* 1989;88:28–31.
17. Culpepper MI, Niemann KM. High school football injuries in Birmingham, Alabama. *South Med J* 1983;76:873–878.
18. Powell JW, Schootman M. A multivariate risk analysis of selected playing surfaces in the National Football League: 1980 to 1989.

An epidemiologic study of knee injuries. *Am J Sports Med* 1992;20(6);686–694.
19. Skovron, ML, Levy IM, Agel J. Living with artificial grass: a knowledge update. Part 2: epidemiology. *Am J Sports Med* 1990;18:510–513.
20. Torg JS, Quedenfeld T. Effect of shoe type and cleat length on incidence and severity of knee injuries among high school football players. *Res Q* 1971;42:203–211.
21. Lambson RB, Barnhill BS, Higgins RW. Football cleat design and its effect on anterior cruciate ligament injuries: a three-year prospective study. *Am J Sports Med* 1996;24(2):155–159.
22. Torg JS, Stilwell G, Rogers K. The effect of ambient temperature on the shoe-surface interface release coefficient. *Am J Sports Med* 1996;24:79–82.
23. Heidt RS, Dormer SG, Cawley PW, et al. Differences in friction and torsional resistance in athletic shoe-turf suface interfaces. *Am J Sports Med* 1996;24:834–842.
24. Cahill BR, Griffith EH. Exposure to injury in major college football: a preliminary report of data collection to determine injury exposure rates and activity risk factors. *Am J Sports Med* 1979;7:183–185.
25. Blyth CS, Mueller FO. Football injury survey: III. Injury rates vary with coaching. *Phys Sportsmed* 1974;2(11):45–50.
26. Torg JS, Quedenfeld TC, Burstein A, et al. National football head and neck injury registry report on cervical quadriplegia 1971–1975. *Am J Sports Med* 1977;7:127–132.
27. Torg JS, Truex R, Quedenfeld TC, et al. The national football head and neck injury registry: report and conclusions 1978. *JAMA* 1979;241:1477–1479.
28. Watkins RG. Neck injuries in football players. *Clin Sports Med* 1986;5:215–247.
29. Irrgang JJ, Miller MD, Johnson DL. Football injuries. In: Fu FH, Stone DA, eds. *Sports injuries: mechanisms, prevention, treatment.* Baltimore: Williams and Wilkins, 1994:349–374.
30. Gieck J, McCue FC.Fitting of protective football equipment. *Am J Sports Med* 1980;8:192–196.
31. Shields, CL, Zommar VD. Analysis of professional football injuries. *Contemp Orthop* 1982;4:90–95.
32. Blevins FT, Hayes WM, Warren RF. Rotator cuff injury in contact athletes. *Am J Sports Med* 1996;24:263–267.
33. Cox JS. The fate of the acromioclavicular joint in athletic injuries. *Am J Sports Med* 1981;9:50–59.
34. Clancy WG Jr, Brand RL, Bergfeld J. Upper trunk brachial plexus injuries in contact sports. *Am J Sports Med* 1977;5:209–216.
35. Marker LB, Klareskov B. Posterior sternoclavicular dislocation: an American football injury. *Br J Sports Med* 1996;30:71–72.
36. Zarins B, Prodromos LC. Shoulder injuries in sports. In: Rowe CR, ed. *The shoulder.* New York: Churchill Livingstone, 1988:411–433.
37. Perlmutter GS, Leffert RD, Zarins B. Direct injury to the axillary nerve in athletes playing contact sports. *Am J Sports Med* 1997;25:65–68.
38. Miller MD, Johnson DL, Fu FH, et al. Rupture of the pectoralis major muscle in a collegiate football player: use of magnetic resonance imaging in early diagnosis. *Am J Sports Med* 1993;21:475–477.
39. Speer KP. Personal communication, 1996.
40. Kenter K, Behr CT, Warren RF, O'Brien SJ, Barnes R. Acute elbow injuries in the National Football League. *J Shoulder Elbow Surg* 1999;9:1–5.
41. Meese MA, Sebastianelli WJ. Periostitis of the upper extremity. *Clin Orthop* 1996;324:222–226.
42. Andrish JT, Bergfeld JA,Walheim JA. Prospective study on the management of shin splints. *J Bone Joint Surg Am* 1974;56A:1697–1700.
43. Ward WG, Sekiya JK, Pope TL. Traumatic ossifying periostitis of the ulna masquerading as a malignancy in a football player: a case report and literature review. *Am J Sports Med* 1996;24:852–856.
44. Ellsasser JC, Stein AH. Management of hand injuries in a professional football team: review of 15 years of experience with one team. *Am J Sports Med* 1979;7(3):178–182.
45. Retig AC, Ryan R, Shelbourne KD, et al. Metacarpal fractures in the athlete. *Am J Sports Med* 1991;17:567–572.
46. Riester JN, Baker BE, Mosher JF, Lowe D. A review of scaphoid fracture healing in competitive athletes. *Am J Sports Med* 1985;13:159–161.
47. Raab DJ. Fischer DA, Quick DC. Lunate and perilunate dislocations in professional football players: a five-year retrospective analysis. *Am J Sports Med* 1994;22(6):841–845.
48. McCue FC, Mayer VI, Moran DJ. Gamekeeper's thumb: ulnar collateral ligament rupture. *J Musculoskeletal Med* 1988;5(12):53–63.
49. Frank CS, Woo S, Andriacchi R, et al. Normal ligament: structure, function, and composition. In: Woo SL-Y, Buckwalter JA, eds. *Injury and repair of the musculoskeletal soft tissues.* Park Ridge, IL: American Academy of Orthopaedic Surgeons, 1988:103–128.
50. Woo SL, Inoue M, McGurk-Burleson E, et al. Treatment of medial collateral ligament injury: II. Structure and funcion of canine knees in response to differing treatment regimens. *Am J Sports Med* 1987;15:22–29.
51. Fumich RM, Fink RJ, Hanna GR. Offensive lineman's thumb. *Phys Sportsmed* 1983;11:113–115.
52. Weiland AJ, Lister GD. Volar fracture dislocations of the 2nd and 3rd carpometacarpal joints associated with acute carpel tunnel syndrome. *J Trauma* 1976;16:672–675.
53. Ferguson AJ, McMaster JH, Stanitski CL. Low back pain in college football linemen. *J Sports Med Physical Fit* 1974;2:63–69.
54. McCarrol JR, Miller JM, Ritter MA. Lumbar spondylolisthesis in college football players: a prospective study. *Am J Sports Med* 1986;14:404–406.
55. Batts M. Etiology of spondylolisthesis. *J Bone Joint Surg* 1939;21:879–884.
56. Hitchcock HH. Spondylolisthesis: observation on its development, progression, and genesis. *J Bone Joint Surg* 1940;22:1–16.
57. Hoshina H. Spondylolysis in athletes. *Physician Sportsmed* 1980;3:75–78.
58. Jackson DW. Low back pain in young athletes: evaluation of stress reaction and discogenic problems. *Am J Sports Med* 1979;7:364–366.
59. McCarrol JR, Miller JM, Ritter MA. Lumbar spondylolisthesis in college football players: a prospective study. *Am J Sports Med* 1986;14:404–406.
60. Semon RL, Spengler D. Significance of lumbar spondylolysis in college football players. *Spine* 1981;6(2);172–174.
61. Tewes DP, Fischer DA, Zamberletti F, Powell J. Lumbar transverse process fractures in professional football players. *Am J Sports Med* 1995;23:507–509.
62. Day AL, Friedman WA, Indelicate PA: Observations on the treatment of lumbar disk disease in college football players. *Am J Sports Med* 1987;15(1):72–75.
63. Renstom P. Tendon and muscle injuries in the groin area. *Clin Sports Med* 1992;11:815–833.
64. Stenger A. Bo's hip dislocates stellar athletic career. *Phys Sportsmed* 1991;19:17–18.
65. Cooper DE, Warren RF, Barnes R. Traumatic subluxation of the hip resulting in aseptic necrosis and condrylolysis in a professional football player. *Am J Sports Med* 1991;19:322–324.
66. Moorman CT, Warren RF, Hershman E, et al. Traumatic hip subluxation in American football. Presented at AOSSM 22 annual meeting, June 1996.
67. Karpos PA, Spindler KP, Pierce MA, Shull HJ. Osteomyelitis of the pubic symphysis in athletes: a case report and literature review. *Med Sci Sports Exerc* 1995;27:473–478.
68. Ryan JB, Wheeler JH, Hopkinson WJ, et al. Quadriceps contusions: West Point update. *Am J Sports Med* 1991;19:299–304.
69. Ciuflo JV, Zarins B. Biomechanics of the musculotendinious unit: relation to athletic performance and injury. *Clin Sports Med* 1983;2:71–86.
70. Jackson DW, Feagin JA. Quadriceps contusions in young athletes. *J Bone Joint Surg Am* 1973;55A:95–105.
71. Colosimo AJ, Ireland ML. Thigh compartment syndrome in a football athlete: a case report and review of the literature. *Med Sci Sports Exerc* 1992;24:958–963.
72. Whitesides TE, Haney TC, Morimoto K, Harada H. Tissue pres-

sure measurements as a determinant for the need of fasciotomy. *Clin Orthop* 1975;113:43–51.
73. Rovere GD, Haupt HA, Yates CS. Prophylactic knee bracing in college football. *Am J Sports Med* 1987;15:111–116.
74. Albright JP, Powell JW, Smith W, et al. Medial collateral ligament knee sprains in college football: effectiveness of preventive braces. *Am J Sports Med* 1994;22:12–18.
75. Hanson BL, Ward JC, Diehl RC. The preventive use of the Anderson Knee Stabler in football. *Physician Sportsmed* 1975; 13:75–81.
76. Hewson GF, Mendini RA, Wang JB. Prophylactic knee bracing in college football. *Am J Sports Med* 1986;14:262–266.
77. Teitz CC, Hermanson RK, Kronmal RA, et al. Evaluations of the use of braces to prevent injury to the knee in collegiate football players. *J Bone Joint Surg Am* 1987;69A:2–9.
78. Grace TG, Skipper BJ, Newberry JC, et al. Prophylactic knee braces and injury to the lower extreniity. *J Bone Joint Surg Am* 1987;70A:422–427.
79. Sitler M, Ryan J, Hopkinson W, et al. The efficacy of prophylactic knee brace to reduce knee injuries in football: a prospective randomized study at West Point. *Am J Sports Med* 1990;18: 310–315.
80. Indelicato PA, Herinansdorfer J, Huegel M. Nonoperative management of complete tears of the medial collateral ligament of the knee in intercollegiate football players. *Clin Orthop* 1990; 256:174–177.
81. Derscheid GL, Garrick JG. Medial collateral ligament injuries in football: nonoperative management of grade I and grade II sprains. *Am J Sports Med* 1981;9:365–368.
82. Jones RE, Henley MB, Francis P. Nonoperative management of isolated grade III collateral ligament injury in high school football players. *Clin Orthop* 1986;213:137–140.
83. Bradley JP. ACL injuries: the NFL experience. Presented at the 1996 NFL Physicians Society Meeting, Palm Harbour, FL, 1996.
84. Noyes FR, Barber-Westin SD. Posterior cruciate ligament allograft reconstruction with and without a ligament augmentation device. *Arthroscopy* 1984;10:371–382.
85. Parolie J, Bergfeld JA. Long term results of nonoperative treatment of PCL injuries in the athlete. *Am J Sports Med* 1986; 13(1);35–38.
86. Kaeding C, Bergfeld JA. Personal communication, 1996.
87. Bergfeld JA, Edelson RH, Parker RD, et al. Biomechanical analysis of posterior cruciate ligament reconstruction: comparison of tibial tunnel versus anatomic posterior tibial fixation of the bone-patellar tendon-bone graft. Presented at AOSSM, Toronto, Canada, 1995.
88. DeHaven KE. Meniscus repair in the athlete. *Clin Orthop* 1985;198:31–35.
89. Barrick EF, Jackson EB. Prophylactic intramedullary fixation of the tibia for stress fracture in the professional athlete. *J Orthop Trauma* 1992;6:241–244.
90. Slauterbeck JR, Shapiro MS, Liu S, Finerman GA. Traumatic fibular shaft fractures in athletes. *Am J Sports Med* 1995; 23:751–754.
91. Guise ER. Rotational ligamentous injuries to the ankle in football. *Am J Sports Med* 1976;4:1–6.
92. Boytim MJ, Fischer DA, Neumann L. Syndesmotic ankle sprains. *Am J Sports Med* 1991;19:294–298.
93. Taylor DC, Englehardt DL, Bassett FH. Syndesmosis sprains of the ankle: the influence of heterotopic ossification. *Am J Sports Med* 1992;20:146–150.
94. Veltri DM, Pagnani MJ, O'Brien SJ, et al. Symptomatic ossification of the tibiofibular syndesmosis in professional football players: a sequela of the syndesmotic ankle sprain. *Foot Ankle Int* 1995;16(5):285–290.
95. Miller CD, Shelton WR, Barrett GR, et al. Deltoid and syndesmosis ligament injury of the ankle without fracture. *Am J Sports Med* 1995;23:746–750.
96. Rodeo SA, O'Brien S, Warren RF, et al. Turf toe: an analysis of metatorsalphalangeal joint sprains in professional football players. *Am J Sports Med* 1990;18:280–285.
97. Ward WG, Bergfeld JA. Fluoroscopic demonstration of acute disruption of the fifth metatarsophalangeal sesamoid bones. *Am J Sports Med* 1993;21:895–897.
98. Browne JE. Foot injuries in the NFL. Presented at the 1996 NFL Physicians Society Meeting, Palm Harbour, FL, 1996.
99. Lossee GM. Ankle injuries in the NFL. Presented at the 1996 NFL Physicians Society Meeting, Palm Harbour, FL, 1996.
100. American Academy of Neurology. Practice parameter: the management of concussion in sports (summary statement). Report of the Quality Standards Subcommittee. *Neurology* 1997;48: 581–585.
101. Wilberger JE. Minor head injuries in American football: prevention of long term sequelae. *Sports Med* 1993;15:338–343.
102. Maroon JC, Steele PB, Berlin R. Football head and neck injuries: an update. *Clin Neurosurg* 1980;27:414–429.
103. Paul JJ, Fine K, Driscoll J, Walters F, Malekzeedah S. A randomized prospective assessment of the efficacy of the ProCap football helmet liner. Presented at the AOSSM annual meeting, Orlando, FL, June 1996.

CHAPTER 41

Golf

Thomas J. Noonan and William J. Mallon

Golf is often regarded as a relatively safe sport because of its seemingly benign nature. Until recently, reports of injury in golf were relatively rare. It has been well established, however, that both professional and amateur golfers experience numerous injuries. It has been estimated that over 50% of touring professionals have sustained some injury that prevented them from playing competitively for 3–10 weeks (1). On average, a professional golfer suffers two injuries per year (1). This is easily imaginable, considering the hundreds of balls that these elite golfers must hit daily to stay competitive. However, even in the casual golfer, injury is common (2). In these cases it is likely due to poor swing mechanics in addition to overuse.

Among male professional golfers, McCarroll and Gioe (1) found lower back injuries to be most common, followed by left wrist, left shoulder, and left knee injuries. Among female professional golfers, left wrist injuries were most common, followed by lower back, left hand, and left knee injuries. In total, left wrist and lower back injuries had nearly the same incidence. Left hand, left shoulder, and left knee injuries occurred with similar incidence and were next most frequent (Table 41–1).

Regarding the recreational golfer, Mallon and Colosimo (3) have also published a report based on a large body of data from letters written to Mallon for a golfing medical column. They reported low back injuries to be the most common by a large margin, followed by left elbow injuries. Left shoulder and left wrist injuries were next most common and occurred with nearly equal frequency (Table 41–2).

McCarroll and colleagues (2) also studied amateur golfers. They found that in males low back injuries were most common, followed by elbow, hand or wrist, shoulder, and knee injuries. In females the elbow was most commonly injured, followed by lower back, shoulder, hand or wrist, and knee. This study did not specify the side injured (Table 41–3).

When comparing handicaps, the golfers with the lowest ones had a slight but significant increase in injury rate (2). The frequency of injury was also higher in golfers who were older than 50 as compared with their younger counterparts (2).

To better understand the origin of the various injuries associated with golf, it is necessary to be familiar with the basic mechanics of the golf swing. The swing is usually considered in several phases: setup and address, backswing, transition between backswing and downswing (forward swing), forward swing, and follow-through.

The setup merely refers to the time at which golfers grip the club and align themselves in the proper stance. The backswing begins with the takeaway. As the club is swung back, the shoulders rotate away from the target. The lower back and thoracic spine perform this rotation. The head seems to remain stationary, which is somewhat illusory. For this to be the case, the cervical spine must counterrotate in the direction opposite that of the shoulder turn. At the top of the backswing in a right-handed golfer, the left wrist is radially deviated and forearm pronated, the right wrist is dorsiflexed and radially deviated and forearm supinated, the right shoulder is abducted and externally rotated, and the left shoulder is forward flexed slightly but mainly undergoes maximal cross-body adduction (3,4).

The transition movement is probably the most critical phase in determining the outcome of a golf shot. Among professional golfers, it is controversial how the forward swing is initiated. It is usually considered to be a movement of the lower body before the upper body. This can be rotation of the hips back toward the target, sliding the hips toward the target, or sliding the knees and ankles toward the target. The result of any of these

---

T. J. Noonan: Charlotte Orthopaedic Specialists, Charlotte, North Carolina 28207.

W. J. Mallon: Duke University Medical Center, Durham, North Carolina 27710.

TABLE 41–1. Injuries among professional golfers

	Men (192)	Women (201)	Totals (393)
Left wrist	31 (16%)	63 (31%)	94 (24%)
Lower back	48 (25%)	45 (22%)	93 (24%)
Left hand	13 (7%)	15 (8%)	28 (7%)
Left shoulder	21 (11%)	6 (3%)	27 (7%)
Left knee	14 (7%)	12 (6%)	26 (7%)
Left elbow	6 (3%)	9 (5%)	15 (4%)
Left thumb	10 (5%)	3 (2%)	13 (3%)
Feet	4 (2%)	9 (5%)	13 (3%)
Cervical spine	9 (4%)	3 (2%)	12 (3%)
Right wrist	3 (2%)	9 (5%)	12 (3%)
Ribs	6 (3%)	6 (3%)	12 (3%)
Right elbow	8 (4%)	3 (2%)	11 (3%)
Right shoulder	1 (1%)	9 (5%)	10 (3%)
Thoracic spine	8 (4%)	0 (0%)	8 (2%)
Ankles	2 (1%)	6 (3%)	8 (2%)
Groin	2 (1%)	3 (2%)	5 (1%)
Left hip	4 (2%)	0 (0%)	4 (1%)
Head	2 (1%)	0 (0%)	2 (1%)

From McCarroll JR, Gioe TJ. Professional golfers and the price they pay. *Phys Sports Med* 1982;10:54–70.

TABLE 41–3. Injuries among amateur golfers

	Men (584)	Women (124)	Totals (708)
Lower back	210 (36%)	34 (27%)	244 (35%)
Elbow	190 (33%)	44 (36%)	234 (33%)
Lateral	160 (27%)	34 (27%)	194 (27%)
Medial	30 (5%)	10 (8%)	40 (6%)
Hand and wrist	124 (21%)	18 (15%)	142 (20%)
Shoulder	64 (11%)	20 (16%)	84 (12%)
Knee	52 (9%)	14 (11%)	66 (9%)
Neck	26 (5%)	2 (2%)	28 (4%)
Hip	18 (3%)	4 (3%)	22 (3%)
Ribs	16 (3%)	6 (5%)	22 (3%)
Ankle	8 (1%)	10 (8%)	18 (3%)
Foot	12 (2%)	0 (0%)	12 (2%)
Head	12 (2%)	0 (0%)	12 (2%)
Thigh	8 (1%)	0 (0%)	8 (1%)
Face	6 (1%)	0 (0%)	6 (1%)
Abdomen	4 (1%)	0 (0%)	4 (1%)
Calf	4 (1%)	0 (0%)	4 (1%)
Forearm	0 (0%)	2 (2%)	2 (0%)

From McCarroll JR, Rettig AC, Shelbourne KD. Injuries in the amateur golfer. *Phys Sports Med* 1990;18:122–126.

movements, as the upper body is held back, is to increase the torque on the lower back and thoracic spine (3).

During the downswing, the left arm reverses its movement of cross-body adduction and returns to a position approximating the setup position. Both wrists change slightly from ulnar deviation to radial deviation. This is often called the "release" in medical writing, but that is a misnomer and is not considered how professionals release the clubhead. The release, which occurs from midbackswing, through impact, and into the follow-through, consists of rapid forearm rotation. At midbackswing, the left arm is internally rotated at the shoulder and pronated at the forearm. The right arm is in the opposite position of external rotation and supination.

TABLE 41–2. Injuries among recreational golfers

	Men (1160)	Women (249)	Totals (1409)
Lower back	617 (53%)	111 (45%)	728 (52%)
Left elbow	273 (24%)	68 (27%)	341 (24%)
Lateral	131 (11%)	49 (20%)	180 (13%)
Medial	44 (4%)	19 (8%)	63 (4%)
Left shoulder	101 (9%)	10 (4%)	111 (8%)
Left wrist	71 (6%)	35 (14%)	106 (8%)
Left ankle	34 (3%)	7 (3%)	41 (3%)
Vision problems	28 (2%)	6 (2%)	34 (2%)
Right hip	13 (1%)	4 (2%)	17 (1%)
Left hip	10 (<1%)	4 (2%)	14 (1%)
Right knee	7 (<1%)	3 (1%)	10 (<1%)
Left knee	6 (<1%)	1 (<1%)	7 (<1%)

From Mallon WJ, Colosimo AJ. Acromio-clavicular joint injury in competitive golfers. *J South Orthop Assoc* 1995;4(4):277–282.

Through impact and into follow-through, the arms reverse their anatomic positions. At mid-follow-through in high-caliber golfers, the left arm is close to the left flank and externally rotated, with the left forearm supinated. At that time the right arm is approaching cross-body adduction, internally rotating, and the forearm is pronating. Shortly after impact, both the left and right arm are straight for the only time during the golf swing (3,5).

Therefore the performance of a golf swing necessitates a considerable range of motion of many joints of the body. In addition, this occurs at high speeds with clubhead velocities of over 100 miles per hour generated in less than a fifth of a second (6). It comes as no surprise, then, that golf is associated with a large number of skeletal injuries. We will now present a more in-depth discussion of some of the more common maladies.

LOW BACK INJURIES

The lower back is among the most common site of injuries among golfers. This can be explained in part by the evolution of the modern golf swing. The classic swing used a flatter swing plane with a large hip and shoulder turn with the hips rotating almost as much as the shoulders. The follow-through found the golfer in an upright-I position. In contrast, the modern swing restricts the hip turn, thereby generating torque in the back and shoulders, yielding higher clubhead speed. In addition, the follow-through is often characterized by a hyperextended back (reverse-C position), although this position is now less popular among good players than it was in the 1960s and 1970s, when it was espoused by Jack

Nicklaus and Johnny Miller (7). The reverse-C position leads to greater rotation and hyperextension of the lumbar spine in the modern swing and is a potential cause of low back injury.

Beyond the mere range of motion required, a golf swing causes large forces to be generated in the lumbar spine. Lateral bending force, shear force in the anteroposterior direction, compression force, and torsional force are all developed during a golf swing. Hosea and colleagues (7) evaluated these forces in four professional and four amateur golfers. The amateurs developed approximately 80% greater peak lateral bending and shear loads than the professionals. The amateurs averaged a peak shear load of 560 N, while the professionals peaked at 329 N. For comparison, peak shear loads in men during rowing and during a squat weight lifting movement were 848 N and 690 N, respectively (8,9).

Compression of the lumbar spine was eight times body weight during a golf swing. The torque at the L3-4 motion segment during a golf swing averaged 85.2 Nm for amateurs and 56.8 Nm for professionals.

Hosea and colleagues also studied the myoelectric activity that is present during a golf swing. The amateurs reached 90% of their peak muscle activity, compared with 80% for the professionals. The professionals displayed a discrete on-off firing pattern when compared with the amateurs.

In early backswing, the left external oblique and, to a lesser degree, the left rectus abdominus and left paraspinal muscles were active. From the transition through impact, the muscles on the right side of the trunk, especially the right external oblique, are active. The right and left paraspinals fired nearly symmetrically during this phase, demonstrating their stabilizing action (7).

The loads on the lumbar spine during a golf swing may predispose a golfer to a number of conditions that may cause back pain: muscle strain injury, herniated nucleus pulposus, spondylolysis, and facet arthropathy with associated spinal stenosis (10–12). The forces required to cause disc disruption in cadaveric studies are similar to those measured by Hosea and colleagues. Adams and Hutton (10) showed disc prolapse with loads of 5448 N, whereas Hosea and colleagues showed compression forces in excess of 6000 N in the golfer. Although discs are made to function under compressive loads, they lose water and proteoglycans with age, which directly affects their viscoelastic properties. This in turn causes increased loading of the facets and other posterior vertebral structures, which can lead to the development of back pain.

The facets in the lumbar spine are oriented to resist shear force. They are capable of resisting one third to one half of the shear force; the discs absorb the remainder. Peak shear loads as measured by Hosea and colleagues approached 600 N, which is similar to experimental forces (570 ± 190 N) necessary to produce fractures of the pars interarticularis in cadavers (13,14). The shear forces may lead to spondylolysis.

SHOULDER

Though the shoulder is not positioned in golf as it is in overhead sports, the joint is nevertheless susceptible to injury in golfers. Certainly, overuse may be causative, as a professional may perform 2000 or more shoulder rotations per week (15). This volume of repetitions can cause tissues to break down faster than they can be repaired. A variety of shoulder conditions may ensue that are both age- and swing-related.

The older golfer faces the problems of the degenerative aging process, which include muscular atrophy, decreased vascularity, and breakdown of articular cartilage. As a result, these golfers are likely to suffer from impingement, rotator cuff tears, and glenohumeral and acromioclavicular arthritis. The younger golfer, on the other hand, is more apt to suffer from instability or pure overuse. This may lead to rotator cuff tendinitis and posterior capsulitis (15).

Swing mechanics also contribute to the occurrence of shoulder disorders in the golfer. These usually relate to the lead arm (the left arm in a right-handed golfer). At the top of the backswing, the lead arm is in slight forward flexion and maximal cross-body adduction, a very unusual position. This position is known to increase the stress across the acromioclavicular joint, and one study has shown a high incidence of problems in that joint among competitive golfers (16).

During the forward swing, the scapular muscles play a major role, as they provide a stable base for the shoulder. If they are weak, a scapular lag can result, causing generalized pain and putting the shoulder at a higher risk for injury (15).

During follow-through, the lead arm is horizontally abducted and externally rotated. This may cause internal impingement, although this has not yet been reported as a common problem among golfers.

Rotator cuff muscles may also suffer from pure overuse, as they play a critical role in the golf swing. Jobe and colleagues (17) studied shoulder muscle activity during a golf swing using electromyography. They found that the subscapularis fires throughout the golf swing bilaterally. Supraspinatus and infraspinatus fire at a lesser level, again bilaterally. They also found that the latissimus dorsi and pectoralis major contributed significantly in power generation, whereas the deltoid is relatively quiet throughout the swing. These results suggest that strengthening of these muscle groups may protect against injury as improper conditioning can lead to undue fatigue and increased susceptibility to muscle strain injury and rotator cuff tendinitis.

ELBOW

Despite the fact that golfer's elbow refers to medial epicondylitis, lateral epicondylitis is a more common finding (2). In a right-handed golfer this is usually found in the lead (left) arm. Less commonly, medial epicondylitis is found in the right arm (6,12) and may be associated with ulnar nerve symptoms. True radial tunnel syndrome is rare in golfers but may occasionally be caused by epicondylar spurring or calcification. Degenerative spurs and loose bodies with resultant catching and locking may also be rarely found.

Several factors relate to elbow injuries in golf. Overuse certainly plays a major role. Repetitive play can lead to lateral elbow pain in the lead arm and medial elbow pain in the following arm (18–21). Age also plays a role; the incidence of elbow injuries increases in frequency in golfers aged 35–55 years (22).

Finally, swing mechanics play a role in elbow injury. Near and through impact, high forces are exerted by the forearm extensors of the lead arm and the forearm flexors of the trail arm. When the forces are repeated hundreds to thousands of times per week, inflammation and ensuing degeneration may occur at the origin of these muscle groups, leading to the aforementioned syndromes (23).

There has been some consideration for the use of graphite shafts to prevent elbow and wrist injuries in golfers and to allow golfers with those injuries to continue playing golf. The hypothesis is that the graphite will absorb the shock of impact and divots more fully, preventing stress from reaching the wrist and elbow. No scientific studies have yet been done to confirm this, and it remains only a conjecture.

WRIST

Wrist injuries are fairly common in golf. The left wrist is injured with much more frequency than the right in the right-handed golfer. Considering the demands of the golf swing on the wrists, this is not surprising. During the swing of a right-handed golfer, considerable right wrist motion is required in the flexion/extension plane (103°) as well as in the plane of radial and ulnar deviation (45°) (11). The left wrist undergoes a smaller amount of flexion and extension (71°) but more radial and ulnar deviation (46.5°) (24). The biomechanics of the wrist nearing impact were discussed in detail earlier. Rotation of the forearms from middownswing to mid-follow-through occurs at speeds approaching 1500 radians/minute among top players. In addition, the range of motion required of the wrist in the golf swing exceeds the functional range of motion of the joint (25). Both of these factors may play a role in wrist injury in the golfer.

Tendinitis is the most common wrist injury in the golfer (26). This is due to repetitive microtrauma, which leads to inflammation and chronically to fibrosis (27). Because of the large number of tendons crossing the wrist, many forms of tendinitis are possible in the golfer.

De Quervain's disease is due to inflammation of the abductor pollicis longus and extensor pollicis brevis tendons as they pass through the first dorsal compartment of the wrist (28). Several aspects of the golf swing may predispose to this condition. At impact, the left wrist assumes an ulnar deviated position that places a strain on these tendons. Also, at the top of the backswing, the higher handicapped golfer is prone to early release of the hands, whereby the golfer allows the wrists to lose their cocked position. This allows the left wrist to abruptly ulnarly deviate while the left thumb is fixed in position between the right hand and the golf club.

Extensor carpi ulnaris tendinitis is characterized by tenderness over the sixth dorsal compartment of the wrist (28). The placement of the wrist into radial deviation at the top of the backswing and then subsequent forceful motion into ulnar deviation at impact may predispose to this condition.

Rupture of the extensor carpi ulnaris tendon sheath can occur when a sudden volar flexion, ulnar deviation, and forearm supination movement combination is applied to the wrist (29). This has been reported in golfers (29,30) as the result of the clubhead striking the ground or an obstruction such as a tree trunk or root. With complete disruption of the ulnar restraint of the sixth dorsal compartment, activation of the extensor carpi ulnaris may lead to volar dislocation of the tendon.

Tendinitis of the flexor carpi radialis is characterized by pain and tenderness over the volar radial aspect of the wrist (31,32). The pain is usually at the distal aspect of the flexor carpi radialis tendon where it passes through a fibro-osseous sheath, the flexor carpi radialis tunnel. The flexor carpi radialis tendon crosses the scaphoid tubercle and scapho-trapezial-trapezoid joint and inserts at the base of the second and third metacarpal and the trapezium. Repetitive volar wrist flexion against resistance (33), as occurs in the golf swing in the lead arm, is considered to be the etiology of flexor carpi radialis tendinitis.

Tendinitis of the flexor carpi ulnaris is fairly common among golfers (27). In the right-handed golfer, it is found most often in the right hand, perhaps because of the large amount of flexion and extension required of the right wrist during the golf swing (23). Flexor carpi ulnaris tendinitis is marked by painful wrist motion and tenderness over the tendon sheath.

Stenosing tenosynovitis of the digital flexors presents with pain, locking and triggering of the involved digit. It is due to thickening of the A1 pulley with associated synovitis. It has been speculated that this can occur as a result of mechanical irritation upon the pulley (27).

Intersection syndrome has been recognized rarely in golfers. It is a tendinitis that is 4–5 cm proximal to

Lister's tubercle (34). The etiology is uncertain, but it is thought to involve a bursa that is found at the intersection of the abductor pollicis longus, extensor pollicis brevus, and radial wrist extensors. The condition presents with localized pain, tenderness, crepitus, and swelling of the distal forearm. Overrolling of the wrists at the completion of the golf swing was felt to be causative in at least one professional golfer (14).

Fractures, on the whole, are seldom seen in golf. However, fracture of the hook of the hamate has been noted on many occasions in the golfer. Torisu (35) first reported this injury. In this case severe pain occurred after a routine swing with a pitching wedge. The reported mechanism was a direct force of the butt of the club against the hook of the hamate. This injury has also been noted after striking behind the ball (16,20,36) as well as striking a golf ball on hard ground (35). Symptoms of a hook of the hamate fracture include ulnar-sided wrist pain, weakness of grip, pain with gripping, and ulnar nerve paresthesias (36,37,38). Physical findings include pain to palpation over the hypothenar eminence, painful abduction and adduction of the small finger against resistance, and painful flexing of the ring and little fingers (37).

SUMMARY

Despite golf's reputation as a safe sport, there is a myriad of injuries that may be encountered in the golfer. The most common of these include injuries to the lower back, shoulder, elbow, and wrist. These injuries are due to overuse as well as to the biomechanics of the golf swing. Effective treatment of a golf-associated injury requires a thorough understanding of the etiology of the problem and its relationship to the biomechanics of the golf swing.

REFERENCES

1. Stark HH, Jobe FW, Boyes JH, et al. Fracture of the hook of the hamate in athletes. *J Bone Joint Surg Am* 1977;59:575–582.
2. McCarroll JR, Gioe TJ. Professional golfers and the price they pay. *Phys Sports Med* 1982;10:54–70.
3. McCarroll JR, Rettig AC, Shelbourne KD. Injuries in the amateur golfer. *Phys Sports Med* 1990;18:122–126.
4. Mallon WJ, Colosimo AJ. Acromio-clavicular joint injury in competitive golfers. *J South Orthop Assoc* 1995;4(4):277–282.
5. Cochran A, Stobbs J. *The search for the perfect swing.* Philadelphia: Lippincott, 1968:44–93.
6. Hogan B, Wind HW. *Five lessons: the modern fundamentals of golf.* New York: AS Barnes, 1957:100–106.
7. Stover CN, Wiren G, Topaz SR. The modern golf swing and stress syndromes. *Phys Sportsmed* 1976;4:42–47.
8. Hosea TM, Gatt CJ, Gertner E. Biomechanical analysis of the golfers back. In: Stover CN, McCarroll JR, Mallon WJ, eds. *Feeling up to par: medicine from tee to green.* Philadelphia: FA Davis, 1994.
9. Hosea TM, Boland AL. Rowing injuries. *Postgrad Adv Sports Med* 1989;3(2):1–17.
10. Hanssen TH, et al. The load on the lumbar spine during isometric strength testing. *Spine* 1984;9:710.
11. Adams MA, Hutton WC. Mechanics of the intervertebral disc. In: Ghosh P, ed. *The biology of the intervertebral disc,* vol 2. Boca Raton, FL: CRC Press, 1988:39–71.
12. Kirkaldy-Willis WH: Pathology of pathogenesis of lumbar spinal stenosis. In: Brown FW, ed. *Symposium on the lumbar spine.* St. Louis: Mosby, 1981:16–20.
13. Wiesel SW, Bernini P, Rothman RH. *The aging lumbar spine.* Philadelphia: WB Saunders, 1982:23–29.
14. Cryon BM, Hutton WC. The fatigue strength of the lumbar neural arch in spondylolysis. *J Bone Joint Surg Br* 1978;60:234.
15. Hutton WC, Stott JRR, Cyron BM. Is spondylolysis a fatigue fracture? *Spine* 1977;2:202.
16. Jobe FW, Pink MM. Shoulder pain in golf. *Clin Sports Med* 1996;15(1):55–63.
17. Carter PR, Eaton RG, Littler JW. Ununited fracture of the hook of the hamate. *J Bone Joint Surg Am* 1977;58:583–588.
18. Jobe FW, Moynes DR, Antonelli DJ. Rotator cuff function during a golf swing. *Am J Sports Med* 1986;14(5):388–392.
19. Stover CN, Mallon WJ. Management and prevention of golf injuries. *J Musculoskel Med* 1992;9:55–72.
20. Batt ME. Golfing injuries: an overview. *Sports Med* 1993;16:64–71.
21. Stark HH, Jobe FW, Boyes JH, et al. Fracture of the hook of the hamate in athletes. *J Bone Joint Surg Am* 1977;59:575-582.
22. Purley M. Golf injuries. *Golf* 1993;35(10):112–113.
23. Kohn HS. Prevention and treatment of elbow injuries in golf. *Clin Sports Med* 1996;15(1):65–83.
24. Cahalan TD, Cooney WP, Tamaj K, et al. Biomechanics of the golf swing in players with pathologic conditions of the forearm, wrist, and hand. *Am J Sports Med* 1991;19:288–293.
25. Chao EYS, Tamai K, Cahalan TD, et al. Biomechanics of the golf swing as related to club handle design. In Rekow ED, ed. *Biomechanics in sports: A 1987 update,* vol 6. New York: American Society of Engineers, 1987:107–111.
26. Palmer AK, Werner FW, Murphy D, et al. Functional wrist motion: a biomechanical study. *J Hand Surg [Am]* 1985;10:39–46.
27. Murray PM, Cooney WP. Golf-induced injuries of the wrist. *Clin Sports Med* 1996;15(1):85–109.
28. Kiefhaber TR, Stern PJ. Upper extremity tendinitis and overuse syndromes in the athlete. *Clin Sports Med* 11: 39–56, 1992.
29. Wolf T. Injuries and physical complaints caused by golf. *Sportverletzung Sportschaden* 1989;3:124–127.
30. Osterman A, Moskow L, Low D. Soft tissue injuries of the hand and wrist in racquet sports. *Clin Sports Med* 1988;7:329–348.
31. Golfer's wrist [editorial]. *Br Med J* 1977;2:1622.
32. Bishop AT, Gabel G. Flexor carpi radialis tendinitis: I and II. *J Bone Joint Surg* 1994;76A:1009–1018.
33. Fritton JM, Shea FW, Goldie W. Lesions of the flexor carpi radialis tendon and sheath causing pain at the wrist. *J Bone Joint Surg Br* 1968;50:359–363.
34. Greenberg AB, Regan DS. Pathologic anatomy of the forearm: intersection syndrome. *J Hand Surg [Am]* 1985;10:299–302.
35. Wood M, Dobyns JH. Sports related extra-articular wrist syndromes. *Clin Orthop* 1986;202:93–102.
36. Torisu T. Fracture of the hook of the hamate by a golf swing. *Clin Orthop* 1972;83:91–94.
37. Norman A, Nelson J, Green S. Fractures of the hook of the hamate: radiographic signs. *Radiology* 1985;154:49–53.
38. Bishop AT, Beckenbaugh RD. Fracture of the hamate hook. *J Hand Surg [Am]* 1988;13:135–139.
39. McCarroll JR, Mallon WJ. Epidemiology of golf injuries. In: Stover CN, McCarroll JR, Mallon WJ, eds. *Feeling up to par: medicine from tee to green.* Philadelphia: FA Davis, 1994.

CHAPTER 42

Ice Hockey

Robert J. Johnson

INTRODUCTION

Ice hockey was once considered a regional phenomenon, the national sport of Canada and the passion of the northern tier of the United States. Now, the presence of professional hockey in such places as Dallas, Texas, Phoenix, Arizona, and Tampa, Florida, has resulted in rapid growth in interest and participation in hockey. In fact, there were almost 27,000 teams with 368,000 players registered with USA Hockey in 1995–1996, a number that is growing at a rate of 10% per year (1).

Women's hockey has exhibited rapid growth. The gold medal performance by the U.S. women's hockey team in their first Olympic experience in Nagano in 1998 both underscores and inspires this growth. During the winter of 1995–1996 there were 38 women's team participating in high school hockey in Minnesota. During the 1999–2000 season more than 100 teams competed at the high school level in Minnesota. The growth of women's intercollegiate hockey parallels this interest.

Each sport is associated with specific injury characteristics that are unique to that sport. The ice hockey injury data that have been collected for many years provide the sports medicine practitioner with a sound basis for understanding the risks and types of injuries occurring on the ice.

Risks for injury in hockey include the rules and nature of the game, the surface and environment in which the game is played (an ice surface surrounded by rigid boards marking the boundaries of play), and the equipment (hockey stick and puck) that are used in the conduct of the game (2). Skating velocity in senior amateur hockey players has been measured at 30 miles per hour (mph), while youth hockey players at the Peewee (age 12–13) level may skate at speeds up to 20 mph. Falling and sliding velocities on the ice have been measured at 15 mph. The puck weighs 6 ounces. When it is struck at maximum velocity (90–120 mph), the force at impact may reach 1250 pounds. Even youth hockey players can shoot the puck with velocities of 50 mph. The act of skating involves vertical, lateral, and posterior reaction forces measured at 1.5–2.5 times body weight, 50 pounds, and 150 pounds, respectively.

This discussion will present injury trends in the sport of ice hockey to be supplemented with a discussion of head injury, spine injury, and special problems that are unique to hockey.

MUSCULOSKELETAL INJURY

Interpreting the available information about injuries in hockey must be done carefully, since the terminology that is used to explain injury frequency and to define injury differ from study to study. Generally, injury has been defined as any musculoskeletal problem that caused an athlete to miss a practice or game.

Epidemiologic data on hockey injury dwells almost exclusively on the acute injury. Very few reports deal with overuse injuries. Those that have looked at these two classifications report a preponderance of acute injuries (80–85.4%) compared to overuse injuries (14.6–20%) (3–5).

To date, very little data have been gathered on injuries to women who play ice hockey. In all likelihood, injury patterns in women's hockey will be different, since the rules strictly limit person-to-person contact. Many of the injuries to women have been gathered from those participating on boys' or men's teams.

INCIDENCE

The incidence of hockey injury has been presented in different formats. Some investigators have described injury incidence as a percentage of players who are

R. J. Johnson: Primary Care Sports Medicine, Minneapolis, Minnesota 55408.

TABLE 42–1. *Injuries per 1000 athletic exposures*

Sport	Overall	Practice	Game
Soccer	8.64	5.34	20.48
Football	6.54	4.00	39.13
Basketball	6.10	4.90	10.68
Ice hockey	5.80	2.21	18.11

TABLE 42–3. *Injury rate by level of play*

Level of play	Practice rate	Game rate
Squirt (age 9–10) (6)	1.2	—
Peewee (age 11–12) (6)	2.2	—
Bantam (age 13–14) (6)	2.5	10.9
Junior A (age 17–19) (7)	3.9	96.1
College (age 18–21) (8)	2.3	84.3
Swedish elite (age 19–33) (9)	1.4	78.4

injured over the course of a season. Others have used the concept of player-hours or player exposures to describe injury rate. This term is consistent with data collected on other sports, permitting comparisons among sports.

In an evaluation of youth sport injury (ages 14–20 years), ice hockey had the highest injury rate, calculated at 8.6 injuries per 10,000 hours of activity (6). This compares to soccer, wrestling, and basketball with 6.6, 6.3, and 3.5 injuries per 10,000 hours, respectively. This study was conducted in Switzerland, thus lacking a comparison to American football.

Data from the 1994–1995 National Collegiate Athletic Association (NCAA) injury surveillance system offers perspective of the relative risk of hockey compared to other men's collegiate sports (Table 42–1) (7).

On the basis of NCAA injury data, soccer has the highest overall and practice injury rate. Football causes more game-related injuries than the other sports. Though hockey has the lowest practice-related injury rate, there tends to be an intermediate risk of game-related injuries in comparison to other men's sports. The large discrepancies between practice- and game-related injury rates for football and hockey reflect the physical nature of the games and the reduced emphasis on contact/collision during practice sessions.

A landmark study by Sutherland highlighted the significant differences in injury rate among various age groups, which directly reflect the speed, skill, and intensity of the game at various levels of hockey (Table 42–2) (8).

For each level the hockey player advances from youth to college, the risk increases by tenfold, leveling off between the college and professional levels. A small pilot study conducted by the Mayo Clinic reflects a similar pattern of increased injury risk with increasing age and skill (Table 42–3) (9).

At all levels of competition the chance of injury in a game is many times higher than the chance of injury during practice. In most studies of college or elite teams, about one fourth to one third of all injuries occur in practice. However, since time spent in practice far exceeds time spent in competition, the risk of injury during games may be up to 29 times greater than injury risk during practice.

Lorentzon presents an interesting perspective to consider the incidence of hockey injury as they occurred at the Swedish elite level (10). In practice, a player is expected to have one minor injury every 5 years, one moderate injury every 15 years, and one major injury every 37 years. The risk rises dramatically during games. A player can expect three minor injuries every year, one moderate injury every 2 years, and one major injury every third year.

The various studies and their level of competition can be seen in Table 42–4. The different measures of injury rate can be seen by reviewing the table. Nevertheless, general trends of injury risk can easily be determined.

Little information is available about injuries to women. Voaklander and colleagues gathered data on male and female ice hockey injuries based on injury presentations to two emergency departments in Canada (11). Male injury rates were 168 injuries per 1000 participants (5.9 injuries per 1000 player-hours), and women's injury rates totaled 201 injuries per 1000 participants (11.9 per 1000 players-hours). Injured women were younger (mean age: women 18.2, men 23.8), had more upper extremity injuries than men (women 38%, men 25%), and, after excluding checking, had fewer injuries caused by collisions (women 22%, men 25%). Unfortunately, the actual numbers of women who played and presented with injury were very small. With the boom in women's hockey in North America at both the high school and college levels, more representative data should be forthcoming.

As with other collision sports, catastrophic injuries in hockey are rare. Brain injury and cervical spine injury will be considered in some detail later in the chapter. Of value, however, is the comparison of catastrophic injury rates between two collision sports of football and hockey. Hockey's catastrophic injury rate is reported as 2.55 per 100,000 participants compared to football at 0.68 per 100,000 participants (12). In Ontario, hockey was the leading cause of significant, serious injury, ac-

TABLE 42–2. *Injury rate per player per year*

Level	Rate
Youth	0.02
High school	0.20
College	2.48
Professional	3.00

TABLE 42-4. *Incidence*

Level	Overall	Practice	Game	Miscellaneous
Brust et al. (15) (youth)	35 per 100 players	1 every 4 hours	1 every 7 hours	Severe: 1 every 34 hours Peewee/Bantam
Gerberich et al. (21) (youth)	75 per 100 players 5 per 1000 hours			
Bjorkenheim et al. (51) (9–18 yr)	9%			Those under age 12 had virtually no injuries (54 teams)
Gerberich et al. (17) (high school)	75 per 100 players			Head and neck injuries were 22% of total number of injuries
Smith et al. (16) (high school)		$n = 1$	$n = 26$	3 varsity and junior varsity teams (26 games for each team)
Hayes et al. (22) (college)	1.17 injuries per team per game			9 American college teams 21 Canadian college teams
NCAA (7) (college 1994–1995)	5.8 per 1000 player exposure	2.21 per 1000 player exposure	18.11 per 1000 player exposure	
NCAA (23) (college 1995–1996)	7.44 per 1000 player exposure	2.94 per 1000 player exposure	24.07 per 1000 player exposure	
Pelletier et al. (14) (college)			19.95 per 1000 player-games	Varsity level players (6 seasons)
Stuart et al. (3) (Junior A) <19	9.4 per 1000 player hours	37% 3.9 per 1000 player hours	58% 96.1 per 1000 player-hours	
Lorentzon et al. (18) (Swedish national)			79.2 per 1000 player game-hours	2 seasons (1984 and 1985)
Molsa et al. (19) (Finnish professional level)		23%	76%	
(national level)	5.8 per 1000 player-hours	1.4 per 1000 player-hours	66 per 1000 player game-hours	
(Division I level)	5.1 per 1000 player exposure	1.6 per 1000 player-hours	36 per 1000 player game-hours	
Jorgensen et al. (4) (Danish pro-elite)	0.9 injuries per player per season 4.7 per 1000 player-hours	1.5 per 1000 player-hours	38 per 1000 player-hours	
Lorentzon et al. (10) (Swedish elite)		24.2% 1.4 per 1000 player-hours	75.8% 78.4 per 1000 player game-hours	3-year study
Petterson et al. (20) (Swedish elite)		5.4% 2.6 per 1000 player-hours	68.9% 74.1 per 1000 player game-hours	(1986–1990) Injury rate 29 times higher in game
Hornof et al. (25) (Czech elite)	29.6 per 1000 players per year	45%	55%	1967
Biener et al. (52) (general population)		30%	70%	1973
Tegner et al. (5) (Swedish elite)		26%	74% 53 per 1000 player game-hours	12 teams 1981–1989
Sutherland (8)				Published 1976
(youth)	0.02 per player per year			
(high school)	0.20 per player per year			
(college)	2.48 per player per year			
(professional)	3.0 per player per year			
Stuart et al. (9)				1993–1994
(Squirt)		1.1 per 1000 hours	0	
(Peewee)		2.2 per 1000 hours	1.8 per 1000 hours	
(Bantam)		2.5 per 1000 hours	10.9 per 1000 hours	
(Junior A)		3.9 per 1000 hours	96.1 per 1000 hours	
(college 18–21)		2.3 per 1000 hours	84.3 per 1000 hours	
(Swedish elite)		1.4 per 1000 hours	78.4 per 1000 hours	
Smith et al. (13)				Ontario
(adult)	16%	5%	95%	Sports and leisure activities
(youth)	10%	12%	88%	
Lindquist et al. (26) (general population)	Injury rate (general) = 22.5 per 1000 inhabitants Soccer (38.9%) > BB/VB/handball (10.9%) > Bandy/hockey (9.2%)			Community recreational injury
Voaklander (53) (recreational/old-timer)				
>18			12.3 per 1000 player exposure	
>30			12.0 per 1000 player exposure	

counting for 15% of all serious injury, followed by basketball responsible for 9% of all catastrophic injury (13).

In summary, the chance of injury in games is many, many times higher than the chance of injury during practice. Injury risk in youth hockey is very low and doesn't seem to pose a significant risk until one competes at the high school level or beyond age 15. The higher the level of hockey at which one competes, the greater the injury risk. Data are incomplete regarding women's hockey.

INJURY SEVERITY

The research on the relative severity of hockey injuries is somewhat confusing, since severity definitions vary considerably. Generally, minimal or nuisance injuries are those that do not keep the athlete from a practice or game. In many reports, nuisance injuries were not even recorded. Minor injuries are generally regarded as those that prevent players from practicing or competing from 1 to 7 days. Moderate injuries keep players off the ice from 8 to 24 days. Major injuries are those that do not allow players to practice or compete for more than 25 days. Injuries that are categorized as severe are characterized as injuries, usually to an extremity, that cause disability. Catastrophic injury criteria require permanent disability or fatality. Table 42–5 summarizes many of the injury severity studies and groups the injuries as closely as possible to the most similar injury classifications. By far, most of the injuries are either minor or nuisance (minimal) injuries. The only level of competition that failed to show a significant difference among minor and moderate injury level is reflected in the NCAA surveillance data in which the frequency of minimal, minor, and moderate injury are nearly identical. Overall, major injuries are far less common and severe and catastrophic injuries are very rare.

In summary, the injuries that are experienced by hockey players of all levels generally result in absence from practice or competition less than 1 week.

INJURY TYPES

Evaluation of the injury statistics for the types of injuries that are incurred while playing the sport suffers the same shortcomings as other injury data. Categorizing inconsistencies from study to study make injury compar-

TABLE 42–5. Injury severity

Level	Minimal (<1 day)	Minor (2–7 days)	Moderate (8–24 days)	Major (>25 days)	Severe (limit/ permanent)	Catastrophic (permanent/ disabilities/ fatal)
Brust et al. (15) (youth)	56%	27%	11%	6%		
NCAA (7) (college 1994–1995)	2.64 per 1000 player exposure	1.48 per 1000 player exposure	1.58 per 1000 player exposure		0.01 per 1000 player exposure	
NCAA (23) (college 1995–1996)	2.81 per 1000 player exposure	2.58 per 1000 player exposure	2.05 per 1000 player exposure		0	0
Stuart et al. (3) (Junior A)		58%	36%	6%		
Molsa et al. (19) (national) (Division I)		80% 63%	16% 28%	4% 9%		
Lorentzon et al. (10) (Swedish elite)	not recorded	72.6%	19.0% (8–30d)	8.4% (>30d)		
Petterson et al. (20) (Swedish elite)	60.6%	34.6%	3.7%	1.1%		
Tegner et al. (5) (Swedish elite 1981–1989)		61.1%	22.3%	8.8%		

isons difficult. Nevertheless, injury trends can be determined.

With the exception of a single study of Junior A level hockey (3) and a single study of college hockey (14), contusions are the most commonly reported injury type. In Junior A hockey, strains and lacerations occurred with similar frequency (25% and 24%, respectively). Pelletier's study of college hockey injury demonstrated sprains outnumbered contusions 31% to 21%. Studies of youth hockey show some discrepancies regarding fracture frequency. In Stuart and Smith's small youth hockey study (9), fully 29% of the recorded injuries are fractures. An earlier report from Brust and colleagues (15) yielded only a 6% fracture rate, while the rate of sprains and strains in these two youth hockey studies are almost identical. No other study, college or professional, reported a fracture incidence higher than 14% of all reported injuries. Table 42–6 summarizes injury types from youth through the professional ranks. Though included in the summary, head injury will be considered as a separate issue.

SITE OF INJURY

Because of different site-of-injury groupings, comparisons are somewhat difficult. Many studies did not separate extremity injuries into individual categories, that is, shoulder, elbow, and so on. Rather, these sites were considered upper extremity injuries. Similar site groupings occur for the lower extremities, back, and head. In spite of these inconsistencies, general comparisons are valid.

Youth hockey consistently established the upper extremity as the most commonly injured site, having more than double the frequency of lower extremity injuries (7,15,16).

TABLE 42–6. *Injury type*

Level	Contusion	Sprain	Strain	Fracture	Dislocation	Laceration	Abrasion	Head Injury
Stuart et al. (9) (Squirt) (Peewee) (Bantam)	36%	21%		29%		7%		
Brust et al. (15) (youth)	50%	6%	13%	8%	4%	2%	8%	9%
Smith et al. (16) (high school)	37%	22.2%	14.8%	7.4%	3.7%	11.1%		
Bjorkenheim et al. (51) (9–18 yr)	[contusions, sprains, lacerations = 50%; most fx UE (30 of 32) {clavicle, hand, forearm}]							
NCAA (7) (college 1994–1995)	1.29 per 1000 player exposure	1.38 per 1000 player exposures	0.92 per 1000 player exposures	0.34 per 1000 player exposures	0.22 per 1000 player exposures	0.49 per 1000 player exposures	0.02 per 1000 player exposures	0.66 per 1000 player exposures 10 with concussion
NCAA (23) college 1995–1996	1.79 per 1000 player exposure	1.52 per 1000 player exposure	1.29 per 1000 player exposure	0.39 per 1000 player exposure	0.27 per 1000 player exposure	0.50 per 1000 player exposure	0.13 per 1000 player exposure	18 mild 5 moderate 0 severe 0.42 1995–1996
Pelletier et al. (14) (college)	21%	31% (sprain/dislocation)	11.3%	10.2%		13%		7.5%
Stuart et al. (3) (Junior A)	18%	16%	25%			24%		
Lorentzon et al. (18) (Swedish national)	36.8%	31.6%	15.8%	10.5%		5.3%		
Molsa et al. (19) (Finnish professional)	38.8%	39.7%		8.0%		11.2%		
Jorgensen et al. (24) (Danish elite)	46%	26%	14%	14%				
Petterson et al. (20) (Swedish elite)	43.4%	12%	9.5%	2.5%		26%		0.8%
Voaklander (53) (recreational/old-timer)								
>18	26%	35%		8%	3%	28%		
>30	24%	47%		9%	2%	16%		

TABLE 42-7. Injury site

Level	Knee	Shoulder	Groin	Back	Head/face	C-spine (neck)	UE	LE	Trunk
Stuart et al. (9) (Squirt)(Peewee)(Bantam)		22%		7%	7%	7%			
Brust et al. (15) (youth)					23.2%		19.3% (arm)	17.3%	17.4%
Gerberich et al. (21) (youth)					22%	25%			
Bjorkenheim et al. (51) (9–18 yr)					10%		55%	19%	
Gerberich et al. (17) (high school)							42.4%	17.3%	
Smith et al. (16) (high school)	14.8%	11.1%	11.1%	7.4	11.1%		33.3%	37.0%	
NCAA (23) (college 1995–1996)	MCL most common; ACL uncommon		0.86 per 1000 player exposures	0.46 per 1000 player exposures	1.08 per 1000 player exposures	0.17 per 1000 player exposures	2.3 per 1000 player exposures	1.81 per 1000 player exposures	
Pelletier et al. (14) (college)	18.6%	14.9%			17.6%	10.6%			
Stuart et al. (3) (Junior A)		20%		6%	2%	1%	28%	25%	
Biasca et al. (27) (professional)	40%	20%	15%	10%					
Hornof et al. (25) (Czech elite 1967)					37.1% (no helmets)		21.9%	35.7%	
Tegner et al. (5) (Swedish elite)				11.4%	39.2%		17.6%	31.6%	
Biener (52) (general population)					42%		11%	21%	
Voaklander (53) (recreational/old-timer)					30%		24%	34%	12%

Upper and lower extremity injuries occur in high school hockey with nearly equal frequency (16,17).

At all levels of professional hockey, the lower extremity tended to be injured more often than the upper extremity (10,18–20). Study has suggested that the knee has caused up to 40% of all absenteeism due to hockey injury (18).

Sifting through the differences in reporting head, neck, and facial injuries proves most difficult, since this site is either recorded as a single site or grouped as head/face or head/neck, separate from concussions and cervical spine injuries. Youth hockey showed head and face injury rates ranging from 7% to 23.2% (6,15,16). High school hockey is associated with an injury rate of 22% to the head and neck (including facial injuries) (21). Head and neck injury rates in college are intermediate in frequency but significantly less than extremity injury rates (7,14). Interpretation of the rate of head and face injury frequency is complicated by the fact that some studies were done before mandatory helmet use and voluntary face mask use and others were done after these safety features were instituted. Consequently, the frequency rates have a broad range of values. Some clarification will occur in the head/spine injury sections of this chapter.

At all levels of hockey the shoulder is the most common site of upper extremity injury (7,8,14,22,23). Daly finds that 45% of professional hockey players compete with asymptomatic abnormalities of the acromioclavicular joint or distal clavicle (24). The knee, particularly the medial collateral ligament, is the most common lower extremity site of injury. Anterior cruciate ligament injuries are uncommon in hockey (18).

Table 42–7 summarizes the results of pertinent studies of the sites of injury.

In summary, the most frequent site of injury depends upon the level of hockey in which one participates. For those in youth hockey the upper extremity is at greatest risk. At the college level the injury rates of the upper extremity and the lower extremity are quite similar. At levels beyond youth, high school, and college the lower extremity is the most frequently injured site. At all levels the shoulder and knee seem to be the joints that are most often injured.

MECHANISM OF INJURY

The range of studies dealing with hockey injury is much more consistent in identifying injury mechanisms. Universally, at all levels of hockey, both those in which the body check is legal or those in which it is illegal (under age 10), the most common mechanism is collision between players, both checking and incidental collision. Ranking behind player-player collision is a player's collision against the boards. See Table 42–8 for a summary of mechanism of injury.

With rare exceptions (19,20), injury caused by the player's use of the stick ranks behind player-player and player-board collisions.

Puck-related injuries range from a low of 5.3% to a high of 17%; both the low and the high rates occur within the professional ranks. Skate-related injuries usually account for 5% or less of all injuries.

Fortunately, most of the series that record injury mechanisms have documented the number of injuries associated with illegal (penalized) play, either an illegal check or a violation of the rules (charging, boarding, elbowing, roughing, slashing). In youth hockey 16–66% of injury-causing collisions (player, boards, sticks) are due to foul play (15–17). At the college level, 10–24.5% of the injuries are a result of illegal play (7,14,23).

At the professional level the number of injuries that are blamed on foul play varies widely. In Finland only 9% of injuries were caused by illegal action (19). Compare this to the Swedish elite level, in which 39% were related to penalized activity (10). These wide ranges reflect either markedly different styles and philosophies of hockey or, more likely, different data-gathering techniques.

In summary, most hockey injuries are a result of player-player or player-board collisions. Illegal or rough play is a significant factor at most levels of play.

PLAYER POSITION AND INJURY

The player's position affects the injury risk. The safest position on the ice is goalie. At the youth level of hockey few actual numbers are available. Generally, the comments are of a more subjective quality, implying that the goalie has the least number of injuries on a team (15,16). Specifically, Brust and colleagues recorded that 7% of all injuries in their study were experienced by goalies. When recorded, the difference in injury rates for forwards and defensemen differ greatly, probably due to small sample sizes that characterize youth hockey studies. One study suggests that the number of injuries suffered by forwards and defensemen is equal (16). Another shows that forwards have 59% of the injuries and defensemen have only 15% (15).

The studies of the relationship between position and injury among college hockey players are very consistent. As in youth hockey, the goalie is the safest position during play. The injury rate for goalies ranges from 5.5% to 9% (7,14,23). Those who play defense in college endure 16.5–31% of reported injuries, and forwards play the riskiest position, with 60–66% of injuries (7,14,23).

There are broad differences at the professional level in injury frequency. The goalie position reflects this variation. The Swedish national team recorded no goalie injuries over the time injuries were studied (10). No goalie injuries occurred in the study of Junior A hockey (8). The maximum injury frequency for professional

TABLE 42–8. Injury mechanism

Level	Player-player (checking)	Player-boards	Player-stick	Puck	Skate	Other	Foul play
Stuart et al. (9) (Squirt) (Peewee) (Bantam)	50%		n = 1	n = 2	n = 1		
Brust et al. (15) (youth)	86% (games) Legal check: 20%						66% (illegal check 39%) (violation 27%)
Gerberich et al. (17) (youth)	45%	34%	22%				26%
Boileau et al. (54) (Quebec) (Bantam)	46% minor injury 75% major injury						
Bjorkenheim et al. (51) (9–18 yr)	most common						32%
Smith et al. (16) (high school)	20/27	9/29	8/20	3/27	1/27		
Hayes et al. (22) (college)							15.5%
NCAA (7) (college 1994–1995)	2.72 per 1000 player exposures	0.73 per 1000 player exposures					2.81/1000 Yes 20.16/1000 No (player exposure)
NCAA (23) (college 1995–1996)	2.84 per 1000 player exposures	1.22 per 1000 player exposures	0.96 per 1000 player exposures			1.12 per 1000 player exposures	
Pelletier et al. (14) (college)	44.6%						
Stuart et al. (3) (Junior A)	51%		14%	11%			
Park et al. (55) (Junior B)	48%		12%	17%			24.5%
Lorentzon et al. (18) (Swedish national)	42.1%	10.5%	0%	5.3%	5.3%		
Molsa et al. (19) (Finnish professional)	44.3%	10.3%	14.6%	7.9%			9%
Lorentzon et al. (10) (Swedish elite)	32.9%	6.6%	11.8%	14.5%	2.6%		39%
Petterson et al. (20) (Swedish elite)	23.9%	7.2%	26.1%	16%	2.1%		
Tegner et al. (5) (Swedish elite)	24%	9.7%	25.5%	11.2%	1.5%		
Hornof et al. (25) (Czech elite 1967)	82.1%	16.6%					
Biener et al. (52) (general population)	17%		25%	17%			
Environics (28)							19% adult 16% youth

TABLE 42-9. Position

Level	Forward	Defense	Goalie
Brust et al. (15) (youth)			Most likely 37%
Bjorkenheim et al. (51) (9–18 yr)	F = D	F = D	Least
NCAA (23) (college 1995–1996)	60.9%	30%	9%
Pelletier et al. (14) (college)	66%	16.5	5.5%
Hayes et al. (22) (college 1970–1971)	61%	41%	7%
Stuart et al. (3) (Junior A)	134 per 1000 player-hours	87 per 1000 player-hours	0
Park et al. (55) (Junior B)	67.5%	30%	2.5%
Lorentzon et al. (18) (Swedish national)	125 per 1000 player game-hours	50 per 1000 player game-hours	0
Molsa et al. (19) (Finnish professional)	54.5%	31.2%	5.8%
Jorgensen et al. (4) (Danish elite)	F = D	F = D	1/2 frequency of other positions
Lorentzon et al. (10) (Swedish elite)	71.8 per 1000 player game-hours; 73% minor, 21% moderate, 6% major	107.8 per 1000 player game-hours; 55% minor, 30% moderate, 15% major	39.2 per 1000 player game-hours; 83% minor, 17% moderate, 0% major
Petterson et al. (20) (Swedish elite)	36%	57%	7%

goalies is only 7% (18). The injury results regarding forwards and defensemen are mixed. In studies of Swedish elite teams, defensemen had more injuries than forwards (25,26). Finnish national and Swedish national teams recorded more injuries in forwards (10,25,26). Forwards and defensemen on the Danish elite teams had equal numbers of injuries (18). See Table 42-9 for details.

In summary, at all levels of competitive hockey, the fewest injuries occur to goalies. Although the data are somewhat inconsistent, generally, forwards experience more injuries than do defensemen.

INJURY AND PERIOD OF PLAY

Intuitively, one would expect more injuries in the third period, possibly because of fatigue. A single youth hockey study that evaluated the time at which game injuries occurred showed an increasing number of injuries through the first and second periods with 45% of the injuries occurring in the third period (15).

Data for high school hockey are unavailable.

Studies of college hockey find the greatest number of injuries occurring in the second period. First- and third-period injury rates are quite varied (7,14,23).

With one exception, studies of European professional teams have the highest injury rate in the second period (10,18–20,25). See Table 42-10 for details.

Junior A hockey, which has injury patterns that frequently deviate from those of other levels, shows a pattern of the highest injury rate in the third period, with the first and second periods being equal (8).

In general, the second period is the riskiest period for injury in college and professional hockey. In the small numbers reported for youth hockey, the third period sees the most injuries.

TABLE 42-10. Period of injury

Level	First period	Second period	Third period
Brust et al. (15) (youth)	Increasing →	→	45%
NCAA (23) (college 1995–1996)	21 injuries	66 injuries	53 injuries
Pelletier et al. (14) (college)	27.1%	35.6%	26.6%
Stuart et al. (3) (Junior A)	75 per 1000 player-hours	75 per 1000 player-hours	135 per 1000 player-hours
Lorentzon et al. (18) (Swedish national)	2 injuries	11 injuries	6 injuries
Pforringer W et al. (32) (West Germany national)	45 injuries	71 injuries	45 injuries
Molsa et al. (19) (Finnish professional)	30 injuries	35 injuries	60 injuries
Tegner et al. (5) (Swedish elite)	31%	38%	28%
Petterson et al. (20) (Swedish elite)	20%	31.5%	21.5%

INJURIES TO THE HEAD AND FACE

The frequency and distribution of injuries to the head and face have been altered by equipment changes, including almost universal use of helmets and the broad use of some form of face mask. Before 1975 injuries to the face and head were the most common in hockey. The NCAA mandated use of face masks during the 1977–1978 hockey season (27). In addition to helmet use, the Canadian Standards Association required that full masks be worn in all minor hockey leagues starting in 1978. The professional leagues began requiring helmets for all those coming into the professional ranks after 1981. Since the helmet and face mask have been used, experts estimate injury cost savings greater than $10 million (28). By 1988 no eye injury was recorded for an athlete wearing a face mask (29). In fact, Pashby estimated that the combination of helmet and face mask use has reduced the incidence of facial injury by 70% (30). Even with helmets, facial injuries are common. Most, however, are lacerations; one series showed them to represent 71% of all facial injuries (31).

Facial injuries are caused by the stick 39% of the time and by the puck 30% of the time (29). Fewer than half of the players in this study wore some kind of facial protection. Older players tended to wear facial protection less than younger players. Those who wore full masks were protected from injury to the nose and above. Masks did not adequately protect the lower face, mouth, or neck. Players who wore half-visors had the same injury incidence and distribution of injury as those who wore no facial protection at all. Fortunately, in this same series, most facial injuries were considered minor.

Head injuries, especially concussion, are of major concern in a sport such as hockey in which collision with another player is an expected part of the game. Most concussions occur as a result of collisions (32). Helmet use has resulted in a decline in the incidence of concussion. Rule changes, especially making checking from behind a violation, has further contributed to this drop. Witness the change in concussion incidence in youth hockey over the years (32). In 1974 the incidence of concussion in youth hockey (ages 5–14) was 2.8 per 1000 player-hours. By 1985 this number had dwindled to 1.5 per 1000 player-hours. By 1990 the rate was a paltry 0.5 per 1000 player-hours. Also noted is the increased incidence of concussion with increasingly higher levels of play (32). Beyond the youth level (incidence of 0.5 per 1000 player-hours), high school hockey players have concussions at a rate of 2.7 per 1000 player-hours, and elite amateur-level hockey players have a rate of 6.6 per 1000 player-hours (32).

A simple example of the effect of helmets on concussion rate hails from a study of intramural hockey games in which helmeted players had a concussion rate of 3.8% while nonhelmeted players experienced a rate of 8.3% (32). A second study that reflected the safety value of helmets was done in Quebec (33). There, the researchers compared consultations for head injuries from leagues requiring helmets with those not requiring helmets. The helmeted league accounted for 15.4% of the consultations. The nonhelmeted league accounted for 42%.

Among Swedish elite hockey players, 22% of the players reported having at least one concussion.(34) The researchers calculated a risk of 5% per player per year. In this series, checking or boarding was responsible for most of the concussions. As a result, these players averaged 6 days of absence from practice and games.

In summary, since the use of helmets has become widespread, concussion rates have declined. The higher the level of hockey, the greater the risk of concussion.

SPINE INJURY

In a review of spine fractures in sports conducted over a 7-year period, ice hockey accounted for 3% of the 1447 fractures (35). This is less than the rates that occur in skiing and tobogganing (5%) and snowmobiling (10%).

Before 1980 spinal injury in hockey was a very rare occurrence (36). Between 1966 and 1993, however, 241 cases of hockey-related spinal injury were reported through SportsSmart Canada, formerly known as the Committee on Prevention of Spinal Cord Injuries Due to Hockey (36) (Fig. 42–1). Anecdotal reports of more cervical spine injuries continue to accumulate, adding to these numbers. These data reflect major injuries to the spine involving fracture or dislocation with or without injury to the spinal cord or nerve roots. Minor neck and back strains and sprains were not included in the report. Of the 241 injuries, six occurred in Europe, 18

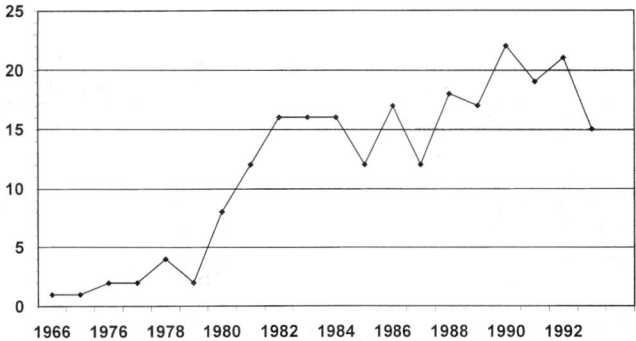

FIG. 42–1. Annual number of spinal injuries in hockey. (From Tator CH, Carson JD, Edmonds VE. New spinal injuries in hockey. *Clin J Sports Med* 1997;7(1):17–21.)

in the United States, and the remainder in Canada. The lower numbers from the United States may represent a failure to report to the Canadian organization. Since 1982 there were an average of 16.8 major spinal injuries per year in hockey. 1990 represented the year with the most injuries reported ($n = 22$). The median age of those with spinal injury was 18, and the mean was 20.7. The age group with the highest number of spinal injuries was age 16–20, reporting 51.9% of all the recorded injuries.

The most common mechanism of injury was a push or check from behind (36.6%) creating an axial load to the cervical spine during a collision with the boards. Slightly over 22% were a result of a legal push or check followed by an axial load to the cervical spine. Slightly over 20% followed a tripping violation; 16.3% occurred as a result of sliding along the ice and striking the boards. The axial load occurred against the boards over 70% of the time. A collision of player against player caused 14.3% of the cervical spine injuries.

Far and away, the most common site of spinal injury is at the cervical level, accounting for 89.1%, followed by lumbosacral injury of 3.3% and thoracic spinal injury 2.8% of the time. The C5-6 level is the most common level of injury (36).

Most of the injuries (170 of 241) are game-related injuries (36). Burst fractures and fracture-dislocations are the most common type of fracture pathology (36).

The spinal injury affected the spinal cord 65.7% of the time with resultant neurologic deficit. Slightly over 9% of spinal injuries resulted in damage to one or more nerve roots without cord injury. Over 50% of those with spinal cord injury had permanent deficits. Half of that 50% with permanent deficits had no preservation of motor or sensory function below the level of injury.

Eight of the 241 spine-injured hockey players died as a result of their injuries, usually from the complication of respiratory failure (36).

Compared to American football, spinal cord injury with quadriplegia is three times greater in ice hockey (27).

The sharp increase in spinal injury beginning in 1980 (see Fig. 42–1) has corresponded to the widespread use of head and facial protection provided by helmets and masks. Some experts have intimated that the increase is due to a rougher style of play fostered by the improved protection. Observers also believe that officials have been more permissive with rough play for this same reason: the hockey player wears a suit of armor. LaPrade evaluated this possibility and concluded that there was no qualitative evidence to support the notion that helmets and face masks are the cause of increased spinal injury (12).

Rule changes to reduce the risk of spinal injury have been implemented. Checking from behind has been singled out for stricter rule enforcement, with more severe penalties applied for this violation. Interference, or checking a player who is not in control of the puck, has also been implemented. USA Hockey has moved the goal line farther from the boards to permit more room for play behind the net. These rules may have had a positive effect on this devastating injury, since the number of spinal cord injuries has decreased in the last 3-year period evaluated by Tator and his colleagues (36,37).

MEDICAL RISKS

Medical problems that affect athletes in other sports may affect hockey players in a similar fashion. Case reports of these medical problems merit consideration.

Individual case reports discuss blunt, concussive impact from the puck leading to cardiac arrest and sudden death (38–40). This trauma has been termed commotio cordis (39) or contusio cordis (38). Maron reviewed 25 such deaths (40). All are related to being struck by a puck or baseball. In retrospect, the trauma created by the missile (puck) was not considered extraordinary. Twelve collapsed immediately; 13 were conscious only for a short time. Seven of the 25 actually wore chest protection of some sort. The exact mechanism is uncertain. Those for which a postmortem report was included showed a puck-shaped contusion of the myocardium (39).

Another special medical problem involves indoor air quality within ice arenas. Case reports involving entire teams and groups of spectators center on the byproducts of combustion of the propane fuel that is burned in the engine of the ice-resurfacing machine known as the Zamboni (41–43). Toxicity associated with nitrogen dioxide (NO_2) and carbon monoxide (CO) intoxication has been reported. Indoor air quality standards in Minnesota require NO_2 levels less than 0.5 ppm. CO levels should be less than 50 ppm.

At low levels of NO_2 (2.5–5.0 ppm) increased pulmonary resistance can occur. At moderate levels (50 ppm), cough, hemoptysis, dyspnea, and chest pain occur. Levels greater than 100 ppm can cause pulmonary edema leading to bronchiolitis obliterans. In one situation attack rates of NO_2-induced respiratory illness affected 82% of the members of one team and 72% of the other (41). A second incident involved 70% of one team and 56% of the members of the other. Eighty-one percent of cheerleaders of the first two teams were affected, along with 62% of one school's band members. In this situation the Zamboni was found to be malfunctioning. Complicating this malfunction included closure of the passive vents to conserve heat during particularly cold weather. Exhaust fans were also turned off. Two days after the games were played, NO_2 levels were still measured at 4 ppm.

Carbon monoxide absorption is 3–4 times higher during exertion (43). CO levels of 1% are typically found in the nonsmoker. Levels of 4% can affect driving skills, levels of 5–10% affects visual skills, and levels of 10–20% cause headache and difficulty breathing. Coma occurs at levels of 50–60%.

A report from Wisconsin recorded both CO and NO_2 intoxication at an ice arena (42). Air quality measurements at this rink showed NO_2 levels of 1.5 ppm and CO levels of 150 ppm.

In spite of the presence of more than 800 ice arenas in the United States, only three states have indoor air quality standards for indoor ice rinks that are monitored regularly (41).

MISCELLANEOUS INJURY REPORTS

Unique to hockey has been the occurrence of abdominal wall muscle tears reported in ten of 11 elite hockey players who were unable to play because of groin pain (44). All presented atypically. Ultimately, all were surgically explored and were found to have tears in the floor of the inguinal ring. These were either repaired directly or reinforced with mesh. All subsequently returned to hockey without groin symptoms. This represents a form of "sportsmen's hernia."

The number of groin injuries in hockey is fairly substantial. Though most are injuries of the hip adductors, a unique subset of groin problems is outlined by Lacroix (45). This small series highlights some of the diagnostic dilemmas posed by hockey players with groin pain. Eleven professional hockey players presented with atypical refractory pain accompanied by paresthesias referred to the lower abdomen. Thorough investigation failed to yield a diagnosis. Surgical exploration revealed tears of the external oblique aponeurosis and external oblique muscle with ilioinguinal nerve entrapment. Surgical repair resulted in full restoration of function and a return to the professional ranks.

Boot-top tendon lacerations involving the anterior tibial tendon, extensor hallucis longus, and extensor communis tendon have been reported (46). This is caused by the skate blade. If the tongue of the skate is worn properly under the shin guards, that area will be protected. Hockey fashion sometimes dictates that the tongue be worn outside the shin guards, rendering the anterior ankle susceptible to injury.

Traumatic rupture of the abdominal wall due to blunt trauma from the puck or stick has been reported, albeit rarely (47).

Direct injury to the axillary nerve has been reported in hockey players (48). Of the 11 injuries reported, two occurred in hockey players as a result of collisions. Ten of the eleven returned to full, unrestricted activity. Though this is a rare cause of shoulder dysfunction, this diagnosis should be included in the differential diagnosis.

RULE CHANGES AND EFFECTS ON INJURY INCIDENCE

Rules have been implemented to make hockey a safer sport. One such rule has been to penalize checking from behind, since it is often implicated in serious injury. Watson and colleagues evaluated the impact of a stricter checking-from-behind penalty on injury rates and player behavior (37). The results showed a fourfold increase in checking-from-behind penalties compared to the number before the rule was implemented. This also resulted in a decrease in the incidence of neck, head, and back injuries. There was no effect on the frequency of other penalties.

In a second study, Watson and colleagues evaluated the effect of the type of ice surface on injury incidence (38). They considered injury data from games conducted on ice surfaces of three different sizes. Standard ice surface size was 17,000 square feet; large was more than 17,000 square feet; and small was less than 17,000 square feet. The data led them to the conclusion that ice surface size has a significant effect on injury rate, the fewest injuries occurring on the large surfaces and the most injuries on the small surfaces. There is no correlation between aggressive penalties and ice surface size.

Youth hockey has experimented with a tournament system using fair-play rules. Roberts and colleagues studied the fair-play concept to see its effects on injury rate and penalty frequency (50). In this system, teams are awarded points. The point system is as follows:

win = 13 points
tie = 7 points
loss = 0 points
less than 6 penalties = 1 point
greater than 12 penalties = −2 points

incentive points:
1 point for each period won
1 point for highest total shots on goal
1 point for shutout

Any player who receives more than five penalties in a game is suspended for the next tournament game. Round-robin games employed the fair-play rules. Championship round games did not. The results showed a significant improvement in safety as a result of the fair-play rules. The injury rate during fair-play games was 4.5 injuries per 1000 athletic exposures; regular-play games had an injury rate of 32.3 injuries per 1000 player exposures. There were 7.1 penalties per game during fair-play and 13 penalties per game during regular play. Penalties related to rough play and injury were four times more common in regular-play games.

SUMMARY

Ice hockey is a popular, rapidly growing sport which is played by all age groups internationally. Injury patterns differ depending upon the level of competition. It behooves the sports medicine practitioner to be familiar with the injury patterns and training demands to better serve these athletes.

REFERENCES

1. USA Hockey. *1995–1996 USA Hockey data.* Colorado Springs, CO: USA Hockey.
2. Sim FH, Simonet WT, Melton LJ, Lehn TA. Ice hockey injuries. *Am J Sports Med* 1987;15(1):30–40.
3. Stuart MJ, Smith A. Injuries in Junior A ice hockey: a three-year prospective study. *Am J Sports Med* 1995;23(4):458–461.
4. Jorgensen U, Schmidt-Olsen S. The epidemiology of ice hockey injuries. *Br J Sports Med* 1986;20(1):7–9.
5. Tegner Y, Lorentzon R. Ice hockey injuries: incidence, nature and causes. *Br J Sports Med* 1991;25(2):87–89.
6. deLoes M. Epidemiology of sports injuries in the Swiss organization "Youth and Sports" 1987–1989: injuries, exposure and other risks of main diagnoses. *Int J Sports Med* 1995;16(2):134–138.
7. National Collegiate Athletic Association. *Injury Surveillance System: 1994–1995 men's ice hockey.* Overland Park, KS: National Collegiate Athletic Association, 1995.
8. Sutherland GW. Fire on ice. *Am J Sports Med* 1976;4:264–269.
9. Stuart MJ, Smith AM, Nieva JJ, Rock MG. Injuries in youth ice hockey: a pilot surveillance strategy. *Mayo Clin Proc* 1995;70:350–356.
10. Lorentzon R, Wedren H, Pietila T. Incidence, nature, and causes of ice hockey injuries: a three-year prospective study of a Swedish elite ice hockey team. *Am J Sports Med* 1988;16(4):392–396.
11. Voaklander DC, Brison RJ, Quinney HA, et al. Ice hockey injuries treated in two emergency departments. *Clin J Sports Med* 1994;4(1):25–30.
12. LaPrade RF, Burnett QM, Zaraour R, Moss R. The effect of the mandatory use of face masks on facial lacerations and head and neck injuries in ice hockey: a prospective study. *Am J Sports Med* 1995;23(6):773–775.
13. Smith MD. Violence and injuries in ice hockey. Clin J Sports Med 1991;1(2):104–109.
14. Pelletier RL, Montelpare WJ, Stark RM. Intercollegiate ice hockey injuries: a case for uniform definitions and reports. *Am J Sports Med* 1993;21(1):78–81.
15. Brust JD, Leonard BJ, Pheley A, Roberts WO. Children's ice hockey injuries. *Am J Dis Child* 1992;146:741–747.
16. Smith Am, Stuart MJ, Wiese-Bjornstal DM, Gunnon C. Predictors of injury in ice hockey players: a multivariate multidisciplinary approach. *Am J Sports Med* 1997;25(4):500–507.
17. Gerberich SG, Murray K, Aamoth G, Priest JD, Madden M, Finke R. An epidemiological study of high school ice hockey injuries. *Childs Nerv Syst* 1987;3(2):59–64.
18. Lorentzon R, Wedren H, Peitila T, Gustavsson B. Injuries in international ice hockey: a prospective, comparative study of injury incidence and injury types in international and Swedish elite ice hockey. *Am J Sports Med* 1988;16(4):389–391.
19. Molsa J, Airaksinen A, Nasman O, Torstila I. Ice hockey injuries in Finland: a prospective epidemiologic study. *Am J Sports Med* 1997;25(4):495–499.
20. Petterson M, Lorentzon R. Ice hockey injuries: a 4-year prospective study of a Swedish elite ice hockey team. *Br J Sports Med* 1993;27(4):251–254.
21. Gerberich SG, Priest JD, Grafft J, et al. Injuries to the brain and spinal cord: assessment, emergency care, and prevention. *Minn Med* 1982;65:691–696.
22. Hayes D. The nature, incidence, location and causes of injury in intercollegiate ice hockey. Thesis, University of Waterloo, Ontario, Canada 1972.
23. National Collegiate Athletic Association. *Injury Surveillance System: 1995–1996 men's ice hockey.* Overland Park, KS: National Collegiate Athletic Association, 1996.
24. Daly PJ, Sim FH, Simonet WT. Ice hockey injuries: a review. *Sports Med* 1990;10(3):122–131.
25. Hornof Z, Napravnik C. Analysis of various accident rate factors in ice hockey. *Med Sci Sports Exerc* 1973;5:283–286.
26. Lindqvist KS, Bjurulf P, Timpka T. Injuries during leisure physical activity in a Swedish municipality. *Scand J Soc Med* 1996;24(4):282–292.
27. Biasca N, Trentz O, Bartolozzi AR, Simmen HP. Review of typical ice hockey injuries: survey of the North American and Hockey Canada versus European leagues. *Unfallchirurg* 1995;98(5):283–288.
28. Environics Research Group. Economic costs of sport, fitness and recreation-related injuries in Ontario, 1986. *Report of the Ontario Sports Medicine and Safety Advisory Board,* vol 2. Toronto: Ministry of Tourism and Recreation, 1987:217–301.
29. Rampton J, Leach T, Therrien Sa, Bota GW, Rowe BH. Head, neck, and facial injuries in ice hockey: the effect of protective equipment. *Clin J Sports Med* 1997;7(3):162–167.
30. Pashby TJ. Eye injuries in Canadian hockey: III. Older players now most at risk. *Can Med Assoc J* 1979;121:643–644.
31. Deady B, Chevrier L, Brison RJ. Head, face and neck injuries in hockey: a descriptive analysis. *J Emerg Med* 1996;14(5):645–649.
32. Honey CR. Brain injury in ice hockey. *Clin J Sports Med* 1998;8(1):43–46.
33. Laflamme P, Laliberte D, Maurice P. Hockey injuries: consultations in a hospital center in Quebec. *Can J Public Health* 1996;87(4):240–243.
34. Tegner Y, Lorentzon R. Concussion among Swedish elite ice hockey players. *Br J Sports Med* 1996;30(3):251–255.
35. Reid DC, Saboe L. Spine fractures in winter sports. *Sports Med* 1989;7(6):393–399.
36. Tator CH, Carson JD, Edmonds VE. New spinal injuries in hockey. *Clin J Sports Med* 1997;7(1):17–21.
37. Watson RC, Singer CD, Sproule JR. Checking from behind in ice hockey: a study of injury and penalty data in the Ontario University Athletic Association Hockey League. *Clin J Sports Med* 1996;6(2):108–111.
38. Hoppe UC, Erdmann E. Contusio cordis: too seldom diagnosed. *Med Klin* 1997;92(7):444–446.
39. Kaplan JA, Karofsky PS, Volturo GA. Commotion cordis in two amateur ice hockey players despite the use of commercial chest protectors: case reports. *J Trauma* 1993;34(1):151–153.
40. Maron BJ, Mueller FO, Kaplan JA, Poliac LC. Blunt impact to the chest leading to sudden death from cardiac arrest during sports activities. *N Engl J Med* 1995;333(6):337–342.
41. Hedberg K, Hedberg C, Iber C, et al. An outbreak of nitrogen dioxide-induced respiratory illness among ice hockey players. *JAMA* 1989;262(21):3014–3017.
42. Epidemiologic notes and reports: nitrogen dioxide and carbon monoxide intoxication in an indoor arena—Wisconsin, 1992. *MMWR* 1992;41(21):383–385.
43. Levesque B, Dewailly E, Lavoie R, et al. Carbon monoxide in indoor ice skating rinks: evaluation of absorption by adult hockey players. *Am J Public Health* 1990;80(5):594–598.
44. Simonet WT, Sim L, Saylor HL III. Abdominal wall muscle tears in hockey players. *Int J Sports Med* 1995;16(2):126–128.
45. Lacroix VJ, Kinnear DG, Mulder DS, Brown RA. Lower abdominal pain syndrome in National Hockey League players: a report of 11 cases. *Clin J Sports Med* 1998;8(1):5–9.
46. Simonet WT, Sim L. Boot-top tendon lacerations in ice hockey. *J Trauma* 1995;38(1):30–31.
47. Zaunschirm G, Steiner E. Traumatic rupture of the abdominal wall: a rare injury in ice hockey. *Sportverletz Sportschaden* 1989;3(4):187–188.
48. Perlmutter GS, Zarins B, Leffert RD. Direct injury to the axillary nerve in athletes playing contact sports. *Am J Sports Med* 1997;25(1):65–68.
49. Watson RC, Nystrom MA, Buckolz E. Safety in Canadian junior ice hockey: the association of ice surface size and injuries and

aggressive penalties in the Ontario hockey league. *Clin J Sports Med* 1997;7(3):192–195.
50. Roberts WO, Brust JD, Leonard B, Hebert BJ. Fair-play rules and injury reduction in ice hockey. *Arch Pediatr Adolesc Med* 1996;150:140–145.
51. Bjorkenheim JM, Syvahuoka I, Rosenberg PH. Injuries in competitive junior ice hockey: 1437 players followed for one season. *Acta Orthop Scand* 1993;64(4):459–461.
52. Biener K, Muller P. Les accidents du hockey sur glace. *Can Med* 1973;14:959–962.
53. Voaklander DC, Saunders LD, Quinney HA, Macnab RBJ. Epidemiology of recreational and old-timer ice hockey injuries. *Clin J Sports Med* 1996;6(1):15–21.
54. Boileau R, Marcotte G, Trudel P. Bernard D. Rapport finale sur l'application d'une strategy d'intervention visant a dimunuer le nombre de blessures et d'actes d'aggression au hockey a la Division Bantam: rapport final Remis au Fonds FCAR. Quebec City: Laval University, 1990:1–62.
55. Park RD, Castaldi CR. Injuries in junior ice hockey. *Phys Sports Med* 1980;8(2):81–90.

CHAPTER 43

Lacrosse and Field Hockey

Leslie S. Matthews and Jeffrey B. Yurkofsky

INTRODUCTION

Both lacrosse and field hockey place constant demands on the body, requiring the combination of running and cutting movements in the lower extremity with upper extremity strength and coordination. Consequently, the two sports share similar injury types and mechanisms but also have unique, sport-specific injuries that are secondary to the inherent differences between the two sports. This chapter presents the epidemiology of lacrosse and field hockey injuries with emphasis on injury types, mechanism, and prevention.

LACROSSE

History

A truly "American game," lacrosse has its roots in the native American Indian groups (1–3). First described in 1636 by the Jesuit missionary Jean de Brebeuf (4), the game originally had strong religious and cultural ties and was often played for a continuous 2-to 3-day period over a "playing field" of many miles. From its inception lacrosse was played with a stick with a netted loop at one end, which reminded early viewers of a crosier (hence the name "la crosse," a symbol of pastoral office). Lacrosse has undergone substantial changes, evolving from being called "a madman's game" by the New York Tribune in 1868 (2) to its modern epithet of "the fastest game on two feet." Lacrosse is now an organized sport that is played extensively at the scholastic, collegiate, club, and professional levels. Although historically thought of as an East Coast "prep" sport, lacrosse has greatly expanded its appeal throughout this country as well as internationally. Domestically, the game is under the guidance of the Lacrosse Foundation, which is housed, along with the Lacrosse Hall of Fame, on the campus of The Johns Hopkins University in Baltimore, Maryland. Although lacrosse is no longer an Olympic event, international competition, known as the World Games, has flourished since 1960 and is played every 4 years with strong U.S., Canadian, U.K., and Australian support. The World Games were played in 1994 in Manchester, England, and the 1998 Games were played in Baltimore, Maryland.

Women's lacrosse, an offshoot of the men's game, originated in England in the 1890s and became popular in U.S. schools and colleges in the 1920s. The women's game displays features similar to those of the men's game, the largest difference being that no deliberate physical contact is allowed in women's lacrosse, although sticks may be checked. The U.S. Women's Lacrosse Association was founded in 1931, and under its guidance, women's lacrosse has flourished at the high school and collegiate levels.

Injury Demographics

Men's Lacrosse

Lacrosse shares with other high-speed contact sports a relatively high rate of injury, although isolated studies on lacrosse (5–7) have shown it to be associated with a low incidence of serious injury. When studying an entire lacrosse team over a full season, Nelson and colleagues (8) noted that 85% of the team's players sustained some form of injury but that only 20% of those injuries were serious enough to cause missed practice or game time. In 1982 the National Collegiate Athletic Association (NCAA) developed the Injury Surveillance System (ISS) to provide data and report on injury trends in collegiate football. Since then the ISS has expanded to 16 sports, combining data from a representative cross-

---

L. S. Matthews and J. B. Yurkofsky: Department of Orthopaedic Surgery, The Union Memorial Hospital, Baltimore, Maryland 21218.

section of its participating Division I, II, and III schools. ISS has data on men's lacrosse from the 1986–1987 season through the 1995–1996 season. Injury rates are defined as the ratio of the number of injuries per 1000 athlete exposures.

The overall injury rate in men's lacrosse (1987–1996 seasons) was reported as 5.7 (per 1000 athlete exposures). This ratio places lacrosse in the middle tier of surveyed collegiate sports; the rate is less than those for spring football, wrestling, women's gymnastics, and men's and women's soccer but similar to those for men's and women's basketball, ice hockey, and men's gymnastics. The men's lacrosse injury rate during practice was 3.8; that during games was 15.6. These rates, combined with the fact that there are far fewer games than practice exposures, indicate that 44% of lacrosse injuries occur during game situations and 56% of injuries occur during practice. Breakdown of collegiate injury rates by division showed equal rates for practice (3.8) among Division I, II, and III schools. Game injury rates were 14.4, 17.9, and 16.0, respectively. Further analysis of collegiate injury rates shows the preseason injury rate to be 5.9, that during the regular season to be 5.5, and, interestingly, that during the postseason to be 2.9. The rates for home versus away injuries were similar: 15.9 and 15.2, respectively. More injuries occurred on artificial turf (18.3) than on natural grass (14.4).

Anatomically, most men's lacrosse injuries occur in the lower extremity (upper leg, knee, and ankle); the second most frequently inured area is the shoulder (7). Most injuries are minor sprains, strains, and contusions. Approximately 70% caused fewer than 7 days of missed practice; the remaining 30% caused more than 1 week of missed practice. This statistic again places men's lacrosse in the middle tier of surveyed collegiate sports.

The percentage of injuries requiring surgery in men's lacrosse was 5.2% (twelfth of 16) with a rate of 0.29 (tenth of 16), placing lacrosse at the lower end of the middle tier of surveyed sports. Putting this in perspective by comparing the 16 participating sports, women's gymnastics has the highest overall percentage (8.9%) of injuries requiring surgery as well as the highest rate (0.84) of injuries requiring surgery.

The most common mechanism of injury is noncontact incidents (e.g., rotational injuries), followed by body-to-body contact with another player, contact with the ball or stick, and contact with the playing surface. Overall, there is a roughly 50/50 division of contact versus noncontact mechanisms (see the section entitled "Mechanism of Injury" for more details).

Women's Lacrosse

The NCAA has also published data on women's lacrosse for the 1986–1997 seasons in the same format as that for men's lacrosse (9). Again, injury rates are expressed as the number of injuries occurring per 1000 athlete exposures. The overall injury rate for women's lacrosse, combining practice and game injuries, was 4.2, placing women's lacrosse in the lowest tier of surveyed sports. As in men's lacrosse, women's lacrosse showed higher game than practice injury rates: 7.2 and 3.5, respectively (7,9). Given the higher number of practices, these data indicate that 68% of the injuries occurred during practice and 32% occurred during games. These percentages are similar to, but overall higher than, those for men's lacrosse: 56 and 44%, respectively. This high practice injury percentage places women's lacrosse third in the sports ranking; only spring football and men's and women's gymnastics have higher injury percentages during practice situations. However, these percentages may be misleading; in looking at rates and total numbers, women's lacrosse is consistently positioned in the lowest tier for injuries among the surveyed sports.

In Divisions I, II, and III, women's lacrosse practice injury rates were 3.4, 3.5, and 3.6, respectively, and game injury rates were 7.0, 6.0, and 7.2, respectively. The preseason injury rate was 4.5, the regular season rate was 3.9, and the postseason rate was 2.4. Injury rates for home and away games were 6.0 and 7.7, respectively. Again, as in men's lacrosse, artificial surfaces showed higher injury rates than natural surfaces: 8.0 and 6.6, respectively.

Anatomically, women's lacrosse injuries were similar to those of men's lacrosse in that the most commonly injured area was the lower extremity (ankle, knee, and upper leg) (7,9). However, noticeably absent in women players are shoulder injuries. This may be related to the lower level of contact (specifically, checking) in women's lacrosse (Fig. 43–1). As in men's lacrosse, most injuries are strains, sprains, and contusions, most (74%) of which caused fewer than 7 days of missed time; 26% caused 7

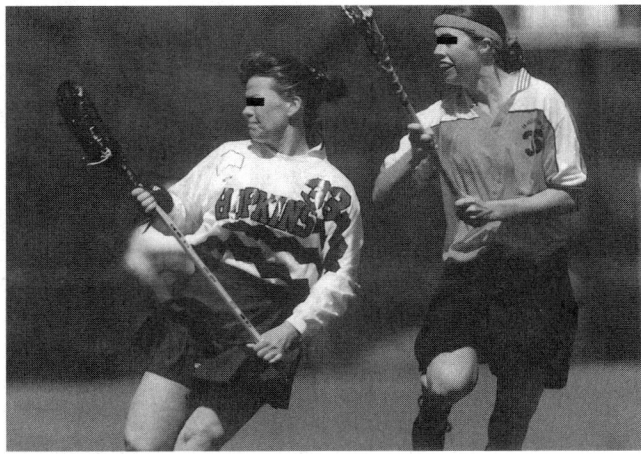

FIG. 43–1. Women's lacrosse prohibits the use of checking, probably resulting in fewer shoulder injuries than are seen in men's lacrosse. (Photo courtesy of David Preece.)

or more days of missed practice or game time. This statistic places lacrosse once again in the lowest tier of surveyed sports.

Women's lacrosse ranks last with ice hockey in the percentage of all injuries requiring surgery (4.1%) and has the lowest injury rate requiring surgery (0.17). As in men's lacrosse, most injuries are classified as noncontact; however, in women's lacrosse this percentage is much higher (approximately 70%) than the roughly 50% noncontact injury percentage in men's lacrosse (7,9).

Types of Injuries

As mentioned previously, the highest incidence of injury occurs in the lower extremity (upper legs, knees, ankles). This may be attributed to a combination of factors: the high-speed running, cutting, and sudden change of direction (Fig. 43–2) combined with the potential for stick, ball, playing surface, and body contact. The lack of protective equipment on the lower extremity may also contribute to the high rate of lower extremity injuries. Lower extremity injuries tend to be more of the lesser type of injury—that is, sprains, strains, and contusions—although more severe injuries (e.g., ankle fractures, ligament and meniscal tears, and stress fractures) do occur.

In general, the upper extremity, shoulder girdle, face, and head are well protected; however, shoulder injuries rank right below lower extremity injuries in the NCAA surveys. Upper extremity injuries also tend to consist of less severe sprains, strains, and contusions; the shoulder tends to be the area that suffers the most severe injuries, including clavicle fractures, shoulder subluxations and dislocations, and acromioclavicular joint separations. Despite well-padded glove protection, hand injuries are still common, probably the result of stick contact with the gloved hand.

Other injuries typical of contact sports also occur, including concussions (although not common) and low back pain and injuries, data that have been substantiated by both NCAA and independent studies (7,8). Low back pain and injuries generally tend to occur in attackmen and midfielders, most likely attributable to the twisting, dodging, and contact required of these players. Midfielders sustain the highest number and most severe injuries, probably because of their open-field play and high involvement in the game. Interestingly, goalies sustain the lowest number of injuries (4,7).

To the authors' knowledge, no reports (other than the NCAA ISS data) detail the types of injuries and their breakdown by position. It is the authors' experience that, in general, women's lacrosse teams sustain fewer and less severe injuries than do men's lacrosse teams. This view is supported by the NCAA reports. Despite the low incidence of head and facial injuries in women's lacrosse, several recent articles have called attention to the lack of protective headgear and the potential for severe eye injury and have documented ocular trauma among women's lacrosse players (10,11). Despite the availability of approved eyewear, use of such protection at this time remains optional for U.S. Women's Lacrosse games and/or internationally sanctioned games and represents an area of potential improvement with minimal intrusion onto the spirit of the woman's game.

The potential for injury to officials and spectators during competitions should be mentioned. Lacrosse balls can travel at high speeds, up to 100 mph. Errant shots have been reported to strike inattentive spectators. Barriers behind goals or restricted seating could reduce or eliminate this problem, and game officials should be made aware of this potential danger. Injuries to officials can occur from inadvertent contact with players or their sticks and from passed, deflected, or shot balls.

Mechanisms of Injury

It is convenient to organize lacrosse injuries into noncontact and contact injury patterns; the latter category includes body-to-body, stick-to-body, ball-to-body, and body-to-playing-surface injuries.

Noncontact Injuries

Lacrosse, like all field sports, requires constant running in the form of sudden acceleration, deceleration, and cutting. As a consequence, a certain amount of noncontact injuries can be expected to occur. Noncontact injuries represent the most common injury mechanism in both men's and women's lacrosse. In the 1995–1996 NCAA statistics, 172 of 341 men's injuries (approxi-

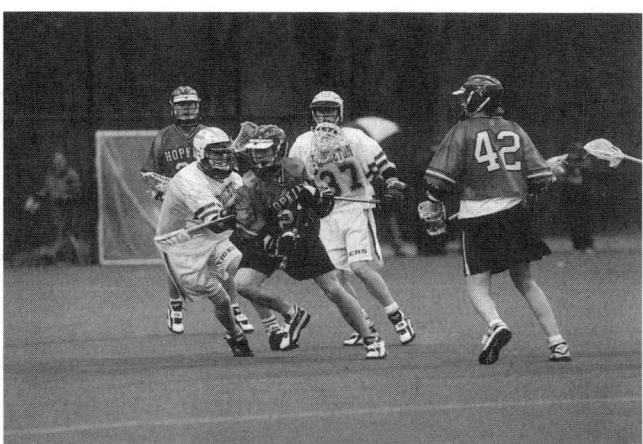

FIG. 43–2. Typical high-speed running, cutting, and changing direction contribute to the high number of lower extremity injuries in lacrosse. (Photo courtesy of David Preece.)

mately 50%) and 144 of 206 of women's injuries (approximately 70%) were classified as noncontact injuries (7). This percentage of noncontact injuries correlates with the authors' experience. Most of these injuries occurred in the lower extremity and consisted of ligamentous injuries of the knees and ankles, muscle strains, shin splints, and stress fractures. Nelson and colleagues (8) also report a high incidence of ankle sprains in men's lacrosse. Most ligamentous knee injuries occur from noncontact mechanisms.

It should be noted that lacrosse tends to be free from the common overuse injuries such as epicondylitis that are seen in the upper extremity in stick or racquet sports such as tennis and golf. Also, unlike other throwing-type sports, lacrosse players do not seem to suffer from bicipital or rotator cuff tendinitis or other inflammatory conditions. This is because of the excellent leverage afforded by the lacrosse stick. The result of this biomechanical advantage is the creation of high-speed shots without subjecting the upper extremity (shoulder and elbow) to excessive arcs of motion, acceleration, deceleration, and their associated stresses. The fluidity of the lacrosse stroke appears advantageous to the upper extremity. The concern often seen in Little League baseball about prolonged or repetitive play among small and growing children appears less justified in lacrosse because of this apparent lack of overuse-type syndromes.

Contact Injuries

Body-to-Body Contact

Body contact is allowed in men's lacrosse but is prohibited in the women's game. This accounts for the higher number of body-to-body contact injuries seen in the men's game. For the 1995–1996 season, NCAA injury data listed body-to-body contact injury rates of 1.53 (99 of 341 injuries) and 0.22 (11 of 206) for men's and women's lacrosse, respectively (7,9). Body-to-body contact can vary from simple shield-blocking to high-velocity contact and checking (Fig. 43-3). Despite this potential for high-velocity contact, the lacrosse player's equipment is not necessarily designed to protect the athlete during this type of collision. Consequently, players delivering and receiving the blow are both at risk for serious injury.

Although lower extremity injuries predominate statistically, it is the upper extremity that tends to sustain injury from body-to-body contact. In particular, shoulder girdle injuries occur quite commonly (Fig. 43-4). Shoulder pads are mandatory in men's lacrosse except for goalkeepers; however, they are not designed to protect the shoulder region from contact in the way that, for example, football pads are designed. These contact injuries often manifest themselves in the form of acromi-

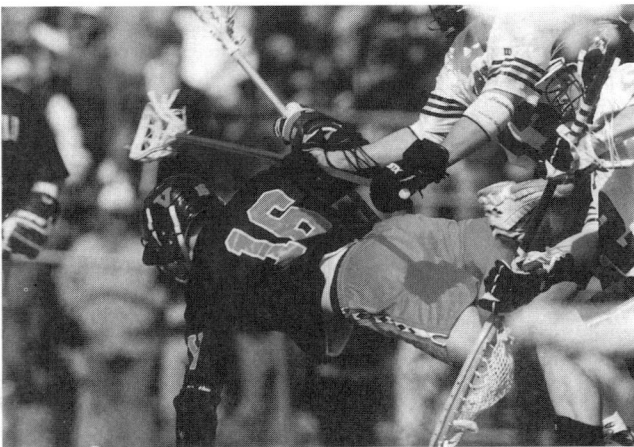

FIG. 43-3. High-velocity checking occurs in men's lacrosse. (Photo courtesy of David Preece.)

oclavicular joint separations and clavicle fractures. Contact shoulder injuries typically outnumber other upper extremity contact injuries 2:1.

In lacrosse, stationary picks, such as those seen in basketball, are legal; cross-body-blocking (in which another player's feet leave the ground) is illegal. As a result, lacrosse picks and checks occur in a more upright, and therefore more exposed, position, using the head, neck, and shoulder regions and putting these areas at risk for injury. Most injuries in the head and neck region tend to be concussions, which are usually grade 1 injuries (12). The lacrosse helmet probably contributes somewhat to this incidence. It is loose-fitting, vented, and constructed of a much more flexible material than is a football helmet. It is designed to protect the cranium from blows from the lacrosse stick, and it appears to be effective in achieving this result. However, despite its

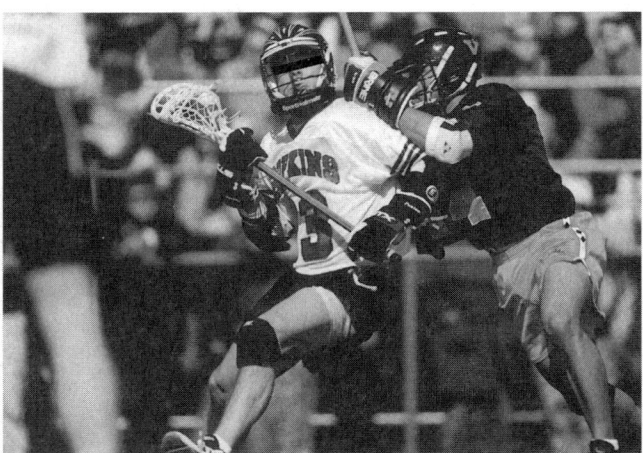

FIG. 43-4. Despite the use of protective shoulder pads, blows to the shoulder girdle can result in injury. (Photo courtesy of David Preece.)

approval by the National Operating Committee on Standards for Athletic Equipment (NOCSAE), the helmet does not appear as effective in protecting from high-speed collisions to the head region. On the other hand, unlike football helmets, the lacrosse helmet does not appear to be a potential weapon according to injury reports (7). In the NCAA 1995–1996 report, only 8 of 341 injuries were directly attributable to contact with or from the helmet (7). In any event, given the design of the lacrosse helmet, those who strike other players with their heads place themselves in great jeopardy, and coaches and trainers alike should make players aware of this at an early stage of lacrosse development.

In general, noncontact injuries produce meniscal and ligamentous injuries about the knee with greater frequency than do contact mechanisms. However, knee injuries that are secondary to contact are almost invariably the result of an illegal block. This factor tends to support the low incidence of posterior cruciate ligament injury compared with anterior cruciate ligament and medial collateral ligament injury. When contact injuries about the knee do occur, they tend to be serious multiligamentous injuries, and often surgical intervention is necessary or advised.

In lacrosse, chest and rib cage injuries tend to predominate over abdominal injuries. Because blocking and checking are often done in a more upright position, it can be surmised that it is the upper torso and thoracic region that absorb the blunt of the blow, rather than the abdominal region. One case of pancreatitis has been reported (6), supposedly linked to a direct blow to the abdomen; splenic injuries are rare. Rib cage injuries usually occur as contusions and fractures, but sometimes as multiple fractures, for two reasons: the rib cage is afforded little protection by standard lacrosse equipment, and upright blocking techniques seem to predispose this area for injury. The authors are aware of one case of pulmonary contusion and hemothorax in an All-American attackman as a result of body contact. Although they are obviously extremely rare, the potential for pneumothorax or other clinically significant mediastinal injuries must be recognized to avoid disastrous consequences.

Stick-to-Body Contact

The hand and shoulder girdle regions are the areas most commonly injured from stick-to-body contact. Although protective equipment used in lacrosse to shield the shoulder and hand is designed specifically to provide coverage to these areas, injuries to these areas still occur regularly, and often seriously, in the form of fractures. Fractures in the shoulder girdle region most commonly result from illegal checks. Fractures of the clavicle and, rarely, the first rib have been seen despite the use of protective gear in the form of shoulder pads.

Fractures of the forearm may also occur from direct stick-to-body contact. While controlling the ball, an offensive player will routinely carry the stick and ball in one hand and use the free arm in a protective posture as a shield in front of the body to ward off blows from the defensive player (Fig. 43–5). This position leaves the free arm exposed and, if not protected, vulnerable to single- or both-bone forearm fractures. Both-bone forearm fractures, isolated ulna shaft fractures, and radial shaft fractures have all been seen as a result of these conditions.

Fractures of the hand are usually the result of stick-to-body contact. It is the authors' opinion that since rules restricting the alteration of the palms and fingers of protective gloves have been enforced, hand injuries are less common. Hand and finger fractures and injuries are seen in women's lacrosse as well because no protective gloves are worn. The injury rate for hand injuries is still much higher in men's than women's lacrosse, reflecting the nature of contact despite protection. In men's lacrosse in particular, the thumb is the most commonly injured digit. Orthoplastic splints for hand fractures are approved and can be worn inside a player's glove, allowing an earlier return to competition.

Eye and facial injuries resulting from stick-to-body contact are less frequent in men's than women's lacrosse because of the protective headgear worn by men. On occasion, certain portions of the stick may be able to penetrate between the slips of the face mask and cause injury, usually the result of an illegal check. Rimel and colleagues (13) have reported a stick injury to the parietal area of the head resulting in an epidural hematoma requiring craniotomy and hematoma evacuation. This player was wearing a lacrosse helmet, although at a time before use of NOCSAE-approved protective helmets was required. Finally, brightly colored mouthguards are

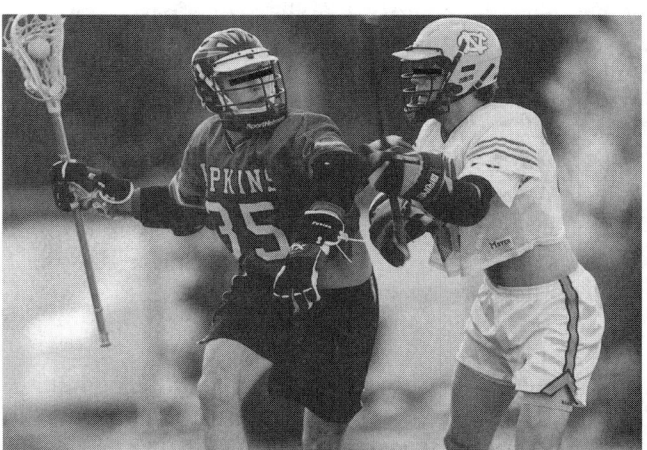

FIG. 43–5. Typical protective posture of an attackman using his forearm to protect against opposing blows, thus predisposing this area to injury. (Photo courtesy of David Preece.)

now mandated by NCAA rules for all players. Bright colors are worn so that compliance may be monitored more readily by officials. Compliance with this rule and extension to interscholastic and club competition will undoubtedly serve to reduce the risk of dental injury in players.

Soft-tissue injuries are the hallmark of stick-to-body contact. These injuries may be from one isolated blow to an unprotected area or from multiple and repeated blows to the same area. Chronic repetitive injury is notoriously common in attackmen, who routinely use their arms to ward off defensive blows. In addition to the more commonly seen contusions and occasional hematomas, several players have developed myositis ossificans in the humeral region as a result of chronic repetitive blows to this area; these players missed substantial playing time as a result. With the high frequency of soft-tissue injuries, especially in the arm area, mandatory protective arm pads from the deltoid to the cuff of the lacrosse glove should be implemented.

Ball-to-Body Contact

The combination of a hard rubber composition ball propelled at high speeds at a large exposed body surface area makes ball-to-body contact a frequent and potentially serious mechanism of injury. It is estimated that 10% of lacrosse injuries result from this mechanism.

Injuries to the neck and throat are potentially the most serious. Nelson and colleagues (14) reported on one player who sustained a blow to the neck that struck the carotid sinus region and caused syncope, bradycardia, and hypertension. This resolved with nonoperative treatment. However, the potential for serious airway injury or other injury in the neck region emphasizes the need for on-field personnel (coaches, trainers, and physicians) to be familiar with basic life support measures in the event of a catastrophic injury. Since 1983 it has been mandatory for all goalkeepers to wear a protective throat shield, which is suspended from the lower portion of the face mask of the helmet.

Facial lacerations and eye injuries occur in men's lacrosse despite the use of a protective helmet and face mask. The nature of the helmet contributes to this fact. The somewhat loose fit of the lacrosse helmet will, on occasion, allow a shot that strikes the mask to displace the mask forcefully against the face, causing the mask itself to lacerate or injure the face. The use of a four-point chin strap should help to prevent the majority of these injuries.

Women's lacrosse also has its share of facial injuries secondary to the lack of head or face protective gear. The 1995–1996 injury data support a higher incidence of eye and nasal injury in women's lacrosse than in men's lacrosse (9). A total of ten injuries were reported (five ocular and five nasal) in women compared with no injuries reported in these areas for men. Although the mechanism was not described for these injuries, ball contact and inadvertent stick contact are the usual culprits. Although it is generally true that ball speeds in the women's game tend to be slower than that in men's lacrosse, recent reports have called attention to the presence of potentially severe ocular injuries (10,11). There is a push to implement protective eyewear for women's lacrosse, a goal that the authors share.

Testicular injuries can occur as a result of a direct blow by a lacrosse ball. Although required for the goalkeepers, protective cups are not required for other positions. It would seem prudent for both offensive and defensive players who are at greatest risk for ball-to-body injury—that is, those players who spend a large amount of time at and around the goal area—to wear protective cups.

Body-to-Playing-Surface Contact

Lacrosse shares with other field sports the potential for contact with the playing surface, which undoubtedly results in a variety of injuries (Fig. 43–6). As more and more artificial surfaces are being used for practice and game situations, new types of problems unique to these surfaces have emerged. As mentioned previously, injury rates for both men and women are higher on artificial surfaces than on natural grass. The 1995–1996 data for men's lacrosse recorded a rate of 4.95 for natural grass compared with 5.51 for artificial surfaces (7). Corresponding data for women were 3.62 and 4.59, respectively. It should also be mentioned that other surfaces used for practices, such as gym floors, also significantly contribute to injuries seen in both men and women: 5.46 and 4.48, respectively (1995–1996 season data) (7).

Abrasions, or turf burns, have the potential to become

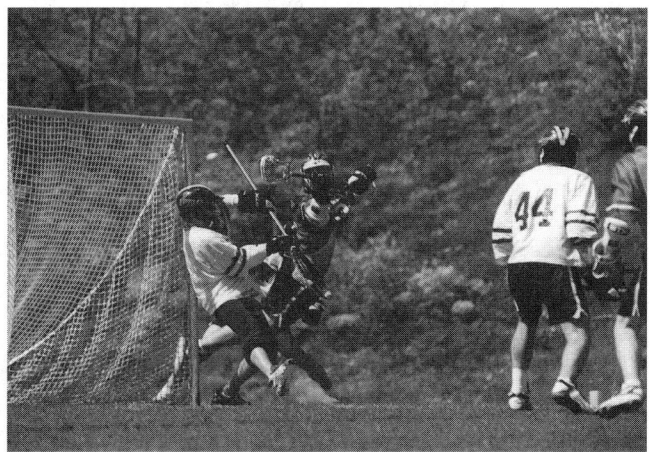

FIG. 43–6. Shot-making aerial acrobatics can result in exciting goals, but at the price of exposing the body to hard contact with the playing surface. (Photo courtesy of David Preece.)

substantial problems in lacrosse. Because lacrosse is a spring sport in which players usually wear shorts, little or no lower extremity protection is afforded by the uniform itself. Consequently, falls or skids, especially on artificial surfaces, can result in deep abrasions with the potential for secondary infection if untreated. Preventive measures can play a large role in reducing the morbidity. The application of thin layers of petroleum gel to bony prominences or the placement of thin stockinglike material or tube gauze can decrease friction and serve as a protective barrier. The authors have noted that play on artificial surfaces has increased the incidence of traumatic prepatellar and olecranon bursitis in lacrosse players. Standard care of these injuries, including aspiration, pressure dressings, antiinflammatory medications, and protective padding, can usually suffice. Close attention to these injuries for the development of septic bursitis is mandatory.

Common injuries will also result from players falling or being knocked to the playing surface, regardless of the surface type. Perhaps the most unavoidable of all types of injuries is the fall on the outstretched arm, as it is a general reflexive action. Wrist fractures, elbow dislocations, acromioclavicular joint separations, and glenohumeral dislocations can all occur from this type of injury mechanism. Although certainly not as prevalent in the women's game because of the lack of legal body contact, falls are still a common occurrence and injury mechanism.

Conditioning and Injury Prevention

Conditioning in lacrosse should be tailored to the specific attributes of the game: speed, agility, strength, and endurance. Both preseason and postseason conditioning programs are typically implemented at the collegiate level. Preseason workouts generally emphasize endurance, strength, and agility training. Particular emphasis is and should be placed on the upper extremity and shoulder girdle region as well as on the lower extremity. Endurance training and strength training for the lower extremity are often accomplished through running programs consisting of short-distance, interval, and long-distance training. Off-season conditioning usually consists of running programs (20–25 miles per week) combined with weight room training three times per week. Goalkeepers specifically train to improve foot speed and hand-eye coordination. Jumping rope and racquetball are often added to the regimen for this position.

During the regular season, frequent practices and full-field scrimmages foster endurance training. Strength training continues with weight-training programs. Speed conditioning is gained during practice and scrimmages, and with the addition of short-distance sprinting programs and interval training techniques. The ultimate goal is to fine-tune the team's overall conditioning to achieve a peak performance on game day.

Although training approaches for female lacrosse players are similar to those for their male counterparts, the female training program does not appear to have the same focus on specific upper and lower extremity strengthening regimens. Endurance training emphasizes long-distance running during the off-season, supported by regular season participation in practices and full scrimmages. Short-distance and interval-type programs are emphasized during the season to improve speed.

Although conditioning programs cannot eliminate the amount of injuries that occur in men's and women's lacrosse, the authors strongly feel that they are a key component for injury prevention. Having the male or female lacrosse player in optimal shape and conditioning should be emphasized at all levels of play.

Conclusions

Lacrosse has been shown to be a relatively safe sport compared with other field sports. However, this fact should not reduce the effort to improve the game, whether it be through equipment changes or modifications or through specific rule changes. Recently, lacrosse has made substantial strides by making the use of mouthguards and shoulderpads mandatory and by prohibiting the alteration of gloves. The use of protective eyewear in women's lacrosse, as evidenced by several recent studies (10,11), represents an area in which new rules may have an impact on injury prevention. These changes have been and continue to be supported by the authors. Continuing to improve equipment, coaching, officiating, and conditioning can only lead to an improved game and a lower incidence of injury. Ultimately, this manifests itself through a meaningful cooperation between coaches, trainers, team physicians, and the governing members of the game.

FIELD HOCKEY

History

Field hockey is believed to have been a feature of many of the earliest civilizations. Depictions of the sport have been uncovered in ancient Egyptian tombs and from ancient Greek and Roman finds as well (15). Its more recent organized form is traced to club teams that were organized in the English schools of the 19th century, where, despite the Victorian era's restrictions on women's sports, field hockey became a very popular sport for women. Organized men's field hockey is also traced to strong British origins, with its international spread easily traced across the once vast British Empire, especially in India. Men's international field hockey competition began in 1895; organized women's international competition did not emerge until the 1970s. Similarly, men's field hockey as an Olympic event predates women's field hockey Olympic competition by approximately 70 years (1908 and 1980, respectively). In the United States, women's field hockey thrives at scholastic and collegiate levels. Men's field hockey is much less popular, most games occurring only on the international circuit.

Injury Demographics

The NCAA ISS has compiled data for women's collegiate field hockey (hereinafter termed "field hockey") from its participating Division I, II, and III schools for the 1986–1987 through 1996–1997 seasons (16). The overall injury rate for field hockey (combined practice and game) was 5.5 per 1000 athlete exposures, placing field hockey in the middle tier of surveyed collegiate sports. Comparable rates are reported for sports such as men's lacrosse, men's and women's basketball, and ice hockey. As for all surveyed collegiate sports in the ISS, overall injury rates and percentages were higher for games than for practices: 9.4 and 59% (games) versus 4.2 and 41% (practices), respectively. Both practice and game rates place field hockey in the middle tier of surveyed sports. In Divisions I, II, and II, injury rates were 3.9, 4.0, and 4.8, respectively, for practices and 9.6, 9.2, and 9.0, respectively, for games. The preseason injury rate was 7.5, the regular season rate was 4.9, and the postseason rate was 4.0. The injury rates for home and away games were similar: 9.6 and 9.5, respectively. As in both men's and women's lacrosse, the rate of injury was higher for artificial surfaces than for natural turf: 10.5 and 9.3, respectively.

As is seen in men's and women's lacrosse, lower extremity injuries, particularly to the upper leg, knee, and ankle, account for the majority of injuries seen in field hockey. Statistics for the 1995–1996 NCAA ISS field hockey season showed that the lower extremity (upper leg through foot region) accounted for 179 of 302 injuries recorded from the cross-sectioned sample of teams (16). Again, as in women's lacrosse, field hockey records a low incidence of shoulder and upper extremity injuries. One notable difference is the occurrence of finger and hand injuries, which tends to be higher in field hockey than in women's lacrosse. Most injuries tend to be minor strains, sprains, and contusions. Field hockey has the lowest ranking of surveyed sports: 77% of the injuries caused fewer than 7 days of missed practice or game time; only 23% of injuries caused 1 week or more of missed time. Correlating this statistic with injury severity rates gives field hockey an injury rate of 1.2 per 1000 athlete exposures, placing field hockey 14th of the 16 surveyed sports. However, in examining the percentage of injuries that required surgery, field hockey placed in the middle tier (ninth of 16) of sports with 5.6% of injuries requiring surgery; these percentages were similar to those reported for women's soccer, baseball, and men's basketball. The overall injury-requiring-surgery rate was 0.29, equaling men's lacrosse as the tenth of 16 surveyed sports. Once again, most injuries occur secondary to noncontact mechanisms, followed by contact with the stick or ball, the playing surface, and another player.

Types of Injuries

As in lacrosse, lower extremity injuries (upper leg, knee, and ankle) predominate in field hockey; noticeably absent are upper extremity injuries, except for those of the hand. These findings are attributed to the nature and style of play in field hockey. Most of the action occurs at the ground level, and no deliberate contact or checking is allowed. The hands are particularly vulnerable, as they are in constant contact with the stick and sustain blows mainly from inadvertent stick contact from opposing players (Fig. 43–7). Although field hockey does require the use of shin guards, these are the only lower extremity padding or protection. Given the nature of the hard ball that is used, shin guards offer only some protection and only in a limited region. Although most lower extremity injuries consist of strains, sprains, and contusions, some are more severe, such as ankle fractures, knee ligament injury, and meniscus tears. Of particular concern is the number of patella injuries, usually from direct ball contact. Of 39 reported knee injuries from sampled schools, 13 were injuries to the patella and/or patella tendon.

In field hockey, the lower back has been an area of concern for the development of low back strain and mechanical back symptoms. The demands of dribbling, shooting, and passing in a semicrouched position have

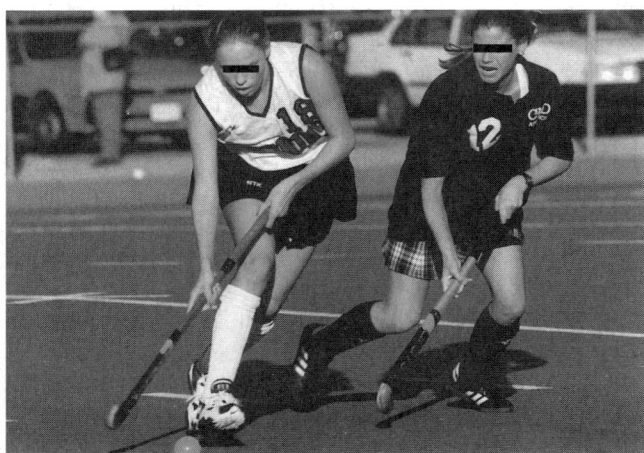

FIG. 43–7. The location of the hands on the field hockey stick predisposes them to injury from inadvertent contact. (Photo courtesy of David Preece.)

been examined. In one study, energy expenditure, heart rate, and subjectively perceived exertion increased in seven male English field hockey players (17). A survey of 81 players showed that 53% reported experiencing low back pain (17). Examination showed a rate of compression of 0.4 mm/min during one 7-minute timed trial, reportedly higher than that seen in other activities (17). The conclusions of this study were that field hockey tends to produce physiologic strain and spinal loading in excess of that associated with orthodox motion. Whether these effects are cumulatively deleterious is not known. Rates of low back injury reported in the 1996–1997 field hockey (16) and 1995–1996 women's lacrosse (9) data were similar, 0.21 and 0.20, respectively, despite the semicrouched posture seen in field hockey and the more upright posture of lacrosse players. These data, however, do not reflect the overall incidence of low back pain.

In the upper body, the area of most concern for injury, after the hand, is the head. No headgear is required, and the ball, although traveling at speeds less than those seen in lacrosse, is extremely hard and unforgiving. Most head injuries consist of lacerations or concussions, and most of the latter (14 of 15 in the 1996–1997 season) are grade-1 injuries (16). Mouthguards are required and aid in reducing dental injuries.

Analysis of injuries by position shows that most positions, with the exception of the goalie, are at relatively equal risk. On the basis of the 1996–1997 data, forwards and defense or sweepers show a trend toward sustaining more injuries (16). As mentioned previously, noncontact injuries still tend to occur more frequently than do contact injuries. Ball handling, shooting, and going after loose balls are the three most common ways in which injuries occur.

Mechanisms of Injury

The mechanisms of injury in field hockey are similar to those of lacrosse and have been categorized as noncontact and contact mechanisms.

Noncontact Injuries

As in women's lacrosse, noncontact injuries in field hockey occur more frequently than contact injuries. Data from the 1996–1997 season (16) show that 160 of 303 injuries (53%) were noncontact in origin. As we stated previously, most noncontact injuries (usually sprains, muscle strains, shin splints, and occasionally stress fractures or tendinitis) involve the lower extremity and are secondary to the running, cutting, accelerating, and decelerating inherent to all field sports.

Field hockey does involve the use of the upper extremity, but most shoulder activity occurs with the arm in only mild to moderate abduction and usually does not require excessive external rotation. These factors, combined with the lack of deliberate contact, help in large part to prevent a higher occurrence of shoulder problems in field hockey players.

Contact Injuries

Body-to-Body Contact

Although deliberate contact with another competitor is illegal in field hockey, incidental and inadvertent yet severe contact can occur during any game. Compared with women's lacrosse, field hockey tends to produce higher rates of injury for all types of contact, including body-to-body contact. Again, as in women's lacrosse, data from the 1996–1997 season (16) indicate that injury from contact with another competitor represented the least common mechanism of all contact patterns described: 29 of 303 injuries (approximately 10%), with an injury rate of 0.56. This injury rate is almost double the body-to-body contact injury rate for the 1995–1996 women's lacrosse season (0.29) and probably reflects the higher rate contact that is expected to occur in field hockey (9,16).

Both upper and lower extremity injuries can be expected from body contact. These injuries can range from simple contusions to more complex fractures or ligamentous knee injuries; the incidence of these more severe injuries is low, as reflected by the relatively low reported rates of surgery and missed time. As in women's lacrosse, no protective gear, other than shin guards, is commonly worn or required of field hockey players; thus, players in both sports are ultimately at higher risk in the event of high-energy body contact.

Stick-to-Body Contact

Data from the 1996–1997 field hockey season indicate that 36 of 303 injuries were secondary to stick-to-body contact, and injury rate of 0.69 compared with a rate of 0.30 for women's lacrosse during the 1995–1996 season (9,16). As in lacrosse, field hockey disallows deliberate stick checking or contact; injuries in this category usually represent inadvertent contact. Most of these injuries are lower extremity soft-tissue trauma, and occur secondary to opposing players challenging for control of the ball. The location of the ball and the sticks generally favor lower extremity injuries, with the exception of the vulnerability of the hands to inadvertent contact. Overall injuries to the hand and wrist region accounted for 22 of 303 injuries in the 1996–1997 season data, an overall injury rate of 0.43 (16). The same injury rate in women's lacrosse was 0.14 (9); in men's lacrosse, where protective gloves are required and contact is allowed, the injury rate was 0.33 (7). Clearly, this represents an area in which substantial improvement can be made, perhaps

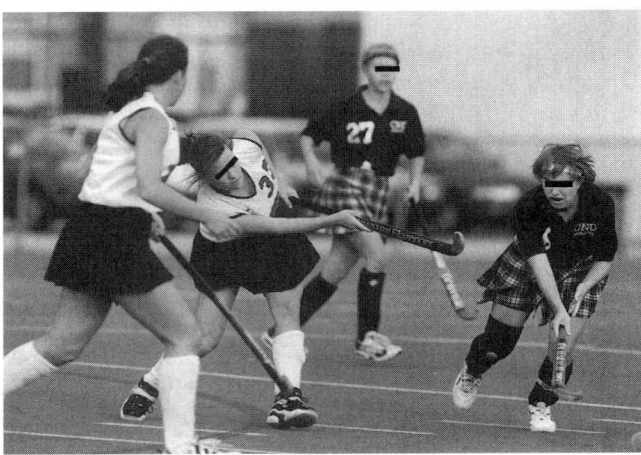

FIG. 43–8. Rules governing high-sticking are in effect to help reduce the potential of serious injury during shots at the goal taken in close proximity to other players. (Photo courtesy of David Preece.)

with the addition of some protective padding to the hand region. Enforcement of the no high-sticking policy ensures that only rarely will sticks cause injury more proximally in the upper extremity (Fig. 43–8).

Ball-to-Body Contact

Ball-to-body contact is the second most common mechanism of injury (the first is noncontact injuries). Data from the 1996–1997 season show that 43 of 303 injuries occurred specifically from ball-to-body contact (16). Contact can occur from both passes and deliberate on-goal attempts; the latter is perhaps the more potentially serious (Fig. 43-9). In comparison with women's lacrosse, field hockey has a higher injury rate: 0.83 and 0.24, respectively (9,16).

Although the speed of the field hockey ball is generally less than that of a lacrosse ball, the former has a harder, less forgiving composition. Certain rules exist to protect the overall speed of the shot and the location of players. High-sticking would certainly generate more ball speed, and rules governing the height of "driven" shots exist to protect exposed players. The addition of an obstruction rule (i.e., players cannot deliberately jump in the path of a driven shot) also helps to protect players. Most injuries will be soft tissue in nature, such as contusions, but serious injury can occur. Blows to the chest wall, neck, throat, and head region all carry the risk of serious injury and should be carefully assessed.

Body-to-Playing-Surface Contact

Body-to-playing-surface injuries are typical of any field sport, regardless of whether contact is allowed. NCAA data from the 1996–1997 season show that this mechanism was responsible for 36 of 303 injuries; this rate of 0.69 was higher than that seen in women's lacrosse (0.48) (9,16). Again, these higher contact injury rates reflect the overall impression of more contact and more severe contact in field hockey than in women's lacrosse. Like lacrosse and other field sports in general, contact with the playing surface (whether natural grass or artificial turf) results in abrasions, contusions, sprains, separations, and (rarely) fractures or dislocations. Field hockey, like lacrosse, shows higher injury rates on artificial surfaces as compared with natural grass.

Conditioning and Injury Prevention

Conditioning for field hockey is similar to that for women's lacrosse. Both tend to emphasize endurance, speed, and lower extremity strength. In the upper extremity, coordination is emphasized to a larger degree than strength.

Running programs, both in-season and off-season, tend to promote both endurance and speed training by emphasizing long-distance, sprint, or interval-type training. Practices and full scrimmages complement this program and aid in the overall development of lower extremity strength and upper extremity coordination. The conditioning and strength programs can only benefit the overall health of the field hockey player and are an essential component to injury prevention.

Conclusions

Field hockey shares with women's lacrosse many features in terms of injury types and mechanisms. Although field hockey appears to involve higher contact injury rates, both sports are generally safe, as is evidenced by

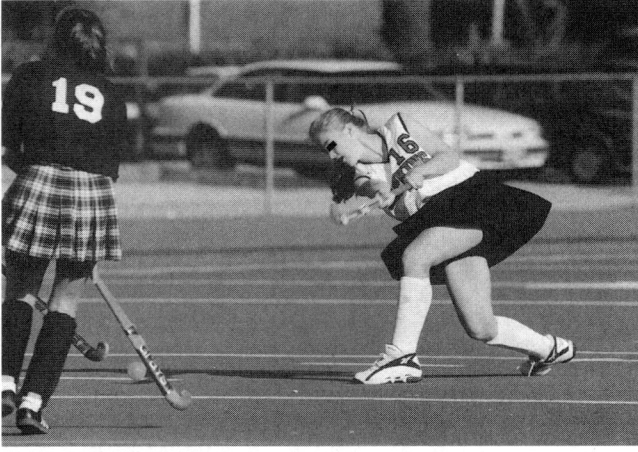

FIG. 43–9. Given the hard composition of the field hockey ball, direct shots on goal can strike opposing players or teammates and result in potentially serious injuries. (Photo courtesy of David Preece.)

the low overall injury rates. Constant scrutiny, aided to a large degree by studies such as the NCAA Injury Surveillance System, can help to identify trends and patterns of injury in these sports. With the combined effort of all those involved with field sports like lacrosse and field hockey, continued improvements can be made in an effort to promote safe, competitive, and entertaining field sports.

REFERENCES

1. Morrill WK. *Lacrosse,* rev ed. New York: Ronald Press, 1966.
2. Scott B. *Lacrosse: technique and tradition.* Baltimore: Johns Hopkins University Press, 1976.
3. Weyland AM, Roberts MR. *The lacrosse story.* Baltimore, Herman, 1965.
4. Matthews LS, Michael RH. Lacrosse. In Fu FH, Stone DA, eds. *Sports injuries: mechanisms, prevention, treatment.* Baltimore: Williams & Wilkins, 1994:469–479.
5. Kulund DN, Schildwachter TL, McCue FC, Gierk JH. Lacrosse injuries. *Phys Sports Med* 1979;7:82–90.
6. Mueller FO, Blyth CS. A survey of 1981 college lacrosse injuries. *Phys Sports Med* 1982;10:86–92.
7. National Collegiate Athletic Association. *Injury Surveillance System: 1995–1996 men's lacrosse.* Overland Park, KS: National Collegiate Athletic Association, 1995.
8. Nelson WE, DePalma B, Gieck JH, et al. Intercollegiate lacrosse injuries. *Phys Sports Med* 1981;9:86–92.
9. National Collegiate Athletic Association. *Injury Surveillance System: 1995–1996 women's lacrosse.* Overland Park, KS: National Collegiate Athletic Association, 1995.
10. Lapidus CS, Nelson LB, Jeffers JB, et al. Eye injuries in lacrosse: women need their vision less than men? *J Trauma* 1992;32:555–556.
11. Livingston LA, Forbes SL. Eye injuries in women's lacrosse: strict rule enforcement and mandatory eyewear required. *J Trauma* 1996;40:144–145.
12. Kelly JP, Nichols JS, Filley CM, et al. Concussion in sports: guidelines for the prevention of catastrophic outcome. *JAMA* 1991;266:2867–2869.
13. Rimel RW, Nelson WE, Persing JA, Jane JA. Epidural hematoma in lacrosse. *Phys Sports Med* 1983;11:140–144.
14. Nelson WE, Crampton RS, McCue FC, Gieck JH. Syncope, bradycardia, and hypotension after a lacrosse shot to the neck. *Phys Sports Med* 1981;9:94–97.
15. Field hockey. In: *The new encyclopaedia Britannica,* 15th ed. Chicago: Encyclopaedia Brittanica, 1986:765.
16. National Collegiate Athletic Association. *Injury Surveillance System: 1996–1997 field hockey.* Overland Park, KS: National Collegiate Athletic Association, 1996.
17. Reilly T, Seaton A. Physiological strain unique to field hockey. *J Sports Med Phys Fitness* 1990;30:142–146.

CHAPTER 44

Martial Arts

Leonard A. Wilkerson

The term "martial arts" means the physical arts that are concerned with the waging of war, but in the 20th century they no longer have a military role. It is said that the study of the martial arts will develop character or higher moral standards. As a result of this change, the martial arts came to mean "the way." An estimated 1.5–2 million Americans (of whom 20% are children) participate in the martial arts with an estimated ratio of 5:1 male to female (1). With such a wide cross-section of Americans participating in an activity about which little is known of the physical forces involved, little thought has been given to potential morbidity and mortality. Information generated from a nationwide computer surveillance of emergency departments and from surveys mailed to martial arts instructors showed that no deaths and no serious weapon injuries were reported. From this information the assertion is often made that "all forms of the martial arts are safe." A review of some of the injuries of the martial arts will show that this information may not necessarily be true.

TYPES OF MARTIAL ARTS

The two most common martial arts that are practiced in the United States are karate (meaning "the way of the empty hand") and tae kwon do (meaning "foot, hand, way"). Tae kwon do is an exhibition sport in the Olympics and has been since 1988, and it appears that it will become an official Olympics sport in the year 2000. Other martial arts are aikido ("the way of harmony"), jujitsu ("compliance techniques"), judo ("compliant way"), and kung fu ("skill, art," a form of Chinese self-defense art, like karate). Hapkido is a Korean martial art that is very similar to aikido (Japanese) that includes kicks and hand strikes.

L. A. Wilkerson: Cigna HealthCare of Tennessee, Memphis, Tennessee 38119.

In our society people seem to gravitate to the martial arts for various reasons. There is an increased desire to know self-defense, while others join to improve cardiovascular fitness, flexibility, and improved self-esteem. Some join for structured exercise program, whereas others want the artistic expression or have a need to compete.

INJURY TRENDS IN MARTIAL ARTS

To understand better the injury trends in tae kwon do tournaments, consider that each round lasts 2 minutes. The fighter might fight a new opponent in a single or double elimination or might fight three 2-minute rounds in a single elimination. Karate usually has 3-minute rounds and, like tae kwon do, can be either single elimination or three 3-minute rounds. In both tournaments kicks to the head are allowed, as well as to the trunk, but not to the back. Punches to the head are prohibited in tae kwon do, although in some karate tournaments, contact to the head with the hands is allowed, but it is supposed to be controlled. Tournaments are otherwise full-contact. In tae kwon do chest protectors are worn, shin and full-arm pads, foot pads, and a groin guard, as well as a head protector. Optional are a mouthguard and hand covers. In karate there is usually no chest protector, but shin and forearm pads are worn. Optional are foot pads, and a groin protector is worn. Gloves are prohibited in some tournaments. It has been found that wearing protective gear will decrease morbidity. Protective gear is available for the forearms, hands, chest, shins, and feet. Wearing a mouthpiece and a groin protector is strongly recommended, and in tae kwon do head protection is worn, which will be discussed in more detail in the coming pages. The injury rate per 100,000 participants in various sports is listed in Table 44-1 (2).

Injuries have been found to be of a higher incidence in the tournament situation. McLatchie and colleagues

TABLE 44-1. *Injury rate per 100,000 participants of various sports*

Sport	Rate	Sport	Rate
Basketball	188.0	Wrestling	26.0
Football	167.0	Sledding	24.6
Aquatic activities	46.0	Dancing	18.8
Lacrosse	39.5	Martial arts	16.9

From Birrer RB, Halbrook SP. Martial arts injuries. *Am J Sports Med* 1988;16:408–410, with permission.

(3) reported that some form of injury occurs an average of once in every four contests, with incapacitating injury severe enough to cause withdrawal from competition occurring once in every tenth contests. Bierer and Bierer surveyed 6347 athletes, finding that 59% of injuries were sustained in tournament settings and 41% in nontournament settings. They also found that injury rate and experience are inversely proportional (1,4,5). This is confirmed by Stricevic and colleagues (6), who reported that punches have a higher injury ratio than do kicks and that protective gear for hands, head, chest, and limbs decreased the morbidity. Injuries are classified into three groups: injuries to the head and face, injuries to the trunk, and injuries to the limbs. In all studies (1–4,7) the most common injuries were contusions, bruises, sprains, and strains. Orthopedic injuries result from direct impact, repetitive action, or ballistic and torsional maneuvers. Serious injuries seen are concussions, paralysis, and visceral rupture (5). Table 44-2 lists injuries at two national tae kwon do tournaments broken down by site of injury, as listed above. Table 44-3 is a summary of the injuries by anatomic site reported as percentages.

HEAD INJURIES

Common injuries to the head and neck appear to be lacerations, epistaxis from a nose blow, and periorbital hematomata, which can occur from an accidental strike in the face, usually with a fist or from a high kick. There have been cases of corneal abrasion as a result of a scratch from a toenail or brushing by the eye with the toes. Concussion is seen more commonly from a high kick or a spinning kick. If the athlete is knocked out, it is important to consider a possible cervical spine injury. Cervical spine injuries commonly are overlooked because associated head injuries and loss of consciousness seem to absorb all the attention. McLatchie (8) reports a fatality from a spinning hook kick to the face. The victim was immediately incapacitated, fell backward onto a hard wood floor, and died within 24 hours at a local hospital. Postmortem examination revealed an occipital skull fracture, bilateral acute subdural hematomata, contusions of the frontal and temporal lobes, and hemorrhage and herniation of the brainstem. A back-

TABLE 44-2. *List of injuries at two national tae kwon do tournaments*

Site of injury	Adult	Junior
Head and neck		
Hematoma, contusion	9	17
Laceration	6	7
Mandible, TMJ strain, R/O fracture	3	10
Epistaxis, R/O fracture	4	6
Concussion without LOC	0	8
Neck strain, R/O fracture	1	6
Nasal fracture/dislocation	3	1
Loss of consciousness	3	1
Teeth avulsion	0	2
Corneal abrasion	0	1
Diplopia, R/O orbital fracture	0	1
Totals	29	60
Upper extremity		
Digit, hand strain, R/O fracture	5	8
Metacarpal fracture	2	3
Digit fracture/dislocation	2	0
Nail avulsion	0	2
Forearm contusion	0	1
Totals	9	14
Lower extremity		
Foot contusion	1	2
Digit sprain, R/O fracture	1	2
Contusion, hematoma	6	2
Knee contusion/synovitis	0	2
Knee strain	1	0
Shin hematoma	0	1
Ankle strain	1	0
Foreign body	1	0
Digit fracture	0	1
Laceration	0	1
Totals	11	11
Groin		
Contusion, hematoma	2	5
Adductor strain	0	2
Totals	2	7
Torso		
Abdominal contusion	0	1
Solar plexus concussion	0	2
Costochondral separation	1	0
Low back spasm	0	1
Lumbosacral contusion, R/O fracture	0	1
Spinal cord contusion, R/O fracture	0	1
Totals	1	6
Other		
Panic reaction	0	3
Insulin reaction	0	1
Totals	0	4
Totals, all injuries	52	102
Grand total: 154		

From Oler M, Tomson W, Pepe H, et al. Morbidity and mortality in the martial arts: a warning. *J Trauma* 1991;31(2):251–253, with permission.

TABLE 44-3. *Summary of injuries by anatomic site (reported as percentages)*

	Percentage of adult presentations ($n = 47$)	Percentage of junior presentations ($n = 91$)	Combined presentations ($n = 138$)
Head and neck	49	54	52
Upper extremity	21	14	17
Lower extremity	23	13	17
Groin	4	8	6
Torso	2	7	5
Other (systemic)	0	4	3
Totals	99 (rounding error)	100	100

From Oler M, Tomson W, Pepe H, et al. Morbidity and mortality in the martial arts: a warning. *J Trauma* 1991;31(2):251–253, with permission.

spinning kick or back hook kick cannot necessarily be thrown with control because if it is thrown too slowly, the opponent will kick the other opponent possibly in the back, and if it is thrown with proper speed, it cannot be controlled to decrease the impact. In central Florida, masters tournaments have disallowed the back hook and back-spinning kicks to the head because of a potential injury and allow front leg kicks to the head, such as a round kick, only in controlled fashion. This change markedly decreases the chance of serious injury.

How protective is headgear in the martial arts? Headgear prevents most soft tissue injuries to the face, that is, lacerations, abrasions, and soft tissue injuries to the ear or scalp. Unfortunately, headgear is not as protective to the brain as many believe in the martial arts. There now seems to be a movement in the United States toward mandatory headgear. Rhulen Insurance Company of New York, one of the largest insurers of the martial arts in the United States, has informed its policyholders that headgear is now required if insurance is to be in force during free-sparring. Because of this, mandatory headgear has now reached the tournament circles and many schools and associations. From this movement, instructors and students are led to believe that they are protected and that they can prevent serious head injuries, but this is not the case.

Studies from neurosurgical literature (9–12) have compared peak acceleration of blows to the head, with and without headgear, using punches both to the front and the side of the head. These punches were with bare hand, safety-chuck hand protectors, and 10-ounce boxing gloves. Kicks also were delivered to the head, with and without headgear, using bare feet and safety-kick padding. These studies showed that for bare karate-style equipment, punches to the side of the head produced greater peak accelerations than kicks to the front and side. Kicks produced greater acceleration than did punches to the front side of the head. Safety equipment for hands or feet failed to soften or lessen peak accelerations with or without headgear. The subjects in the study perceived that safety equipment for hands or feet was protection for the wearer rather than for the opponent.

Unequivocal evidence exists that repeated brain injury of concussive or even subconcussive force results in characteristic patterns of brain damage and a steady decline in the ability to process information efficiently (13). Furthermore, the effects of repeated blows to the head, whether punch or kick, are cumulative; although some blows may be more severe than others, none is trivial, and each has the potential to be lethal. Blunt head blows cause shearing injury to nerve fibers and neurons in proportion to the degree to which the head is accelerated, and these acceleration forces are impacted to the brain. Blows to the side of the head tend to produce greater acceleration forces than those to the face, whereas those to the chin (which acts as a lever) produce maximal forces (10,13). Shearing of blood vessels may lead to bleeding within the brain and skull, creating a subdural hematoma, or bleeding within the brain, which can produce intracerebral hematoma with rapid death. Headgear and protective padding to the hands and feet may lessen the force of brain acceleration, which seems to decrease the chance of a fatal bleed but increases nerve fiber shearing. Thus extra padding may reduce the chances of death, but it will not prevent brain damage due to tearing of brain substance.

Punch-drunk syndrome—or, more appropriately, dementia pugilistica—is a traumatic encephalopathy that may occur in anyone who is subjected to repeated blows to the head from any cause (10). It has also been recognized in football players, rugby players, soccer players, and wrestlers. The characteristic symptoms and signs include the slow onset of an increasingly euphoric personality; the person cries easily and has little insight into his or her deterioration. Speech and thought become progressively slower. Memory deteriorates considerably. There may be mood swings, intense irritability, and sometimes truculence leading to violent behavior.

Cheerfulness is the commonest prevailing mood, however, with bouts of depression. Also tremor and difficulty in speaking are common.

INJURY TO EXTREMITIES

Injuries to the extremities are numerous and include strains, sprains, fractures, dislocations, and tendon avulsions. The most common injury is hematoma to the forearm, thigh, shin, calf, and dorsum of the foot. In tournament situations in which kicking is below the belt, hematoma to the quadriceps often will cause the competitor to retire from competition. Dislocation of the proximal interphalangeal joints occurs when punches are poorly executed. Laceration of the fingers occurs from scratches if gloves are not worn (2,6). A common question asked is, Do karate and tae kwon do experts have increased incidence of osteoarthritis in their hands? This problem was studied in the United Kingdom (5), where karate is an established sport. The hands and wrists of 22 karate instructors who had practiced the sport for a minimum of 5 years were examined and X-rayed. There was no evidence that practice of the sport predisposed to the early onset of chronic tenosynovitis or osteoarthritis. Four activities seemed to have the greatest potential for damage (5): doing push-ups on the knuckles, repeated punching of a firm target, sparring, and breaking objects. The metacarpal phalangeal joint may have a chronic synovitis from the wood-breaking techniques. In the hand, avulsion of the extensor tendons of the distal fingers or dislocation of the proximal interphalangeal joints can also occur from hitting hard objects using a "spear finger" technique.

Elbow dislocations have been seen, mostly posterior. Supracondylar and intracondylar humeral fractures are rare but can occur. Tendinitis of medial/lateral humeral epicondyles is common. In the shoulder, 95% of dislocations are anterior, with 5% posterior. Acromioclavicular sprain is seen if a fall or roll is inaccurately executed. The knee is vulnerable in most sports. In the martial arts, especially karate and tae kwon do, in which the ballistic and twisting moves are the rule, injury is usually from hyperextension, rotation, flexion, valgus, or varus clipping. Injuries vary from meniscal and ligament injuries, patellar tendinitis, patellar subluxation or dislocation, and femoral epiphyseal fracture to Osgood-Schlatter disease. Knee dislocation is very rare and a true emergency. Hematoma can occur in any of the extremities, and is the most common injury, as previously stated, with the quadriceps the most common site. In all studies (3,6,7,14) contestants had to stop fighting secondary to the pain. A late complication of hematoma is myositis ossificans. Ankle sprain and fractures are seen, just as in any contact or collision sport. Injuries to the great toe, second toe, and fifth toe is common and may lead to osteoarthritis in later years.

INJURIES OF THE TRUNK

Injuries of the trunk are common in the martial arts. Many martial artists aim at the region of the solar plexus surrounding the coeliac ganglion. This blow causes the classic winding of the opponent, leaving him or her vulnerable for further attack. A blow to the solar plexus produces transient inspiratory difficulty with spontaneous recovery in 20–40 seconds. In tae kwon do, chest protectors are worn to disperse the penetration of the blow. Tae kwon do practitioners kick 80% of the time, as opposed to punching. In karate, however, chest protectors are not worn. Karate instructors believe that they decrease the student's ability to control the blow and thus decrease the discipline. Damage to the chest is usually by direct kick or punch. Costochondritis, rib fracture, and even pneumothorax have been seen. There have been three reported cases of death from anterior chest trauma from these types of blows. The roundhouse kick, also called round kick, to the trunk can damage the vulnerable liver, spleen, kidney, and pancreas. Testicular injury usually occurs from an uncontrolled kick and many times will cause the forced retirement of the competitor. Groin guards markedly decrease this risk. Although there can be some pain, usually the competitor can continue to fight after a time out. The most common trunk injuries therefore are to the ribs, mainly from punches; the solar plexus, which are from kicks or punches and have the potential to cause pancreatitis; and the testes.

Some deaths have occurred from the martial arts. In one case a spinning kick hit an opponent in the face, knocking him out, and on hitting the floor he expired. Three cases of deaths from anterior chest trauma have been reported (3):

1. A 26-year-old Caucasian male (Korean tae kwon do stylist) was practicing kumite (free-sparring) with his instructor when he received a kick to the left lower lateral aspect of the anterior chest (Fig. 44–1). The patient was seen in the emergency room with fixed dilated pupils and had an isoelectric electrocardiogram, apnea, and cyanosis with bruise marks on the left anterior chest. External cardiac compression and endotracheal manual ventilation were performed. Administration of intracardiac adrenaline resulted in ventricular fibrillation, which subsequently converted to a ventricular tachycardia. In view of the prolonged dilation of the pupils, rescue efforts were stopped, and the patient was pronounced dead. Gross anatomic diagnosis revealed pulmonary edema and congestion, liver ecchymosis, rib fracture (fifth left), and aspirated food within the trachea, hypopharynx, and lungs. At autopsy the suggested cause of

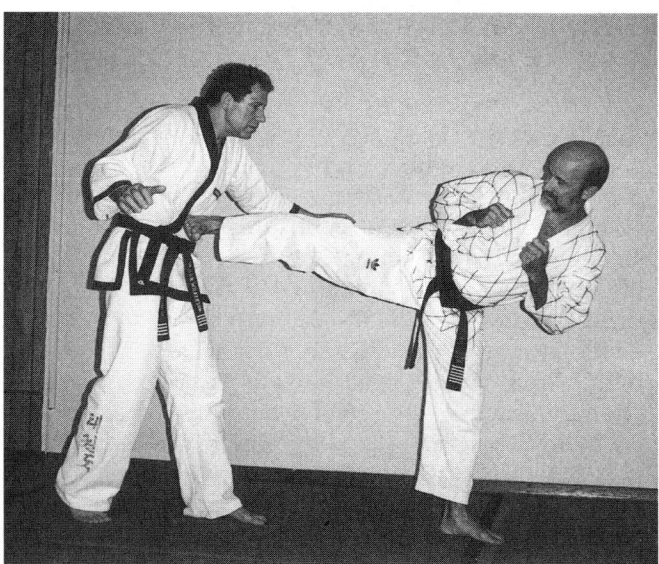

FIG. 44–1. Side kick to left lower lateral aspect of the anterior chest (case study no. 1).

death was aspiration and asphyxia secondary to the blow to the chest.

2. An 18-year-old Caucasian male (kempo stylist) was participating in his fifth bout of a competitive free-sparring tournament when he received a blow or multiple blows to the midsection (Fig. 44–2) that apparently ruptured his spleen. Later that evening the patient began to vomit and was in severe pain. He was transported to a hospital, where he was admitted with an admission diagnosis of a ruptured spleen. An exploratory laparotomy and splenectomy were subsequently performed. However, the patient expired within 1 hour after surgery. Gross and microscopic examination of the heart, liver, and spleen showed that the epicardium was normal, and the coronary vessels showed no lesions. Moderate numbers of myelocytes, occasional collections of lymphocytes, and a few polymorphonuclear cells were present in the interstitial tissue. Considerable numbers of atypical lymphocytes with moderately large nuclei and varying amounts of cytoplasm were found in the sinusoids and portal areas. A microscopic diagnosis of infectious mononucleosis involving the heart, liver, and spleen was determined from the examination.

3. An 18-year-old black male (Korean tae kwon do stylist) was practicing kumite with an advanced student when he received light contact from a roundhouse kick to the solar plexus (Fig. 44–3). The instructor and another student administered external cardiac compression and mouth-to-mouth resuscitation. Although ambulance attendants continued resuscitative efforts, the patient was pronounced dead on arrival at a local hospital. Autopsy examination revealed the following gross anatomic diagnoses: hemorrhage into the soft tissue around the carotid sinus and vagus nerve at the level of the bifurcation of the innominate artery, multiple areas of ecchymosis in the liver, multiple petechial hemorrhages of all lobes of the lungs, hyperinflation of both lungs, and aspiration bronchitis.

All three of the fatally injured people had been training for less than one year. Free-sparring training should be only for students who have undergone a period of adequate physical conditioning and have demonstrated competence in the basic free-sparring techniques.

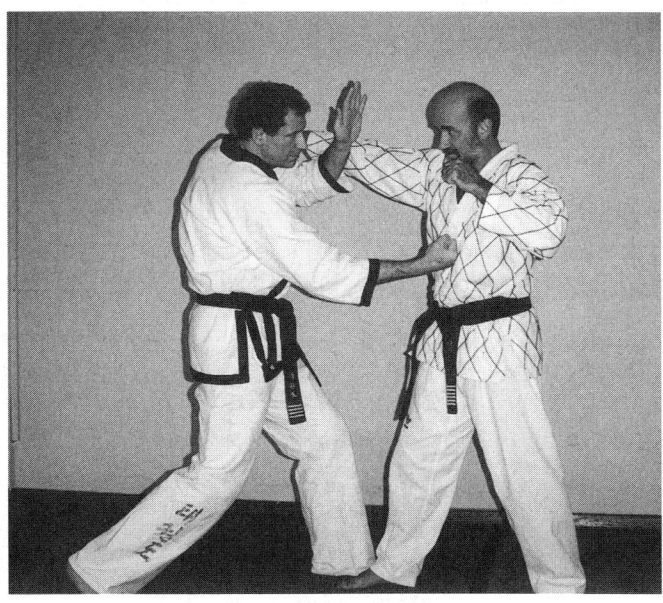

FIG. 44–2. Multiple blows to midsection (case study no. 2).

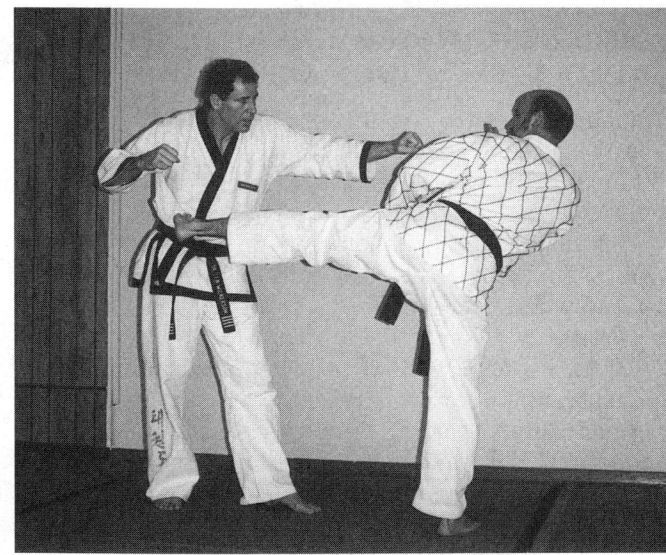

FIG. 44–3. Roundhouse kick to the solar plexus (case study no. 3).

COMMON MEDICAL DISORDERS SEEN IN PARTICIPANTS OF THE MARTIAL ARTS

Studies have shown that a regular exercise program may have a beneficial effect on seizure control. There are no reports of status epilepticus triggered by exercise. It is a difficult decision for physicians, parents, and the martial arts instructor to give permission to the participant. Reservations are based on the following concerns (15):

1. Would a seizure during practice or tournament predispose the athlete to a serious injury, particularly the brain or spinal cord? Most data to date do not support this (15).
2. Would single or cumulative head blow adversely affect seizure control or cause an immediate or early posttraumatic seizure? To date reports suggest that this should not be a concern; however, because of inherent dangers, kicking or punching to the head should be excluded (15).
3. The Committee on Children with Handicaps and Sports Medicine of the American Medical Association recommends that children be allowed to participate in physical education and interscholastic activities, including contact and collision sports, provided that there are (a) proper medical management, good seizure control, and proper supervision and (b) avoidance of situations in which a dangerous fall could occur.

On the basis of the aforecited studies and data, athletes with a seizure disorder may participate. However, when they are ready to participate in sparring, head contact is not allowed. Contact to the trunk (chest and abdomen) must be limited, and a chest protector must be worn.

DISORDERS THAT WOULD DISQUALIFY AN ATHLETE FROM THE MARTIAL ARTS

Standard American Medical Association guidelines on participation in strenuous contact of collision sports should be followed. Of note, athletes with a skin infection such as boils, herpes, impetigo, and scabies should be disqualified until the condition is no longer contagious. Acute illnesses need individual evaluation so as not to worsen the illness or put others at risk at being in contact with a contagious individual.

If the participant wants to do the martial arts for self-defense, fitness, or flexibility, without ever participating in full-contact sparring, then some of the disqualifying conditions merit individual assessment, allowing some individuals to train only in a noncontact environment.

THE PHYSICIAN'S RESPONSIBILITY AT A KARATE OR TAE KWON DO COMPETITION

Among the physician's duties at a martial arts competition is the examination of the competitors before the competition on request by officials. Many times the officials will not make such a request. The physician is to administer first aid, while circulating on the floor during simultaneous sparring matches, which could be in any multiplication of rings going on at the same time. The fighting area should be inspected to ascertain that adequate flooring is used. The physician treats any minor injuries that are received, such as lacerations, strains, and sprains. It is best to refer serious injuries to a hospital. When requested, the physician advises the referees as to the fitness of a competitor to continue in a competition.

Some of the injuries that would exclude further participation are fractures; concussions that result in disorientation and amnesia, certainly if there is any loss of consciousness; ocular injuries when sight is impaired, including periorbital injuries (i.e., hematoma and lacerations); and certain cases of testicular injury when recovery is not rapid, and scrotal hematoma is present (3,8).

REFERENCES

1. Oler M, Tomson W, Pepe H, et al. Morbidity and mortality in the martial arts: a warning. *J Trauma* 1991;31:251–253.
2. Birrer RB, Halbrook SP. Martial arts injuries: the results of a five-year national survey. *Am J Sports Med* 1988;16:408–410.
3. McLatchie GR, Davies JE, Caulley JH. Injuries in karate: a case for medical control. *J Trauma* 1980;20(11):956–958.
4. Birrer RB, Birrer CD, Son DS, et al. Injuries in TaeKwon-Do. *Phys Sportsmed* 1981;9(2):97–103.
5. Crosby AC. The hands of karate experts: clinical and radiological findings. *Br J Sports Med* 1985;19:41–42.
6. Stricevic MV, Patel MR, Okazaki T, et al. Karate: historical perspective and injuries sustained in national and international tournament competitions. *Am J Sports Med* 1983;11:320–324.
7. Birrer RB, Birrer CD. Martial arts injuries. *Phys Sportsmed* 1982;10(6):103–108.
8. McLatchie GR. Analysis of karate injuries sustained in 295 contests. *Injury* 1976;8:132–134.
9. *Preparticipation physical evaluation.* Joint publication of American Academy of Family Physicians, American Academy of Pediatrics, American Medical Society of Sports Medicine, American Osteopathic Academy of Sports Medicine, American Orthopaedic Society for Sports Medicine, 1992.
10. Adams WM, Bruton CJ. The cerebral vasculature in dementia puglistica. *J Neurol Neurosurg Psychiatry* 1989;52:600–604.
11. Corsellis J, Brutan CJ, Freeman-Brouse D. The aftermath of boxing. *Psychol Med* 1975;3:270–303.
12. Martland HS. Punch-drunk. *JAMA* 1928;19:41–42.
13. Schwartz ML, Hudson AR, Fernie GR, et al. Biomechanical study of full-contact karate contrasted with boxing. *J Neurosurg* 1986;64:248–252.
14. McLatchie GR. Karate and karate injuries. *Br J Sports Med* 1981;15:84–86.
15. Mellion MD, Walsh WM, Shelton GL, eds. *The team physician's handbook.* Philadelphia: Hanley & Belfus, 1990.

CHAPTER 45

Oar Sports

Jo A. Hannafin and Timothy M. Hosea

Rowing is one of the original sports of the modern Olympiad and has continued to expand in popularity over the last 20 years. Rowing was introduced as Olympic event for heavyweight men in 1900 and for heavyweight women in 1976 and was expanded to include participation by lightweight men and women in the 1996 Olympic Games in Atlanta. Participation in the sport of rowing is traditionally thought to be limited to athletes in private high schools and colleges; however, this is no longer the case. Rowing programs now exist across the United States for high school, college, and masters athletes, mirroring the increased interest and opportunities for competition on local, national, and international levels.

The majority of injuries that occur in the sport of rowing are overuse injuries. Abrupt alterations in training level, alterations in technique or type of boat rowed, and the increasing volume of training being undertaken by national and international athletes contribute to these overload injuries. To best understand and treat these injuries, a thorough understanding of the sport is essential.

Oarsmen and oarswomen can be characterized by the types of boats they row (Fig. 45–1), the use of a single oar (sweep rowing) or two oars (sculling), and the weight class in which they participate. In international competition lightweight male rowers average 72.5 kg, and lightweight female rowers average 59 kg, while heavyweight men and women average 92 kg and 79 kg, respectively. In sweep rowing, each athlete uses a single oar that enters the water on the port or starboard side of the boat (Fig. 45–2); in sculling, each athlete uses two oars. Rowing is an unusual sport in that the athletes do not face the finish line, but sit "backwards" in the boat. The athlete sits on a sliding seat facing the stern of the boat with the feet anchored in sneakers attached to the foot stretcher. The athlete begins at the finish, with the legs fully extended and the oar or sculls at waist height. The recovery or slide phase begins with movement of the hands away from the body toward the stern of the boat, followed by forward flexion at the hip. The legs slowly begin to bend until a compressed position of approximately 120–130 degrees of knee flexion is reached. During the recovery phase, potential energy is stored in the legs, back, and arms in preparation for the drive phase of the stroke, which is explosive in nature. During the drive phase the oars enter the water at the catch, followed by leg and back extension to propel the boat through the water during the drive (Fig. 45–3). In sweep rowing, there is considerable trunk rotation during the catch and early drive phases of the rowing stroke in addition to the compressive loads demonstrated in the spine in both sweep and sculling. The forces generated during the phases of the rowing stroke are concentrated in different regions of the arms, chest, back, and legs.

Myoelectric analysis has demonstrated that at the catch, the rectus femoris and thoracic paraspinal muscles fire nearly simultaneously, initiating the drive phase of the stroke. As the knees and hips extend during the drive, the gluteus maximus and hamstrings fire, controlling the drive and stabilizing the pelvis. The power generated by the legs is transferred through the back and shoulders to the oar. The back acts as a braced cantilever and provides an additional source of power by extending. This is demonstrated by the marked increase in L3 paraspinal activity shortly after the catch which is maintained through the drive phase of the stroke, reflecting the corresponding increase in the lumbar loads (Fig. 45–4).

The force that is generated by the back and legs is then transmitted to the oar through the shoulders, which are stabilized by the latissimus dorsi and serratus anterior. With peak acceleration of the oar at middrive, these muscles function maximally and in unison. During the latter part of the drive, the rectus femoris continues to fire, keeping the knees extended as the arms pull the

---

J. A. Hannafin and T. M. Hosea: Orthopaedic Surgery and Sports Medicine, Hospital for Special Surgery, New York, New York 10021.

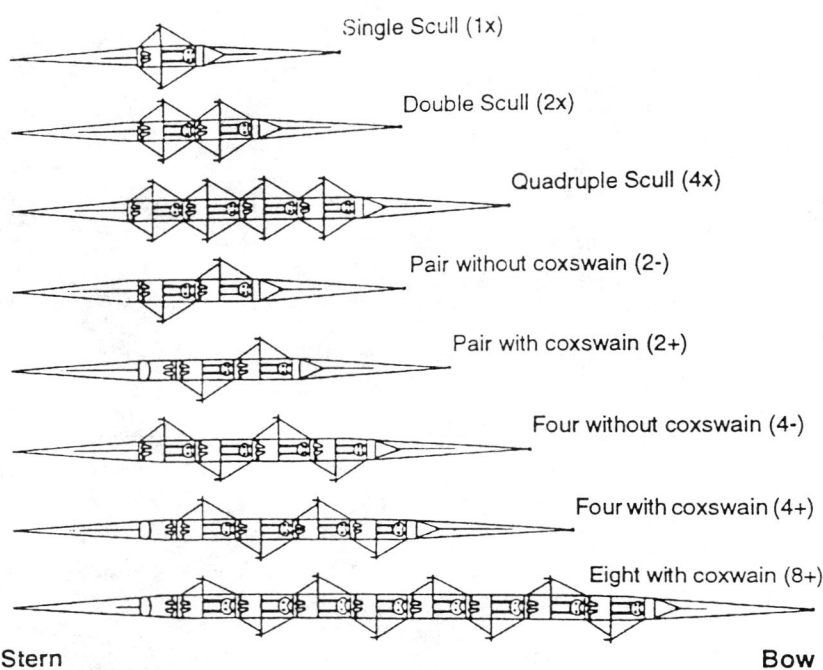

FIG. 45-1. The variety of sculling and sweep boats that are rowed for recreation and competition. Sweep rowers use a single oar; scullers use two smaller oars.

oar into the body. At the finish, the aforementioned major muscle groups generate minimal activity. The rectus abdominis and external oblique fire to stabilize and flex the trunk, which is now in extension. During the recovery there is little or no activity of the paraspinal musculature. The compressive load on the lumbar spine is balanced by the anterior musculature and the posterior passive restraints. The medial hamstrings fire submaximally to flex the knee and initiate the movement of the seat up the slide. Detailed discussions on oar sports can be found in Chapters 47 and 54 of the companion volume in this series, *Exercise and Sport Science*.

ROWING INJURIES

Injuries in rowing occur most frequently in the knee, lower back, rib cage, shoulder, and upper extremity and are seen during periods of intense training and racing (1). When an athlete presents with an injury, it is therefore critical to ascertain a description of recent training, to determine whether the injury occurred during sweep or sculling, and to determine whether the injury can be related to on-water training, ergometer training, weight lifting or cross-training (running, stadiums, cross-country skiing). It is also important to review the mechanics of the rowing stroke and to elicit symptoms that may be referable to specific phases of the rowing stroke.

The preparticipation exam should evaluate the range of motion, strength, and flexibility necessary for participation in sweep rowing or sculling, while evaluation of an acute or overuse injury will be more specific and focused on the region in question. It is important to evaluate the joints that are proximal and distal to the site of injury because of the complexity of the rowing stroke and interrelationship of the arms and trunk, trunk and back, and back and legs. It is often helpful to simulate rowing technique on an ergometer to determine whether a correctable biomechanical abnormality is contributing to the injury being evaluated.

The treatment of specific injuries has been outlined elsewhere and will not be discussed in detail in this section. However, alterations in training or technique that are specific to the sport of rowing will be reviewed in the treatment of specific injuries. When injuries occur as part of ergometer or on-water training, it may be necessary to decrease the intensity or duration of training. In mild injuries it is generally possible to continue to train with a decreased work load or duration of exercise while applying principles of stretching, strengthening, ice, and nonsteroidal antiinflammatory drugs (NSAIDs). It may also be possible to modify the equipment being used by the athlete to diminish the load, to alter the functional range of motion, or to modify the stress seen by the athlete. The load necessary to drive the oar through the water can be modified by changing the length or stiffness of the oar or by alteration of the inboard/outboard ratio. The height and position (toe in versus toe out) of the foot stretchers can be modified to decrease or increase knee flexion angles and to modify tibial rotation. Exposure to rotational stresses on the lumbar or thoracic spine can theoretically be modified by changing the sweep rower from port to starboard; however, this is less often a practical consideration, as athletes may have a natural predilection for rowing on

OAR SPORTS / 533

stop training in the face of injury; therefore the principles of active rest and cross-training are critical in successful treatment of these athletes. It is equally important to educate the athlete and to provide viable alternatives for training to allow rapid resolution of symptoms and return to sport.

Back

Low back pain is a common complaint in the rowing population. Howell's study of elite lightweight female rowers revealed an 82.2% incidence of low back pain compared to an age- and sex-matched incidence in the general population of 20–30% (2). Stallard stated, "Backache is suffered by almost all those in serious rowing training nowadays" (3). Our review of two intercollegiate programs revealed the lower back as the second most common area injured (1).

Kinetic and myoelectric analysis of the lower lumbar spine reveals significant loading of the lumbar spine with each stroke. The back functions as a braced cantilever during the rowing stroke and is a major contributor to the generation of the total linear velocity of the oar. These forces are similar with sculling and ergometer rowing (4). Sweep rowing adds a torsional and lateral bending stress to the shear and compression components of the sculling stroke. At the catch there is a rapid generation of force at the oar. This force accelerates to a peak near the middrive and tapers to the finish. This pattern is similar for both men and women. The anterior shear load at the L3–4 segment mirrors the resistance applied to the oar (Figs. 45–5, 45–6). The peak of the anterior shear load affecting the L3–4 motion segment averaged 848 N for the males and 717 N for the women. These are essentially the same for both sexes when normalized for body weight.

The trunk moves from approximately 30 degrees of flexion at the catch to 28 degrees of extension at the finish. While both sexes finished the rowing stroke with

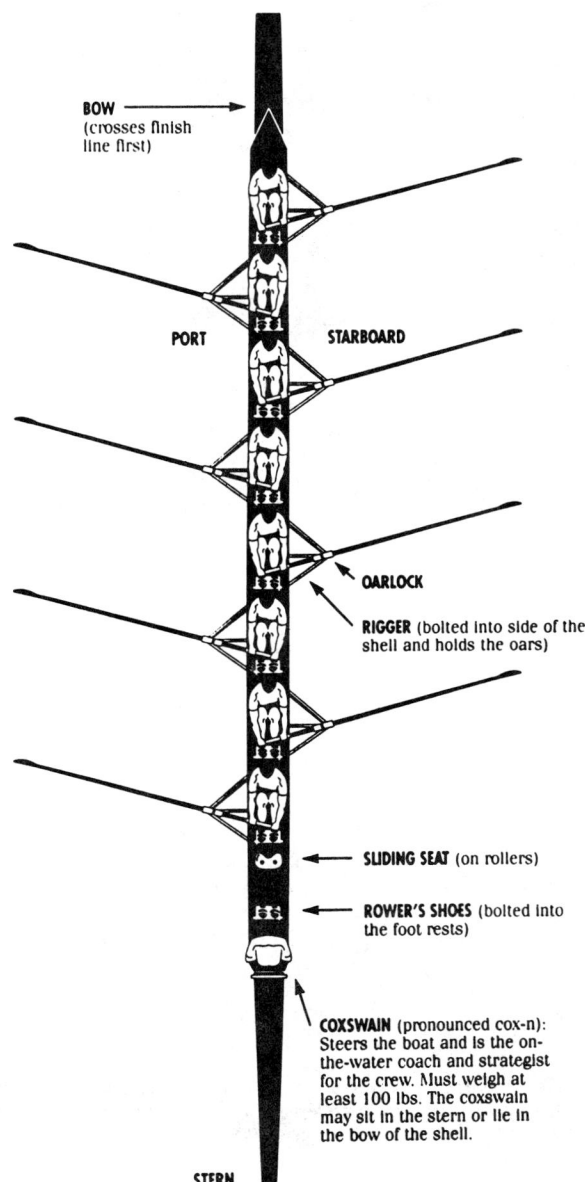

FIG. 45–2. A diagrammatic representation of an eight-oared shell. The bow crosses the finish line first. (Adapted with the permission of U.S. Rowing.)

either the starboard or port side. If these modifications are not successful, it may be necessary to discontinue on-water training if the symptoms fail to improve or worsen with continued training. It is necessary to discontinue ergometer or on-water training for more severe injuries, including disc disease and stress fractures of the ribs, as continuation of training will not allow healing and resolution of symptoms. It is important for the physician to recognize that this is a group of athletes who routinely experience the pain associated with lactate overload to compete successfully. It is virtually impossible to advise a competitive oarsman or oarswoman to

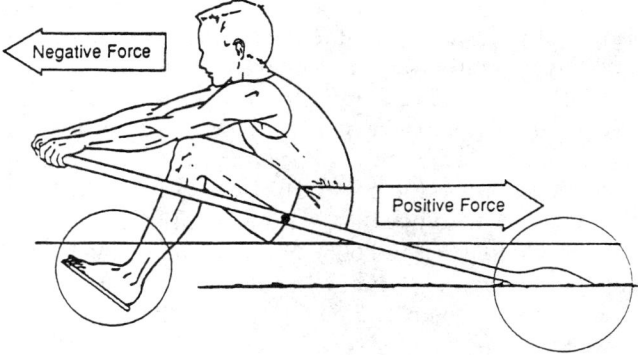

FIG. 45–3. The athlete pictured has initiated the drive phase of the rowing stroke and is accelerating the oar through the water using the arms, back, and thighs.

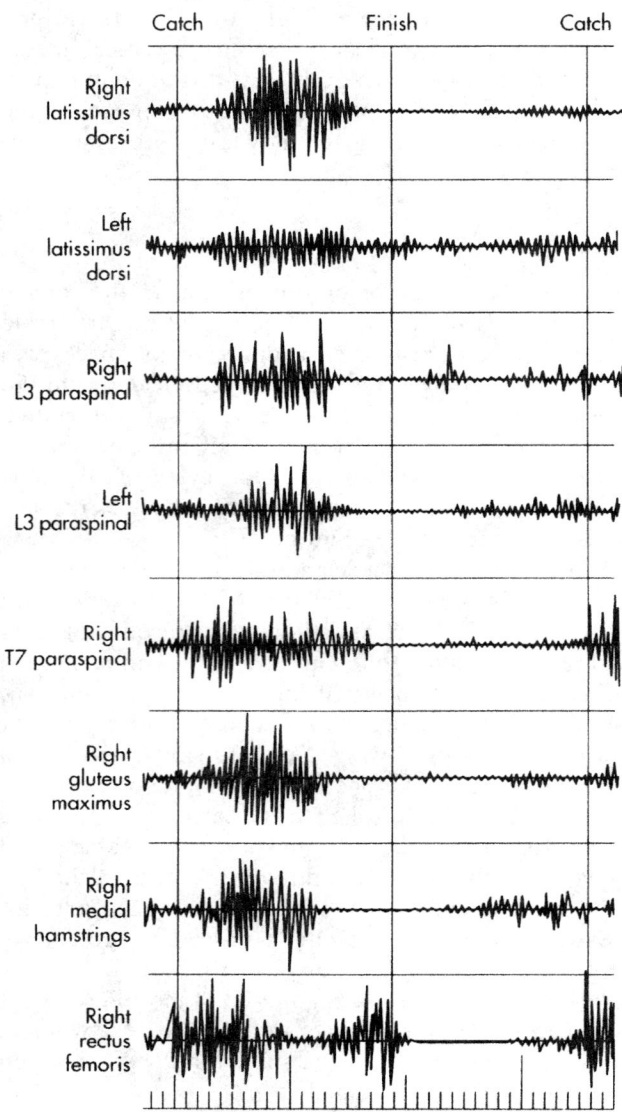

FIG. 45-4. EMG activity during the rowing stroke. The activity of the lumbar paraspinal muscles increases as the shear load of the lumbar spine increases, to a peak in the middrive phase of the rowing stroke.

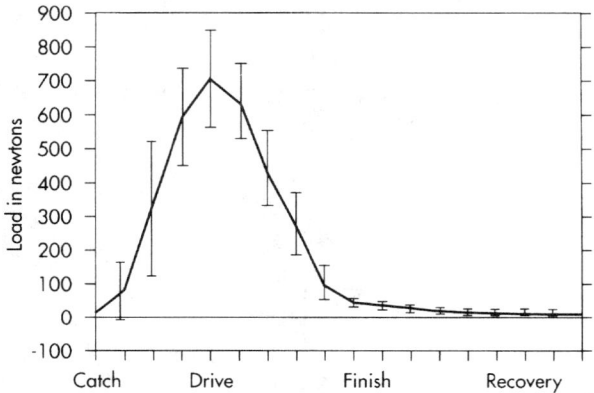

FIG. 45-5. The anterior shear loading pattern of the L3-4 motion segment of the lumbar spine during the rowing stroke. This demonstrates the rapid increase following the catch, to a peak at the middrive followed by a tapering to the finish.

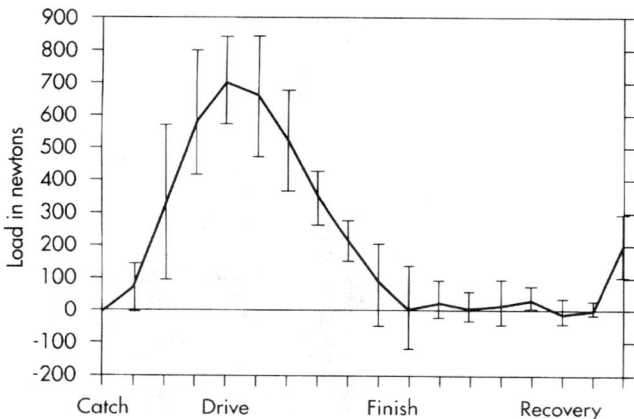

FIG. 45-6. The load generated at the oar during the rowing stroke as measured by a strain gauge. The rapid acceleration is related to the leg drive that peaks at middrive.

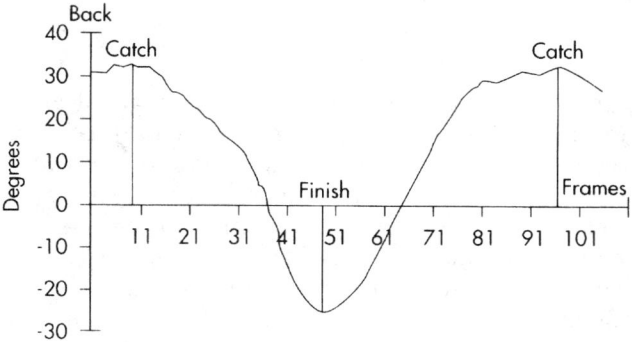

FIG. 45-7. A typical example of the trunk motion during a rowing stroke, with approximately 30 degrees of flexion at the catch and smooth progression to extension at the finish and return to the flexed position at the catch.

essentially the same amount of extension, the men demonstrate a greater flexion angle of the trunk at the catch (Fig. 45-7). Compression of the L3-4 motion segment averaged 3919 N for the men and 3330 N for the women. The peak compression load occurs in the latter part of the drive phase as the upper torso passes over the pelvis into the extended position. At this point the peak compression load averaged 6066 N for the men and 5031 N for the women, or, when normalized for body weight, 7 times for the men and 6.85 times for the women.

The mechanics of the rowing stroke with its repetitive, cyclical, and intense loading of the lumbar spine explain the increased incidence of lumbar spine injuries in the rowing population. The loads generated with the rowing stroke are similar to those that have been shown to produce pathologic changes in cadaveric specimens. While the spinal motion segment is well suited to resist compression, as the disc degenerates and loses its shock-absorbing capability it becomes susceptible to injury and also transfers significant load to the facets and posterior structures. The facets are well oriented to resist shear forces and, when combined with compression, resist half to one third of the corresponding shear force, with the intervertebral disc resisting the balance. The peak shear loads in the rowing stroke averaged 848 N for the men and 717 N for the women, or greater than the peak shear loads of 570 ± 190 N which produced fractures of the pars interarticularis in cadaveric specimens (5). Thus the rowing stroke puts considerable pressure on the posterior elements of the spine, which may result in bony injury of the lumbar spine.

Although the rowing stroke subjects the lumbar motion to significant mechanical loads, it is important to consider all etiologies of the lower back pain in the differential diagnosis (Table 45–1). Back pain in the rowing population can be described as mechanical (lumbar strains or muscular spasms), discogenic, spondylogenic, or, in the master rower, related to facet arthropathy.

Mechanical lower back pain is generally localized to the lumbar area. It is associated with significant muscle spasm and may begin gradually with episodic exacerbation. Quite often, especially in the adolescent or collegiate rower, this ill-defined low back pain and spasm without radicular symptoms signal early disc degeneration or herniation. This pain is generally exacerbated by activity and relieved by rest and NSAIDs. Prevention must include a comprehensive trunk strengthening program, use of proper rowing technique, and thorough warm-up and stretching before the workout.

Discogenic back pain refers to disorders of the intervertebral disc, which result in nerve root irritation and sciatica. However in the older rower, facet arthropathy may also cause sciatica. A herniated nucleus pulposis most commonly occurs in the third decade. Often a "snap" or "pop" will be felt in the lumbar region with associated lower back pain. Within 24–48 hours, leg pain develops with an appropriate dermatome specific physical findings (Table 45–2). A herniated disc typically occurs in the lower lumbar motion segments. A L3–4 herniation produces a L4 radiculopathy with pain radiating into the posterior lateral thigh across the patella and anteromedial leg. Weakness of the quadriceps and, in chronic cases, atrophy are present. The knee deep tendon reflex is diminished, and the sensation is diminished over the anteromedial thigh. The L4–5 motion segment affects the L5 nerve root with associated pain radiating down the posterolateral thigh and anterolateral leg. Weakness of the extensor hallux longus and anterior tibialis may be present. A L5–S1 herniation affects the S1 nerve root. This results in pain radiating down the posterolateral aspect of the thigh and leg, decreased sensation along the lateral heel and foot, weakness of planter flexion with associated atrophy of the soleus and gastrocnemius, and a decrease in, or absence of, the ankle deep tendon reflex.

Treatment for discogenic low back pain includes cessation of rowing, active rest as tolerated, local modal-

TABLE 45–1. *Etiologic factors in low back pain*

I. Congenital disorders
  A. Facet tropism (asymmetry)
  B. Transitional vertebra
    1. Sacralization of lumbar vertebra
    2. Lumbarization of sacral vertebra
II. Tumors
  A. Benign
    1. Tumors involving nerve roots or meninges (e.g., neurinoma, hemangioma, meningioma)
    2. Tumors involving vertebrae (e.g., osteoid osteoma, Paget's disease, osteoblastoma)
  B. Malignant
    1. Primary bone tumors (e.g., multiple myeloma)
    2. Primary neural tumors
    3. Secondary tumors (e.g., metastases from breast, prostate, kidney, lung, thyroid)
III. Trauma
  A. Lumbar strain
    1. Acute
    2. Chronic
  B. Compression fracture
    1. Fracture of vertebral body
    2. Fracture of transverse process
  C. Subluxated facet joint (facet syndrome)
  D. Spondylolysis and spondylolisthesis
IV. Toxicity
  A. Heavy metal poisoning (e.g., radium)
V. Metabolic disorders (e.g., osteoporosis)
VI. Inflammatory diseases (e.g., rheumatoid arthritis, ankylosing spondylitis)
VII. Degenerative disorders (e.g., spondylosis, osteoarthritis, herniated disc, herniated nucleus pulposus, spinal stenosis—nerve root entrapment syndrome)
VIII. Infections
  A. Acute (e.g., pyogenic disc space infections)
  B. Chronic (e.g., tuberculosis, chronic osteomyelitis, fungal infection)
IX. Circulatory disorders (e.g., abdominal aortic aneurysm)
X. Mechanical causes
  A. Intrinsic (e.g., poor muscle tone, chronic postural strain, myofascial pain, unstable vertebrae)
  B. Extrinsic (e.g., uterine fibroids, pelvic tumors or infections, hip diseases, prostate disease, sacroiliac joint infections and sprains, untreated lumbar scoliosis)
XI. Psychoneurotic problems (e.g., hysteria, malingering, compensatory low back pain—"green poultice" syndrome)

From Keim HA, Kirkaldy-Willis WH: Low back pain. Clin Symp 1980;32(6):8. Copyright © 1980 CIBA-GEIGY Corporation, all rights reserved; with permission.

TABLE 45-2. *Clinical features of herniated lumbar discs*

L3-4 disc; L4 nerve root

Pain	Lower back hip, posterolateral thigh, across patella, anteromedial aspect of leg
Numbness	Anteromedial thigh and knee
Weakness	Knee extension
Atrophy	Quadriceps
Reflexes	Knee jerk diminished

L4-5 disc; L5 nerve root

Pain	Sacroiliac region, hip, posterolateral thigh, anterolateral leg
Numbness	Lateral leg, first webspace
Weakness	Dorsiflexion of great toe and foot
Atrophy	Minimal anterior calf
Reflexes	None, or absent posterior tibial tendon reflex

L5-S1 disc; S1 nerve root

Pain	Sacroiliac region, hip, posterolateral thigh/leg
Numbness	Back of calf; lateral heel, foot, and toe
Weakness	Pantarflexion of foot and great toe
Atrophy	Gastrocnemius and soleus
Reflexes	Ankle jerk diminished or absent

From Boden SD, Wiesel SW, Laws ER, et al. *The aging spine.* Philadelphia, WB Saunders, 1991.

ities, NSAIDs, and on occasion antispasmodic medication. Patients with a documented neurologic deficit should be followed very closely. If there is no resolution or improvement of the deficit, or if radicular pain persists after 14 days of treatment, further work-up is indicated.

Lumbar spine radiographs are obtained to rule out other pathology such as spondylolysis, infection, tumor, segmental instability, or fracture. The next diagnostic modality for discogenic low back pain is magnetic resonance imaging (MRI), which is an excellent means for imaging disc pathology, although a false positive rate of 22% has been reported (6). However, the "gold standard" for defining the lumbar spinal canal pathology is the myelogram in conjunction with a metrizamide computed tomography (CT) scan.

In general, individuals with a disc herniation do well with conservative management. Once the acute symptoms have subsided and the pain and neurologic symptoms have largely resolved, a comprehensive rehabilitation begins, starting with hamstring and lumbosacral stretching exercises associated with instruction in body mechanics, progressing to William's flexion and abdominal strengthening exercises. McKenzie lumbar extension exercises are an essential component of the rehabilitation of disc herniation. In those individuals with a persistent, symptomatic lumbar radiculopathy, epidural cortisone injections may be warranted (7). However, if the neurologic deficit persists or progresses despite conservative management, and if it correlates with the objective findings on physical examination as well as diagnostic studies, surgical intervention may be indicated. For individuals with persistent radicular and lower back symptoms but no clearly defined neurologic deficits and negative diagnostic studies, continued conservative management is indicated. Surgical intervention is never indicated in the absence of a clear-cut anatomic lesion.

Spondylolysis is a defect of the pars interarticularis and in most cases represents a stress-type injury caused by repetitive loading of the lumbar spine. The rower usually presents complaining of lower back pain, generally without sciatica. This pain is localized over the pars, lateral to the midline, and is exacerbated by hyperextension of the lumbar spine. There are no neurologic deficits. Radiographs should include the lumbar posterior oblique view, which optimizes identification of the pars defect. Often when radiographs are inconclusive, a single-photon emission computed tomography bone scan will provide a sensitive tool for visualizing the defect (8).

Symptomatic individuals should follow a comprehensive back program with an emphasis on lower extremity and trunk stretching as well as strengthening. While the person is symptomatic, rowing should be avoided. For individuals with resistant symptoms and a positive bone scan, bracing may be helpful.

Facet joint arthropathy is the result of aging and minor trauma. Rowers with degenerative facet changes initially complain of vague back pain without radicular symptoms. As the process develops, the pain is described as deep, dull, and aching. It may be referred to the lumbosacral region, buttocks and upper thighs. It is generally exacerbated by ambulation and relieved by sitting.

Physical examination may reveal a loss of normal lumbar lordosis with a decreased lumbar range of motion. Significant paraspinal spasm may be present, and pain is elicited by palpation over the affected facet joints. The neurologic examination reflects the level of the motion segment involvement with associated nerve root compression. However, if the facet hypertrophy is extensive, the nerve root exiting one level below may be involved, thus presenting a complex clinical picture. Imaging studies, including radiographs, CT scan, MRI, and myelogram with a metrizamide CT scan will be helpful in defining the pathology. Limitation of activity, NSAIDs, and a lumbar support will generally provide relief. With cessation of symptoms, a trunk and hamstring stretching and strengthening program should be instituted.

Low back pain in the rowing population is common and directly related to loads placed on the lumbar spine while participating in this activity. Management includes accurate diagnosis and appropriate management with an emphasis on maintaining the aerobic performance of the rower while rehabilitating the lower back injury.

Ribs and Thorax

Pain associated with the rib cage is a common complaint in the rowing population. The vast majority of these injuries are rib stress fractures. Studies of collegiate rowing programs and the Canadian national rowing team revealed that rib stress fractures make up approximately 10% of all rowing injuries (8,9). Stress fractures of the ribs have been associated with throwing (10,11), golfing (12), rowing (13,14), canoeing (15), and swimming (16). While the vast majority of rib stress fractures reported in the literature involve the first rib, the ribs primarily affected in rowers are the fifth through ninth.

Biomechanical analysis of the ribs predicts that the greatest bending moments occur at the middle third of the rib in its posterior lateral segment. This is the site of the majority of fractures in the rowing population. It has been proposed that the opposing actions of the serratus anterior and the external oblique muscles are the major contributors to the development of the stress fracture (17). The serratus anterior muscle originates at the medial border of the scapula and inserts into the anterolateral aspect of the first through ninth ribs (Fig. 45–8). It interdigitates with the origin of the external oblique muscle on the fifth through ninth ribs. By using wire electrodes, the serratus anterior muscle was found to fire maximally at the catch phase of the rowing stroke. This activity continued through the drive phase of the

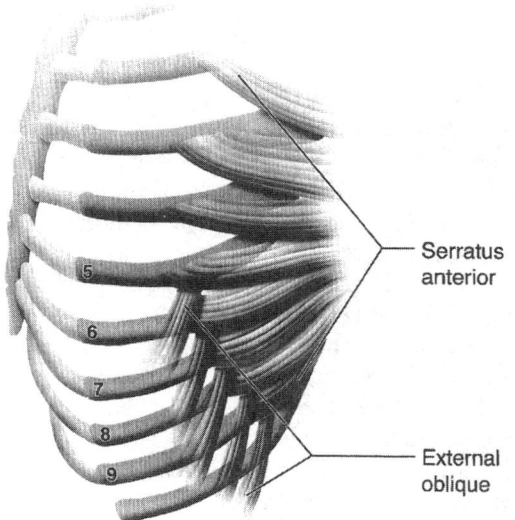

FIG. 45–8. Diagram of the anatomy of the serratus anterior and external oblique muscles showing the interdigitation of these muscles on the fifth to ninth rib. (From Karlson KA. Rib stress fractures in elite rowers. *Am J Sports Med* 1998; 26(4):516.)

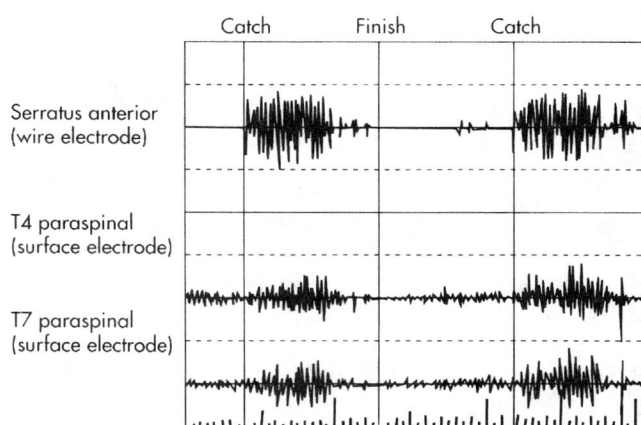

FIG. 45–9. EMG activity of the serratus anterior and thoracic musculature during the rowing stroke. The activity of the serratus anterior is maximal during the drive phase, corresponding to the stabilization of the scapula allowing the transfer of power to the oar.

stroke and "turned off" at the finish (Fig. 45–9). The activity of this muscle stabilizes the scapula, allowing transfer of the power generated by the legs to be transmitted to the oar.

The external oblique muscle has been found to increase the lateral segment bend of the rib by pulling it inward and downward. It is assumed to fire maximally at the finish of the rowing stroke when the shoulders are behind the hips and the scapulae are fully retracted, with the serratus anterior muscle firing eccentrically (18). The opposing action of these two muscles results in a repetitive bending force on the middle segment of the rib. With intense training and increasing loads, this on-and-off firing pattern results in a fatigue mode of stress loading and may result in a rib stress fracture.

Rib stress fractures generally occur during periods of intense training, with a relatively low stroke rate and a high load per stroke. This generally occurs during the fall and winter training when the rowers spend a lot of time doing long steady-state rows on the water and spend a significant length of time on the rowing ergometer. As with stress fractures in other locations, the rib stress fracture generally presents with a vague ill-defined thoracic discomfort before progressing to an obviously painful stress fracture. Recognizing the insidious onset and changing the rib stress patterns at that time may prevent the onset of the acute stress fracture. The stress fracture presents with sharp, stabbing pain that is exacerbated by coughing, deep breathing, and changing position. It has been accompanied by winging of the scapula. The pain is generally discretely localized over the affected rib in the posterior lateral corner, and radiates to the anterior axillary line. Pain is also reproduced with thoracic compression as well as stressing the serratus anterior muscle on the affected side.

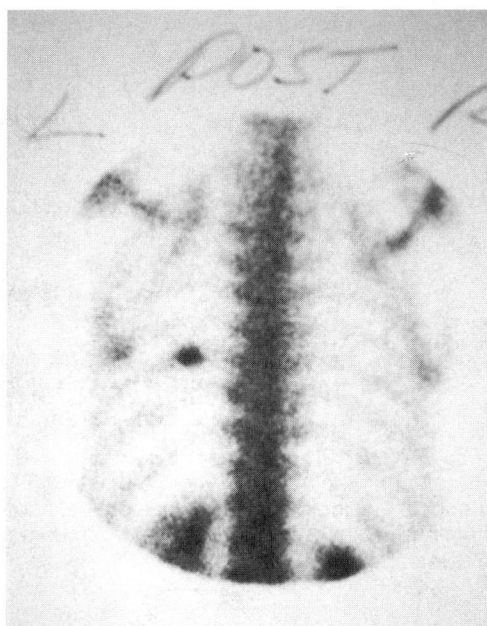

FIG. 45–10. Bone scan of a rib stress fracture.

Diagnosis is confirmed by a bone scan that identifies the increased uptake in the rib (Fig. 45–10). Occasionally, the acute stress fracture may be seen in routine radiographs, but generally, the radiographs become positive late in the healing process when the fracture callus becomes visible. We have seen one case of a hypertrophic nonunion following an unrecognized stress fracture (Fig. 45–11). Rib stress fractures generally heal within 6–8 weeks. With the onset of symptoms the rower should cease all activities until he or she is comfortable with activities of daily living. This generally takes 5–7 days. At this point the rower continues to avoid rowing activities and begins cross-training to maintain aerobic fitness, using devices such as the bicycle ergometer and stairmaster machines. Running and impact-loading activities tend to exacerbate the discomfort and are to be avoided during the early healing period. As the fracture heals and the rower becomes less symptomatic, training on the rowing ergometer is allowed, with minimal resistance and at a relatively high stroke rate. The rower then progresses with slowly increasing resistance and lowering stroke rate as tolerated until able to resume normal training activities.

Symptomatic relief is provided with analgesics and NSAIDs. The use of a TENS unit has been helpful on occasion, while rib belts have not been helpful in our experience. It is currently recommended that exercises such as push-ups and pull-ups that stress the rib cage and strengthen the scapular stabilizers be instituted to prevent this injury.

Shoulder and Upper Extremity

Impingement syndrome is a common injury in oarsmen and oarswomen. Development of subacromial impingement can be related to training errors, poor technique, and asymmetry of the strength and flexibility of the shoulder and periscapular musculature or can be secondary, resulting from excessive glenohumeral laxity.

Technical errors that may predispose the rower to development of impingement syndrome include overreaching at the catch to achieve increased stroke length and "shooting the tail," which involves rapid acceleration of the legs without appropriate coupling of the back and shoulder musculature. Overreaching at the catch involves increased glenohumeral forward flexion, coupled with excessive scapular protraction, which, when coupled with a tight posterior capsule, results in anterior-superior translation of the humeral head that may predispose to development of subacromial impingement. Excessive strength training of the deltoid, pectoralis, and subscapularis without concomitant strengthening of the teres, infraspinatus, supraspinatus, rhomboids, serratus, and trapezius during land-based training may also be provocative. Treatment of impingement syndrome includes the short-term use of NSAIDs, ice, physical therapy to include attention to abnormalities in capsular flexibility, and a well-designed strengthening and conditioning program that is designed to treat the specific deficits noted on physical exam, including the rotator cuff, serratus, rhomboids, latissimus, and middle trapezius. Symptomatic glenohumeral subluxation can frequently be controlled with appropriate strength training and technique modification; however, surgical stabilization may be necessary in more extreme cases. Modification of the height of the rigger and alteration of the

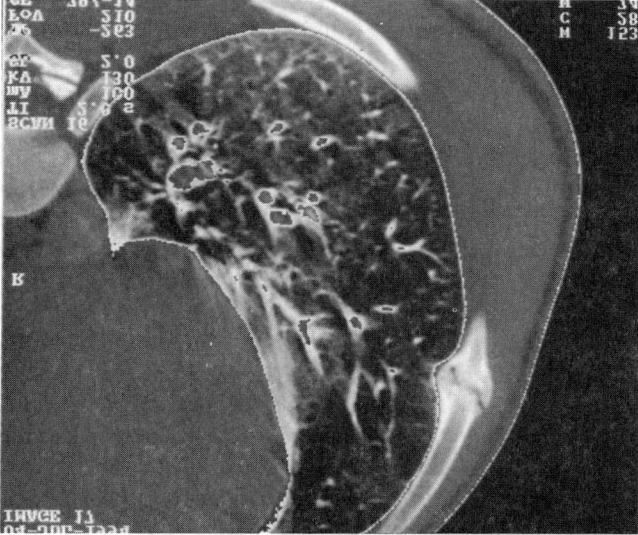

FIG. 45–11. CT scan of a hypertrophic nonunion in a 20-year-old intercollegiate male rower.

inboard/outboard ratio of the oar may be helpful in allowing the athlete to continue to train and compete. The athlete should be evaluated by the coach or trainer to diminish technique errors, including overreaching at the catch, excessive scapular protraction, and loss of the obligatory linkage between arms, back, and legs resulting in shooting the tail.

Elbow and Wrist

Medial epicondylitis is more common in scullers and athletes training extensively on the rowing ergometer and is related to a premature break in the extended elbow during the drive, resulting in compensatory hyperflexion of the wrist and overload of the flexor-pronator origin. Lateral epicondylitis is seen more commonly in sweep rowing, particularly involving the inside hand, which undergoes repetitive dorsiflexion to feather the oar at the end of each stroke (Figs. 45–12A, 45–12B). This injury can also be related to the size of the oar handle, placing the female athlete with a smaller grip size at increased risk. Recent advances have been made in the form of exchangeable oar handles of varying size and grip surface design, permitting the athletes to customize their oars. These injuries have thus become less common in the elite athlete but continue to be seen in collegiate, club, and masters rowers secondary to training errors or equipment misfit. Treatment of epicondylitis in the rower follows the same principles as treatment in other athletes, including the use of NSAIDs; physical therapy modalities, including iontophoresis or phonophoresis; improvement of the strength, endurance, and flexibility of the forearm musculature; and correction of training errors. The use of injectable corticosteroids is not advocated in this population.

Extensor tenosynovitis was first described in a group of elite oarsmen by Williams (19) but occurs with equal frequency in men and women. Extensor tenosynovitis, also known as crossover tendinitis, involves the area of crossover of the abductor pollicis brevis and the extensor pollicis brevis. This overuse injury presents with pain and crepitus, and symptoms can be reproduced by repetitive wrist dorsiflexion. Treatment consists of ice, functional wrist splinting, iontophoresis or phonophoresis, and technique modification. Adaptive splinting may be used to allow that athlete to continue to train but must be carefully designed and padded to avoid skin breakdown. Corticosteroid injection may be helpful for the athlete who does not respond to initial conservative treatment. Surgical intervention has been reported but is infrequently needed (19). It is not often necessary to remove the athlete from on-water training if appropriate splinting and technique modification are undertaken.

Knee

The sport of rowing places extremely high loads on the patellofemoral joint secondary to the repetitive flexion-extension of the knee that occurs during on-water and ergometer training as well as land based training which may involve hill running, Olympic-style lifting, and plyometric training for the lower extremities. Compressive patellofemoral pain and lateral facet syndrome may present following transition to winter land training or following resumption of on-water speed work in the early spring. Iliotibial band friction syndrome is most commonly observed during the fall season, wherein distance or endurance training predominate, but can also be seen with any significant increase in training intensity. Genu valgum, femoral anteversion, and external tibial torsion may predispose to patellofemoral pain, whereas genu varum may predispose to the development of iliotibial band friction syndrome. Evaluation of the strength and flexibility of the hamstrings, quadriceps, and hip flexors should be performed and focal strength or flexibility deficits addressed. Hamstring flexibility plays a critical role setting the appropriate body angle during the recovery phase, which is critical in subsequent application of power and appropriate body linkages during the drive phase of the stroke. Treatment of anterior knee pain in the rower is directed toward correction of abnormal patterns of muscle weakness or inflexibility. To reach this goal, it may be necessary to temporarily modify training with a decrease in hill running, stair climbing, open chain knee extension exercises, and plyometric training until symptoms resolve. Patellar bracing

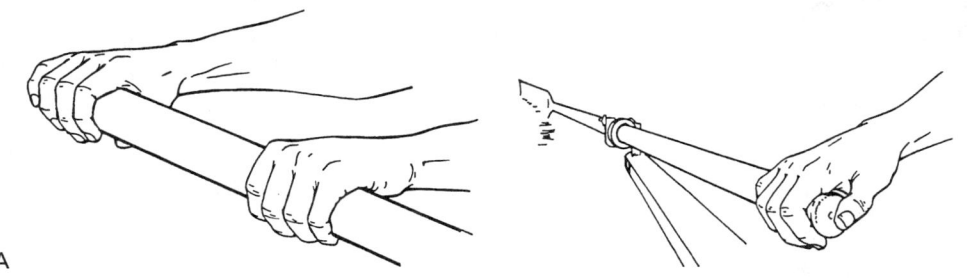

FIG. 45–12. A: The sweep grip is demonstrated here. Repetitive wrist dorsiflexion at the end of the rowing stroke may result in the development of lateral epicondylitis and crossover tendinitis. **B**: The sculling grip is demonstrated here.

or taping may provide short term assistance in the treatment of lateral facet syndrome particularly in athletes with patellar hypermobility. Modifications in the foot stretcher can be made to alter patellofemoral mechanics: A decrease in knee flexion angle at the catch can be achieved by raising the height of the foot stretcher, whereas functional knee varus or valgus can be modified by alteration of the toe in or toe out of the sneakers. Front or back stops can be placed on the track of the sliding seat in the boat or on the ergometer to limit the arc of knee flexion and extension.

MEDICAL CONDITIONS IN ROWERS

Exercise-Induced Bronchospasm

Exercise-induced bronchospasm (EIB) is seen in 15–20% of elite oarsmen and oarswomen; the incidence in high school, collegiate, and masters rowers is unknown. There is no known influence of gender on the development of EIB, and the treatment of EIB in rowers is similar to the treatment in other athletes. Environmental factors may play an increased role in the rower, however, as rapid changes in temperature can occur while the athlete is on the water. In addition, these athletes often train and compete at a significant distance from medical personnel and must therefore be well educated in the preventive use of inhaled medication and in early recognition of symptoms. Inhaled beta-2-agonists such as albuterol are permissible in international rowing competition but must be registered in advance of competition.

Dermatologic Concerns Specific to the Rower

The most common sites of dermatologic problems are the hands, calves, and buttocks. The development of blisters on the palms and palmar surface of the fingers is common in athletes who are new to the sport of rowing. Significant callosities will subsequently develop in response to training. If these callosities become hypertrophic, blisters will develop deep to the callus and can result in a localized skin slough. Athletes must be reminded to maintain optimal thickness of the callus with the use of a pumice stone. Acute blisters should be allowed to resolve spontaneously and should be padded or taped to allow continued training. The prophylactic use of hand taping has not been shown to be beneficial and may promote blister formation at the tape edges. Gloves are not generally used, as the proprioceptive sense of oar position in the hand is critical in fine control of the oar.

Track bite is a focal loss of skin in the area where the calves contact the tip of the track on which the seat glides. These soft tissue erosions can easily become infected and are treated with aggressive local care and padding of the point of contact. Skin ulcerations can also occur on the buttocks in the gluteal crease secondary to repetitive chafing during the rowing stroke. The design of some rowing ergometer seats also results in local chafing with the transition to endurance style winter training on the ergometer. Careful attention to personal hygiene and early treatment of focal skin irritation is successful in treatment of these skin conditions. Local application of Vaseline or ointment to the area of potential chafing may prevent the development of these painful sores.

REFERENCES

1. Hosea TM, Boland AL, et al. Rowing injuries. *Postgrad Adv Sports Med* 1989;3:1.
2. Howell D. Musculoskeletal profile and incidence of musculoskeletal injuries in lightweight female rowers. *Am J Sports Med* 1984; 2:278.
3. Stallard MC. Backache in oarsman. *Br J Sports Med* 1980;14:105.
4. Lamb DH. A kinematic comparison of ergometer and on water rowing. *Am J Sports Med* 1989;17:367.
5. Cryon BM, Hutton WC. The fatigue strength of the lumbar neural arch in spondylosis. *J Bone Joint Surg* 1978;60B:234.
6. Boden SD, Davis DO. Abnormal lumbar spine MRI scans in asymptomatic subjects: a prospective investigation. *J Bone Joint Surg* 1990;72A:403.
7. Jackson DW, Retting A, Wiltse LL. Epidural cortisone injections in the young athletic adult. *Am J Sports Med* 1980;8:239.
8. Collier BD, Johnson RP, et al. Painful spondylosis or spondylolisthesis studies by radiography and single-photon emission computerized tomography. *Radiography* 1985;154:207.
9. Bachus R. Personal communication, 1996.
10. Curran DB, Kelly DA. Stress fracture of the first rib. *Am J Orthop* 1966;8:16.
11. Gurtler R, Pavlov H, Torg JS. Stress fracture of the ipselateral first rib in a pitcher. *Am J Sports Med* 1985;13:277.
12. Lord MJ, Ha KI, et al. Stress fracture of the ribs in golfers. *Am J Sports Med* 1996;24:118.
13. Holden D, Jackson D. Stress fractures of the ribs in female rowers. *Am J Sports Med* 1985;13(5):342.
14. Brukner P, Khan K. Stress fracture of the neck of the seventh and eighth ribs: a case report. *Clin J Sports Med* 1996;6:204–206.
15. Maffuli N, Pintore E. Stress fracture of the sixth rib in a canoeist. *Br J Sports Med* 1990;24:247.
16. Taimela S, Kajala UM, et al. Two consecutive rib stress fractures in a female competitive swimmer. *Clin J Sports Med* 1995;5:254.
17. Karlson K. Rib stress fractures in elite rowers: a case series and proposed mechanism. *Am J Sports Med* 1998;26(4):515–519.
18. Mier A. Action of the abdominal muscles on the rib cage in humans. *J Appl Physiol* 1985;58:1438.
19. Williams J. Surgical management of traumatic non-infective tenosynovitis of the wrist extensors. *J Bone Joint Surg* 59B:408, 1977.

CHAPTER 46

Running

Karl B. Fields and Steven G. Reece

INTRODUCTION

Running boomed in popularity as a sport in the United States in the 1970s. Numerous influences contributed to this, foremost being Kenneth Cooper's book *Aerobics*, which prescribed a simplified system for attaining physical fitness that relied heavily on aerobic sports, specifically running. Shortly after the publication of *Aerobics*, Frank Shorter won the Olympic marathon in 1972. This victory captured the imagination of Americans and triggered a dramatic increase in the number of marathons held throughout the country. Another influential work published in 1977 was James Fixx's *The Complete Book of Running*, a practical how-to guide for novices to the sport.

Although enthusiasm for running has waned, the running movement has not died. Studies suggest that 40–50 million Americans run at least 2–3 days per week for fitness. The popularity of running has continued for many reasons, the principal one being health benefits. Runners consistently score high in overall assessments of general health. Now newer studies demonstrate that physical fitness level best predicts longevity, showing specifically that people who are in very good to excellent health have a reduced risk of death from cardiovascular disease and cancer. In addition, for most individuals running is the fastest way to reach and maintain a high fitness level.

For years the medical establishment discouraged running because of the potential risks. Perhaps the myth that was perpetuated the most was that running led to degenerative joint disease. Greater knowledge of sports medicine and better data about cardiovascular benefits have changed the negative impression that many physicians historically held toward running. Studies assessing runners compared to inactive counterparts indicate that runners do not face an increased risk of degenerative joint disease and, in fact, have lower levels of overall musculoskeletal disability.

While health benefits draw many people to running, injury problems sidetrack many others. Prospective analysis suggests that approximately 40–60% of runners have a significant injury each year. Patterns and frequency of injury differ and depend on age, experience, physical characteristics, and type of running, that is, competitive track and field athletes, cross-country racers, recreational road racers, and people who run purely for fitness. For example, high school level women's cross-country has a high injury rate, with as many as 60% of the individuals injured for up to 5 days during a cross-country season. This is in contrast to jogging 2 miles three times a week for recreation, where the stress threshold is low enough that injury would be quite uncommon. For this reason, injury risk needs to be assessed on the basis of the individual athlete and the type of running he or she wishes to pursue.

TRAINING SCHEDULE OF RUNNERS

Excessive or improper training can be linked at least temporally to most running injuries. The physician who is evaluating a runner needs to ask about training to decide whether this is a factor. Few runners would trust a physician who does not establish his or her credibility by demonstrating some knowledge of the type of training that a runner pursues. A basic concept of training is that the athlete must gradually but progressively stress the biological system to improve. Unfortunately, a thin line exists between overtraining and maximal training, so overuse injuries predominate as the major risk for runners.

A key concept of a successful training program is

K. B. Fields: Family Practice Center, Greensboro, North Carolina 27401.

S. G. Reece: Family Practice Specialists, Richmond, Virginia 23235-4730.

periodization: the division of training into different phases. For example, runners who want to succeed at racing a distance of 1 mile or longer must establish a baseline of endurance strength. Typically, the runner might divide training into 3 months of slower, long runs to establish overall endurance and strength. A second period, also lasting 3 months, would emphasize a combination of strength training and steadily increasing speed work that approaches the race pace for the event in which he or she plans to participate. A final, shorter phase, approximately 1–2 months, would emphasize running at faster than race pace with less total volume of training. The greater speed and intensity of this final phase helps the runner to reach a peak performance.

Another aspect of training is the progressive increase in total work. Training overload allows the body to become accustomed to running different distances. For example, even an elite class 10-kilometer runner in excellent condition would hesitate to enter a marathon without having done a number of runs longer than 2 hours to get accustomed to the type of stress that is encountered over a 26-mile distance. Training overload leads to performance improvement and adaptation of the musculoskeletal system. Whether the performance improvements arise secondary to circulatory changes, enzymatic or chemical inducements, or even adaptations of the nervous system remains a topic of investigation of numerous exercise physiology studies. However, one key concept has emerged: Increased distance must be achieved slowly to avoid injury.

Training needs to be tailored to the type of event. Logically, the training for a 1500-meter race differs dramatically from preparation for a marathon race. Running rapidly around a track requires muscle groups to adapt for high-velocity turns. By contrast, running a cross-country course may require runners to become very comfortable with uneven surfaces and numerous hills.

Several common workouts, however, are incorporated in the training schedules of most competitive runners regardless of the specific event. The first of these is the interval workout, in which the runner completes a specific distance repetitively at an approximate pace. The rest period between each repetition remains fixed. The runner typically will limit the number of repetitions the basis of his or her ability to stay close to 90% of the chosen pace for the entire workout. These workouts can vary by recovery or by pace to maximally stress the VO_2 max system or to mix the training stress between aerobic and anaerobic metabolism. Fartlek or "speed play" is a variant on the theme of interval training in which the runner uses bursts of speed that are unmeasured and untimed. This helps the runner gauge effort by feel not the watch. Other aspects of speed training include techniques such as hurdling, starting, or running turns.

For distance runners a second type of workout is a tempo run. This run totals 18–20 minutes, usually at a slightly slower pace than the runner's best 10-kilometer racing pace. The idea behind tempo runs is to condition runners to tolerate a race pace. One of the physiologic considerations is whether this will allow runners to increase what is termed the lactate threshold. In other words, runners can exercise longer without by-products of muscle metabolism limiting their performance. These workouts differ from what are termed maximal pace workouts, which are designed to be shorter and to emphasize a running rate that is faster than that typically used in a race. The maximal pace workouts generally are used in the final phase of sharpening for race performance.

For runners who race distances of 10 kilometers or more, long, slower distance runs become an important part of training. These runs primarily stress the slow twitch (aerobic) muscle fibers and result in an athlete who can endure long workouts without excessive fatigue. Muscle cell adaptation and enzyme induction may be two of the physiologic changes that occur with this training. In addition, runners doing longer mileage or more intense high-quality workouts need to incorporate planned recovery runs. These represent easy efforts at a pace of no more than 50% of maximum and no more than 10–15% of the runner's total weekly running mileage.

In taking a history from a runner, a key feature of determining whether the individual's training is flawed is to review the specific workouts. Runners with too frequent interval workouts, tempo runs, or long-distance runs may be excessively stressing their system and be expected to break down with injury. In addition, some runners never use recovery runs and therefore may underperform or be unable to recover from minor injuries, regardless of their total mileage.

ETIOLOGY OF RUNNING INJURIES

A number of factors have been identified as etiologic variables in running injury. The most prominent of these is training error, with absolute mileage being the best predictor of who becomes injured. Runners who consistently log more than 40 miles per week have higher injury rates. Runners who consistently run 7 days per week without a rest day are injured more than those who take periodic rest days. Other factors, such as intensity of workouts or specific changes in training schedule, seem likely to increase injury risk, but less evidence exists for their association. Also, a competitive orientation appears to play a factor as elite runners and highly competitive runners have significant rates of the more serious injuries.

A second etiologic factor for running injuries is the anatomic makeup of the individual. A prospective association of most anatomic variants with running injury remains elusive. Cowan (1) did demonstrate a strong association of arch height with lower extremity injury in a group of soldiers. In that study, individuals with a soft tissue arch height greater than 3.14 cm had a markedly elevated risk of lower extremity injury, whereas those with a flattened arch actually had a lower risk of injury. Other studies have looked at enlarged Q-angles (quadriceps tracking angles) as a factor in development of patellofemoral stress syndrome (PFSS). Evaluations of genu valgum, genu varum, genu recurvatum, and other rotational abnormalities of lower extremities have not conclusively shown an association with higher injury rates. Leg length inequality has been cited in a number of studies that were retrospective reviews of injured runners. However, prospective studies to date have not demonstrated this as a predictor of running injury. At best, the research linking running injury to anatomic makeup has led to mixed results, and studies have not determined the degree of significance of any anatomic factor.

Functional running form errors receive most of the blame for running injury in the lay press. The primary error that has been noted is excessive pronation of the hindfoot or midfoot. Most clinicians evaluate this before giving recommendations for treatment. In addition, a number of running shoes purport to provide motion control, and studies of orthotic devices demonstrate the ability of these to lessen the degree of pronation. Nevertheless, studies confirming excessive pronation as a key factor in running injury remain quite limited.

Extrinsic factors at one time were given much of the blame for running injuries. These generally related to inadequate shoe support or using the wrong type of shoe. However, over the last two decades the emergence of numerous shoe options for every runner, regardless of anatomic makeup, gender, or size, has lessened the number of individuals with poor footwear. However, without question, the wrong shoe may cause certain individuals to alter their running form in such a way that injury would seem more likely. The shift over the last two decades in the frequency pattern of stress fractures to the tibia rather than the metatarsals may suggest that shoes, while providing adequate protection for the foot, transfer the force higher up the lower extremity. Other extrinsic factors that contribute to running problems include the surface on which the runner trains. Asphalt, tracks, grass, and concrete have quite different resistances to impact, and so the cumulative stress to the biologic system would not be the same for a runner training on one type of surface versus another. Each surface stresses different muscle groups based on camber, unevenness, and variability of terrain.

A good predictor of injury in most sports is a history of a prior injury. This seems to be the case for running as well. This brings into question the concept of kinetic chain dysfunction. If the anatomic and physiologic system of the runner is intact, the force of footstrike dissipates by transfer from the foot to the lower extremity through the pelvis to the trunk. With normal stress transfer over this distribution, no one anatomic area reaches the point of stress overload. A runner coming back from injury may not return to the same pattern, and clinical evaluations have indicated that runners with a prior injury may have residual changes such as a more limited range of motion of a previously injured joint. Theoretically, this would change the biomechanics of the individual. If the altered form results in an interruption of the kinetic chain, then excess force may accrue to some anatomic area, leading to higher injury risk at that location. In addition, weakness of a muscle that had prior inflammation may change the energy absorption potential and thus the protection that is given to a specific anatomic area. Typically, muscle absorbs up to 80% of impact with less going to bone and other tissue. Another example of how muscle dysfunction could promote injury is a weakened vastus medialis oblique (VMO) muscle that may not control patellar tracking as well as one of normal strength. Laboratory evaluation confirms this and also shows that muscle strength affects form in that strengthening of the tibialis posterior muscle appears to lessen the degree of pronation that is observed in runners. Before this type of science can reach clinical relevance, specific types of kinetic chain dysfunction require better description, quantification, and linkage through prospective studies with specific injuries.

Psychological factors seem a logical area for study regarding running injuries. Since overtraining appears to be a major factor in many injuries, does the individual psyche contribute to the tendency to overtrain or inappropriately train? These questions have been asked in smaller trials, and some evidence points to association of type A behavior with running injury, particularly recurrent injury. A compulsion to run and increased personal stressors may affect running injury. However, attempts to identify a particular personality type for the injured runner have not demonstrated a clear pattern. With limited studies to date, care association of psychological stress to injury risk requires more investigation.

ANATOMIC LOCATION AND TYPES OF RUNNING INJURY

A number of large series have evaluated both the types and locations of injuries experienced by runners. These studies agree that the knee typically accounts for more injuries than any other anatomic location. Following the knee, the lower leg, ankle, and foot account for the next highest frequency of running injuries. The hip, thigh, and low back experience smaller numbers of problems. These injury patterns vary depending on the type of running and the age of the patient. However, gender differences that determine injury location relationships have typically been noted in studies to date, though women do appear to have a higher risk of patellofemoral stress syndrome (PFSS).

The incidence of injury to the hip, thigh, hamstring, lower back, pubic symphysis, and other anatomic locations varies in the literature but always ranks as less frequent than the common problems listed above. However, individuals with prior orthopedic injury may demonstrate a different pattern than is typically seen in studies. For example, surveys of lower back problems among runners show that approximately half of the injuries are new but the other half relate to a flair of a chronic back problem. Thus a study with a number of patients with prior low back pain may overestimate this as a running-related injury.

The anatomic location of running injuries has remained relatively constant in studies conducted over the last three decades. However, the location of stress fractures has changed. Historically, metatarsal stress fractures predominated in athletes. Now tibial shaft stress fractures are the most common type, with fibular, tarsal bone, and metatarsal occurring less frequently. On rare occasions femoral shaft, femoral neck, tibial plateau, pelvic, and sacral stress fractures develop in runners. Theories explaining the changed locations of stress fractures speculate about differences in shoes, reduced use of spikes, changes in training regimens, nutrition, or other factors not yet identified.

In general, younger runners may have a greater risk for muscular strains, particularly of the hamstrings or quadriceps. "Shin pain" from a variety of causes ranks as the top injury in high school age cross-country. This may relate to inexperience, but perhaps these soft tissue injuries relate to greater intensity training or faster speed workouts than would be typical of older runners. Martin and Morgan (2) identified one other specific change in injury patterns in that runners over the age of 40 who participate in road races have a strong tendency toward Achilles tendon and calf injuries. In fact, these were the most common injuries described in this age group. Since this injury information arose from a competitive group, the injury risk to the calf and Achilles tendon may be more specifically related to those who tend to race and would be expected to be doing faster-paced runs than the general population. Another general observation from multiple studies suggests that competitive runners show a greater incidence of strains and stress fractures when they are compared with recreational runners and individuals who only occasionally participate in a race.

In fact, the most common specific injuries correlate quite well among various studies that included distance runners, fitness runners, and individuals who participate in road races. Invariably, PFSS ranked as the most common injury of runners. Following this, five other conditions occurred with variable frequency but were consistently among the top six injuries. These include iliotibial band syndrome, medial tibial stress syndrome (either with or without tibial stress fracture), Achilles tendinitis, plantar fasciitis, and patellar tendinitis. Stress fractures make up approximately 10% of the total number of running injuries.

REVIEW AND TREATMENT APPROACH FOR THE MOST COMMON INJURIES

Patellofemoral Stress Syndrome and Patellar Tendinitis

Patellofemoral stress syndrome ranks as the most common injury among runners, often referred to as runner's knee. PFSS encompasses any of a variety of entities characterized by anterior knee pain. Multiple predisposing factors, such as extensor mechanism malalignment, quadricep muscle imbalance, abnormal patellar tracking, patellar instability, increased Q-angle, a tight lateral retinaculum, inflexible hamstrings, extremes of genu valgum and genu varus, and excessive pronation, have been implicated in this condition.

Runners often present with anterior knee pain exacerbated by downhill work and prolonged sitting with knees in a flexed position ("theater sign"). Mild swelling and crepitus often accompany this syndrome. The runner's knee may occasionally give way but seldom demonstrates mechanical locking. Physical examination includes evaluation of alignment, stance, and gait to check for the aforementioned predisposing factors. A running gait that shows excessive pronation, excessive knee motion, particularly in a horizontal plane or what is sometimes called an S-shaped tracking of patellar contraction, may provide additional reasons to suspect the diagnosis.

Examination often reveals quadriceps atrophy usually involving the vastus medialis oblique on the affected side. A small effusion may be present. Range-of-motion testing demonstrates patellar crepitus. Pain is often reproduced with patellar compression testing. Patellar apprehension testing may reveal patellar instability. Further examination of the extensor mechanism often shows increased Q-angle and tight lateral retinacular structures. Hamstring tightness may exist as well.

X-ray examination is reserved for cases that are severe, that are associated with effusions, or in which the diagnosis remains in doubt. Special radiologic techniques such as computed tomography (CT) or magnetic resonance imaging (MRI) tend to exaggerate the findings and rarely change the treatment plan.

Differential diagnosis of anterior knee pain can be divided by age of the population. In younger runners this includes Osgood-Schlatter disease, Sinding-Larson-Johansson syndrome, osteochondritis dissecans of the femur or patella, and referred pain from Legg-Calve-Perthes disease or slipped capital femoral epiphysis. Bone tumors or hematologic malignancies should be considered in unusual cases, particularly in childhood. Even though these are quite rare, their presentation may be unexplained knee or bone pain. The older running population also experiences osteoarthritis and systemic inflammatory diseases as a cause of anterior knee pain. In both age populations, patellar tendinitis commonly occurs.

Patellar tendinitis more commonly affects jumping athletes; hence the common term "jumper's knee." However, runners may develop this condition, and certain workouts may stress the patellar tendon more than typical training. Quadriceps tendinitis also arises in runners, particularly those who have been doing workouts requiring quadriceps extension such as hill running or hurdling. Knee capsular strains, retinacular inflammation, and unusual causes such as patellar stress fracture are other possible diagnoses.

The runner with patellar tendinitis initially complains of anterior knee pain after exercise. This often progresses to pain with exercise and ultimately to pain at rest. Physical examination reveals tenderness at the inferior pole of the patella and may reveal extensor mechanism malalignments as previously discussed. Typically, radiographs are not needed.

Treatment of both PFSS and patellar tendinitis begins with control of inflammation followed by a consistent program of quadriceps strengthening. Ice, particularly after activity and for pain relief, along with judicious use of nonsteroidal antiinflammatory drugs (NSAIDs), sufficiently deals with the inflammation. Runners need not stop training unless the pain is severe enough to cause a limp with running. Instead, runners should reduce the training load during the initial phase of treatment by avoidance of speed work, downhill running, and hard training surfaces. Typically, mileage is reduced by about 50%, and this increased steadily by 10% per week over the following 4–5 weeks.

Quadriceps-strengthening exercises should emphasize the VMO muscle. Straight leg raises in either a lying or sitting position are effective, particularly if the foot is externally rotated to isolate the VMO. Bent knee extension, squats, and modified lunges must be done carefully to avoid aggravating the injury by limiting total knee flexion to 45 degrees. Athletes with tight hamstrings are given therapeutic stretching, and all athletes should be advised to begin warm-up activities gradually so that both the hamstring and quadriceps mechanisms can function optimally before running at normal training pace.

The most popular bracing used for these conditions are patellar tendon straps. These straps relieve tension at the patellar tendon origin and change the angle of patella tracking, thus providing symptomatic relief. Knee sleeves with horseshoe patellar stabilization pads can benefit those who have excessive lateral tracking by restoration of more normal tracking. McConnell taping techniques have stood the test of several clinical trials. However, McConnell taping requires experience and consistent application to be effective.

Orthotic inserts help runners who have abnormal knee tracking associated with significant pronation. For less severe pronators, inexpensive felt antipronation pads or commercial inserts may effectively correct the gait abnormality and obviate the need for customized devices. Recalcitrant cases of PFSS and patellar tendinitis may require surgical repair, although ten-year follow-ups of surgical versus nonsurgical therapy fail to show a difference in functional or anatomic outcome.

Iliotibial Band Syndrome

Iliotibial band (ITB) syndrome is an inflammatory process that occurs on the lateral aspect of the knee. It is thought to be secondary to friction of the ITB over the lateral femoral condyle during knee flexion. Runners describe sharp pain during the late swing phase of gait and at footstrike. Frequently, the pain varies quite dramatically with different running paces and can be triggered by downhill running, speed running, or sloped surfaces.

The anatomic factors that are most commonly implicated are genu varum and unequal leg lengths. In addition, the excessively pronated foot that leads to increased tibial rotation has also been cited. In spite of these retrospectively observed associations, one of the few large cohort studies of ITB syndrome did not find anatomic variants to be contributors. In fact, this study demonstrated that weekly running mileage and maximum normalized breaking force appeared to be good discriminators of the condition. Other investigators have noted that friction with the ITB occurs only during weight bearing and at approximately 30 degrees of knee flexion.

Often the examination for iliotibial band syndrome is remarkably negative. Occasionally, point tenderness of the lateral femoral condyle or pain elicited by stressing the knee through various degrees of flexion helps to confirm the diagnosis. Ober's test demonstrates whether excessive iliotibial band tightness exists, but it has limited usefulness. Radiographs are not indicated unless the diagnosis seems suspect.

The differential diagnosis should include popliteus tendinitis and lateral meniscus injury. A tender popliteus muscle and tendon can be palpated in the popliteal fossa, and further stress tests by modified lunges with internal rotation of the foot will produce pain. Lateral meniscal pathology is brought out by McMurray's testing with a reproducible click or pain along the lateral joint line.

Treatment of ITB syndrome is often frustrating. Stretches of the ITB have been described in various standing or seated positions. In essence, the athlete needs to feel the stretch to know whether this is effective. Lateral leg lifts in straight and bent leg positions may help to strengthen the tensor fascia lata muscle, offering some benefit. Ice and short-term use of NSAIDs with or without corticosteroid injection into the small bursa just beneath the ITB at the level of the femoral condyle can help to lessen inflammation. Physical therapists may offer transverse friction massage and additional stretches and exercise regimens. The efficacy of modalities such as phonophoresis or iontophoresis for treatment of ITB remains to be firmly established, though such modalities are often prescribed to hasten symptomatic relief. Surgical release can improve symptoms in the most extreme cases, and the surgical literature describes the posterior aspect of the ITB as being more tightly adherent to the lateral knee structure than in the typical athlete.

Runners can continue to train by modifying workouts. One simple modification is to stay on flat, nonbanked surfaces. Variable-paced workouts may limit the degree of knee flexion at the point of footstrike and thus reduce symptoms. A review of gait abnormalities such as excessive pronation or "cross-over strides" may reveal that certain functional changes need to occur before the runner can lessen his or her risk of injury. Simple neoprene knee sleeves often symptomatically benefit runners by keeping the area warm and/or by changing the degree of knee flexion during the running gait, which lessens the likelihood of symptoms.

Cross-training with bicycling, stairmaster, or other nonimpact activities allows the maintenance of cardiovascular conditioning without exacerbating ITB symptoms.

Medial Tibial Stress Syndrome, Shin Pain, and Tibial Stress Fracture

Medial tibial pain and pain around the shin commonly trouble runners. The lay term "shin splints" is nonspecific and does not describe the type of conditions that occur, which include inflammatory problems such as tibialis posterior tendinitis, anterior tibialis tendinitis, peroneal tendinitis, and soleus inflammation. Moderate MTSS more often occurs in young or inexperienced runners who start with mild symptoms and continue to run through the pain. More experienced runners typically have pain that is localized at the juncture of distal and the medial third of the tibia. This pain can radiate up and down the shins, and sometimes the runner may complain of swelling and persistent aching that occurs with daily activity as well as exercise.

More severe medial tibial stress syndrome must be considered a tibial stress fracture until the condition is excluded. In fact, the condition may be a continuum starting with soft tissue inflammation and evolving to stress fracture. In the severe case the runner usually experiences pain that does not go away with rest. The pain persists with walking and becomes worse with even moderate activity, such as walking up steps. Often the individual notes pain at night, and this, in particular, increases the likelihood of a stress fracture.

When runners also complain of numbness or weakness in the foot, the diagnosis of compartment syndrome should be entertained. Compartment syndromes can affect any of the four compartments of the leg, including the deep posterior compartment, which gives symptoms that are similar to those of MTSS. Anterior tibialis inflammation that persists suggests an anterior compartment syndrome, and lateral shin pain, particularly for runners who may have been running on banked surfaces, suggests inflammation of the peroneal compartment.

The examination for mild MTSS or shin pain may point to a specific diagnosis. For example, stressing a given tendon may cause pain, whereas the tibia may not be tender to palpation. Swelling in tendinitis may localize over the tendon sheaths rather than the medial tibial border. For moderate MTSS, swelling may extend up and down the medial aspect of the tibia. When swelling localizes to the distal third of the tibia and tenderness is more marked at one location, the diagnosis of stress fracture becomes paramount. A functional test called the "one-leg hop test" may suggest a stress fracture if the runner is unable to hop on the affected leg 10 times without significant pain. In addition, vibration with a tuning fork may cause pain.

After physical evaluation, radiographs of the tibia may reveal haziness along the border or the presence of a stress fracture characterized by callus formation. Bone scans for MTSS tend to light up an inflammatory response along the medial aspect of the tibia, as opposed to the findings of a stress fracture that tends to localize to one area. Additional testing, such as CT or MRI, may be utilized in cases in which the diagnosis is difficult to establish although a stress fracture is strongly suspected.

Treatment of MTSS depends on the severity of symptoms. For mild tendinitis the athlete should control the inflammation with ice massage and a 1- to 2-week course of NSAIDs. Specific exercises to strengthen the involved muscle groups can include walking on the heels, walking on the toes, walking backwards, and specific weight exercises. Occasionally, a compression wrap may make the shin area feel more comfortable. In a mild case the runner may be able to continue training at a reduced level during treatment. When the runner is unable to train, a substitute aerobic activity such as swimming is usually tolerated.

Moderate MTSS requires a minimum of 2 weeks away from running. Individuals with this injury warrant a more careful look at factors such as anatomic alignment or excessive pronation. Arch pads or orthotics may help individuals with biomechanic problems. Good control of pronation should be established, and shoes should be chosen for motion control. When the runner does return to activity, hills and speed work should be avoided. In addition, the total training volume should be decreased to approximately 50% of normal and gradually increased by 10–15% per week until symptoms resolve. Mild stretching activities are useful for the individual muscle groups that are involved.

In cases of severe MTSS, application of a long air splint should be considered whether tibial stress fracture has been documented or not. Since it has not been established whether severe MTSS evolves into tibial stress fractures, no evidence proves that this approach prevents stress fractures. However, many individuals find significant symptomatic relief with compression of the shins that can best be accomplished with this type of splint. A return to running activities within 10 days to 2 weeks of starting on the air splint is possible in many runners. Other treatment is the same as for mild or moderate MTSS. During the 10 days to 2 weeks in when the individual cannot run, cross-training with other aerobic activity generally is well tolerated.

For documented tibial stress fractures, the same approach is used. A number of studies have shown that 10–14 days of an air splint will allow runners with distal tibial stress fractures to resume activity. When a runner with a documented tibial stress fracture returns to activity, this should be limited to no more than one third of the preinjury training distance and should all be done on a level, soft surface such as a track. In addition, when the runner begins workouts, they should be no more frequent than every other day, and both the distance and frequency should increase gradually (10–20% per week) unless symptoms dictate that a longer period of non-weight bearing is necessary.

A more cautious approach is warranted for patients with a tibial stress fracture that is higher than the junction of the distal and medial third of the tibia. These individuals may require a prolonged period of non weight bearing before beginning any running. In addition, those with a horizontal lucency, particularly on the higher anterior tibia, may have a high risk of stress fracture. This condition has been referred to as the "dreaded black line" and represents an area of nonunion of the tibia. This particular stress fracture has required surgical stabilization in a number of athletes and may take as long as a year to heal in others. Additional radiologic testing with CT allows the clinician to determine the degree of healing taking place.

Further attention should be paid to the individual who develops a stress fracture. Poor health habits should be screened. These include a diet that is insufficient in calcium, vitamins, or total calories. In addition, the quest for thinness and perfection can lead to severe stresses, and the physician should consider the possibility of an eating disorder. The presence of the female triad is a particular concern that can suggest modifying treatment and attention to psychological as well as physical concerns.

For any individual in whom the diagnosis seems likely to be compartment syndrome rather than MTSS, further diagnostic evaluation is warranted. Compartment syndrome can be diagnosed by simple, percutaneous catheter measurements in an outpatient setting. When exercise pressures are dramatically higher than rest pressures, the runner warrants evaluation for possible fasciotomy.

Achilles Tendon and Calf Injuries

The gastrocnemius and soleus complex in the calf, along with their common attachment through the Achilles tendon, form the musculotendinous complex that allows the runner to have forceful pushoff. Without an efficient pushoff the runner cannot achieve a normal airborne, or "float," phase of the gait cycle. With any unilateral weakness of this complex, the gait becomes uneven. Unequal pushoff may also occur from severe pain in the Achilles or calf.

Injury in this area most often involves the actual Achilles tendon. Excessive speed work, in particular, stresses the Achilles such that inflammation of the tendon is often the earliest sign of overtraining. In fact, runners often refer to the Achilles as their thermometer. When a light squeeze of the Achilles produces pain, the runner realizes that he or she has overtrained.

Symptoms of Achilles injury range from persistent pain to pain with light activity or, in mild cases, to pain from more strenuous activity such as running up hills. Individuals may note swelling or crepitation. Examination may verify this with point tenderness located either at the insertion of the tendon or anywhere along its length. Palpable nodules along the tendon suggest the possibility of a partial Achilles rupture. The nodules often represent torn fibers that have rolled back on themselves to form a nodular area in which there is excessive synovial fluid and inflammatory change. Complete tendinous rupture, though uncommon in the running population, will present with pain and often an audible pop. The exam shows a palpable gap at the insertion site, retraction of the gastrocnemius complex, and a positive Thompson sign (lack of foot plantar flexion when gastrocnemius is provoked by squeezing the calf with the knee flexed).

Treatment for mild tendinitis may require only a reduction in activity, icing, and a course of antiinflammatory medications. Heel cups or other types of heel lifts help to relieve symptoms and can improve the runner's ability to walk or run. In general, for mild tendinitis the decision to allow the runner to continue training on a reduced schedule hinges on running with good form and continuing progress with healing.

Moderate or severe tendinitis requires variable periods of rest along with ice and NSAIDs. Runners can often substitute activities such as biking or swimming without worsening irritation to the tendon. Partial tears and severe tendinitis may respond further to ultrasound, massage, and formal physical therapy treatments. For moderate to severe cases and chronic symptoms, strengthening exercises are indicated for both the gastrocnemius and soleus. Heel raises with the knees in extension effectively exercise the gastrocnemius complex, while heel raises with the knees in slight flexion more selectively strengthen the soleus complex. Complete tears of the Achilles tendon in the competitive athlete should typically proceed to surgical repair.

Most runners stretch the Achilles tendon while training. However, during a phase of acute inflammation, stretching should be used carefully so as to not worsen the condition. This is particularly true when a partial tear exists, as excessive stretching may increase the amount of tissue injury.

Use of corticosteroid injection around the Achilles has not been conclusively proven to produce Achilles rupture. However, because of a theoretical concern about weakening tissue and easier breakdown with injection of corticosteroid substances near a weight-bearing tendon, the standard of care in the United States suggests that injection is to be avoided. Significantly, no studies indicate that steroid injections improve outcomes for Achilles tendonitis. Currently, pathologic evaluation of Achilles and other chronic tendon injuries indicate that the inflammatory phase of the injury is short. Chronic injury shows tissue breakdown more consistent with the term tendinosus. The key to tissue healing may require a totally new approach, since persistent use of antiinflammatory medication makes little sense from a pathologic perspective. Other alternative therapies for tendonitis, including cool laser treatments, prolotherapy, acupuncture, subcutaneous injections of low molecular weight heparin, and topical antiinflammatory agents lack conclusive proof of efficacy.

Many Achilles tendon and calf injuries occur higher in the leg and involve the gastrocnemius muscle or the plantaris muscle. Runners injure both locations with moderate frequency. Plantaris rupture occurs as a sudden pop with a sharp, searing pain, usually in the midcalf area. The individual may note swelling and point tenderness of variable degree afterward. The disability from plantaris rupture generally resolves over 7–14 days without significant residual weakness. Treatment involves icing, NSAIDs, and relative rest. If pain is severe for 1–2 days, the individual may feel more comfortable with crutch-assisted ambulation. Heel lifts may also lessen the pain that is experienced with walking.

More serious calf muscle injury occurs when the broad musculotendinous attachment of the gastrocnemius muscle ruptures. The popular name for this condition, "tennis leg," relates to the tendency of this injury to occur with forceful pushoff. An individual who experiences tennis leg usually feels a sharp pain and may or may not hear a pop. The gastrocnemius area, most often along the medial head, develops discoloration and significant swelling. The individual limps with an antalgic gait and is unable to push off or bear weight comfortably. The same treatment approach as in plantaris injury generally helps in gastrocnemius tears. Because of the greater amount of swelling in this larger muscle group, a compression wrap may make the individual more comfortable. Most runners will require several days of crutch walking and a few weeks of strengthening before regaining normal stride length to resume running activities. Substitute aerobic activities such as biking or swimming help to maintain overall conditioning. Calf-strengthening exercises, particularly those that emphasize heel raises, should resume as soon as the individual can comfortably pursue them. Physical therapy and the use of electrical stimulation or other modalities can help to speed the resolution of difficult cases.

After significant injury to the gastrocnemius–soleus–Achilles complex, repeat assessment of the runner's gait is helpful to detect any form of breakdown that has developed as a result of the injury. Training under a coach and modifying workouts until normal form has returned may help the runner to avoid recurrent injuries. Rehabilitation programs emphasizing eccentric strengthening appear as efficacious as any treatment approach for calf and Achilles injuries.

Plantar Fasciitis

Medial heel pain develops as a symptom in many runners, typically following excessive training or after a vigorous race effort. A classic symptom of plantar fascial inflammation is debilitating pain on the first step out of bed each morning. During training, a runner may note severe symptoms for the first several steps that gradually lessen and start resolving 5–10 minutes into the run. Depending on the degree of injury, the pain (often described as dull and nagging) recurs shortly after completion of the run or after a delay of several hours. The pain is not present if the individual is lying down but will recur in a lancinating fashion with weight bearing after a period of inactivity. The symptoms can be aggravated by standing persistently on hard floors. Individuals may note a difference in symptoms depending on the type of footwear that is worn. Shoes with an added soft heel cup often provide symptomatic relief.

Physical examination demonstrates pain along the medial insertion of the plantar fascia into the calcaneus. The pain can be experienced farther up into the longitudinal arch as well. Extension of the great toe may increase the symptoms. A negative calcaneal squeeze test and absence of tenderness with application of a vibrating tuning fork to the calcaneus differentiates plantar fasciitis from a calcaneal stress fracture. Palpable pain at the point of the os calcis more commonly suggests a bruised heel syndrome in which the fat pad splits and no longer offers cushion to the heel. A small percentage of plantar fascial symptoms are triggered by entrapment of the calcaneal branch of the medial plantar nerve.

Certain anatomic features may predispose to plantar fasciitis. Individuals with cavus feet seem more likely to be affected. In addition, individuals who pronate excessively create a torque on the plantar fascia that causes inflammation and sometimes a plantar fascial rupture. Tightness of the Achilles tendon may also play a role, as the plantar fascia serves as a bridge to help transfer the contraction from the great toe through the foot and Achilles–gastrocnemius complex to give the runner forceful pushoff. Since this fibrous tissue plays a crucial role in the muscular function of the foot and calf, most individuals cannot maintain normal running form with moderate to severe plantar fasciitis.

Treatment of plantar fascial injuries often frustrates both patients and physicians. Response can be slow in spite of various modalities. Ice massage or immersion of the heel in ice water plus NSAIDs helps to eliminate inflammation. Toe flexion and arch exercises, stretching, and massaging the foot by rolling it over a soda bottle have been used to strengthen the longitudinal arch and lessen symptoms. Functional-type activities may exercise the area more effectively. These include heel walking, toe walking, walking backwards, and doing some running drills barefoot on grass or soft surfaces while trying to reestablish normal form.

For moderate to severe inflammation, corticosteroid injection is often needed to obtain symptom relief. Some physicians hesitate to use injection because of the fear of rupture of the plantar fascia, but rupture may actually lead to quicker resolution of symptoms; complete rupture mimics the surgical release that is used in recalcitrant cases. The major precaution with corticosteroid injection of the plantar fascial insertion is not to induce fat pad atrophy with superficial and/or frequent injections. In the absence of an adequate fat pad, the individual may have a persistently painful heel even after the plantar fascial inflammation lessens.

Different supports, such as heel cups, low dye strapping with moleskin and tape, various padded heel inserts, and temporary orthotics or arch pads, provide symptomatic relief for a number of individuals. For people with more significant biomechanic abnormalities, such as excessive pronation or high arches, custom orthotics hasten resolution of symptoms in approximately 75% of cases. Shoe change may help. While heavier and slower runners may prefer a more supportive shoe, the competitive runner often needs a lighter, more flexible shoe to reestablish normal arch motion.

Recent studies have examined the role of night splints in resolution of symptoms. Night splints place the foot and ankle at a neutral position with slight extension of the great toe. The individual wears the splint each night until symptoms resolve (approximately 16 weeks if the night splint is effective). Not all studies have shown a good response to this treatment, but the therapy can be utilized as a helpful adjunct to other treatment modalities.

As with most injuries, rest has been prescribed as a key component in the resolution of plantar fasciitis. In the authors' experience runners rarely resolve the condition any more rapidly with rest than with continued training as long as their running form and biomechanics remain unchanged. Virtually all runners find that they do have to reduce total mileage and speed work until symptoms lessen. Whether the individual rests or continues a training program, substitute aerobic activity helps to maintain cardiovascular conditioning. In addition, generalized weight strengthening exercises for the lower extremities may lessen the time necessary to return to peak training form. Runners who return to training and feel that their form has changed should have either a formal biomechanic assessment or evaluation by experienced coaches to evaluate their running gait.

SYMPTOMS INDICATIVE OF LESS COMMON RUNNING INJURIES

Recurrent Knee Effusions

Runners with recurrent effusions may have intraarticular pathology. In adolescent and younger runners, osteochondritis dissecans should be ruled out. This condition is secondary to vascular insufficiency to a portion of the osteochondral cartilage arising from either the medial or lateral femoral condyle. Whether this results from a high-impact injury or overuse remains to be established. The treatment for these conditions is surgery and postoperative rehabilitation.

Persistent knee effusions may also represent aggravation of prior injuries. Knee instability, persistent swelling, or severe pain can be the first sign of breakdown of a previous surgical repair. Attritional meniscal tears, regardless of prior history, may develop in the older running population and present with a knee effusion.

Other rare entities in the differential diagnosis of knee effusions include tibial plateau stress fractures and systemic collagen vascular disease.

Medial Arch Pain

The medial portion of the arch provides a primary spring for the pushoff phase of running. This area is anchored by the navicular, which forms a keystone for arch function. Excessive pronation or ligamentous breakdown of the arch will increase stress to the navicular and can result in navicular stress fracture. Diagnosis requires MRI, CT, or bone scan. The navicular does not heal as consistently as other stress fractures; strongly consider avascular necrosis and nonunion when treatment or healing is delayed. Initial treatment consists of non–weight-bearing casting or splinting. Open reduction and internal fixation with bone grafting is necessary if conservative measures fail.

Other injuries that cause medial arch pain include tibialis posterior tendinitis, insertional tears of either the flexor digitorum or flexor hallucis longus tendons, spring ligament sprain, and plantar fasciitis.

Groin Pain

Consistent groin pain merits evaluation because of the serious nature of femoral neck stress fractures. Examination reveals antalgic gait with decreased internal rotation of the hip. Plain radiographs, if taken early, are often negative. Bone scan, MRI, or CT is needed to confirm diagnosis. Treatment of nondisplaced fractures demands non weight bearing with or without immobilization. Extensive and displaced fractures require internal fixation.

In prepubescent runners the differential includes Legg-Calve-Perthes disease and slipped capital femoral epiphysis. Conversely, older runners develop groin pain as an early symptom of osteoarthritis. Groin pain may also be due to referred symptoms from conditions such as osteitis pubis, stress fractures of the pubic symphysis or pelvic ring, chronic adductor strains, and tendon injuries such as snapping hip syndrome. "Gilmore's groin, or what is now commonly called a sports hernia, may cause inguinal area pain.

Chronic Forefoot Pain

Metatarsal inflammation, particularly behind the second metatarsal head, remains a common problem to runners doing speed work or excessive distance training. Diagnosis is confirmed by palpation on the plantar surface of the foot, with pain greatest proximal to the second or occasionally third or fourth metatarsal heads. Persistent pain or swelling requires ruling out a metatarsal stress fracture. Adolescents with chronic metatarsalgia may develop avascular necrosis of the second metatarsal head (Freiberg's disease). Plain radiographs reveal squaring of the metatarsal head and sclerotic changes consistent with avascular necrosis. In addition to ice and NSAIDs, placement of metatarsal pads often alleviates symptoms.

Other common forefoot problems include injuries of the great toe, such as degenerative joint disease, hallux rigidus, and bunions; sesamoid injuries, either bruising, contusion, or stress fractures; lancinating pain, particularly between the third and fourth toes, characterizing thickening of the digital nerve known as Morton's neuroma; and stress fractures involving the metatarsal bones.

Hip Pain, Posterior Thigh Pain, and Sciatica

A complex of symptoms affect the hip, posterior thigh, and sciatic nerve. Runners who complain of sciatica more commonly have piriformis syndrome or another injury of the hip or upper hamstrings rather than ruptured discs. However, a thorough evaluation to eliminate a herniated disc as a cause for sciatica should be completed.

Pain to palpation in the deep buttocks area that reproduces radicular symptoms down a sciatic nerve distribution suggests a diagnosis of piriformis injury. Further evaluation, including stretches that stress the piriformis muscle, may increase symptomatology and further confirm accurate differentiation from discogenic pathology. Treatment for piriformis injuries includes a piriformis stretching program and hip external rotator muscle strengthening, a reduction of the training schedule, and avoidance of speed work and downhill runs. Physical therapy or injection at the musculotendinous insertion of the piriformis can hasten resolution of chronic symptoms.

Hamstring injuries, particularly at the proximal insertion, can cause spasm that leads to sciatic radiation. The powerful hamstring complex is most susceptible to injury when it is eccentrically contracted while fatigued or improperly warmed up before activity. Physical exam shows tenderness and decreased strength and flexibility and can show ecchymosis with partial and/or complete muscular tears. Radiographs can be used to rule out pubic ramus stress fracture and ischial avulsion fracture. Treatment requires rest, ice, compression, and elevation (RICE) and nonsteroidal antiinflammatory drugs (NSAIDs) followed by physical therapy and appropriate modalities. During recovery the runner should keep the hamstring warm by wearing running tights or a compressive wrap. Grade III hamstring strains (tears) often heal with underlying bands of scar tissue that can require surgical release.

Less common problems around the hip include gluteus medius/minimus injury, greater trochanteric bursitis, sacral stress fractures, and snapping hip syndrome.

Miscellaneous Conditions

Changes in bone architecture may cause pain or compress nerves. One example of this is Haglund's deformity ("pump bump"). This bony exostosis off the posterior calcaneus results from repetitive stress and motion at the Achilles tendon insertion. Treatment involves shoe modification, orthotics, and ultimately surgical excision if conservative measures fail.

Accessory naviculars can be injured by excessive pronation and cause significant medial arch pain in runners. Orthotics may relieve pressure on accessory navicular bones; however, surgical excision is often required.

Tarsal tunnel syndrome is a neuropathy of the distal portion of the tibial nerve due to excessive foot pronation and resultant pressure on this nerve as it passes through the tarsal tunnel. Examination reveals pain and numbness of the plantar aspect of the foot, usually the medial aspect of the great and second toe, along with weakness of plantar flexion of the toes. On physical exam, Tinel's sign over the tarsal tunnel reproduces pain along the nerve's distribution; NCV/EMG confirms the diagnosis. Treatment measures include RICE and NSAIDs and the use of arch pads or orthotics to block excessive pronation. Intractable cases require surgical decompression.

Another common nerve entrapment in the foot involves the medial calcaneal branch of the tibial nerve. Injury to this nerve mimics plantar fasciitis and should be considered in the differential of medial heel/foot pain.

GENERAL CONSIDERATIONS AND THE TREATMENT OF RUNNING INJURIES

During the initial phase running injuries are best treated by successful control of inflammation. This generally requires the use of a great deal of ice. Virtually all these anatomic areas will respond to application of ice, particularly if pain occurs around a joint or bony structure. Probably nothing better relieves the pain in PFSS or plantar fasciitis than liberal application of ice for periods of approximately 10 minutes at a time. For certain muscular injuries, low back pain, and other conditions, heat plays an adjunctive role, and the physician should carefully consider when to use this modality.

Use of medications helps to speed the process of healing. NSAIDS have a role, but this role is short term and probably should be limited to 1–2 weeks. When pain persists much longer than this, additional considerations about diagnosis or appropriate treatment should be entertained. Short bursts of oral cortical steroids are used for a number of injuries and may effectively control inflammation but carry the concomitant risk of corticosteroid use, particularly repeated too often. Injectable corticosteroids often benefit specific injuries but do not have a useful role in weight-bearing tendons because of concern about tendon rupture.

During the acute phase of injury, rehabilitation and substituted aerobic activity require careful prescription, as the wrong types of activity may worsen the given injury. A key assessment during the acute phase is the degree to which the injury affects the biomechanic function of the runner. Should the runner not show significant biomechanic breakdown or limping during gait, she or he can generally return to a reduced and modified training program. In particular, some aspects of training will aggravate certain injuries more. For example, hill training logically stresses the Achilles tendon and would be inappropriate for someone with this injury. Downhill running, on the other hand, often aggravates PFSS symptoms more than level or uphill running does and should be avoided in individuals troubled with this condition.

During the subacute phase when the runner returns to activity, part of the follow-up includes an analysis of what modifications he or she has made of the training schedule. For example, the runner who returns to speed work too quickly may return an injury to a previously severe level. In addition, training in certain locations may stress specific muscle groups. A runner with hip pain who performs interval workouts around curves requires a lot more involvement of the piriformus muscle than would be the case for someone running on a road with very few turns. In this situation a track workout would clearly be inappropriate for the recovering runner, who might do the same type of workout on a road course marked off to allow the interval training.

A key concept in the treatment of almost every injury is a reduction of stress. This generally means a reduction of mileage. A good principle for most injuries is to take the individual who is able to return to training and suggest that the first week of returning to training occur at 50% of the runner's normal training mileage. For milder injuries that would be expected to heal in 2–3 weeks, the rate of increase after that first week of training might be as much as a 20% return to normal mileage per week. For more significant injuries the rate at return to normal training mileage should progress at approximately 10% weekly. In addition to reducing mileage, careful assessment of whether the individual ever uses rest days may lead to this as a part of an ongoing recommendation. In particular, when a runner returns from an injury such as a stress fracture in which cumulative impact may be important, the return to running may best occur on an every-other-day basis until significant progress has been made in healing the injury.

Another common consideration would be the reason why a runner has frequent injuries. In particular, if the injury suggests that training location may play a role, a change in training surface may be appropriately recommended. Softer surfaces certainly reduce impact. Uneven surfaces may aggravate specific type of injuries. Too many sessions on a track may aggravate hip rotators, abductors, adductors, and other muscle groups that help to stabilize the runner for running sharply around turns.

SUMMARY

Running ranks among the most popular participant sports for adults wishing to maintain overall fitness. The key advantage of running as a fitness exercise is that the time of total exercise to reach a high fitness level is low. Association of a higher fitness level with longevity has stimulated interest from the American College of Sports Medicine and other groups to encourage more vigorous aerobic activity on a daily basis. Running also helps individuals lose weight and gain self-esteem. The completion of running goals gives positive feedback and contributes to individuals continuing with the sport. Additional studies that show decreased disabilities of runners rather than an increase in osteoarthritis and other chronic problems have not been fully appreciated by the lay public or the medical community. A renewed emphasis in sports medicine is to use these positive outcomes to encourage people about the health aspects of aerobic sport rather than the potential negative aspects of injury.

Running injuries remain a complex problem. No one cause has been found that explains why some runners have frequent injuries. However, training errors seem to be the most frequent factor identified in most studies. Anatomic problems appear to play a role, but their true contribution remains to be established. Prospective association of anatomic changes with injuries remains limited. In addition, assessments of the kinetic chain, biomechanic evaluations, and analysis of running form have not been sufficiently developed as a clinical tool to predict injury. Smaller studies that have suggested these associations are certainly provocative, but additional work needs to be done before too many of these factors can be taken into account in treating runners. Other factors, including body composition, medical illnesses, and psychological makeup, may be significant contributors to running injuries, but studies to determine this will need to include larger groups of runners than have been evaluated to date and will need long-term follow-up.

Injury complicates the lives of those who use running for fitness or competition. Most runners who train consistently will average one significant injury every 1–2 years. However, a disproportionate number of these injuries probably occur in runners who run excesssive mileage or who never take rest days. In addition, speed work including races or too frequent interval workouts may be a factor in injury. Fortunately, in spite of the high injury rate, running injuries rarely lead to long-term disability. Most injuries are overuse injuries, can be treated without surgery, and in many cases can be successfully treated while the runner pursues a reduced training schedule. Understanding the principles of training and recovery may help the physician to play a role in keeping the runner active during the acute, subacute, and recovery phases of the injury. In addition, appropriate rehabilitation exercises, such as stretching when indicated for given injuries and modifications of training, may allow the runner to have a lower risk of recurrent injury.

REFERENCES

1. Cowan D, Jones BH, Robinson JR. Foot morphologic characteristics and risk of exercise-related injury. *Arch Fam Med* 1993; 2(7):773–777.
2. Martin PE, Morgan DW. Biomechanical considerations for economical walking and running. *Med Sci Sports Exerc* 1992;24(4): 467–473.

BIBLIOGRAPHY

Chang PS, Harris RM. Intramedullary nailing for chronic tibial stress fractures: a review of five cases. *Am J Sports Med* 1996;24(5): 688–692.

Clement DB, Taunton JE, Smart GW, McNicol KL. A survey of overuse running injuries. *Phys Sports Med* 1981;9(5):47–58.

D'Ambrosia R. Orthotic devices in running injuries. *Clin Sports Med* 1985;4(4):611–618.

D'Ambrosia R, Drez D Jr. *Prevention and treatment of running injuries*. Thorofare, NJ: Charles B. Slack, 1982.

Donatelli R, Hurlbert C, Conaway D, et al. Biomechanical foot orthotics: a retrospective study. *J Orthop Sports Phys Ther* 1988;10(6): 205–212.

Eller DJ, Katz DS, Bergman AG, et al. Sacral stress fractures in long-distance runners. *Clin J Sporst Med* 1997;7(3):222–225.

Frey C. Footwear and stress fractures. *Clin Sports Med* 1997;16(2): 249–257.

Guten GN. *Running injuries*. Philadelphia: WB Saunders, 1997.

Jacobs R, Bobbert MF, Schenau GJ. Function of mono- and biarticular muscles in running. *Med Sci Sports Exerc* 1993;25(10):1163–1173.

James SL, Bates BT, Osternig LR. Injuries to runners. *Am J Sports Med* 1978;6(2):40–50.

Kannus V. Evaluation of abnormal biomechanics of the foot and ankle in athletes. *Br J Sports Med* 1992;26(2):83–89.

Kilmartin TE, Wallace WA. The scientific basis for the use of biomechanical foot orthoses in the treatment of lower limb sports injuries: a review of the literature. *Br J Sports Med* 1994;28(3):180–184.

Komi PV. The musculoskeletal system. In: Dirix A, Knuttgen HG, Tittel K, eds. *The Olympic book of sports medicine,* vol 1. Oxford, England: Blackwell Scientific Publications, 1988:15–39.

MacIntyre J, Lloyd-Smith R. Overuse running injuries. In: Renstrom PAFH, ed. *Sports injuries: basic principles of prevention and care.* Cambridge, MA: Blackwell Scientific Publications, 1994:139–160.

Mann RA. Running sports: biomechanics of running. In: Mack R, ed. *American Academy of Orthopaedic Surgeons symposium on the foot and leg in running sports.* Chicago: Year Book Medical Publishers, 1982:1–29.

Mellion MB, Walsh WM, Shelton GL. *The team physician's handbook,* 2nd ed. Philadelphia: Hanley & Belfus, 1997.

Nigg BM. Biomechanics as applied to sports. In: Harries M, Williams C, Stanish WD, Micheli LJ, eds. *The Oxford textbook of sports medicine.* New York: Oxford Medical Publications, 1994:94–111.

Ounpuu S. The biomechanics of walking and running. *Clin Sports Med* 1994;13(4):843–863.

Sallis RE, Massimino F. *ACSM's essentials of sports medicine.* St. Louis: Mosby, 1997.

Stanton P, Purdam C. Hamstring injuries in sprinting: the role of eccentric exercise. *J Orthop Sports Phys Ther* 1989;March:343–349.

Vixie DE. Orthotics and shoe corrections. In: Mack R, ed. *American Academy of Orthopaedic Surgeons symposium on the foot and leg in running sports.* Chicago: Year Book Medical Publishers, 1982: 76–79.

CHAPTER 47

Skiing

Antero Natri and Robert J. Johnson

INTRODUCTION

Alpine, or downhill, skiing has become an increasingly popular recreational sport during the last few decades all over the world. Recently, it has been estimated that approximately 15 million people are skiing in the United States and up to 200 million worldwide (1,2). The demographic characteristics of downhill skiers and the technical quality of the equipment they use have changed during recent decades. At its inception in the United States, skiing attracted a well-conditioned group of participants, but the sport now attracts a broad spectrum of individuals, including many with little athletic experience. Boots, bindings, skis, and ski-restraining devices have significantly changed the characteristics of the ski–skier coupling system. Furthermore, modern snowmaking, trail design, and trail grooming have also dramatically altered the nature of skiing environment (3,4).

However, in skiing, as in other sports, there is a certain inherent risk of injury. In the 1960s tibia fractures and ankle sprains were common. During the past 20 years, with the rapid development in skiing-related equipment, including ski boots and bindings, the above-mentioned injuries have decreased significantly, by as much as 90% (5). Indeed, one of the primary design objectives of ski boots and bindings has been to protect the skier from tibia and ankle fractures. Today, modern bindings, when properly mounted, adjusted, and maintained, provide excellent protection against all below-knee injuries. Unfortunately, despite advances in equipment design, modern ski bindings are obviously incapable of protecting the knee. It has been observed since the early 1980s that the incidence of severe knee injuries usually involving the anterior cruciate ligament (ACL) has increased alarmingly (3,6), and this trend continues today (7). The rate of severe knee sprains has tripled since 1980. Today, complete tears of the ACL are definitely the most significant medical problem in skiing and are occurring in epidemic proportions (7–10).

In this chapter we summarize the incidences of common alpine skiing injuries and discuss their prevention.

THE EPIDEMIOLOGY OF THE ALPINE SKIING INJURIES

Incidence of Injuries

The incidence of injuries in alpine skiing has decreased from about 5–8 injuries per 1000 skier days before the 1970s (11) to about 3–4 injuries per 1000 skier days during the early 1980s (12,13) and to 2–3 injuries per 1000 skier days in the late 1980s and early 1990s (7,8,14,15). It is believed that efforts to reduce the risk of skiing injuries has resulted from improvements of the ski-boot-binding system and from education (5).

On the other hand, the incidence of severe knee injuries has increased dramatically since the early 1980s (3,6,8), and today the complete rupture of the ACL is clearly the most common serious medical problem in alpine skiing (7). Although the medial collateral ligament (usually grade I or grade II sprains) is the most frequently injured structure of the knee in skiing, the ACL is injured in approximately 20% of all skiing injuries (7,15,16).

Johnson and colleagues studied prospectively the injury trends of downhill skiing in Sugarbush ski area in Vermont (United States) between 1972 and 1997 using a

---

A. Natri: Section of Orthopaedics, Department of Surgery, Tampere University Hospital, University of Tampere, and Tampere Research Centre of Sports Medicine, Tampere, Finland.

R. J. Johnson: Department of Orthopaedics and Rehabilitation, Sports Medicine Division, The University of Vermont, College of Medicine, McClure Musculoskeletal Research Center, Burlington, Vermont, 05405-0084.

TABLE 47-1. Incidence of alpine skiing injuries between 1972 and 1997 (regression estimates) at Sugarbush, Vermont (N = 14,982)

	MBDI, 1972	MBDI, 1997	% Change	r^2	p
All injuries	228	436	48	0.50	<0.01
Upper body injuries	516	854	40	0.29	<0.01
Lower leg injuries			87	0.90	<0.01
Twist injuries	1,904	16,120	88	0.76	<0.01
Bend injuries	1,664	11,908	86	0.85	<0.01
All fractures	1,571	2,795	44	0.37	<0.01
Tibia fractures	4,186	34,593	88	0.74	<0.01
Nonspiral tibia fractures	9,275	78,516	84	0.70	<0.01
Spiral tibia fractures	11,372	174,141	94	0.80	<0.01
Clavicular fractures	36,916	14,147	−38	0.27	<0.01
Metacarpal phalangeal ulnar collateral ligament injuries	2,037	6,448	68	0.54	<0.01
All knee sprains	1,193	1,412	16	N.S.	N.S.
Grade I and II knee sprains	1,444	4,251	66	0.56	<0.01
Grade III knee sprains	5,857	1,722	−240	0.74	<0.01

N.S., not significant

case control study design. They evaluated 14,982 injuries reported to injury clinics operated in the base lodges of a moderate-sized northern New England ski area. During that time, approximately 5,098,000 skier-visits occurred at the ski area.

Most previous studies reported injuries per 1000 skier days to indicate the injury rate, but rather than change from the base (1000) to 10,000 or 1,000,000 skier days for relatively rare injury groups, the investigators have chosen to indicate the incidence in terms of mean days between injuries (MDBI), which is calculated by dividing the number of skier visits by the number of injuries (3). The higher the MDBI number, the lower the injury rate. The MDBI for each injury group was fitted to an exponential curve as follows:

$$\text{MDBI} = (a)e^{(b)\text{YR}}$$

where a and b are coefficients determined by regression analysis, YR is the study year, and e is the universal constant (2.7182).

The percent change in the MDBI between years 1 and 25 was calculated as follows:

$$\% \text{ change in MDBI} = 1 - (\text{MDBI initial}/\text{MDBI final}) \times 100$$

Tests of significance for r^2 were two-tailed.

TABLE 47-2. Distribution of the ten most common injuries in 1972 and 1993 at Sugarbush, Vermont

1972 (Total injuries: 335)	n	%	1993 (Total injuries: 331)	n	%
1. Knee sprain	67	20.0	1. Knee sprain	99	29.9
2. Ankle sprain	32	9.6	2. Thumb sprain	27	8.2
3. Laceration	26	7.8	3. Laceration	26	7.9
4. Leg contusion	23	6.9	4. Shoulder contusion	14	4.3
5. Thumb sprain	23	6.9	5. Concussion	14	4.3
6. Tibia fracture	22	6.6	6. Leg contusion	13	3.9
7. Shoulder contusion	17	5.1	7. Shoulder dislocation	12	3.6
8. Knee contusion	14	4.2	8. Metacarpal fracture	11	3.3
9. Ankle fracture	12	3.6	9. Knee contusion	10	3.0
10. Boot top contusion	12	3.6	10. Humerus fracture	10	3.0
	248	74.2%		236	71.4%

This table demonstrates the rank order of the ten most frequent injuries treated in the clinic at the Sugarbush, Vermont, ski area during the 1971–1972 and 1992–1993 ski seasons, a season early in our study and a relatively recent one in which the number of injuries was nearly the same. Although knee sprains were number one in occurrence during both seasons studied, the frequency of ankle fractures and sprains and tibia fractures were dramatically reduced by 1993, and they no longer rate in the group of the ten most frequent injuries. Ankle sprains accounted for 1.3%, ankle fractures 1.0%, and tibia fractures 1.6% of all injuries during the 1992–1993 season.

Injury Trends

Overall Incidence

During 25 years of study of skiing injuries at Sugarbush, we observed a 48% decline in the overall injury rate ($r^2 = 0.50$, $p < 0.01$) (Table 47–1). Most of this decline can be attributed to a reduction in the incidence of lower leg injuries (below the knee), which decreased by 87% ($r^2 = 0.90$, $p < 0.01$) (Table 47–1).

During the years 1987–1994 of the Sugarbush study (17), the most common injuries were a contusion of the knee in children, a sprain of the ulnar collateral ligament of the thumb in adolescents, and a grade III sprain of the anterior cruciate ligament in adults.

Lower Extremity Injuries

The study shows that tibia fractures and ankle sprains had the greatest decline: 88% and 92%, respectively (Tables 47–1 and 47–2).

In knee injuries, grade I and grade II knee sprains (minor to moderate damage, usually involving the medial collateral ligament (MCL), are also down, in this case by 66% ($r^2 = 0.56$, $p < 0.01$). However, serious (complete disruption of at least one ligament) grade III knee sprains, usually involving the ACL, increased by 240% ($r^2 = 0.74$, $p < 0.01$). This is the strongest, largest, and most significant negative trend identified in the study (Table 47–1). On the basis of regression analysis the percentage of knee sprains classified as severe climbed from 17% to 61.7% during the 25-year period. As of January 1998, severe ACL sprains accounted for 21% of all reported injuries at Sugarbush, Vermont, during the 1997–1998 season. It is remarkable that the study of ski injuries from 1982 through 1993 at Jackson Hole, Wyoming (15), revealed that knee sprains in general accounted for 30% of all injuries and ACL injuries accounted for 16% of all injuries, rates that are very similar to our data, presented in Tables 47–3 and 47–4.

Upper Body Injuries

Overall, upper body injuries declined 40% ($r^2 = 0.29$, $p < 0.01$) during the study. Lacerations and metacarpal phalangeal ulnar collateral ligament thumb injuries showed significant declines: 64% ($r^2 = 0.51$, $p < 0.01$) and 68% ($r^2 = 0.54$, $p < 0.01$), respectively. The only negative trends within the fracture group were among upper body injuries. Clavicle and trunk fractures were up by 38% ($r^2 = 0.27$, $p < 0.01$) and 202% ($r^2 = 0.22$, $p < 0.05$), respectively. Together, these two injury groups in 1994 included more than one third of all fractures but only 5% of all injuries.

The long-term trends reported from the Sugarbush study through 1994 showed that the rate of concussions increased 48% in children and 37% in adolescents (not found to be significant in either groups), the rate of head injuries increased 66% in children and 5% in adolescents (not found to be significant in either group), and the rate of spinal injuries increased 130% in children and 407% in adolescents ($p < 0.01$) (17). The primary reason for the lack of significant changes for concussions and other head injuries and spinal injuries in children was the relatively small numbers of these injuries in the study.

KNEE INJURY MECHANISMS IN ALPINE SKIING

The exact mechanism of injury may be difficult for a skier to recall because of the associated speed and the complexity of events occurring during a typical fall. From interviews with injured skiers and, more recently, with the aid of videotapes of skiers experiencing ACL injuries, the most common ACL injury mechanisms in alpine skiing have been identified (5,10,16,18).

They can be divided into the following categories:

1. Valgus–external rotation (Fig. 47–1): In the classic forward fall, in which the medial edge of the tip of the ski engages the snow, the skier is propelled forward by his or her downhill momentum, and the lower leg is abducted and externally rotated in relation to the thigh. The long moment arm of the ski creates considerable magnitudes of torque about the knee. If the adverse forces are not eliminated by release of the binding or removal of the ski edge from the snow, then the primary

TABLE 47–3. *Knee sprains expressed as a percentage of all injuries, 1974–1997, at Sugarbush, Vermont*

Years	Percentage
1974–1976	21.9
1977–1979	20.0
1980–1982	21.3
1983–1985	22.9
1986–1988	28.2
1989–1991	24.3
1992–1994	29.1
1995–1997	31.3

TABLE 47–4. *ACL sprains expressed as a percentage of all injuries, 1973–1998, at Sugarbush, Vermont*

Years	Percentage
1973–1975	3.3
1976–1978	4.3
1979–1981	5.8
1982–1984	10.8
1985–1987	14.4
1988–1990	13.7
1991–1993	16.7
1994–1996	20.4
1997	18.0
1998	21.0

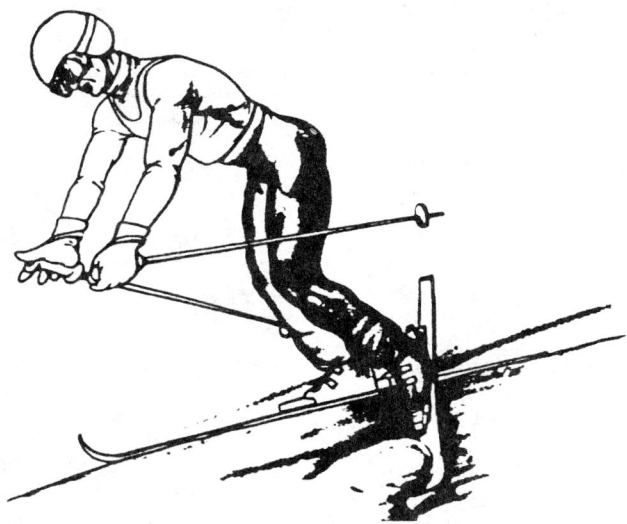

FIG. 47-1. The valgus–external rotation knee injury mechanism in skiing. (Reprinted with permission from Feagin JA Jr, ed. *The crucial ligaments: diagnosis and treatment of ligamentous injuries about the knee.* New York: Churchill Livingstone, 1988.)

ligament that is injured in such a fall is usually the medial collateral; however, in approximately 20% of these cases the ACL is also torn.

2. Boot-induced anterior drawer mechanism (Fig. 47-2): In this injury mechanism the ACL is damaged when the top of the ski boot drives the tibia forward, producing an anteriorly directed force on the tibia relative to the femur (an "anterior drawer maneuver") that can result in disruption of the ACL. This can occur when the skier who has become airborne lands on the tail of the uphill ski, slightly off balance to the rear, with the upper body leaning backward and the knee in full extension (5).

3. Flexion-internal rotation ("phantom foot mechanism") (Fig. 47-3): In this injury the skier typically loses balance, becomes positioned well back on the skies with knees flexed past 90°, has most of the weight on the tail of the downhill ski, and places his or her uphill arm backward. No weight is placed on the uphill ski, and the upper body faces the downhill ski; this positioning results in sudden internal rotation of the hyperflexed knee. If the magnitude of this moment is sufficient, the ACL is injured. This has been termed the phantom-foot injury mechanism because it results from edging of that portion of ski extending behind the foot. This injury mechanism is believed to be the most common and insidious ACL injury scenario in alpine skiing today (5).

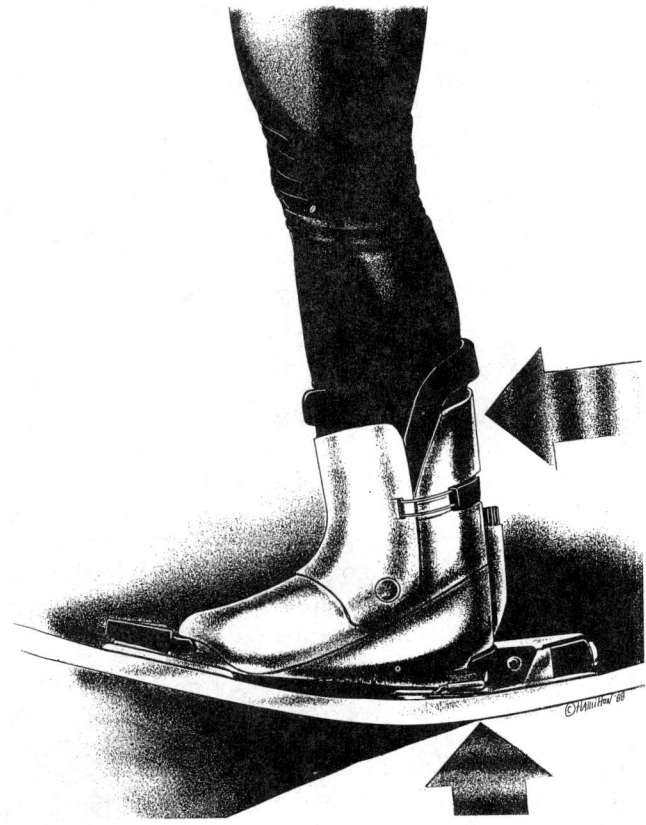

FIG. 47-2. The boot-induced anterior drawer knee injury mechanism in skiing. (Reprinted with permission from *The American Journal of Sports Medicine,* Vol. 23, No. 5, 1995, p. 533.)

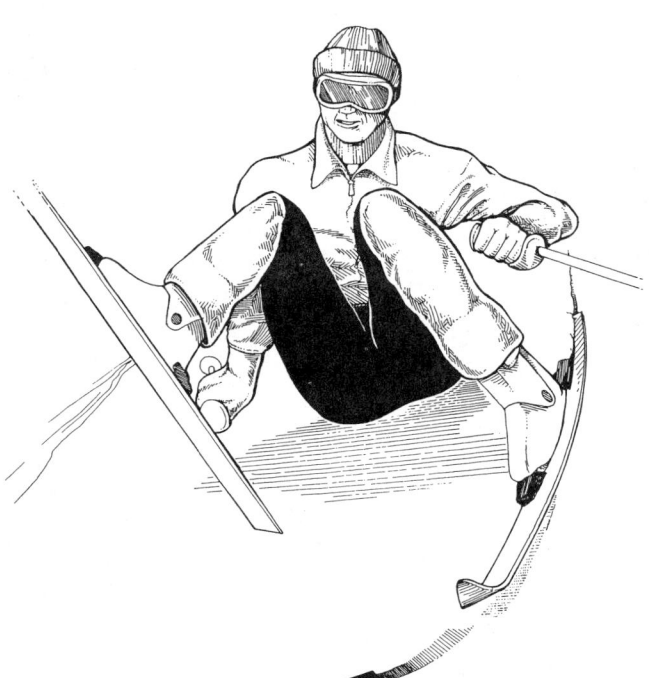

FIG. 47-3. The flexion–internal rotation ("phantom foot") knee injury mechanism in skiing. (Reprinted with permission from *The American Journal of Sports Medicine,* Vol. 23, No. 5, 1995, p. 532.)

4. Other suggested knee ligament injury mechanisms: A mechanism involving hyperextension or a combination of hyperextension and internal rotation may result in disruption of the anterior cruciate ligament (19). In our experience this mechanism is very rare. Some researchers (20) believe that another mechanism occurs when skiers are down and sliding with the principle axis of the ski perpendicular to the long axis of the body and the skier's direction of travel. At that point, the skier can suddenly catch the outside edge of the downhill ski; this creates a sudden jerk that lifts the tibia up suddenly and therefore puts the knee in internal rotation, resulting in an ACL disruption. It has also been proposed that a forceful quadriceps contraction may injure the ACL as the skier is trying to regain balance when he or she is off balance to the rear (21). The quadriceps muscle acts to translate the tibia anteriorly relative to the femur, if the knee is near extension (22). Although the ACL is influenced by the forces produced by the thigh muscles, there is some doubt as to whether a forceful quadriceps contraction alone can disrupt the ACL (23,24). In fact, a quadriceps muscle contraction acts to unload the ACL when the knee is flexed beyond 50–60° (25).

SPECIFIC INJURY RISK FACTORS

Gender

Although the overall risk of suffering a skiing injury is similar for females and males (26,27), it has been reported that the risk for severe knee injury in downhill skiing is higher for females than for males. Ellman and colleagues (28) found that female ski racers were six times more likely than males to sustain a severe knee injury. According to Ekeland (26) and Shealy and colleagues (27), females have about twice the knee injury rate of males. Stevenson and colleagues (29) found that among competitive skiers, the proportion of females to males sustaining a knee injury was 2.3 to 1. In addition, females were 3.1 times more likely to have sustained an ACL disruption than were their male counterparts. A study by Järvinen and colleagues (30) found that female skiers had a higher propensity to sustain ACL injuries by the phantom foot mechanism than did male skiers.

These results suggest that there are important anatomic as well as behavioral differences between male and female skiers. Today the high rate of noncontact ACL injuries in female athletes has become a prominent and controversial subject in many sports events (31). The suggestions for possible causative factors include gender differences in knee joint laxity, ligament or muscle strength, conditioning, endurance, femoral notch dimensions, or anatomy or even the effect of estrogen level (31–34). Huston and Wojtys (33) found that female athletes demonstrated more anterior tibial laxity than their male counterparts and significantly less muscle strength and endurance. The female athletes took significantly longer to generate maximum hamstring muscle torque during isokinetic testing. Further investigations are necessary to elucidate the variables resulting in the difference in the risk of ACL injuries between the sexes.

Age

The study from Sugarbush (17) showed that the overall rate of injury in children was 59% higher than that in adults. The study by Blitzer and colleagues (35) found that for all injuries combined, children under 11 years of age had the same rate of injury as adults. But foot and ankle injuries were more common in younger children. They had also more head and spine injuries than adults. Sherry and colleagues (36) reported that children are more prone to serious ski injuries than are adults—in particular, tibial fractures.

The high rate of tibia fractures sustained by children may indicate that they use poor-quality equipment and/or do not adjust their bindings properly (37,38). The bindings that children use tend to be adjusted higher than is recommended (35,39). It is recommended that parents provide modern equipment and make sure that the bindings are mounted, adjusted, and tested according to American Society of Testing and Materials (40) standard ski shop practices.

Skill Level

It has been estimated that a low skill level is the biggest single risk factor in skiing (26). Shealy (14) reported that the rate of injury of beginner skiers is ten times that of advanced skiers. Ekeland and colleagues (41) reported that beginners were six times more at risk for a lower extremity equipment-related injury than were skiers of higher skiing abilities. Blitzer and colleagues (35) reported that children with less skill or experience had a higher incidence of injuries than did more experienced skiers or the control population. Greenwald and Toelcke (42) found that isolated ACL injuries occurred much more often in advanced skiers than in beginners, while ACL rupture coupled with other soft tissue injury, particularly to the MCL, were significantly more common in beginners.

INJURY PREVENTION

Equipment

Bindings

Many reports have developed a clear relationship between the function of the binding release and boot and the incidence of lower leg injuries such as tibia and ankle fractures (11,43–47).

The alarming increase in the incidence of knee sprains since the late 1970s and early 1980s (7) has led many to suggest a connection between modern ski bindings and knee injuries. Binding-related injuries have been mentioned as being due to improper design, installation, adjustment, and maintenance (3,48). However, according to Ettlinger and colleagues (5), no statistically significant relationship has been found in any study between the quality or type of the binding and the increase in severe knee sprains. The events that lead to an ACL tear can be more subtle than those that lead to a lower leg fracture, so in most ACL injury scenarios, neither the binding nor the skier is forewarned.

The intended protective purpose of the release properties of the best binding systems is and always has been directed toward the prevention of midshaft tibial injuries where the ski acts as a lever to bend or twist the tibia, and thus there has never been any intent to prevent injuries to the knee. It would certainly be wonderful if modern boot–binding systems could protect against serious knee injuries, but there is no evidence that they can, and it is not clear that such protection is even feasible at this point.

Nevertheless, there may be some evidence that knee injuries produced by valgus stress and external rotation applied to the knee (MCL and combined MCL and ACL sprains) (see Fig. 47–1) may be prevented by properly adjusted and properly functioning modern bindings (49,50).

Both the International Standards Organization and the American Society for Testing and Materials (ASTM) have defined standard release settings for alpine ski bindings based on age, body weight, and skier type, and these should be closely followed. Standard ski shop practices have also been defined by ASTM. These should be followed to ensure that bindings that have been set to manufacturers' specifications and international standards are in fact functioning as they were intended. Only with release checks by trained shop mechanics using torque wrenches can appropriate binding function be assured. Only trained shop mechanics following ASTM standards shop practices should mount, set, and test bindings. Skiers should be discouraged from mounting and adjusting their own equipment if safe and reliable function is to be obtained.

Countries where standard shop practices are not in force should be encouraged to adopt them, since it has been well established that appropriately functioning modern bindings can greatly reduce the risk of most tibia and ankle injuries.

Skiing Boots

In the boot-induced mechanism of ACL injury (see Fig. 47–2), the design of the boot (rigid shell posteriorly with a fixed forward-lean angle) may directly contribute to injury. Years ago, boot tops were more flexible and allowed plantar flexion of the ankle, making such an injury mechanism less likely (4,18). In the future boots may be available that will allow plantar flexion of the ankle when loads exceed the levels necessary for productive control, decreasing strain on the ACL. A system that is sensitive to tibial displacement relative to the femur could possibly reduce these injuries. No such system currently exists, and it is not clear how one would function.

Helmets

Even though the long-term trends for head injuries in children and adolescents have not been found to be significant, they are nevertheless alarming (17). Several reports have documented that helmets may be beneficial, particularly for children and adolescents (41,51,52).

It is important to continue to reevaluate the potential benefits of wearing a helmet while skiing. A large helmet may increase the risk of an injury of the cervical spine, but a lightweight helmet with a diameter that is not substantially greater than the diameter of the skier's head could provide protection for the head while minimizing the problems associated with heavier helmets (17).

Although helmets can prevent head injury in impacts of up to 15 miles per hour, they would not necessarily reduce the incidence of severe injury in accidents occurring at higher speed. There is also concern that the use of helmets may encourage more reckless behavior, such as skiing faster and closer to trees. This behavior change induced by wearing a helmet may actually increase the risk of head injury in a segment of the skiing population.

Ski Poles

The rupture of ulnar collateral ligament of the metacarpophalangeal joint of the thumb (skier's thumb) is considered one of the most frequent injuries in skiing (as high as 20% of all ski injuries) (4,38,53). This injury is sustained when the skier attempts to break a fall with the hand still grasping the ski pole handle (4). It is noteworthy that snowboarders have very few injuries to the ulnar collateral ligament of the thumb because they do not grasp a ski pole.

To prevent skier's thumb, it is recommended that skiers avoid use of safety strap or gripping the poles outside the strap, since often the key feature of the injury is that the skier retained the pole in the hand at the moment of impact (4). The pole should be discarded before the skier places his or her hand in the snow to break a fall or attempt to recover during a fall.

Education

Using videotapes of skiers actually sustaining ACL sprains and the data associated with more than 1,900 ACL injuries observed in a 25-year study, we have identified two common mechanisms of ACL injury: the boot-induced and phantom foot mechanisms (see Figs. 47–2 and 47–3). An intervention study was designed to determine whether training could help to reduce the risk of ACL sprains (5,10). During the 1993–1994 ski season, the on-slope staff from 20 ski areas participated in a training program that involved viewing videotaped scenes in which ACL injuries occurred. The program used the technique of guided discovery, "a process in which subjects are presented with carefully selected stimuli intended to lead them to discover the mechanisms of ACL injury on their own" (5). In this way, participants develop an inner awareness of the situations that lead to ACL injury. The program was composed of three parts: avoiding high-risk behavior, recognizing potentially dangerous situations, and responding quickly and effectively. The professional skiing staff from 22 other ski areas who did not undergo the training served as a control group. Data concerning ACL injuries were collected from both groups for the three seasons between 1991 and 1994, and 179 serious knee sprains were evaluated. Any injury that was referred to as a grade II or III ACL sprain or a grade III knee sprain was included in the ACL count. Serious knee sprains declined by 62% among trained patrollers and instructors compared with the two previous seasons, but no decline occurred in the control group (5,10).

Following publication of the initial study, the study group was monitored for two subsequent seasons, and the reduction in the numbers of ACL injuries continued to be lower than the historic control level by better than 50%. A cost analysis of the ACL Awareness Training program proved that it is extremely effective from the standpoint of health care costs (5). To our knowledge, no other intervention has been shown to be as effective in reducing the incidence of ACL injury.

Bracing

In recent years a significant number of prophylactic or functional knee braces have become available that allegedly protect knee ligaments during physical activity. However, the use of these braces to decrease the risk of knee ligament injuries remains controversial, because present information reveals that available braces provide little or no control of knee laxity in anteroposterior direction (54,55). Only during application of very low forces can these braces resist anterior motion of the tibia relative to the femur (56). Moreover, Wojtys and colleagues (54) found that most braces appear to consistently slow hamstring muscle reaction times at the voluntary level, which could result in an increased risk of knee ligament injury. Thus functional or prophylactic knee braces cannot be relied on to protect the anterior cruciate ligament, whether intact or surgically reconstructed. The suggested proprioceptive benefits of knee braces may be more important than their mechanical stabilizing potential (57).

CONCLUSION AND RECOMMENDATIONS

There can be no doubt that the risk of lower extremity injury other than that of the knee has been reduced by the use of modern skiing equipment that is properly mounted, adjusted, and maintained. It is important that skiers seek trained shop mechanics who follow ASTM or similar shop practices for yearly or even more frequent checks to be certain that their equipment is functioning properly. Untrained individuals, including the skier himself or herself, should not perform these services if safety is to be assured.

There is no single or simple way to prevent ACL injuries. The knee and the forces that lead to ligament disruption are complicated. Education seems to hold as much promise as any other method to reduce the incidence of severe knee sprains. The apparent difference in the incidence of ACL injuries in males and females and the effects of conditioning on ACL strength deserve further study. Many people within the sports medicine community have devoted their careers to treating ACL injuries. Now is the time to commit more resources to preventing ACL injuries. Everyone with a professional or personal interest in sporting activities, including physicians, coaches, and physical therapists, needs to contribute to this knowledge base.

ACKNOWLEDGMENTS

This work was supported by the Medical Research Fund of the Tampere University Hospital, Tampere, Finland and Yrjö Jahnson Foundation Grant No. 3836.

REFERENCES

1. Burns TP, Steadman JR, Rodkey WG. Alpine skiing and the mature athlete. *Clin Sports Med* 1991;10:327–342.
2. Chissell HR, Feagin JA Jr, Warme WJ, et al. Trends in ski and snowboard injuries. *Sports Med* 1996;22:141–145.
3. Johnson RJ, Pope MH. Epidemiology and prevention of skiing injuries. *Ann Chir Gynaecol* 1991;80:110–115.
4. Kannus P, Johnson RJ. Downhill skiing injuries: trends to watch for this season. *J Musculoskel Med* 1991;8:13–32.
5. Ettlinger CF, Johnson RJ, Shealy JE. A method to help reduce the risk of serious knee sprains incurred in alpine skiing. *Am J Sports Med* 1995;23:531–537.
6. Natri A, Järvinen M, Kannus P, et al. Changing injury pattern of acute anterior cruciate ligament tears treated at Tampere University Hospital in 1980s. *Scand J Med Sci Sports* 1995;5:100–104.

7. Johnson RJ, Ettlinger CF, Shealy JE. Skier injury trends: 1972 to 1994. In: Johnson RJ, Mote CD Jr, Ekeland A, eds. *Skiing trauma and safety: Eleventh International Symposium, ASTM STP 1289*. Philadelphia: American Society for Testing and Materials, 1997:37–48.
8. Johnson RJ, Ettlinger CF, Shealy JE. Skier injury trends 1972–1990. In: Johnson RJ, Mote CD Jr, Zelcer J, eds. *Skiing trauma and safety: Ninth International Symposium, ASTM STP 1182*. Philadelphia: American Society for Testing and Materials, 1993:11–22.
9. Paletta GA, Warren RF. Knee injuries and alpine skiing. *Sports Med* 1994;17:411–423.
10. Ryder SH, Johnson RJ, Beynnon BD, Ettlinger CF. Prevention of ACL injuries. *J Sports Rehab* 1997;6:80–96.
11. Johnson RJ, Pope MH, Ettlinger CF. Ski injuries and equipment function. *J Sports Med* 1974;2:299–307.
12. Shealy JE. Overall analysis of NSAA/ASTM data on skiing injuries for 1978 through 1981. In: Johnson RJ, Mote CD Jr, eds. *Skiing trauma and safety: Fifth International Symposium, ASTM STP 860*. Philadelphia: American Society for Testing and Materials, 1985:302–313.
13. Johnson RJ, Ettlinger CF, Shealy JE. Skier injury trends. In: Johnson RJ, Mote CD Jr, Binet M-H, eds. *Skiing trauma and safety: Seventh International Symposium, ASTM STP 1022*. Philadelphia: American Society for Testing and Materials, 1989:25–31.
14. Shealy JE. Comparison of downhill ski injury patterns: 1978–81 vs. 1988–90. In: Johnson RJ, Mote CD Jr, Zelcer J, eds. *Skiing trauma and safety: Ninth International Symposium, ASTM STP 1182*. Philadelphia: American Society for Testing and Materials, 1993:23–32.
15. Warme WJ, Feagin JA Jr, King P, et al. Ski injury statistics, 1982 to 1993, Jackson Hole ski resort. *Am J Sports Med* 1995;23:597–600.
16. Johnson RJ. Prevention of cruciate ligament injuries. In: Feagin JA Jr, ed. *The crucial ligaments*. New York: Churchill Livingstone, 1988:349–356.
17. Deibert MC, Aronsson DD, Johnson RJ, et al. Skiing injuries in children, adolescents, and adults. *J Bone Joint Surg* 1998;80-A:25–32.
18. Elmqvist LG, Johnson RJ. Prevention of cruciate ligament injuries. In: Feagin JA Jr, ed. *The crucial ligaments*, 2nd ed. New York: Churchill Livingstone, 1994:495–505.
19. Feagin JA, Lambert KL, Cunningham RR, et al. Consideration of the anterior cruciate ligament injury in skiing. *Clin Orthop* 1987;216:13–18.
20. Chambat P, Siegrist O, Neyret Ph, Millon J. ACL rupture mechanism during skiing. Twelfth International Symposium on Ski Trauma and Safety, May 4–10, Whistler, British Columbia, Canada, 1997, Abstract no 57.
21. McConkey JP. Anterior cruciate ligament rupture in skiing: a new mechanism of injury. *Am J Sports Med* 1986;14:160–164.
22. Beynnon B, Howe JG, Pope MH, et al. The measurement of anterior cruciate ligament strain in vivo. *Int Orthop* 1992;16:1–12.
23. Chiang AL, Mote CD Jr. Translations and rotations across the knee under isometric quadriceps contraction. In: Johnson RJ, Mote CD Jr, Zelcer J, eds. *Skiing trauma and safety: Ninth International Symposium, ASTM STP 1182*. Philadelphia: American Society for Testing and Materials, 1993:62–74.
24. Aune AK, Schaff P, Nordsletten L. Contraction of knee flexors and extensors in skiing related to the backward fall mechanism of injury to the anterior cruciate ligament. *Scand J Med Sci Sports* 1995;5:165–169.
25. Aune AK, Cawley PW, Ekeland A. Quadriceps muscle contraction protects the anterior cruciate ligament during anterior tibial translation. *Am J Sports Med* 1997;25:187–190.
26. Ekeland A. The knees are in danger in skiing [Editorial]. *Scand J Med Sci Sports* 1995;5:61–63.
27. Shealy JE, Johnson RJ, Ettlinger CF. Gender- and age-related skiing injury patterns. Abstract in the 11th International Congress on Ski Trauma and Skiing Safety, Voss, Norway, April 23–29, 1995. *Scand J Med Sci Sports* 1995;5:111.
28. Ellman B, Holmes E, Jordan J, McCarty P. Cruciate ligament injuries in female alpine ski racers. In: Johnson RJ, Mote CD Jr, Binet M-H, eds. *Skiing trauma and safety: Seventh International Symposium, ASTM STP 1022*. Philadelphia: American Society for Testing and Materials, 1989:105–111.
29. Stevenson H, Webster J, Johnson R, Beynnon B. Gender differences in knee injury epidemiology amongst competitive alpine ski racers. *Iowa Orthop J* 1998;18:64–66.
30. Järvinen M, Natri A, Laurila S, Kannus P. Mechanisms of anterior cruciate ligament ruptures in skiing. *Knee Surg Sports Traumatol Arthrosc* 1994;2:224–228.
31. Ireland ML, Gaudette M, Crook S. ACL injuries in the female athletes. *J Sports Rehab* 1997;6:97–110.
32. Arendt E, Dick R. Knee injury patterns among men and women in collegiate basketball and soccer. *Am J Sports Med* 1995;23:694–701.
33. Huston LJ, Wojtys EM. Neuromuscular performance characteristics in elite female athletes. *Am J Sports Med* 1996;24:427–436.
34. Liu SH, Al-Shaik RA, Panossian V, et al. Estrogen affects the cellular metabolism of the anterior cruciate ligament: a potential explanation for female athletic injury. *Am J Sports Med* 1997;25:704–709.
35. Blitzer CM, Johnson RJ, Ettlinger CF, Aggeborn K. Downhill skiing injuries in children. *Am J Sports Med* 1984;12:142–147.
36. Sherry E, Korbel P, Henderson A. Children's skiing injuries in Australia. *Med J Aust* 1987;146:193–195.
37. Ungerholm S, Gustavsson J. Skiing safety in children: a prospective study of downhill skiing injuries and their relation to the skier and his equipment. *Int J Sports Med* 1985;6:353–358.
38. Bouter LM, Knipschild PG. Causes and prevention of injury in downhill skiing. *Phys Sportsmed* 1989;17:81–94.
39. Ungerholm S, Gierup J, Gustavsson J, Lindsjo U. Skiing safety in children: adjustment and reliability of the bindings. *Int J Sports Med* 1984;5:325–329.
40. *Annual book of ASTM standards*. Philadelphia: American Society for Testing and Materials, 1985.
41. Ekeland A, Holtmoen A, Lystad H. Lower extremity equipment-related injuries in alpine recreational skiers. *Am J Sports Med* 1993;21:201–205.
42. Greenwald RM, Toelcke T. Gender differences in alpine skiing injuries: a profile of the knee-injured skier. In: Johnson RJ, Mote CD Jr, Ekeland A, eds. *Skiing trauma and safety: Eleventh International Symposium, ASTM STP 1289*. Baltimore: American Society for Testing and Materials, 1997:111–121.
43. Spademan R. Lower-extremity injuries as related to the use of ski safety bindings. *JAMA* 1968;203:445–450.
44. Eriksson E. Ski injuries in Sweden: a one year survey. *Orthop Clin North Am* 1976;7:3–9.
45. Johnson RJ, Ettlinger CF, Campbell RJ, Pope MH. Trends in skiing injuries: analysis of a 6-year study (1972 to 1978). *Am J Sports Med* 1980;8:106–113.
46. Ettlinger CF, Johnson RJ. The state of the art in preventing equipment-related alpine ski injuries. *Clin Sports Med* 1982;1:199–207.
47. Johnson RJ, Ettlinger CF. Alpine ski injuries: changes through the years. *Clin Sports Med* 1982;1:181–197.
48. Ekeland A, Nordsletten L. Equipment related injuries in skiing: recommendations. *Sports Med* 1994;17:284–287.
49. Hauser W. Experimental prospective skiing injury study. In: Johnson RJ, Mote CD Jr, Binet M-H, eds. *Skiing trauma and safety: Seventh International Symposium, ASTM STP 1022*. Philadelphia: American Society for Testing and Materials, 1989:18–24.
50. Hull ML. Analysis of skiing accidents involving combined injuries to the medial collateral and anterior cruciate ligaments. *Am J Sports Med* 1997;25:35–40.
51. Sandegård J, Ericson B, Lundqvist S. Nationwide registration of ski injuries in Sweden. In: Johnson RJ, Mote CD Jr, eds. *Skiing trauma and safety: Eighth International Symposium, ASTM STP 1104*. Philadelphia: American Society for Testing and Materials, 1991:170–176.
52. Lystad H, Thoresen I. Head injuries in alpine skiing: can they be prevented? Paper presented at the 10th International World Congress on Ski Trauma and Skiing Safety, Zell am See, Austria, May 17–21, 1993.
53. Asikainen P, Lüthje P, Järvinen M, et al. Downhill skiing injuries and their cost at a Finnish skiing area. *Scand J Med Sci Sports* 1991;1:228–231.

54. Wojtys E, Kothari S, Huston L. Anterior cruciate ligament functional brace use in sports. *Am J Sports Med* 1996;24:539–546.
55. Beynnon B, Johnson RJ, Fleming BC, et al. The effect of functional knee bracing on the anterior cruciate ligament in the weightbearing and nonweightbearing knee. *Am J Sports Med* 1997;25:353–359.
56. Beynnon BD, Pope MH, Wertheimer CM, et al. The effect of functional knee braces on strain on the anterior cruciate ligament in vivo. *J Bone Joint Surg* 1992;74-A:1298–1312.
57. Németh G, Lamontagne M, Tho KS, Eriksson E. Electromyographic activity in expert downhill skiers using functional knee braces after anterior cruciate ligament injuries. *Am J Sports Med* 1997;25:635–641.

CHAPTER 48

Soccer

Lawrence L. Golusinski, Jr.

INTRODUCTION

More than 40 million individuals around the world participate in soccer. The sport is enjoyed by both genders and every age. With such a large following, soccer is responsible for a large number of sports injuries. Many investigators have studied soccer and its related injuries. These studies have attempted to describe the patterns and causes of soccer injuries. Many of these studies are difficult to compare because of their different populations, definitions of injury, and study methodologies.

Because soccer has enjoyed its greatest popularity in Europe, most published studies come from researchers in those countries. Some of these reports attempt to describe the percentage of sports injuries that are attributable to soccer. While such information may be useful in these individual countries or in countries with similar sports participation, one must be careful not to apply the data to countries where the percentage of soccer participants may be different from that in the countries studied. Soccer injuries may cause up to 40–55% of all sports injuries, depending on the location of the study (1,2).

Studies have employed different definitions of injuries. Most definitions include two elements: The injury must be a medical problem that occurs during the play of soccer, whether game or practice, and the injury must result in time lost from subsequent competition or practice. If the injury occurred during a game, most definitions require that either the participant leave the game or play is stopped because of the injury. Some definitions have also included adverse social or economic effects in determining whether a medical complaint is considered an injury. However, while time lost from competition or practice may be useful in helping define increasingly serious injuries, minor injuries requiring treatment on the field or in the treatment room and not resulting in time lost from play might not get included. It is important to include even these minor injuries, as they utilize medical resources and may affect player performance.

Several different methodologies have been used to study and describe soccer-related injuries. A number of studies use insurance data or visits to the sports medicine clinic or hospital as a basis for sampling. While these are readily available data, retrospective studies based on insurance claims or visits to a physician underestimate the number of injuries, since many injuries may be self-treated or treated by the coach or trainer. These studies overestimate the severity of injuries, as a disproportionate number of players with serious injuries may present to the physician's office or hospital. A number of prospective studies are reported in the literature. These use various mechanisms: information gathered from trainers and coaches, on-site evaluation by physicians of players seeking medical assistance, and even aggressive seeking out of potentially injured players during matches. While labor intensive, these studies probably provide a more accurate description of soccer-related injuries, since acute and chronic, mild and severe cases will all be seen. However, even these studies are fraught with some bias, owing to the players' differences in reporting symptoms and seeking evaluation. Finally, many soccer injuries are reported in the literature as case reports. While important contributions to the body of knowledge about soccer-related injuries, these do not allow for the calculation of incidence rates or relative risk for injuries and should serve as the basis for continuing study.

With these different methodologies, investigators have found incidence rates to be as low as 0.66 per 1000 playing hours (1) and as high as 32 per 1000 playing hours (3). The majority of studies place the incidence rate between 4 and 20 per 1000 playing hours.

Most (50–65%) soccer injuries are mild, resulting in less than one week of time lost from play; the remainder

---

L. L. Golusinski, Jr.: Department of Family and Preventive Medicine, Emory University School of Medicine, Altanta, Georgia 30306.

are split between moderate (20–40%), resulting in 1 week to 1 month of time lost from play, and severe (10–30%), resulting in more than 1 month of time lost from play (4,5). The vast majority of reported soccer injuries are sprains, strains, and contusions. Fractures account for fewer than 10% of injuries (6,7). Most injuries (70–90%) are acute, while 10–30% are overuse or chronic injuries (5,8). These overuse injuries often happen in the preseason period, occurring more frequently during practice, while traumatic injuries occur during games (9).

HEAD AND NECK INJURIES

Injuries to the head and neck make up approximately 4–22% of soccer-related injuries (4,7,8,10–13). These include abrasions, contusions, lacerations, fractures, eye injuries, and acute and chronic brain injury.

Abrasions, contusions, and lacerations make up more than half of the injuries to the head and neck. However, these do not usually result in time lost from play (8,10).

Soccer is responsible for acute fractures of the nasal bones, mandible, and orbital wall. These are usually due to impact with another player but may also be due to impact with the ground, ball, or goalposts (14,15). Nasal fractures account for about two thirds of facial fractures. Zygomatic and mandibular fractures together make up about one third of facial fractures (16). Mandibular fractures are associated with mucosal lacerations, lost or fractured teeth, and concussion (17). Soccer players make up as many as 30% of orbital blowout fractures due to sporting activity (15).

Injuries to the eyes make up a small percentage of soccer injuries. However, when such trauma occurs, its severity may often necessitate hospitalization. Periorbital injuries, such as orbital blowout fractures, hyphema, and corneal abrasions, are most common. Uveitis, retinal edema, angle recession, glaucoma secondary to intraocular bleeding, retinal tear, and rupture of the globe all occur. Injuries may be caused by the ball or by another player's body parts, such as head, fingers, elbows, or foot. Some injuries are caused by shattered glass from prescription eyewear. Foreign bodies and lime used to mark the playing field may cause corneal abrasions or conjunctivitis. Fortunately, despite their initial severity, soccer-related eye injuries do not cause permanent decreases in visual acuity (18–22).

Acute neck injuries may include cervical muscle strains, fractures to the cervical spine, cervical disk herniation, central cervical cord syndrome, and brachial plexus injuries (23). Chronic arthritic changes in the cervical spine attributable to repetitive minor trauma from heading the ball have been described. These degenerative changes occur at an earlier age and more frequently than in controls. Heading the ball does not seem to contribute to these radiographic findings, but former players who believe that they frequently headed the ball have been found to have a tendency to have more complaints of pain and stiffness later in life (24).

Acute brain injuries, primarily concussions, make up about 1–3% of soccer injuries (11,12,25) or between 0.14 and 0.6 concussions per 1000 athlete exposures (13,26). Men are more likely to sustain concussions than are women (12,13). Deaths are extremely rare and when they occur are usually due to collision with a goalpost (27,28). The most common mechanisms of injury for concussions are collision with another player, collision with the ground, and unintentional contact with the ball. Grade I concussions make up the vast majority of these acute injuries (12,13). Chronic brain injury due to heading the ball has probably caused the most worry in regard to soccer injuries to the head and neck. Some studies have shown abnormal electroencephalograms, computerized tomography, magnetic resonance images, and neuropsychiatric studies in soccer players (29–34). Other studies have not shown such abnormalities (16,26). Differences between these studies may be due to lack of control groups and to confounding variables such as alcohol use and previous brain injury. In one study of elite soccer players, almost 90% of men and over 40% of women reported having a previous head injury with over half of the men and more than one-third of the women reporting a previous concussion (12). A 1996 study that addressed these deficiencies found that age when soccer playing was begun, length of time playing, and frequency of heading were not correlated with symptoms of chronic brain injury (24,26). Only the history of a previous concussion was associated with symptoms of chronic brain injury. No studies conclusively show a correlation between heading the ball and long-term sequelae.

INJURIES TO THE SHOULDER, ARM, WRIST, AND HAND

Upper extremity injuries make up 3–30% of soccer injuries (4,7,8,10). The majority of these are due to lacerations, contusions, sprains, and strains, with less than half being attributable to fractures and dislocations (7,8). Most fractures and dislocations involving the forearm and wrist, including scaphoid fractures and distal radius fractures, are due to a fall onto an outstretched hand. Only one fifth of distal radius fractures are caused by the ball hitting the wrist (35–37). Falls may also result in clavicle fractures and shoulder dislocations, usually anteriorly, although posterior dislocations have been described. Players are at risk for hand injuries such as dislocations of the proximal interphalangeal joints, phalangeal fractures, and carpal and metacarpal fractures. Falls are the primary cause of carpal fractures, specifically scaphoid fractures, although hyperextension injuries of the wrist caused by blocking the ball also have been described (35). Player contact is more often the cause of metacarpal fractures (38,39). Because they may use their hands during play, goalkeepers also sustain injuries to the ulnar collateral ligament of the thumb and are at higher risk of hand injuries in general (40). More serious degloving injuries have been described in goalkeepers who have gotten their rings caught on a hook in the nets (41).

INJURIES TO THE TRUNK AND BACK

Five to eleven percent of soccer injuries occur to the torso (4,7,8,11). Injuries to the back may occur in up to 14% of patients (25). In adolescents back pain may be due to spondylolysis secondary to stress fractures of the pars interarticularis.

Abdominal injuries are not uncommon. These usually consist of contusions to the abdominal wall or damaged kidneys. Less commonly, they may involve the spleen, small intestine, pancreas, and liver. Rib fractures may be associated with up to one quarter of intraabdominal injuries (42).

INJURIES TO THE PELVIS

Groin pain may occur in 13% of soccer players (43) while 5–8% of soccer injuries are to the groin (44,45). Its etiology may be difficult to elucidate, as many injuries and conditions may cause groin pain. Strains of the iliopsoas, adductors, rectus abdominis, and rectus femoris may all cause pain (43,46,47). Bony problems such as stress fractures to the femoral neck and anterior iliac crest, avascular necrosis, and avulsion fractures may also occur. Other surgical and medical problems such as hernia, nerve entrapment, appendicitis, and prostatitis must be considered in evaluating groin pain. An increasingly recognized cause of groin pain is Gilmore's groin, also known as sports hernia or athletic pubalgia. This musculotendinous injury in the area of the inguinal canal affects primarily men and presents as insidious groin pain without a clinical hernia (44).

Trauma to the testicles from the soccer ball or stray kicks also occurs and may require operative intervention. Such trauma may result in a scrotal or intratesticular hematoma or may result in rupture of the testicle (48).

INJURIES TO THE LEG, KNEE, ANKLE, AND FOOT

The vast majority of injuries in soccer are to the lower extremities. Studies have found a range of 60–90% of soccer injuries occurring in the hip, thigh, knee, leg, ankle, and foot (4,7,8,10,11). In most studies, the knee and the ankle are the most common sites of injury (4,7). In other studies, the thigh is most commonly injured, followed by the knee and ankle (8,11).

Knee injuries account for 16–25% of all soccer injuries (4,7,8,10,11,49). The most common knee injury is a collateral ligament sprain, composing about 40% of all knee injuries (49). Among college men, meniscal tears and patella/patella tendon injuries are the next most common injuries, contributing to 16% of knee injuries. Anterior cruciate ligament tears make up about 10% of knee injuries in men. In college women, meniscal injuries and anterior cruciate ligament tears are the second most common injuries, each making up about 20% of all knee injuries. Posterior cruciate ligament tears are relatively uncommon in both genders, contributing to about 3% of all knee injuries (49). Decreased knee extension strength is associated with an increased risk of noncontact injuries but not contact injuries. This difference may be due to ligamentous laxity or inadequate rehabilitation of previous injuries (9,43). Chondral delamination injuries to the knees are being described more frequently in soccer players with symptoms of pain, effusion, and joint line tenderness (50).

Ankle injuries are the second most common injury reported in the soccer epidemiology literature. Between 13% and 26% of soccer injuries involve the ankle (4,6–8,10,11). The vast majority of these are lateral ligament sprains. The dominant leg is most often affected, and almost half of ankle injuries occur in previously injured ankles (9). Repetitive ankle sprains may result in ankle impingement due to either osteophytes or fibrous bands forming between the tibia or the fibula and the talus (51). Subluxation or dislocation of the peroneal tendons (52) and rupture of the posterior tibialis and flexor hallucis brevis tendons may also occur (53).

Other foot injuries, such as plantar fasciitis, metatarsal phalangeal joint sprains, and fractures to the tarsals, metatarsals, and phalanges, may occur. Stress fractures of the second and fifth metatarsals are the most common stress fractures in soccer players.

Depending on the study, thigh injuries constitute 10–45% of soccer injuries (6–8,11). Some studies indicate that the majority of these injuries are contusions while other studies report the majority to be muscle strains. Contusions may occur in the shins and may result in acute compartment syndrome. Compartment syndrome may also occur with exertion and noncontact injuries (54,55).

Fractures of the lower extremity occur in about 3% of soccer injuries (7,8). However, although infrequent, fractures of the tibia and fibula account for a significant time missed from play. Most fractures of the tibia are caused by a slide tackle (56). Soccer players are also at risk for stress fractures of the leg, usually of the tibia and fibula (57).

The lower extremities are also subject to chronic injuries. Studies have reported increased incidence of osteoarthritis of the hip (58), knee (59,60), and ankle (61). Former soccer players have a higher incidence of radiographic evidence of osteoarthritis of the knee. In addition to their higher frequency, these changes occur at an earlier age than in controls. While much of this increase may be due to the sequelae of meniscal injury and subsequent meniscectomy, up to 41% of knees without meniscectomies may have degenerative changes. Fortunately, the vast majority (70%) of these knees with degenerative radiographic changes are asymptomatic (60). Muscle strains are often considered chronic overuse injuries when reported in the soccer literature. Quadriceps strains, adductor strains, hamstring strains, and Achilles tendinitis may occur (39). These may be associated with muscle tightness in these muscle groups.

OTHER INJURIES

Soccer may also be the cause of a number of nonmusculoskeletal injuries. Heat illness has been found to be the cause of 4.5% of soccer injuries (11). Less commonly, soccer may cause skin infections. There have been reports of group A streptococcus skin infections following an indoor soccer tournament (62) and aeromonas hydrophila wound infections following contamination of a wound with water from a brook bordering the playing field (63). Contact dermatitis caused by shin guards has been described (64).

INJURY TRENDS

Variations with Age

Most studies agree that younger players, those less than 12 years old, sustain fewer injuries than players older than 12 years old (4,7) Such injuries are also less serious (3,61) and may more commonly affect the head and upper extremity (65). The increase in body size and strength with increasing age, resulting in increased body and ball momentum, may be the cause of the more serious injuries in older players, while lower skill levels in younger players, resulting in more falls, poor heading technique, and illegal contact with the ball, may be the cause of the higher proportion of head and upper extremity injuries (25,65). Injury rates then increase with increasing age, peaking in some studies in the late teens (6) and in other studies in the twenties (4,7). Older players incur more muscle strains, while younger players sustain more contusions (65). Among adolescents, boys who are skeletally mature but muscularly weak may be at a higher risk of injury (66). Players who are skeletally immature may develop Sever disease or calcaneal apophysitis (67).

Gender

Men have the greatest absolute number of soccer injuries, owing to the larger number of men participating in the sport. However, using calculations based on exposures or hours played, studies show that the injury rate for women is higher than that for men (68). The incidence of injury in outdoor play in women is usually described as being twice that of men in studies comparing the genders. This difference does not seem to be present when the incidence of injuries in indoor play is studied. Studies of indoor soccer have shown approximately equal incidences for both genders (4,10). The age at which the most injuries occur differs between men and women, with women having higher injury rates at lower ages (4).

The types of injuries also vary between the sexes, with men suffering more ankle injuries and women suffering more muscle contusions (4). Patterns of overuse differ, with men suffering from adductor and Achilles tendinitis (9) and women having more iliotibial band syndrome and medial tibial stress syndrome (69). In addition, one study has suggested that women are at higher risk of traumatic injury during the menstrual and premenstrual portions of their cycles and may be at lower risk when using oral contraceptives (70).

Of great concern is the finding that anterior cruciate ligament injuries occur at almost twice the frequency in women as in men (49,69). In addition, tears of the meniscus have also found to occur more frequently in women (49). However, this finding may be confounded by the high association of meniscus tears with anterior cruciate ligament tears. The mechanism of injury also differs for women with fewer contact injuries and more noncontact injuries (49).

Variations with Level of Play, Location of Play, and Position

As one would expect, injuries are more frequent as the intensity of play increases. Studies have shown that the incidence of injuries is higher during games than during practices (71). Injuries may occur almost twice as frequently during games (72). Players at higher levels of play are almost twice as likely to incur injury as those at lower levels of play (6).

Despite being the fewest in number on the field, goalkeepers suffer more injuries than players in other positions in outdoor soccer (2,73). These injuries are more often of the head and upper extremities. In indoor soccer, however, goalkeepers may experience fewer injuries than field players (4,10).

Some studies have shown higher injury rates in outdoor soccer as compared to indoor soccer (65). Other studies have shown the indoor soccer to have as high as six times the injury rate of outdoor soccer (4,10,73). It is thought that the confined field size, surrounding walls, and fast-paced nature of indoor soccer may contribute to the higher rate of injury.

PREVENTION OF INJURIES

The majority of injuries may be caused by factors that may be altered to minimize the risk of injury. These factors include joint instability, muscle tightness, inadequate rehabilitation, lack of training, playing field, equipment, and rules violations (43). Attempts to prevent soccer injuries may be made in two ways: primary prevention and secondary prevention. Primary prevention of injuries seeks to prevent the initial occurrence of injuries. Such prevention may address the player, the field and equipment, and the rules.

A general conditioning program for participants may help to prevent injury. Teams with more hours of practice have been found to have lower rates of traumatic injuries during practice. However, the benefit from more practice time does not seem to protect against overuse injuries during practice (72). Studies comparing preseason and in-season incidence rates show the latter to be decreased, suggesting the benefit of training and conditioning (9,74). Likewise, injuries have been found to be more common in the second half of games and higher in the final rounds than in the qualifying rounds of tournaments (3,8,75), suggesting that fatigue may play a factor in injuries. A training and conditioning program may help to prevent this as well. Conditioning programs should address specific body parts in which poor body mechanics have been shown to be related to ankle, knee, and back injuries (76). Players with tight muscles are more likely to suffer from strains (43). Warm-ups focusing on stretching frequently injured muscles may help to prevent acute strains. Likewise, cool-downs may help to prevent future injury by decreasing muscle tightness as well. Stretching during warm-ups and cool-downs should include adequate stretching of all of the muscles of the lower extremity, with a special focus on the adductors, a muscle group in which tightness has been associated with injury (43). In addition to stretching during a conditioning program, one study suggests that inclusion of a proprioceptive training program may reduce the incidence of anterior cruciate ligament tears (77).

Equipment and the playing field play a role in primary prevention of soccer injuries. Failure to use shin guards has been related to the lower leg injuries (43). Shin guards decrease the force transmitted to the lower leg (78) and may help reduce the frequency and severity of minor injuries such as contusions and abrasions as well as more severe fractures (56,79). Those shin guards that distribute the force of the impact along the length of the guard, are more compliant and increase the contact time during impact, and are thicker and longer provide the most protection, especially at higher impact forces (79). As many as 13% of injuries have been attributed to poor footwear (43). Inadequate shoes, especially when used with screw-in cleats, have been related to injuries as well (65). Players and coaches should be educated in the consistent use of appropriate shinguards and proper footwear. Men should use protective athletic cups to avoid testicular trauma. The American Dental Association has recommended the use of mouthguards (80). These protect the teeth and reduce the incidence of concussion (81). The American Academy of Pediatrics has recommended that polycarbonate lenses be worn as protective eye equipment (67). Poor field conditions, such as rough or slippery surfaces, and sprinkler heads and other foreign objects have also been related to as many as a quarter of injuries (43). Efforts should be made to maintain safe field conditions, and the playing pitch should be inspected before play to try to minimize dangerous conditions. Goalposts have caused head injuries and even deaths (27). To prevent such injuries, goalposts should be secured to the ground and covered with padding. Such padding has been shown to decrease goalpost injuries to players (82).

In multiple studies, both players and referees have related that up to one third of injuries are caused by fouls (5,8,43,74). The player causing the foul may be likely to be more seriously injured, as measured by time missed from play (43). Given the high percentages of injuries that occur during fouls, referees should take care to enforce the rules of play, and coaches should encourage players to play accordingly. Proper coaching in heading may also reduce head injuries resulting from poor technique.

Secondary prevention attempts to prevent reinjury or further damage to an already injured player. Minor injuries often precede moderate and severe injuries within a season (9,61), and close to half of injured players may report a similar injury in the year before a specific injury (5). More than half of players with previous injuries may have residual symptoms. Mechanical instability and ligamentous laxity have been found in up to 25% of previously injured knees and ankles (69). This has prompted study of rehabilitative efforts to prevent reinjury, and some studies of ankle injuries have suggested that a physical therapy program may decrease the rate of reinjuries. In addition, taping and bracing have been shown to be effective in preventing subsequent injuries (74). Use of an ankle stirrup orthosis has been shown to decrease the incidence of reinjury of ankles, though not the incidence of primary injury (83). Most studies indicate that such bracing does not negatively impact performance; however, player reaction to and acceptance of such protective equipment varies. Ankle rehabilitation has been recommended for players with sprained ankles prior to return to play. In addition, those with more severe injuries should wear an ankle stabilizing orthosis for 6–12 months after the injury to prevent recurrence (84).

Such primary and secondary prevention methods have reduced soccer injuries up to 75% in some studies (65).

REFERENCES

1. de Loës M. Epidemiology of sports injuries in the Swiss organization "Youth and Sports" 1987–1989. *Int J Sports Med* 1995; 16:134–138.
2. Stokes MA, McKeever JA, McQuillan RF, et al. A season of football injuries. *Irish J Med Sci* 1994;163:290–293.
3. Nillson S, Roass A. Soccer injuries in adolescents. *Am J Sports Med* 1978;6:358–361.
4. Lindenfeld TN, Schmitt DJ, Hendy MP, et al. Incidence of injury in indoor soccer. *Am J Sports Med* 1994;22:364–371.
5. Nielsen AB, Yde J. Epidemiology and traumatology of injuries in soccer. *Am J Sports Med* 1989;17:803–807.
6. Inklaar H, Bol E, Schmikli SL, et al. Injuries in male soccer players: team risk analysis. *Int J Sports Med* 1996;17:229–234.
7. Kujala UM, Taimela S, Antti-Poika I, et al. Acute injuries in soccer, ice hockey, volleyball, basketball, judo and karate: analysis of national registry data. *BMJ* 1995;311:1465–1468.
8. Lüthje P, Nurmi I, Kataja M, et al. Epidemiology and traumatology of injuries in elite soccer: a prospective study in Finland. *Scand J Med Sci Sports* 1996;6:180–185.
9. Ekstrand J, Gillquist J. Soccer injuries and their mechanisms: a prospective study. *Med Sci Sports Exerc* 1983;15:267–270.
10. Putukian M, Knowles WK, Swere S, et al. Injuries in indoor soccer: the Lake Placid Dawn to Dark Soccer Tournament. *Am J Sports Med* 1996;24:317–322.
11. Kibler WB. Injuries in adolescent and preadolescent soccer players. *Med Sci Sports Exerc* 1993;25:1330–1332.
12. Barnes BC, Cooper L, Kirkendall DT, et al. Concussion history in elite male and female soccer players. *Am J Sports Med* 1998; 26:433–438.
13. Boden BP, Kirkendall DT, Garrett WE. Concussion incidence in elite college soccer players. *Am J Sports Med* 1998;26:238–241.
14. Tanka N, Hayashi S, Amagasa T, et al. Maxillofacial fractures sustained during sports. *J Oral Maxillofac Surg* 1996;54:715–719.
15. Jones NP. Orbital blowout fractures in sport. *Br J Sports Med* 1994;28:272–275.
16. Frenguelli A, Ruscito P, Biccioto G, et al. Head and neck trauma in sporting activities. *J Craniomaxillofac Surg* 1991;19:178–181.
17. Emshoff R, Schöning H, Röthler, et al. Trends in the incidence and cause of sport-related mandibular fractures: a retrospective analysis. *J Oral Maxillofac Surg* 1997;55:585–592.
18. Burke MJ, Sanitato JJ, Vinger PF, et al. Soccerball induced eye injuries. *JAMA* 1983;249:2682–2685.
19. Orlando RG. Soccer-related eye injuries in children and adolescents. *Phys Sportsmed* 1988;16:103–106.
20. MacEwen CJ. Sport associated eye injury: a casualty department survey. *Br J Ophthalmol* 1987;71:701–705.
21. MacEwen CJ. Eye injuries: a prospective survey of 5671 cases. *Br J Ophthalmol* 1989;73:888–894.
22. Jones NP. Orbital blowout fractures in sport. *Br J Sports Med* 1994;28:272–275.
23. Tysvaer AT. Head and neck injuries in soccer. *Sports Med* 1992; 14:200–213.
24. Sortland O, Tysvaer, Storli OV. Changes in the cervical spine in association football players. *Br J Sports Med* 1982;16:80–84.
25. Schmidt-Olsen S, Jørgensen U, Kaalund S, et al. Injuries among young soccer players *Am J Sports Med* 1991;19:273–275.
26. Jordan SE, Green GA, Galanty HL, et al. Acute and chronic brain injury in United States national team soccer players. *Am J Sports Med* 1996;24:205–210.
27. Injuries associated with soccer goalposts: United States, 1979–1993. *MMWR Morb Mortal Wkly Rep* 1994;43:153–155.
28. United States Consumer Product Safety Commission summary reports. National Electronic Injury Surveillance System: 1990 through 1992, Washington, DC, US Consumer Product Safety Commission, 1993.
29. Tysvaer AT, Storli OV. Soccer injuries to the brain: a neurologic and electroencephalographic study of active football players. *Am J Sports Med* 1989;17:573–578.
30. Sortland O, Tysvaer AT. Brain damage in former association football players. *Neuroradiology* 1989;31:44–48.
31. Tysvaer AT, Løchen EA. Soccer injuries to the brain: a neuropsychologic study of former soccer players. *Am J Sports Med* 1991; 19:56–60.
32. Tysvaer A, Storli O. Association football injuries to the brain: a preliminary report. *Br J Sports Med* 1981;15:163–166.
33. Matser EJ, Kessels AG, Lezak MD, et al. Neuropsychological impairment in amateur soccer players. *JAMA* 1999:282:971–973.
34. Matser JT, Kessels AG, Jordan BD, et al. Chronic traumatic brain injury in professional soccer players. *Neurology* 1998:51:791–796.
35. Green JR, Rayan GM. Scaphoid fractures in soccer goalkeepers. *J Okla State Med Assoc* 1997;90:45–47.
36. Lawson GM, Hajducka C, McQueen MM. Sports fractures of the distal radius: epidemiology and outcome. *Injury* 1995;26:33–36.
37. Jaddad FS, Manktelow ARJ, Dorrell JH. Radial head dislocation with radial shaft fracture. *Injury* 1995;26:502–503.
38. Curtin J, Kay NR. Hand injuries due to soccer. *Hand* 1976;8:93–95.
39. McMaster WC, Walter M. Injuries in soccer. *Am J Sports Med* 1978;6:354–357.
40. Hunt M, Fulford S. Amateur soccer: injuries in relation to field position. *Br J Sports Med* 1990;24:265.
41. Scerri GV, Ratcliffe RJ. The goalkeeper's fear of the nets. *J Hand Surg* 1994;19:459–460.
42. Bergquist D, Hedelin H, Karlsson G, et al. Abdominal injury from sporting activities. *Br J Sports Med* 1982;16:76–79.
43. Ekstrand J, Gillquist J. The avoidability of soccer injuries. *Int J Sports Med* 1983;4:124–128.
44. Renstrom P, Peterson L. Groin injuries in athletes. *Br J Sports Med* 1980;14:30–36.
45. Ekstrand J, Hilding J. The incidence and differential diagnosis of acute groin injuries in male soccer players. *Scand J Med Sci Sports* 1999;9:98–103.
46. Mozes M, Papa MZ, Zweig A, et al. Iliopsoas injury in soccer players. *Br J Sports Med* 1985;19:168–170.
47. Gilmore J. Groin pain in the soccer athlete: fact, fiction, and treatment. *Clin Sports Med* 1998;17:787–793.
48. Altarac S, Marekovic Z, Kalauz N, et al. Testicular trauma sustained during football. *Acta Med Croatica* 1993;47:141–143.
49. Arendt E, Dick R. Knee injury patterns among men and women in collegiate basketball and soccer: NCAA data and review of the literature. *Am J Sports Med* 1995;23:694–701.
50. Levy AS, Lohnes J, Sculley S, et al. Chondral delamination of the knee in soccer players. *Am J Sports Med* 1996;24:634–639.
51. McCarroll JR, Schrader JW, Shelbourne KD, et al. Meniscoid lesions of the ankle in soccer players. *Am J Sports Med* 1987;5: 255–257.
52. Karlsson J, Eriksson BI, Swärd L. Recurrent dislocation of the peroneal tendons. *Scand J Med Sci Sports* 1996;6:242–246.
53. Inokuchi S, Usami N. Closed complete rupture of the flexor hallucis longus tendon at the groove of the talus. *Foot Ankle Int* 1997;18:47–49.
54. Fehlandt A, Micheli L. Acute exertional anterior compartment syndrome in an adolescent female. *Med Sci Sports Exerc* 1995; 27:3–7.
55. Moyer RA, Boden BP, Marchetto PA, et al. Acute compartment syndrome of the lower extremity secondary to noncontact injury. *Foot Ankle Int* 1993;14:534–537.
56. Boden BP, Lohnes JH, Nunley JA, et al. Tibia and fibula fractures in soccer players. *Knee Surgery, Sports Traumatology, Arthroscopy* 1999;7:262–266.
57. McBryde AM. Stress fracture in athletes. *J Sports Med* 1976; 3:212–217.
58. Lindberg H, Roos H, Gärdsell P. Prevalence of coxarthrosis in former soccer players: 286 players compared with matched controls. *Acta Orthop Scand* 1993;64:165–167.
59. Roos H, Lindberg H, Gärdsell P, et al. The prevalence of gonarthrosis and its relation to meniscectomy in former soccer players. *Am J Sports Med* 1994;22:219–222.
60. Chantraine A. Knee joint in soccer players: osteoarthritis and axis deviation. *Med Sci Sports Exerc* 1985;17:434–439.
61. Inklaar H. Soccer injuries: incidence and severity. *Sports Med* 1994;18:55–73.
62. Falck G. Group A streptococcal skin infections after indoor association football tournament [Letter]. *Lancet* 1996;3447:840–841.
63. Davis PJ, Stirling AJ. Aeromonas hydrophila wound infection

associated with water immersion: an unusual football injury. *Injury* 1993;24:633–634.
64. Sommer S, Wilkinson SM, Dodman B. Contact dermatitis due to urea-formaldehyde resin in shin-pads. *Contact Dermatitis* 1999;40:159–160.
65. Keller CS, Noyes FR, Buncher CR. Medical aspects of soccer injury epidemiology. *Am J Sports Med* 1987;15:230–237.
66. Backous DD, Friedl KE, Smith NJ, et al. Soccer injuries and their relation to physical maturity. *Am J Dis Child* 1988;142:839–842.
67. Injuries in youth soccer: a subject review. American Academy of Pediatrics. Committee on Sports Medicine and Fitness. *Pediatrics* 2000;105:659–661.
68. Engström B, Johansson C, Törnkvist H. Soccer injuries among elite female players. *Am J Sports Med* 1991;19:372–375.
69. Brynhildsen J, Ekstrand J, Jeppsson A, et al. Previous injuries and persistent symptoms in female soccer players. *Int J Sports Med* 1990;11:489–492.
70. Möller-Nielsen J, Hammar M. Women's soccer injuries in relation to the use of the menstrual cycle and oral contraceptive use. *Med Sci Sports Exerc* 1989;21:126–129.
71. Hoff GL, Martin TA. Outdoor and indoor soccer: injuries among youth players. *Am J Sports Med* 1986;14:231–233.
72. Ekstrand J, Gillquist J, Möller M, et al. Incidence of soccer injuries and their relation to training and team success. *Am J Sports Med* 1983;11:63–67.
73. Sullivan JA, Gross RH, Grana WA, et al. Evaluation of injuries in youth soccer. *Am J Sports Med* 1980;8:325–327.
74. Inklaar H. Soccer injuries II: aetiology and prevention. *Sports Med* 1994;18:81–93.
75. Hawkins RD, Fuller CW. Risk assessment in professional football: an examination of accidents and incidents in the 1994 World Cup finals. *Br J Sports Med* 1996;30:165–170.
76. Watson AW. Sports injuries in footballers related to defects of posture and body mechanics. *J Sports Med Phys Fitness* 1995;35:289–294.
77. Caraffa A, Cerulli G, Projetti M, et al. Prevention of anterior cruciate ligament injuries in soccer. A prospective controlled study of proprioceptive training. *Knee Surg Sports Traumatol Arthrosc* 1996;4:19–21.
78. Bir CA, Cassatta SJ, Janda DH. An analysis and comparison of soccer shin guards. *Clin J Sports Med* 1995;5:95–99.
79. Francisco AC, Nightingale RW, Guilak F, et al. Comparison of soccer shin guards in preventing tibia fracture. *Am J Sports Med* 2000;28:227–233.
80. American Dental Association. Mouth protectors and sports team dentists. *J Am Dent Assoc* 1984;109:84–87.
81. Tompson BD. Protection of the head and neck. *Dent Clin North Am* 1982;26:659–667.
82. Janda DH, Bir C, Wild B, et al. Goal post injuries in soccer: a laboratory and field testing analysis of a preventive intervention. *Am J Sports Med* 1995;23:340–344.
83. Surve I, Schwellnus MP, Noakes T, et al. A fivefold reduction in the incidence of recurrent ankle sprains in soccer players using the Sport-Stirrup orthosis. *Am J Sports Med* 1994;22:601–606.
84. Thacker SB, Stroup DF, Branche CM, et al. The prevention of ankle sprains in sports. A systematic review of the literature. *Am J Sports Med* 1999;27:753–760.

CHAPTER 49

Swimming

James C. Puffer

Swimming is one of the most popular sports in the United States. Participants compete at almost every level, including young age group swimmers, interscholastic and collegiate athletes, elite or Olympic-level athletes, and a growing number of master athletes. Participation requires considerable upper and lower body strength as well as excellent cardiopulmonary fitness. Although many people consider swimming a safe, noncontact sport, it is not free from injuries or medical problems. Given that the average swimmer may spend at least 4 hours in the pool daily, swimming approximately 10,000 yards per day, 5 days per week, using approximately 15 strokes per pool length and breathing every other stroke, this will produce 1,200,000 arm movements, 600,000 cervical spine rotations, and 1,200,000 lumbar rotatory movements each year. Additionally, stroke-specific stresses are placed on a number of other anatomic structures. While the shoulder, knee, and spine are the most frequently injured anatomic structures, this chapter will take a head-to-toe approach to the assessment of injuries in swimmers and the special problems that they may encounter.

SHOULDER

The shoulder is the most commonly injured joint in the swimmer (1). The incidence of shoulder injury has been reported to vary from as low as 3% to as high as 67% (1–3). A survey of age group, senior development, and national team athletes demonstrated that the incidence of interfering shoulder pain varied by the skill level of the population studied, with 10% of the age group population to 26% of the national team athletes demonstrating shoulder pain (4). The incidence increased with time in the sport, and the use of hand paddles, weight training, stretching, and kick board use as well as other resistance activities were found to aggravate shoulder pain. Kennedy and Hawkins (5) coined the classic term *swimmer's shoulder* to describe the inflammatory rotator cuff tendinitis that is frequently seen in swimmers, but we now know that shoulder pain in this population is a complex entity that may have many different etiologies.

The shoulder was inadequately designed to withstand the repetitive overhead motion to which it is subjected in swimming. It is a mobile joint with little bony support, as only 20% of the surface of the humeral head comes into contact with the glenoid fossa. While the glenoid labrum increases contact area, primary stability in the shoulder is provided by both dynamic and static stabilizers. Static stabilization is provided by the form of the glenohumeral ligaments and shoulder capsule, while dynamic support is supplied by the rotator cuff musculature, which acts as a force couple with the deltoid during overhead motion. The primary responsibility of the rotator cuff is to adduct and to center the head of the humerus in the glenoid fossa during this motion. The scapular stabilizers—the serratus anterior, the trapezius, and the rhomboids—are important for fixing the scapula against the thorax and providing a stable platform for normal glenohumeral joint mechanics. Failure or fatigue of any of these stabilizers can result in disruption of the subtle mechanisms that are responsible for providing shoulder stability during the overhead motion and result in the vicious cycle of repetitive microtrauma, inflammation, secondary impingement, and repeated microtrauma.

Repetitive tensile overload of the rotator cuff can and does occur in the swimmer. Kennedy and Hawkins have described this phenomenon as "wringing out" (5). Rathbun and MacNab have eloquently demonstrated in a cadaver model that as the arm is brought into adduction and extension, the rotator cuff—primarily the supraspinatus—is stretched over the convex surface of the humeral head and the microvasculature is compromised

---

J. C. Puffer: Department of Family Medicine, UCLA School of Medicine, Los Angeles, California 90095-7087.

(6). This repeated microtrauma can result in the development of an inflammatory response and the subsequent development of pain. As the rotator cuff fails, its ability to center the humeral head and to maintain stability in the glenohumeral joint is lost, and the humeral head begins to migrate superiorly. This results in secondary impingement of the cuff beneath the coricocromial arch, adding further insult.

Although secondary impingement can certainly result from overuse as described above, it can also result from shoulder instability. It is important to note that swimmers, by and large, have lax shoulders. Whether this is a result of many years of repetitive training or whether those with inherently lax shoulders tend to migrate to this sport is open to question, but needless to say, it is critical to distinguish clinical instability from laxity. The former will almost always result in development of significant problems, while the latter usually does not. While all types of atraumatic instability can be seen in a swimmer's shoulder, it is not uncommon to see a large number of swimmers with shoulder pain who have frank multidirectional instability. The hallmark of this disorder is abnormal inferior glenohumeral ligament laxity without labral detachment.

Given the increasing number of older swimmers who are participating both recreationally and competitively in this sport, it is not unusual to see evidence of primary impingement in older athletes with shoulder pain. This is almost always due to acromioclavicular joint disease or significant bony pathology on the undersurface of the acromion process.

The evaluation of the swimmer's shoulder is relatively straightforward. Usually, the athlete will present with a history of pain during the late recovery phase and early catch phase of the stroke. The pain may be aggravated with hand paddles, weight training, or use of kick boards with the arm in a forward-flexed position. A painful arc of movement between 60° and 120° of abduction will be demonstrated, and exquisite tenderness over the supraspinatus or the long head of the biceps tendon will be appreciated. Considerable weakness will be demonstrated in the supraspinatus when tested against resistance. A positive impingement sign will usually be present with either the Neer or Hawkins impingement maneuver. Subtle signs of instability should be carefully assessed during the physical examination. Although radiographs may be of little benefit in the initial evaluation of the young swimmer, they are critically important in evaluating bony pathology in the older swimmer.

The treatment plan is relatively straightforward and is directed at reducing inflammation, maintaining cardiovascular fitness, and subsequently achieving strength, balance, and a return to normal stroke mechanics. We have described a progressive rehabilitation program for injuries of overuse that modifies activity and directs rehabilitation on the basis of the severity of symptoms (7). Milder forms of overuse may be treated with a relative reduction in mileage, the use of nonsteroidal antiinflammatory drugs (NSAIDs), and an appropriately directed rehabilitation program. More severe forms of overuse, which result in pain that compromises performance, should result in a brief period of complete rest along with the appropriate control of inflammation and subsequent rehabilitation.

The careful assessment and rehabilitation of shoulder pain in most swimmers will result in resolution of this problem with an appropriately directed treatment regimen. Occasionally, surgery will be required in difficult cases that fail to respond to conservative therapy or in instances in which pain can be attributed specifically to either labral injury secondary to instability, frank instability, or bony abnormalities that result in primary impingement. The most critical factor, however, in treating swimmer's shoulder, is preventing it in the first place. Workload increases should be sensible and gradual. A balanced strength and conditioning program is the cornerstone of any well-designed competitive program, and workouts should be designed to avoid the deleterious effects of the excessive use of hand paddles and other resistive exercises for the shoulder. Selective swimmers may benefit from stroke analysis to correct stroke deficiencies.

ELBOW

Elbow problems are uncommon in the swimmer. When they do occur, they are almost always the result of the extreme elbow-up position during the catch phase of the stroke. Some have likened this to "reaching over a barrel" (8). This results in the development of a lateral epicondylitis. Pain can be appreciated over the extensor carpi radialis brevis and the extensor communis aponeurosis. Treatment should be directed at reducing inflammation with the use of ice and NSAIDs, but, more important, alteration of stroke mechanics is critical in preventing recurrence of this problem, as is appropriate forearm extensor strengthening.

HAND

Hand injuries are uncommon in the swimmer. Lacerations on the dorsum of the hand can be inflicted by hand paddles used by teammates during practice. Occasionally, metacarpal fractures can be incurred during the finish of the backstroke event as the dorsum of the hand forcibly strikes the wall.

BACK

Long neglected, the back is gaining increasing recognition as an important structure that can be injured in the swimmer. This is primarily due to new positions that are used to propel the body above water. While all spinal structures are at risk during swimming, the biomechanics of specific strokes predispose particular structures to increased risk. The freestyle and backstroke increase lumbar torque forces, thereby increasing lumbar segmental axial rotation most. These forces place the annulus fibrosis at jeopardy. Although body roll can minimize forces across individual lumbar segments with proper stroke mechanics, paradoxically, the elite swimmer probably subjects these segments to greater force per stroke (9).

The breaststroke and butterfly stroke accentuate lumbar extension and place the back in repeated exaggerated lordosis. These two strokes place the lumbar facets at particular risk because of the exaggerated undulation that increases sagittal plane motion. While the breaststroke has traditionally been characterized by linear horizontal plane motion, recent advances in the stroke that have increased sagittal plane motion by emphasizing undulatory movement have increased the risk for back pain in these stroke specialists. While not common, spondylolysis can occur in swimmers who participate predominantly in the breaststroke and butterfly events.

Thoracic spine injury occurs much less frequently than lumbar spine injury, but when it does occur, it usually manifests as facet dysfunction, particularly with the freestyle and backstroke events because of the great degree of increased segmental rotatory motion at thoracic segments. On the other hand, the repetitive extension that is required in the butterfly and breaststroke events may result in repetitive facet compression, distraction, and sheer force, which would result in inflammation and subsequent development of pain. Cole and Eagleston described the forces that are responsible for the development of thoracic spine facet joint dysfunction (9). During the pull phase, the compressive forces are generated by the ipsilateral latissimus dorsi, scapular retractors, and long thoracic spinal extensor musculature. Ipsilateral thoracic spinal muscle groups produce an extension to counter the flexion of the latissimus dorsi. The contralateral thoracic spinal musculature stabilizes the thoracic spine, preventing untoward lateral flexion during the pull-through phase of the stroke. Passive distraction forces affect the ipsilateral facet during the recovery phase because of the activation of the ipsilateral scapular protractors, relaxation of the scapular retractors, inactivation of the latissimus dorsi, and relative relaxation of the thoracic spine extensor musculature.

The costovertebral joints may also be injured. This may be due to repetitive chest wall and rib motion as well as repetitive arm elevation and subsequent tension on the ribs. Faulty stroke mechanics resulting in increased rotation through the thoracic spine may also contribute to costovertebral joint pain, particularly at the thoracolumbar junction, which acts as a transitional zone from spine rotation to flexion and extension.

The cervical spine is subject to repetitive continuous motion during breathing. The significant rotation that is required for breathing to the side in the freestyle stroke can result in annular as well as facet joint injuries. In the breaststroke and butterfly events, which result in extension of the neck, the posterior cervical elements are placed at risk, thereby resulting in potential cervical facet pain. Repetitive cervical extension can also increase intradiscal pressure, placing the intravertebral disk at risk. The backstroke requires stabilization of the cervical segments in the relatively neutral position to decrease drag. While cervical segmental abnormalities are minimized because of the stroke mechanics, muscular strain resulting from this dynamic stabilization is increased in both the cervical capital and cervical flexor and extensor groups.

It is important to appreciate that peripheral joint dysfunction can result in a cascading series of motion alterations throughout the spinal axis, which can result in spinal dysfunction. This most typically occurs at the cervicothoracic and thoracolumbar transition zones because they represent the junction between the more mobile and less mobile sections of the spine. To illustrate this, appreciate that a swimmer with shoulder pain may not fully abduct and extend the arm as would normally be expected during recovery, resulting in decreased body roll. This would result in increased lumbar segmental motion and an abnormally low head position from which to breathe. The cervical spine would compensate with cervical extension and rotation, facilitating an increased range of motion in the upper and midcervical segments. This might ultimately result in painful and hypomobile segments in the lower cervical spine as well as compensatory hypermobility in the upper thoracic spine and hypomobility in the lower thoracic spine.

This underscores the complete assessment of the swimmer who presents with back pain. Back pain secondary to peripheral joint dysfunction must be distinguished from primary spinal dysfunction secondary to repetitive overuse or faulty stroke mechanics. Therapy must be targeted at correcting segmental motion abnormalities, reduction of inflammation, and spinal stabilization.

Before leaving the subject of back pain, it is important to discuss idiopathic scoliosis. While the incidence of idiopathic scoliosis is approximately 2%, Becker described an incidence of idiopathic scoliosis of 6.9% in 336 age group swimmers; 16% of these swimmers had a functional scoliosis without a rib hump, the lateral curvature occurring to the hand-dominant side of the body (10). These findings highlight the repetitive torsional motion of this sport and the repetitive forces that are placed on the thoracic and lumbar spine as described above.

KNEE

Knee pain in swimmers is almost exclusive to the breaststroker. This is due to the repetitive whip kick that these swimmers use to propel themselves through the water. While knee pain in this population can be due to a variety of causes, the three most common etiologies are repetitive chronic stress of the medial collateral ligament, patellofemoral dysfunction, and medial synovial plica syndrome. Kennedy and Hawkins demonstrated in a group of world-class breaststrokers that of those with knee problems during their competitive years, 46% continued to have problems an average of 15.5 years later (11).

Repetitive chronic stress occurs to the medial collateral ligament during the breaststroke kick. It has been demonstrated in cadaver models that force increases geometrically in the medial collateral ligament during the propulsive phase of the breaststroke kick (2). Typically, swimmers will present with pain at the origin of the medial collateral ligament or where the superficial fibers of the ligament cross over the upper tibial margin. Pain can be reproduced with valgus–external rotation stress at 20–30° of flexion. Treatment is directed at refraining from the breaststroke kick while reducing the inflammation with NSAIDs.

Patellofemoral dysfunction in the swimmer is similar to that seen in other athletes. Again, the repetitive valgus stress placed on the knee places the patella at risk and, in those predisposed, to lateral tracking of the patella. These athletes will typically present with peripatellar pain and demonstrate vastus medialus obliquus insufficiency, excessive passive patellar tilt, tight lateral structures, and/or abnormal distal extensor mechanism dysfunction. Treatment should be directed at correcting the specific abnormalities that are detected upon physical examination.

Medial synovial plica syndrome is also similar to that seen in other athletes. This excessive medial synovial fold snaps over the medial femoral condyle during the extension phase of the whip kick, resulting in the development of inflammation, hypertrophy, and thickening. Physical examination will demonstrate reproducible pain on palpation of the plica, and extension of the knee in valgus may result in a palpable and audible snap of the plica over the medial femoral condyle. Conservative treatment of this should include relative rest by avoidance of the whip kick, the use of NSAIDs, and, in selected cases, judicious use of injectable corticosteroid. Recalcitrant cases can be treated with surgical excision of the offending plica.

ANKLE AND FOOT

Injuries to the ankle and foot result primarily from either overuse or direct trauma. Heel trauma can occur as a result of forcibly striking the foot during the flip turn. More common is extensor tendinitis, which occurs at the extensor retinaculum as a result of repetitive flexion and extension of the foot during the backstroke and freestyle kicks (8). The treatment of this problem is relatively straightforward, with a decrease in kicking mileage, the use of ice and NSAIDs, gradual stretching, and a return to full kicking as tolerated.

MEDICAL PROBLEMS

While the majority of problems seen in swimmers are orthopedic, swimmers are not immune from specific medical problems. The most common of these is otitis externa (swimmer's ear). This infection of the external auditory canal results from the proliferation of *Escherichia coli,* pseudomonas and proteus species, and fungi. The athlete will complain of a painful ear, and on physical examination pain will be appreciated on motion of the penna and tragus. Otoscopic evaluation will reveal a raw, red, macerated epithelium with considerable squamous debris. Treatment of this entity should consist of careful debridement of the ear with suction and the subsequent use of an otic solution consisting of acetic acid, neomycin, polymixin, and hydrocortisone (12). During treatment, silicone ear plugs can be used to avoid entry of water into the external canal. Prophylaxis of this condition with the use of an acetic acid/Burrow's solution after swimming can be helpful.

Another common but relatively minor problem that is seen in swimmers can be contact dermatitis caused by the neoprene foam that is found on many goggles used by swimmers to protect their eyes during many hours of swimming. This problem will usually be obvious and apparent. The swimmer will present with periorbital swelling, an erythematous rash, and pruritis. The use of the offending goggles should be discontinued. Topical corticosteroids and antihistamines may be employed, and the athlete should switch to using goggles with a nonneoprene rim before returning to the water.

A more serious and debilitating medical condition that deserves mention before completion of this chapter is the phenomenon of overtraining. Given the long hours and many yards to which swimmers are subjected during the course of training, they are at significant risk for the development of the overtraining syndrome. This syndrome is characterized by staleness, fatigue, depression, recurrent upper respiratory tract infection, and sleep disturbance (13). The manifestation of any or all of these symptoms should lead the clinician to a careful evaluation of the athlete's general health to exclude serious underlying pathology. Once more serious disorders have been excluded, the athlete must be treated with a period of relative rest, the initiation of a high-carbohydrate diet, and supportive therapy (14). While most cases respond to this aggressive approach, more serious cases may require intensive psychotherapy and the use of antidepressants.

SUMMARY

Although swimming is generally a safe sport with a low incidence of significant injury, a number of problems present with consistent regularity in the swimmer. These include injuries to the shoulder, knee, and back as well as some relatively common medical problems. The treatment of these problems—and, more important, their prevention—requires cooperation among the athlete, coach, and physician. Careful attention to sensible training programs, prophylactic strength and conditioning programs, and the prompt recognition of specific injuries can provide an environment in which the swimmer's well-being can be guaranteed.

REFERENCES

1. Richardson AB, Jobe FW, Collins HR. The shoulder in competitive swimming. *Am J Sports Med* 1980;8:159–163.
2. Kennedy JC, Hawkins RJ, Krisoff WB. Orthopedic manifestations of swimming. *Am J Sports Med* 1978;6:309–322.
3. Dominguez RH. Shoulder pain in age group swimmers. In: Erickson B, Furberg B, eds. *Swimming medicine,* vol. 4. Baltimore: University Park Press, 1978:105–109.
4. McMaster WC, Troup J. A survey of interfering shoulder pain in United States competitive swimmers. *Am J Sports Med* 1993;21:67–70.
5. Kennedy JC, Hawkins RJ. Swimmer's shoulder. *Phys Sports Med* 1974;2(April):34–38.
6. Rathbun JB, MacNab I. The microvascular pattern of the rotator cuff. *J Bone Joint Surg* 1970;52B:544–553.
7. Puffer JC, Zachezewski J. Management of overuse injuries. *Am Fam Physician* 1988;38(3):225–232.
8. Fowler PT, Regan WD. Swimming injuries of the knee, foot and ankle, elbow and back. *Clin Sports Med* 1986;5(1):139–148.
9. Cole AJ, Eagleston RE. Spine injuries in competitive swimmers. *Sports Med Digest* 1994;16(3):1–3.
10. Becker TJ. Scoliosis in swimmers. *Clin Sports Med* 1986;5(1):149–158.
11. Kennedy JC. Hawkins RJ. Breaststroker's knee. *Phys Sports Med* 1974;2:33–38.
12. Eichel BS. How I manage external otitis in competitive swimmers. *Phys Sports Med* 1986;14(8):108–116.
13. Morgan WP, Brown DR, Raglin JS, et al. Psychological monitoring of overtraining and staleness. *Br J Sports Med* 1987;21:107–114.
14. Puffer JC, McShane JM. Depression and chronic fatigue in athletes. *Clin Sports Med* 1992;11(2):327–338.

CHAPTER 50

Tennis

W. Ben Kibler and T. Jeff Chandler

INJURY ANALYSIS

Analysis of injuries sustained in tennis competition reveals that they are very common, they occur throughout the body, they are relatively mild in disability, and they occur frequently as a result of microtrauma and infrequently from macrotrauma.

Most studies of injury patterns have been done on elite or competitive athletes. Table 50-1 summarizes injury incidence reports from several studies: an international study (1), a U.S. Tennis Association study (2), a Belgian study (3), and a Danish study (4). Table 50-2 shows injury sites from these plus a U.S. study (5). Table 50-3 breaks these injuries into types, either macrotrauma (sprains and fractures) or microtrauma overload. These studies, though limited owing to population studied, population size, and lack of a common definition of injury, are similar in their findings and probably do represent injury profiles in competitive tennis players.

Injury occurrence in competitive tennis players is quite high: 50–90% of players reported an injury in the 12 months before the questionnaire (Table 50-1). These injuries were spread throughout the entire body, reflecting the stresses applied to all parts of the body during tennis (Table 50-2). In general, the injuries tended toward mild disabilities. The only study that closely followed downtime showed that the mean time away from sport was 3.1 weeks, and no player had to give up tennis directly because of the injury (3).

Macrotrauma, such as sprains and fractures, was a causative factor in a minority of tennis injuries. These types of injuries represent an event in which previously normal tissues are rendered immediately abnormal (Fig. 50-1). These injuries occur as a result of an externally applied force, are unpredictable, and are difficult to prevent by conditioning activities.

The major type of injury in tennis players is due to microtrauma repetitive overload (Table 50-3). Injuries in the upper extremity and back are almost exclusively due to overload, while lower extremity injuries are due to overload in half of the cases. Overall, microtrauma injuries account for 65–75% of all injuries seen in these studies.

Microtrauma injuries represent a process of injury in which normal tissues gradually become altered (6,7). These alterations, most of which can be objectively measured, cause the tissues to be unable to respond adequately to sports demands. Decreased performance and overt tissue injury result from these alterations. This process may create adaptations in other tissues as the athlete tries to continue to participate in sport. The athlete may alternate between symptomatic and asymptomatic states, depending on the workload and the intensity and degree of healing of the tissue (Fig. 50-2). The incidence of these injuries may be modifiable with proper conditioning (6–9).

The incidence and distribution of injuries in recreational players is not as well documented. Several general statements can be made about these injuries from anecdotal observations, from injury data in exercising populations (10,11), and from research on overload injuries (6,12). First, older athletes have a tendency to have an increased incidence of overload injuries, especially rotator cuff tendinitis, elbow epicondylitis, back strain, and Achilles tendinitis. Second, a low skill level, with accompanying poor stroke mechanics, also increases injury incidence in certain areas of the body. Third, the relative decrease in flexibility that is seen in more sedentary or older populations may be a risk factor for increased injury. Finally, the incidence of macrotrauma injuries does not seem to be as high, since the forces and loads are usually not as high. All of these generalities point to a predominance of microtrauma

---

W. B. Kibler: Lexington Sports Medicine Center, Lexington Clinic, Lexington, Kentucky 40507.

T. J. Chandler: Division of Exercise Science, Sport, and Recreation, Marshall University, Huntington, West Virginia 25755.

TABLE 50-1. Injury incidence

Study	Total players	Players with injury (%)	Total number of injuries
International			
English	17	11 (64.7)	14
Swedish	13	12 (92.3)	18
United States	33	18 (54.5)	27
Total	63	41 (65.1)	59
USTA	34	22 (64.7)	26
Belgian	127	110 (87)	167
Danish	88	68 (77.2)	81

TABLE 50-3. Injury type

	Macrotrauma (%)	Microtrauma (%)
Overall (USTA + U.S.)	33	67
Overall (international)	31	69
Overall (Belgian)	24	76
Overall (Danish)	29	71
Individual: shoulder	6	94
Individual: back	25	75
Individual: knee	42	58
Individual: foot and ankle	48	52

overload as the main mechanism of injury in recreational tennis players.

This chapter will review current concepts on the pathophysiology of microtrauma overload injuries in tennis to provide a scientific framework for evaluating, treating, and rehabilitating these injuries.

PATHOLOGY IN MICROTRAUMA OVERLOAD INJURIES

Pathologic specimens from several different areas reveal a characteristic picture of a long-standing process of injury (7,13). There are many blood vessels and a large amount of poorly organized, undifferentiated tissue, indicating a lack of organized healing to normal tissue. There are very few inflammatory cells, indicating chronicity and lack of an ongoing attempt to heal the tissue through the normal process of tissue regeneration. This tissue has not responded and probably cannot respond to normal biologic signals for repair and recovery, collagen orientation, or maturation (7). This failed healing response has been termed angiofibroblastic tendinosis, reflecting the pathological picture of a degenerative lesion to a lower order of maturation (7,12).

These changes have their genesis in the effect that overload exerts on cells. Cellular effects include decreased enzyme levels, alteration in mitochondrial size, changes in RNA transcription, alterations in calcium release and uptake, and changes in myofibril attachment to the sarcomere cytoskeleton (13,14). Recent evidence suggests that mechanical tensile load on the tissue is the most important factor in these changes (15). In muscle and muscle–tendon injuries, the exact mechanism is fiber and fibril strain that occurs during lengthening of an activated muscle (16). Implied in this description is that the load causing the lengthening is important only as a relative load compared to the muscle's or tissue's ability to protect itself against the strain generated by the load. Normal loads on weakened or fatigued muscles or tissues, a relative force overload, are as capable of causing excessive strain as supranormal loads acting on normal muscles or tissues, an absolute force overload.

Vascular or hormonal changes also participate in microtrauma causation. Probably all of these factors are involved to varying degrees. The net result is cellular contents that are incapable of making matrix of normal quality and quantity (7,12).

These cellular alterations are expressed on a tissue level as overt tissue injury or nonovert tissue adaptations, such as inflexibility, weakness, or inability to absorb loads. These adaptations may not produce clinical symptoms but do reduce performance (8) and may act as risk factors for producing injuries (9,10,17).

MODEL FOR MICROTRAUMA INJURY CAUSATION

It appears that many factors may affect the process of microtrauma injury causation. A direct one-to-one cause-and-effect relationship can rarely be established between one particular anatomic or physiologic factor and a specific diagnosis (18).

We use a modification of Meeuwisse's (18) model of multifactoral causation in microtrauma injuries (Fig. 50-3). Intrinsic risk factors (age, inflexibility, lack of strength, previous injury, lack of endurance) that are part of the athlete's musculoskeletal base create a predisposed athlete. This athlete then interacts with the inherent demands of the sport (biomechanical requirements, metabolic requirements, strength, agility) and other extrinsic factors (equipment, playing conditions, environment) to produce a susceptible athlete. This athlete is not normal or optimally efficient but is functioning. An inciting event, such as more athletic exposure, different equipment, more intense participation, a change in training, or a change in technique, may lead

TABLE 50-2. Injury site

	International (%)	USTA (%)	Belgian (%)	U.S. (%)
Shoulder	7 (22)	4 (15)	21 (13)	(14.1)
Elbow	26 (6.3%)	1 (4)	10 (9)	(10.4)
Back	4 (12.5)	2 (8)	31 (18.5)	(22.3)
Knee	4 (12.5)	5 (19)	33 (20)	(18)
Ankle and foot	6 (18)	7 (27)	26 (15.5)	(18)

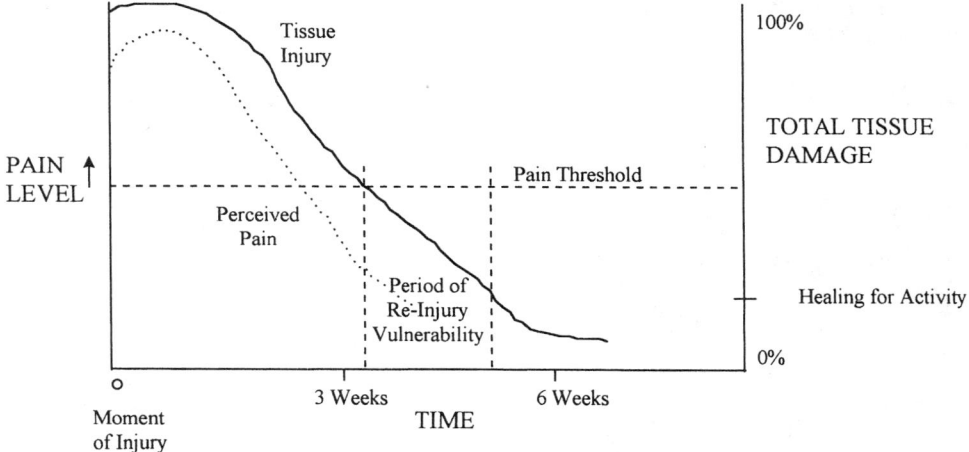

FIG. 50-1. Graphic representation of an acute macrotraumatic injury. The tissues are acutely injured, healing takes place along a predictable curve, and the athlete returns to play when healing has occurred.

to overt injury and symptom production. This has been termed a transition event (Fig. 50-4) (7).

IMPLICATIONS OF THE INJURY MODEL

This model has several implications for the evaluation and treatment of tennis injuries. First, the clinician should have a working knowledge of the demands inherent in tennis, on either a competitive or a recreational level. Second, there must be a good profiling of the athlete's musculoskeletal base to discover any deficits in flexibility, strength, or endurance that may exist. Third, there must be a search for any transition conditions that may have caused the overt symptoms. Fourth, injury evaluation should include not only the source of clinical symptoms, but also any tissue alterations that may be associated with or causing the symptoms. Finally, this model directs attention to conditioning the athlete's musculoskeletal base in light of the inherent demands to reduce the population of predisposed athletes (8,17,18).

INHERENT DEMANDS IN TENNIS

Several studies have evaluated the biomechanical and physiologic demands that are imposed by the sport of tennis. The demands are highest in magnitude in the competitive athlete but are also present in the recreational athlete.

Biomechanics

Large motions, loads, and forces are seen in many areas of the body, reflecting the whole-body nature of tennis.

Shoulder

Scapular motion around the thoracic wall may be as high as 15 cm, depending on body size. It also rotates through an arc of 65° as the shoulder abducts or forward-flexes to allow the humerus to move freely under the coracoacromial arch. The glenohumeral joint moves

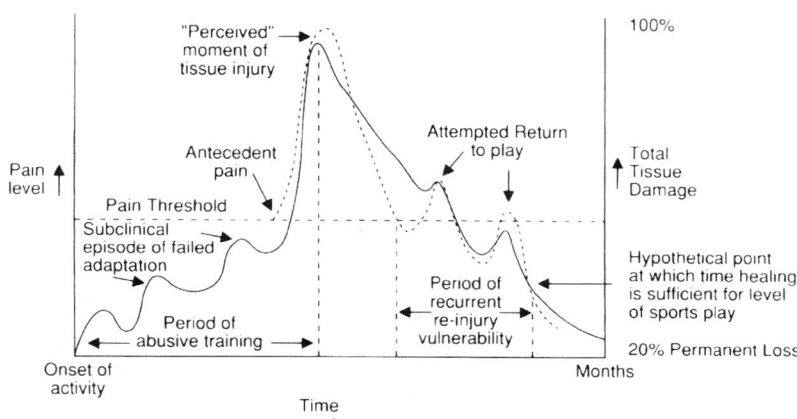

FIG. 50-2. Graphic representation of a chronic microtrauma overload injury. The athlete tries to compete with tissue deficits that do not heal. Eventually, enough tissue damage occurs that play is stopped.

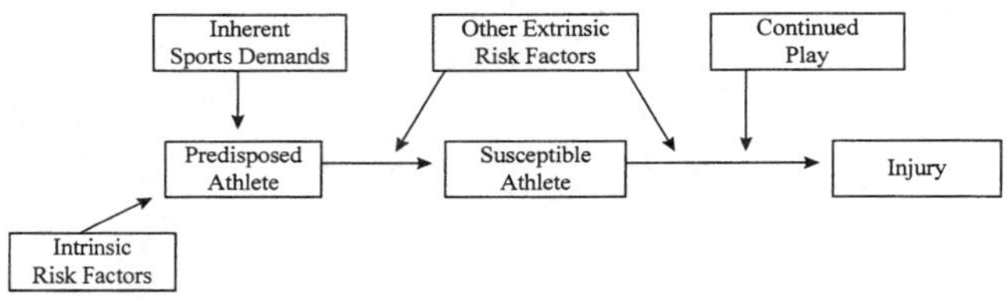

FIG. 50-3. Model of multifactoral causation in microtrauma injuries. Many factors, intrinsic and extrinsic to the athlete and inherent to the sport, create predisposed and susceptible athletes. Continued play or exposure to demands can create injury.

through an arc of 135°, from 55° external rotation to 80° internal rotation. This rotation stays centered in the glenoid, showing that the glenohumeral joint is a true ball-and-socket articulation (19,20).

High rotational velocities are achieved at the shoulder during tennis strokes in skilled athletes (19). Internal rotation velocity averages 1500° per second, horizontal adduction velocity averages 400° per second, and abduction velocity averages 200° per second in the tennis serve. These velocities generate racquet speeds averaging 70 miles per hour and ball speeds averaging 115 miles per hour. Internal rotation in the forehand averages 320° per second and generates racquet velocities of 54 miles per hour and ball velocities of 80 miles per hour. External rotation in the backhand averages 485° per second and generates racquet velocities of 42 miles per hour and ball velocities of 68 miles per hour.

These velocities produce loads on the anterior glenoid labrum of almost two times body weight in acceleration and 2.5 times body weight in deceleration.

Elbow

Elbow flexion/extension is largest in the tennis serve, flexing to around 120° in cocking and extending to 20° in follow-through. Ball impact occurs at 35° flexion. Extension velocity averages 982° per second. Varus/valgus motion is minimal in nonpathologic conditions. Small ranges of motion (20–30°) occur in the forehand and backhand strokes, reflecting the stabilizing nature of the joint in these strokes. Forearm pronation is large, ranging from 40° supination to 50° pronation. This generates a rotational velocity of 347° per second (21).

Wrist

The wrist is subject to large ranges of motion in the deceleration phase of serving. These are largely passively imposed, owing to the wrist's position at the "end of the whip" of the kinetic chain and the large mass of the racquet. The motions range from 35° extension to 45° flexion. Actual motion during the acceleration phase is less, with only 20° total rotation.

Back, Hip, and Trunk

Rotations of the hip and trunk are large in all of the tennis strokes. Rotational arcs average 80° on the serve, 60–90° on the forehand, depending on the stance, and 60° on the backhand. Rotational velocities average 365° per second on the serve, 485° per second on the forehand, and 215° per second on the backhand.

Physiology

Metabolic Demands

The metabolic demands in the sport of tennis have been characterized by Fox and Matthews (22) as being approximately 70% alactic anaerobic, 20% lactic anaerobic, and 10% aerobic. Of course, this varies with the age of the player, the player's skill level, the skill level of the competition, and the style of play. Metabolic speci-

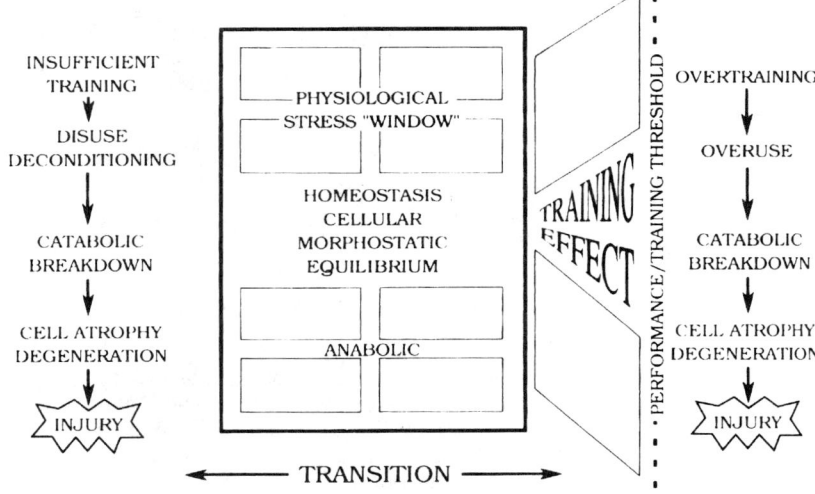

FIG. 50-4. A transition event occurs when too abrupt a change in playing environment occurs. If the musculoskeletal base is unable to withstand the magnitude of the new load, a force overload situation may exist.

ficity in the sport of tennis dictates that the alactic anaerobic energy system is the primary system used in the sport.

The relative duration of each of the three primary energy systems indicates that the first 10–15 seconds of maximal exercise is alactic anaerobic. Because tennis is not a sport of constant maximal exertion, much of the energy in a tennis match comes from the alactic component. Recovery from this alactic anaerobic work, particularly alactic oxygen debt, can take place during low-intensity exercise or short rest periods. Within 20 seconds, 50% of the depleted ATP is replenished; in 40 seconds, 75% is replenished; and in 60 seconds, 87% is replenished (23).

It is likely that playing tennis confers some degree of cardiorespiratory fitness. There is an increasing body of data to suggest that repeated short bursts of energy, such as the metabolic work patterns in tennis, may improve aerobic endurance (24). Particularly for the recreational tennis player, this would depend on whether the individual plays singles or doubles, the level of competition, the initial fitness level of the individual, and the style of play.

Work/Rest Intervals

The large majority of the points in tennis are of relatively short duration. Time study analysis shows that over 80% of the points in professional tennis last less than 20 seconds. On hard courts the average work/rest ratio was 1:3.4 for males and 1:2.7 for females. In recreational athletes the ratio was slightly less, reflecting a less intense game. On hard courts the ratio was 1:2.2 for males and 1:2.3 for females. On clay courts the ratio was 1:1.8 for males and 1:2.1 for females. During the points, the workload is quite high. There is an average of 6.2 changes of direction per point. The average distance run is 22 feet. In an average three-set match consisting of 162 points per match, the player would change directions 1004 times and run over 3500 feet.

Motor Firing Patterns

To meet the biomechanical and metabolic demands inherent in tennis, muscle firing is organized into patterns to generate force, accept loads, and stabilize joints. These patterns involve sequential activation of large force-generating muscles in the legs and trunks, then activation of the smaller stabilizing and regulating muscles of the arm and hand (25). The interaction between the motor organization patterns that link and harmonize several joints and the patterns that control individual joint stability allows a kinetic chain of energy and force development that achieves the high velocities that are required without creating excessive stress on any one segment (19,26). These patterns are well developed in skilled athletes (27,28) but are fragile and tend to become disorganized early in pathologic conditions. In general, the large muscles of the legs, hips, and trunk utilize agonist/antagonist force couples to generate force and rotational momentum and accept loads of running, turning, and jumping, while the smaller muscles of the shoulder and elbow utilize cocontraction force couples to control joint perturbations and regulate forces through each of the segments in the serving or hitting phases of activity. The most common agonist/antagonist pattern is the plyometric, or stretch/shortening activation. This pattern supplies the power that is important in the modern tennis game. Evaluation of injuries and rehabilitation must take into account and restore these patterns (29,30).

MUSCULOSKELETAL BASE EVALUATION

Each athlete brings a definable musculoskeletal base to the demands of tennis. Profiling this base through a preparticipation examination can identify predisposed athletes and suggest conditioning activities to better prepare the athlete for the sport. If the musculoskeletal base is adequate for the specific sport, there will be a decreased chance of overload injuries. If the musculoskeletal base is exceptional for the specific sport, improved performance may well be the result, assuming an adequate skill level in the sport or activity. If the musculoskeletal base is inadequate for the sport, overload injury, fatigue, and decreased performance may well be the result. As the season progresses, injury and decreased performance become more likely.

There are many different approaches to the preparticipation exam. Some are relatively nonspecific, looking mainly at general fitness items (31,32). Others are organized around evaluating anatomic factors that are more important for a given sport (33,34). The tennis preparticipation exam should be comprehensive enough to look at all anatomic areas that are affected by tennis, be able to evaluate tennis specific motions and strength requirements, and be appropriate in complexity for the athlete's age, skill, and competitive level.

The preparticipation exam may be as simple as a sit and reach test for low back flexibility, a shoulder rotation flexibility exam, sit-ups and push-ups for strength, and a 20-yard dash and 1-mile run for endurance. This would be appropriate for young players or as a general screening for recreational players. More specific tests, such as goniometric range of motion of all joints, specific tests for strength around each joint, agility drills and tennis-specific short-duration anaerobic tests, and V_{O_2}max determinations for aerobic endurance, can be performed for more skilled players. This can give a more accurate evaluation of the player's ability to generate the motions and forces necessary to perform well and respond to the motions and loads that are developed in the game (35,36).

Analysis of the results of these exams in tennis players shows that the body of the tennis player adapts to the demands of the game. Some adaptations, such as increased bone density (37), increased tendon size (37), increased endurance (1), and increased muscle strength (38,39), are beneficial for performance. However, some adaptations are biomechanically not beneficial (17,18) and can be considered maladaptations. They include hip rotation inflexibility (2), low back inflexibility (35), back strength imbalance (39), shoulder strength imbalance (38), shoulder internal rotation inflexibility (39,40), elbow inflexibility (12), and forearm pronation contracture (2). These inflexibilities alter joint motion, create extra joint shear forces, transfer loads to distal joints, and break the kinetic chain of force development. They are the most common factors that create the predisposed athlete.

Muscle weakness patterns and muscle imbalances have been identified in "throwing" athletes, including tennis players. In one study on tennis players (38), 24 male and female college tennis players were tested for bilateral shoulder internal/external rotation strength on a Cybex 340 isokinetic dynamometer. Subjects produced significantly ($p < 0.01$) more torque in internal rotation at 60° and 300° per second in the dominant arm than in the nondominant arm. The increase in internal rotation strength may be related to the plyometric action of the tennis stroke. By significantly increasing the strength of the dominant shoulder in internal rotation without subsequent strengthening of the external rotators, muscle imbalances may be created in the dominant arm that could affect the tennis player's predisposition to overload injuries of the shoulder joint.

These flexibility and strength adaptations are important for several reasons. First, they have been demonstrated in players as young as 12–14 years of age (41), indicating that age is not a protective factor. Second, these adaptations are in the exact anatomic places that show high incidences of injury: the shoulder, elbow, and back. Third, posterior shoulder inflexibility has been implicated in possible shoulder injury, and elbow inflexibility has been shown to be a risk factor in lateral epicondylitis.

It may be that these adaptations are local efforts to control the high forces that are applied. However, these adaptations appear to be deleterious to the entire kinetic chain. These appear to create biomechanical inefficiencies and cause functional alterations such that injury risk is higher and optimal performance requires more energy. The demonstration of these adaptations in a large number of active tennis players may raise the question of whether these are "normal" adaptations and should be left alone. We believe that these are statistically "average" but not "normal." Improvement in these adaptations can alter injury risk by improving anatomic stability and movement and can improve tennis performance by improving biomechanical efficiency (40,42). These adaptations should be sought during a comprehensive preparticipation exam and should be aggressively corrected.

INJURY EVALUATION

The Evaluation Process

The evaluation process for acute injuries that occur in tennis should be the same as that for any acute injury. Proper early evaluation, stabilization, protection, and early treatment should be carried out. In the evaluation of overload injuries, several additional points should be observed. This is necessary for the evaluation of overload injuries in any sport, but it is especially relevant in tennis because of the high preponderance of this type of injury.

In evaluation of microtrauma injuries, the clinician often has to play the game of "victims and culprits" (43). The clinician must recognize all of the tissue alterations that exist as a result of the process of pathophysiology. These include local alterations in flexibility or strength, tissue injuries that produce the predominant clinical symptoms, alterations in distant areas of the kinetic chain that may be causing or affecting the local injury, and adaptations that may exist as the athlete continues to play (29). By doing this type of evaluation, the clinician will often find that the source of clinical symptoms (the "victim") is not the sole source of the pathophysiologic changes (the "culprits"). We evaluate injuries on the basis of a framework in which all of the local and distant alterations are categorized into five complexes. These complexes appear to interact with each other in the causation of these microtrauma-moderated injuries, and are all detectable on the clinical level. These complexes also interact with each other in a negative feedback cycle, as shown in Figure 50–5.

The five complexes are:

1. Tissue injury complex: a group of anatomic structures that have overt pathologic change

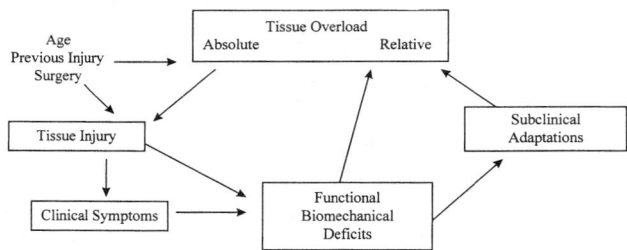

FIG. 50–5. Negative feedback vicious cycle. All of the complexes interact to produce abnormalities that eventually result in clinical symptoms.

2. Clinical symptom complex: a group of overt signs and symptoms that characterize the injury
3. Tissue overload complex: a group of anatomic structures that have clinically detectable change but are not overtly symptomatic
4. Functional biomechanical deficit complex: inflexibilities or strength imbalances that create altered athletic mechanics
5. Subclinical adaptation complex: the substitute actions that the athlete uses to compensate for altered mechanics to maintain performance

The model allows description of most of the abnormalities that may exist in the predisposed or susceptible athlete and emphasizes the multifactoral process that is occurring to produce the eventual clinical symptoms and altered performance. The tissue overload complex is part of the intrinsic risk factors that are present in the predisposed athlete, whereas the functional biomechanical deficits and subclinical adaptations characterize the susceptible athlete. The tissue injury and clinical symptom complexes are part of the overt pathology. Typically, an athlete may cycle as a susceptible athlete for some time before clinical symptoms appear. Prevention of some of these injuries may be possible at this time. Appropriate preparticipation screening can detect the early development of microtrauma-induced tissue overloads and suggest correct rehabilitation before they create overt pathology.

Specific Injury Evaluation Using the Negative Feedback Vicious Cycle

All tennis injuries can be evaluated by using this framework. After proper evaluation, treatment can then proceed by resolving each of the complexes. Treatment principles will be outlined in this chapter.

Rotator Cuff Tendinitis

This specific injury is one of the most common injuries at all activity levels in tennis players.

Tissue overload: posterior capsule, shoulder external rotator muscles, scapular stabilizers
Tissue injury: rotator cuff impingement or tensile stretch, glenoid labrum, anterior capsule
Clinical symptoms: pain over anterior lateral acromion, impingement upon abduction and rotation, glenohumeral subluxation, positive "clunk" or anterior slide test
Functional biomechanical deficit: functional "lateral scapular slide," consisting of inflexibility in internal rotation, muscle strength deficits in shoulder external rotators and scapular stabilizers; in more advanced cases, superior or anterior glenohumeral translation
Subclinical adaptations: "short arming" the throw, alteration of arm position during throwing or lifting, muscle recruitment from anterior shoulder, forearm, or trunk

Treatment should start with resting of the injured tissues. It should continue with strengthening of the scapular stabilizing muscles and progress to closed chain rotator cuff exercises. Treatment of the symptomatic tendinitis may be limited by the associated anatomic instability, so if conservative treatment is not successful in progressing the athlete by 6–8 weeks, further evaluation by computed tomography (CT) arthrogram or magnetic resonance imaging (MRI) should be considered to evaluate possible surgical cases. In these cases the superior surface of the rotator cuff and subacromial space are usually not involved. The pathologic problem will be found in the glenohumeral joint and on the undersurface of the rotator cuff.

In the older tennis athlete the signs and symptoms are more commonly based on actual rotator cuff impingement and degeneration. In these patients the tendinitis has been described as primary compressive because it is caused by direct damage to the cuff. A high percentage will show plain X-ray changes in acromioclavicular joint, subacromial area, or greater tuberosity that are consistent with chronic wear. Tests for instability will usually be normal, but a pattern of strength imbalances similar to those of younger athletes may be present. Conservative treatment may be instituted, especially if there are few indications of muscle tears. However, more complete diagnosis of the anatomic problem by arthrogram, CT arthrogram, or MRI should be considered early in the treatment process so that accurate information about diagnosis, prognosis, treatment options, and return to play can be given.

Actual tearing of the rotator cuff is the end stage of the tendinitis spectrum. In most cases there is a definite history of a painful episode after hitting an overhead or extending the arm. The pain may range from mild to severe, but the condition is usually functionally disabling. Early accurate diagnosis and institution of definite treatment are important to minimize functional deficit. Some small tears may be rehabilitated nonoperatively, but most tears are incompatible with vigorous overhead function. Surgical evaluation and repair should be considered if vigorous activity is contemplated.

Lateral Epicondylitis

"Tennis elbow" is a very common problem in recreational athletes but a rather infrequent one in more accomplished tennis players. This injury occurs almost exclusively as a result of repetitive overload. Pathologic change is seen in the extensor tendon attachments around the lateral epicondyle, especially in the extensor carpi radialis brevis.

Tissue overload: lateral muscle mass, mainly extensor carpi radialis brevis, wrist pronators and extensors, and shoulder external rotators

Tissue injury: same as for tissue overload, plus annular ligament and joint capsule

Clinical symptoms: point tender pain over extensor muscle mass, swelling in varying degree, pain on hitting backhand (usually in recreational athlete)

Functional biomechanical deficit: extensor inflexibility and muscle weakness, decreased range of motion in pronators and supinators, decreased shoulder external rotation strength

Subclinical adaptations: hitting "behind the body," hitting with wrist movement, recruitment of triceps or alteration of position of elbow

Treatment should emphasize improving mechanics and reducing symptoms. A good tennis teaching professional can be of major help in improving mechanics. Rehabilitation starts with decreasing painful activities to reduce stress and antiinflammatory medications in the acute phase. Strengthening exercises should start at the shoulder and proceed distally, with special emphasis on all of the deficits of strength, strength imbalance, and flexibility noted in the exam. Rubber tubing has been found to be a good way to start the strengthening process. Early use of a counterforce brace will decrease the load applied at the site of injury and allow more vigorous rehabilitation. In addition, its use allows earlier return to play.

Steroid injections have been used as treatment in many cases of tennis elbow. It certainly should not be the first form of treatment unless there is an extremely tender, inflamed area. The only major benefit of corticosteroid injections is the antiinflammatory action, so its use should be confined to situations in which active inflammation is present. After injections the patient should refrain from tennis for 10 days. A physical therapy program should be instituted after injection. Repeated injections are deleterious to the tendon and subcutaneous tissues, and they are not recommended.

Failure to respond to conservative treatment will make surgery necessary to regain athletic function. Six to eight weeks of a properly devised and supervised program should be enough to identify the patients who do not respond. If the symptoms and signs remain the same, further modality or rehabilitative treatment is not going to be beneficial in healing the injury. The patient will continue to be in the overload vicious cycle with more deficits and adaptations. Most commonly, the surgical procedure will remove the degenerative granulation tissue and will repair the tendon either side to side or back to bone. Postoperative care includes a period of protection of the repair and gradual rehabilitation along the same lines that are advocated for nonoperative treatment. Return to play averages 3 months.

Medial Epicondylitis

"Medial tennis elbow" is not as common as lateral epicondylitis but is more commonly seen in advanced and competitive players. The pathology appears to be the same, with repetitive tensile microtears eventually giving rise to clinical tears and symptoms.

Tissue overload: forearm flexor mass, biceps, pronator teres, usually absolute overload

Tissue injury: same as for tissue overload, ± medial collateral ligament, ulnar nerve, and/or posterior medial olecranon ("valgus overload complex")

Clinical symptoms: point tender over flexor muscle mass, medial collateral ligament, posterior medial elbow, ± ulnar nerve symptoms

Functional biomechanical deficit: functional pronation contracture, consisting of elbow flexion and pronation inflexibility, tight and weak flexors, and decreased shoulder internal rotation strength

Subclinical adaptations: hitting "behind the body," more overhead serving motion, more wrist snap, more use of shoulder in serving motion

Conservative treatment should be employed first, with rest, alteration of mechanics, and antiinflammatory medicine or modalities. Medial counterforce braces may be beneficial. Treatment of this problem more commonly involves surgical repair. Surgery consists of excision of all degenerative tendon tissue, fasciotomy and debridement of damaged muscle, and either side-to-side or tendon-to-bone repair. Failure of this entity to heal nonoperatively probably reflects the larger peak forces that are generated by the advanced player that can result in more tissue disruption.

Before surgery it is important to differentiate epicondylitis from the valgus overload syndrome, which is common in baseball players but less common in tennis participants. This syndrome is caused by medial collateral ligament deficiency and is characterized by valgus instability, ulnar nerve irritation, and posteromedial bony impingement.

After surgery the repair is protected in a splint for 10–14 days, after which gradual range-of-motion exercises are instituted with protection in a functional brace. Rehabilitation should include muscle strengthening, as advocated for lateral epicondylitis, and restoration of normal flexibility. Before returning to play, the athlete either should have adequate muscular strength to withstand the demands of the power game or should alter the mechanics of the forehand strokes.

Low Back and Trunk Pain

This anatomic area is the site of many tennis-related injuries. Three main types of injuries are seen. The first is located in the posterior midline and is usually associated with the service motion or with straight-ahead activities, such as running to the net or hitting a low volley. The second is in the peripheral musculature of the quadratus lumborum or oblique abdominal muscles; it is associated with change in service motion or with ground strokes. The third is a tear of the rectus abdominis anteriorum, which is associated with hitting overheads or many serves.

Tissue overload: posterior back musculature, hamstrings, and hip rotators
Tissue injury: same as for tissue overload, with the addition of facet joints or sacroiliac joints
Functional biomechanical deficit: tight hamstrings, tight hip rotation and decreased trunk rotation
Subclinical adaptations: alteration of arm motion, excessive thoracolumbar motion, excessive hip and leg rotation

Treatment starts, as usual, with rest. This is especially important in these injuries, because as players try to play through the pain, they may further injure this area. This area is notoriously slow to return to normal function, and further insults slow the process down even more. Also, if this vital area of force transfer is impaired, alteration in the mechanics of the strokes is inevitable, leading to decreased performance and increased injury risk in many areas of the kinetic chain.

Further treatment emphasizes short-term protection with a light lumbosacral corset for pain relief, ice, and modalities. Early range-of-motion exercises are encouraged, with special emphasis on trunk rotation. Strengthening of both the flexor/extensor muscles and the trunk rotators must be complete before return to play.

If proper recognition and correction of the underlying musculoskeletal deficits are not accomplished as part of the rehabilitation process, the acute back strain may become chronic, with much more difficulty in returning to top performance.

Some tennis players will present with acute back pain and radicular symptoms. These should be managed as any nerve impingement.

Leg Muscle Strains

Acute muscle strains or acute exacerbation of chronic muscle strains may occur in any of the leg muscles, but they seem to be most common in the adductors (groin strain), the medial head of the gastrocnemius ("tennis leg"), and the hamstrings.

All of these may seem to be acute injuries, but a substantial proportion of them are acute exacerbations of chronic injuries. The chronic injury may be mildly symptomatic or overtly asymptomatic but still capable of creating a functional biomechanical deficit. Before initiation of treatment, it is important to inquire about previous injuries or prodromal symptoms and to check for anatomic deficits.

The difference between examining for acute hamstring strains and chronic hamstring strains may be seen in the evaluations. In the acute hamstring strain, the following complexes are observed:

Tissue overload: origin/insertion of hamstring or muscle tendon junction
Tissue injury: medial or lateral hamstring, secondary to mechanical disruption, varying degrees of inflammation
Clinical symptoms: point tenderness, swelling and/or bruising, mass
Functional biomechanical deficit: none
Subclinical adaptations: none

In the chronic hamstring strain, the following complexes are observed:

Tissue overload: same as acute
Tissue injury: same as acute plus fibrosis
Clinical symptoms: point tenderness, diffuse over leg, reinjury
Functional biomechanical deficit: hamstring inflexibility, quadriceps/hamstring muscle imbalance, adductor inflexibility, hip extensor weakness
Subclinical adaptations: shortened stride, shortened kick, use of hip extensors and gastrocnemius

Treatment of all the strains follows the same pattern. Ice should be used for early edema control. Support with conforming neoprene wraps helps to decrease further injury and allows early muscle use. Severe tears with large muscle damage, especially in the gastrocnemius, quadriceps, or hamstrings, should be splinted in a stretched position for 7–10 days, as this position has been shown to maintain maximal muscle tension and decrease scar contracture. Early massage will reduce edema and fibrous adhesions. Stretching exercises are instituted as soon as pain allows, followed by strengthening. Concentric power usually returns early, but eccentric power returns more slowly. Return to play should occur only after eccentric power has returned and any deficits have been corrected.

Achilles Tendinitis

Achilles tendinitis is not very common in tennis players but is disabling when it occurs. It usually occurs when playing surfaces are changed, as in going from hard courts indoors to soft courts outdoors in the spring. It may also occur when playing intensity increases, as in attending a tennis camp.

Tissue overload: gastrocnemius/soleus muscle or muscle tendon junction
Tissue injury: Achilles tendon, along its course or at its distal tendon bone attachment.

Clinical symptoms: point tenderness, ± knot, stiffness after rest
Functional biomechanical deficit: inflexibility in dorsiflexion, weak plantar flexors
Subclinical adaptations: shortened stance, less push-off

This injury is often prolonged in its treatment. In addition to standard antiinflammatory modalities, brace protection and stretching are advocated. Soft court surfaces may actually exacerbate the symptoms on return to play if the gastrocnemius is still tight and unable to absorb the applied load.

Achilles tendon rupture is relatively common in tennis players, especially among older players. Unfortunately, this is often underdiagnosed. Classically, patients feel a "pop" or feel that they have been struck in the leg. Plantar flexion may still be present owing to tibialis posterior activity, but the patient cannot stand on the toes and cannot "power off" the foot. The most sensitive test is the Thomas test, in which manual compression of the calf fails to produce passive plantar flexion of the foot.

Treatment of Achilles tendon ruptures may be surgical or nonsurgical. In active tennis players, surgical treatment allows secure repair, accurate coaptation of tendon tissue, minimal immobilization, and earlier onset of rehabilitation. This set of circumstances usually leads to earlier and more complete return to athletic function (44).

Ankle Sprains

Just as in other sports in which running, cutting, and stopping and starting are major demands, ankle sprains are the most common macrotrauma injury in tennis players. Twisting forces, especially in plantar flexion, account for most of the injuries.

Treatment for the large majority of acute ankle sprains should be conservative. Relative rest, protection, commonly in a pneumatic splint and only rarely in a cast, and ice are first-line modalities. Early protected range of motion and strengthening can be started as symptoms abate. Most ankle sprains tend to be treated too nonchalantly, with return to play when symptoms are gone. The reinjury rate within 1 year in these circumstances is around 70%. Inadequate treatment of the acute ankle sprain leads to the chronic ankle sprain syndrome, which has a more complex evaluation and is more difficult to rehabilitate. Therefore treatment should ensure good ligamentous stability, full flexibility, good plantar flexion and eversion strength, and proprioceptive retraining before return to play.

In the acute ankle sprain, the following complexes are observed:

Tissue overload: none
Tissue injury: anterior talofibular, fibulocalcaneal ligaments
Clinical symptoms: pain, swelling, point tender area
Functional biomechanical deficit: none
Subclinical adaptations: none

In the chronic ankle sprain, the following complexes are observed:

Tissue overload: plantar flexors, evertors
Tissue injury: same as above, plus ankle capsule
Clinical symptoms: recurrent sprains, locking of joint
Functional biomechanical deficit: plantar flexion inflexibility and weakness
Subclinical adaptations: running on heels, decreased stride length

Surgical treatment of ankle sprain problems is recommended in three special cases. One case is the loose or detached osteochondral fragment from the talar bone. Arthroscopic techniques are usually adequate to remove this piece of bone. The second case is soft tissue impingement in the anterolateral gutter. This impingement may take the form of "meniscoid" tissue or other types of scar tissue that may get trapped between the bones. Arthroscopic debridement has been very successful in this case as well. The final case is the chronically unstable ankle with functional instability, a positive anterior drawer test, some varus instability, and a failure of conservative treatment. A combination of an arthroscopic debridement of intraarticular scar and a modified Bronstrom-type repair of the lateral ligaments and retinaculum works well in most cases. In cases in which the lateral ligaments are too thin for plication, reconstruction with a portion of the peroneus brevis does well.

Plantar Fasciitis

Plantar fasciitis is common among athletes who run as part of their sport. The classical findings are of pinpoint tenderness over the insertion of the plantar fascia into the calcaneus, pain on first arising or after sitting, and return of symptoms during activity. Differential diagnostic possibilities include stress fractures of the calcaneus and impingement of the posterior tibial or medial calcaneal nerves. X-ray demonstration of an inferior calcaneal heel spur is not necessary for the diagnosis and is actually often misleading. In most cases the spur is of secondary importance, since it is not the cause of the pain.

Treatment is directed toward relieving the painful symptoms with the use of "arch aid" counterforce braces, modalities, rest, and medication. Athletes with plantar fasciitis have been shown to have deficits in flexibility and strength in the ankle plantar flexors that affect the onset of the symptoms and the outcome of the treatment. These deficits can be categorized into the following deficits:

Tissue overload: plantar flexor muscles, plantar fascial insertion at heel, foot intrinsic muscles

Tissue injury: plantar fascial attachment at heel

Clinical symptoms: point tenderness at base of calcaneus, worse in and/or after running

Functional biomechanical deficit: plantar flexor inflexibility and weakness, creating functional pronation

Subclinical adaptations: running on toes, shortened stride length, foot inversion

Correction of these deficits speeds the recovery process and allows for normalization of strength for running and jumping.

Surgical treatment, consisting of debridement of the damaged tissue and releasing the involved plantar fascia, is necessary in 10–15% of the cases. Recovery after such surgery is good but can be prolonged because of the important role of the heel pad and the plantar fascia in absorbing loads about the foot.

PRINCIPLES OF REHABILITATION

Adequate rehabilitation is the key to restoration of athletic function after injury. Most of the common tennis injuries can be successfully treated by nonsurgical means. In some athletes' and coaches' minds this implies that little rehabilitation must be done. On the contrary, this group of repetitive microtrauma overload injuries requires the most precise rehabilitation because of the nature of the pathogenesis of the injury. The outline of this process has been presented for each of the injuries. Several other points need to be emphasized (29,30).

The negative feedback vicious cycle may be used to guide rehabilitation as well. As has been demonstrated, there may be significant abnormalities in surrounding and supporting tissues in addition to the abnormalities causing symptoms. A complete and accurate diagnosis of all of the abnormalities by the process that has been outlined above is the first prerequisite for proper rehabilitation.

The second prerequisite is satisfactory completion of all phases of rehabilitation. The first is the acute phase, in which new clinical symptoms are reduced and tissue injury is controlled and started toward healing. The second is the recovery phase, in which tissue injury is healed, tissue overloads are reduced, and the functional biomechanical deficits are normalized. The third is the functional phase, in which all of the previous gains are directed toward elimination of the subclinical alterations and functional progressions for sports-specific and kinetic chain-specific activities are instituted.

The final prerequisite is a clearly defined set of criteria for return to play. This should include normalization of all of the parts of the negative feedback vicious cycle and completion of tennis functional progressions.

INTERVENTION STRATEGIES FOR INJURY PREVENTION

It is an enticing thought that since many of these injuries proceed through a rather long process of gradual damage before producing clinical symptoms, recognition of athletes in the preclinical stages could be accomplished and adequate steps could be undertaken to prevent further progression. It is also enticing to think that if all the sports-specific demands could be identified, then skill training programs could be designed to stay within certain limits, or "doses," and conditioning programs could be designed to optimize the musculoskeletal base for a particular sport. Research along these lines is proceeding, and early evidence points to support for these thoughts. Most of the research concerning tennis has already been presented. Reviews of the role of subclinical adaptations in injury causation and the role of strengthening in injury prevention point to positive results from improvement of these important parameters (6,8). Because of these findings, interventional strategies should be actively pursued in tennis injury work.

Identification of muscle weaknesses and inflexibilities can best be approached through a sports-specific preparticipation examination (35,36). By testing specific anatomic areas with tests that are relatively specific for the sport or activity, a profile of musculoskeletal readiness for play can be identified. Conditioning programs based on correcting deficits and strengthening areas of high demand can then be constructed. These have shown promise in decreasing injury (8). Fine-tuning of both the examination process and the conditioning programs will allow better results in the future.

This process of "prehabilitation," or prospective conditioning, is also important in young elite athletes who have the prospect of more intensive play as they get older. Studies have shown that adaptive changes occur as a result of playing sports in tennis players as young as 12–13 years of age (41). Injuries are not prevalent in this age group but are seen with high incidence in the 15- to 18-year-old group. It is surmised that the younger athlete's adaptive changes may be creating biomechanical deficits that predispose the athlete to injury with continued increased use. The areas of injury in the players (the shoulder, back, and knee) correspond with the areas of demonstrated inflexibility and weakness. Much work is now being directed toward defining the proper exercise dose in the young athlete to prevent such adaptations and defining the most appropriate conditioning programs, given the age and physical limitations in these athletes.

CONDITIONING FOR TENNIS

Due to factors such as the length of the season, the musculoskeletal maladaptations that occur with the sport, and the sport-specific injury patterns, it is necessary to discuss the sport-specific aspects of conditioning for tennis. A conditioning program for tennis can be divided into the following areas: prehabilitation (the correction of musculoskeletal maladaptations that may predispose the tennis player to injury), resistive training, and, finally, sprint/interval, footwork, and speech training.

Prehabilitation

Prehabilitation exercises would consist of exercises to correct musculoskeletal deficits found in a preparticipation evaluation of the tennis player. At the elite level, such exercises are important both to prevent injury and to improve performance. At the recreational level, these exercises are important to prevent injury and to allow the player to continue to enjoy and benefit from the sport of tennis. Typical goals of a prehabilitation program might be as follows:

1. To improve internal rotation range of motion on the dominant arm
2. To improve external rotation strength and endurance
3. To improve the strength of the scapular stabilizing musculature
4. To improve low back and hamstring flexibility
5. To correct any individual weaknesses in terms of strength and range of motion

Resistive Training

Resistive training for the tennis player is an important goal if the player is interested in preventing injuries and improving performance. Resistive training includes not only weight training, but also drills for abdominal strength, medicine ball drills for total body strength, and calisthenic exercises. By improving strength, power is increased, which is becoming an increasingly important component of tennis. Also, short-term endurance is increased, which is of tremendous importance to the tennis player. Conditioning with medicine balls has the advantage of conditioning the entire kinetic chain in a way that promotes improved power in the tennis stroke.

Sprint/Interval, Footwork, and Speed Training

As was previously mentioned, the sport of tennis is generally played in short bursts of activity. Interval training in the off-season progressing to shorter bursts of activity as the tennis season approaches is likely the best way to train for tennis. Interval training can provide an aerobic base that can be maintained by sprint training during the season. It is possible that extensive aerobic training during the season would interfere with the production of strength and power. Particularly for competitive tennis players, training in 10- to 20-second bursts is more specific to tennis performance than running long distances. By training in shorter bursts for long periods of time, the aerobic energy system will be utilized during the recovery process between exercise bouts, which is the same way it is used in a tennis match, that is, recovery between points.

One problem that often arises with competitive tennis players is that there is no off-season in which to condition. The best answer is found in the concept of periodization (8,23,36). By carefully planning the competitive year and by choosing the times of the year when the player wants to be at his or her best, a schedule of conditioning can be incorporated into this plan. Typically, there will be an off-season, a preseason, and an in-season leading to a peak. After a peak, there should be some time of active rest, when the athlete is allowed time to recover from intense competition. An athlete who would like to peak twice in a period of 4–6 weeks will not likely have the opportunity for active rest or for going into an off-season phase.

REFERENCES

1. Kibler WB, McQueen C, Uhl TL. Fitness evaluations and fitness findings in competitive junior tennis players. *Clin Sports Med* 1988;7:403–416.
2. Kibler WB, Chandler TJ. Racquet sports. In: Fu F, Stone R, eds. *Sports injuries: mechanisms, prevention, and treatment.* Baltimore: Williams & Wilkins, 1994:531–550.
3. Verspeelt P. A review of tennis related injuries in Flemish high-level tennis players. In: Krahl H, Pieper HG, Kibler WB, Renstrom P, eds. *Tennis: sports medicine and science.* Dusseldorf: Rau, 1995:47–51.
4. Winge S, Jorgenson U, Nielson L. Epidemiology of injuries in Danish championship tennis. *Int J Sports Med* 1989;10:368–371.
5. Hutchinson MR, Laprade RF, Burnett QM. Injury surveillance at the USTA boys' tennis championships: a 6 year study. *Med Sci Sports Exerc* 1995;7:826–830.
6. Butler D, Siegel A. Alterations in tissue response: conditioning effects at different ages. In: Leadbetter WB, Buckwalter JA, Gordon SL, eds. *Sports induced inflammation.* Rosemont IL: American Academy of Orthopaedic Surgeons, 1990:713–731.
7. Leadbetter WB. Cell-matrix response in tendon injury. *Clin Sports Med* 1992;11:553–578.
8. Chandler TJ, Kibler WB. Muscle training in injury prevention. In: Renstrom P, ed. *Sports injuries, principles of prevention and care.* London: Blackwell, 1993:252–261.
9. Ekstrand J, Gillquist J. The avoidability of soccer injuries. *Int J Sports Med* 1983;4:124–128.
10. O'Connor FG, Howard TM, Fiessler CM, et al. Managing overuse injuries: a systematic approach. *Phys Sports Med* 1997;25:88–113.
11. Baquie P, Brukner P. Injuries presenting to an Australian sports medicine centre: a 12-month study. *Clin J Sports Med* 1997;7:28–31.
12. Nirschl RP, Elbow tendinosis/tennis elbow. *Clin Sports Med* 1992;11:851–869.
13. Kannus P, Jozsa L. Histopathological changes preceding spontaneous rupture of a tendon. *J Bone Joint Surg* 1991;73:1517–1525.
14. Kibler WB. Pathophysiology of overload injuries around the elbow. *Clin Sports Med* 1995;14:447–456.
15. Teague BN, Schwane JA. Effect of intermittent eccentric contraction on symptoms of muscle microinjury. *Med Sci Sports Exerc* 1995;27:1378–1384.
16. Lieber RL. Friden J. Muscle damage is not a function of muscle force but active muscle strain. *J Appl Phys* 1993;74:520–526.

17. Knapik JJ, Bauman CL, Jones BH, Harris JM. Preseason strength and flexibility imbalances associated with athletic injuries in female collegiate athletes. *Am J Sports Med* 1991;19:76–81.
18. Meeuwisse WH. Assessing causation in sport injury: a multi-factoral model. *Clin J Sports Med* 1994;4:166–170.
19. Kibler WB. Biomechanical analysis of the shoulder during tennis activities. *Clin Sports Med* 1995;14:79–86.
20. Matsen FA, Harryman DT, Sidles JA. Mechanics of glenohumeral instability. *Clin Sports Med* 1991;10:783–788.
21. Kibler WB. Clinical biomechanics of the elbow in tennis: implications for evaluation and diagnosis. *Med Sci Sports Exerc* 1994;26:1203–1206.
22. Fox EL, Matthews DK. *Interval training*. Philadelphia: WB Saunders, 1974.
23. Fleck SJ, Kraemer WJ. *Designing resistance training programs*. Champaign, IL: Human Kinetics, 1987.
24. Pollock ML, Fox JH, Fox SM, *Health and fitness through physical activity*. New York: Wiley and Sons, 1990.
25. Nichols TR. A biomechanical perspective on spinal mechanisms of coordinated muscular action: an architectural principle. *Acta Anat (Basel)* 1994;151:1–13.
26. Elliott BC. Tennis strokes and equipment. In: Vaughn CL, ed. *Biomechanics of Sport*. Boca Raton FL: CRC Press, 1989: 263–288.
27. Giangarra CE, Conroy B, Jobe FW, Pink M. EMG and cinematographic analysis of elbow function in tennis players. *Am J Sports Med* 1993;21:394–399.
28. Glousman R, Jobe FW, Tibone JE. Dynamic EMG analysis of the throwing shoulder with glenohumeral instability. *J Bone Joint Surg* 1988;70:220–226.
29. Kibler WB, Chandler TJ, Pace BK. Principles of rehabilitation after chronic tendon injuries. *Clin Sports Med* 1992;11:661–673.
30. Kibler WB. Shoulder rehabilitation: principles and practice. *Med Sci Sports Exerc* 1998;30(4)(suppl):540–550.
31. *The preparticipation physical evaluation* [Monograph]. Minneapolis, MN: Physician and Sports Medicine Publishing, 1996.
32. Smith DM. Preparticipation physical evaluations. *Sports Med* 1995;18:293–299.
33. Kibler WB. *The sport preparticipation examination*. Champaign, IL: Human Kinetics, 1990.
34. *U.S. Tennis Association Tennis Profiling Exam*. Key Biscayne, FL: U.S. Tennis Association, 1994.
35. Kibler WB, Chandler TJ, Uhl TL. A musculoskeletal approach to the preparticipation exam. preventing injury and improving performance. *Am J Sports Med* 1989;17:525–531.
36. Kibler WB, Chandler TJ. Sport specific conditioning. *Am J Sports Med* 1994;22:424–432.
37. Krahl H, Michaelis U, Pieper HG. Stimulation of bone growth through sports. *Am J Sports Med* 1994;22:751–757.
38. Chandler TJ, Kibler WB, Kiser AM, Wooten BP. Shoulder strength, power, and endurance in college tennis players. *Am J Sports Med* 1992;20:455–458.
39. Ellenbecker TS. Rehabilitation of shoulder and elbow injuries in tennis players. *Clin Sports Med* 1993;14:87–105.
40. Silliman FJ, Hawkins RJ. Current concepts and recent advances in the athlete's shoulder. *Clin Sports Med* 1991;10:693–705.
41. Kibler WB, Chandler TJ. Musculoskeletal adaptations and injuries associated with intense participation in sports. In: Cahill BR, Pearl AJ, eds. *Intensive participation in children's sports*. Chicago: American Academy of Orthopaedic Surgeons, 1993.
42. Kibler WB, Chandler TJ, Roetert EP. Shoulder range of motion in elite tennis players. *Am J Sports Med* 1996;24:279–285.
43. MacIntyre JG, Lloyd-Smith DR. Overuse running injuries. In: Renstrom PA, ed. *Sports injuries: basic principles of prevention and care*. Cambridge, MA: Blackwell, 1993.
44. Kibler WB. Diagnosis, treatment, and rehabilitation principles in complete tendon ruptures in sports. *Scand J Med Sci Sports* 1997;7:119–129.

CHAPTER 51

Volleyball

Lee Rice and Allen Richburg

INTRODUCTION

In 1895 William G. Morgan, a YMCA physical fitness director, invented volleyball in Holyoke, Massachusetts. Volleyball, originally called mintonette, was intended to be a slower, less strenuous form of basketball. The sport was slow to gain popularity until 1947, when the Fédération Internationale de Volley-Ball (FIVB) was formed (1). Volleyball became an Olympic sport in 1964, and over the last three decades the game has blossomed into one of the world's most popular participation sports. Currently, over 200 countries are members of the FIVB, and there are an estimated 200 million volleyball players in the world (1–5).

Through the 1960s, 1970s, and 1980s, volleyball evolved into a fast-paced game of speed, power, and agility. In the 1960s the Japanese were the masters of complex setting and high-speed hitting schemes. As power increased and technique improved, the ball speeds have approached 80 miles per hour. Another innovation in the 1960s was the Czechoslovakian school of defending and receiving high-speed serves or spikes ("kills") with the outstretched arms instead of passing the ball with the fingers. With increasing ball speeds, players are required to move more rapidly to hit the ball. Another major change in the evolution of the game occurred in the 1970s, when a rule change allowed the athletes to step over the middle line under the net (4). This rule change prevented the game from being stopped so often and increased the pace of the game. It also subjected the athletes to more trauma under the net. Ballistic jumping to attack, block, or serve occurs multiple times in a game. The players train hard to gain strength, speed, and endurance so that they are able to explosively move vertically and horizontally to hit the ball. With the advent of a faster, more powerful game, and as the competition has improved, interest in the game has increased. As the sport is progressing, a better understanding of its specific acute and overuse injuries is occurring. The team physician must understand volleyball rules, terminology, body movements, and demands of the sport to fully comprehend the multiple types of injuries these athletes receive.

There are six basic volleyball skills in which the athletes have different biomechanics subjecting them to injuries: serving, passing (serve reception), setting, attacking, blocking, and defending ("digging") (Figs. 51–1 through 51–4). With blocking, attacking, and jump serving, a high power jump begins the maneuver, subjecting the athlete to patellofemoral and Achilles tendon problems. When the player is in the air during a block, the fingers and shoulders are extended and vulnerable to trauma and strains. The block and attack both usually involve landing at the net, where there could be a collision with an opponent, since the players feet are allowed to cross the line under the net. This is a frequent cause of ankle, foot, and knee injuries. The attack and serve both involve high-velocity overhead arm movements, which often cause acute or overuse shoulder and back injuries. Defending often requires a player to dive with an outstretched arm, "digging" the ball up from nearly hitting the floor. This maneuver may cause trauma to the hand, wrist, elbow, shoulder, knee, and head. Passing and setting involve using the fingers, hands, and arms to precisely deliver the ball to a teammate for the attack ("spike"). Fingers are the most commonly injured body part during the pass and the set in volleyball. Additionally setters often develop back problems due to chronic repetitive hyperextension of the lumbar spine.

Several studies were done in the 1980s and 1990s on the incidence of volleyball injuries (1,2,6–14) (Table 51–1). There is an estimated overall injury incidence ranging from 0.67 to 2.3 per 100 hours of play (7,13). Most of these injuries are minor injuries (12). The inci-

---

L. Rice and A. Richburg: San Diego Sports Medicine, San Diego, California 92120.

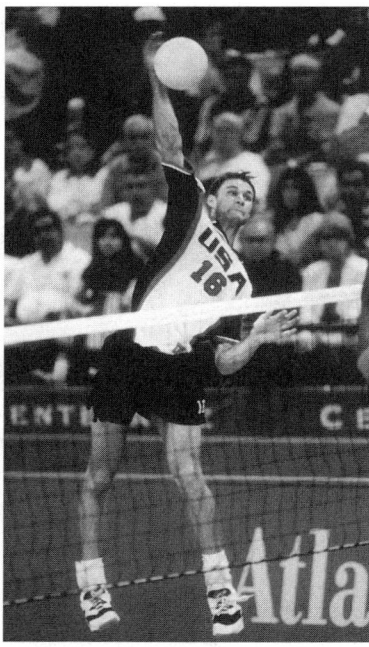

FIG. 51–1. A powerful spike may have biomechanics similar to that of the serve.

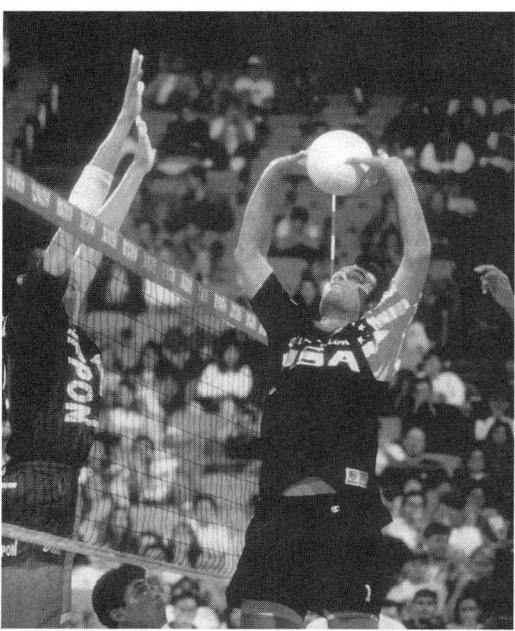

FIG. 51–3. The setter often sets the ball on the second volley with the fingers extended and the back hyperextended for the offensive spike.

dence of injuries requiring special medical attention or a player to miss one or more days of play ranges from 1.5 to 3.8 per 1000 hours of play (6,7). School-age children (8–17 years old) injure themselves more during practice, whereas highly competitive and elite athletes injure themselves up to four times more during competition (7,9). Over the last 10 years the popularity of volleyball has increased, resulting in better competition and therefore a greater training demand. This has resulted in a greater number of overuse injuries. Therefore the

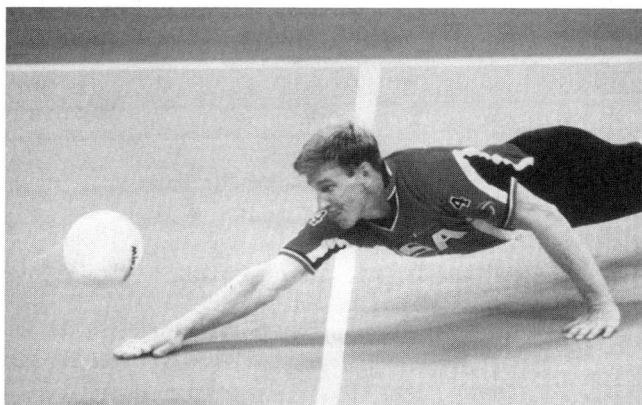

FIG. 51–2. Diving for the ball, or "digging," is often required to defend against the opponent's possible scoring volley. This subjects the digger to possible wrist, elbow, shoulder, and head trauma with the floor or another player.

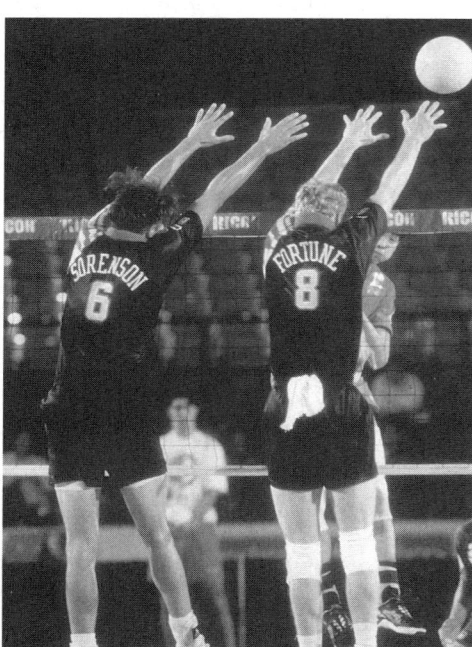

FIG. 51–4. Defending the spike requires high jumping at the net with arms above the head and fingers extended. This potentiates the risk of injuries under the net and finger injuries.

TABLE 51-1. Body part injury location

Study	Total number of injuries	Ankle and foot (%)	Knee (%)	Shoulder (%)	Finger, hand, and wrist (%)	Back (%)	Head (%)	Misc. (%)
Ho (1996)	*	44	11	22	6	8	4	5
Rice and Anderson (1994)	222†	20	19	16	14	18	6	7
Watkins and Green (1992)	46	35	30	2	22	17		
Schafle et al. (1990)	154	18	11	8	10	14		
Lohmann et al. (1988)	242	34	10		59			

* 10-year NCAA Division III university volleyball injuries.
† 10-year National Volleyball Team injuries reported to the team physician.

team physician may see up to 40–50% of volleyball injuries resulting from repetitive trauma (6).

Even though volleyball is a noncontact sport, it is considered a high-risk sport by some (7). The competitive player endures up to 150 maximal effort explosive jumps and multiple powerful volleys in a game. This, plus extensive pregame training, is a setup for many acute and overuse injuries. Approximately 60% of injuries occur at the net, either blocking or spiking. Of these injuries the majority are acute finger or ankle injuries and overuse knee or shoulder injuries (6). The beginning volleyball player is more likely to suffer finger injuries and contusions, whereas the elite athlete suffers a higher percentage of ankle, knee, shoulder, and low back injuries. Injury risk factors for volleyball include jumping, landing, contact under the net or with a teammate, hand contact with the ball during a spike or block, hardness of the playing surface, shock absorbency of the shoes, and level of physical conditioning (4,12,13).

More volleyball injuries are seen as more competitors enter the sport and the competition increases. With increased competition comes a demand to spend more time training. Two-player sand volleyball and the lucrative professional "beach tour" have also given an incentive to train harder and have brought many new players to the sport. The influx of players has increased the sports medicine physician's interest in the many acute and overuse injuries of volleyball. The team physician should develop sports-specific preventive mechanisms, training strategies, and treatment protocols to improve athletic performance. This chapter will detail many of the common injuries of volleyball in an attempt to assist the team physician in prevention, diagnosis, and treatment of volleyball injuries.

ANKLE AND FOOT INJURIES

The volleyball team physician will see many acute ankle sprains. Approximately one ankle sprain per 1000 player hours will occur, resulting in 20–50% of all volleyball injuries (2,5,8). This is the most common injury in most studies and one of the most debilitating to the player's need to perform multiple explosive jumps in a game. Recurrent sprains, ankle instability, syndesmosis injury, chronic synovial impingement, osteochondral fracture, and fibular physis disruption are among the complications (1). Explosive jumping or awkward landing may cause Achilles tendon rupture, os trigonum fracture, peroneal tendon dislocation, or multiple other foot fractures. Repetitive jumping may cause retrocalcaneal bursitis, Achilles, posterior tibial, and peroneal tendinitis. In addition, repetitive jumping may also cause stress fractures of the metatarsal or navicular bones, plantar fasciitis, and Morton's plantar neuroma.

The most important step in diagnosis is the history. Approximately 90% of acute ankle sprains are inversion injuries. Often players will roll their ankle after a jump, landing on an opponent's foot under the net or off balance on their own supinated foot. With this type of injury the foot is usually in a plantar flexed position that first stresses the anterior talofibular ligament as the inversion occurs. The next ligament stressed is the calcaneofibular ligament, followed by the posterior talofibular ligament as the inverted foot moves from plantar flexion to dorsiflexion. Moderate to severe inversion injuries may also involve sprains to the interosseous ligament between the distal tibia and fibula. An eversion injury is less common and usually less serious, because the deltoid ligament is a much larger structure. However, significant deltoid ligament injuries may heal slowly and keep the athlete out of action for an extended period of time. The severity of the injury is important to assess immediately after the injury. Important considerations are the mechanism of injury; whether or not the player was able to continue to play, walk, or bear weight immediately after the injury; and previous history of injury.

Examination of the injured ankle and foot should consist of appearance, range of motion, stress testing, strength testing, and neurovascular status. Radiographs are recommended if a fracture, dislocation, or unstable ankle mortise is suspected. Clinically, one must distinguish between a grade I (microtrauma), grade II (partial tear), and grade III (complete tear) injury of the involved ligaments. After the proper grade of ankle sprain is diagnosed, the appropriate treatment may ensue.

Early treatment of all ankle sprains consists of rest, ice, compression, elevation, and early aggressive rehabilitation. Grade I and II ankle sprains can all be treated conservatively. Return to competition with a significantly injured ankle will delay healing and may lead to further injury. Crutches may be needed for a few days to partially bear weight on a painful ankle. Ice treatment beginning within the first 24 hours has been shown to decrease the number of days before return to function by about 50% (15). Compression and elevation help to decrease pain and swelling. A removable walking cast or air splint/cast may allow earlier protected weight bearing while protecting the injured ligaments from mechanical stress.

Early rehabilitation is an essential part of treatment to facilitate a rapid recovery and prevent reinjury. It should first consist of range-of-motion exercises. As soon as the player has adequate range of motion, work on regaining proprioception should begin with exercises such as drawing the alphabet with the toe. Then, when the player can bear weight, balance exercises on the affected ankle can begin. The physical therapist or athletic trainer can begin proprioception exercises using a balance board or tilt board. A progression from partial weight bearing to full weight bearing, to jogging, to running, to running figure eights, to sports-specific activities may proceed rapidly. Grade I sprains generally improve well enough for return to play within a week or two. Grade II ankle sprains usually improve within 2–6 weeks. Grade III ankle sprains require either immobilization or surgery and should be evaluated by an orthopedic surgeon. Debate continues among orthopedic surgeons about the proper indications for surgical repair of grade III sprains.

An ankle injury prevention program has been found to reduce the incidence of acute ankle sprains twofold over a 2-year period. The injury program consisted of an injury awareness session, technical training on proper jumping mechanisms, and balance board training (2). Recurrent ankle sprains and ankle instability are complications of ankle sprains. Recurrent ankle sprains are four times more likely to occur than a first-time injury. Therefore ankle braces worn for 6–12 months after an acute injury may prevent recurrent sprains (2,8,9) and the risk of developing instability. In addition, ankle braces may prevent contact-related lateral ankle injury (16).

Eversion ankle sprains make up only 10% of all ankle sprains in volleyball players. This injury occurs when a player lands off balance on a dorsally flexed foot, causing external rotation and eversion. Most eversion ankle sprains are mild injuries to the deltoid ligament, but if there is significant force, the anterior tibiofibular ligament and interosseous membrane may become involved. This causes more pain with lateral rotation of the foot and tenderness over the deltoid and anterior tibiofibular ligament. Proximal fibular fractures, medial malleolus fractures, and mortise instability are more common with this type of sprain. This type of high ankle sprain is called a syndesmotic ankle sprain. High ankle sprains cause increased pain when standing, when walking on the ball of the foot, and during takeoff from a jump. Treatment principles are similar to lateral ankle sprains, but recovery is generally prolonged.

In jumping sports, persistent ankle symptoms occasionally occur after an ankle sprain. If this occurs, reevaluation of the athlete may reveal chronic conditions such as synovial impingement syndrome of the ankle, peroneal tendon strain, posterior tibial tendinitis, chronic ankle instability, painful os trigonum, stress fractures of the fibula or navicular, or osteochondritis dissecans. Most of these chronic problems cause pain with pushoff and landing during a jump. Synovial impingement syndrome usually involves the anterolateral synovium, resulting in tenderness under the anterior talofibular ligament. If adequate physical therapy and nonsteroidal antiinflammatory drugs (NSAIDs) have failed, the mature player may benefit from a corticosteroid injection into the joint space. Two to four weeks of immobilization for severe cases of the above conditions may be necessary. If symptoms persist, ankle arthroscopy may be indicated.

Peroneus longus, brevis, and tertius muscles function to evert and plantar flex the foot. The volleyball player uses these muscles during ballistic lateral jumping and lateral shuffling. Inflammations and strains of these tendons are frequently associated with inversion ankle sprains and overuse injuries. Symptoms are usually localized to the lateral ankle where the peroneal brevis and tertius tendons insert on the proximal fifth metatarsal, over the cuboid bone where the peroneus longus turns medially, the peroneus muscle bellies, or the origin of the peroneus brevis and tertius on the distal lateral fibula. Treatment consists of relative rest with stretching, icing, strengthening, physical therapy, proprioception training, and NSAIDs. Ballistic lateral jumping may rarely cause acute peroneal tendon rupture or dislocation over the lateral malleolus, both of which need to be surgically repaired.

The os trigonum is an accessory bone on the lateral tubercle of the posterior talus found in 10% of the population. The tubercle may fracture with extreme plantar flexion that may occur with jumping. It may also become acutely stressed if a player lands on the foot of another player, forcing him or her to fall backward in extreme plantar flexion. The athlete acutely presents with posterior lateral ankle pain and decreased range of motion. This injury must be suspected if posterior ankle pain is provoked with passive hyperextension and active flexion of the great toe. Radiographs confirm the diagnosis. Treatment of a nondisplaced acute fracture generally includes immobilization for 4–6 weeks. If the fracture is widely displaced or becomes chronically symptomatic, excision may be appropriate.

Achilles tendinitis, retrocalcaneal bursitis, posterior tibial tendinitis, peroneal tendinitis, and stress fractures of the metatarsals or navicular are some of the most common overuse injuries of the foot. Tendonopathies and fractures are diagnosed by history of the pain and tenderness over the structure involved. As the problem worsens, the athlete may notice pain after an event or practice, then during practice, that progresses to pain throughout the day exacerbated by practice.

Achilles tendinitis may present with thickness, crepitus, and pain with active plantar flexion over the distal tendon at the insertion on the calcaneus. Retrocalcaneal bursitis may be confused with Achilles tendinitis. With retrocalcaneal bursitis, pain is often worse with jumping while wearing shoes than when the shoes are taken off because the heel rubs against the back of the shoe. Careful palpation of the bursae, either deep or superficial to the distal Achilles tendon, elicits pain. In addition, the bursa is often inflamed and edematous, and the Achilles tendon is pain free. Both problems respond well to relative rest, icing, proper shoes, Achilles tendon stretching, NSAIDs, and physical therapy. A heel lift may also decrease the tendon pull and decrease the pain. A slow graded return to a normal exercise program guided by the athletic trainer and coach is the cornerstone in preventing recurrence.

One of the most dramatic injuries in jumping sports is an Achilles tendon rupture. This seems to occur more frequently if the tendon is tight from tendinitis or a poor warm-up (11). Acute onset of pain in the back of the leg after a forceful pushoff or landing, which has been described as feeling like getting shot, is often the history. There is usually a palpable defect 2–6 cm above the Achilles insertion on the calcaneus. Also noted is severe weakness or the inability to actively plantar flex the foot. The Thompson squeeze test is positive when the relaxed calf is squeezed in the prone athlete with the knees bent at 90° and a significant difference in plantar flexion of the normal ankle is noted. Treatment is either a long-leg cast with the knee in 45° of flexion and the ankle in gravity equinus or surgical repair. Orthopedic consultation is recommended.

Acute and stress fractures are not uncommon injuries in volleyball players. Bone tenderness should prompt a radiograph in the athlete. Supination injuries of the ankle may result in avulsion fractures or spiral fractures of the distal fibula with or without an accompanying fracture of the medial malleolus. Pronation injuries may result in avulsion fractures of the medial malleolus or fractures anywhere along the fibula. In addition, twisting injuries to the ankle may result in subtle avulsion and chip fractures of the proximal metaphysis of the fifth metatarsal, lateral process of the talus, posterior tubercle of the talus, osteochondral dome of the talus, or anterior process of the calcaneus. Whether to treat these fractures conservatively or surgically depends on the stability of the ankle mortise and the amount of displacement. Most of these fractures do very well with conservative management. If the diagnosis or treatment is in doubt, orthopedic consultation is advised.

Landing from a high jump onto another player's foot may result in a strong adduction and plantar flexion force to the fifth metatarsal, resulting in fracture at the junction between the diaphysis and metaphysis. This potentially season-ending injury is the result of a fracture between the insertion of the peroneus brevis and tertius tendons where there is poor vascularization. This fracture, commonly called a Jones fracture, has a high rate of nonunion, especially if the athlete tries to come back too early or does not comply with the recommended treatment of at least 4 weeks of non-weight-bearing immobilization followed by graduated weight-bearing immobilization for another 4 weeks or until radiographic evidence of full healing is present. This athlete should be referred to an orthopedic surgeon, and if not healed by 12 weeks, a decision to operate should be made (17).

Stress fractures of the foot in volleyball players are common. Metatarsal and navicular stress fractures are the most common (1,4). Usually, by the time the player complains, there has been pain for a number of days that has slowly gotten worse and is now affecting play. Physical examination reveals tenderness over the bone involved with subtle edema. Radiographs are often negative if taken within 3–4 weeks of the onset. At that time a bone scan may show the injury. After 3–4 weeks, cortical thickening may be seen on the plain films. Further jumping or running by the athlete may lead to an acute event in which the athlete may feel the bone completely fracture. The athlete will heal within 4–8 weeks with a firm-soled shoe and cessation of jumping and running. Play may resume when the athlete is pain free and evidence of healing is noted on the radiograph. A careful history must be taken to rule out potential causes of osteoporosis such as corticosteroid use, eating disorders, and amenorrhea. If osteoporosis is suspected, a DEXA scan for bone mineral density should be completed. The athlete should consume a minimum of 1000–1200 mg of calcium per day and have other factors corrected that may lead to osteoporosis.

Pain at the bottom of the foot during pushoff or landing is another common complaint. Three common problems associated with plantar foot pain are plantar fasciitis, Morton's neuroma, and sesamoiditis. Plantar fasciitis presents with arch pain that is worse in the morning or at the beginning of play, tenderness at the plantar fascia's origin on the calcaneus, and tight heel cords. Treatment consists of icing, NSAIDs, doughnut heel pads or arch supports, calf stretching, and night stretching, massaging the plantar fascia, injection, and physical therapy. Morton's neuroma is characterized by pain between the third and fourth toes due to constrictive footwear. Less frequently, the neuroma can occur between the second and third toes or the fourth and fifth toes. This is aggravated by accumulative jumping trauma and can be very painful. Treatment includes shoes with more cushion and a wider toe box, relative rest, metatarsal pads, corticosteroid injection, and physical therapy. Surgical resection of the neuroma is a last resort. Sesamoiditis presents with pain under the metatarsal phalangeal joint of the great toe. There is often local tenderness, edema, and pain with passive dorsiflexion of the foot. Treatment is conservative with relative rest, ice, massage, physical therapy, NSAIDs, and shoe padding orthotics. Occasionally, corticosteroid injection is beneficial, but a sesamoid stress fracture must be ruled out by radiographs and bone scan if suspected. Surgical excision of the sesamoid bone may be indicated if conservative treatment fails.

KNEE AND LEG INJURIES

Complex hitting and spiking schemes in which multiple players jump before one hits the ball are common offensive strategies that have greatly increased the demand for repetitive jumping. Up to 40% of high-level volleyball players will get "jumper's knee," or patellar tendinitis (18). Other common overuse injuries of the lower extremity include patella femoral syndrome, tibial periostitis, tibial stress fractures, iliotibial band syndrome, semimembranosis tendinitis, and prepatella bursitis. In the younger athlete the team physician will often see Osgood-Schlatter disease (tibial tuberosity apophysitis) due to sliding on the knees or repetitive jumping. The more mature athlete may have joint pain complaints due to osteoarthritis. Multiple acute injuries also occur. Ligament sprains and tears, along with muscle strains, are the most frequent acute injuries. Of these a rupture of the anterior cruciate ligament is of the most common and devastating, owing to chronic instability or long rehabilitation after surgery.

Volleyball is a high-risk sport for patellar tendinitis (jumper's knee) because of the demand of repetitive ballistic jumping on a hard surface (1,4,11,14,19–21). The strongest jumper with poor biomechanics will have a higher risk for patellar tendinitis (21,22). This injury occurs more frequently in women, on hard playing surfaces, and during actual game play in upper-level players (13). This problem is seen less in sand volleyball competitors (19). Patellar tendinitis can be debilitating to the overworked volleyball player. The natural progression of the problem begins with anterior knee pain after exercise, then pain at the beginning of exercise, followed by pain throughout and after exercise. A rare complication is patellar tendon rupture. There is usually tenderness of the distal patella pole, but there may be tenderness anywhere along the patellar tendon. Radiographs may show calcifications in the tendon or spurring of the distal patella. Treatment includes a workout with less jumping, a slow progressive warm-up, regular stretching, and quadricep strengthening. Ice, NSAIDs and physical therapy are also often needed. In severe cases, when jumping has to be stopped until the athlete is pain free, a gradual progression back should start with stationary bicycling, followed by running on a soft surface or mini-trampoline, and then a slow return to graded jumping drills in practice.

Patellofemoral syndrome is a common injury resulting from repetitive jumping, maltracking of the patella, or degenerative changes to the patellofemoral joint. This is diagnosed by complaints of knee pain during jumping, going down stairs, knee extension exercises, and prolonged sitting. Physical examination will elicit pain under the patella. The team physician may also notice decreased tone or atrophy of the vastus medialus oblique muscle (VMO), infrapatellar crepitus, Q-angle greater than 13°, overpronation, and effusion. Treatment includes relative rest with an aggressive VMO-strengthening program, ice, NSAIDs, a knee sleeve with a lateral buttress, and arch support if there is excessive pronation (1,13,23).

Traumatic injuries to the ligaments and cartilage of the knee are common and occur more frequently in players during competition who are playing at the net (18). The mechanism of injury and the immediate signs and symptoms are the most important diagnostic indicators. A history of hearing or feeling a "pop" during a valgus twisting injury followed by the sensation of an unstable knee strongly suggests an anterior cruciate ligament (ACL) tear. An accurate diagnosis is most likely to be made if the athlete is examined immediately after the injury before an effusion develops. The team physician should first examine the noninjured knee and then observe the injured knee for deformity or ecchymosis. Next palpation should be done, looking particularly for effusion (suggests internal derangement), tenderness over the patellar tendon, tenderness over the collateral ligaments and joint line tenderness (meniscal tears). Lachman's test is preferred for ACL testing. Varus and valgus stress tests the lateral collateral and medial collateral ligaments, respectively. The McMurry test, Apley test, and ability to squat test appraise the menisci. Relaxation of the patient during the exam is very important. Once a diagnosis is made, appropriate treatment consists of a knee brace if there is instability, crutches if the patient is unable to bear weight, early physical therapy, and orthopedic follow-up depending on the injury. Ice, NSAID's, compression, elevation, and sometimes analgesic pain medicine may be necessary.

A popping sensation is not always synonymous with an ACL tear. Athletes will often describe a popping sensation if they suffer a patellar subluxation. The mechanism for this injury is a strong quadriceps contraction with a flexed leg with valgus stress. Risk factors for this injury are a poorly developed VMO muscle, a large Q-angle, and others similar to those for the previously mentioned patellofemoral syndrome. With a patellar subluxation there will be medial retinaculum pain and apprehension with lateral patellar stress. An athlete with patellofemoral syndrome may have some apprehension, but the condition does not result from an acute injury. Treatment for patellar subluxation includes rest until the athlete is relatively pain free, VMO strengthening, ice, NSAIDs, a patellar stabilization brace, and correction of overpronation. Surgical treatment for refractory cases is an arthroscopic lateral retinaculum release and/or patellar tendon transfer.

A common cause of lateral knee pain from overtraining is iliotibial band syndrome. The athlete usually has sharp lateral knee pain during knee flexion with varus stress and walking down a slope or stairs. There is usually point tenderness over Gerdy's tubercle, the lateral femoral epicondyle, or the fibular collateral ligament from iliotibial band friction. A tight iliotibial band predisposes an athlete to this syndrome; therefore stretching is the cornerstone to preventing and treating this problem unless there is a biomechanical etiology.

Another important cause of insidious knee pain in the jumping athlete is osteochondritis dissecans. This is due to trauma causing avascular necrosis of the subchondral bone and 75% of the time involves the medial femoral condyle. Aching knee pain is usually worse with weight-bearing exercise and jumping. Physical examination is usually nonspecific. Radiographs show a characteristic half-moon defect in the subchondral bone. Since the prognosis is variable, the athlete should be referred to an orthopedist. Young athletes have a better prognosis and are usually recommended non-weight-bearing immobilization or active weight-bearing modification. Arthroscopic surgery to remove the necrosed fragment or drill the defect to facilitate revascularization may be recommended.

Vigorous overtraining can cause shin splints, stress fractures, gastrocnemius muscle strains, and compartment syndrome of the leg. The most frequently occurring problem when athletes start a vigorous running or jumping program is shin splints. This is also called medial tibial stress syndrome and is due to periostitis, myositis, or musculotendinitis, typically along the distal third of the medial tibia. The athlete may have tenderness, swelling, warmth, or elevation of the periostium. However, severe point tenderness, edema, tuning pain, and a painful hop test suggest a stress fracture. Radiographs are typically negative, and a technetium bone scan has limited specificity because an inflamed periostium will show diffuse uptake. A true stress fracture, however, will show intense uptake. Severe stress fractures will show the ominous "horizontal black line," usually on the midshaft of the anterior tibia. Treatment varies with the severity of symptoms. If no fracture exists, then a reduction in jumping and running, calf stretches, ice massage, backward-walking warm-up, NSAIDs, and antipronation orthotics or taping will usually help. If symptoms persist or pain increases, cessation of running and jumping may be required for 2 weeks. If a stress fracture is evident, a short-leg walking cast for 4–6 weeks may be recommended. Occasionally, if there is a suspected nonunion with an anterior horizontal black line on radiograph, placement of a tibial rod may allow an earlier return to play.

If symptoms persist out of proportion to the training injury, if there is numbness, or if there is significant pain with passive range of motion, then the team physician must consider an exertional chronic compartment syndrome. In addition to medial tibial stress syndrome, the differential includes a gastrocnemius strain that usually will reveal point tenderness in the area of injury. If exertional compartment syndrome is suspected, then the location of symptoms will locate the compartment in which pressures should be measured during exercise and during cool-down. If specific surgical criteria are met, then a fasciotomy should be completed.

SHOULDER INJURIES

Most shoulder injuries in volleyball are due to overuse. However, occasionally, a player may sustain a traumatic shoulder dislocation, rotator cuff tear, or glenoid labral tear. Players who have multidirectional instability or ligamentous laxity are the most likely to suffer a shoulder subluxation or dislocation with blocking or diving. Other traumatic shoulder injuries in volleyball are very rare, whereas overuse injuries like chronic shoulder impingement, tendonopathies, and chronic instability are so common that many volleyball players will have some form of these problems during their career (11). Another common condition that is unique to volleyball players and other overhand sports is infraspinatus atrophy. Each of these common shoulder problems is discussed below.

Repetitive overhead hitting, performed in spiking and serving, may cause rotator cuff tendinitis, bicep tendinitis, or subacromial bursitis—all part of the shoulder impingement syndrome. This is an overuse injury that may be associated with a type II or III acromion (anterior inferior acromion beaking) and glenohumeral instability. The athlete will complain of shoulder pain with overhead hitting and with raising the arm above 80–120° and will often have shoulder pain at night. Physical examination may reveal tenderness of the supraspinatus insertion on the greater tuberosity of the humerus, in the subacromial region, or of the long head of the bicep in the bicepital groove. There is usually pain without true weakness during isolated testing of the rotator cuff muscles, and there are usually positive Neer's and Hawkin's impingement signs. Treatment includes ice, relative rest, stretching, physical therapy, and NSAIDs. A subacromial corticosteroid injection may be helpful, depending on the severity and chronicity of the impingement as well as the response to other conservative measures. Arthroscopic subacromial decompression is warranted when conservative treatment has failed and the player wants to continue the sport. Prevention of the injury includes balance of shoulder flexibility (24), strengthening of rotator cuff muscles, training modifications, and biomechanical modification of overhead hitting techniques.

Chronic impingement syndrome may increase the athlete's vulnerability to an acute tear of the rotator cuff. The supraspinatus, infraspinatus, subscapularis, and teres minor muscles are often acutely stressed with blocking or diving to make a save. With maximum flexion of the arm, the force is transmitted to the rotator cuff. The most common area for a tear is at the attachment of the supraspinatus muscle on the humerus. Isolated supraspinatus provocation testing is done by having the athlete elevate the internally rotated arm against downward resistance while held at 90° abduction and 45° forward flexion. Radiographs may show signs of chronic calcific rotator cuff tendinitis, subacromial space narrowing, and subacromial spurring. Partial or complete rotator cuff tears and glenoid labral pathology can generally be diagnosed with magnetic resonance imaging (MRI). Open surgical, arthroscopic, and combined procedures are available for repair of the rotator cuff and subacromial decompression. Complete surgical recovery is usually 2–4 months until return to competition. Prevention and rehabilitation consist of a graduated rotator cuff range of motion, stretching and strengthening regimen, and reconditioning of contiguous and related muscle groups.

The same mechanism that is responsible for rotator cuff injuries may also cause tears of the glenoid labrum. This is especially true for forces resulting in anterior–posterior humeral head transition. The athlete experiences pain and clicking with glenohumeral motion as the humeral head moves across the torn labrum. There may be associated weakness of the rotator cuff muscles. "Crank" and "clunk" tests may be positive. An MRI scan often shows the lesion. Conservative treatment including relative rest and rehabilitation should be attempted before consideration of surgical arthroscopic labral debridement or repair.

Traumatic shoulder dislocation or subluxation may occur during a block, diving, or an awkward overhand serve. The most common mechanism is a strong posteriorly directed horizontal force applied to the hand when the arm is abducted and externally rotated as the rotator cuff and pectoralis major muscles are becoming fully contracted. This results in an anterior dislocation. Posterior dislocations may occur with a posteriorly directed glenohumeral force. After an acute dislocation the athlete will experience pain and will not be able to move the glenohumeral joint, the arm generally being held at the side. A sulcus sign or other soft tissue deformity will be present. Neurovascular status should be assessed before and after reduction. An immediate on-the-court reduction will minimize the athlete's discomfort and may decrease the risk of neurovascular compromise. This should be attempted only by an experienced clinician who is able to determine the safety and appropriateness of the procedure. Any loss of pulse warrants emergent vascular and orthopedic consultation. If there is extreme pain or crepitus with manual reduction or the diagnosis is in question, there may be a fracture of the humeral neck, scapula, or clavicle, and emergent radiographs are warranted. Postreduction radiographs are recommended. In the emergency room, prereduction radiographs are beneficial for confirming the exact diagnosis and for medical-legal reasons. Commonly seen are Hill-Sachs and bony Bankart fractures, which are a reason for continued pain after reduction and may lead to an increased risk for future surgical repair for instability. Postreduction treatment includes wearing a sling for comfort for 3–7 days, after which range-of-motion exercises and physical therapy should begin. Patients with chronic instability or recurrent dislocations should be referred for orthopedic consultation for consideration of surgical repair.

Suprascapular neuropathy ("volleyball shoulder") occurs in the dominant shoulder of approximately 15% of high-level volleyball players (4,25). Isolated, painless atrophy and weakness of the infraspinatus muscle are usually the presenting problem (26) (Fig. 51–5). There is usually no associated pain or change in performance, but there is a notable decrease in shoulder external rotation strength. Causative actions for this are thought to be the deceleration phase of the serve and spike and possibly the defensive reception (4,26–28). During these

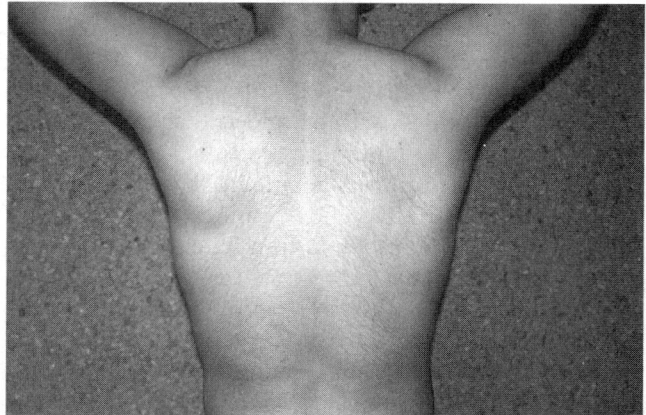

FIG. 51–5. Right infraspinatus atrophy is evident in this athlete. This often painless injury is common among volleyball players.

activities there is contraction of the infraspinatus and a stretch or compression of the suprascapular nerve at the suprascapula notch (SSN), the spinoglenoid notch (SGN), or the lateral edge of the scapular spine. Entrapment at the SGN is most common. Pain may be associated with suprascapular nerve entrapment at the SSN, which usually causes supraspinatus muscle atrophy. Pain is more likely associated with compression of the nerve by a ganglion cyst or a resulting impingement syndrome. Electrophysiologic studies should be done to confirm the diagnosis. If the diagnosis is still in question, one might consider an MRI to visualize the anatomy of the periscapula region. If there are pain, pallor, and decreased pulses, MRI angiography should be considered to rule out a posterior circumflex humeral artery aneurysm, which is occasionally found in volleyball players (29). Good treatment results have been seen with stretching and strengthening the remaining infraspinatus and teres minor muscles and teaching follow-through on the serve to decrease trauma caused by the deceleration phase. Surgery is indicated if pain is associated with compression of the nerve by a ganglionic cyst, space-occupying mass, or stretching neuropathy. In most cases cessation of volleyball will alleviate the problem, and the infraspinatus will recover. After surgery pain in often relieved, but the infraspinatus muscle rarely recovers (27).

ELBOW INJURIES

Common elbow injuries in volleyball players are lateral epicondylitis, olecranon bursitis, and triceps tendinitis. Setting the ball requires repetitive contraction of the extensor muscles of the forearm as the ball is precisely placed for the spike. Inflammation and pain at the origin of the extensor complex on the lateral epicondyle are treated with relative rest, stretching, strengthening, icing, modalities, oral or topical NSAIDs, a forearm compression strap, and occasionally corticosteroid injection. Prevention measures include adequate warm-up, conditioning, and stretching of the wrist extensor muscles.

Olecranon bursitis occurs with repetitive or acute trauma to the elbow during diving to save the ball. Superficial pain and swelling occur over the olecranon. Treatment includes ice, NSAIDs, compression, and protective padding. Aspiration may be necessary but should be used judiciously, as nonhealing fistulous traits and/or infection are not uncommon complications. Rarely, a chronic fibrous bursitis may require surgical excision. Prevention includes elbow pads and technique improvement.

Triceps tendinitis occurs with repetitive elbow extension that occurs with setting, spiking, and serving. The athlete usually experiences a gradual onset of elbow pain at the insertion of the tricep. Treatment is conservative and similar to that for lateral epicondylitis along with activity modification. Prevention includes strengthening, stretching the triceps, and an adequate warm-up period before the practice or game.

HAND AND WRIST INJURIES

Acute hand and wrist injuries are very common in volleyball. Also, overuse vascular injuries to the dominant hand occur in up to one third of high-level volleyball players (30). Finger sprains are by far the most common and are probably underrecorded in most studies because players often do not report minor sprains of the phalanges. During the block, fingers are outstretched and vulnerable to being jammed by a high-speed spike. A sprained finger may pose a significant performance problem for a setter, since setting the ball requires extremely deft control from the fingertips. Specific proximal interphalangeal splints or distal interphalangeal taping may help to prevent finger injury (31). Buddy taping the sprained finger to the adjacent finger for support and comfort will help to keep a player in the game. Finger dislocations are also common and occur by the same mechanism as finger sprains. An experienced physician or athletic trainer may attempt relocation immediately after the accident if the diagnosis is certain. Radiographs are recommended postreduction if there is any significant deformity noticed after a sprain or if severe localized pain or swelling persists. If a fracture involves more than 30% of the articular surface or is more than 2 mm displaced, orthopedic consultation for surgical fixation should be considered. Pain, swelling, and stiffness will be helped by ice, NSAIDs, and buddy taping. Practice should consist of limited hitting and blocking during the acute phase. Molded padding may allow a quicker return to play. Pain may persist for 2–3 months after a severe phalangeal sprain or dislocation.

An avulsion of the extensor tendon at the distal interphalangeal joint (DIP) may occur when a player is hit on the end of the finger with a volleyball. This injury causes an inability to extend the DIP and a flexion deformity called a mallet finger. The joint should be splinted in extension for 6–8 weeks. The athlete should be reminded of the importance of keeping the finger in extension at all times. Return to play with an extension splint may be permitted. Persistent volar subluxation of the DIP or fracture involving 30% or more of the joint space may require surgical intervention.

Multiple other hand and wrist fractures may occur, especially in blocking or diving for balls. Suspected fractures should be radiographed and treated as indicated for the particular fracture. Injury-specific braces may facilitate a faster return to play. Particular injuries to be aware of after a fall on the outstretched hand include distal radius fractures, scaphoid fractures, triangular fibrocartilage complex tear, and scapholunate dissociation. Each of these areas should be carefully examined.

If distal radius or anatomic snuffbox tenderness or deformity is noted in the wrist, radiographs should be completed to rule out fractures or carpal dislocations. A negative initial radiograph with persistent anatomic snuffbox tenderness warrants aggressive follow-up because of the high risk of avascular necrosis of a fractured scaphoid bone. A short-arm thumb spica cast should be applied for 2 weeks, followed by repeat scaphoid radiographs. If radiographs are negative but there is persistent anatomic snuffbox tenderness, a bone scan may locate the fracture. With persistent pain a cast or splint should be considered for 2–4 weeks or until the athlete is pain free. Complex or nonhealing scaphoid fractures and scapholunate dissociation should be managed with orthopedic consultation.

BACK INJURIES

The majority of back injuries in volleyball are due to lumbar extension and rotation during a powerful spike or serve. Most injuries involve either a sprain of the paraspinous or sacroiliac ligaments or a strain of the paraspinous muscles. Stress fracture of the pars interarticularus or spondylolysis may occur because of repetitive hyperextension. Occasionally, a player may injure the cervical or lumbar region during a dive if there is a collision or if the player has not warmed up adequately.

Evaluation of back pain includes a history of the mechanism of injury and aggravating factors. Palpation of the spine and surrounding musculature, range-of-motion testing, and a complete neurologic exam including assessment of gait and a straight leg raise should be completed. Radiographs are warranted if there is bone tenderness or a neurologic deficit. With either severe pain or a positive unilateral straight leg raise and progressing neurologic deficit an MRI may be required to confirm a herniated nucleus pulposus impinging on the nerve roots and/or thecal sac.

Treatment and prevention for most back sprains and strains include an extensive stretching and strengthening program concentrating on torso and hamstring flexibility, torso strength, and biomechanical alterations. In addition, training modifications, ice, NSAIDs, physical therapy modalities, gravity traction, and gentle manipulation therapy may be helpful in getting the athlete back to optimal play. Pelvic stabilization exercises are essential.

Spondylolysis may be either a familial disease or a result of repetitive microtrauma to the pars interarticularus. Spondylolysis may be painful and lead to a spondylolisthesis or subluxation of the spine. A spondylolisthesis of less than 25% may be treated symptomatically with avoidance of aggravating factors, flexibility, and strengthening. Competitive play should be halted until evidence of healing is seen on radiographs and there has been no pain for 6 weeks.

SKIN INJURIES

Many skin problems can affect the volleyball player's performance. Painful blisters and calluses may form after many hours in improperly fitting shoes. Subungal hematomas may also form during jump and sprint training, especially in new shoes. Sole burns may occur in sand volleyball players during a hot summer day tournament. Fungal and plantar wart infections may also affect play if not properly treated. Finally, the team physician should be prepared to care for lacerations of the chin, eyebrow, and forehead that may occur after a collision.

LIFE-THREATENING INJURIES

The team physician should be aware of a multitude of injury possibilities. In volleyball life-threatening injuries rarely occur. Head and neck injuries may occur if two players collide. The majority of head injuries are low-grade concussions or minor lacerations. High ball velocities can cause a concussion or a fractured nose in the unfortunate defender. In addition, there is a rare case report of a physically fit male suffering a traumatic myocardial infarction after getting hit in the chest with a volleyball (32). A high level of suspicion, a timely diagnosis, and accurate follow-up are needed for these rare serious volleyball injuries. Trainers and team physicians should have current CPR certification. Disaster plans should be in place and well known. It is the medical team's responsibility to make sure that appropriate equipment and supplies are available at courtside or in the training room. Each player's medical history and preparticipation exam findings should be accessible for all practices and competitions.

REFERENCES

1. Ho SSW. Basketball and volleyball. In: Reider B, ed. *Sports medicine: the school age athlete,* 2nd ed. Philadelphia: WB Saunders, 1996:659–689.
2. Bahr R, Lian Ø, Bahr IA. A twofold reduction in the incidence of acute ankle sprains in volleyball after the introduction of an injury prevention program: a prospective cohort study. *Scand J Med Sci Sports* 1997;7:172–177.
3. Fédération International de Volleyball (FIVB). *X–press.* Lausanne, Switzerland: 1994;47(Jan):1.
4. Ferretti A. *Volleyball injuries: a color atlas of volleyball traumatology.* Italy: Fédération International de Volleyball, 1994.
5. Watkins J. Injuries in volleyball. In: Renstrom PAFH, ed. *Clinical practice of sports injury prevention and care,* vol 5 of the *Encyclopaedia of sports medicine.* Oxford: Blackwell Scientific Publications, 1994:360–374.
6. Aagaard H, Jorgensen U. Injuries in elite volleyball. *Scand J Med Sci Sports* 1996;6:228–232.
7. Backx FJG, Beijer HJM, Bol E, Erich WBM. Injuries in high–risk persons and high–risk sports: a longitudinal study of 1818 school children. *Am J Sports Med* 1991;19(2):124–130.
8. Bahr R, Bahr IA. Incidence of acute volleyball injuries: a prospective cohort study of injury mechanisms and risk factors. *Scand J Med Sci Sports* 1997;7:166–171.
9. Bahr R, Karlsen R, Lian Ø, Øvrebo RV. Incidence and mechanisms of acute ankle inversion injuries in volleyball. *Am J Sports Med* 1994;22(5)595–600.

10. Lohmann M, Holmich P, Overback–Pedersen A. *Danish EH–Lass Project.* Copenhagen: Herleu Hospital, 1988.
11. Rice EL, Anderson KL. Volleyball. In: Fu FH, Stone DA, ed. *Sports injuries: mechanisms, prevention and treatment.* Baltimore: Williams & Wilkins, 1994:689–700.
12. Schafle MD. Common injuries in volleyball, treatment, prevention, and rehabilitation. *Sports Med* 1993;16(2):126–129.
13. Schafle MD, Requa RK, Patton WL, Garrick JG. Injuries in the 1987 national amateur volleyball tournament. *Am J Sports Med* 1990;18(6):624–631.
14. Watkins J, Green BN. Volleyball injuries: A survey of injuries in Scottish National League male players. *Br J Sports Med* 1992;26(2):135–137.
15. Rubin AL. Ankle ligament sprains. In: Sallis RE, Massimino F, ed. *ACSM's essentials of sports medicine.* St. Louis: Mosby, 1997:450–453.
16. Sitler M, et al. The efficacy of semirigid ankle stabilizer to reduce acute ankle injuries in basketball. *Am J Sports Med* 1994;22(4):454–461.
17. Yu WD, Shapiro MS. Fractures of the fifth metatarsal careful identification for optimal treatment. *Phys Sportsmed* 1988;26(2):47–64.
18. Ferretti A, Papandrea P, Conteduca F, Mariani PP. Knee ligament injuries in volleyball players. *Am J Sports Med* 1992;20(2):203–207.
19. Briner WW, Kacmar L. Common injuries in volleyball. *Sports Med* 1997;24(1):65–71.
20. Ferretti A. Papandrea P, Conteduca F. Knee injuries in volleyball. *Sports Med* 1990;10(2):132–138.
21. Richards DP, Ajemian SV, Wiley JP, Zernicke RF. Knee joint dynamics predict patellar tendinitis in elite volleyball players. *Am J Sports Med* 1996;24(5):676–683.
22. Lian Ø, Engebretsen L, Øvrebo RV, Bahr R. Characteristics of the leg extensors in male volleyball players with jumper's knee. *Am J Sports Med* 1996;24(3):380–385.
23. Jackson MD, Moeller SL, Hough DO. Basketball injuries. In: Sallis RE, Massimino F, ed. *ACSM's essentials of sports medicine.* St. Louis: Mosby, 1997:558–570.
24. Kugler A, Kruger–Fronke M, Reiringer S, et al. Muscular imbalance and shoulder pain in volleyball attackers. *Br J Sports Med* 1996;30(3):256–259.
25. Côelho Gonçalves TD. Isolated and painless (?) atrophy of the infraspinatus muscle. *Arq Neuropsiquiatr* 1994;52(4):539–544.
26. Montagna P, Colonna S. Suprascapular neuropathy restricted to the infraspinatus muscle in volleyball players. *Acta Neurol Scand* 1993;87:248–250.
27. Fédération International de Volleyball. Third World Symposium of Sports Medicine Applied to Volleyball, Paris, Oct. 5–7, 1995.
28. Tengan CH, Oliveira ASB, Kiymoto BH, et al. Isolated and painless infraspinatus atrophy in top–level volleyball players. *Arq Neuropsiquiatr* 1993;51(1):125–129.
29. Reekers JA, den Hartog BMG, Kuyper CF, et al. Traumatic aneurysm of the posterior circumflex humeral artery: a volleyball player's disease? *J Vasc Interv Radiol* 1993;4:405–408.
30. Rosi G, Pichot O, Bosson JL, et al. Echographic and doppler screening of the forearm arteries in professional volleyball players. *Am J Sports Med* 1992;20(5):604–606.
31. Benalglia PG, Sartorio F. Ingenito R. Evaluation of a thermoplastic splint to protect the proximal interphalangeal joints of volleyball players. *J Hand Ther* 1996;9:52–56.
32. Grossfeld PD, Friedman DB, Levine BD. Traumatic myocardial infarction during competitive volleyball: a case report. *Med Sci Sports Exerc* 1993;25(8)901–903.

CHAPTER 52

Water-Skiing

Peter I. Sallay

INTRODUCTION

Water-skiing is a relatively young sport invented by an 18-year-old daredevil named Ralph Samuelson shortly after World War I. Samuelson first had the notion to ski on the water's surface in 1922 (1). He initially fashioned makeshift skis out of barrel staves. After failing in several attempts, he tried snow skis, which didn't work either. Finally, realizing that he needed a wider board to enlarge the surface area, he fabricated skis out of 9-inch-wide pine boards. He boiled the tips of the skis to curve the ends upward, thus preventing the tips from being submerged in the water. Using leather straps to hold his feet to the boards, he successfully skied behind a boat on Lake Pepin in Minnesota on July 2, 1922. In 1925 Samuelson completed the first ski jump, using a half-submerged dock as a ramp. In the same year Fred Waller from Long Island, New York, invented and patented the "Dolphin Akwa Skees." Unaware of either Samuelson's or Waller's accomplishments Don Ibsen and his colleagues in Bellevue, Washington, were frustrated that they could not continue snow skiing in the warmer months. To prolong the ski season, they began to ski on water in 1928 (2,3). The first national skiing organization, the American Water Ski Association (AWSA), was established in 1939 by Dan Hains and Bruce Parker. The first National Water Ski Championships were held in Long Island, New York, that same year. During World War II Dick Pope organized the first water ski show at Cypress Gardens, Florida. It subsequently became the world's most popular ski show.

The original equipment was crude and inefficient, with tennis shoes serving as bindings attached to wooden skis. Through the 1960s skis were made of wood with low rubber boot bindings. In the 1970s skis were fabricated from fiberglass, and a higher boot binding was designed to exert greater control over the ski. Recent modifications have included composite substrates such as polymer foam forming a core with any combination of plastic, carbon graphite, aluminum, and fiberglass forming the outer skin. Modern competitive bindings are fabricated from neoprene rubber fabric and have various straps to firmly fix the foot to the ski. This gives the competitive skier greater control over the ski. A quick-release binding, resembling that of a snow ski boot, has recently been introduced. The boot is rigid and is attached to ski with a pressure-sensitive release. Although in theory this design may reduce torsional injury, no studies have compared this to older designs.

Although most skiing is done at an informal, recreational level, organized events are well established. Professional and amateur competitions are organized at the local, national, and international levels. There were 821 sanctioned water-ski tournaments held nationwide in 1994–1995 (AWSA, unpublished data) including classic three-event, collegiate, show, barefoot, kneeboard, speed, disabled, and recreational events. In 1995 water-skiing became a Pan American Games sport, and it is currently under consideration as an Olympic sport. In the last few years selected events have been nationally televised on cable sports networks, reaching half a billion viewers.

Historically, water-skiing competitions consisted of three main events: slalom skiing, trick skiing, and ski jump (4). A slalom ski course consists of six buoys and two end gates. A successful pass entails skiing through both gates and around each buoy as fast as possible without falling. Trick skiing involves the skier performing tricks in a straight-line path behind the boat. The skier attempts to perform as many tricks as possible in 20 seconds in two consecutive runs. During a ski jump, the boat will accelerate the skier toward a ramp. The skier will use the forward velocity to propel himself or herself as far as possible before

---

P. I. Sallay: Methodist Sports Medicine Center, Indianapolis, Indiana 46202.

landing in the water. Each competitor is allowed three passes. The world record jump is over 61 meters (220 feet) and was set by Sammy Duvall in 1993 (4). Other nontraditional events have been gaining in popularity in recent years. Beginning in the early 1980s, international barefoot competitions were held annually. In 1985 Tony Finn of San Diego invented the sport of wakeboarding (3). A wakeboard is a flat, lightweight board fabricated from composite materials that resembles a cross between a surfboard and a snowboard. Recently, wakeboarding and barefoot skiing have gained in popularity, mainly because of the individual's ability to increase the repertoire of more complex and exciting tricks.

EPIDEMIOLOGY

Water-skiing has enjoyed increasing popularity over the last decade. There are an estimated 17 million recreational enthusiasts nationwide (3). Unfortunately, water-skiing has been known to be a hazardous sport. National injury statistics are collected in a database by the U.S. Coast Guard at the Department of Transportation in Washington, D.C. The Boating Accident Report Database contains data on reported recreational boating accidents (5). States and jurisdictions with federally approved numbering systems submit data. Current regulations require the operator of any recreational vessel to file a Boating Accident Report if an accident results in loss of life, personal injury requiring medical treatment (beyond first aid), property damage (including damage to the vessel) exceeding $500, or disappearance of a person indicating injury or death. Hummel and Gainor reported that in 1979 there were 46 deaths and 24,000 injuries related to boating accidents nationwide. In 1994 there were 6906 accidents resulting in 784 fatalities and 4084 injuries (6). The total reported property loss was $25,190,200. In the same year seven deaths and 305 injuries were directly attributed to a water-skier falling. The other two injury categories that may also include a proportion of skiing-related trauma were propeller injuries (13 deaths, 126 injuries) and collision with an object (70 deaths, 588 injuries). The database is limited in that it does not capture data on every accident. Many accidents go unreported because of ignorance and difficulty in enforcing the law. Also federal regulations do not require reporting on private waters or on state waters in Alaska. Additionally, unlike downhill snow skiing, in which most skiers are confined to a specific patrolled area, water-skiing is practiced in a large number of unpatrolled lakes. In these areas injuries are less likely to be reported. Although only a small percentage of nonfatal accidents are reported, it is likely that nearly all fatalities are included in the database.

The AWSA national safety committee records injury statistics for sanctioned events. There is a designated safety director at all AWSA-sanctioned events. It is his or her responsibility to ensure compliance with safety measures and to maintain a record of all injuries. This database provides more accurate information because the number of skiers and the number of exposures are known and more than 90% of the tournaments are included. Also the injuries are more directly related to the act of skiing rather than environmental hazards, driver error, or other boats. The composite statistics for 1990–1996 reveal that there were 1311 injuries in 240,913 skiers during 543,497 runs for an injury to exposure ratio of 0.22% (AWSA, unpublished data). A complete statistical summary appears in Table 52–1. The injury-to-exposure ratio has dropped consistently from the 1992–1993 season from 0.3% to 0.17% in 1995–1996, presumably from enhanced safety efforts among coordinators and skiers.

FACTORS CONTRIBUTING TO INJURIES

Injuries observed during recreational water-skiing are related to various factors. Stanislavljevic and colleagues thought that three primary factors were involved in most water-skiing related injuries (7). The first involved the boat, the driver, and the speed of the boat. The second was the condition of the water. The last was the ski equipment and the ability of the individual. On the basis of the data presented in their study, they concluded that most injuries occurred when boats were driven by relatively inexperienced drivers at speeds exceeding the skill level of the skier. They also noted that six of the seven injuries occurred in skiers wearing high top boot bindings. The bindings were thought to anchor the foot

TABLE 52–1. *AWSA injury statistics, 1990–1996*

Year	No. of tournaments	No. of skiers	Rides	Injuries	% injured
1990–1991	616	42,429	100,000	259	0.26
1991–1992	644	41,756	103,680	252	0.24
1992–1993	596	32,600	66,340	198	0.30
1993–1994	858	43,190	100,604	263	0.25
1994–1995	824	37,947	86,998	189	0.22
1995–1996	821	42,991	85,875	150	0.17
Totals	4,359	240,913	543,497	1311	0.22

to the ski during a fall, thereby creating excessive torque on the lower extremity, producing severe injuries to the soft tissue and bone. Romano and colleagues also noted that distances are difficult to judge at high speeds, preventive conditioning programs are rare, and there is a lack of widespread education and safety programs (2). Hummel and Gainor found that all four fatalities in their series of 26 injuries occurred in individuals who were not wearing life vests (6). They recommended the routine use of Coast Guard-approved personal floatation devices and avoiding heavy boat traffic, rough water, and marginal daylight.

An alarming number of injuries seem to be related to ignorance and irresponsible behavior. According to the U.S. Coast Guard statistics for 1995, 296 accidents were related to passenger or skier behavior. This includes inattention, reckless driving, and hazardous skiing. Six hundred fifty-one mishaps were related to operator inexperience. Finally, alcohol was a primary cause of an accident in 286 cases. This last statistic is likely to be underreported because of the legal implications for the operator.

CLASSIFICATION OF RECREATIONAL WATER-SKIING INJURIES

Romano and colleagues first suggested a classification for water-skiing injuries in 1962 (2). They subdivided all injuries into four main groups: collisions, falls, tow rope entanglements, and propeller injuries. Each category can be further subdivided as shown in Table 52–2.

Some of the severest injuries result from collisions. Paterson reported two cases of skiers who were too close to the shoreline in shallow water sustaining cervical spine injuries after colliding with sandbars (8). Romano and colleagues reported a similar case of an individual who was attempting a shoreline landing (2). As he approached the shore, his skis struck bottom, causing him to pitch forward onto his head. He died instantly from a cervical spine fracture dislocation. Paterson recommended avoiding high-speed perpendicular approaches to the shoreline to avoid coming into contact with submerged obstacles, which could result in serious head and neck injury (8). Head injury can also occur as the result of collision with a disengaged ski. The severity can range from lacerations and dental trauma to severe head injury (2).

Fractures of the extremities resulting from collisions with objects in the water or boat docks have been reported by several authors (2,6,8,9). Fractures of the lower extremity seem to predominate in most series, although upper extremity fractures can also occur. Romano and colleagues commented that misjudging the distance and colliding with the dock was the most frequent cause for injury (2). They noted that bumper-type fractures occurred in the femur or lower leg, depending on the height of the dock.

In a review of 26 water-skiing mishaps, Hummel and Gainor reported that nearly half of the injuries occurred as a result of a fall into unobstructed water (6). Ligamentous trauma is common and is similar to other athletic injuries (6). Knee injuries reported include meniscal injuries, medial collateral ligament sprain, anterior cruciate ligament tears, combined ligament injury, and, most severe, knee dislocation (2,6,7). Romano and colleagues reported one case of a young male who suffered a knee dislocation with arterial damage that eventually resulted in amputation (2). Dislocation of the shoulder is thought to be relatively common and is related to sudden traction applied to the abducted shoulder by the tow rope. Two cases of hip dislocation, one anterior and one posterior, have also been reported (2,7). The vast majority of these noncontact injuries have a common mechanism of injury. Typically, the ski tip becomes transiently submerged, resulting in a rapid torsion force on the foot. This violent force is then transmitted to the lower extremity via the binding. Stanislavljevic and co-authors believe strongly that high boot top skis designed for competition are responsible for a significant proportion of these injuries, particularly in less experienced skiers (7).

Myotendinous strains are commonplace in many sports, including water skiing. Strain injury to the hamstrings, plantaris, biceps, rotator cuff, hand flexor tendons, and adductors have been reported (2,6,8,10,11). Blasier and Morawa (10) and Sallay and colleagues (11) have documented a peculiar injury to the proximal hamstring musculature. Sallay and colleagues commented that unlike more common strain injuries, these injuries tended to be more severe and potentially disabling (11). They reported on 12 novice and elite skiers who sustained partial or complete disruption of the proximal hamstring attachment. The injury mechanism was identical in the two groups, though the skiing activity during injury was different. Five of six novice skiers were in-

TABLE 52–2. *Classification of injury*

Collision (dock, floating objects, skis)
    Fractures of the extremities
    Head injury (including dental injury)
    Cervical spine injury
Fall into water (noncontact)
    Ligamentous injury: ACL, MCL, knee dislocation, shoulder dislocation, hip dislocation
    Soft tissue strains: adductors, hamstrings
    Hydrotrauma: rectal and vaginal douches, otic trauma
Tow rope entanglement
    Skin avulsion
    Upper extremity fractures
Struck by boat
    Blunt force injury
    Propeller injury

jured during a submerged water takeoff, whereas all elite skiers were injured during falls. The injury occurred because of rapid trunk flexion with the knee extended. This resulted in disruption of the proximal attachment of the hamstring muscles (Fig. 52–1). Convalescence was prolonged, and five patients were chronically disabled from vigorous sporting activities. The authors suggested preventing injury by properly instructing novice skiers on the technique of submerged takeoff, avoiding skiing if fatigued, and implementing a stretching and strengthening program for all skiers.

A number of articles have dealt with injuries resulting from high-pressure jets of water forced into the body's orifices. The most frequently reported injury is the "vaginal douche" (12–15). The mechanism of injury is either failure to elevate from a crouch position or falling backward with the legs in abduction (8,14). A similar injury to the rectum can occur in men and women. The spectrum of injury includes damage to the broad ligament, partial cervical or uterine avulsion, traumatic abortion, salpingitis, and peritonitis (14). The injury can easily be avoided by wearing shorts or a wetsuit (12–15). A similar mechanism can also force water into the ear and sinus cavities (2,16). The mildest injury results in chemical otitis (swimmer's ear), perhaps the most common otic malady. However, more significant injury can occur from the concussive effect of the water (2,8,16). Lindeman noted that tympanic membrane perforation is most common, but incus and/or stapes dislocation and round window membrane rupture can also occur (16). In addition to conductive hearing loss, a small number of cases are complicated by sensineuronal loss. Sinusitis commonly occurs in a similar manner, owing to water forced into the nasal and oral cavities. One severe injury has been reported to result in pneumocephalus secondary to a column of air trapped behind a water jet being forced across the cribiform plate (17).

The tow rope can be a source of significant injury. Entanglement of an extremity by the rope has been reported to cause burns, lacerations, degloving injuries, finger amputation, and upper extremity fracture (2,6). Hummel and Gainor report one case of rope entanglement causing skull fracture and subsequent death by drowning (6). Most injuries result from poor communication between the skier and the driver. If the skier is not prepared and the rope is not untangled, injury occurs as the boat rapidly takes the slack out of the line. The driver and the skier should always check to make sure the tow rope is fully visible and untangled before takeoff. The skier should signal the driver when he or she is ready.

The last category of injury—being struck by a boat—is perhaps the most mutilating. Injury can result from blunt force trauma when a skier is hit by a boat. This can result in head injury, fractures, and drowning. Other injuries occur as a result of propeller lacerations. Mann reported 32 such injuries over a 15-year period (18). Twenty ended in death, and five patients of 12

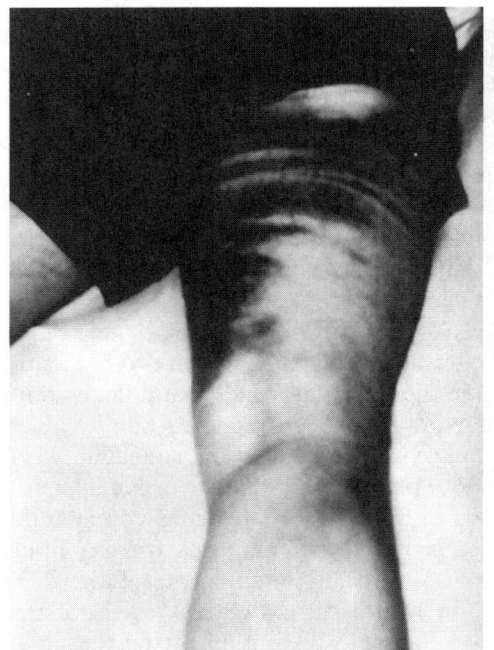
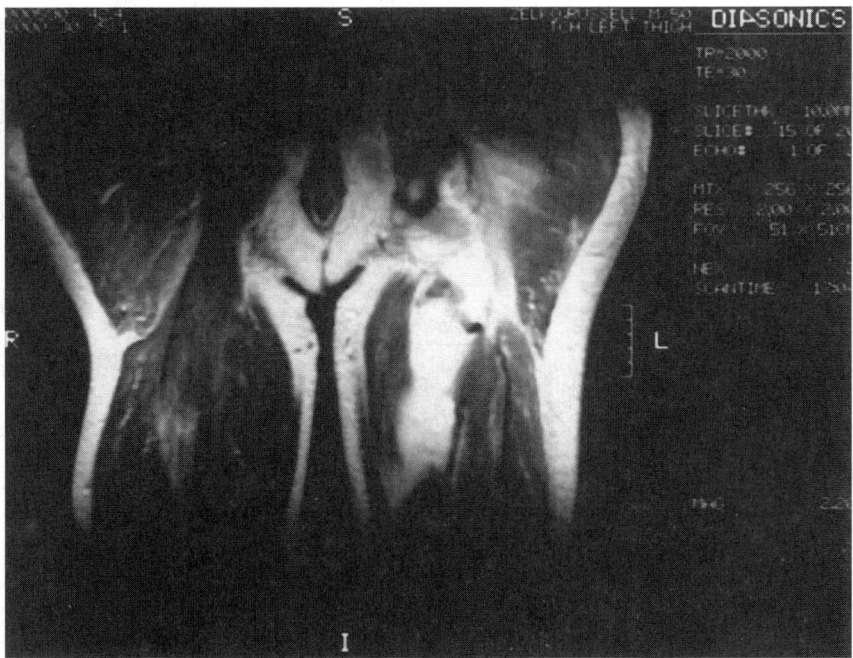

FIG. 52–1. A: Extensive ecchymosis and swelling in the posterior thigh of a 50-year-old skier injured during takeoff. **B:** A sagittal magnetic resonance image demonstrating complete disruption of the proximal hamstring from the ischium on the right.

surviving individuals sustained amputation of an extremity. Bacterial contamination, typically *Pseudomonas species,* was a problem in the majority of cases. Because of their severity these injuries were likened to battlefield wounds. Mann recommended legislation to require safer propellers and the presence of a third person observer in the boat to identify a fallen skier.

INJURIES IN TOURNAMENT SKIING

As was previously mentioned, the AWSA keeps a record of all injuries occurring in sanctioned events. The spectrum of injury is somewhat different than what has been reported in recreational skiers. Far less severe injury, including death, occurs at the elite level, presumably because of the controlled environment and safety regulations. Carder (unpublished data) has studied the incidence and severity of tournament water-skiing over a three year period (1991–1993). The incidence of all injuries in sanctioned three-event tournaments during the study period was 232.5 per 100,000 exposures, and the incidence of severe injury was 32.6 per 100,000 exposures. There were no deaths during the study period. The most common injuries were knee injuries, followed closely by back/neck injury, facial trauma, and rib contusions. The most common severe injuries were knee injuries, shoulder injuries, and lower extremity fractures. The jump event had the highest injury rate, with 52% of all injuries (65% of severe injuries), followed by slalom with 46%, and trick with 2%. In tournament jump competition male skiers are allowed to ski up to 35 miles per hour off of a ramp that is 5.5 feet above the water. Tremendous forces are sustained during takeoff and landing, increasing the risk of injury. In general slalom, speeds are same or higher because of the slingshot effect when the skier crosses the path of the boat; however, the distance that one falls is considerably less. In contrast, the boat speed for trick skiing is considerably slower, allowing the skier to perform as many tricks as possible in the allotted time.

The author noted that the young adult categories (17- to 34-year-olds) had the highest injury rate, particularly in the jump event. Ability level seemed to have a bimodal distribution when related to injury risk. The highest rates were among the most experienced skiers followed closely by the least experienced. Skiers of intermediate ability seem to have a lower risk of injury because they ski well enough to avoid beginners' injuries but are not skilled enough to ski at high speeds or attempt more dangerous tricks.

SUMMARY

Water-skiing is an exciting sport that is gaining popularity among both recreational enthusiasts and elite competitors. This sport is associated with severe injury, including death. Recreational skiers are particularly at risk for severe injury due to inexperience or negligence. Table 52–3 list some basic dos and don'ts for recreational skiers. An awareness of basic safety considerations and common sense should prevent most potential injuries.

TABLE 52–3. *Guidelines for safe skiing*

Don'ts
- Don't ski in shallow water or water of unknown depth.
- Don't consume alcohol while driving or skiing.
- Don't ski at night.
- Don't wrap the rope or bridle around any part of your body.
- Don't ski near docks or floating objects.
- Don't ski in congested areas.
- Don't attempt perpendicular landings in shallow water or close to shore.
- Don't ski without proper instruction.
- Don't ski without an approved PFD.
- Don't ski when you are fatigued.

Dos
- Do have a person in the boat, other than the driver, to monitor the skier.
- Do ensure the tow rope is not tangled prior to takeoff.
- Do hold up a ski as a signal that you have fallen.
- Do return to a fallen skier quickly.
- Do ski within the limits of your ability.
- Do warm up before skiing.
- Do wear shorts or a wetsuit.
- Do use equipment appropriate for your skill level.

Adapted from Romano RL, Burgess EM, Andrews CB. Medical implications of water-skiing. *Clin Orthop* 1962; 23:140–145.

ACKNOWLEDGMENTS

The author would like to thank John Carder, M.D. for supplying his data on tournament ski injuries and Leon Larson for sharing AWSA injury statistics.

REFERENCES

1. Stephens R. The good father. *Waterski* 1997;19:45–48.
2. Romano RL, Burgess EM, Andrews CB. Medical implications of water-skiing. *Clin Orthop* 1962;23:140–145.
3. Stephens R. We take you on a ride through 75 years of water sking. *Waterski* 1997;19:31–43.
4. Leggett SH, Kenney K, Eberhardt T. Applied physiology of water-skiing. *Sports Med* 1996;4:262–276.
5. U.S. Coast Guard. *Boating statistics: 1994–1995.* Document P16754.8. Washington, DC: U.S. Department of Transportation, 1995.
6. Hummel G, Gainor BJ. Water-skiing related injuries. *Am J Sports Med* 1982;10:215–218.
7. Stanislavljevic S, Irwin RB, Brown LR. Orthopedic injuries in water-skiing: etiology and prevention. *Orthop* 1978;1:125–129.
8. Paterson DC. Water-skiing injuries. *Practitioner* 1971;206: 655–660.
9. Banta JV. Epidemiology of waterskiing injuries. *West J Med* 1979;130:493–497.
10. Blasier RB, Morawa LG. Complete rupture of the hamstring

origin from a water skiing injury. *Am J Sports Med* 1990;18:435–437.
11. Sallay PI, Friedman RL, Coogan PG, Garrett WE. Hamstring injuries among water skiers. *Am J Sports Med* 1996;24:130–136.
12. McCarthy GF. Hazards of water-skiing. *Med J Aust* 1969;1:481.
13. Morton DC. Gynaecological complications of water-skiing. *Med J Aust* 1970;1:1256–1257.
14. Rudoff JC. Vulvovaginal water-skiing injury. *Ann Emerg Med* 1993;22:1072.
15. Smith BL. Vaginal laceration caused by water skiing. *J Emerg Nurs* 1996;22:156–157.
16. Lindeman RC. Temporal bone trauma and facial paralysis. *Otolaryngol Clin North Am* 1979;12:403–413.
17. David SK, Guarisco JL, Coulon RA. Pneumocephalus secondary to a high-pressure water injury to the nose. *Arch Otolaryngol Head Neck Surg* 1990;116:1435–1436.
18. Mann RJ. Propeller injuries incurred in boating accidents. *Am J Sports Med* 1980;8:280–284.

CHAPTER 53

Weightlifting (Strength-Power Activities)

Richard T. Herrick

For the uninitiated, a group that includes most medical professionals, one first needs to define the various types of weightlifting so that we can speak the same language when discussing problems encountered by those who lift weights.

"Weightlifting" is the specific name of a very ancient sport, the first recorded mention of which is in a 5000-year-old Chinese text describing lifting tests for prospective soldiers. It is also called "Olympic lifting." As Olympic lifting, it has been competed ever since the inception of the modern Olympics in 1896 and is practiced competitively in over 100 countries around the world; it is best known, of course, when it is competed during the Olympics. At one time, weightlifting or Olympic lifting included three competitive lifts: the press, the snatch, and the clean and jerk (Fig. 53–1). The press was eliminated after the 1972 Olympics, not only because it has been indicted as one of the primary causes of back problems in weightlifting, but also to shorten the program and thereby also significantly shorten the lengths of the various competitions. This not only was good for those who watch or judge the competition, but also enabled the lifters to concentrate on two lifts. Since then the two remaining lifts, the snatch and the clean and jerk, have improved immensely with regard to the amount of weights lifted. Women have had weightlifting world championships since 1987 and will compete for the first time in the Olympics in Sydney in 2000.

The essence of weightlifting is to get the weight overhead, using very specific techniques, the snatch being done in one motion and the clean and jerk in two motions. See Chapter 60 on the physiology of weightlifting in the companion volume *Exercise and Sport Science* as well as Chapter 39 on the biomechanics of weightlifting for a complete description.

The object, of course, is to lift the most weight; however, considerable speed and technique, in addition to strength, are needed to enable the lifter to get the weight overhead and then control it to complete the lift. There is obviously an element of strength involved, but more than any other weight training or weightlifting event, Olympic lifting requires a considerable amount of technique, repetitious training, speed, and production of power.

Powerlifting, by contrast, is much more dependent on brute strength, although of course it requires proper technique as well. Powerlifting is not competed in the Olympics, but it has been competed in the World Games ever since their inception in 1967, and in the Western world, it is competed by more participants than Olympic lifting (weightlifting). Powerlifting includes three lifts: the squat, the bench press, and the dead lift (Fig. 53–2). None of these is performed strictly overhead, and speed or quickness is not of the essence, at least to the extent that it is in Olympic weightlifting.

Powerlifting was initially competed in Austria around 1860 and included the squat and the dead lift. The bench press was added around the end of the 1920s and supplanted other "odd lifts." Powerlifting is competed in over 80 countries around the world, usually in three-lift meets, but it may also be competed as single-lift meets, especially the bench press, which at this time has its own world championship as well. As in Olympic weightlifting, winners in powerlifting contests are determined not only by the maximum weight that is lifted in three attempts in each of the lifts, but also by the total of the two or three lifts, depending on the sport being competed.

Bodybuilding is also a competitive sport, competed around the world in over 150 countries. Like powerlifting, it is competed in the World Games but not in the

R. T. Herrick: Herrick Orthopaedic Clinic, Opelika, Alabama 36802.

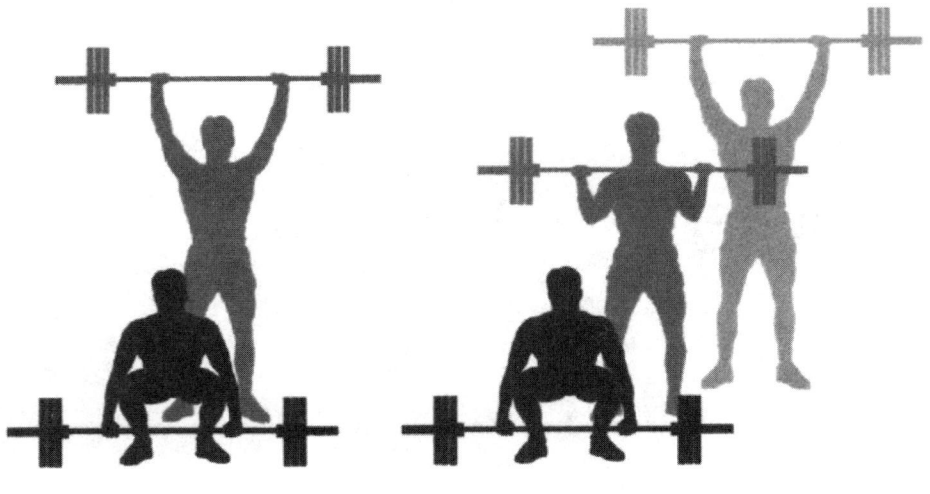

FIG. 53-1. The snatch and the clean and jerk lift.

Olympic Games. The essence of this sport is to exhibit the body and to be able to display the enhanced appearance, encompassing size, symmetry, shape, and striation of defined muscle, with as little subcutaneous tissue as possible and the ability to display these various muscles in both mandatory poses and freestyle posing. In this respect, bodybuilding is judged more as an expository competition than by amount of weight lifted, although of course these are intimately related.

All three sports—Olympic weightlifting, powerlifting, and bodybuilding—are competed in various body weights, with eight body weights for men in Olympic weightlifting and seven for women. Powerlifting has eleven body weights for men and ten for women. Bodybuilding can be and is often divided among various weight classifications, although in the past it was also competed in various height classifications within both men's and women's individual competition and pairs competition. In pairs competition the pairs are composed of one man and one woman competing simultaneously as a team.

Weight training is essentially the utilization of weights to ultimately produce an enhanced appearance, as in body sculpting, or, if it becomes competitive, in bodybuilding. However, the other aspect, one that is probably more widespread, especially among competitive athletes, is sport-specific weight training, in which various exercises are developed to enhance the abilities of an athlete competing within a specific sport other than Olympic weightlifting, powerlifting, or bodybuilding. All these utilize both free weights and weight machines of various types; frequently, a combination of both is utilized.

Competition in all these sports is carried out on vari-

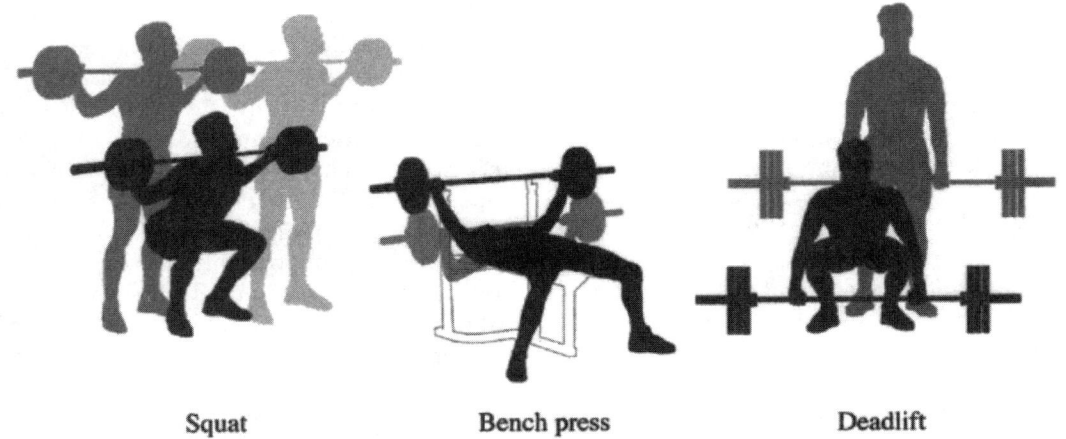

FIG. 53-2. The squat, bench press, and dead lift.

ous levels, up to the epitome of the Olympic competition and world championships for Olympic lifting and the World Games competition and world championship competition for powerlifting and bodybuilding. Each of these sports is also competed on a regional level, such as the North American championships and European championships; these competitions are usually based on continents, but other regions may be combined as well, as in the Pan American and British Commonwealth championships. Each of these is also competed within each nation, not only in national or open championships, both men's and women's, but also in collegiate championships, high school and/or teenage championships, junior championships, and masters championships. The university games sometimes include powerlifting and/or weightlifting and include collegiate champions from around the world.

Masters championships in these sports are for those who are at least 35 years of age. In weightlifting and powerlifting, they are competed within various weight categories in addition to age group categories, usually in five-year increments.

Each of these sports has its own international federation. The primary international federation for bodybuilding is the International Federation of Bodybuilding (IFBB), although there are several organizations, especially within the United States, that have various types of state, regional, and national championships.

The international organization for weightlifting is the International Weightlifting Federation (IWF), which has only one recognized national federation within each of the member countries; these national federations determine which competitors go to the world championships.

The international organization for powerlifting that is recognized by the International World Games Association, and thereby also by the General Assembly of International Federation of Sports, is the International Powerlifting Federation (IPF). There are a few other "international federations," but these comprise many fewer countries, and a vast majority of their members are from the United States and a few other English-speaking countries. To further confuse the situation, there are at least 14 "national federations" of powerlifting within the United States, but only one, USA Powerlifting, is recognized by the International Powerlifting Federation.

Additionally, the bench press is competed in the Paralympics, and although it was originally called "weightlifting," since it fell under the aegis of various sports within the Olympic movement, the specific sport has recently been named, more appropriately, the bench press. It has its own set of rules, differing somewhat from those competed under the guidance of the International Powerlifting Federation. There is, of course, some crossover, not only among the rules but also among competitors, and there are many judges who referee a number of these sports.

There are various levels of doping control (drug testing) within these sports organizations. The most widespread and sophisticated testing is done in Olympic lifting and to a slightly lesser extent powerlifting and then bodybuilding, but the sophistication of the testing is gradually increasing in all these sports, as is the number of competitors being tested on a regular basis, not only at competition, but also incorporating more out-of-competition testing.

As the sophistication of doping control has improved, the use of anabolic steroids, initially widespread, slowly decreased. Changes in the incidence and types of injuries over the last 30 years are due not only to the increased amount of weight being utilized, but also to the adverse effects of anabolic steroids and stimulants and to the increased sophistication of dietary assistance and training programs. Furthermore, each of the individual sports has specific signature injuries that, although they can occur in any of the sports, are more prevalent in one than in the others.

Olympic weightlifters, for instance, share many more shoulder problems with athletes in racquet sports and swimmers than bodybuilders or powerlifters do, and although Olympic lifters seem to have a higher incidence of knee injuries than do powerlifters or bodybuilders, neither have the number of knee injuries seen in contact sports such as football, basketball, and wrestling. Some injuries, especially shoulder injuries or significant knee injuries in the Olympic lifter, can frequently be devastating enough that the athlete can no longer compete at an elite level; however, she or he can then successfully compete in either powerlifting or bodybuilding because of the different nature of the sports.

Because each of these activities uses the various muscles in the joints differently, the medical professional who is to not only recognize the injury, but also guide the athlete through the appropriate rehabilitation process, whether it requires surgery or not, must be well aware of the intricacies of the various activities to which the athlete desires to return. Only in this way can the medical professional help the patient athlete make good decisions. This is regardless of the age of the athlete, since each of these sports has competitive members into the ninth decade of life.

Also, since some of the more devastating injuries in lifters are not orthopedic, all who care for lifters must be aware of them and be prepared to rapidly diagnose and refer the lifter. These injuries include subarachnoid hemorrhage (1), tetraplegia (2), stroke (3), aortic dissection (4), external iliac artery stenosis (5), myocardial infarction (6,7), pulmonary embolism (8), spontaneous pneumothorax (9), and effort thrombosis (10–16).

Likewise, the incorporation of aerobic exercise into their rehabilitation programs is different among the various sports and activities, since various types of aerobic exercises, although they may be indicated in the initial rehabilitation of the injury, are contraindicated once the athlete has reached the point at which he or she starts to train sports specifically. For instance, it has been shown that there is a definite increase in knee problems in powerlifters who incorporate running into their training program to any great extent, and, to a lesser extent, in Olympic weightlifters. Similarly, an athlete who is going to be returning to Olympic weightlifting should not incorporate much of a swimming program, since this would intensify the overhead work being done by the athlete, which can also be detrimental.

Although weight training and weight lifting have become some of the fastest-growing forms of exercise in the United States and throughout the world, there is a dearth of information about specific injuries sustained in these activities, their treatment, including rehabilitation, and, perhaps more important, their prevention. More than 45 million Americans train with weights regularly (17). Fortunately, serious injuries rarely occur; in 1995, the most recent year for which statistics are available, emergency room visits for weight training injuries totaled 56,400 out of more than 5.4 million visits for all sports (18).

An exhaustive study of the literature, aided by three computer-assisted searches, located fewer than 100 articles pertaining to strength-power injuries, and some of the information that was found is considered erroneous in light of current research (17,19–31).

The various maladies that were reported included the following injuries attributed to strength-power activities: wrist fractures (32); musculocutaneous nerve compressions (33,34); ulnar neuritis (35); pectoralis tears (36–38); shoulder impingement syndromes, including coracoacromial ligament pain and bicipital and rotator cuff tears; ruptured biceps (distal) (39–42); ruptured triceps (43–45); osteolysis of the distal clavicle (46–49); acute digital ischemia (50); patellar tendon tears (51,52); meniscal tears; patellofemoral syndrome; knee ligament tears (53); myositis ossificans (54); neck fracture, both direct trauma and indirect avulsion (55); lumbar spondylolysis (19,56–67); undefined elbow pain, including brachialis muscle and aconeous muscle strains (68); and elbow instability/dislocations (69,70). Most of the articles that cited episodes of lower back pain and spondylolysis incriminated the military or overhead press, an activity that has virtually been eliminated since the standing or overhead press was discontinued as a competitive lift in 1972 (19,27).

Fitzgerald and McLatchie, through clinical and radiological studies, found degenerative joint disease (osteoarthrosis), caused by lifting, primarily in the lower extremity joints of 20% of their subjects (71). The incidence was much greater in Olympic weightlifters; however, that percentage was no larger than the occurrence of osteoarthrosis in the general population of the age group studied. Others imply that there may be a relationship between lifting and osteoarthritis (71,72).

Some of the early orthopedic literature (71) stated that deep-knee bends with weights, especially heavy squats, were injurious to the ligaments of the knees and could increase an individual's injury potential. Unfortunately, this misconception is often quoted and still perpetuated by well-meaning but ill-informed physicians, coaches, and trainers (17). Subsequent studies have refuted this idea (73,74). In fact, Karpovich and colleagues concluded that deep-knee bends with weights (i.e., squats) would improve knee stability, provided that the placement of the foot caused no undue lateral rotational effects on the knees (75). Also, little predictive relationship exists between knee stability measurements and the incidence of knee injuries. According to Tipton and colleagues, the junction strength of bone–ligament–bone is increased with exercises training and decreased with immobilization (76). The strength of repaired ligaments, at least in male animals, increases with interstitial cell-stimulating hormone (ICSH), testosterone, and strength training and decreases with adrenocorticotrophic hormone (ACTH), thyroxine, and immobility. Tipton and colleagues add that their findings reinforce the specificity of exercise concept and suggest that junction strength changes depend on the type of exercise performed and not solely on the time devoted to exercise, possibly because of the increased flow of blood and healing hormones to the repaired ligaments.

In a biomechanical analysis based on cinematographic data of actual national weightlifting championship competition, Zernicke and colleagues postulated that before the knee fails, the tension at the patellar tendon rupture point is 17.5 times the lifter's weight during dynamic loading conditions when the knee approaches a 90° angle (51).

Most lifters reporting knee injuries caused by weight training incidents ascribed the injuries to a limited number of specific one-time "mistakes." Stone of the National Strength Research Center sought more information about knee trauma and found that most causes of weight training–produced knee pain conform to the ones that are most frequently cited in the literature: inadequate warm-up or stretching, improper or untested technique, and excessive maximum competitive effort (77).

The researchers collected and collated information pertaining to weightlifters and the knee injuries they sustain, hoping to establish possible preventive measures. Questionnaires were distributed over a 3-year period to all elite-class powerlifters and weightlifters after the national and world championship meets of each of the two sports.

Of over 600 questionnaires sent out, 210 were returned by 176 men and 33 women; all the subjects were proficient at the national and/or international level in weightlifting and/or powerlifting. Data on these lifters included operative notes, orthopedic examination, medical history, training regimen, and rehabilitative measures. The statistical method that was used was multivariate analysis of variance plus the chi-square test (with Yates correction), a format that is designed to handle multiple variables within a limited population. Multiple variables included the biometric data of age, sex, size, lifting specialty, competitive level, and training program, including the number of high intensity sessions per week, as well as the frequency of competition, degree of pain, incidence of injury, and use of medication and/or surgery. Moderate knee pain was defined as that requiring modification of the training program for more than 3 weeks; severe pain was defined as that requiring surgery or altered training for more than 2 months.

The data revealed no significant ($p < 0.05$) relationships between the incidence or amount of knee pain and the number of years in training; the number of high-intensity sessions; the number of competitions per year; or the age, height, or weight of the competitor. Almost all high-caliber lifters experience some degree of pain, patellar tendinitis and ligament strain being most frequently listed as the presumed diagnosis.

Within the group that attributed their knee pain to lifting, a number of powerlifters, both male and female, had moderate pain, but only 8% of the men and none of the women had severe pain (Table 53–1). Both sexes of weightlifters had a significantly higher percentage of pain, but none had severe pain (Table 53–2). The most proficient lifters tended to have a greater frequency of moderate knee pain, regardless of the specific sport in which they participated.

Not all lifters attributed knee pain to lifting. In fact, many had started lifting to rehabilitate injuries that they had sustained in other sports, such as football (75), wrestling (54), and rugby (57). Among the lifters who attributed knee pain to causes other than lifting per se, more powerlifters than weightlifters had severe pain. The leader among other causes listed as reasons for knee pain was football, followed by a smaller, though fairly equal, distribution among vehicular accidents, wrestling, falls, and running injuries.

Pain increased dramatically with the inclusion of running in the training program: 80% of weightlifters who ran and only 7% who did not run experienced pain, while 76% of powerlifters who ran and 53% who did not run felt pain. Running as part of the training program was defined as more than 1 mile per day at a frequency of three or more times per week.

All but four lifters who suffered significant knee injury had undergone knee surgery and had returned to lifting competitively, and two of these are competing in bodybuilding. In conservative treatment, aspirin was the most

TABLE 53–1. *Powerlifters*

	Male (135)		Female (32)	
	Mean	Range	Mean	Range
With knee pain				
Present age (years)	30	17–65	26	18–41
Weight (kg)	94	55–185	65	46–88
Height (cm)	173	130–200	158	148–178
Training:				
Age begun (years)	21	5–55	23	15–38
Months/year	11	4–12	11	4–12
Days/week	4	2–6	3	3–6
Sessions/day	1	1–3	1	1–4
Hours/day	2	1–6	3	1–4
High intensity	3	1–6	2	1–6
Competitions/year	3	1–20	4	3–6
With no knee pain				
Present age (years)	32	16–62	28	20–42
Weight (kg)	95	51–126	55	42–103
Height (cm)	170	155–183	153	138–160
Training:				
Age begun (years)	25	13–52	27	20–39
Months/year	11	6–12	10	3–12
Days/week	4	2–6	4	3–6
Sessions/day	1	1–1	1	1–1
Hours/day	2	1–3	3	1–5
High intensity/week	2	1–7	3	2–6
Competitions/year	3	1–8	4	1–10

$N = 167$.

TABLE 53–2. Weightlifters

	Male (54)		Female (4)	
	Mean	Range	Mean	Range
With knee pain				
Present age (years)	28	14–76	24	23–25
Weight (kg)	94	55–146	85	81–88
Height (cm)	173	150–190	178	175–180
Training:				
Age begun (years)	17	7–28	23	22–24
Months/year	11	10–12	4	2–6
Days/week	4	2–5	2	2–3
Sessions/day	2	1–3	1	1–1
Hours/day	3	1–4	2	1–3
High intensity/week	2	1–3	—	—
Competitions/year	4	1–8	—	—
With no knee pain				
Present age (years)	23	19–30	38	21–49
Weight (kg)	72	51–106	91	59–113
Height (cm)	173	165–185	175	168–188
Training:				
Age begun (years)	19	15–23	19	15–22
Months/year	8	8–11	11	10–12
Days/week	4	3–7	3	3–6
Sessions/day	1	1–3	1	1–1
Hours/day	2	1–3	2	2–2
High intensity/week	2	2–3	4	3–5
Competitions/year	2	1–3	3	2–3

$N = 58$.

commonly used medication, followed by nonsteroidal antiinflammatory drugs (NSAIDs), which not only diminish pain but also decrease inflammation secondary to overuse and injury. Several lifters also routinely used dimethylsulfoxone (DMSO) and other topical liniments, more recently ones containing capsicum (capsaicin).

Although weightlifters seem somewhat more vulnerable to moderate knee injury and powerlifters seem more prone to severe injuries, in both categories proper weight-training techniques, including squats, appear to increase knee stability and therefore to deter knee injury (73). Proper technique (78) requires using the weights safely; positioning them correctly; descending slowly with the torso erect and without a bounce at the bottom; and keeping the head up, the thighs parallel to the floor, and the heels in contact with the floor (79,80). At least two well-trained spotters should assist. Studies conducted by Henja and Rosenburg confirm the lifters' belief in the rehabilitative nature of lifting including squatting (81).

The rehabilitative nature of properly supervised and executed lifting results from exercising specific muscles: the erector spinae of the lower back, the tensor fascia lata, and all gluteal muscles and the quadriceps (73). Likewise, such specificity of exercise (78) appeared to prove beneficial in the rehabilitation of knee injuries from any cause, as was also noted by several responding lifters in the study.

Regarding injuries and the use of anabolic steroids, it should be noted that Hama and colleagues observed "a close interrelationship between collagen content and fibril diameter in the joint capsule" (82), since both increase with increased levels of testosterone in orchiectomized Wistar rats. Whether this finding can be applied to the human lifter is unknown and, of course, is overshadowed by the current furor over the use of anabolic steroids.

Also Wahl and colleagues had identified a definite change within the structure of the collagen in animals that had been given high levels of anabolic steroids (83). Such changes may result from the stress–strain relationship and, as such, could affect the incidence and severity of injuries, especially at the knee. Unfortunately, the difficulty of obtaining information from those who are directly involved (i.e., coaches, physicians, athletes) hampers the application of theory to human subjects. We did not specifically question the athletes about their use of anabolic steroids, but several volunteered that there may be a relationship to their own injury.

Several injuries in lifters have been cited as being related to the use of anabolic steroids; these include ruptured triceps (45,84), ruptured extensor pollicis longus tendon (50,62), ruptured quadriceps tendon (85), ruptured distal biceps tendon (42), aortic dissection (4), sudden death (86), myocardial infarction (6,7), pulmonary embolism (8), and stroke (3).

This research tends to corroborate previously cited studies that indicated that weighted deep–knee bends improve knee stability, that there is little predictive relationship between knee stability measurements and injuries, and that strength training increases both bone–ligament junction and repaired ligament strength. Also, lifters as a group of athletes seem to suffer from no more degenerative knee changes than the general population of a given age group studied. Most notable among the conclusions is the obvious preventive and rehabilitative nature of properly supervised and executed lifting.

A few articles have specifically implicated the use of machines as being responsible for injuries, including quadriplegia (2), acromioclavicular joint stress injuries (87), second rib fracture (88), bilateral glenoid fracture with shoulder dislocation (89), ruptured triceps (84), bilateral avulsion fractures of the olecranon apophyses (90), bilateral upper extremity compartment syndromes (91), manubrium sterni stress fracture (92), suprascapular neuropathy (93), long thoracic neuropathy (94), volar lunate dislocation (95), spontaneous pneumothorax (9), and death (96).

Although the literature is replete with the subjects of prevention, diagnosis, and treatment of sports injuries, very little has been written specifically pertaining to weightlifting injuries.

The study of injuries sustained during training or participation is still in its infancy. Most publications are case reports (97) or include several sports, very few pertaining specifically to powerlifting and/or weightlifting (17,23,24,30). The epidemiologic method has great potential; however, it has not been used enough, at least in weightlifting, for us to find all that information in the extant literature. Unfortunately, the traditional clinical approach of examining each injury in turn or through case series limits the ideological inferences that can be drawn and are frequently biased or misleading (29).

One of the few epidemiologic analyses was of the sports injuries at the 1985 Junior Olympics. Although of interest, this included but five weightlifting athletes being treated, and only two of the injuries were significant enough to produce medical disqualification (26).

Regrettably, the average sports medicine professional knows, and frequently cares, little about the specific sport involved; this is particularly true of weightlifting (27). Weightlifters are reported to have a few medical problems that are specific to weightlifting and/or powerlifting; most injuries are the same as those found in other sports (20). One study noted that the incidence of injuries in weightlifting and weight training is significantly less than that in most other sports, even taking into consideration the fact that fewer athletes are involved in weightlifting, at least in the United States (25).

The evaluation format of any musculoskeletal disorder can best be handled by using the SOAP format—specifically, the Subjective examination, the Objective examination, the Assessment of the situation, and the Plan of treatment (98).

Generally, the goal is to prevent as many as possible of any injuries and, when they occur, to protect the area of injury against further aggravation, at the same time minimizing disuse atrophy of the rest of the body, allowing the athlete to continue training, albeit modified, until the original injury has healed (79,80).

As in all sports medicine injuries the short-term goals include protecting the involved area, decreasing pain and inflammation, increasing the range of motion of the joints, and educating the athlete (99,100). Long-term goals include increasing musculotendinous flexibility (99–101), muscular strength and power, muscular endurance, and maintenance of cardiovascular fitness, as well as restoration of normal biomechanical function, proprioception, balance, kinesthetic awareness, and progressive return to full functional activity. Discharge parameters require reaching the flexibility, strength, and endurance of normalcy to allow the athlete to return to regular training, and, ultimately, unimpeded competition.

Most injuries are of the overuse type (102–106) and can usually be prevented by the use of proper warm-ups, flexibility training, appropriate coaching, periodization of training, and so on, as discussed at length in other chapters.

Acute injuries occur when the athlete has, for one reason or another, lost his or her concentration, tries to do too much too soon, has not completely rehabilitated a previous injury, and/or (rarely) experiences coaching failure.

The relationship of injury to strength and flexibility has been discussed at length in the literature and will be discussed only briefly here. Safe spotting, safety equipment, environmental safety factors, and preparticipation evaluation are likewise discussed elsewhere.

Injury prevention mandates proper warm-up, flexibility training, and balanced strength training (ensuring that the agonists and antagonists are developed simultaneously) carried out under appropriate supervision of a coach who is well versed in the safe techniques of the specific sport for which the athlete is training. Stress and hypertrophy are necessary and can be developed most appropriately by using periodization. Several injuries occur because of poor exercise technique, limited supervision, and/or poor exercise habits, including the failure to include proper warm-up and cool-down procedures as well as flexibility stretching. All these procedures are used by well-trained athletes but occasionally are ignored, usually because of ineffective planning. This is especially true in lifting because of the absolute necessity of balanced strength, power, and flexibility, much more so than in most other sports.

Finally, rehabilitation should start immediately after athlete sustains an injury (107) and should continue until the patient is completely rehabilitated, thereby preventing, in almost all cases, recurrence of similar or related injuries in the future (71,108).

Whether one utilizes a modified proprioceptive neuromuscular facilitation (PNF) technique for stretching or a simple hold-and-relax technique, all of which are discussed at length in the literature, the primary thing to remember is that no stretching should be done ballistically, all methods should be preceded by proper warm-up, and all methods should be used to increase flexibility of the musculature, not of the joint itself (109,110). Only in the case of arthrofibrosis, or stiffness of a joint following injury or disease is the goal to stretch a joint.

In the remainder of this chapter the body is divided into the general areas of chest and back; shoulder; elbow; forearm, wrist, and hand; pelvis, hip, and thigh; knee; and foot and ankle.

One must remember, however, that an injury can and will affect all parts of the body, since all are connected and have a direct influence on the proper functioning of all other portions of the anatomy. In evaluating and treating any injury, those who are responsible for this must take this into consideration and use that knowledge throughout the rehabilitation phase. For example, an ankle sprain must be rehabilitated, but one also must know whether there is a rigid cavus foot and/or hyperpronating foot that could have contributed to the sprain, certainly could complicate the rehabilitation, and may adversely be affected by a leg length discrepancy, tight hamstrings, or even inadequate shoulder flexibility, all of which need to be dealt with appropriately to totally rehabilitate the lifter.

All who are concerned with the care of athletes, especially lifters, must be aware of the possible relationship between injury and the use of anabolic steroids (111). Anabolic steroids are drugs that act like testosterone, the male hormone. Natural testosterone regulates, promotes, and maintains physical and sexual development in normal males. The abuse of anabolic steroids may result in increased body hair, deepening of the voice, decreased sperm production, and abnormal liver function. Many of the masculinizing changes may also occur in the female and are apt to be irreversible once experienced. Their use has been implicated in the production of severe acne, increased atherosclerosis and heart disease, gynecomastia, high blood pressure, and kidney disease. Psychological dysfunction, including uncontrolled aggression, manic-depressive disorder, and paranoia may occur as an effect of anabolic steroid use.

Anabolic steroids promote protein synthesis. They have been used in cancer and other debilitating patients when a deficiency is present, but their use has generally been discontinued because of the potentially severe (liver and heart) side effects associated with high dosages and prolonged usage. The only generally accepted therapeutic uses of anabolic steroids are to bring a testosterone-deficient male back to normal, to treat certain advanced cases of breast cancer, to treat a rare medical condition known as hereditary angioedema, and to stimulate the bone marrow in patients with unusual and rare anemias.

Recent studies have also shown that there is a significant, abnormal, probably pathologic change in both tendons and muscles in athletes who take anabolic steroids (111). These then decrease the tensile strength of the various tissues and thereby undoubtedly increase the chance of injury, especially to the soft tissues, specifically including muscles, tendons, and tendon insertion areas.

CHEST AND BACK

Weightlifting has been implicated in spondylolysis (19,56–67), probably representing a stress fracture of the pars interarticularis as one of the causes of back pain (19,59). Whether this is indeed true remains to be seen. One study showed that over 44% of weightlifters' radiographs were positive for spondylolysis, but no statistical evidence could be found when the age at which training began was studied (56). Although spondylolysis probably does represent a fatigue fracture (112), resulting from repetitive loads on the spine, and other studies show a high incidence and prevalence among those who have lifted for a long period of time, the only real relationship is between those who have back pain and spondylolysis (65). It is known that extreme axial loading of the spine can cause disc damage, but all the studies in the literature are biased in that they were selected on the basis of chronic low back pain (58,63). The incidence may actually be decreasing, since the overhead press is no longer a competed lift (61).

The most common cause of low back pain in any athlete (65,76,113,114), including a lifter, is overuse, resulting in a strain or sprain of the paravertebral muscles and ligaments (66). Most of these can be handled with the usual treatment modalities of rest and ice for 24–36 hours, followed by spray and stretch (114–116), heat and massage, analgesics, and NSAIDs until flexion and strengthening exercises have returned the damaged part to normal. Most reported cases of low back pain are actually due to improper lifting techniques, rather than the sport itself (117). If one suspects a problem in the pars interarticularis and regular X-rays are normal, a bone scan will usually show an early stress fracture. If the scan is abnormal, one must avoid any activities that exacerbate the symptoms until healing occurs, which may take several weeks (118).

When the pain has abated sufficiently, the athlete should initiate stretching of the lumbar muscles, with early strengthening of the abdominal muscles, until normal strength and flexibility have been obtained. If the lifter is a juvenile, one must consider Scheuerman's disease, primarily at the dorsolumbar junction, but even it usually involves simple intermittent aching with no neurologic deficit (100). The abnormalities do not appear to be progressive and should simply be treated symptomatically (112).

If the bone scan is "hot" (119) and the patient continues to have difficulty, one then must consider the use of an anterior-opening Boston brace with zero degrees of lordosis until the patient becomes asymptomatic and there is evidence of healing. At times tomography of the pars may be needed to delineate the presence of stress fractures. While the patient is still in the Boston brace, abdominal strengthening exercises and flexibility exercises of the lumbar spine should be performed daily, and swimming is an ideal method for rehabilitating the back while retaining cardiovascular fitness (120).

If the back pain proves to be due to spondylolisthesis, one must be aware that progressive displacement usually occurs in the younger patient, the greatest danger being between the ages of 9 and 14. If it is a grade I, less than 25% slip, all sports are allowed as soon as the patient is asymptomatic. If the displacement approaches 50%, grade II, all stress-provoking activities should be curtailed until the patient is asymptomatic. The athlete must be watched until he or she is skeletally mature, evaluated at 6-month intervals. Any evidence of progressive slip, but less than 50%, means full-time antilordotic bracing. If the progression is greater than 50%, surgery is usually indicated. Once the patient is skeletally mature, spondylolisthesis is almost inevitably nonprogressive, but any activity, including weight training, that reproduces symptomatology, must be curtailed until the patient is asymptomatic.

Fractures of the cervical spine—in particular, avulsion injuries to the spinous processes—may occur. However, unless they are related to any instability, they may be treated purely on a symptomatic basis, with return to activities as pain allows (55).

If one suspects disc injury, in particular those with neurologic abnormalities, a computed axial tomography (CAT) scan, magnetic resonance imaging (MRI) scan, and/or electrophysiologic studies are indicated. Recurrent and/or persistent neurologic deficits are absolute indications for a referral to an orthopedic surgeon or a neurosurgeon (113).

Once one has ruled out the possibility of either a major skeletal abnormality and/or neurophysiologic injury and has determined that the pain is due to a muscle strain or minimal joint sprain (121), one can then treat the patient conservatively (122) but intensively, utilizing, in addition to the aforementioned modalities, ultrasound, electrostimulation (123), deep tissue massage, iontophoresis (124), NSAIDs, and occasionally, muscle relaxants.

Occasionally, the athlete may develop rib pain (125), often from costochondral separation. This may become chronic, and if it does not respond to activity modification, NSAIDs, and/or phonophoresis, careful steroid injection at the site of separation may be helpful. Rarely is surgical resection ever indicated.

Stress fractures of the rib do occur (88), and the "slipping rib syndrome" is another form of the costochondral separation and are treated similarly (126).

Active trigger points (114,115), which can be found during a careful examination, may be treated by using massage, spray and stretch technique, phonophoresis, transcutaneous electrical nerve stimulation, or even trigger point injections (127). NSAIDs and acetaminophen are also helpful, as are contrast-temperature baths and postural retraining (114,116).

Ruptures of the pectoralis major muscle or tendon are becoming increasingly common, almost always the result of a maximum attempt bench press (36–38). For optimal recovery these need to be surgically repaired after the swelling has resolved. Until that time, they should be treated with ice, compression, a sling, and analgesics but no antiinflammatories, since these may increase bleeding initially.

SHOULDER

The shoulders of lifters incur tremendous amounts of stress, and the best way to prevent injuries to the shoulder include gaining and maintaining flexibility, using "dislocate" exercises, utilizing exact technique, as well as proper warm-up and stretching, and avoiding overtraining (22,128). These problems are especially prevalent in those athletes training for more than one specific sport, such as powerlifting and weightlifting or swimming and weightlifting (28).

Special tests that are supplementary to a standard examination, specific for diagnoses about the shoulder are as follows (129).

A commonly used test for bicipital tendinitis was developed by Yergason. This test is positive if pain at the anterior inner aspect of the shoulder results from the athlete's active attempt to supinate against resistance while the elbow is kept at 90° flexion. Usually, this is associated with tenderness over the long head of the biceps, proximally, but occasionally, distally also.

Lippman's test may produce sharp pain when the biceps tendon is displaced from side to side in the groove at the proximal anterior aspect of the shoulder and then released while the elbow is flexed at 90°. Ludington's test is positive when sharp pain is elicited when the biceps is contracted while the athlete clasps his or her hands behind the head.

The test for a ruptured transverse humeral ligament is positive when the shoulder is abducted and externally rotated, with the examiner's fingers placed along the bicipital groove. The arm is then internally rotated, and the tendon can be palpated snapping into or out of the groove.

If any biceps tendon problems progress to gross rupture, they need to be repaired to enable the athlete to continue to be an active participant (130). This, of course, is also true for large or complete rotator cuff tears.

The Neer test is for impingement syndrome (131), one of the most common problems in shoulders of athletes, including lifters. Flexion of the shoulder will cause the rotator cuff tissues to abut against the anterior third of the acromion if the arm is in the anatomic position and against the coracoacromial ligament if the humerus is internally rotated. Some people call this the "empty beer can test" for obvious reasons. Another method is to flex the humerus to 90°, then forcibly internally rotate it to drive the greater tuberosity under the coracoacromial ligament.

The apprehension test for glenohumeral dislocation or subluxation is performed by slowly abducting and externally rotating the humerus while the athlete is in a relaxed supine position. If the athlete will not allow the examiner to carry this motion to its extreme or is very apprehensive about the motion, this is a positive sign. Posterior glenohumeral subluxation also has an apprehension test, carried out by transmitting a posterior force with the humerus held in various angles of flexion and internal rotation, but this normally is a result of a fall rather than lifting.

If the shoulder problem persists for more than just a few days, radiographic evaluation should be done to rule out fractures, osteolysis of the distal clavicle (48), and other problems. Occasionally, tomography, MRI or CAT scanning, or even bone scanning is necessary to complete the radiographic examination (132).

Most impingement syndromes, whether isolated or associated with other problems, can be treated by stretching the tight structures about the rotator cuff and strengthening the internal and external rotator musculature until there is balanced strength about the shoulder. The exercises described by Jobe are the ones that are most frequently utilized and are successful in most cases (133) when done religiously and, if necessary, accompanied by various physical therapy modalities of phonophoresis, iontophoresis, and so on (134).

Occasionally, decompression has to be done at the subacromial area and/or the acromioclavicular joint. This is often done openly but can sometimes be done arthroscopically (135). The test for a complete tear of the supraspinatus tendon is the "drop arm test." This is positive if the athlete is unable to lower his or her arm slowly and smoothly from a position of 90° abduction.

With condensing osteitis of the clavicle, there is sclerosis and usually enlargement of the medial end of the clavicle, with a normal sternoclavicular joint (136). These can usually be treated symptomatically with NSAIDs, restraint of training within the confines of symptoms, and then gradual return to weight training when the bone scan is negative, if it is "hot" initially, and symptoms permit (137).

With osteolysis of the distal clavicle (46), with or without arthrosis, if conservative management is unsuccessful (138), resection of the distal clavicle usually produces a complete cure (49,139). With this resection, open or arthroscopically, the coracoclavicular ligaments must be intact, after which the athlete can return to regular activities (47,140).

Occasionally, there are inferior spurs in the distal end of the clavicle that not only are the result of arthritis of the acromioclavicular joint, but also impinge on the subdeltoid bursa area to the extent that it simultaneously causes an impingement. If this is treated appropriately, often with injection (7,141), and quickly enough, rotator cuff tears may be prevented. If symptomatic treatment for several months is unsuccessful, surgical debridement, often arthroscopically, is indicated. Whenever one is uncertain about the diagnosis and the patient does not respond appropriately to conservative care, bone scans and/or thermography are sometimes helpful (142).

Some of the exercises that seem to be implicated in the impingement problems and that need to be avoided during rehabilitation of the shoulder are the military press, dumbbell press, incline press, triceps extension, pull-downs, flies, pullovers, and behind the neck press.

Heavy weight training has been implicated as the cause of the "snapping scapula," usually due to scapulothoracic bursal inflammation (87). This injury usually responds to conservative care but occasionally must be treated with excision of the bursa or of a rarely found osteochondroma at the inferior surface of the scapula.

An increasingly commonly diagnosed problem in athletes, especially those involved in weight training or competitive lifting, is entrapment neuropathies of the long thoracic nerve (11), axillary nerve at the quadrilateral space, and supraspinatus and infraspinatus branches of the suprascapular nerve (143,144). Again, intensive conservative care, utilizing physical therapy modalities, are usually successful; however, if symptoms persist, and especially if electrodiagnostic studies are positive (93,145), these may be decompressed surgically (146,147), usually with very good results and quick return to athletic activities (148). Resection of the transverse scapular ligament is usually an effective treatment, but one must explore the spinoglenoid notch if there is any question of both branches of the nerve being compressed (149). Any ganglia need to be excised (150).

The thoracic outlet syndrome (TOS) can occur in athletes but rarely requires surgical intervention (151). There are several types of thoracic outlet syndrome, and they may, if left untreated, progress to effort thrombosis of the subclavian vein as well as pain, numbness, tingling, weakness, and atrophy of the musculature (152). This is a difficult diagnosis to prove objectively, since even the most sophisticated tests are frequently normal, even when the limb is placed in the provocative position. Thermography can often prove invaluable in proving the presence of thoracic outlet syndrome.

The Adson maneuver can sometimes be used to confirm the presence of thoracic outlet syndrome. This is done by having the athlete hold his or her breath in deep inspiration while fully extending the neck and turning the chin toward the side being examined. The examiner can palpate the radial pulse, checking for any obliteration or dampening. One must ensure that there is lack of symmetry, since this test is frequently positive in asymptomatic shoulders. This should be considered positive only if there is simultaneous exacerbation of the symptoms.

The Allen's maneuver consists of holding the arm in full flexion and abduction while the neck is extended and the hand is supinated. Obliteration of the radial pulse and/or reproduction of the symptoms suggests that the pectoralis minor is compressing the neurovascular bundle.

The costoclavicular syndrome can be tested with the exaggerated military position by having the athlete sit, holding the shoulders back and downward with the arm in 30° of abduction and extension, following which the patient takes a breath and holds it. Dampening or obliteration of the radial pulse with exacerbation of symptoms denotes a positive test.

Another diagnostic exam is the claudication test, in which the patient exercises the forearm by opening and closing his or her hands rapidly for 60 seconds. If there is a vascular occlusion above the brachial (upper arm) level, this exercise is tolerated for only a few seconds. Dampening of the radial pulse concurrently with exacerbation of the symptoms can also be used to screen for TOS (153).

Most patients with this phenomenon can be rehabilitated by using flexibility exercises, various modalities of physical therapy including deep tissue massage, and specific strengthening exercises. Rehabilitation frequently requires at least 4–6 weeks to achieve significant results. Muscle relaxants occasionally help, as do NSAIDs or even the use of a TENS unit. Deep breathing exercises, lateral neck stretching, pectoralis stretching, and scalene stretch exercises are necessary. Also one needs to strengthen the serratus anterior, the shoulder abductor muscles, and the midtrapezius, utilizing shoulder shrugging, the lower trapezius, and erector spinae muscles.

Only if intensive prolonged therapy is unsuccessful would one suggest the possibility of first rib resection, but these have been successful, even in lifting athletes (154,155).

If all the aforementioned problems have been eliminated, and/or ruled out, radionuclide imaging (bone scans) may be helpful, since an osteoid osteoma can be found by using three-phase bone scanning and cannot usually be seen otherwise (137).

Effort thrombosis of the upper extremity is being increasingly diagnosed and may be more prevalent in the dehydrated lifter (10,11,156). If present, this must be treated expeditiously to minimize long-term morbidity (10,14). Thrombolytic therapy may help (13), but frequently, surgical release is needed (15,16), sometimes requiring stent insertion (10).

Powerlifters frequently fracture their humeral shafts while squatting (157), and most should be internally fixed (158), since almost absolute anatomic restoration is needed to be able to continue to compete (159). These injuries may actually be similar to those of grenade throwers (160).

Much of chronic pain in the athlete's shoulder actually relates to the myofascial pain syndrome (fibromyalgia), which exhibits trigger points (161). This can occur once one has injured the musculature with either an acute injury and/or repetitive chronic strain of the muscle, producing intramuscular and perimuscular adhesions. With careful examination one can frequently find several trigger points, the most common of which is at the infraspinatus muscle at the back of the shoulder blade (127). They are found also in the subscapularis, rhomboids, and teres minor and major, and even the superior latissimus dorsi muscle may occasionally be involved. Treatment of the trigger points include the spray and stretch technique, contrasting heat and ice, deep tissue massage, NSAIDs, and occasional injection into the trigger point itself. The presence of trigger points can usually be documented, if necessary, by using thermography.

ELBOW

Elbow injuries are common in athletes who participate in throwing or overhead sports, including, of course, weightlifting (142). The acute traumatic form of injury includes both fractures and dislocations. Early reduction of the dislocation can be done, often without anesthesia, if it is done almost immediately after the injury occurs. Caution should be used, however, since these injuries are occasionally associated with neurovascular injuries, which must be documented before the reduction (162). Reduction should be done, of course, only by individuals who are trained and competent in doing so, and all reductions need to be followed by appropriate radiographic evaluation to verify the anatomic position of the elbow joint, as well as to rule out any associated fracture (163). The integrity of the medial collateral elbow ligaments should be evaluated during forced valgus in pronation and in neutral forearm rotation (164).

If significant laxity is found, the ligaments should be repaired by using an isometric ligament reconstruction. Various fractures can occur about the elbow with a dislocation, including the radial head, the coronoid process, and the condyles or medial epicondyle. Frequently, what appears to be an elbow dislocation can be a supracondylar fracture, the treatment of which is significantly different from the treatment of a dislocation and which must always be considered in all elbow injuries of this type. Early protected range of motion of a dislocated elbow in an athlete is absolutely necessary for complete range of motion following the injury, which is even more important to the weight lifter. Common complications are partial ankylosis and heterotopic ossification, which may reduce the full range of motion. Recurrent dislocations are rare but may require surgical reconstruction. Occasionally, surgical repair may be indicated for acute medial disruption of the elbow (165), but this is rarely needed in lifters.

Isolated medial epicondyle fractures, especially in young athletes, frequently require internal fixation (87). Similarly, isolated radial head and/or neck fractures and supracondylar fractures may require open reduction and internal fixation.

The olecranon apophysis (tip of the elbow) may be avulsed, usually in the skeletally immature, usually because of sudden contracture of the triceps, and, if left untreated, may migrate, adhering to the distal humerus, resulting in limitation of motion of the elbow. This likewise requires surgical treatment (90).

Many soft tissue injuries occur about the elbow in athletes, especially in lifters, including lateral epicondylitis and medial epicondylitis, either of which may be associated with either radial or ulnar nerve dysfunction (166). Most of these occur because of heavy repetitive forearm activity, and approximately 10% of patients with one of these injuries will suffer in multiple areas (the so-called mesenchymal syndrome, such as at both elbows, and/or shoulders, carpal tunnel syndrome, etc.). Both medial and lateral epicondylitis present with tenderness and pain about the bony prominences on the respective side of the elbow. Posterior tennis elbow (olecranon-triceps tendinitis) frequently occurs just proximal to the olecranon tip. Modified rest is the best method of treatment to control the inflammation, avoiding activities that cause an increase in the symptomatology while treating the cause. The usual methodologies of ultrasound, iontophoresis, deep frictional massage, NSAIDs, and liniments, as well as specific flexibility exercises, help the athlete return to normal activity as quickly as possible. Theoretically, all of these are the result of angiofibroplastic changes at the point of inflammation, usually producing incomplete rupture that does not require surgical treatment. Persistent weakness and/or pain after local injection (12) and/or intensive, prolonged therapy for several weeks are the primary indications for surgery. These may also be associated with loose bodies within the elbow joint, large spurs that continue to irritate the soft tissues surrounding them, and/or cartilaginous injury to the various aspects of the elbow joint, which frequently cannot be seen on routine X-rays. Triceps tendinitis is more frequently associated with osteocartilaginous loose bodies, which usually require removal, which may be done arthroscopically. The various problems that may be dealt with arthroscopically include loose body removal, treatment of osteochondritis dissecans, synovectomy for nonspecific synovitis, excision of osteophytes, or evaluation and treatment of otherwise undiagnosed painful elbows (167). Symptoms of postfracture problems, especially of the radial head and/or capitellum, may be relieved by simply removing adhesions and/or doing a synovectomy with debridement or trimming of the involved areas of the cartilage and bone, usually arthroscopically (168).

Snapping of the medial head of a hypertrophic triceps muscle may produce ulnar dislocation with symptoms of cubital tunnel syndrome (169). This must be differentiated from cubital tunnel syndrome due to a ruptured triceps (71).

Following surgery to the elbow, either arthroscopic or open, return to athletic endeavors is contingent on the procedure that was used, the problem being treated, and how quickly the patient is able to return to a full range of motion, with flexibility and strength and endurance of the elbow at least 80% of the opposite before resumption of weight training. Even in lifters, one must remember that full strength of the dominant arm is usually at least 5–10% greater than in the opposite arm, and this must be considered in determining when the athlete may return to training.

Rupture of the triceps insertion at the olecranon, once originally considered a rare injury, is now being more commonly seen in lifters (43). The snatch and the bench press have been implicated more frequently than other lifts. Triceps rupture may present as a cubital tunnel syndrome, and almost always, the lifter, in retrospect, has had problems with tendinitis around the distal triceps tendon for several weeks, or even months, before the final rupture. For the athlete to continue in athletics, these must be repaired surgically (84).

Another soft tissue injury about the elbow that is being seen more frequently in lifters is rupture of the distal insertion of the biceps brachii tendon, on the radius (40,41). These also should be repaired surgically to return to elite-caliber weightlifting (39). Unrepaired distal biceps ruptures may also be implicated in later shoulder problems (11).

The cubital tunnel syndrome, is essentially irritation or compression of the ulnar nerve at the medial aspect of the elbow. This can be due to an overuse syndrome, especially when associated with lack of full flexibility of the elbow, an anatomic variation, a partial rupture of the surrounding soft tissues producing significant inflammatory response, or even direct trauma to the nerve itself. Most of these, when diagnosed early and treated appropriately, may be treated nonsurgically utilizing a long arm splint, NSAIDs, and megavitamin therapy. If the problem is associated with an anatomic variant, it frequently requires surgical release, following which, after the patient has recovered full range of motion and strength, lifting can be resumed without difficulty. The ulnar nerve should probably not be transferred submuscularly in a lifter, at least not as a primary procedure, unless there is excessive perineural scarring.

A relatively rare problem is the "Popeye syndrome": brachial artery entrapment as a result of muscular hypertrophy, in which the lacertus fibrosus, a prolongation of the biceps tendon, can entrap the brachial artery at the cubital fossa at the elbow, producing pain, weakness, and occasionally, "coldness" or paresthesia. Surgical division of the lacertus fibrosis produces cure (170).

Lateral elbow pain with tenderness along the anconeus muscle can be caused by either a compartment syndrome of the muscle itself (68) due to overuse, and/or compression of the musculocutaneous nerve (33) or the lateral antebrachial cutaneous nerve between the biceps aponeurosis and brachialis fascia (87). If a compartment syndrome is present, surgical fasciotomy is usually necessary. If caught soon enough, these may be treated adequately, using rest, ice massage, phonophoresis, and so on. Compartment syndrome in the biceps and triceps have also been reported in lifters, in which passive stretching of the involved muscles causes severe pain and muscle weakness with normal pulses and sensation. This syndrome is treated similarly to that of the anconeus (34).

FOREARM, WRIST, AND HAND

Stress fractures of the shaft of the ulna have been reported in lifters (171) and, if suspected, must be X-rayed. They may be diagnosed early, using bone scans and/or thermography, and can usually be treated by splint immobilization until healing has occurred, after which slow return to lifting is usually possible without difficulty (172). Any suspected fracture or dislocation, especially of the forearm, wrist, or hand, needs to be X-rayed and examined by a physician who is well versed in problems with this part of the anatomy (173).

The scaphoid fracture is one of the most common wrist fractures, frequently occurs because of overuse, as well as with a single acute injury, and may be associated with a scapholunate dissociation. This latter problem is even further complicated by the fact that the dissociation may be dynamic, in which case routine X-rays do not show the problem. Carpal bone fractures may not be apparent radiographically for 10–14 days after the injury. Sometimes an occult fracture can be diagnosed by using CAT scans, tomograms, or bone scans. A good screening test for whether a fracture may or may not be involved is the use of therapeutic, not diagnostic, ultrasound. If there is no significant increase in pain around the area of suspected fracture while the ultrasound is being used, slowly increased up to its maximum, the chance of a fracture being present is very small. Treatment of a scaphoid fracture and/or acute scapholunate dissociation requires immobilization for several weeks—occasionally months—and may require surgical repair, especially if displaced.

Forearm compartment syndromes due to lifting have also been reported and can usually be diagnosed by noting forearm pain occurring with passive dorsiflexion or palmar flexion of the wrist or fingers (91). They must be treated with rest and NSAIDs. If there is no positive response within several hours, surgical decompression is necessary. They may also be diagnosed by using slit-catheter compartment pressure transducers.

There are several areas in the forearm and wrist in which nerve entrapment may occur, usually because of overuse, and that can be sustained by lifters. These five tunnels include the radial, pronator, cubital, carpal, and ulnar at the wrist (Guyon's canal).

Entrapment of a nerve can be caused by a mechanical compression within the confined anatomic spaces, such as narrow, fibrous passages, canals, tunnels, or unusually thick peritendinous tissue pressing the nerve against bone or ligament. Prompt diagnosis and treatment produces quick recovery, but if the problem is prolonged and/or severe, it may require surgical decompression. Endoscopic carpal tunnel release may help the lifter return to training more quickly than the open technique.

Entrapment of the radial nerve along the proximal radius by the supinator muscle is frequently called the resistant tennis elbow. The point of entrapment is actually 2 or 3 inches distal to the lateral epicondyle of the humerus, the pain is usually nocturnal, and it usually occurs after physical exertion. Marked tenderness over the compressed areas is the most helpful diagnostic sign, another diagnostic test being the long finger resistance test, in which there is a significant increase in pain over the area of the nerve when the examiner resists active extension of the long finger by the patient. Wrist pain can also occasionally be caused by this, since the interosseous nerve has branches going into the carpal bones. Treatment includes elimination of the offending mechanism, splintage, NSAIDs, iontophoresis, phonophoresis, and so on. If pain continues, exploration and neurolysis of the radial nerve are indicated, following which return to athletic endeavors is usually possible, but recovery is often prolonged.

The pronator syndrome is one in which the median nerve is entrapped as it enters the pronator tunnel in the forearm (40,174–177). This entrapment can cause pain on the volar surface of the forearm that is increased by activity and occasionally associated with reduced sensibility in the thumb, index, and long finger. Often, in addition to the pain, there is at least subjective weakness of grasp and clumsy, awkward movements of the fingers, accompanied by paresthesia. A test for determining the exact location of this nerve compression includes resistance to elbow flexion, in which the elbow is held in 120–135° flexion, reproducing the symptoms (176). Resistance to flexion of the long finger flexor superficialis implies median nerve compression at the flexor superficialis arcade at the proximal forearm. Electromyelographs (EMG) may help to confirm the diagnosis; however, these are frequently normal even when there is severe pain and do not usually help localize the entrapment lesion. In addition to avoiding activities that cause the symptoms, modalities of physical therapy can be used, sometimes in addition to a long arm splint, to try to avoid surgical decompression. If surgery is necessary, there are usually no long-term deficits (87,177).

The anterior interosseous syndrome is characterized by weak pinch, often associated with a dull, vague ache in the volar forearm, preceding any motor loss. The incomplete syndrome is more frequent, and rest and physical therapy modalities are usually successful; however, if there is no recovery either clinically or with electrophysiologic tests, after 8–12 weeks, surgical decompression is indicated. Stress EMGs may be of help in these various neuropathies but can usually be done successfully only by those who are well trained in this specific testing modality. Rarely, the pronator syndrome may be associated with a persistent median artery and is usually exacerbated by any exercise of the volar forearm muscles, especially with forceful pronation of the forearm, which is so frequently used in lifting. Bilateral fracture-separations of the distal radial epiphyses (growth plates) have been reported in the adolescent lifter (32).

More frequently, in the adult lifter the problems consist of scaphoid impaction, triquetral-hamate impaction, sometimes producing a carpal boss (178), and occult ganglia. There is usually point tenderness over the wrist, but routine X-rays are usually normal. An MRI or ultrasound can sometimes show an occult ganglion (179). The usual treatment is splinting and/or steroid injection and NSAIDs for at least 2 or 3 weeks. Occasionally, a cheilectomy of either of the surfaces and/or synovial debridement is necessary and may be done arthroscopically. If there has been a scapholunate dissociation, in addition to immobilization for several weeks, at least 6 months of protection should be considered before return to intensive weight-training (180).

The triangular fibrocartilage complex at the ulnar aspect of the wrist can be injured with either repetitive injuries and/or an acute single episode. If they are diagnosed immediately and immobilized for several weeks, they may heal without the necessity of surgical intervention. If there are persistent problems, the patient should be examined by an upper extremity specialist and may require special stress X-rays, MRI, tomography, bone scans, arthrograms or even arthroscopic examination, and occasionally surgical debridement, usually arthroscopically.

Other sports-related extraarticular wrist syndromes include the various types of tendinitis and nerve compression problems. DeQuervain's disease (stenosing tenosynovitis of the first extensor compartment of the wrist) is an inflammation of the tendons of the abductor pollicis longus and extensor pollicis brevis as they pass through the fibro-osseous canal at the level of the radial styloid. If there is an audible squeak (43) or crepitus with a positive Finkelstein test (pain with the patient grasping the thumb with his or her fingers and with passive ulnar deviation of the wrist, with stress applied by the examiner to the metacarpal of the index finger), one can be assured of the correct diagnosis, but there may be a concurrent basilar joint arthrosis or intersection syndrome. In the earlier stages, the inflammation may resolve as a result of avoidance of the aggravating activity, using a splint, NSAIDs, and various modes of therapy, including iontophoresis and/or phonophoresis. Direct injection of a long-acting steroid may produce dramatic improvement but is not a substitute for protection and preventive measures. If frank thickening of the roof of the first dorsal compartment occurs, this may lead to actual stenosis of the fibro-osseous canal. When this occurs, nonoperative treatment is generally ineffective and surgical decompression is indicated. Any associated ganglia, if present, should be excised.

Tenosynovitis occurs in the other dorsal compartments of the wrist, including the sixth dorsal compartment composing the extensor carpi ulnaris, which is the most common of the other sites (181). This is occasionally associated with calcific deposits. The radial wrist extensors in the second dorsal compartment may be the next most common, and treatment is identical to the treatments described above. Tenosynovitis of the fourth and fifth extensor compartments is relatively uncommon; if it occurs, an anatomic abnormality should be suspected.

Involvement of the third dorsal compartment (extensor pollicis longus), directly adjacent to Lister's tubercle, may be the result of exostosis formation from a healed distal radius fracture or simple degenerative changes around the area due to overuse. If a bony abnormality is revealed radiographically, early operation to remove the exostoses or simply reroute the tendon before tendon rupture should be seriously considered.

The intersection (or crossover) syndrome is characterized by localized pain, tenderness, crepitus, and soft tissue swelling over the radiodorsal aspect of the distal forearm, approximately 4–8 cm proximal to Lister's tubercle. This crepitus, which in some instances may be more like a squeak, is usually present on both direct palpation and during wrist motion. It may be both audible and palpable and is frequent in lifters. Nonoperative treatment is usually successful, as was previously discussed, and operative exploration is rarely necessary. If surgery is necessary, it should be followed by prolonged protection from any aggravating stress.

Recurrent subluxation of the extensor carpi ulnaris tendon is usually characterized by a painful snap over the dorsoulnar aspect of the wrist, particularly with forearm rotation. Most cases have been associated with a single traumatic episode, and the pathologic lesion is a recurrent subluxation due to a disruption of the ulnar wall or septum of the sixth dorsal compartment fibro-osseous sheath. On supination with the wrist in ulnar deviation, the tendon displaces, often with an audible snap, when moved in the ulnar and palmar direction. On pronation it relocates into its normal sulcus. Closed treatment by immobilization with the forearm in pronation and the wrist in radial deviation may be appropriate; however, if the patient presents after recurrent painful episodes, surgical reconstruction is advised.

Flexor carpi ulnaris tendinitis is relatively common, is usually associated with chronic repetitive trauma, and may be bilateral and frequently associated with calcific deposits. Nonoperative treatment is usually curative, but the injury may require operative intervention if it is very severe.

Flexor carpi radialis tendinitis is less common, but if it is recalcitrant, surgery should be considered; if operation is required, the fibro-osseous tunnel should be decompressed. Digital flexor tenosynovitis at the wrist area produces acute pain of the stabbing or burning type, and may be associated with tenderness or irritability of the median nerve all the way up as far as the axilla. There are frequent signs of autonomic dysfunction. Electrodiagnostic procedures are usually normal, but there is usually a palpable fullness just proximal to the flexor crease of the wrist, which may occur after a hyperextension injury of the wrist or after chronic repetitive digital flexion, all of which can easily occur in lifting. Recovery, whether operative or nonoperative treatment is required, may be surprisingly prolonged.

Linburg's syndrome is associated with an anomaly of the flexor tendons. The patient presents with vague complaints of pain over the radiovolar aspect of the distal forearm, with subjective tightness and occasionally cramping of the thumb. The characteristic sign of this syndrome is inability to flex the thumb fully while at the same time extending the index finger, or even, rarely, the long finger. This condition is caused by an anomalous tendon slip, a musculotendinous slip, or, infrequently, an adhesion of the flexor pollicis longus. This tendon slip usually inserts into the tendon of the profundus muscle or thickened adjacent tenosynovium of the index finger and occasionally of the third digital flexor. If the condition persists after a trial of conservative treatment, excision of the anomalous tendon slip is warranted. Recovery is rapid.

Extraarticular ganglion cysts or anomalous muscles may also occur, especially the extensor digitorum brevis manus. The symptoms usually resolve with rest, protection, and the usual methods of physical therapy but may at times require surgical excision or decompression, respectively (182).

There has been at least one reported instance of a spontaneous rupture of the extensor pollicis longus tendon in a patient who had taken several months of anabolic steroids. Of course, this type of injury needs to be repaired surgically (62).

Thrombosis or aneurysm of the ulnar artery of the wrist may occur but is usually associated with repeated blunt trauma. The most appropriate treatment is not well established, but it may be necessary to seriously consider revascularization by excision of the thrombosed segment and reconstruction by a reversed vein graft. Simple Guyon's canal decompression or excision of the thrombosed arterial segment or aneurysm has also been found to be helpful.

Neuropathies of the hand do occur in weight training, the most common of which is the carpal tunnel syndrome (44). Usually, it is related to digital flexor tenosynovitis, the clinical features of which typically include numbness and/or tingling of the radial three and one-half fingers that is particularly worse at night. There may be some subjective weakness or tightness of digit flexion, and the pathognomonic clinical findings are a positive Tinel's sign of the median nerve at the wrist and positive Phalen's test (183). Frequently, electrophysiologic tests are negative.

Avoidance of activities that cause symptoms, especially repetitive flexion, a splint, NSAIDs, and even megavitamin therapy can produce resolution if the problem is caught soon enough and there is no adhesion formation. If the electrophysiologic tests are positive and/or the patient does not respond within a very few weeks to the usual aforementioned therapeutic modalities, there may be a positive response to injection of a steroid into the tunnel itself, but these frequently produce only temporary relief, and surgical decompression may be indicated. If surgery is required in a lifter, the surgeon may want to seriously consider lengthening the flexor retinaculum or volar carpal ligament rather than simple division, as is usually done. Endoscopic release may allow the athlete to return to lifting more quickly.

Guyon's canal syndrome (compressive neuropathy of the ulnar nerve within the wrist) affects the ulnar one and a half digits, with or without ulnar intrinsic weakness. Occasionally, the findings may be restricted to the deep motor branch of the nerve with atrophy or weakness of the interossei in the complete absence of sensory symptoms, but this syndrome is frequently associated with severe pain. Treatment is the same as that for carpal tunnel syndrome.

Other, less well-known neuropathies include those of the superficial radial nerve, the dorsal sensory branch of the ulnar nerve, and the posterior interosseous nerve about the wrist. Most commonly, perineural fibrosis from direct contusion is responsible, but since the latter condition may persist despite efforts to avoid wrist hyperextension stresses, frequently seen in lifters, neurectomy of the terminal portion of the posterior interosseous nerve may be required if injection(s) and/or the various physiotherapy modalities are unsuccessful.

Ganglia may also occur along the flexor sheath of the fingers at the level of the proximal phalanx; they are usually very small, tender masses and are not associated with snapping or clicking. Trigger finger(s) (stenosing tenosynovitis of the finger flexor tendons) usually occur at the level of the junction of the palm and finger, with the complaint often of pain at the level of the proximal interphalangeal joint, but the primary difficulty is a swelling of the tendon within the fibro-osseous sheath, usually at the first annular pulley. If these do not respond to rest, with a splint, antiinflammatories, iontophoresis, and/or phonophoresis, they may require surgical release, which may be done percutaneously. Similarly, a ganglion of the flexor sheath in the finger may be cured, if it does not respond to more conservative care, by trephination (puncturing) of the ganglion itself. If there is any recurrence, these may be removed surgically (184).

If there is any suggestion of fracture of the fingers or hand, X-rays are indicated. If the X-rays are negative, one must be aware of various other problems, including mallet finger (disruption of the extensor tendon at the distal interphalangeal joint producing a drooped finger), a volar plate tear of the proximal interphalangeal joint, a boutonniere deformity (inability to fully extend the PIP joint), and/or collateral ligament tears, partial or complete. Each of these can usually be treated with appropriate splintage and protection, but they frequently take several weeks to heal before the athlete may return to activities that require full flexion or extension of the joints. Occasionally, they are associated with small avulsion fractures but, unless there is significant subluxation of the joint, do not require surgical intervention. If one suspects the possibility of a tear of any of these structures, the fingers need to be splinted until they are seen by a physician who is trained in the care of hand injuries. One of the more difficult problems occasionally seen in athletes, including lifters, is an initially incomplete injury that, when treated inadequately, becomes a chronic, complete injury requiring surgical reconstruction. Once reconstruction is required, there is usually some loss of motion; therefore this is to be avoided, unless absolutely indicated. The minimum time for splintage of injuring one of the small joints is 6–8 weeks, but this may frequently extend to several months.

Direct crushing injury to the fingers, especially to the nailbeds, occasionally occurs in lifting and must be dealt with appropriately and quickly for optimal recovery. Any subungual hematoma should be decompressed, and if there is a suggestion of an underlying fracture or nailbed injury, the athlete should see a physician for exploration and repair as soon as possible.

Calluses are frequently torn, significantly reducing the lifter's ability to handle weights efficiently and safely. All calluses should be kept pared down to help minimize tearing. If tearing does occur, the loose skin should be removed, and the base of the tear should be cleansed, dressed with antibiotic cream, and protected until healing is complete.

PELVIS, HIP, AND THIGH

Most injuries to weightlifters in this area consist of muscle strains, which occur when the tension capacity of the muscle–tendon unit is not adequate to meet the demands (101). These most frequently involve biarticulate muscle structures, the hamstring group consisting predominantly of type II fibers being the most commonly involved. The dual innervation of the semitendinosus and biceps femoris may contribute asynchrony of firing and fatiguing properties, which may increase the probability of injury (185). Muscles that have been strengthened, preconditioned, or warmed up and acclimated to activity through specific muscular action are less likely to be strained. This follows the specificity of training theory, in that eccentric training needs to be used for eccentric activities, high-speed work for high-speed activities, and so on.

The actual location of the injury is usually at the muscle–tendon junction. Whether the stretch is applied proximally or distally as to the location of the injury and the force required for the injury to occur seem to make no difference, and it presents primarily as an inflammatory condition. For this reason most preventive measures include strengthening and stretching the muscles, with a good warm-up before the workout and use of periodization to prevent overuse or overworking the muscles involved. Most recurrent injuries are the result of inadequate rehabilitation, which implies, in addition to poor flexibility, inadequate muscle strength and/or endurance, dyssynergic muscle contraction, insufficient warm-up or stretching before exercising, or a return to activity before complete rehabilitation (186). Imbalance in strength of the quadriceps as compared to the ipsilateral hamstring muscles and/or a weak hamstring muscle group on one side compared to the other have been most frequently implicated in hamstring injuries (187).

A reduction in strength may be associated with fatigue. An excessive amount of running may actually increase the chance of hamstring injury, in particular if the running shoe is inadequate or inappropriate for that particular athlete's foot.

In a mild first-degree strain, the athlete is usually not aware of the injury until after cooling down. The usual therapeutic regimen for such injuries consists of ice packs and rest, with stretching and strengthening slowly, over several days. Second- and third-degree strain injuries usually produce symptoms that are known immediately and are primarily a painful pop, snap, or tearing sensation in the back of the thigh. After a few days, ecchymosis may be seen on the back of the thigh that may, with time, descend all the way to the back of the knee or below.

Immediate treatment for these injuries includes not only crushed ice, immobilization, and compression with elastic wraps, but also NSAIDs and analgesics as needed. Ambulation should not be started until the swelling and tenderness begin to subside. When ambulation is started, crutches should be used until normal pain-free walking is possible. At that time, very gentle, pain-free stretching of the hamstring muscles may be initiated. Gentle massage, ultrasound, and/or electrical stimulation may be started after 48–72 hours but should never be used if it is associated with a significant increase in pain. After strengthening has started, ultrasound and gentle friction massage may be helpful in aiding the resolution of adhesions within the muscle. When adequate strength, power, and endurance have been achieved, such that the legs are essentially equal in strength and endurance, jogging may be begun, as may low-intensity weight training. Following the return to athletic endeavors, stretching before the workout after a warm-up period and then stretching again in the cooldown period are recommended.

If there is any suggestion of any bony hip or pelvic injury, X-ray examination is indicated (175). Fractures may occur at the inferior pubic ramus or elsewhere and may be invisible on routine X-rays but obvious on radionuclide bone scans. Once a fracture has been identified, the treatment is rest. This does not mean inactivity but limiting activities to any that do not reproduce the pain until there is complete healing radiographically.

Avulsion of the pectineus muscle has been reported as a cause for persistent medial groin pain (188). Since the action of the pectineus is to flex, adduct, and medially rotate the hip, this muscle is extensively used when one attempts to squat. The wider the stance, the more strain is applied to this muscle; and the greater the load the lifter lifts, the greater the strain. Symptoms include a tearing sensation along the inner thigh, with swelling of the inguinal area. The injury usually responds to rest, antiinflammatories, and the other modalities mentioned. Occasionally, there is enough avulsion that myositis ossificans develops; if suggested, a CAT scan can reveal its presence. If the mass is large enough to interfere with activity, it may need to be removed, but its excision should be postponed until the region has a cold bone scan, indicating inactivity of the mass. MRI technique may be another possibility as an adjunctive diagnostic aid in such problems (189).

Another cause of groin pain in athletes, including lifters, is the "sports hernia" (190), which sometimes must be repaired surgically, after which competition is almost always unaffected. Quadratus femoris tendinitis has been reported to cause groin pain (191) and usually responds to conservative treatment but may be prolonged. Osteitis pubis can also present as groin pain, and there may be a need to be injected before it finally allows return to competition (192).

The hip is a very stable joint, generally, but may be injured during lifting (193). Stress fractures can occur but are unusual in weight-training athletes. The avulsion fractures that may occur in the teenage years rarely occur in the skeletally mature individual. Pinpoint tenderness and pain will be found in the stress fracture or avulsion fracture, but radiographs may initially appear normal. Stress fractures of the anterior iliac crest can be treated by rest, weight-bearing relief, and avoiding stressful non-weight-bearing positions. Avulsion fractures of the anterior superior iliac spine may require internal fixation and/or casting.

One of the most common areas of pain about the hip involves the greater trochanteric bursa. This lies between the tendon of the gluteus maximus at the posterolateral surface of the greater trochanter. The major cause of this bursitis relates to the iliotibial band into which the gluteus maximus muscle inserts. Imbalance between the adductor and abductor muscles may produce difficulty here, as would excessive posterolateral heel wear on a shoe or even repeated adduction of a limb. Ober's test is usually positive, and resisted abduction will increase the symptoms. Treatment is usually symptomatic, utilizing ultrasound, diathermy or iontophoresis, NSAIDs, gait and posture training, flexibility, and the appropriate footwear retrofitted with the necessary orthoses. As with other types of bursitis, this may respond to acuscope therapy, deep friction massage or, occasionally, injection of steroids but will very rarely require any kind of surgery.

Ischial bursitis can also occur between the tuberosity of the ischium and the gluteus maximus, occasionally associated with pain radiating into the hamstring muscles. Iliopectineal bursitis occurs over the anterior aspect of the hip joint and is usually caused by tight iliopsoas muscle. The pain is caused by tensing the iliopsoas muscle during forced flexion or flexing it during hip extension. Tenderness will usually be found on palpation of the inguinal area, and there is occasionally referred pain at the anterior thigh and/or knee. Diathermy, ultrasound, or the like is usually successful, combined with stretching the iliopsoas muscle.

The rectus femoris muscle may be strained, as may the hamstrings, but the symptoms are anterior rather than posterior. As with the hamstring strains, immediate treatment includes ice and compression with an elastic wrap and should be used as long as it is effective. After this, contrast baths using heat and ice combined with ultrasound, cross-frictional massage, and flexibility exercises should be started, but not before the fifth day after the injury because of risk of hemorrhage. On about the third day after injury, the athlete starts submaximal isometric exercises; after 2 weeks, more aggressive training, including increased flexibility exercising and full running, may be indicated.

The piriformis syndrome is an irritation of the sciatic nerve as it passes underneath or through the piriformis muscle in the buttock area. The athlete complains of deep, localized pain in the posterior aspect of the hip or buttock near the sciatic notch, and there may be some numbness and tingling down the leg. The most significant finding implicating this will be that both active external rotation with resistance and a passive stretch into internal rotation will reproduce the pain. Initial treatment includes ice, rest, and NSAIDs with mild stretching and contract/relax exercises, possibly the modified PNF technique, in the side-lying position, followed by deep massage as healing occurs.

Occasionally, an athlete will complain of severe, sharp, searing pain along the lateral aspect of the thigh, essentially at the junction between the anterior and posterior musculature of the thigh. Sometimes the pain is so severe that the athlete cannot continue with his or her activities and may even require crutches for ambulation. This is most frequently seen in squatting movements and may occur anywhere along the thigh from the level of the iliac crest distally to the area of the lateral femoral condyle. It is usually associated with exquisite tenderness, moderate swelling within a few hours, and discoloration after a day or so. Treatment consists of rest, ice, NSAIDs, and, if necessary, muscle relaxants if there is so much spasm that the patient is unable to sleep. Flexibility exercises should be resumed within 72 hours of the injury, ambulation as possible within pain tolerance, and contrast baths started after 48–72 hours.

A rare cause of upper leg pain reported in a bodybuilder is external iliac artery stenosis (5), which needs to be treated by a vascular surgeon.

KNEE

Since an injury to the knee can be one of the most devastating injuries to an athlete, most people assume that the incidence of knee injuries in weight training is significantly higher than the incidence of injuries in other portions of the anatomy and/or greater than that in other sports. Several studies have now shown that there is not an increased incidence of knee injuries in lifters; in fact, long-term lifting probably protects the knee such that there are fewer knee problems in weightlifters than in the general population (23). Although Olympic weightlifters suffer a higher incidence of knee problems than powerlifters, powerlifters seem to have more severe injuries, possibly because of the nature of the sport itself (24). Furthermore, weight training appears to be a deterrent to knee injuries in other athletic endeavors. Exercises that extend the range of motion of the knee joint appear to strengthen, rather than weaken, the medial collateral ligaments and most likely the other ligaments as well. Loading of the knee joint actually improves congruity, thus providing greater knee stability, which may protect against shear forces (74). Knee stability appears to be greater in powerlifters and weightlifters.

Possible causes of injury while performing squats, snatches, and of course the clean and jerk, include inadequate warming up or stretching, using improper technique, trying a new or unfamiliar technique, performing maximum efforts during competition, and, when attempting one final repetition, cheating to complete the repetition while training to exhaustion or failure (69).

Most knee problems in lifters consist of tendinitis or bursitis. These include quadriceps tendinitis, or patellar tendinitis, often called jumper's knee (194). Most of these are due to a functional stress overload, occasionally following a single traumatic incident, and may be related to working out on hard surfaces as opposed to ones that have an intermediate degree of elasticity, that is, wood. Treatment includes avoiding activities that cause an increase in the pain and tenderness; the usual modalities of iontophoresis, phonophoresis, and the like; NSAIDs; and, in particular, flexibility exercises that are specifically directed toward the quadriceps (195). Similarly, there is an increased incidence in athletes with hyperpronated feet; therefore it behooves those who care for athletes to make sure they are wearing appropriate footwear. Also, deep tissue massage, contrast baths, whirlpool therapy, and the like are very helpful.

The deep infrapatellar bursa may become hypertrophic and/or inflamed (196), usually responds to conservative care, occasionally needs to be injected, and rarely needs to be excised to effect a permanent cure.

Meniscotibial (coronary) ligament sprain can also be a cause of knee pain, as a primary source or a residual source of pain long after a meniscus or collateral ligament sprain has healed (53). Injury to these ligaments are most likely to occur with excessive knee rotation; indeed, one of the diagnostic maneuvers is to rotate the foot on a supine patient with the knee flexed at 60°. At this point, the coronary ligament can be considered the primary lesion when the meniscal and collateral ligament tests are negative and only the rotation test is positive (197). Treatment includes friction massage and NSAIDs.

Torn menisci and/or ligamentous injury involving the medial or lateral collateral ligaments, or anterior and/or posterior cruciate ligaments must always be considered when there is an acute onset of pain, especially when it is associated with a snap or pop, swelling either immediately or within just a few hours, and inability to put the knee through a full range of motion and/or ambulate without pain. Radiographic evaluation and orthopedic consultation are indicated in these instances. If there is any point tenderness at any part of the joint and/or increased pain with varus or valgus stress or a suggestion of instability with any of the various maneuvers, the athlete should be placed on crutches; the knee should be iced, ace-wrapped, and immobilized with a splint; and the athlete should be referred appropriately.

A complete knee examination should include not only the knee itself but the adjacent joints as well, specifically the hip and ankle. Once you have determined the status of the hip and ankle, then you can complete the knee examination. Initially, simple observation should show whether there is any swelling, whether effusion or synovitis or even a hemarthrosis. Usually, a hemarthrosis occurs very rapidly, within a matter of minutes or a couple of hours after the injury. A reactive synovitis and/or excessive synovial fluid collection within the joint usually requires several hours, sometimes even days, to occur, and the history can often answer this question. One should then observe whether there is any pain or tenderness, especially around the patella, whether it is located at the superior or inferior poles, and whether there is any patellar instability. One should determine whether there is any tenderness at the undersurface of the patella, whether there is apprehension sign with attempted subluxation of the patella, usually laterally, though it may occur medially as well. If there is tenderness in the midportion of the patella, one has to suspect the possibility of patellar fracture. Of course, one needs to check to make sure that the extensor mechanism is intact, by having the patient do a straight leg raise, and to make sure there is no extensor lag. Frequently, within the first hour or two after injury, though not usually after a day or two has passed, one can palpate a defect in either the patellar tendon or quadriceps tendon if indeed one is torn, especially if more than 50% is involved. After one has determined whether there is any joint pain and has noted exactly the area of the pain, the examination should include both varus and valgus stress of the knee joint while in full extension, at 20 or 30°, and again at approximately 80 or 90°.

If the pain is not severe enough to produce significant muscle spasm, one can then do the McMurray test to determine the possibility of meniscal tear by simultaneously rotating, producing a valgus stress, and compressing the joint, initially medially and then laterally, while palpating the particular meniscus being tested with the opposite hand. A significant snap, click, or "thunk," at the same time reproducing the primary pain, is indicative of a possible meniscal tear. Of course, one should always examine the opposite, uninjured knee for comparison in doing any of these tests and be aware of any previous injuries that may have produced residual abnormal signs.

The most opportune time to do the knee examination is immediately after the injury, before the onset of muscle spasm and effusion or hemarthrosis. Once a very muscular athlete has developed any of these, it usually is necessary to do the examination under anesthesia.

One must check the anterior drawer and posterior drawer and sag tests while stabilizing the foot and of course comparing with the opposite side.

The jerk test may be helpful if pain allows and is done by stabilizing the tibia with the patient in the supine position and attempting to anteriorly displace the tibia while in less than full extension.

The pivot shift test similarly determines the presence or absence of rotary instability, whether anteromedial, anterolateral, posterolateral, posteromedial, or a combination thereof, each of which indicates a separate entity having been injured. The exact methodology of doing these tests should be found elsewhere.

Finally, the Lachman test is performed by gently attempting to anteriorly displace the tibia, while gently rotating it, taking care to make sure the quadriceps is completely relaxed, to determine the probable presence or absence of cruciate ligament damage.

If there is any question of possible internal derangement, various imaging modalities may be helpful, including, routine X-rays, stress X-rays, arthrography, CAT scans, and now especially MRI examinations (198). All of these, however, are only adjuncts, the physical examination being the most important before the knee is examined arthroscopically.

Should the knee ultimately undergo surgery, the exact nature of rehabilitation is determined by the findings and the surgical procedures necessitated thereafter.

If the problem is only one of a very small tear of a meniscus, the tear may be excised arthroscopically, and the athlete may return to full activity as soon as pain allows. If the meniscus has to be repaired but this can be done arthroscopically, range of motion usually starts within a few days, but no stress should be applied to the knee for at least 6–8 weeks. With ligamentous repairs, it takes at least 6–8 weeks before any real stress can be applied, and if a cruciate ligament has to be repaired and/or reconstructed, the rehabilitation phase is often between 6 and 12 months.

Even if a devastating knee injury has occurred, if it is diagnosed adequately and cared for appropriately, one can usually expect the athlete to return eventually to full activity. If the injury necessitates knee reconstruction, however, it is very difficult for a weight lifter to return to elite competition, because of the necessity of full squatting, which frequently is lacking after knee reconstruction, in spite of adequate rehabilitation.

One must remember that knee pain may be due to hip or pelvis pathology and of course may be due to back injury involving the nerve roots as well.

Another cause of knee pain is subsartorial entrapment of the saphenous nerve (199). This nerve originates from the L-3 and L-4 nerve roots and courses posteromedially within the femoral triangle to enter Hunter's canal, from which it extends to reach its subcutaneous position medial to the knee. The nerve may be compressed either within the subsartorial canal or where it exits the fascial opening, particularly during strong contractions of the surrounding musculature, as may occur with knee extensions or squats. Symptoms include throbbing aching, to the extent that it eventually interferes with sleep and lessens when the athlete arises and walks briefly, with only minimal pain during the day. Sensory testing may demonstrate diminished light touch and hyperesthesia to pinprick, from the level of the medial tibial condyle around the infrapatellar region to the superior aspect of the medial malleolus. Knee pain may be elicited by firm palpation of the anteromedial thigh about 10 cm proximal to the medial joint line, and manual percussion may produce a Tinel's sign. If the injury is caught early enough, NSAIDs, ice massage, and appropriate stretching exercises as well as other physical therapy modalities may be sufficient. An injection over the painful site may be necessary for complete relief. Rarely is surgery indicated.

Partial and complete ruptures of the quadriceps tendon, patellar tendon, gastrocnemius muscles, and distal insertions of the hamstrings about the knee have all been reported and usually require surgery (51). Small, minor muscle tears and/or ligament tears are usually treated conservatively (nonoperatively) with rest, protection, and the usual physical therapy modalities, including NSAIDs, ultrasound, and massage therapy. Complete tears must be repaired and/or reconstructed surgically for the athlete to be able to return to training and competition and to minimize degenerative arthrosis in the future. Postoperative recovery takes several weeks, even months.

Compartment syndromes of the calf and thigh have been reported in lifters and are treated identically to those of the upper extremity: avoidance of activities that cause increased pain, ice, massage, NSAIDs, and avoidance of compression (200).

If there is persistent pain, increased swelling, and diminishing function, especially with normal vascularity, prompt referral for surgery is necessary to avoid eventual significant morbidity.

FOOT AND ANKLE

Injuries to the foot and ankle are exceedingly common in sports, and although they may seem to be prosaic, they can be devastating to the athlete if they are treated inadequately. The ankle sprain is probably the single most common injury in sport, but it is relatively infrequent in weightlifting (201). Weightlifters occasionally have ankle sprains and foot sprains, but most of the injuries consist of overuse problems, frequently associated with biomechanical abnormalities (23).

Since the foot is composed of 26 bones and 30 major synovial joints, innumerable combinations of injuries are possible. Most of the problems in the foot are due to various pathomechanics of the foot, the most common of which is hyperpronation. Others are related to an equinus deformity, essentially a limitation of dorsiflexion of the ankle of less than 10° while the subtalar joint is in neutral and the knee fully extended.

As with most other injuries, especially of the chronic overuse type, a proper flexibility program, appropriate warm-up before the workout, and appropriate footwear mitigate the vast majority of these injuries (202).

The foot has three major functions: shock absorption, ground-shape accommodation, and formation of a rigid lever for propulsion or lifting. The majority of athletes exhibit some sort of foot-related postural instability, the most common being excessive pronation. These frequently contribute to strained arches, shin splints (medial tibial syndrome), and Achilles tendinitis. Excessively supinated feet are not nearly as common; this condition typically occurs in high-arched and rigid feet, which are therefore unable to effectively pronate.

In a foot in which there is significant biomechanical abnormality, flexibility, proper warm-up and training technique, and orthotic devices can prevent many of these problems from occurring (203). A functional orthotic is necessary in the treatment of foot symptomatology occurring as a result of biomechanical foot imbalance. These are designed to control pathomechanical disorders in the foot and leg by maintaining the foot in an approximately neutral position. Because most commercially made devices are mass produced, they cannot be expected to correct a biomechanical imbalance within the foot. The treatment approach therefore must be the fabrication of a functional orthotic device by a professional who is trained and experienced specifically in treating athletes. Few athletic trainers and/or orthopedic surgeons are trained in doing so and must depend on a clinical pedorthist or a podiatrist for this service (24).

One of the most potentially devastating injuries of the foot and ankle is an Achilles tendon rupture. Although these can occur as an avulsion of the tendon from the calcaneus, this usually occurs in youngsters and requires an open reduction to reestablish the length of the tendon. Most Achilles tendon tears occur below the musculotendinous junction, just proximal to the insertion, and can usually be diagnosed by using the Thompson test. This test is performed with the patient lying prone, with both the hips and knees in extension and the feet freely overhanging the end of the table. Simultaneous medial and lateral compression of the gastrocnemius bellies is performed, attention being paid to judging the symmetry of the plantar flexion of the foot compared to the contralateral extremity. A positive Thompson test is judged by reduced plantar flexion as indicative of rupture of the gastrocnemius—soleus complex. Frequently, one can palpate a defect; however, after some time, this could be filled with hematoma and very difficult to ascertain. Most authorities agree that a ruptured Achilles tendon in an athlete must be repaired, since, while conservative care may allow healing, there is significant loss of pushoff.

If there is any question of a partial tear of the Achilles tendon, which can sometimes be diagnosed by palpating a thickening in the tendon, usually anterior to the tendon in the area of the retrocalcaneal fat pad, ultrasound or an MRI can help to elucidate the situation. If there is a partial tear, it should be short-leg casted for 3 or 4 weeks in a plantar flexed position for protection. This is then followed by gentle stretching and massage until a full range of painless motion is attained. If the tenderness is at the inner or medial aspect of the Achilles tendon, a medial wedge can be inserted into the footwear to decrease the stress on the medial aspect of the tendon fibers; this should be maintained until the tenderness is gone. If the tenderness persists, exploration of the tendon may be necessary. If the tendon ruptures and is repaired, it often takes as long as 6 months before high-performance individuals can return to participation. In the interim they are placed on a nongravity exercise program, such as swimming or bicycling, with the extremity plantar flexed for several weeks.

Haglund's disease, caused by tenting of the Achilles tendon over the bony prominence of the calcaneus, causes pain and attritional changes in the tendon and may predispose to rupture of the tendon. Most of these, when caught early, can be treated with the usual modalities of ultrasound, massage, antiinflammatories, and a heel lift. If they persist, they may require a partial excision of that prominence of the calcaneus at the posterior superior aspect to prevent further attrition and possible tear. This can sometimes be done endoscopically, significantly shortening the recovery period.

Ankle sprains are by far one of the most common injuries to athletes, and although they do not occur quite as frequently in lifting as in other sports, they can significantly shorten the lifter's competitive life if treated inadequately.

According to the most widely accepted system of classification for ankle sprain, in a grade I sprain, there is a partial interstitial tear in the ligamentous structures. In a grade II sprain, there is an incomplete but more severe tear in the ligament, with gross stability of the joint retained. A grade III classification implies potential gross instability of the joint. Whenever an ankle sprain in a lifter is suspected, X-rays should be done to rule out the possibility of fracture or subluxation. Most sprains involve the lateral ligamentous structures, specifically the anterior talofibular ligament, the calcaneofibular ligament, and the posterior talofibular ligament, in that order. Occasionally, the deltoid ligament on the medial aspect of the joint may be involved. A good examination always includes an anterior and posterior drawer test, since instability may be solely in one of these two directions, mandating more intensive treatment.

Regardless of the type, ice, compression and elevation should be started immediately, and the patient should be placed on NSAIDs, with non weight bearing for the first 24–72 hours, depending on the severity. At that time reexamination is performed, and if there is no gross instability, the lifter is provided with a splint to prevent undue inversion and eversion but to allow active dorsiflexion and plantar flexion, and contrast baths can be instituted, followed by ice massage.

Grade I sprains usually heal sufficiently to allow return to athletics in a few days or a couple of weeks when the athlete is pain free, albeit with a splint for protection for a while. Grade II sprains usually take 3 or 4 weeks, possibly longer, until the athlete can return to unrestricted athletic endeavors. Treatment is essentially the same as that for a grade I sprain. Treatment of a grade III sprain involves immobilizing the ankle for a few days, after which the athlete can bear weight painlessly in a removable brace, but no athletic endeavors are permitted until the athlete is completely rehabilitated. This implies range of motion equal to that of the other ankle, inversion/eversion, dorsiflexion, and plantar flexion, without pain or evidence of instability and/or pain with stress and the standing hop test.

The final phase of rehabilitation, regardless of the grade, involves the ankle balance exercise board, various types of which are on the market. These are used to develop proprioception and can also be used to increase power building. As soon as proprioception has returned, in addition to full range of motion without pain, no swelling, tenderness, and strength equal to the opposite uninjured ankle, the athlete is ready to return to unlimited athletic activity (204).

Rarely is an open surgical procedure indicated, and only if there is a positive drawer sign is a cast, usually removable, used; then only for 3 or 4 weeks, following which the aforementioned rehabilitation procedures are instituted.

If the ankle is grossly dislocated, some physicians will repair the ligaments directly, but most simply immobilize the ankle for 3–5 weeks, followed by splintage and gradual controlled development of range of motion, strength, endurance, and so on.

Occasionally, usually when an ankle has been inappropriately rehabilitated, there may be persistent instability for as long as 1 or 2 years after the injury. If this proves to be the case, even under anesthesia, a direct repair of the ligaments with reefing and/or reconstruction is indicated.

If the athlete has to undergo either open repair and/or reconstruction of the lateral ligaments of the ankle, the recovery period is prolonged, usually taking between 6 and 12 months, but the athlete is normally able to return to lifting at the same level as before the injury. Most reconstructive ankle surgeons now start early motion after repair and/or reconstruction; however, full weight bearing, even with protection, usually takes several weeks. The repair and/or reconstruction must be protected from unusual inversion or eversion for at least 6 or 8 weeks, and most require 3 months before the ligaments may be stressed significantly. In the meantime, rehabilitation includes not only regaining flexibility, strength, and endurance, but also maintaining cardiovascular fitness and preventing as much disuse atrophy of the musculature as possible.

Chronic, persistent synovitis following an ankle sprain is frequently caused by thickened tissue within the ankle joint (205) and sometimes can be treated conservatively, but if a diagnostic injection gives only temporary relief, arthroscopic debridement will usually be required to produce full recovery.

Unfortunately, if the injury involves osteocartilaginous damage of the joint, especially a part of the weight-bearing area such as the talar dome, which has been reported to be fractured during weight training (206), the outlook is worse. Even though these injuries can often be cared for arthroscopically, the long-term results, after 2–3 years, show decreased range of motion and increased arthrosis, which probably inhibit the athlete from continuing his or her lifting career.

Occasionally, the superficial peroneal nerve may be injured with an ankle sprain (201). This is one of the causes of persistent pain following ankle sprain, in spite of a stable ankle with all other signs of recovery positive. By increasing the length of the nerve by as little as 6–8%, one can produce a temporary insult to the extent that the nerve no longer functions correctly. In inversion injury to the ankle (the most common type), one can stretch the nerve much more than that, with the injury located anywhere from 12 to 20 cm proximal to the tip of the lateral malleolus on the lateral side of the calf. Most of these will recover with the use of ultrasound and such treatments and occasionally injections; only rarely do they need to be decompressed surgically.

There may be some pain over the dorsal aspect of the ankle, since the inferior retinaculum may produce an impingement over the deep peroneal nerve. Although this occurs more frequently in runners, it can occur in any athlete who wears shoes that are too tight across the top. Only infrequently is surgery necessary, with the usual modalities such as ultrasound, massage, antiinflammatories being sufficient to allow healing to occur while the nerve is protected with a doughnut-shaped or U-shaped felt pad.

Acute ruptures of the peroneal sheath and/or peroneal tendon subluxation at the outside or lateral aspect of the ankle also occur. Although these injuries are most common in skiers, they can occur in any athlete who twists the ankle. The injury must be diagnosed and usually surgically repaired acutely; otherwise, reconstruction is indicated. Unfortunately, the results of surgical treatment for chronic recurrent subluxation are inconsistent, and a significant amount of disability and morbidity may occur. If one suspects this diagnosis, indicated by significant pain, tenderness, and swelling over the retinaculum at the front of the ankle, the best treatment is to apply a splint, have the patient be non weight bearing, and have the patient return for reexamination in 2 or 3 days. By this time, the pain and swelling should have subsided so that the patient can actively dorsiflex the foot; this is all that is usually required to dislocate the peroneal tendons to make the diagnosis (201).

The posterior tibial tendon at the medial aspect of the ankle may develop tendinitis, which usually occurs with pain on the medial aspect of the ankle or foot at the talonavicular joint, at which the posterior tibial tendon may rub against the prominent navicular, causing inflammatory tendinitis. In this case the athlete should be non weight bearing and be provided with antiinflammatory medication. Phonophoresis and/or iontophoresis and so on may clear up the problem, but if it persists for several weeks, one may need to decompress the tendon, sometimes arthroscopically, before it ruptures. An acute rupture can occur but is usually preceded by chronic symptoms and more frequently involves an accessory navicular, which may need to be removed if the tendinitis persists. If rupture occurs, the tendon must be repaired to allow the lifter to return to competition, and orthoses must be used, regardless of the treatment required otherwise.

Plantar fasciitis and/or partial rupture of the plantar fascia may also produce pain in the heel or at the longitudinal arch; it is usually related to inappropriate footwear, hyperpronated foot, or a cavus, rigid foot (203). Most of the time these injuries may be treated with the usual physical therapy modalities as well as flexibility exercises, antiinflammatories, and appropriate orthoses. A rupture or strain of the plantar fascia is usually treated conservatively and only very rarely requires any kind of surgical intervention.

The lateral tarsometatarsal joint at the midfoot can also develop problems with a strain and/or sprain of the ligaments or muscles in this area (202). Usually, these injuries can be treated with immobilization for a few days, followed by appropriate orthotic support in a well-constructed shoe and the usual therapy modalities, including NSAIDs. With persistent problems a CT scan may show disruption, particularly the ligaments on the plantar surface. Again, these can usually be treated with antiinflammatory medication, a flexibility program, and appropriate orthoses in the shoe. Surgery is not indicated for minimal subluxation that is not obvious on a routine X-ray. If one suspects a tarsometatarsal problem, a pivot-shift type of test, while doing the flexion–extension maneuver to pronate the foot, exacerbates the pain in the area where the point of maximum tenderness is located. In the acute stage, 3 weeks of immobilization in a walking cast, followed by conservative rehabilitation program, is usually sufficient to avoid a long-term problem.

A problem associated with forefoot pain is sesamoiditis on the sole of the foot just behind the toes. This occurs after vigorous activity and can actually be extremely disabling and difficult to diagnose. There is characteristic tenderness located beneath the involved sesamoid. Pain exacerbated by passive dorsiflexion of the big toe helps to confirm the diagnosis. When the toe is dorsiflexed, the tender area moves distally as the sesamoid moves distally. This can usually be treated with a horseshoe-shaped felt pad, and the first and second toes are buddy-taped to restrict motion, with elevation, antiinflammatory agents, and the usual physical therapy modalities. These injuries usually resolve without surgical intervention but occasionally may develop a fracture of the sesamoid with nonunion or fibrous union with persistent pain, avascular necrosis, or even arthritic changes in the joint. Any of these may require surgical treatment of the sesamoid but should be treated conservatively for several months before any surgery.

Tarsal tunnel syndrome, or compression of the posterior tibial nerve at the level of the ankle just distal to the medial malleolus, can also occur in athletes (201), including lifters (207). Clinically, there is pain at the medial heel, medial arch, or sometimes even radiating down the arch of the foot to the level of the metatarsophalangeal joints. Occasionally, there may be a decrease in touch sensation, and there is usually a positive Tinel's sign at the area of the posterior tibial nerve under the retinaculum. Occasionally, there may be compression of the branch of the nerve that goes through the abductor hallucis longus, producing pain and weakness, without a Tinel's sign, often with normal electrophysiological studies. Most of these will resolve with appropriate footwear, retrofitted with the necessary orthoses, and the usual modalities of therapy, including iontophoresis and/or phonophoresis, acuscope, and NSAIDs. Rarely, entrapment of the medial calcaneal branch and motor branch to the abductor digiti minimi can occur; these are treated similarly but may require surgical intervention, including a total tarsal tunnel release. These also can occur following surgical release or rupture of the plantar fascia, producing traction on the plantar nerves. If surgery is necessary, recovery frequently takes several months.

Occasionally, there can be compression of the plantar interdigital nerves at the level of the metatarsal heads, commonly called a plantar neuroma or Morton's neuroma. These can be diagnosed by finding tenderness between the metatarsal heads rather than at the metatarsophalangeal joints, with increased pain, numbness, and tingling with manual compression of the metatarsal heads. There may be an associated decreased sensation of the interspace between the toes, usually in the 3–4 interspace, although it may occur in others as well. These are treated similarly to the plantar fasciitis and tarsal tunnel syndromes but with different orthoses. Occasionally, surgery is needed for a cure but may require weeks or even months for recovery.

Any suspected dislocation or fracture of the foot should be treated like those in the hand, though anatomic restoration of displaced fractures is not as important as in the hand. The most common fracture is to the proximal phalanx of the fifth toe and, if undisplaced, is treated with simple buddy-taping to the adjacent fourth toe until it is no longer symptomatic. If there is significant angulation or displacement, these can usually be reduced, closed, and then treated similarly.

Another injury that is frequently seen in lifters includes the subungual hematoma when someone drops a weight on the foot. These need to be treated identically to those in the hand, for similar reasons.

Extensor and flexor tendons may be lacerated or avulsed, as in the hand, but do not need to be reconstructed as frequently as in the hand. Only the great toe needs to retain extension for full function, but all toes need to retain some flexion for balance, pushoff, and so on. Any suspected injuries such as these should be referred to a physician who is well versed in their care.

Blackened nails, frequently associated with tender toes with no known injury, are usually the result of ill-fitting shoes, at least inappropriate ones for that particular foot. This implies the necessity of providing the correct shoe, retrofitted if necessary with the appropriate orthoses.

One should not forget the wheelchair athlete or the Paralympic lifter who, while required to ambulate using an unusual method, is still a true athlete. Also, when treating Paralympic athletes, the medical professional must realize that some of our Paralympic athletes actually compete on a level field with our able-bodied lifters, which even further complicates our relationship with the athlete but also enhances our recognition and appreciation of the lifting athlete, each of whom is in a special, instructive situation and must be dealt with accordingly.

Any medical professional who gets the chance to become acquainted with, treat, and help develop a lifting athlete will find it an extremely rewarding, occasionally frustrating, and always educational experience.

REFERENCES

1. Haykowsky MJ, Findlay JN, Ignaszewki AP. Aneurysmal subarachnoid hemorrhage associated with weight-training: three case reports. *Clin J Sports Med* 1996;6(1):52–55.
2. Shea JM. Acute quadriplegia following the use of progressive resistance exercise machinery. *Phys Sports Med* 1986;14(4):120–124.
3. Frankle MA, Eichberg R, Zachariah SB. Anabolic androgenic steroids and a stroke in an athlete: case report. *Arch Phys Med Rehabil* 1988;69(8):632–633.
4. de Virgilio C, Nelson RJ, Milliken J, et al. Ascending aortic dissection in weight lifters with cystic medial degeneration. *Ann Thoracic Surg* 1990;49(4):638–642.
5. Khaira HS, Awad RW, Aluwihare N, et al. External iliac artery stenosis in a young bodybuilder. *Eur J Vasc Endovasc Surg* 1996;11(4):499–501.
6. Appleby M, Fisher M, Martin M. Myocardial infarction, hyperkalaemia and ventricular tachycardia in a young male bodybuilder. *Int J Cardiol* 1994;44(2):171–174.
7. Huie MJ. An acute myocardial infarction occurring in an anabolic steroid user. *Med Sci Sports Exerc* 1994;26(4):408–413.
8. Gaede JT, Montine TJ. Massive pulmonary embolis and anabolic steroid abuse [Letter]. *JAMA* 1992;267(17):2328–2329.
9. Simoneaux SF, Murphy BJ, Tehranzadeh J. Spontaneous pneumothorax in a weightlifter: a case report. *Am J Sports Med* 1990;18(6):647–648.
10. Cohen GS, Braunstein L, Ball DS, et al. Effort thrombosis: effective treatment with a vascular stent after unrelieved venous stasis following a surgical release procedure. *Cardiovasc Intervent Radiol* 1996;19(1):37–39.
11. Schulte KR, Warner JJP. Uncommon causes of shoulder pain in the athlete. *Orthop Clin North Am* 1995;26(3):505–528.
12. Stahl S, Kaufman T. The efficacy of an injection of steroids for medial epicondylitis. *J Bone Joint Surg* 1997;79A(11):1648–1652.
13. AbuRahma AF, Sadler D, Stuart P, et al. Conventional versus thrombolytic therapy in spontaneous (effort) axillary-subclavian vein thrombosis. *Am J Surg* 1991;161:459–465.
14. Donayre CE, White GH, Mehringer SM, Wilson SE. Pathogenesis determines late morbidity of axillo-subclavian vein thrombosis. *Am J Surg* 1986;152:179–184.
15. Aziz S, Straehley CJ, Whelan TJ, Jr. Effort-related axillo-subclavian vein thrombosis: a new theory of pathogenesis and a plea for direct surgical intervention. *Am J Surg* 1986;152:57–61.
16. Elliott G. Upper-extremity deep vein thrombosis. *Lancet* 1997;349:1188–1189.
17. Reeves RK, Laskowski ER, Smith J. Weight training injuries: I. Diagnosing and managing acute conditions. *Phys Sportsmed* 1998;26(2):67–83,96.
18. *National electronic injury surveillance system: 1995 summary on injuries caused by weight lifting and sports.* Washington, DC: U.S. Consumer Products Safety Commission, 1997.
19. Aggrawal ND, Kaur R, Kumar S, Mathur DN. A study of changes in the spine in weightlifters and other athletes. *Br J Sports Med* 1979;13:58–61.
20. Basford JR. Weightlifting, weight training and injuries. *Orthopedics* 1985;8:1051–1056.
21. Faeth K. Weightlifting injuries: an overview. *U.S. Weightlifting Federation Sports Medicine Manual.* Colorado Springs: U.S. Weightlifting Federation, I:1–19.
22. Gill P. The down side of overhead lifting. *Men's Fitness* 1988;4(3):125.
23. Herrick RT, Stone M, Herrick S. Knee injuries of strength-power athletes. *Iron Sport* 1987;1:41–43.
24. Herrick RT, Stone M, Herrick S. Injuries of strength-power athletes with special reference to the knee. *AMAA Newsletter* 1986;1:12–14.
25. Lander J. Weight training injuries and their prevention. *Strength-Power Update* 1986;1:14–15.
26. Martin RK, Yesalis CE, Foster D, Albright JP. Sports injuries at the 1985 Junior Olympics: an epidemiologic analysis. *Am J Sports Med* 1987;15:603–608.
27. Scott C. Is weightlifting dangerous? *International Olympic Lifter* 1977;4:29,31.
28. Sterling JC, Calvo RD, Holden SC. An unusual stress fracture in a multiple-sport athlete. *Med Sci Sports Exerc* 1991;23:298–303.
29. Walter SD, Sutton JR, McIntosh JM, Connolly C. The aetiology of sports injuries: a review of methodologies. *Sports Med* 1985;2:47–58.
30. Reeves RK, Laskowski ER, Smith J. Weight training injuries: 2. Diagnosing and managing chronic conditions. *Phys Sportsmed* 1998;26(3):54–63.
31. Namey TC, Carek JC. Power lifting, weight lifting, and bodybuilding. In Fu FH, Stone DA, eds. *Sports injuries: mechanisms, prevention, treatment.* Baltimore: Williams & Wilkins, 1994:515–529.
32. Jenkins NH, Mintowt WJ. Bilateral fracture: separations of the distal radial epiphyses during weight-lifting. *Br J Sports Med* 1986;20:72–73.
33. Bassett FH, Nunley JA. Compression of the musculocutaneous nerve at the elbow. *J Bone Joint Surg* 1982;64A:1050–1052.
34. Braddom RL, Wolfe C. Musculocutaneous nerve after heavy exercise. *Arch Phys Med Rehabil* 1978;59:290–293.
35. Dangles CJ, Bilos ZJ. Ulnar nerve neuritis in a world champion weightlifter: a case report. *Am J Sports Med* 1980;8:443–445.
36. Kretzler H, Richardson A. Rupture of the pectoralis major muscle. *J Sports Med* 1989;17:453–458.
37. Mazur LJ, Yetman RJ, Risser W. Weight-training injuries: common injuries and preventative methods. *Sports Med* 1993;16(1):57–63.
38. Liu J, Wu JJ, Chang CY, et al. Avulsion of the pectoralis major tendon. *Am J Sports Med* 1992;20(3):366–368.
39. Agins HJ, Chess JL, Hoekstra DV, Teitge RA. Rupture of the distal insertion of the biceps brachii tendon. *Clin Orthop* 1988;234:34–38.
40. Caldwell GL Jr, Safran MR. Elbow problems in the athlete. *Orthop Clin North Am* 1995;26(3):465–485.
41. Herrick RT. Distal biceps tendinitis resulting in distal insertion rupture. *ASSH Correspondence Newsletter* 1992;85:1–3.
42. Visuri T, Lindholm H. Bilateral distal biceps tendon avulsion with use of anabolic steroids. *Med Sci Sports Exerc* 1994;26(8):941–944.
43. Bach BR, Warren RF, Wickiewicz TL. Triceps rupture: a case report and literature review. *Am J Sports Med* 1987;15:285–289.
44. Howard FM. Controversies in nerve entrapment syndromes in the forearm and wrist. *Orthop Clin North Am* 1986;17:375–381.
45. Stannard JP, Bucknell AL. Rupture of the triceps tendon associated with steroid injections. *Am J Sports Med* 1993;21(3):482–485.
46. Cahill BR. Osteolysis of the distal part of the clavicle in male athletes. *J Bone Joint Surg* 1982;64A:1053–1058.
47. Gruel J, Newman PJ. Distal clavicle osteolysis. *Orthopedics* 1987;10:811–812.
48. Rowe LJ, Cardin A. Post-traumatic osteolysis of the clavicle. *Chiropractic Sports Med* 1987;1:2–7.
49. Scavenius M, Iversen BF, Sturup J. Resection of the lateral end of the clavicle following osteolysis, with emphasis on nontraumatic osteolysis of the acromial end of the clavicle in athletes. *Injury* 1987;18:261–263.
50. Busconi BD, Morgan WJ. Acute digital ischemia in a body builder. *Orthopedics* 1998;21(1):85–87.
51. Zernicke RF, Garhammer J, Jobe FW. Human patellar-tendon rupture: a kinetic analysis. *J Bone Joint Surg* 1977;59A:179–183.

52. Munshi NI, Mbubaegbu CE. Simultaneous rupture of the quadriceps tendon with contralateral rupture of the patellar tendon in an otherwise healthy athlete. *Br J Sports Med* 1996;30(2):177–178.
53. Hammer WI. Meniscotibial (coronary) ligament sprain: diagnosis and treatment. *Chiropractic Sports Med* 1988;2:48–50.
54. Jones BV, Ward MW. Myositis ossificans in the biceps femoris muscles causing sciatic nerve palsy: a case report. *J Bone Joint Surg Am* 1980;62B:506–507.
55. Herrick RT. Clay-shoveler's fracture in powerlifting: a case report. *Am J Sports Med* 1981;9:29–30.
56. Kotani PT, Ichikawa N, Wakabayashi W, et al. Studies of spondylolysis found among weightlifters. *Br J Sports Med* 1970;6:4–8.
57. Dangles CJ, Spencer DL. Spondylolysis in competitive weight lifters. *J Sports Med* 1987;15:624–625.
58. Duda M. Elite lifters at risk for spondylolysis. *Phys Sportsmed* 1987;15:57,59.
59. Granhed H, Morelli B. Low back pain among retired wrestlers and heavyweight lifters. *Am J Sports Med* 1988;16(5):530–533.
60. Greene TL, Hensinger RN, Hunter LY. Back pain and vertebral changes simulating Scheuermann's disease. *J Pediatr Orthop* 1985;5:1–7.
61. Keene JS, Drummond DS. Back pain in the athlete: some common considerations. *Compr Ther* 1985;11:7–14.
62. Kramhoft M, Solgaard S. Spontaneous rupture of the extensor pollicis longus tendon after anabolic steroids. *J Hand Surg* 1986;11:87.
63. Kraus DR, Shapiro D. The symptomatic lumbar spine in the athlete. *Clin Sports Med* 1989;8:59–69.
64. Rossi F. Spondylolyis, spondylolisthesis and sports. *J Sports Med Phys Fitness* 1988;18(4):317–340.
65. Rovere GD. Low back pain in athletes. *Phys Sportsmed* 1987;15(1):105–118.
66. Schafer MF. Low back injuries in athletes. *Sports Med Digest* 1986;8:1–4.
67. Wittmer MJ. Low back pain and the weightlifter. *U.S. Weightlifting Federation Sports Medicine Manual.* Colorado Springs: U.S. Weightlifting Federation, I:40–43.
68. Abrahamsson S, Sollerman C, Soderberg T, et al. Lateral elbow pain caused by anconeus compartment syndrome: a case report. *Acta Orthop Scand* 1987;58:589–591.
69. Durr D. Derrick Crass tries to forget the Olympic crash. *St. Louis Post-Dispatch* 1988 July 10:8F–8C.
70. O'Driscoll SW, Bell DF, Morrey BF. Posterolateral rotary instability of the elbow. *J Bone Joint Surg* 1991;73A:440–448.
71. Fitzgerald B, McLatchie GR. Degenerative joint disease in weight-lifters: fact or fiction? *Br J Sports Med* 1980;14:97–101.
72. Kujala UM, Kettunen J, Paananen H. Knee osteoarthritis in former runners, soccer players, weight lifters, and shooters. *Arthr Rheum* 1995;38(4):539–546.
73. Chandler TJ, Wilson GD, Stone MH. The effect of the squat exercise on knee stability. *Med Sci Sports Exerc* 1989;21:299–303.
74. Giacobbe J. The full squat and its effect on knee stability. *Strength Power Update* 1987;2:3.
75. Karpovich PV, Singh M, Tipton CM. Effect of deep knee bends upon knee stability. *Teor Praxe Til Vvuch* 1970;18:112–115.
76. Tipton CM, Matthes RD, Maynard JA, Carey RA. The influence of physical activity on ligaments and tendons. *Med Sci Sports Exerc* 1975;7:165–175.
77. Stone MH. A theoretical model of strength training. In: *Proceedings of Strength-Power Symposium II,* Auburn University, Alabama, 1981.
78. Hatfield FC. The squat: king of all exercises. *Muscle Fitness* 1983;44:58–63.
79. Roy S, Irvin R. *Sports medicine: prevention, evaluation, management, and rehabilitation.* Englewood Cliffs, NJ: Prentice Hall, 1983.
80. Wilson D. The prevention and care of injuries. *Iron Sport* 1988;1(4):42.
81. Hejna WF, Rosenburg A, Buturusis DJ, Krieger A. The prevention of sports injuries in high school students through strength training. *Nat Strength Conditioning Assoc J* 1982;4:28–31.
82. Hama H, Yamamuro T, Takeda T. Experimental studies on connective tissue of the capsular ligament: Influences of aging and sex hormones. *Acta Orthop Scand* 1976;47:473–479.
83. Wahl LM, Blandau RJ, Page RC. Effect of hormones on collagen metabolism and collagenase activity in the pubic symphysis ligament of the guinea pig. *Endocrinology* 1977;100:571–579.
84. Herrick RT, Herrick S. Ruptured triceps in a powerlifter presenting as cubital tunnel syndrome: a case report. *Am J Sports Med* 1987;15:514–516.
85. David HG, Green JT, Grant AJ, et al. Simultaneous bilateral quadriceps rupture: a complication of anabolic steroid abuse. *J Bone Joint Surg Br* 1995;77(1):159–160.
86. Dickerman RD, Schaller F, Prather I, et al. Sudden cardiac death in a twenty-year-old bodybuilder using anabolic steroids. *Cardiology* 1995;86(2):172–173.
87. Whiteside JA. Musculoskeletal overload problems in the immature recreational athlete: II. The upper extremity. *Sports Med Update* 1995;10(1):16–26.
88. Goeser CD, Aikenhead JA. Rib fracture due to benchpressing. *J Manip Physiol Ther* 1990;13(1):26–29.
89. Heggland EJH, Parker RD. Simultaneous bilateral glenoid fracture associated with a glenohumeral subluxation/dislocation in a weightlifter. *Orthopedics* 1997;20:1180–1184.
90. Schweitzer G. Bilateral avulsion fractures of olecranon apophyses. *Arch Orthop Trauma Surg* 1988;107:181–182.
91. Segan DJ, Sladek EC, Gomez J, et al. Weight lifting as a cause of bilateral upper extremity compartment syndrome. *Phys Sportsmed* 1988;16:73–75.
92. Robertsen K, Kristensen O, Vejen L. Manubrium sterni stress fracture: an unusual complication of non-contact sport. *Br J Sports Med* 1996;30(2):176–177.
93. Agre JC, Ash N, Cameron MC. Suprascapular neuropathy after intense progressive resistive exercise: case report. *Arch Phys Med Rehabil* 1987;68(4):236–238.
94. Schultz JS, Leonard JA Jr. Long thoracic neuropathy from athletic activity. *Arch Phys Med Rehabil* 1992;73(1):87–90.
95. Miller SJ, Smith PA. Volar dislocation of the lunate in a weight lifter. *Orthopedics* 1996;19(1):61–63.
96. George DH, Stakiw K, Wright CJ. Fatal accident with weightlifting equipment: implications for safety standards. *Can Med Assoc J* 1989;140(8):925–926.
97. Smoker J. Injuries: 2. *PL USA* 1989;12(6):27.
98. Saunders HD. Evaluation of a musculoskeletal disorder. In: Gould JA, Davies GJ, ed. *Orthopaedic and sports physical therapy.* St. Louis: Mosby, 1985:169–180.
99. Barton B, Cain S, Fix B, et al. Understanding injury in its relationship to strength and flexibility: part I. *NSCA J* 1986;8(1):14–24.
100. Barton B, Cain S, Fix B, et al. Understanding injury in its relationship to strength and flexibility: part II. *NSCA J* 1986;8(2):14–24.
101. Agre JC. Hamstring injuries: proposed aetiological factors, prevention, and treatment. *Sports Med* 1985;2:21–33.
102. Herring SA, Nilson KL. Introduction to overuse injuries. *Clin Sports Med* 1987;6:225–239.
103. O'Neill DB, Micheli LJ. Overuse injuries in the young athlete. *Clin Sports Med* 1988;7:591–610.
104. Relly JP, Nicholas JA. The chronically inflamed bursa. *Clin Sports Med* 1987;6:345–370.
105. Servi JT. Wrist pain from overuse-detecting and relieving intersection syndrome. *Phys Sportsmed* 1997;25(12):41–44.
106. Riley SA. Wrist pain in adult athletes. *Postgrad Med* 1995;98(1):147–148,151–152,154.
107. Lerner FN. Proteolytic enzymes and aloe gel via iontophoresis reduce the pain of chronic and acute athletic injuries. *Pain Management* 1989;2:29–36.
108. O'Donoghue DH. *Treatment of injuries to athletes.* Philadelphia: WB Saunders, 1980.
109. Baker BE. Current concepts in the diagnosis and treatment of musculotendinous injuries. *Med Sci Sports Exerc* 1984;16:323–327.
110. Gould JA, Davies GJ. Orthopaedic and sports rehabilitation concepts. In: Gould JA, Davies GJ, eds. *Orthopaedic and sports physical therapy.* St. Louis: Mosby, 1985.
111. Michna H. Researches on the architecture of tendons into the problem of the so-called doping with anabolic steroids. Paper

presented at 1984 Olympic Scientific Congress, University of Oregon, Eugene, Oregon, July 19–26, 1984.
112. Browne TD, Yost RP, McCarron RF. Lumbar ring apophyseal fracture in an adolescent weight lifter: a case report. *Am J Sports Med* 1990;18(5):533–535.
113. Mundt DJ, Kelsey JL, Golden AL, et al. An epidemiologic study of sports and weightlifting as possible risk factors for herniated lumbar and cervical disks. *Am J Sports Med* 1993;21(6):854–860.
114. Travell JG, Simons DG. Serratus anterior "stitch-in-the-side." In: Travell JG, Simons DG, eds. *Myofascial pain and dysfunction: the trigger point manual.* Baltimore: Williams & Wilkins, 1983:622–630.
115. Travell JG, Simons DG, eds. *Myofascial pain and dysfunction: the trigger point manual.* Baltimore: Williams & Wilkins, 1983: 636–658.
116. Harvey J, Tanner S. Low back pain in young athletes: a practical approach. *Sports Med* 1991;12(6):394–406.
117. Adams MA, Hutton WC. The effect of posture on the lumbar spine. *J Bone Joint Surg* 1985;67A:625–629.
118. Hunter GR, Culpepper M, Cheung T. A comparison of fifth lumbar torque, shear and compression during two techniques of the Olympic snatch. *NASC J* 1985;7:69.
119. Martire JR. The role of nuclear medicine bone scans in evaluating pain in athletic injuries. *Clin Sports Med* 1987;6:713–737.
120. Jackson CP, Klugerman M. How to start a back school. *J Orthop Sports Phys Ther* 1988;10:1–7.
121. The value of negative thermography. *Neurothermography Electromyography* 1984;2(Spring/Summer):1.
122. Santiesteban AJ. Physical agents and musculoskeletal pain. In: Gould JA, Davies GJ, eds. *Orthopaedic and sports physical therapy.* St. Louis: Mosby, 1985:199–211.
123. Hatfield FC. Electrostimulation. *Muscle Fitness* 1988;49:41,194, 196.
124. Stephen RC, Petelenz TJ, Fay MF, Kapel M. *Understanding iontophoresis.* Salt Lake City: IOMED, Inc. 1988;1–15.
125. Zuelzer W. Managing rib pain in athletes. *Phys Sports Med* 1987;15:44.
126. Groskin S. The radiologic evaluation of chest pain in the athlete. *Clin Sports Med* 1987;6:845–871.
127. Amadio PC. Current concepts review: pain dysfunction syndromes. *J Bone Joint Surg* 1988;7OA:944–949.
128. Burton BL, Dobbins B. 1988. Shoulder injuries: the right way to treat them—and prevent them. *Muscle Fitness* 1988;49:88–90,241,244–246,248.
129. Halbach JW, Tank RT. The shoulder. In: Gould JA, Davies GJ, eds. *Orthopaedic and sports physical therapy.* St. Louis: Mosby, 1985:497–517.
130. Refior HJ, Theermann R. Limits to the durability of the long biceps-tendon in sport. *Int J Sports Med* 1988;9:394.
131. Bigliani LU, Levine WN. Subacromial impingement syndrome (current concepts review). *J Bone Joint Surg* 1997;79A:1854–1868.
132. Newberg AH. The radiographic evaluation of shoulder and elbow pain in the athlete. *Clin Sports Med* 1987;6:785–809.
133. Richards DB, Kibler WB. Sports-related shoulder rehabilitation: an overview of concepts. *J Musculoskel Med* 1997;14(8):44–63.
134. Moore TP, Fritts HM, Quick DC, Buss DD. Suprascapular nerve entrapment caused by supraglenoid cyst compression. *J Shoulder Elbow Surg* 1997;6:445–462.
135. Mendoza FX, Nicholas JA, Rubinstein MP. The arthroscopic treatment of subacromial impingement. *Clin Sports Med* 1987; 6:573–579.
136. Werner SN, Levy M, Bernstein R, Morehouse H. Condensing osteitis of the clavicle. *J Bone Joint Surg* 1984;66A:1484–1486.
137. Holder LE, Michael RH. Unexplained shoulder pain in a weight lifter. *Phys Sportsmed* 1988;16:91–92.
138. Lemos MJ. The evaluation and treatment of the injured acromioclavicular joint in athletes. *Am J Sports Med* 1998;26(1): 137–144.
139. Cook FF, Tibone JE. The Mumford procedure in athletes: an objective analysis of function. *Am J Sports Med* 1988;16:97–100.
140. Ellman H. Shoulder arthroscopy: current indications and techniques. *Orthopedics* 1988;11:45–51.
141. Genovese MC. Joint and soft-tissue injection: a useful adjuvant to systemic and local treatment. *Postgrad Med* 1998;103(2): 125–134.
142. Ireland ML, Andrews JR. Shoulder and elbow injuries in the young athlete. *Clin Sports Med* 1988;7:473–494.
143. Menon J, Gramyk K. Suprascapular nerve neuropathy. Paper presented at the American Society for Surgery of the Hand Annual Meeting, San Antonio, TX, 1987.
144. Pagliano JW. Forearm compartment syndrome due to weightlifting. *Sports Med* Digest 1985;7:6.
145. Padua L, LoMonaco M, Padua R, et al. Suprascapular nerve entrapment: neurophysiological localization in six cases. *Acta Orthop Scand* 1996;67(5):482–484.
146. Alon M, Weiss S, Fishel B, Dekal S. Bilateral suprascapular nerve entrapment syndrome due to an anomalous transverse scapular ligament. *Clin Orthop* 1988;234:31–33.
147. Banerjee T, Fadel JN. Suprascapular nerve entrapment: experience with surgical treatment of twenty patients. *South Med J* 1988;81[Suppl 4]:35.
148. Neviaser TJ, Ain BR, Neviaser RJ. Suprascapular nerve denervation secondary to attentuation by a ganglionic cyst. *J Bone Joint Surg* 1986;68A:627–628.
149. Capra SW, Lovejoy S. Entrapment neuropathies of the supraspinatus and infraspinatus branches of the suprascapular nerve. *South Med J* 1988;81[Suppl 4]:56.
150. Moore RA, Tramer MR, Carroll D, et al. Quantitive systematic review of topically applied non-steroidal anti-inflammatory drugs. *BMJ* 1998;316:333–338.
151. Lutz FR, Gieck JH. Thoracic outlet compression syndrome. *Athl Training* 1986;21:302–309.
152. Smith-Behn J, Althar R, Katz W. Primary thrombosis of the axillary/subclavian vein. *South Med J* 1986;79:1176–1178.
153. Roos DB. New concepts of thoracic outlet syndrome that explain etiology, symptoms, diagnosis and treatment. *Vasc Surg* 1979; 13(5):313–321.
154. Richardson RR, Torres H, Analitis S, Downie J. Traumatic thoracic outlet syndrome: a six case report. *J Neurol Orthop Surg* 1983;4:327–337.
155. Wood VE, Twito R, Verska JM. Thoracic outlet syndrome: the results of first rib resection in 100 patients. *Orthop Clin North Am* 1988;19:131–146.
156. Martinelli I, Cattaneo M, Penzeri D, et al. Risk factors for deep venous thrombosis of the upper extremities. *Ann Intern Med* 1997;126(9):707–711.
157. Horwitz BR, DiStefano V. Stress fracture of the humerus in a weight lifter. *Orthopedics* 1995;18(2):185–187.
158. Wallny T, Sagebiel C, Westerman K, et al. Comparative results of bracing and interlocking nailing in the treatment of humeral shaft fractures. *Int Orthop* 1997;21:374–379.
159. Chiu F-Y, Chen C-M, Lin C-FJ, et al. Closed humeral shaft fractures: a prospective evaluation of surgical treatment. *J Trauma* 1997;43(6):947–951.
160. Kaplan H, Kiral A, Kuskucu M, et al. Report of eight cases of humeral fracture following the throwing of hand grenades. *Arch Orthop Trauma Surg* 1998;117:50–52.
161. Margoles MS. Trigger points and chronic pain. *J Neurol Orthop Med Surg* 1988;9:155–157.
162. Cohen MS, Hastings H. Acute elbow dislocation: evaluation and management. *J Am Acad Orthop Surg* 1998;6:15–23.
163. Berg EE, DeHoll D. Radiography of the medial elbow ligaments. *J Shoulder Elbow Surg* 1997;6:528–533.
164. Olsen BS, Sojbjerg JO, Nielsen KK, et al. Posterolateral the basis kinematics. *J Shoulder Elbow Surg* 1998;7:19–29.
165. Inoue G, Kuwahata Y. Surgical repair of traumatic medial disruption of the elbow in competitive athletes. *Br J Sports Med* 1995; 29(2):139–142.
166. Nirschl RP. Soft-tissue injuries about the elbow. *Clin Sports Med* 1986;5:637–652.
167. Guhl JF. Arthroscopy and arthroscopic surgery of the elbow. *Orthopedics* 1985;8:1290–1296.
168. Andrews JR, St. Pierre RK, Carson WG. Arthroscopy of the elbow. *Clin Sports Med* 1986;5:653–662.
169. Spinner RJ, Goldner RD. Snapping of the medial head of the triceps and recurrent dislocation of the ulnar nerve. *J Bone Joint Surg* 1998;80A:239–247.

170. Biemans RGM. The popeye syndrome: brachial artery entrapment as a result of muscular hypertrophy. *Neth J Surg* 1984; 36:103–106.
171. Chen WC, Hsu WY, Wu JJ. Stress fracture of the diaphysis of the ulna. *Int Orthop* 1991;15(3):197–198.
172. Patel MR, Irizarry J, Stricevic M. Stress fracture of the ulnar diaphysis: review of the literature and report of a case. *J Hand Surg* 1986;11A:443–445.
173. Mosher JF. Current concepts in the diagnosis and treatment of hand and wrist injuries in sports. *Med Sci Sports Exerc* 1985; 17:48–55.
174. Werner CO, Rossen I, Thorngren KG. Clinical and neurophysiologic characteristics of the pronator syndrome. *Clin Orthop* 1985;197:231–236.
175. Shin AY, Gillingham BL. Fatigue fractures of the femoral neck in athletes. *J Am Acad Orthop Surg* 1997;5:293–302.
176. Pagliano JW. Suprascapular neuropathy after resistive exercise. *Sports Med* Digest 1988;10:3.
177. Gainor BJ, Jeffries JT. Pronator syndrome associated with a persistent median artery. *J Bone Joint Surg* 1987;69A:303–304.
178. Fusi S, Watson HK, Cuono CB. The carpal boss: a twenty-year review of operative management. *J Hand Surg* 1995;20B:405–408.
179. Osterwalder JJ, Widrig R, Stober R, Gächter A. Diagnostic validity of ultrasound in patients with persistent wrist pain and suspected occult ganglion. *J Hand Surg* 1997;22A:1034–1040.
180. Louis DS, Hankin FM, Greene TL, et al. Central carpal instability-capitate lunate instability pattern: diagnosis by dynamic displacement. *Orthopedics* 1984;7:1693–1696.
181. Green DP. The sore wrist without a fracture. In: Stauffer, Shannon, ed. *Instructional course lecture*. The American Academy of Orthopaedic Surgeons. St. Louis: Mosby, 1985:303–313.
182. Wood MB, Dobyns JH. Sports-related extra-articular wrist syndromes. *Clin Orthop* 1986;202:93–101.
183. Gibson CT, Manke PR. Carpal tunnel syndrome in the adolescent. *J Hand Surg* 1987;12A:279–281.
184. Kato H, Minami A, Hirachi K, Kasashima T. Treatment of flexor sheath ganglions using ultrasound imaging. *J Hand Surg* 1997; 22A:1027–1033.
185. Malone TR, Garrett WE. Muscle strains: histology, cause and treatment. *Surg Rounds Orthop* 1989;3:43–46.
186. Carstensen EJ. Preventing and managing hamstring injuries. *Phys Sportsmed* 1998;26(1):26.
187. Kujala UM, Orava S, Jarvinen M. Hamstring injuries: current trends in treatment and prevention. *Sports Med* 1997;23(6):397–404.
188. Hyde TE, Danbert RJ. Avulsion of the pectineus muscle in weight lifting. *Chiropractic Sports Med* 1987;1:144–149.
189. Pavlov H. Roentgen examination of groin and hip pain in the athlete. *Clin Sports Med* 1987;6:829–843.
190. Kemp S, Batt ME. The "sports hernia": a common cause of groin pain. *Phys Sportsmed* 1998;26(1):36–44.
191. Klinkert P Jr, Porte RJ, de Rooij TPW, de Vries AC. Quadratus femoris tendinitis as a cause of groin pain. *Br J Sports Med* 1997;31:348–350.
192. Holt MA, Keene JS, Graf BK, Helwig DC. Treatment of osteitis pubis in athletes: results of corticosteriod injections. *Am J Sports Med* 1995;23(5):601–606.
193. Saudek CE. The hip. In: Gould JA, Davies GJ, ed. *Orthopaedic and sports physical therapy*. St. Louis: Mosby, 1985:365,402–407.
194. Ferretti A. Epidemiology of jumper's knee. *Sports Med* 1986;3:289–295.
195. Cook JL, Kahn KM, Harcourt PR, et al. A cross sectional study of 100 athletes with jumper's knee managed conservatively and surgically. *Br J Sports Med* 1997;31:332–336.
196. LaPrade RF. The anatomy of the deep infra-patellar bursa of the knee. *Am J Sports Med* 1998;26(1):129–132.
197. Bloom MH. Differentiating between meniscal and patellar pain. *Phys Sportsmed* 1989;17(8):95,96,101–104,108.
198. Ross G, Champman AW, Newberg AR, et al. Magnetic resonance imaging for the evaluation of acute posterolateral complex injuries of the knee. *Am J Sports Med* 1997;25(4):444–448.
199. Dumitru D, Windsor RE. Subsartorial entrapment of the saphenous nerve of a competitive female bodybuilder. *Phys Sportsmed* 1989;17:116–125.
200. Yessis M. Sports massage and the knee. *Muscle Fitness* 1988; 49:27,182.
201. Adelaar RS, Baxter DE, Herrick RT, et al. Symposium: acute soft tissue injuries below the knee in athletes. *Contemp Orthop* 1986;12:69–74,79–84,86,92,93,97,98,101,106,116,118,120,121.
202. Garrick JG, Requa RK. The epidemiology of foot and ankle injuries in sports. *Clin Sports Med* 1988;7:29–36.
203. McPoil TG Jr, Brocato RS. The foot and ankle: biomechanical evaluation and treatment. In: Gould JA, Davies GJ, ed. *Orthopaedic and sports physical therapy*. St Louis: Mosby, 1985: 313–341.
204. Blievernicht J, Weill R. Training the foot and ankle for optimum performance and prevention of injuries. *NSCA J* 1986;3:32,34.
205. Bassewitz HL, Shapiro MS. Persistent pain after ankle sprain: targeting the causes. *Phys Sportsmed* 1997;25(12):58–68.
206. Mannis CI. Transchondral fracture of the dome of the talus sustained during weight training. *Am J Sports Med* 1983;11(5):354–356.
207. Johnson ER, Kirby K, Lieberman JS. Lateral plantar nerve entrapment: foot pain in a power lifter. *Am J Sports Med* 1992; 20(5):619–620.

CHAPTER 54

Wrestling

William M. Heinz

INTRODUCTION

The sport of wrestling dates back to 3000 B.C. It most likely originated in hand-to-hand combat. Wrestling was extremely popular amongst the ancient Greeks and was the supreme contest of the Olympic Games from 776 B.C. Wrestling was not nearly as popular with the ancient Romans, and after the fall of the Roman Empire, wrestling disappeared in Europe until about A.D. 800. Through the Middle Ages, many styles of wrestling developed. Two styles evolved that ultimately came to dominate international wrestling: Greco-Roman wrestling and freestyle wrestling (1).

Greco-Roman wrestling is so-called because it is thought to be the type of wrestling performed by the ancients. In this form of wrestling, only holds above the waist are permitted, and the legs may not be used in any way to obtain a fall. Greco-Roman wrestling has been a part of the modern Olympic Games since 1896 (2).

International freestyle wrestling is a type of wrestling that is seen in Olympic, international, and AAU competitions. Under international rules, any hold, throw, or trip is permitted as long as it does not endanger the life or limb of the wrestlers. International bouts have a single 5-minute period, with the wrestlers starting on their feet. The match is awarded by a touch-fall, with the victor holding both of his or her opponent's shoulders to the mat simultaneously. If a fall does not occur, the bout is decided on points awarded for takedowns, reversals, escapes, and exposure (3,4).

Intercollegiate freestyle (or scholastic) wrestling is the style that is practiced in U.S. colleges and high schools. It is similar to international freestyle wrestling except that points are awarded for near falls and time advantage (riding time) in addition to takedowns, reversals, and escapes. The collegiate bouts consist of three periods of 3, 2, and 2 minutes, with no rest between periods. High school matches also have three periods, each being 2 minutes long (4,5).

International amateur wrestling is under the supervision of the Fédération International de Lutte Amateur (FILA), or International Amateur Wrestling Federation. In the United States, USA Wrestling is the national governing body that oversees amateur wrestling. It is estimated that between 400,000 and 750,000 wrestlers are involved in the sport every year in the United States (6). At the high school level, 227,596 boys and 1,629 girls participated in wrestling during the 1996–1997 season. In boys' sports this places wrestling sixth in number of participants, behind football, basketball, outdoor track and field, baseball, and soccer (7). At the club and college levels, the total number of wrestlers is unknown but is thought to be between 250,000 and 500,000 individuals each year (6). Wrestling is popular with adolescents because of the pairing of participants of nearly equal weight against each other, thus allowing athletes of all sizes to compete.

WRESTLING INJURIES

Numerous studies have investigated the incidence and types of injuries sustained by wrestlers (8–12). Historically, wrestling has always had a high rate of injuries, and this trend continues (13–15). Comparison of the data in these reports is difficult, as the definition of an injury is not consistent amongst the studies and the time spans covered by the studies varies widely, from two isolated tournaments (9), each spanning 2.5 days, to an ongoing study of collegiate wrestlers that was started in 1982 (16). In addition, several studies evaluated only injuries that occurred in competition, while others grouped injuries sustained in competition with those seen in practice. However, some individual studies are

---

W. M. Heinz: Orthopaedic Associates of Portland, Portland, Maine 04102.

helpful in delineating the injury rate and injury patterns seen in wrestling. Beachy and colleagues conducted an 8-year, prospective, longitudinal study of athletic injuries at a private high school (13). They found wrestling to have the second highest injury rate in male athletes, football having the highest. In their study, they defined an injury as "any athletic complaint that required the attention of the athletic trainer, regardless of the time lost from activity." Under this definition, 1.82 injuries per wrestler were reported, with an injury risk of 0.74 (the number of athletes injured divided by the number of athletes participating in the sport). Of these injuries, 73% occurred during practice sessions. They did not report on exposure data (injuries per 1000 exposures), as the data were not available for all the sports that they studied.

In 1982 the National Collegiate Athletic Association (NCAA) developed the Injury Surveillance System (ISS) to study injury trends in intercollegiate athletics. Injury data are currently collected yearly from a representative sample of NCAA member institutions. A reportable injury in the ISS is defined as occurring as a result of participation in an organized intercollegiate practice or game, requiring medical attention by a team athletic trainer or physician, and resulting in restriction of the student-athlete's participation or performance for one or more days beyond the day of injury. In the ISS the injury rate is a ratio of the number of injuries to the number of athlete exposures. This is expressed as injuries per 1000 athlete exposures. Each athlete exposure is defined as one athlete participating in one practice or contest in which he or she is exposed to the possibility of an athletic injury (14). Data are collected on both practices and games. In addition, the severity of injury and body part injured are reported.

A summary of the ISS analyzed through the 1995–1996 season reports an injury rate of 7.2 injuries per 1000 athlete exposures in wrestling practice and an injury rate of 30.6 in wrestling competitions. The combined practice and game injury rate is 9.6 injuries per 1000 athlete exposures. This places wrestling second in overall injury rate, just behind spring football, which had a rate of 9.8. The NCAA also reports that 39% of all wrestling injuries caused restricted or missed participation for 7 or more days and that 6.1% of all wrestling injuries required surgery.

The ISS report reveals that the knee (24%), shoulder (13%), and ankle (9%) were the three most commonly injured body parts, with sprains (31%), strains (18%), and infections (8%) the most common types of injury (16). In a 5-year study of injuries sustained by a single intercollegiate wrestling team, Snook found a high incidence of knee injuries, shoulder injuries, and skin infections (10). Even though he did not present statistics on the frequency of injury, these data are consistent with the injuries reported in the ISS. This same injury pattern was seen in a 3-year study of intercollegiate wrestling injuries presented by Roy (12).

An injury that is unique to wrestling is the auricle hematoma, or "wrestlers ear." This typically occurs after direct trauma to the external ear and produces a sudden, painless swelling of the ear. If left untreated, this can result in a thickened auricle. With repeated injuries, it may lead to the classic disfigurement known as "cauliflower ear" (Fig. 54–1). This condition was recorded in drawings of ancient Greek wrestlers and is still considered a sign of bravado among wrestlers. It was common in the past for wrestlers to line up after a match to have their ears "needled" by the team physician (17). Many wrestlers avoided this treatment because of the pain involved and their belief that it was not ultimately beneficial. Consequently, ear disfigurement was frequently seen in wrestlers (hence the term *earmarked*). Studies into the pathogenesis of cauliflower ear have shown that the bleeding in the auricle must be subperichondrial to have an adverse effect (18). This hematoma then induces new cartilage formation in the auricle, with the perichondrium acting as a tight casement to hold the developing cartilage in place and leading to the auricular disfigurement.

The treatment of auricular hematomas has involved many different approaches. These include simple aspiration, aspiration with application of bandages or collodion-reinforced molded dressings, incision of the hematoma with evacuation of the clot, and a postauricular incision followed by resection of a portion of the cartilage and application of a cotton bolster dressing (17).

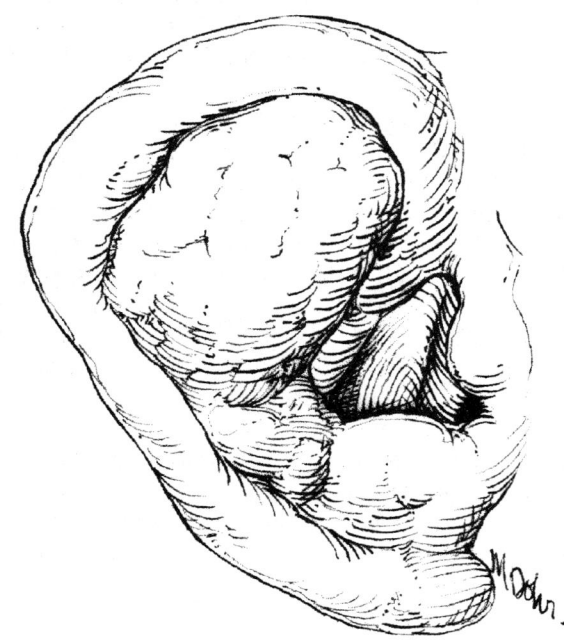

FIG. 54–1. The classic disfigurement known as cauliflower ear.

Griffin advocates opening the wound and complete excision of the newly formed fibroneocartilaginous layer along with the attached perichondrium (19). Mattress sutures are then tied over cotton bolsters to secure the skin in position. He describes excellent results with this method of treatment, which allows the wrestler to resume competition the day after surgery.

Since the late 1960s the NCAA has required wrestlers to wear a protective ear guard during competition. Ear protection is also required at the high school and international levels. The use of protective headgear in practices and competition has lead to a dramatic reduction in the number of auricular hematomas.

The third most common type of injury reported in wrestling is skin infection (16). This accounts for 8–22% of the time loss injuries seen in wrestling at the NCAA level. Examples of common wrestling skin infections include herpes gladiatorum (herpes simplex), tinea corporis gladiatorum (tinea corporis), and impetigo. It is hypothesized that skin infections are spread primarily through skin-to-skin contact and not through infected fomites such as mat surfaces or headgear (20–22). Abrasions or breaks in the skin integrity are thought to allow a pathway of infection among susceptible hosts (21). The use of a protective skin barrier (such as Kenshield Skin Protection) may be helpful in decreasing the skin-to-skin transmission of tinea corporis (23). In addition, intermittent doses of oral itraconazole have been shown to decrease the acquisition and transmission of dermatophytosis in competitive wrestlers (24).

The high rate of infection in wrestling has prompted the NCAA to recommend that "qualified personnel, including a knowledgeable, experienced physician examine the skin over the entire body and hair of the scalp and pubic area of all wrestlers before any participation" (5). On the basis of this examination, any open wounds or infectious skin conditions that are noted that could not be adequately protected should cause the medical disqualification of the wrestler for practice or competition. A similar but not as extensive skin evaluation is required at the high school level.

Among sanctioned competitive sports, wrestling is considered to have one of the highest risks for incidence of neck injuries (25). The NCAA wrestling ISS for 1995–1996 reports an injury rate of 0.43 neck injuries per 1000 athlete exposures (26), placing neck injuries seventh in the rank of most commonly injured body parts. Very rarely do these injuries result in paralysis or a fatality. The rules of wrestling help to prevent these injuries by citing the acts of spearing and slamming as dangerous and therefore illegal maneuvers. Compression-hyperextension injuries to the neck can occur with bridging while attempting to block a fall or pin (Fig. 54-2). These injuries may result in facet sprains, degenerative disc changes, transient brachial plexopathy ("burners"), and/or permanent neurologic loss. The cumulative ef-

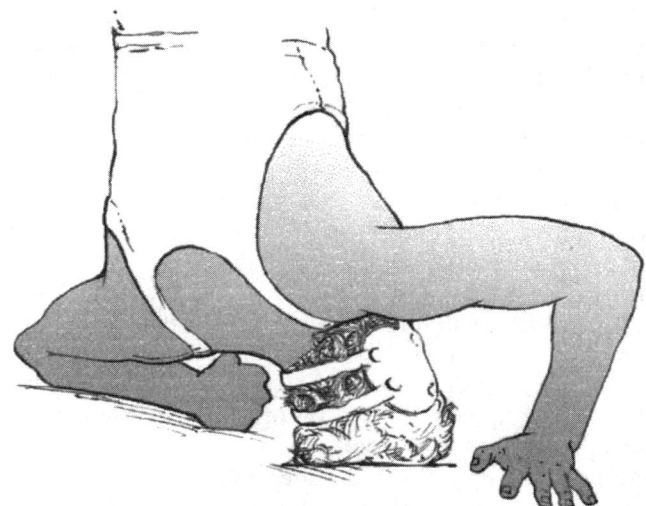

FIG. 54–2. Compression-hyperextension injuries to the neck with bridging while attempting to block a fall or pin.

fects of these injuries are believed to contribute to the degenerative changes that are often seen in the cervical spine of wrestlers long after they retire from the sport (25). A neck exercise program that emphasizes strength and flexibility may be important in decreasing the frequency of neck injuries; however, no studies to date have validated this theory.

WEIGHT LOSS IN WRESTLERS

In the fall of 1997, three collegiate wrestlers collapsed and died after performing workouts that were intended to help them make weight for an upcoming wrestling match. These fatalities were the first deaths reported in wrestling since it became a NCAA sport in 1928 (27) and the first deaths associated with intentional rapid weight loss in interscholastic or collegiate wrestling since national record keeping began in 1982 (28). In all three cases blood chemistries at the time of autopsy showed clear evidence of dehydration. Rapid weight reduction in wrestlers has long been a topic of concern (29–32). Typically, this weight loss is achieved through a variety of potentially harmful methods, including the use of rubber sweat suits, saunas, steam rooms, hot boxes, diuretics, laxatives, self-induced vomiting, spitting, fasting, and severe restriction of food and fluids (33–42). Many national organizations and governing bodies, including the NCAA, the American College of Sports Medicine (ACSM), the American Medical Association, and the National Federation of State High School Associations, have recognized the health risks of this behavior. They have all responded with recommendations and position stands that prohibit or strongly discourage the use of these weight loss practices (14,33,34,43). In spite of the dire consequences, these weight loss methods still persist in the sport of wrestling. It is estimated that 25–95% of wrestlers attempt to cut weight by fasting, food/fluid restriction, and exercising beyond practice (40,41). A smaller but very concerning number of wrestlers use diuretics, laxatives, and/or self-induced vomiting as a weight loss method. Oppliger and colleagues reported that diuretics are used once a month or more by 3–5% of high school wrestlers (44). Stiene found that 16% of high school wrestlers admitted to the use of diuretics at least once a week (41). He noted a significantly higher use of diuretics in high school wrestlers than in college wrestlers (16% versus 5%). This difference was thought to be due in part to the banning of diuretic use by the NCAA, with violations resulting in suspension from competition.

Over the past three decades there has been little change in the prevalence or procedure of weight cycling by high school and college wrestlers (31,33). On a weekly basis, individual wrestlers lose and regain 1.4–9.1 kg (4.0–12% of body weight) in an attempt to make weight (31). This practice may be repeated 15 times in a competitive season and over 100 times in a wrestling career (45). The effects that this weight cycling has on performance or its long-term health risks are not clear. There seems to be a progressive decrease in muscle glycogen levels with repeated weight cycling through the season (45), but it remains unknown whether this actually affects wrestling performance. Adolescent wrestlers have been found to have inadequate energy and protein intake throughout the wrestling season, with resultant diminished protein nutritional status (46). However, despite the changes, these wrestlers were not classified as malnourished, and not all the indices of protein nutritional status, including albumin, were found to have decreased. Housh and colleagues examined the anthropometric growth patterns of high school wrestlers who participated in repeated bouts of weight cycling (47). They found that this behavior does not adversely affect normal anthropometric growth patterns. It has been speculated that weight cycling may reduce resting metabolic rate (RMR), leading to increased fat accretion during subsequent weight gains and contribute to possible long-term obesity or increased risks for coronary heart disease (45). Although studies have shown transient reduction in RMR during weight cycling (48,49), RMR returned to the preseason rate when the weight was regained (49). No longitudinal studies have been done on wrestlers beyond their competitive careers that show that wrestlers are at increased risk for obesity or related health risk factors later in life.

Many wrestlers and coaches believe that dropping weight to compete in a lower weight class will provide an erogenic aid and improve their success in competition. They may also lose weight on a rapid basis to fill voids or weaknesses in their teams' lineups. There has been much investigation into the effects these weight loss practices have on a wrestlers physical performance but little investigation on how these practices affect success on the wrestling mat. Anaerobic performance seems to be the most relevant type of performance to the wrestler. The predominant energy systems used in wrestling are the ATP-PC energy system (which supports static and dynamic strength, peak torque, and anaerobic power) and the intermediate energy system involving anaerobic glycolysis (which contributes to anaerobic capacity and the amount of work performed during continuous or intermittent maximum contractions that last 30–180 seconds) (45,50). It appears that short-term, high-intensity performance (involving the ATP-PC energy system) is unaffected by rapid weight loss (i.e., dehydration) (32,51–53). This is thought to be related in part to the relatively unaffected muscle concentrations of ATP and PC after rapid weight loss (51). The effect of weight loss on performance that relies on anaerobic glycolysis is mixed, depending on the length of time the athlete is tested. A sustained 30-second maximum effort, the typical measure of anaerobic capacity, is not affected by rapid weight loss (53,54). However, performances involving a longer time duration (1–6 minutes), including both sustained and intermittent exercise, are diminished after weight cutting (55–60). This performance after rapid weight loss in wrestlers seems to be influenced by the carbohydrate content of the weight loss diet. If 70% or more of the energy in the weight loss diet is supplied by carbohydrate, anaerobic performance can be maintained, even when the wrestler is fed a hypoenergy diet (55,60,61). The mechanism of this effect is unclear. Short-duration, anaerobic exercise does not typically deplete muscle glycogen stores. However, when exercise is combined with energy restriction over 1–3 days, it is possible that glycogen stores are diminished enough to affect performance (55). It was suggested that changes in the body's acid/base environment that are identified after 3–4 days of a reduced-carbohydrate diet play a role in the reduced anaerobic performance (60,62). This was not confirmed by Rankin and colleagues, who found no change in the resting base excess of wrestlers after 3 days of an energy restriction diet in which 60% of the calories were carbohydrate (55).

Performance supported mainly by aerobic metabolism, including running endurance time and power output at peak oxygen uptake, appears to be adversely affected by rapid weight loss (45). Current studies suggest that anaerobic power and muscular endurance are more important for success in wrestling than are a high maximum oxygen uptake or aerobic endurance (63–66). Wrestlers do not lose weight on an acute basis in an attempt to increase their aerobic endurance. It is their hope that by dropping weight, they will have an increase in strength and power relative to their weight class, thus providing an erogenic aid and increasing their chances for success. Unfortunately, very little scientific investigation has been conducted that either proves or disproves this theory. In a study of high school wrestlers, Parks and colleagues found no difference between the win-loss records of wrestlers who competed in a dehydrated and catabolic state and those of wrestlers who competed in a euhydrated state (67). It should be pointed out that high school wrestling rules allow only 0.5–2 hours from the weigh-in until the start of competition (68). Weigh-in for collegiate matches is now held no more than 2 hours before the start of competition. Before 1998, NCAA wrestlers were allowed 20 hours or more between weigh-in and the start of competition (27). Scott and colleagues found that collegiate wrestlers gained significant amounts of weight (3.7 kg average) during that time period (69). Only one study has actually investigated the success of wrestlers after this cycle of rapid weight loss and rapid weight gain before competition. In it, Horswill and colleagues found that neither the acute weight gain after weigh-in nor the weight discrepancy between opponents influenced success in the first round of a collegiate wrestling tournament (70). With this limited number of studies, no conclusion can be drawn as to the influence that rapid weight loss and subsequent weight gain has on success in wrestling.

A possible adverse effect that rapid weight loss has on wrestlers is a change in their mood states. When the profile of mood states (POMS) is assessed before and after weight loss, the desirable iceberg profile that is normally recognized in elite wrestlers (71) changes after weight loss to a pattern that is commonly seen with overtraining and when athletes become stale (60,72). What effect the rapid weight gain has on restoring the POMS scores to baseline is unknown, nor is it clear whether this change in mood states plays a role in the wrestlers' ultimate success or failure.

The ACSM position stand on weight loss in wrestlers contains a recommendation that the body composition of each wrestler be assessed before the start of the wrestling season (33). From this an appropriate minimal wrestling weight can be determined. The guidelines require medical clearance for males 16 years of age and younger with body fat below 7% or those over 16 years of age with body fat below 5%. Female wrestlers need minimal body fat of 12–14%. Also emphasized in the position stand are guidelines for minimal daily caloric and protein intake. In 1989 the Wisconsin Interscholastic Athletic Association began developing a Wrestling Minimum Weight Program (WMWP) (44,73). This statewide program was put into place and has been fully enforced since the 1991–1992 wrestling season. It includes a minimal weight limit determined by percentage of body fat and a nutrition education program. Oppliger and colleagues reported that after the WMWP was instituted, unhealthy weight loss practices were significantly reduced among Wisconsin high school wrestlers (44). In addition, there was high acceptance and positive response about the WMWP among wrestlers, coaches, administrators, teachers, and parents. This was the first statewide effort to curb excessive weight cutting among high school wrestlers. Many other state associations and governing bodies in wrestling have started to develop minimal weight policies and implement rule changes with regard to weight cutting. A rule change by the NCAA in early 1998 prohibits the use of hot rooms (>79°F), hot boxes, saunas, steam rooms, vapor-impermeable suits, laxatives, emetics, self-induced vomiting, and excessive food and fluid restriction by wrestlers attempting to cut weight (27). It is hoped that with these changes and with the further education of wrestlers and coaches as to safe weight loss methods, the endemic, often extreme, and potentially fatal weight-cutting practices that have long been familiar to wrestlers will be eliminated from the sport.

REFERENCES

1. Wrestling. *Britannica CD,* Version 97. Encyclopaedia Britannica, 1997.
2. Greco-Roman wrestling. *Britannica CD,* Version 97. Encyclopaedia Britannica, 1997.
3. Freestyle wrestling. *Britannica CD,* Version 97. Encyclopaedia Britannica, 1997.
4. Wrestling. *Encarta 96 Encyclopedia.* Redmond, WA: Microsoft, 1993–1995.
5. Benson M, ed.1998 NCAA *Wrestling rules and interpretations.* Overland Park, KS: National Collegiate Athletic Association, 1997.
6. Gary Abbott, director of communication, USA Wrestling. Personal communication, 1998.
7. High school wrestling participation climbs again. *Wrestling USA* 1998;March:45.
8. Strauss RH, Lanese RR. Injuries among wrestlers in school and college tournaments. *JAMA* 1982;248:2016–2019.
9. Lorish TR, Rizzo TD, Ilstrup DM, Scott SG. Injuries in adolescent and preadolescent boys at two large wrestling tournaments. *Am J Sports Med* 1992;20:199–202.
10. Snook GA. Injuries in intercollegiate wrestling: a 5-year study. *Am J Sports Med* 1982;10:142–144.
11. Estwanik JJ, Bergfeld J, Canty T. Report of injuries sustained during the United States Olympic wrestling trials. *Am J Sports Med* 1978;6:335–341.
12. Roy SP. Intercollegiate wrestling injuries. *Phys Sportsmed* 1979; 7:83–94.
13. Beachy G, Akau CK, Martinson M, Olderr TF. High school sports injuries: a longitudinal study at Punahou School: 1988 to 1996. *Am J Sports Med* 1997;25:675–681.
14. *1997–98 NCAA Sports Medicine Handbook,* 9th ed. Overland Park, KS: National Collegiate Athletic Association, 1997.
15. Garrick JG, Requa RK. Injuries in high school sports. *Pediatrics* 1978;61:465–469.
16. *NCAA Injury Surveillance System, 1996–1997 wrestling.* Overland Park, KS: National Collegiate Athletic Association, 1997.
17. Griffin CS. Wrestler's ear: pathophysiology and treatment. *Ann Plast Surg* 1992;28:131–139.
18. Ohlsen L, Skoog T, Sohn S. Pathogenesis of cauliflower ear: an experimental study in rabbits. *Scand J Plast Reconstr Surg* 1975; 9:34–39.
19. Griffin, CS. The wrestler's ear (acute auricular hematoma). *Arch Otolaryngol Head Neck Surg* 1985;111:161–164.
20. Belongia EA, Goodman JL, Holland EJ, et al. An outbreak of herpes gladiatorum at a high-school wrestling camp. *N Engl J Med* 1991;325:906–910.

21. Becker TM. Herpes gladiatorum: a growing problem in sports medicine. *Cutis* 1992;50(8):150–152.
22. Beller M, Gessner BD. An outbreak of tinea corporis gladiatorum on a high school wrestling team. *J Am Acad Dermatol* 1994; 31:197–201.
23. Wroble R, Hand J. Unpublished data.
24. Hazen PG, Weil ML. Itraconazole in the prevention and management of dermatophytosis in competitive wrestlers. *J Am Acad Dermatol* 1997;36:481–482.
25. Wroble RR, Albright JP. Neck and low back injuries in wrestling. *Clin Sports Med* 1986;5(2):295–325.
26. Randall W. Dick, assistant director of sports sciences, National Collegiate Athletic Association. Personal communication.
27. National Collegiate Athletic Association. Immediate wrestling rules changes on weight [Memorandum]. Overland Park, KS: National Collegiate Athletic Association, Jan 13, 1998.
28. Hyperthermia and dehydration-related deaths associated with intentional rapid weight loss in three collegiate wrestlers: North Carolina, Wisconsin, and Michigan, November–December 1997. *MMWR* 1998;47:105–108.
29. Kenny HE. The problem of making weight for wrestling meets. *J Health Phys Ed* 1930;1:24.
30. Doshner N. The effect of rapid weight loss upon the performance of wrestlers and boxers and upon the physical proficiency of college students. *Res Q* 1944;15:317–324.
31. Steen SN, Brownell KD. Patterns of weight loss and regain in wrestlers: has the tradition changed? *Med Sci Sports Exerc* 1990;22:726–768.
32. Tuttle WW. The effects of weight loss by dehydration and withholding food on the physiologic response of wrestlers. *Res Q* 1943;14:158–166.
33. American College of Sports Medicine. Position stand on weight loss in wrestlers. *Med Sci Sports Exerc* 1996;28:ix–xii.
34. American Medical Association, Committee on the Medical Aspects of Sports. Wrestling and weight control. *JAMA* 1967; 201:541–543.
35. Brownell KD, Steen SN, Wilmore J. Weight regulation practices in athletes: analysis of metabolic and health effects. *Med Sci Sports Exerc* 1987;19:546–556.
36. Hursh LM. Food and water restriction in the wrestler. *JAMA* 1979;241:915–916.
37. Ribisl PM. Rapid weight reduction in wrestling. *J Sports Med* 1975;3:55–57.
38. Smith NJ. Weight control in the athlete. *Clin Sports Med* 1984; 3:693–704.
39. Tipton CM, Tcheng TK. Iowa wrestling study: weight loss in high school students. *JAMA* 1970;214:1269–1274.
40. Woods ER, Wilson CD, Masland RP. Weight control methods in high school wrestlers. *J Adolesc Health Care* 1988;9:394–397.
41. Stiene HA. A comparison of weight-loss methods in high school and collegiate wrestlers. *Clin J Sport Med* 1993;3:95–100.
42. Kiningham R, Gorenflo D. Weight loss methods of high school wrestlers [Research abstract]. *Clin J Sport Med* 1997;7:320.
43. NCAA News Release. Overland Park, KS: National Collegiate Athletic Association, Jan 13, 1998.
44. Oppliger RA, Landry GL, Foster SW, Lambrecht AC. Wisconsin minimum weight program reduces weight-cutting practices of high school wrestlers. *Clin J Sport Med* 1998;8:26–31.
45. Horswill CA. Weight loss and weight cycling in amateur wrestlers: implications for performance and resting metabolic rate. *Int J Sport Nutrit* 1993;3:245–260.
46. Horswill CA, Park SH, Roemmich JN. Changes in the protein nutritional status of adolescent wrestlers. *Med Sci Sports Exerc* 1990;22:599–604.
47. Housh TJ, Johnson GO, Stout J, Housh DJ. Anthropometric growth patterns of high school wrestlers. *Med Sci Sports Exerc* 1993;25:1141–1150.
48. Steen SN, Oppliger RA, Brownell KD. Metabolic effects of repeated weight loss and regain in adolescent wrestlers. *JAMA* 1988;260:47–50.
49. Melby CL, Schmidt WD, Corrigan D. Resting metabolic rate in weight-cycling collegiate wrestlers compared with physically active, noncycling control subjects. *Am J Clin Nutr* 1990;52: 409–414.
50. Fox EL. *Sports physiology*, 2nd ed. Philadelphia: CBS College, 1984.
51. Houston ME, Marin DA, Green HJ, Thomson JA. The effect of rapid weight loss on physiological function in wrestlers. *Phys Sportsmed* 1981;9(11):73–78.
52. Greiwe JS, Staffey KS, Melrose DR, et al. Effects of dehydration on isometric muscular strength and endurance. *Med Sci Sports Exerc* 1998;30:284–288.
53. Jacobs I. The effect of thermal dehydration on performance on the Wingate Anaerobic Test. *Int J Sports Med* 1980;1:21–24.
54. Park SH, Roemmich JN, Horswill CA. A season of wrestling and weight loss by adolescent wrestlers: effect on anaerobic arm power. *J Appl Sport Sci Res* 1990;4:1–4.
55. Rankin JW, Ocel JV, Craft LL. Effect of weight loss and refeeding diet composition on anaerobic performance in wrestlers. *Med Sci Sports Exerc* 1996;28:1292–1299.
56. Webster S, Rutt R, Weltman A. Physiological effects of a weight loss regimen practiced by college wrestlers. *Med Sci Sports Exerc* 1990;22:229–234.
57. Smith SA, Williams JH, Ward CW, Davy KP. Dehydration effects on repeated bouts of short-term, high-intensity exercise on college wrestlers. *Med Sci Sports Exerc* 1991;23:S67.
58. Moore BJ, King DS, Kesl L, et al. Effect of rapid dehydration and rehydration on work capacity and muscle metabolism during intense exercise in wrestlers. *Med Sci Sports Exerc* 1992;24:S95.
59. Hickner RC, Horswill CA, Welker J, et al. Test development for study of physical performance in wrestlers following weight loss. *Int J Sports Med* 1991;12:557–562.
60. Horswill CA, Hickner RC, Scott JR, et al. Weight loss, dietary carbohydrate modifications and high intensity, physical performance. *Med Sci Sports Exerc* 1990;22:470–476.
61. McMurray RG, Proctor CR, Wilson WL. Effect of caloric deficit and dietary manipulation on aerobic and anaerobic exercise. *Int J Sports Med* 1991;12:167–172.
62. Greenhaff PL, Gleeson M, Maughan RJ. Diet-induced acidosis and performance of high intensity exercise in man. *J Appl Physiol* 1988;57:580–590.
63. Horswill CA, Scott JR, and Galea P. Comparison of maximum aerobic power, maximum anaerobic power, and skinfold thickness of elite and nonelite junior wrestlers. *Int J Sports Med* 1989; 10:165–168.
64. Cisar CJ, Johnson GO, Fry AC, et al. Preseason body composition, build, and strength as predictors of high school wrestling success. *J Appl Sport Sci Res* 1987;1:66–70.
65. Nagle FJ, Morgan WP, Hellickson RO, et al. Spotting success traits in Olympic Contenders. *Phys Sportsmed* 1975;3(12):31–34.
66. Stine G, Ratliff R, Shierman G, Grana WA. Physical profile of the wrestlers at the 1977 NCAA Championships. *Phys Sportsmed* 1979;7(11):98–105.
67. Parks L, Lampe K, Stiene HA. The Missouri state high school wrestling study [Abstract]. *Clin J Sport Med* 1997;7:320.
68. McGinness FL, ed. *1997–1998 high school wrestling rules*. Kansas City, MO: National Federation of High School Associations, 1997.
69. Scott JR, Horswill CA, Dick RW. Acute weight gain in collegiate wrestlers following a tournament weigh-in. *Med Sci Sports Exerc* 1994;26:1181–1185.
70. Horswill CA, Scott JR, Dick RW, Hayes J. Influence of rapid weight gain after the weigh-in on success in collegiate wrestlers. *Med Sci Sports Exerc* 1994;26:1290–1294.
71. Morgan WP. Test of champions: the iceberg profile. *Psychol Today* 1980;July:92–108.
72. Morgan WP, Costill DL, Flynn MG, et al. Mood disturbance following increased training in swimmers. *Med Sci Sports Exerc* 1988;20:408–414.
73. Oppliger RA, Harms RD, Hermann DE, et al. The Wisconsin wrestling minimum weight project: a model for weight control among high school wrestlers. *Med Sci Sports Exerc* 1995;27:1220–1224.

PART VII

Management of Injuries

CHAPTER 55

Principle-Centered Rehabilitation

P. Gunnar Brolinson and Gary Gray

The magic is not in the medicine, but in the patient's body . . . in the vis medicatrix naturae, the recuperative or self-corrective energy of nature, what the treatment does is to stimulate natural functions or to remove what hinders them.

Miracles, C. S. Lewis, 1940

INTRODUCTION

Human behavior is locomotion. Traditionally, medical training has emphasized the viscera, which conveys the impression that human behavior is a composite of visceral functions. As clinicians interested in sports medicine rehabilitation, we understand that the ultimate instrument of human action and behavior is the neuromusculoskeletal system. Most of the efferent output from and sensory input to the central nervous system is from the musculoskeletal system.

The neuromusculoskeletal system continually challenges our body's homeostatic mechanisms. Indeed, the total economy of the body is constantly tuned to the high and variable requirements of the neuromusculoskeletal system. These concepts are especially important in the rehabilitation of the injured athlete. We recognize that because of what we choose to do and how we choose to do it, the human framework is vulnerable to the compressive forces of gravity, which may be amplified in the performance of sport. As a species, we are truly "gravitationally challenged."

We recognize that the most important symptom of disturbed motor function is pain. Pain is present as a signal to reduce movement in the injured tissue so as to prevent structural damage. As sports medicine clinicians interested in structural evaluation, diagnosis, treatment, and rehabilitation, we must learn to identify dysfunctional patterns and seek to guide our patients in neuromusculoskeletal behavioral patterns that are less costly biomechanically and more favorable to health and efficient function.

THE PRINCIPLE-CENTERED APPROACH

Principles are natural laws that are, for the most part, intuitively obvious. We hope that by introducing you to principles rather than practices and describing the principles behind some of the practices, we will better prepare you to handle the current challenges of sports medicine rehabilitation as well as the unknown challenges of the future. We hope to be able to prepare you to handle each patient and the situations that are unique to each patient. This approach will tend to orient you away from a particular treatment protocol or algorithmic approach to the rehabilitative process and will provide you with a philosophic approach that we hope will allow your patients to have outstanding functional outcomes.

Inherent in this process is the understanding of the concept of treatment thinking versus preventive thinking. As sports medicine clinicians, we want to avoid falling into the trap of treating symptoms. Instead we want to produce an evaluation and programming process that prevents the injury from recurring.

We hope to identify the root cause of the injury and to orient the rehabilitative process to attack the root cause, rather than simply treating the symptom of the injury. This process can be thought of as the Functional Analysis Rehabilitative Method. In other words, our rehabilitative method is guided by our comprehensive functional analysis and understanding of the pathomechanics of sports injury. We must deal with the natural laws that govern successful (or unsuccessful) function of the neuromusculoskeletal system in the performance of sport in our gravitationally challenged environment.

P. G. Brolinson: Sports Care, Toledo, Ohio 43615.
G. Gray: Gary Gray and Associates, Adrian, Michigan 49221.

If we violate these natural laws with impunity, dysfunction and/or injury will occur. However, for peak performance, athletes must often function at the threshold of (and sometimes beyond) these natural laws. The more physiologically aligned our athletes are with these basic principles, the less the opportunity there will be for injury and the greater the chance for success.

Albert Einstein once said, "The significant problems we face cannot be solved by the same level of thinking that created them." In a rehabilitative sense, the problems that our patients face in function cannot be solved at the same level of function that created them. We must be able to transform our patients to a new level of function to successfully reintegrate them into sports-related activities and prevent reinjury.

THE FUNCTIONAL EVALUATION

To treat dysfunction, we must first understand function. We often recognize athletes by their walking or running gait, golf swing, pitching motion, forehand tennis stroke, or other particular sport-related movements. Every individual acquires highly characteristic motor patterns during growth and development. As sports medicine clinicians, we sometimes identify "functional pathology," recognizing that characteristic motor patterns have been altered under the influence of injury, fatigue, and/or abnormal compensations. Joints are not only mechanical organs but also sensory organs, providing proprioceptive feedback to the central nervous system and, in cases of dysfunction, also nociceptive information. The processing of this altered information by the central nervous system may ultimately alter motor patterns and produce injury or dysfunction. Therefore injury may result from inappropriate or excessive demand being placed on a gravitationally, biomechanically, and/or metabolically challenged locomotor system.

Somatic dysfunction frequently develops in the human neuromusculoskeletal system in the course of adapting to the relentless force of gravity. The athlete's ability to adapt is additionally challenged by the particular demands of his or her sport. Somatic dysfunction is defined as impaired or altered function of related components of the somatic (body framework) system: skeletal, arthrodial, and myofascial structures and related vascular, lymphatic, and neural elements. We recognize the importance of somatovisceral and visceral-somatic reflexes and understand the neuromusculoskeletal system in that it not only influences but also reflects the quality of function and/or pathology of other organs and systems.

We must concentrate on developing a comprehensive yet basic philosophic approach to the injured athlete. As we noted above, to treat dysfunction, we must first understand function. Because of the needs and requirements of developing full-spectrum functional neuromuscular rehabilitative environments, we must develop the ability to be accurate in reproducing a functional profile of the injured segments as well as the relationship of these segments to the whole. Practical and consistent functional testing tools allow for the ability to measure and assess components of function. Measurement tools that provide objective data assist us in designing as well as progressing the therapeutic environment. These specific pieces of evidence that constitute the components of function help us to determine where functional success ends and failure begins. A functional profile fulfills the need to objectively measure function, communicate function, and therefore direct rehabilitative conditioning efforts while documenting efficacy and improvement.

The most important feature of any testing protocol is safety. Adherence to specific protocols helps to reduce the possibility of harm or danger to the athlete who is being tested. We therefore test at subthreshold levels of function and demonstrate success before threshold levels are evaluated. The clinician logically and safely progresses the individual patient through the appropriate spectrum of tests. Functional testing may include, but not be limited to, such things as balance tests, balance reach tests, excursion tests, lunge tests, step tests, and hop tests. The ultimate goal of functional testing is to determine the threshold boundaries of successful function and not to introduce failure or potential harm. Functional tests should be governed by a set of standardized rules that allow for the appropriate quantification of specific functional activities. Testing assists the examiner in designing and implementing specific rehabilitative exercises, depending on the needs of each individual. Tests should be designed to complement each other as well as to provide a comprehensive profile of the threshold function. Tests can be plane dominant, joint dominant, and/or activity dominant and can be used to complement other appropriate orthopedic, neurologic, and radiographic tests as well as other indicated diagnostic tests. Meaningful testing leads to meaningful intervention and allows for the opportunity to provide appropriate and specific functional, rehabilitative, and conditioning environments. Documentation should be clear and concise, using clear and consistent terminology to describe functional movements and positions.

Comprehensive descriptions of various approaches to functional profiling are beyond the scope of this chapter. However, in general, we must remember the following rules and guidelines:

1. Make it safe.
2. Test for a reason.
3. Make meaningful measurements.
4. Test subthreshold before testing threshold.
5. Give consistent and appropriate verbal and visual cues.

6. Modify and vary functional tests as appropriate.
7. Compare side to side, part to part, and time to time.
8. Create an appropriate testing environment as well as standard protocols, including the use of reference vectors to allow clinicians to adequately communicate with each other as well as injured patients.
9. Remember to make it simple and fun!

To give you an example of the type of testing we are talking about, we will use balance testing. Some simple tools are necessary to perform the testing. These include tape, a goniometer, incremental steps, a yardstick or meterstick, a stopwatch, measuring tape, and a functional knowledge of the kinetic chain (Fig. 55–1). Balance tests measure the time an individual can maintain balance on one leg. An unlimited number of timed balance tests are available, as balance time is challenged by various head, arm, trunk, and leg positions and motions. Visual feedback can be varied, and any number of positions and motions can be combined to challenge balance time.

Balance reach tests measure the distance an individual can reach with arms or the opposite leg to challenge the ability to balance on one leg. Measurements can be made along any of the testing vectors at any specified height to determine what reach distance can be achieved while maintaining balance.

Balance tests are designed to test central balance and peripheral balance along with balance in various positions and with various motions. All planes of balance are tested. Balance reach tests can also challenge balance while measuring reaches to failure, reaches per time, and time per reaches (Figs. 55–2 and 55–3).

THE REHABILITATIVE ENVIRONMENT

As we begin to approach the strategy for the design of a functional rehabilitative process for our injured athletes, it is useful to think of the locomotor system as a kinetic chain. Some things that are part of this chain include, but are not limited to, the joints, muscles, bones, and proprioceptors that help to guide our patients in successful athletic activities. We must therefore begin to appreciate that there is a strange relationship between the cause and the cure of injuries. The ultimate goal of rehabilitation of an injured athlete is to return the injured individual back safely to the activity that directly contributed to the injury. In general, athletes enjoy having the opportunity to return, in a successful and pain-free manner, to the activity that originally caused their pain.

Therefore a vital component of the functional rehabilitative environment will actually be the causative activity. Therein lies the challenge of rehabilitation: to transform the cause into the cure. This transformation is the rehabilitation. Through rehabilitation we must transform the injured tissue into tissue that successfully deals with the loads and motions of the causative activity. We must reintegrate the injured tissue into a more effective and efficient functional chain reaction system.

For this transformation and reintegration to occur and be successful, a logical progression of clinically controlled techniques that are symptom and performance directed must be accomplished. Intelligent management of these techniques requires and is based on a strong biomechanical understanding of the kinetic chain and the pathophysiology of injury.

Central to the understanding of kinetic chain muscle function in the locomotor system is understanding the concept of an oxymoron: a unique combination of two incongruent qualities that are juxtaposed to form a more meaningful concept. To wit, the integrated use of opposite words provides an understanding synergistically that is greater than the combined understanding of each word used in an isolated manner. "Functional oxymo-

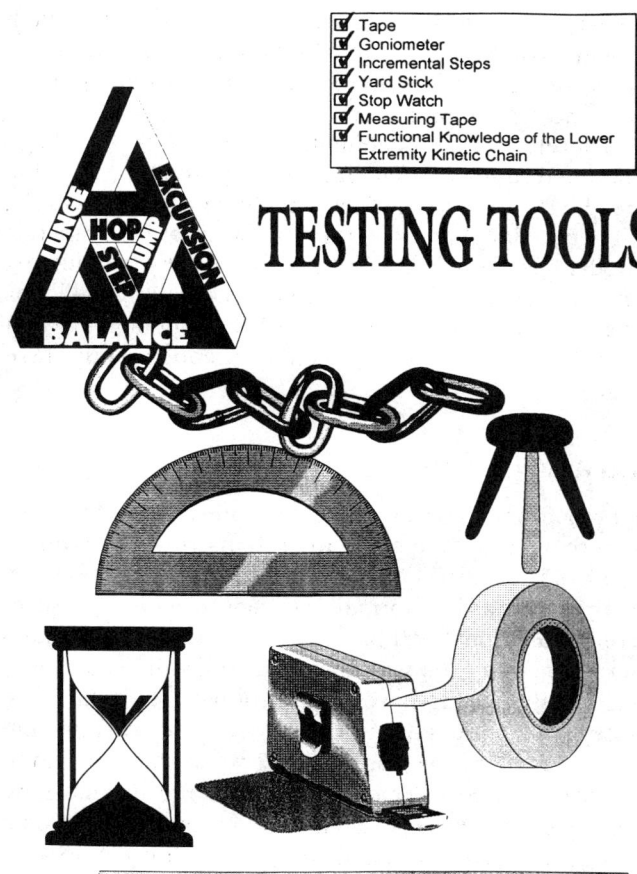

FIG. 55–1. Tools necessary to perform balance testing. (Reprinted from Gray GW, *Chain Reaction Festival, 1996. Lower Extremity Functional Profile, 1995.* Adrian, Mich.: Wynn Marketing, Inc., in cooperation with Gary Gray and Associates Physical Therapy Clinic, Inc.)

BALANCE TESTS

Measurement: Time Balanced

Unilateral Stance Balance With:
➤ Eye/s open/closed
➤ Head Position/Motion
➤ Arm/s Position/Motion
➤ Trunk Position/Motion
➤ Balance Leg Position/Motion
➤ Opposite Leg Position/Motion
➤ Any Combination of Above

BALANCE REACH TESTS

Measurement: Distance Reached

Unilateral Stance Balance Reaching With:
➤ Bilateral Arms
➤ Ipsilateral Arm
➤ Contralateral Arm
➤ Opposite Leg

Arm Reach Directions

All 8 Reference Vectors
(If Arm Reach Not On Vector Indicate Reach Height-Also Indicate Counter Balance Status)

Opposite Leg Reach Directions

➤ All 8 Reference Vectors
  (Except Lateral)
➤ Medial Rotation
➤ Posterior/Medial Rotation

Other Measurements:

➤ Reaches to Failure
➤ Reaches/Time
➤ Time/Reaches

FIG. 55-2. Balance tests. (Reprinted from Gray GW, *Chain Reaction Festival*, 1996. *Lower Extremity Functional Profile*, 1995. Adrian, Mich.: Wynn Marketing, Inc., in cooperation with Gary Gray and Associates Physical Therapy Clinic, Inc.)

rons" provide us with the necessary foundation to design and manage biomechanically reactive rehabilitative environments (e.g., "causative cure").

The isolation of a soft tissue in an integrated system begins to describe the concept of "integrated isolation" (another functional oxymoron). Initially, one must isolate the involved tissue to fully understand the site of injury, the extent of injury, and the effect of injury. Concurrently, one must appreciate the actual function of the involved tissue and how its integration into the function compensation system allowed for the excessive mechanical loading of the tissue and the resultant injury.

To determine the integrated isolated function of this tissue in the kinetic chain, what this tissue does in real life must be practically comprehended. To what forces does the tissue react? What joints and motions does the tissue decelerate, stabilize, and accelerate? In what planes and with what other tissues does it function? How does the tissue dynamically integrate its isolated function? These are all questions that must be answered to appreciate the causes and compensations resulting in tissue failure in order to design the appropriate functional environment for rehabilitation, transform the injured tissue into healthy tissue, and then reintegrate it into the functional system.

Therefore the rehabilitative strategy is to design the environment to facilitate the appropriate reaction of the target tissue functionally and progressively, with functional exercises and appropriate therapeutic modalities. This is controlled clinically by modulating the stress and strain of the activity, controlling the joints that dominate the activity, and determining in what plane the action and reaction predominantly take place.

COMPENSATIONS

Compensations occur in the neuromusculoskeletal system that allow us to adapt to both internal and external stressors (Table 55-1). Some compensations can be normal; others are abnormal and can be indicative of or create functional pathology. Part of the difficulty in determining which is which demonstrates the cause-and-effect relationship between functional activity and the resultant compensations. Gravity, ground reaction, and momentum are the primary drivers for functional compensations. Footwear and various orthotic interfaces are examples of extrinsic environments that a functional system can react with and compensate for. Compensations can be caused by interacting with various forms of equipment, therapeutic or otherwise, as well as types of terrain (e.g., playing fields).

Structural malalignment abnormalities are examples of intrinsic causes of compensations. Intuitively, the strength, endurance, and flexibility of the connective

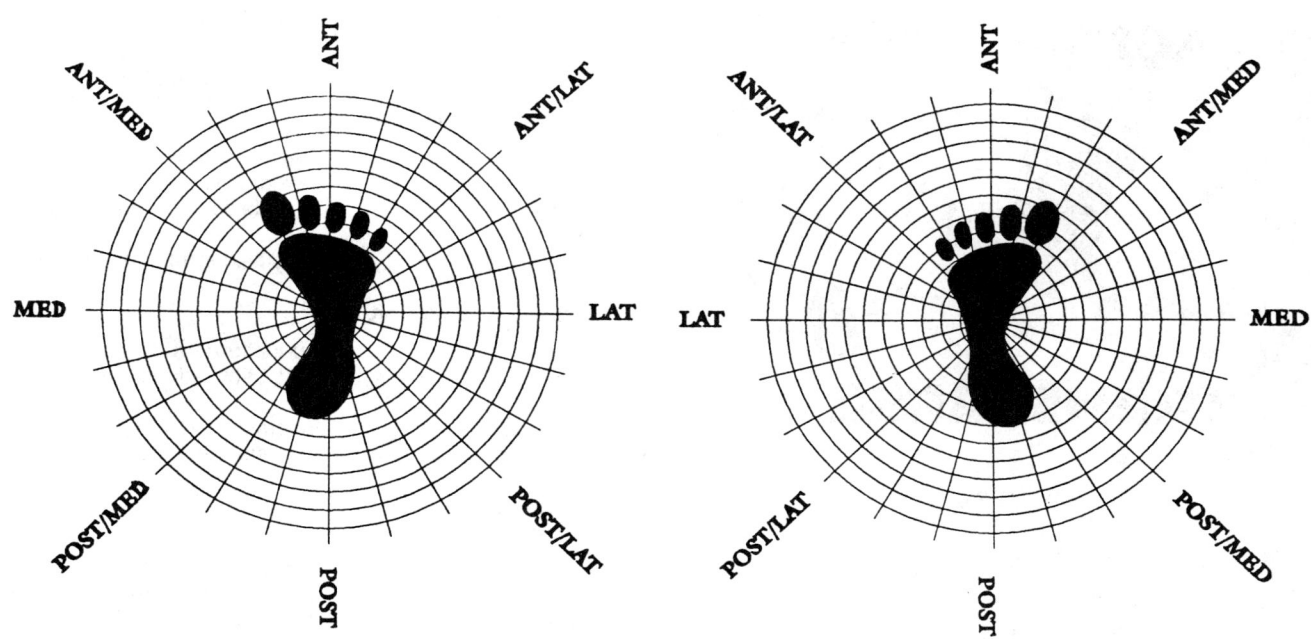

FIG. 55-3. The Lower Extremity Functional Profile uses vectors on the floor to reference the start of a test and the direction of a test. There are eight vectors that are 45° apart. An individual to be tested is oriented on the vectors in reference to the lower extremity that is being tested and in reference to the direction of the test. Please refer to each test for the specific rules of start position and testing direction. (Reprinted from Gray GW, *Chain Reaction Festival, 1996. Lower Extremity Functional Profile, 1995.* Adrian, Mich.: Wynn Marketing, Inc., in cooperation with Gary Gray and Associates Physical Therapy Clinic, Inc.)

tissue have a direct effect on the compensation of the linkage system. Additionally, balance and other neuromuscular considerations, such as proprioceptive ability and muscle tone, have a dramatic effect on function and functional compensation. Determining the actual cause or causes of the compensation and what relationship the compensation has to the contribution of excessive mechanical loads to the involved tissue is the major task of the biomechanical evaluation. Understanding the potential causes and resultant compensation is based on the biomechanics of function and the timing of function. This understanding allows for more effective treatment of the causes of the injury and the resultant compensations, as well as the symptoms (pain).

TABLE 55-1. *Causes of compensation*

Forces	Extrinsic causes	Intrinsic causes
Gravity	Equipment	Structural
Ground reaction	Footwear	Connective tissue
Momentum	Orthotic interface	Neurologic
External	Terrain	Balance

Reprinted from Gray GW, Chain Reaction Festival, 1996. Lower Extremity Profile, 1995. Adrian, Mich.: Wynn Marketing, Inc., in cooperation with Gary Gray and Associates Physical Therapy Clinic, Inc.

PLANES OF MOTION

It is important to remember that all motion at all joints involves the three planes—sagittal, frontal, and transverse—with appropriate neuromuscular control. Generally, each joint will have a dominant plane of motion for a given activity. However, injury can occur in a nondominant plane. A typical example is the knee joint, which is primarily a sagittal plane–dominant joint but is often injured in the transverse or frontal plane. An understanding of these planes of motion allows us to intelligently design rehabilitative environments (Fig. 55-4, Tables 55-2 and 55-3).

REAL-WORLD MUSCLE FUNCTION

Clinicians typically describe muscle function in three ways: concentric, eccentric, and isometric. We think of a concentric muscular contraction as a functional shortening of the muscle while it contracts. Eccentric contraction is a functional lengthening of the muscle while it contracts. Isometric contraction is a stabilizing force during which neither shortening nor lengthening of the muscle occurs.

As we begin to understand the real-world function of muscles and groups of muscles, we begin to understand that muscles may function concentrically at one

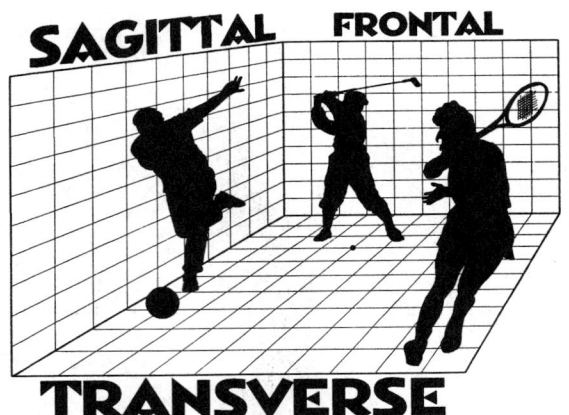

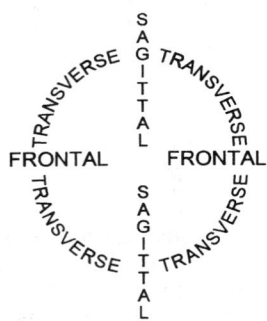

FIG. 55-4. Planes of motion. (Reprinted from Gray GW, *Chain Reaction Festival, 1996. Lower Extremity Functional Profile, 1995.* Adrian, Mich.: Wynn Marketing, Inc., in cooperation with Gary Gray and Associates Physical Therapy Clinic, Inc.)

TABLE 55-2. *Multiplane joint motion*

Joint	Plane		
	Sagittal	Frontal	Transverse
Pronation			
Hip	Flexion	Adduction	Internal rotation
Knee	Flexion	Abduction	Internal rotation
Ankle	Plantar flexion/ dorsiflexion		Adduction/ abduction
STJ		Eversion	Abduction
MTJ	Dorsiflexion	Inversion	Abduction
Supination			
Hip	Extension	Abduction	External rotation
Knee	Extension	Adduction	External rotation
Ankle	Dorsiflexion/ plantar flexion		Abduction/ adduction
STJ		Inversion	Adduction
MTJ	Plantar flexion	Eversion	Adduction

Abbreviations: STJ, subtalar joint; MTJ, midtalar joint
Reprinted from Gray GW, Chain Reaction Festival, 1996. Lower Extremity Profile, 1995. Adrian, Mich.: Wynn Marketing, Inc., in cooperation with Gary Gray and Associates Physical Therapy Clinic, Inc.

TABLE 55-3. *Lower extremity joint motions within the planes*

Joint	Motion
Sagittal Plane Motion	
Hip	Flexion/extension
Knee	Flexion/extension
Ankle	Dorsiflexion/plantar flexion
Subtalar	
Midtarsal	Dorsiflexion/plantar flexion
Frontal Plane Motion	
Hip	Abduction/adduction
Knee	Abduction/adduction
Ankle	
Subtalar	Inversion/eversion
Midtarsal	Inversion/eversion
Transverse Plane Motion	
Hip	Internal rotation/external rotation
Knee	Internal rotation/external rotation
Ankle	Abduction/adduction
Subtalar	Abduction/adduction
Midtarsal	Abduction/adduction

Reprinted from Gray GW, Chain Reaction Festival, 1996. Lower Extremity Profile, 1995. Adrian, Mich.: Wynn Marketing, Inc., in cooperation with Gary Gray and Associates Physical Therapy Clinic, Inc.

joint and eccentrically or isometrically at another joint or in another plane at the same joint at the same time. This occurs within the kinetic chain, reacting with and against gravity, ground reaction, and momentum, in multiple planes of motion. This concept of chain reaction muscle function is best summed up in the term "econcentric." This concept of econcentric muscle function allows clinicians to understand the causes and compensations of both acute and overuse injuries and gives us an enhanced ability to determine the appropriate econcentric reaction of the injured tissue to facilitate healing and enhance function.

To intelligently rehabilitate injuries, we must know not only what the affected tissue is doing during the activity that contributed to its breakdown, but also what it does, when it does, and why it does. As we previously noted, we must also know how the involved tissue is integrated into the entire kinetic chain system.

PRONATION AND SUPINATION

Understanding pronation and supination gives us a head start in our thought process to determine potential causes of dysfunction and the resultant symptoms. Understanding functional chain reaction pronation and supination gives us the ability to begin to determine which dynamic compensations are normal and which are abnormal. This also allows us to understand the integrated isolated function of the involved tissue with the other tissues that synergistically work in the kinetic chain with the symptomatic tissue. This understanding also allows us to begin to take advantage of the concept of econcentric muscle function.

Pronation is a collapsing of the chain, and supination is a regirding of the chain. Pronation is shock absorption; supination is propulsion. Pronation is a reaction caused by the effects of gravity and ground reaction forces. Supination is a reaction resulting from pronation. Pronation succumbs to gravity, whereas supination overcomes gravity. The transformation of pronation into supination is the key to the success of the locomotor system in sport movement. Pronation and supination occur at all joints and in all planes of motion of the locomotor system.

Remember that pronation and supination many times have more to do with the timing of motions at certain joints and in certain planes than with the actual amount of motion of the joint. Pronation is dominated by eccentric (deceleration) muscle function. Supination is dominated by concentric (acceleration) muscle function. Therefore the transformation of pronation into supination is dominated by isometric (stabilizing) and econcentric muscle function: a deceleration of motion at one joint and the acceleration of motion at another joint or in another plane, all at the same time.

THE REHABILITATIVE PROCESS: FUNCTIONAL FEEDING

It is imperative that the rehabilitative environment reflect the strategy of providing a calibrated and progressive stress, functionally controlled motions, and reasonable reactive responses. The strategy must be based on a biomechanical understanding of the neuromuscular system, the demands of sport, and the pathophysiology of injury. The environment must be proprioceptively enriched. The appropriate functional chain reaction depends on the plane dominance of the exercise activity, along with the joint dominance. The injured tissue response needs to be predicted and evaluated with reference to its ability to decelerate, stabilize, and accelerate specific functional motions.

Functional chain reaction rehabilitation must be based on performance while being sensitive to symptoms. All components of the kinetic chain that are able to contribute to the success of the injured tissue must be integrated and progressively rehabilitated as part of this process. This is known as functional feeding. Depending on the symptoms of the trauma, along with the resultant abnormal components of function, the rehabilitative environment may initially emphasize planes of movement that the injured structure does not dominate, at joints where the soft tissue does not have a direct control, to functionally integrate without artificially isolating and stressing the symptomatic tissue. This is the initial and early exercise strategy of a functional rehabilitative process. A nonfunctional approach may try to initially isolate the injured tissue with inappropriate stretching techniques, exercises, and nonphysiologic application of stress in an artificially designed nonfunctional environment. This may inhibit the ability of the involved tissue to heal successfully.

REHABILITATIVE STRATEGY

This functionally feeding chain reaction rehabilitative strategy can be thought of as a "spectrum" rather than "phases" of rehabilitation. Motion, stability, flexibility, and strength are facilitated concurrently and not independently. Comprehensive functional spectrum therapy begins with function and ends with function. Progression within the exercise and therapeutic environment is based on performance and symptoms, not on some artificial timeline (i.e., compass directed, not time directed).

The rehabilitative and evaluative environment are one and the same. The spectrum of reactive environments is designed to enhance healing in the injured tissue by facilitating the appropriate joint and limb kinematics within specific planes of motion at specific joints with appropriate plane and joint dominance.

Some basic rehabilitative and training strategies include creating an environment for healing and improvement that is both fun and safe. As clinicians we must manage that environment and become the most integral part of it. We must remember to make designs functional and progress through a functional spectrum continuum, providing multiple environments and experiences along the way. We must learn to introduce controlled instability and work consciously with our injured patients to reestablish functional pattern movements in a repetitive fashion, ultimately making the conscious subconscious.

Almost counterintuitively, we may initially ask our patients to load eccentrically and move rapidly to take advantage of inherent tissue elasticity and energy storage, then gradually slow the motion down to fully rehabilitate the injured tissue, remembering that it is in the transverse plane that most loading occurs. We must remember to initially orient away from symptoms or dysfunctions while specifically attacking and treating root biomechanical causes, as well as abnormal compensations. We must not forget to involve multiple joints and complimentary planes, isolating the injured tissue in an integrated fashion. When appropriate, we must then begin to react the entire kinetic chain and, as we do so, to provide specific, achievable, and modifiable goals. All the while, we must think proprioceptively and understand the difference between exercising and training, recalling that exercises may not always be functional; however, training is always functional.

We must take advantage of gravity, momentum,

ground reaction force, center of body weight, and muscle movements as complimentary forces. We must constantly seek and test functional balance thresholds and treat muscles as functionally linked structures while understanding and appreciating the differences between normal and abnormal compensations. We must design home exercise programs that are reasonable and home workable, while remembering at all times to be encouraging and uplifting. By "home workable," we mean activities that are safe, fun, goal oriented, and retestable.

Functional stretching is an important component of the rehabilitative environment. In creating a stretching program, we must begin to utilize gravity, body weight, and ground reaction to minimize control but maximize balance while creating the safest, most effective functional stretching techniques. To do this, contract/relax techniques can be used.

We must orient the joints and muscles to be stretched in their position of function at the time when the greatest degree of flexibility is required from the tissue being stretched. We must also remember to orient the body into the most functional position possible, then consider all three planes of motion of the joint or muscle to be stretched. Some type of active warm-up (such as light jogging in place) before the stretching program is also important and may help to facilitate this activity.

SUMMARY: THE SUCCESS IMPERATIVE

Successful rehabilitation depends on the ability to functionally take advantage of just the right amount of motion, at just the right joint, in just the right plane, in just the right direction, at just the right time. A basic principle of functional rehabilitation is always to allow the patient to be successful and to allow this success to ultimately transform into the ultimate goal of returning the athlete to his or her sport. However, we must remember that the athlete's health and safety are our primary concern. Our ability to successfully return athletes to the environment of sport is based on the integrative findings of the comprehensive biomechanical examination and an in-depth understanding of the pathophysiology of injury as well as the loads and motions of the particular sport.

We must be always mindful that the examination, diagnosis, and treatment of the injured athletic injuries is a dialogue between two human beings, including physical, physiological, and psychological linkages. This is a complex transaction that, when skillfully performed, can have a profound and long-lasting effect. The clinician who is interested in neuromusculoskeletal medicine quite literally has at his or her fingertips an extensive document of the patient's history, including indications of general health and the extent of structural adaptation to the environment, as well as challenges produced in the pursuit of sport.

> Criticize yourself once in a while and see what you may be doing wrong. Never criticize others . . . it only stirs resentment. Speak no ill of anyone and all the good you know of everyone. Do not judge a person too soon . . . God waits until the end.
> Harvey Penick, legendary golf pro

BIBLIOGRAPHY

Buser B, Tortland P. The common compensatory pattern. *VNECOM OP:P;* University of New England, College of Osteopathic Medicine, Department of Osteopathic Principles and Practice, unpublished video presentation, September/May 1990.

Covey SR. *Principle-centered leadership.* New York: Simon and Schuster, 1992.

Covey SR. *First things first.* New York: Simon and Schuster, 1994.

Gray GW. *Chain reaction festival.* Adrian, Mich.: Wynn Marketing, Inc., in cooperation with Gary Gray and Associates Physical Therapy Clinic, 1996.

Gray GW. *Lower extremity functional profile,* Adrian, Mich.: Wynn Marketing, Inc., in cooperation with Gary Gray and Associates Physical Therapy Clinic, 1995.

Korr IM. Osteopathic principles for basic scientists. *J Am Osteopath Assoc* 1987;87(7):513–515.

Korr IM. Principles of osteopathic manipulation: a rationale (part I). *Osteopath Ann* 1984;12:10–26.

Korr IM. Proprioceptors and somatic dysfunction. *J Am Osteopath Assoc* 1975;74(3):638,509.

Korr IM. Somatic dysfunction, osteopathic manipulative treatment, and the nervous system: a few facts, some theories, many questions. *J Am Osteopath Assoc* 1996;86(2):109–114.

Korr IM, Taylor A. Still Memorial Lecture: research and practice a century later. *J Am Osteopath Assoc* 1974;76(1):362–370.

Lewit K. Interpretation of the motor system. *Mich Osteopath J* 1988;53(1):6.

Ward RC et al. *American Ostepathic Association: Foundations for Osteopathic Medicine.* Baltimore: Williams & Wilkins, 1997.

Worth RM. *Discussion: the neurobiologic mechanisms in manipulative therapy.* New York: Plenum Press, 1978:371–373.

CHAPTER 56

Athletic Taping

Brent S. E. Rich and Brent C. Mangus

Athletic taping is used as an injury prevention technique or as an adjunct mechanism to prevent excessive movement related to an injury. This is accomplished by applying the athletic tape in such a manner as to biomechanically prevent the injured body part from being placed in a compromising position. Athletic taping is contraindicated when restricted range of motion might lead to decreased function and cause further injury. In those cases a more rigid form of stabilization may be indicated. Taping is also not recommended over open wounds, over active infection, or in the presence of a skin allergy.

The effectiveness of athletic taping as an injury prevention method has been researched and compared to bracing for prevention of injury, movement capabilities, and other factors (1–3). It has been demonstrated that both athletic taping and bracing have positive effects on the prevention of injury, both allow movement in the necessary planes, and both are effective for athletes recovering from an ankle injury (4,5). Although it has been demonstrated that preventive ankle taping before practice or competition loses a good part of its stabilizing value within the first 10–15 minutes after application, their many coaches, athletic trainers, and athletes remain very committed to this practice (6). Other body parts, such as the wrists or fingers, are also routinely taped, and it is believed that these tapings maintain their functional protection longer. Although some research conclusions will point to one technique being better than another, not enough conclusive work has been completed to make a definite decision as the best method to use in all situations. Cost is a variable in the decision between taping and bracing. Financially, it is more cost-effective to brace than to tape an athlete for an entire season. These decisions are made on an individual and institutional basis.

B. S. E. Rich and B. C. Mangus: Arizona Orthopaedic and Sports Medicine Specialists, Phoenix, Arizona 85044.

There is speculation that athletic taping decreases the muscular strength of the involved area (7). This has never been reliably proven, nor is there significant impairment of normal range of motion. Additionally, it has been suggested that athletes develop a psychological dependence on the external support. This may occur on an individual basis, but the significance of harmful effects is difficult to determine. A rehabilitation program is indicated if weakness or psychological dependence is noted.

The most accepted purpose of athletic taping is to provide assistance to the athlete for the return to activity after a minor injury. When applied appropriately, athletic tape provides stability and support to an injured structure. This added benefit might allow the athlete to return to play before the area has returned to preinjury status. Athletic taping does not preempt an appropriate or comprehensive rehabilitation plan that includes flexibility, strengthening, proprioception, endurance, and sports-specific exercises and, if indicated, pharmacologic therapy. The athlete should not rely on prophylactic taping to prevent further injury.

Preventive taping is a learned process that requires a level of expertise to understand the fundamental concepts that are involved in the placement of tape and how each strip can be most effective in the entire taping procedure. Additionally, a high level of skill needs to be attained to be able to complete a taping procedure so that it is functional and will not cause problems for the athlete. The application of athletic tape is both an art and a science. The science component can be learned through coursework or study. However, the art of preventive taping must be perfected through practice and continued performance of the skill, incorporating competent feedback from a trained professional. In the hands of a qualified athletic trainer, it may look as though taping is an easy skill to acquire or that any attempt at preventive taping would be helpful. This is not the case. Incorrectly applied tape may predispose the athlete to injury or cause severe blisters to form.

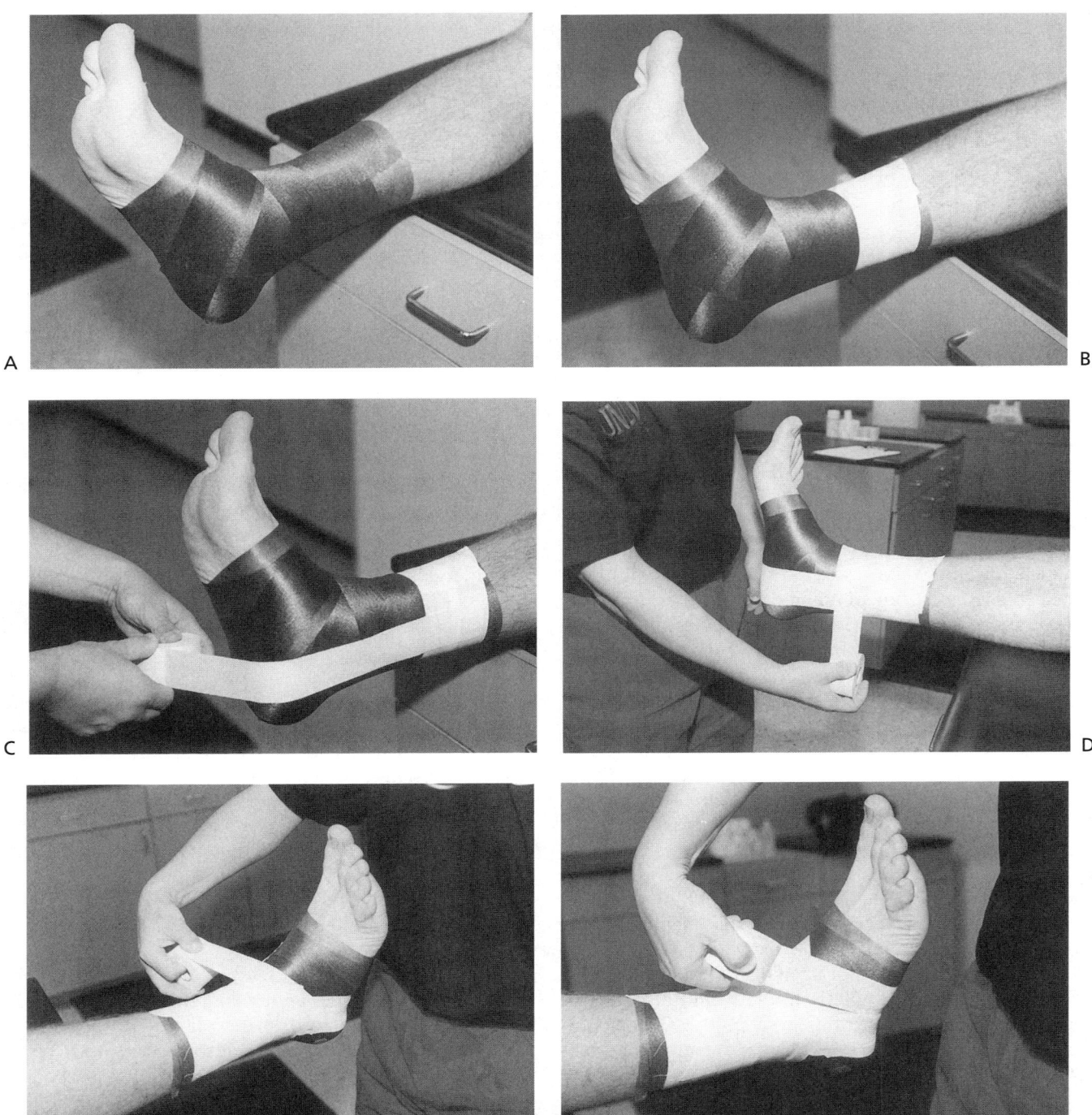

FIG. 56–1. Preventive ankle taping procedure. **A**: Prewrap. **B**: Anchor strips. **C**: Stirrups. **D**: Locking strips. **E**: Figure eight (start). **F**: Figure eight (finish).

Additionally, athletes must not assume that the tape will prevent injury in all situations. Preventive taping of an athlete is not a procedure that should be taken lightly by the coach, athlete, or health care provider.

The general principles of athletic taping are as follows:

1. Place the athlete in an appropriate position that he or she can maintain during the procedure.
2. Select a comfortable table height and position that is appropriate for the health care provider to minimize strain and fatigue.

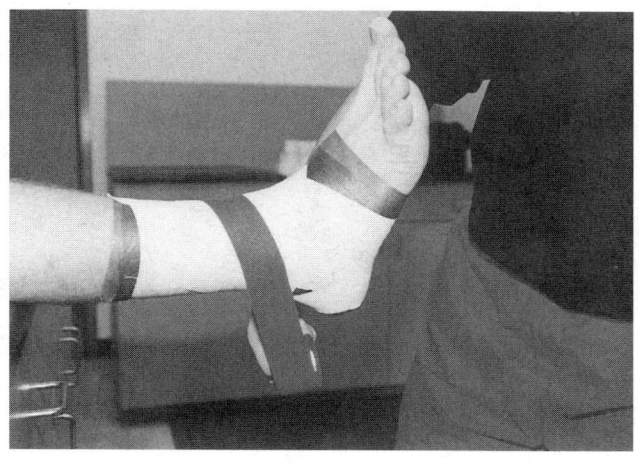
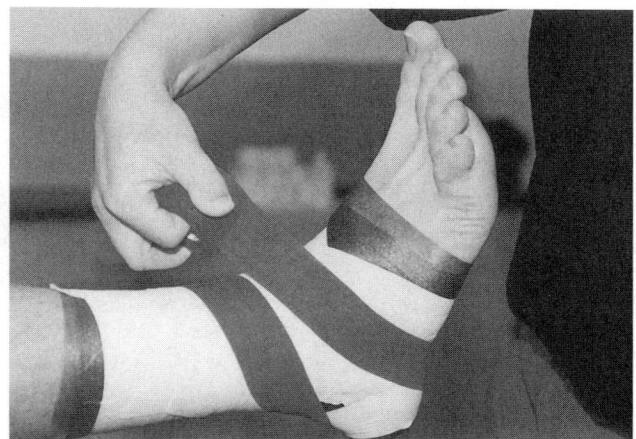
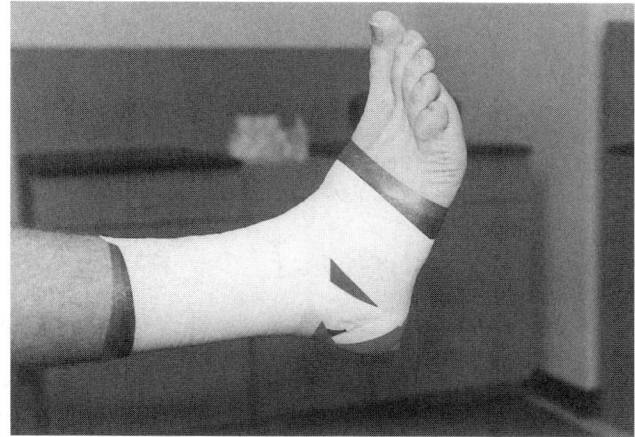
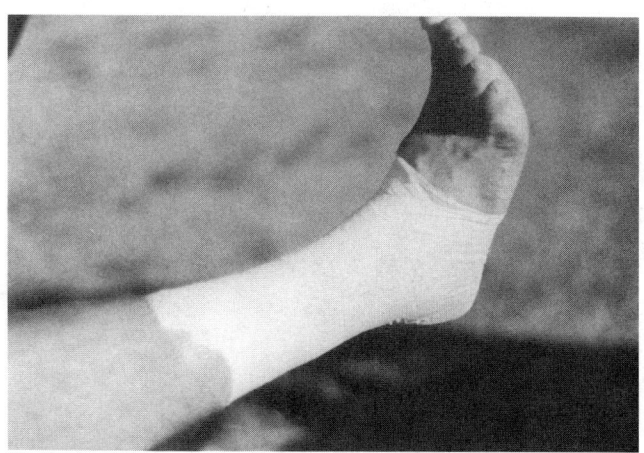

FIG. 56–1. *Continued.* **G**: Heel lock (start). **H**: Heel lock (finish). **I**: Applying closing strips to limit blisters. **J**: Ankle taping completed.

3. Select the appropriate type and width of athletic tape for the area in question.
4. Apply the athletic tape to a dry and clean area that is at body temperature. It is inappropriate to apply tape immediately after cryotherapy or hydrotherapy or if there is perspiration at the site.
5. Apply the athletic tape directly on the skin or on underwrap that has been placed on the skin with tape adherent to prevent slippage.
6. Use protective pads or underwrap on areas that may be subject to friction blisters.
7. Apply the tape in a firm yet smooth, wrinkle-free fashion to prevent skin blister or impair circulation or normal movement of muscles and tendons underneath the tape. Avoid excessive pressure over bony prominences. Monitor for tingling, numbness, decreased tactile sensation, or impairment of distal venous return.
8. Position the body part in a biomechanical fashion to prevent injury, support bony anatomy, and allow appropriate range of motion.
9. Tear or break the tape in an extended or stretched fashion to avoid folded edges.
10. Teach the athlete the appropriate method to remove the tape with tape cutters or specially designed scissors.
11. Clean the skin adequately of tape residue, and tend to any blisters or skin abrasions as indicated.

Specific taping procedures are outlined below.
Following is the preventive ankle taping procedure:

1. Use adherent and prewrap to hold the procedure in place and reduce skin damage (Fig. 56–1A).
2. Anchor strips begin the procedure (Fig. 56–1B).
3. Stirrups are applied from medial to lateral, holding the foot in a neutral position (Fig. 56–1C).
4. Locking strips help to hold the stirrups in place (Fig. 56–1D).
5. Figure eights begin from the lateral side of the foot, traverse medially to go around the ankle, and are finished by completing the figure eight on the anterior

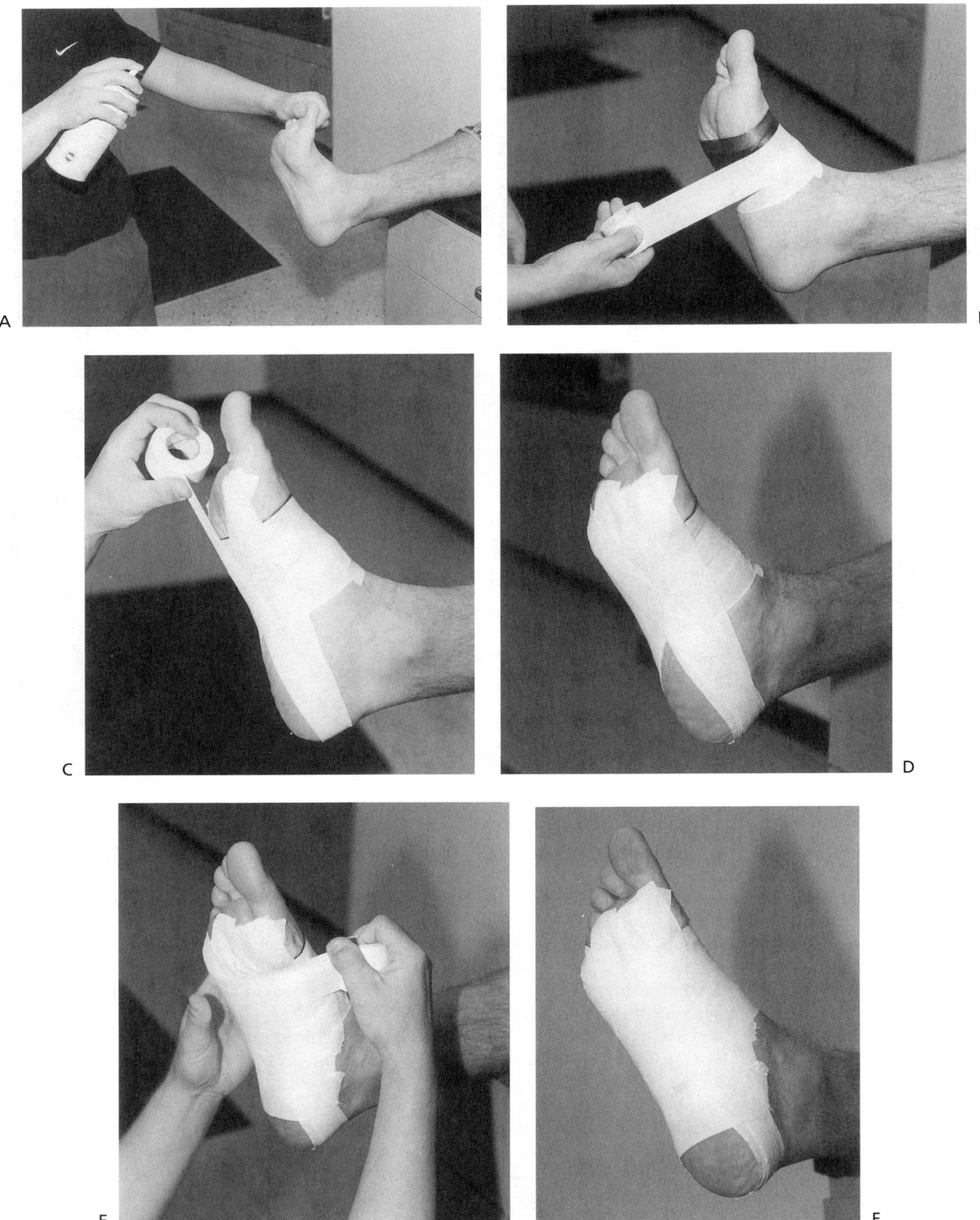

FIG. 56–2. Longitudinal arch taping procedure. **A**: Apply tape adherent. **B**: Anchor strips. **C**: Figure eight (start). **D**: Figure eight (finish). **E**: Finishing strips (plantar surface). **F**: Longitudinal arch taping completed.

ankle. These are used to help control excessive inversion joint movement (Figs. 56–1E and 56–1F).
6. "Heel locks" help to maintain a neutral position of the subtalar joint (Figs. 56–1G and 56–1H).
7. Closing strips act to maintain the integrity of the procedure and eliminate holes or gaps in the tape that might lead to blisters or cuts. Close from the distal to proximal so that the tape will not roll when the athlete puts his or her socks on (Fig. 56–1I).
8. The procedure is completed (Fig. 56–1J).

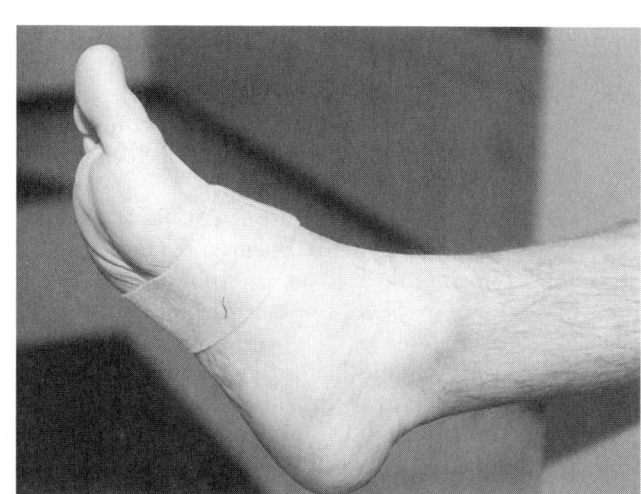
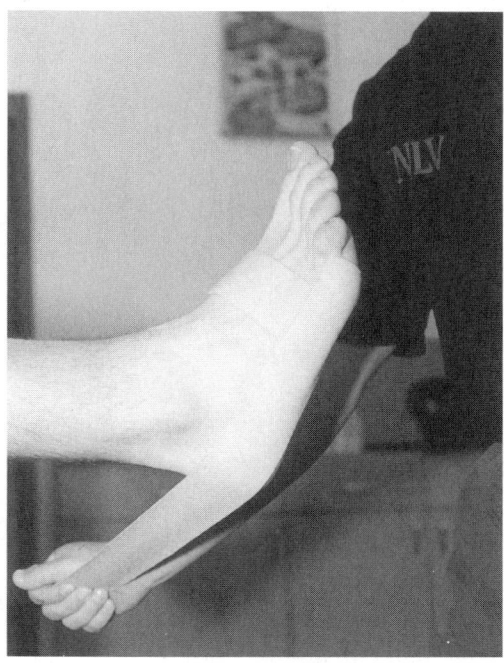
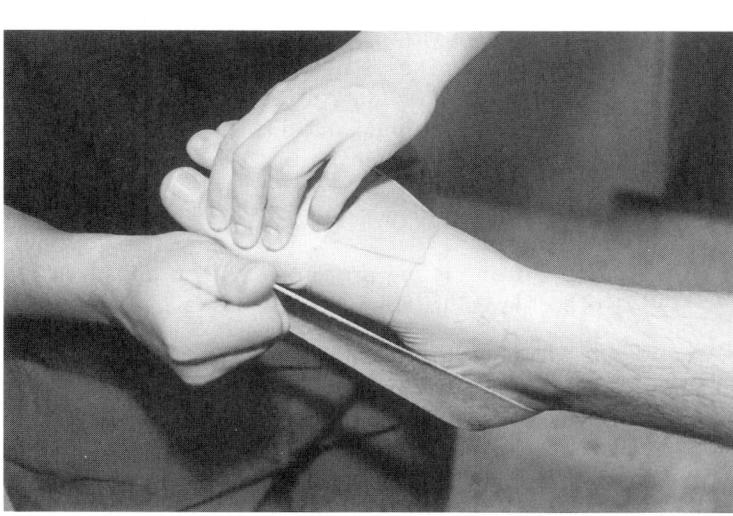
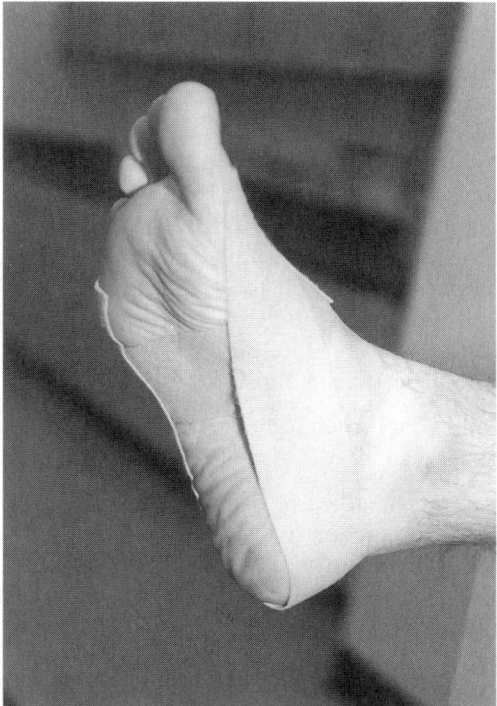

FIG. 56–3. "Low-dye" arch taping procedure. **A**: Apply moleskin (distal metatarsals). **B**: Apply moleskin (laterally). **C**: Apply moleskin (lateral to medial). **D**: Moleskin.

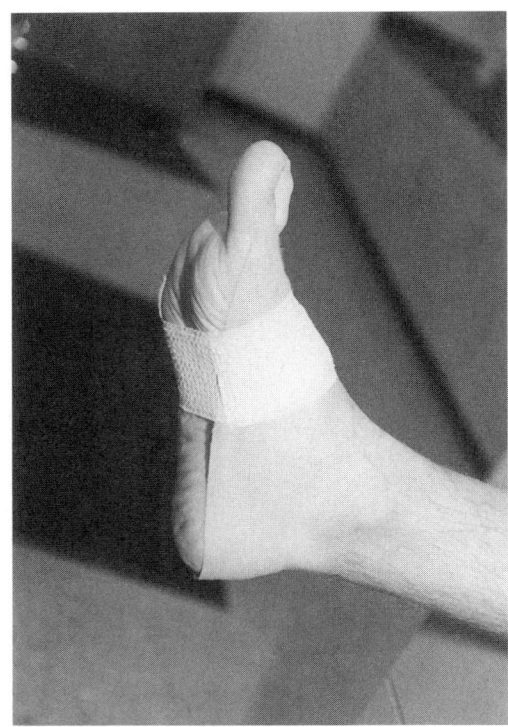

FIG. 56–3. *Continued.* **E**: "Low-dye" arch taping completed.

The longitudinal arch taping procedure is as follows (Fig. 56–2):

1. Tape adherent is applied (Fig. 56–2A).
2. Anchor strips begin the procedure and give the building strips to follow a good base of support (Fig. 56–2B).
3. Figure eight strips are applied to alternating directions starting from medial and moving laterally on the plantar surface of the foot. (Figs. 56–2C and 56–2D).
4. Finishing strips are applied across the plantar surface of the foot (lateral to medial directions of pull) to add support to the figure eight strips applied directly to the foot (Fig. 56–2E).
5. The procedure is finished (Fig. 56–2F).

Following is the modified "low-dye" arch taping procedure (Fig. 56–3):

1. Use spray adhesive to hold the strapping in place.
2. Place an anchor strip of 2-inch moleskin directly on the skin around the distal metatarsals (Fig. 56–3A).
3. Use a second piece of 2-inch moleskin starting from the lateral border of the foot near the fifth digit and pulling around the calcaneous and to the base of the first metatarsal. Note: As you pull the moleskin to the first metatarsal, use the opposite hand to gently push the forefoot into a pronated position (Figs. 56–3B, 56–3C, and 56–3D).
4. Finish by securing the strapping with cover strips (Fig. 56–3E).

The Achilles tendon taping procedure is as follows (Fig. 56–4):

1. Use adherent and prewrap to hold the procedure in place and reduce skin damage (Fig. 56–4A).
2. Begin the procedure with anchor strips just below the point where the triceps surae and the Achilles tendon attach, and wrap around the arch of the foot (Fig. 56–4B).
2a. Use elastic tape, cutting and splitting the end of the tape enough to completely surround the athlete's lower leg. Have the athlete plantar flex the foot (Fig. 56–4C).
2b. Apply the split portion of the elastic tape to the athlete, and stretch the tape as you unroll it so that there is a similar tape-splitting technique near the toes (Fig. 56–4D).
2c. Repeat this procedure if you think that it is necessary to add the extra support (Fig. 56–4E).
3. Finish with a cover of stretch tape, which can be done in a continuous fashion up the lower leg (Fig. 56–4F).
4. If the athlete has an ankle injury also or will feel more secure with the entire ankle taped, have the athlete bring the ankle and foot into a neutral position, and apply preventive ankle taping as outlined above (Fig. 56–4G).

The turf toe taping procedure is as follows (Fig. 56–5):

1. Begin with adhesive spray on the ball of the foot and great toe to provide a better base of support for the procedure (Fig. 56–5A).
2. Start with anchor strips around the arch of the foot.
3. Stability strips are placed from the plantar surface around the medial border and on the dorsal surface (Fig. 56–5B).
4. Reinforcing strips start from the proximal great toe (dorsal and plantar surfaces) and for an "X" over the metatarsalphalangeal (MP) joint of the great toe (Fig. 56–5C).
5. Complete the procedure by finishing with arch strips (Fig. 56–5D).

Following is the preventive thumb and wrist taping procedure (Fig. 56–6):

1. Use adherent and prewrap to hold the procedure in place and reduce skin damage.
1a. Have the athlete place the hand in the thumb-up, fingers-extended position.
2. Apply anchor strips around the wrist (Fig. 56–6A).
3. With a roll of 1-inch tape, begin at the wrist and bring the tape up, circling the thumb and returning to the opposite side of the wrist (Fig. 56–6B).

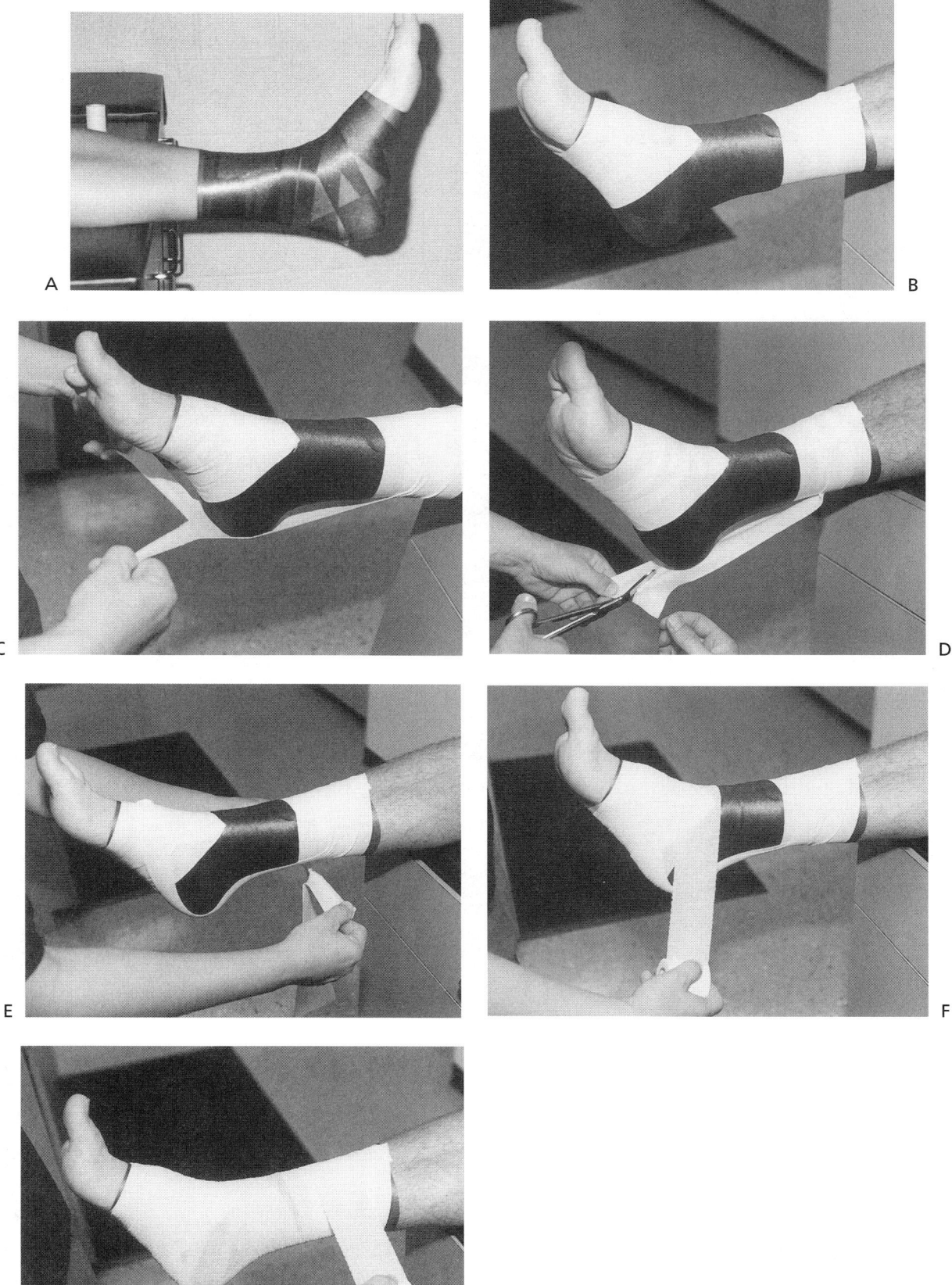

FIG. 56–4. Achilles tendon taping procedure. **A**: Apply prewrap. **B**: Anchor strips. **C**: Split tape around lower leg. **D**: Tape splitting. **E**: Repeat as necessary. **F**: Apply cover of stretch tape. **G**: Achilles taping completed.

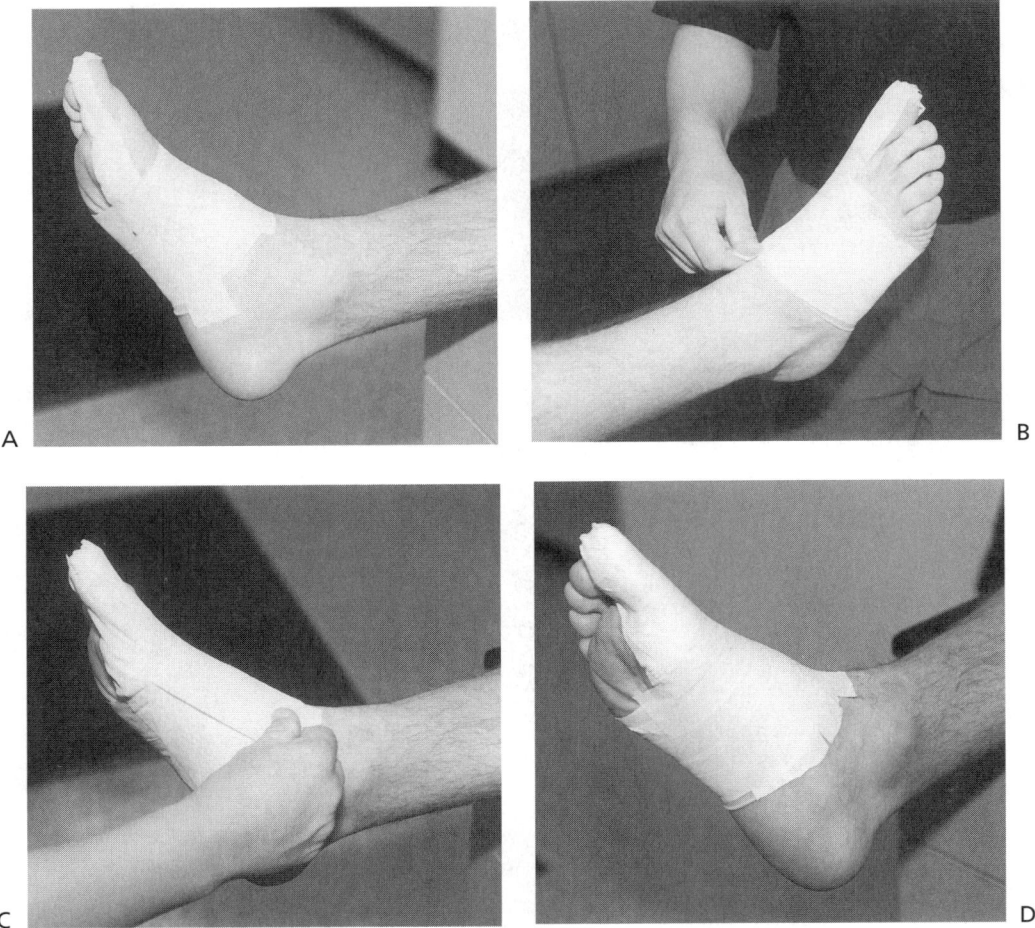

FIG. 56–5. Turf toe taping procedure. **A**: Anchor strips. **B**: Stability strips. **C**: Reinforcing strips. **D**: Turf toe taping completed.

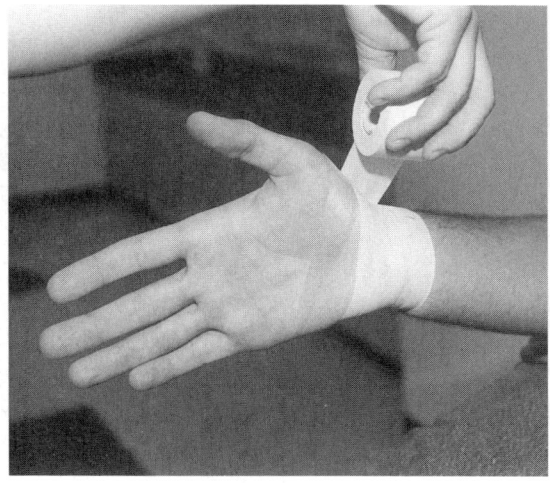
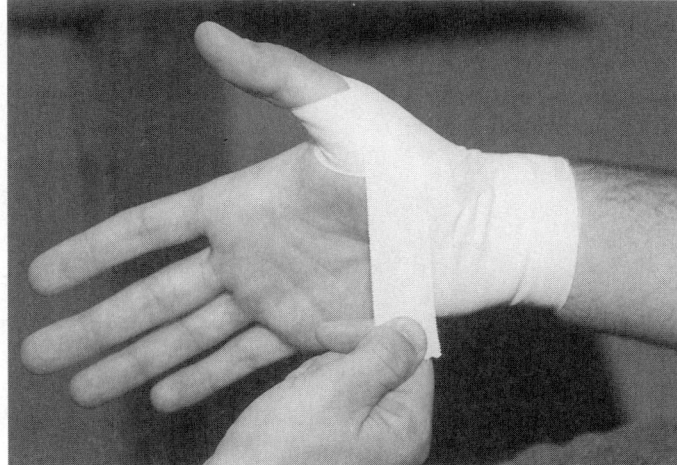
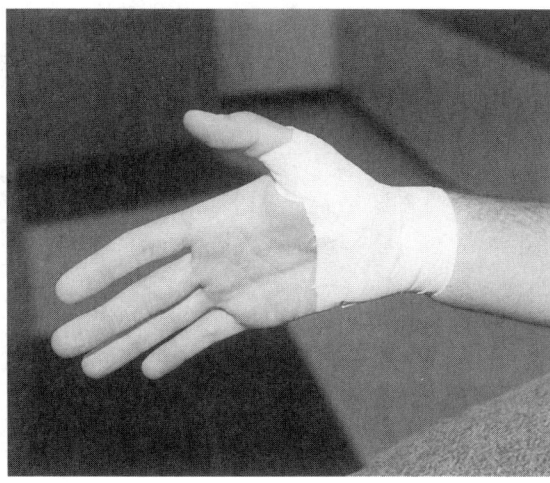

FIG. 56–6. Preventive thumb and wrist taping procedure. **A:** Anchor strips (fingers extended). **B:** Encircle thumb. **C:** Thumb taping completed.

3a. Alternate these strips beginning at the base of the thumb and placing alternating strips about one half of the tape width as you move distally.
3b. Apply these strips until the interphalangeal joint is covered. Leave the tip of the thumb exposed, and monitor for adequate blood flow to the thumb (Fig. 56–6C).
4. Closing strips can be applied over the thumb to restrict thumb abduction.
5. The wrist can then be preventively taped at this point. Wrist taping can be completed without application of the thumb taping procedure if restriction of thumb movement is not required.

The preventive wrist taping procedure is as follows (Fig. 56–7):

1. Have the athlete position the hand in the same manner as for the thumb taping procedure.
2. Begin with prewrap and anchor strips as demonstrated.
3. Apply figure eights, alternating directions of pull. A good hint here is to pinch the tape at the spot it passes nearest the thumb (Figs. 56–7A and 56–7B).
4. The procedure can be finished by applying finishing strips around the wrist to the comfort of the athlete (Figs. 56–7C and 56–7D).

The steps in applying a hip spica are as follows (Fig. 56–8):

1. Have the athlete stand with the affected leg in a semiflexed position. It is easiest to have the athlete place the heel on a 2-inch wedge.
2. For best results, have the athlete wear tight-fitting shorts under the spica to be applied.
3. Begin with the 6-inch elastic wrap on the medial thigh, and go around the thigh so that the direction of pull is to the midline (Fig. 56–8A).
4. Pull the elastic wrap medially up and around the waist, bringing it back to the thigh, and follow the same pattern until the elastic wrap is completely ap-

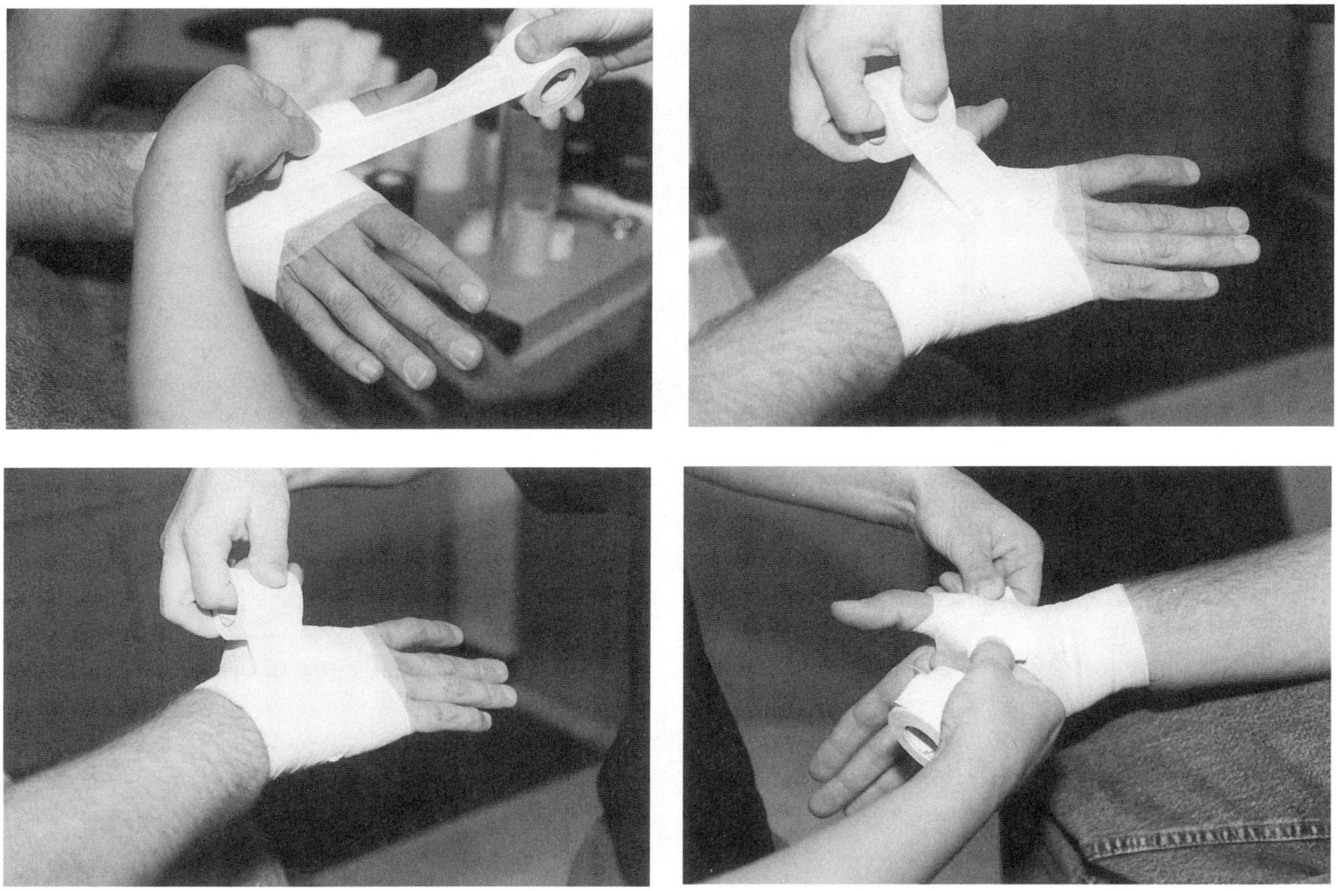

FIG. 56–7. Preventive wrist taping procedure. **A**: Pinch tape as it passes thumb. **B**: Encircle thumb. **C**: Finishing strips. **D**: Finishing strips. Wrist taping completed.

plied (Fig. 56–8B). (Note: If the athlete has a hip flexor strain when applying this wrap, have the athlete bend at the waist to help bring the hip flexors into a more flexed position.)

5. Complete the procedure with a set of finishing strips to hold the wrap in place on the thigh (Fig. 56–8C).

The steps in applying a shoulder spica are as follows (Fig. 56–9):

1. An elastic wrap 6 inches wide and double long in length is the most effective means for applying the shoulder spica (Fig. 56–9A).

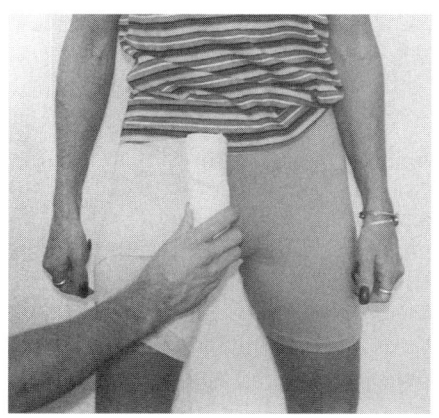
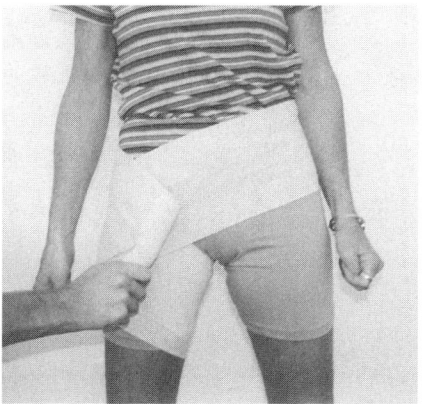
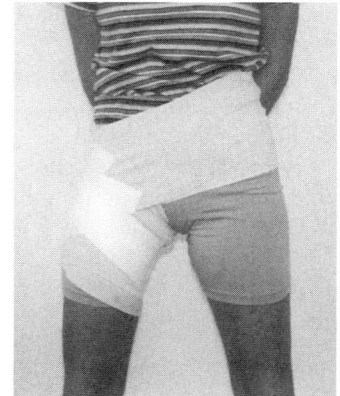

FIG. 56–8. Hip spica taping procedure. **A**: Six-inch lateral wrap around thigh. **B**: Wrap to midline. **C**: Hip spica completed.

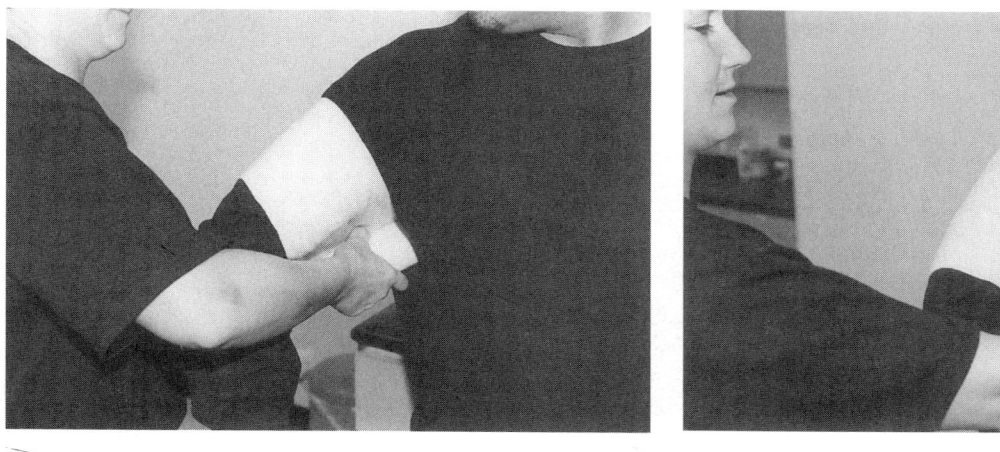

FIG. 56–9. Shoulder spica taping procedure. **A**: Six-inch elastic wrap around upper arm. **B**: Pull lateral to medial. **C**: Figure eight around body. **D**: Shoulder spica completed.

2. Begin the spica on the humerus, and pull the wrap from lateral to medial, which will assist in keeping the arm close to the body (Fig. 56–9B).
3. Proceed to use the elastic wrap in a figure eight pattern, using the upper arm and body as the reference points (Fig. 56–9C).
4. Standard white tape is adequate to hold the end of the elastic wrap in place at the end of the spica wrap (Fig. 56–9D).

REFERENCES

1. Gross MT, Bradshaw MK, Ventry LC, Weller KH. Comparison of support provided by ankle taping and semirigid orthosis. *J Orthop Sports Phys Ther* 1987;9:33–39.
2. Frankey JR, Jewett DL, Hanks GA, Sebastianelli WJ. A comparison of ankle-taping methods. *Clin J Sport Med* 1993;3:20–25.
3. Paris DL. The effects of the Swedo-O, New Cross, and McDavid ankle braces and adhesive ankle taping on speed, balance, agility, and vertical jump. *J Athl Training* 1992;27:253–256.
4. Gross MT, Lapp AK, Davis JM. Comparison of Swedo-O-Universal ankle support and Aircast support-stirrup orthoses and ankle tape in restricting eversion-inversion before and after exercise. *J Orthop Sports Phys Ther* 1991;13:11–19.
5. Gross MT, Ballard CL, Mears HG, Watkins EJ. Comparison of DonJoy ankle ligament protector and Aircast Sport-stirrup orthoses in restricting foot and ankle motion before and after exercise. *J Orthop Sports Phys Ther* 1992;16:60–67.
6. Pfeiffer RP, Mangus BC. *Concepts of athletic training*, 2nd ed. Boston: Jones & Bartlett, 1997:221.
7. Ferguson AB. The case against ankle taping. *Am J Sports Med* 1973;1:46–47.

CHAPTER 57

PRICE: Management of Injuries

Brent S. E. Rich

Injuries occur during athletics. With that as the starting premise, prevention, recognition, and management of injuries become the next steps. The purpose of this chapter is to define the management of injuries by using the PRICE concept (i.e., protection, rest, ice, compression, and elevation) (1).

PROTECTION

Protection is necessary both before and after injury. Protection from injury before athletic endeavor involves intrinsic and extrinsic measures. Intrinsic measures begin long before competition. Preseason conditioning programs institute the principle of *prehabilitation*. Like its counterpart, rehabilitation, which is the restoration of an injured area to preinjury status, prehabilitation is preventative medicine that anticipates the types of injuries that may occur and develops strategies against them. This is accomplished by the team physician, the athletic trainer, the strength and conditioning coach, and the coaching staff working together, implementing the principles of flexibility, strength, power, speed, endurance, and development of sports-specific skills. The use of these variables differs with individual sports. General health guidelines, including proper nutrition, adequate rest, and avoidance of overtraining, also protect against injury and illness.

Equipment and protective devices provide an extrinsic method of protection. They are allowed and in many cases required to prevent injury. Required devices must meet recognized standards in design and fabrication that have developed over time. Prior medical injuries, some of them catastrophic with accompanying legal ramifications, often lead to equipment modification. The helmet in football is an example. By contrast, some equipment is optional, such as the prophylactic knee or ankle brace. Though they are made with protective principles in mind, research may be lacking in regard to potential benefit and universally accepted validity. Individuals who have had prior medical injuries may be more susceptible to reinjury. Athletes playing in certain positions (e.g., offensive linemen in football) may also be prone to certain types of injuries (e.g., medial collateral ligament sprains). In such cases, protective equipment (e.g., prophylactic knee braces) may be suggested. In any event, equipment should be designed with specific protective principles in mind and constructed so as not to cause harm to the individual, teammates, or an opposing player.

After injury the use of devices to restrict movement of the injured area may be necessary. Splints, braces, crutches, slings, and other immobilizers will decrease painful range of motion and thereby limit further discomfort. Limiting painful movement is the first step in the recovery after injury.

REST

Impatience is a trait that athletes, coaches, athletic trainers, and sports medicine practitioners frequently demonstrate when an athlete is ill or injured. Return-to-play questions are often asked before the diagnosis is even made. The human body is remarkably efficient in its reparative ability, but it must obey healing principles. For example, when a muscle is traumatized, there is a biochemical response leading to swelling, redness, warmth, and pain (2). Swelling occurs from torn arteries, veins, and capillaries and from release of intracellular fluid from damaged cells. Redness and warmth result from increased blood flow and the release of cellular enzymes initiated by the inflammatory or healing response. Pain results from tissue anoxia and the release of bradykinin and prostaglandins that are part of the

---

B. S. E. Rich: Arizona Orthopaedic and Sports Medicine Specialists, Phoenix, Arizona 85044.

inflammatory reaction. After the initial cellular response has occurred, regeneration and remodeling complete the healing process (3).

In the PRICE philosophy, rest is defined in terms of absolute or relative rest (4). The need for absolute rest depends on the severity of the injury. Absolute rest means decreased initiation of muscle contractions while limiting flexibility and proprioceptive action to allow healing. If rest is used at all, the degree of absolute rest should be limited to lessen atrophy and deconditioning. Examples include bed rest, crutch use for a lower extremity injury, and the use of a sling for an upper extremity injury. Relative rest should be used when the injury is not severe and should be initiated shortly after the inflammatory response subsides. Relative rest is designed to allow the injured area to continue to heal while preventing deconditioning. The use of an aircast for an ankle sprain while allowing walking or running is an example.

With relative rest, the injured area is kept from full functional activity, but the unaffected body parts may continue to exercise. For example, riding a stationary bicycle is allowed when one is recovering from a rotator cuff injury. Rehabilitative principles such as flexibility, movement through a pain-free range of motion, initiation of muscular contraction (e.g., isometric exercises), and proprioceptive activities are encouraged. The goal is to minimize deconditioning, decrease the length of time for return to sports-specific activities once the area is further healed, and allow partial participation based on symptoms. The physician, physical therapist, or athletic trainer must individualize the use of absolute and relative rest. Healing to the point of return to functional activity differs between athletes.

ICE

Cryotherapy can alter the cellular response after injury. At the macroscopic level, after initial vasoconstriction, vasodilation occurs. The degree of vasodilation and bleeding can be decreased by the application of cold. At the microscopic level, the intensity of the inflammatory response and the amount of extracellular extravasation of fluid are markedly decreased by ice application. By interrupting the inflammatory response and limiting the degree of bleeding, recovery time is accelerated. Metabolic demands for oxygen are decreased when the tissues are cooled. In turn, the tissues can better survive the demands of the inflammatory response. Additionally, cryotherapy decreases nerve conduction velocity and muscle spasm, thereby decreasing pain. All of these effects allow the athlete to return to functional activity faster after tissue insult (4).

Cold can be rendered in many forms, including ice water immersion, refreezable chemical gel packs, ice massage, aerosol sprays (ethyl chloride), or, most commonly and preferred, crushed ice in a plastic bag. Though there is no universal rule as to how long ice should be applied, it is generally recommended that it be left on initially for 20–30 minutes after acute injury. Depending on the severity of injury and the degree of bleeding, ice may be reapplied for 20 minutes after the area has rewarmed for 2 hours. Repeat application is indicated on an individual basis.

No universally accepted standard for the use of ice after injury has been established, though limiting its use after the first 24–72 hours followed by the application of heat has been reported in the medical literature. Most important, ice should be used as long as there is active swelling, and heat should not be used during the acute inflammatory response. Contraindications to the use of ice after injury include cold hypersensitivity, Raynaud's disease, and other circulatory impairments. Nerve impairment has also been reported after application of cold near a superficial nerve. If there is any question as to persistence of the inflammatory reaction or if there is continued bleeding with initiation of activity, ice remains the rule.

COMPRESSION

Compression limits the degree of bleeding after injury and provides a splint, which disallows movement of the injury body part. Additionally, compression will disperse swelling, allowing the lymphatic and circulatory system to reabsorb local tissue fluid. Circumferential wrapping from distal to proximal overlapping the bandage by one half its width is the accepted standard. A standard ace bandage works well if it is kept snug but not tight. Avoidance of a tourniquet effect is important. Felt or foam cutouts may be used to form around irregular or bony prominence to add additional compression. Pneumatic compression devices may also be used if available. Palpation of a normal distal pulse after application is recommended.

The length of compression varies depending on individual circumstances. In general, compression is used in the first few days or until the active bleeding has subsided. If numbness, tingling, or increased pain occurs as a result of the compression, it must be loosened to prevent tissue anoxia or other damage. Compression might be indicated after the generation of muscle contractions following a period of rest to decrease any bleeding that may occur.

ELEVATION

In combination with rest, ice, and compression, elevation will decrease tissue swelling and the acute inflammatory response after injury. Gravity can be used to advantage by decreasing extravasation of blood and intracellular fluid into the adjacent tissues. Ideally, elevation above the level of the heart is most effective, though any degree of elevation will help to decrease dependent swelling and will be beneficial. Care to prevent impingement on bony prominences and compression of superficial nerves by appropriate padding is also indicated. For a lower extremity injury, elevation of the foot of the mattress by placing pillows or books under the mattress is preferred to placing the extremity on pillows because of the degree of movement one makes during sleep. For an upper extremity injury, elevating the arm on pillows or sleeping in a chair or upright position may be necessary.

SUMMARY

The first principles to be universally used after injury are PRICE: protection, rest, ice, compression, and elevation. If these principles are understood and utilized immediately after trauma, the degree of the acute inflammatory response can be limited, leading to earlier healing, a quicker return to range of motion, a faster return to normal strength and proprioception, and a more rapid return to functional and sports-specific activities.

REFERENCES

1. Shirley ME. Initial injury management: P-R-I-C-E-S. In: Mellion MB, ed. *Sports medicine secrets*. Philadelphia: Mosby, 1994: 321–323.
2. Roy S, Irvin R. *Sports medicine prevention, evaluation, management, and rehabilitation*. Englewood Cliffs, NJ: Prentice-Hall, 1983:125–127.
3. Pfeiffer RP, Mangus BC. *Concepts of athletic training,* 2nd ed. Boston: Jones & Bartlett, 1998:89–93.
4. Shelton GL. Comprehensive rehabilitation of the athlete. In: Mellion MB, Walsh WM, Shelton GL, eds. *The team physician's handbook,* 2nd ed. Philadelphia: Hanley & Belfus, 1997.

Subject Index

Page references for figures are followed by an *f*, and page references for tables are followed by a *t*.

A

Abdominal curls, following abdominal injuries, 368, 368*f*
Abdominal injuries, 353–371. *See also specific injuries*
  diaphragmatic, 358, 359*f*
  hernias, 359*f*, 359–362
  to hollow organs, 357*f*, 357–358
  to liver, 356*f*, 356–357, 357*t*
  muscular, 362–364
    ice hockey and, 510
  osteitis pubis, 364–367, 365*f*, 366*f*
  pancreatic, 358, 358*f*
  rehabilitation following, 367–368, 368*f*, 369*t*, 370, 370–371, 371*f*
  splenic, 353–354, 354*f*–356*f*, 354*t*–356*t*, 356
Absence seizures, 266
Abstinence, to circumvent drug testing, 171–172
Accessory navicular injury, running and, 550–551
"Accessory testicles," 378, 378*f*, 459
Achilles bursitis, cycling and, 465
Achilles tendinitis
  cycling and, 465
  tennis and, 585–586
  volleyball and, 595
Achilles tendon, taping procedure for, 659, 659*f*
Achilles tendon injuries
  running and, 547–548
  ruptures
    football and, 489
    volleyball and, 595
    weightlifting and, 628–629
Acne, exacerbation of, 236, 236*f*
Acquired hernia, 360
Acromial apophysitis, 400
Acromial process, avulsion fractures of, 417
Acromioclavicular injuries
  football and, 481
  martial arts and, 528
Active rewarming, for hypothermia, 316–317
Acute renal failure, exercise-induced, 306, 306*f*
Adolescents, female, scoliosis in, 103
Adson maneuver, 619
Adulterants, to circumvent drug testing, 172
Aerobic performance, of female athletes, 95–96
Age
  skiing injuries and, 557
  soccer injuries and, 566
Aikido, 525. *See also* Martial arts
Air quality, in ice arenas, 509–510
Airway, opening, 24, 26*f*
Alcohol
  abuse of, 141–142, 142*t*
  hypothermia and, 315

prohibition by major sports organizations, 183*t*
Aldosterone, renal function and, 300, 300*t*
All-American Girls' Baseball League, 94
Allen's maneuver, 619
Allopurinol, renal effects of, 301, 301*t*
Altitude training, for blood boosting, 297
Amateur Sports Act (1978), 223
Amateur wrestling, international, 637
Amenorrhea, 106–107
American Athletic Association of the Deaf, 116
American College Health Association, Athletic Medicine Section of, 5
American College of Sports Medicine (ACSM), 5
  position paper on alcohol use of, 141
American Medical Association (AMA), Committee on Medical Aspects of Sports of, 5
American Medical Society for Sports Medicine (AMSSM), 6
American Orthopaedic Society for Sports Medicine, 5
Americans with Disabilities Act (ADA) (1990), 6, 54, 115, 223
  application to sports, 224
Amphetamines
  abuse of, 152
  testing for, 168–169
Anabolic-androgenic steroids (AASs)
  abuse of, 133–136, 134*t*, 135*t*, 153
    in weightlifting, 614, 616
  prohibition by major sports organizations, 181*t*–182*t*
  renal effects of, 301*t*, 301–302
  testing for, 164–165, 166*t*, 169
Anaerobic performance, of female athletes, 96–97
Anaphylaxis, 261
  exercise-induced. *See* Exercise-induced anaphylaxis (EIAna)
Anconeus muscle injury, weightlifting and, 621
Androstenedione, abuse of, 144–146
Andry, Nicholas, 4
Anemia, 293–295
  iron-deficiency, 294–295
    in female athletes, 108
  sports, 294
Anesthetics, prohibition by major sports organizations, 184*t*
Angioedema, 261
Ankle deformities, in athletes with cerebral palsy, 124
Ankle injuries. *See also specific injuries*
  avulsion injuries, 423

football and, 488–489
soccer and, 565
swimming and, 574
volleyball and, 593–594, 595
weightlifting and, 628–630
Ankle sprains
  due to dance, 472–473
  football and, 488
  skiing and, 554*t*, 555
  tennis and, 586
  volleyball and, 593–594
  weightlifting and, 629–630
Anorexia athletica, 105, 105*t*
Anorexia nervosa. *See also* Eating disorders
  diagnostic criteria for, 185, 186*t*
  in female athletes, 104*t*, 104–106
Anterior cruciate ligament (ACL) injuries
  in female athletes, 99, 100, 101
  football and, 486–487
  in skeletally immature athletes, 391–392
  skiing and
    mechanisms of injury and, 556*f*, 556–557
    prevention of, 557–559
    risk factors for, 557
    trends in, 555, 555*t*
  tears, imaging of, 63–64, 64*f*, 78
  volleyball and, 596
Anterior interosseous syndrome, weightlifting and, 622
Antiepileptic drugs (AEDs), 267
Apophyseal injuries, 391
Apophysitis. *See* Traction apophysitis
Arch
  pain in, medial, running and, 549–550
  taping procedures for
    longitudinal, 656*f*, 658
    modified "low-dye," 657*f*–658*f*, 658
Architectural Barriers Act (1968), 223
Arthritic disorders
  athletes with, 126
  cycling and, 464
  in female athletes, 103
Artificial turf
  football injuries and, 478–479
  lacrosse injuries and, 518–519
Association for Intercollegiate Athletics for Women (AIAW), 94
Association Internationale Medico-Sportive (AIMS), 4
Asthma, 273–278
  exercise-induced. *See* Exercise-induced asthma (EIA)
Athletes
  female. *See* Female athletes
  physically challenged. *See* Physically challenged athletes; Wheelchair athletes

responsibility to protect own health, 52–53
young. *See* Child athletes
Athlete's foot, 231–232
Athlete's heart, 251–258
  clinical examination for, 253
  echocardiography with, 255–257
  electrocardiogram with, 253–255, 254*f*–256*f*
  in female athletes, 255
  historical background of, 251–252
  hypertrophic cardiomyopathy versus, 257
  physiology of, 252–253
Athletic pseudoanemia, 294
Athletic pseudonephritis, 302–303, 303*f*
Athletic taping. *See* Taping procedures
Athletic trainers, health-related values, attitudes, and beliefs of, 211–212
Atrial fibrillation, with athlete's heart, 254
Atrial natriuretic peptide (ANP), renal function and, 300, 300*t*
Attitudes, health-related. *See* Sport, health-related values, attitudes, and beliefs in
Auricular hematomas, 30
  wrestling and, 638*f*, 638–639
Autonomic hyperreflexia, in wheelchair athletes, 123
Avicenna, 4
Avulsion injuries, 413–425
  about elbow, 416
  of ankle, 423
  of foot, 423–425
  of hand, 413–415
  of knee, 420–423
  of lumbar spine, 417–418
  of pelvis and hip, 418–420
  of shoulder, 416–417
  of triquetrum, 415
  of ulnar styloid, 415
  of wrist, 415
AXA World Ride '95, 127
Axillary nerve injuries, ice hockey and, 510

B

Back, biomechanics of, in tennis, 580
Back injuries. *See also specific injuries*
  soccer and, 564–565
  swimming and, 572–573
  volleyball and, 600
Back pain. *See also* Low back pain
  cycling and, 459
  swimming and, 573
Baker's cysts, cycling and, 465
Ballance's sign, 353
Baseball, 441. *See also* Major League Baseball (MLB)

669

Baseball (contd.)
  catastrophic injuries in, 325, 326, 328
  head injuries in, 332, 332t, 333t
  overhead throw in. *See* Overhead throw
Basilar skull fractures, with head injury, 340, 340f, 340t, 341f
Basketball. *See also* National Basketball Association (NBA)
  catastrophic injuries in, 324, 325, 329
  head injuries in, 332, 332t, 333t
Beliefs, health-related. *See* Sport, health-related values, attitudes, and beliefs in
Benign exertional headaches, 284
Bent-knee fall-out exercise, 368f
Bergerius, 4
Beta-2 agonists
  prohibited by major sports organizations, 182t
  testing for, 164
Beta-blockers
  prohibition by major sports organizations, 184t
  testing for, 164
Biceps tendon rupture
  football and, 482
  weightlifting and, 620
Bicipital tendinitis, tests for, 617
Bicycling. *See* Cycling
Bindings, for skiing, 557–558
Biofeedback, 198
Biomechanics
  of golf swing, 493–494
  physeal, 383
  of rowing, 531–532, 532f–534f
  of tennis, 579–580
  traction apophysitis due to, 398
Bleeding problems, 296
Blind athletes, 116, 125
  snow skiing for, 126
Blisters, 232t, 234
  in rowers, 540
Blood doping, 297. *See also* Erythropoietin (EPO)
  prohibition by major sports organizations, 183t
Blood glucose (BG), 287
  control of, 287
  exercise guidelines and, 287–290
  low
    exercise-induced, 288, 289, 289t
    hypothermia and, 315
Blood testing, for drug testing, 166t
Bodybuilding, 609–610
Body composition, of female athletes, 94–95, 95–96
  prepubescent, 98, 98t
Body fluid, exercise and, 301
Body temperature
  measurement of, 312–313
  regulation of, 311, 312
Body weight loss
  recommendations for, 189
  in wrestlers, 639–641
Bone
  contusions of, occult, 66–67, 67f
  of female athletes, 95
  fractures of. *See* Avulsion injuries; Fractures; Physeal injuries; Stress fractures; *specific sites of fractures*
  imaging of, 61–67, 62f–67f
Bone mineral density (BMD)
  amenorrhea and, 106, 107
  osteopenia and osteoporosis and, in female athletes, 107–108
Bone scans, 59, 80–81
  of stress fractures, 433, 433t
Boot-top tendon lacerations, ice hockey and, 510
Boston Marathon, 223

Boutonniere deformity, secondary to central slip avulsion injuries, 414
Bowler's callus, 235f
Boxing, head injury and, 348
Brachial artery entrapment, weightlifting and, 621
Bracing
  for skiing, 559
  for stress fractures, 434
Brain injuries. *See* Head injuries
Bromantan
  abuse of, 144
  to circumvent drug testing, 173
Bronchospasm, exercise-induced, in rowers, 540
Brunell, Mark, 199
Bulimia nervosa. *See also* Eating disorders
  diagnostic criteria for, 185, 186t
  in female athletes, 104t, 104–106

C

Calcaneal apophysitis, 408f, 408–409, 409f
Calcaneal tuberosity, avulsion fractures of, 425
Calcaneus, anterior process of, avulsion fractures of, 423–424, 424f
Calf muscle injuries, running and, 548
Calluses, 235, 235f
  in rowers, 540
  weightlifting and, 624
Cancer, testicular, 375
Cardiac disorders. *See* Athlete's heart
Cardiomyopathy, hypertrophic, athlete's heart versus, 257
Cardiovascular emergencies, 27
Carpal tunnel syndrome, in wheelchair athletes, 121
Cartilage, imaging of, 67–74, 68f–74f
Catastrophic injuries, 202. *See also specific injuries*
  in high school and college sports, study of, 321–330
  data collection for, 321–322
  in fall sports, 322t, 322–324, 324t
  in females, 329–330
  in spring sports, 325–326, 326t, 327t
  in winter sports, 324–325, 325t, 326t
  prevention of, recommendations for, 330
Catheterization, to circumvent drug testing, 171
Cauliflower ear, 30, 638f, 638–639
Cealabolil, 172–173
Cerebral concussion, 337t, 337–338
Cerebral contusions, 336
Cerebral hemorrhage, 336, 336f, 337f
Cerebral palsy, athletes with, 116, 123–124
  classification of, 123
  exercise physiology and, 123–124
  prevention and treatment of injuries in, 124
Cerebral Palsy International Sports and Recreation Association, 116
Cervical spine injuries. *See also* Neck injuries
  football and, 322–323
  with head injury, 341
Chain of custody, drug testing and, 158–159, 159t
Cheerleading, catastrophic injuries in, 329
Chest injuries, lacrosse and, 517
Chilblains, 313
Child athletes, 87–91
  advantages of exercise and, 87–88
  epidemiology of injuries in, 88f, 88–89, 89f, 89t

female, 97–98, 98t
  head injuries in, 90
  injuries unique to, 89–90
  intense participation by, 91
  physeal injuries in. *See* Physeal injuries
  strength training of, 90
  traction apophysitis in. *See* Traction apophysitis
Cholinergic urticaria (CU), 261–262
  diagnosis of, 263
  epidemiology of, 263
  pathophysiology of, 263
  prevention of, 264
  treatment of, 264
Chondromalacia patella, cycling and, 462–463, 463f
Chronic traumatic encephalopathy (CTE), 342
Claudication test, 619
Cleats, football injuries and, 479
Clenbuterol, abuse of, 140
Clonic convulsions, 265
Clonic-tonic convulsions, 265
Clothing
  for cycling, 460–461
  for frostbite prevention, 314
Clotting problems, 296–297
Coaches
  experience of, football injuries and, 479
  health-related values, attitudes, and beliefs of, 209, 210
Cocaine
  abuse of, 140–141
  testing for, 168–169
Coffin, Thomas, 224
Cold, 311–317
  body temperature measurement and, 312–313
  body temperature regulation and, 312
  disorders related to, 313t, 313–317
  heat balance and, 311
  thermodynamics and, 311–312
  tolerance of, 312
Collision sports, with epilepsy, 269–270
Common warts, 232t
Communication, of endurance events, 42
Compartment syndromes
  volleyball and, 597
  weightlifting and, 621, 628
Compensations, in neuromusculoskeletal system, 609, 649t
Compliance, with treatment, 201
Compression, in PRICE concept of injury management, 666
Computed tomography (CT), 57–58, 58f
  of bone, 61, 62f, 62–63, 63f, 67
  in brain injury, focal, 336–337
  of cartilage, 71–72, 73f, 74
  of muscles, 80
  of physeal injuries, 387
  with rectus sheath hematomas, 364
  of shoulder, 71–72, 73f
  with splenic injuries, 354, 354t
  of stress fractures, 433
Conditioning
  injury prevention and, in lacrosse, 519
  for tennis, 587–588
Consciousness, loss of, with head injury, 334
Consent, informed, 50–51
  for drug testing, 157–158
Contact dermatitis, 232t
  swimming and, 574
Contact sports, with epilepsy, 269–270
Continued performance enhancement training, 197

Controlled substances, prohibition by major sports organizations, 184t
Convection, heat exchange by, 311
Conventional tomography, 57
Convulsions, definition of, 265
Cooper, Kenneth, 541
Coordination, in athletes with cerebral palsy, 124
Coping, determined, as response to injury, 193–194
Core rewarming, for hypothermia, 316–317
Corn(s), 235
Corneal abrasions, 30
Coronary heart disease (CHD), risk of, exercise and, 87
Coronoid process, avulsion fractures of, 416–417
  of base, 417
  distal, 416
Corticosteroids, prohibition by major sports organizations, 184t
Corticotropin (ACTH), prohibition by major sports organizations, 183t
Costoclavicular syndrome, weightlifting and, 619
Costovertebral joint injuries, swimming and, 573
Creatine monohydrate, abuse of, 144
Cricothyroidotomy, needle, 24, 26, 26f
Cross-country, catastrophic injuries in, 323, 329
Crossover syndrome, weightlifting and, 622–623
Crotch dermatitis, cycling and, 460–461
Cruciate, posterior, avulsion fractures of, 421
Cubital tunnel syndrome, weightlifting and, 620–621
Cycling, 453–469
  bicycle position and, 454–456
  brake levers and, 455
  frame sizing and, 454
  handlebars and, 455
  leg-length discrepancy and, 455–456, 456f
  pedal fore-aft and, 454
  seat and, 454–455
  setup and, 454
  stem and, 455
  head injury in, 334
  medical coverage for races and, 44
  overuse injuries and, 456–467
    causes of, 456–457
    crotch dermatitis, 460–461
    epicondylitis, 458, 458f
    of feet, 465–466
    of female athletes, 467
    of knee and lower leg, 461–465
    low back pain due to, 459
    of male athletes, 466
    neck pain due to, 457
    saddle sores, 378, 378f, 459–460
    scapula syndrome, 457–458
    ulnar neuropathy, 458f, 458–459
  pudendal neuropathy and, 376
  safety for, 453–454
    equipment for, 453–454
    riding style and, 453
  traumatic injuries and, 467–469
    abrasions, 467–468
    clavicle fracture, 468–469
    head injury, 469
    shoulder dislocation, 469
    shoulder separation, 469
Cyclist's palsy, 458f, 458–459
Cyst(s)
  Baker's, cycling and, 465
  epidermal, testicular, 376f
  ganglion, weightlifting and, 623

meniscal, imaging of, 70, 71f
paramensical, imaging of, 70, 72f
Cystic fibrosis (CF), 278

D
Dance, 471–476
  injuries due to
    ankle sprains, 472–473
    flexor hallucis tendinitis, 475
    fractures, 474, 474f
    impingement syndromes, 474f, 474–475, 475f
    pathogenesis of, 471–472, 472f, 473f
    prevention of, 475–476
Dandy, D. J., 6
Darling, E. A., 4
Deadbug, 368f
Deaf athletes, 116, 126
  World Games for the Deaf and, 115
Death, sudden, preperformance physical examination and, 12–13
Deaths, 202
  in baseball, 326, 327t
  in basketball, 326, 326t, 329
  cardiac. See Athlete's heart
  in cheerleading, 329
  in cross-country, 329
  in football, 322, 322t
  in ice hockey, 326, 326t
  in lacrosse, 326, 326t, 327t, 329
  in martial arts, 528–529, 529f
  in pole vault, 328
  in skiing, 326, 326t
  in soccer, 329
  in swimming, 326, 326t, 329
  in tennis, 326, 327t
  in track, 326, 327t, 329
  in volleyball, 329
  in winter sports, 324
Decubitus ulcers, in wheelchair athletes, 121
Deep venous thrombosis (DVT), 296–297
DeLorme, Thomas, 5
Dementia pugilistica, 527–528
DeMont, Rick, 139
De Morbis Artificum (Ramazzini), 4
Denial, as response to injury, 193, 194
Dental injuries, 31
DeQuervain's disease
  golf and, 496
  weightlifting and, 622
Dermatitis
  contact, 232t
    swimming and, 574
  crotch, cycling and, 460–461
  seborrheic, 232t
Dermatologic problems, 231–237, 232t. See also specific problems
  exacerbations of underlying conditions, 236–237
  infectious, 231–234
    in wrestlers, 639
  mechanical and physical, 234–236
  in rowers, 540
  ulceration, cycling and, 459
  volleyball and, 600
  in wheelchair athletes, 120–121
Designer drugs, to circumvent drug testing, 172–173
Determined coping, as response to injury, 193–194
Diabetes mellitus
  type 1, 287–291
    exercise in, See Type 1 diabetes, exercise in
  type 2, 288t
Diagnostic peritoneal lavage (DPL), with splenic injuries, 353–354, 355t
Diaphragmatic rupture, 358, 359f

Diazepam, for cardiovascular emergencies, 27
Didrickson, Babe, 94
Diffuse brain injury, 334, 337t, 337–338
  mechanism and pathophysiology of, 338–339
"Digging," in volleyball, 591, 592f
Disability, 221–227
  elite athletes with, 223–225. See also Paralympics; Wheelchair athletes
  future directions for, 226–227
  historical perceptions of, 221–223
  legislation on, 223
  recreational sport and physical activity for people with, 225–226
    empowerment and, 225–226
    mind-body-spirit integration and, 226
    therapeutic value of, 226
Disabled Sports USA (DS/USA), 116
Disc herniations, rowing and, 535–536, 536t
Discus throw, catastrophic injuries in, 329
Distress, as response to injury, 193, 194
Diuretics
  to circumvent drug testing, 173
  prohibited by major sports organizations, 182t–183t
  renal effects of, 301, 301t
  testing for, 165, 166t, 169
Dolan, Tom, 273
Dopamine, for splenic injuries, 28
Doping, 152. See also Drug abuse
Doping control. See also Drug testing
  of endurance events, 42
Double PCL sign, 70, 71f
Drawer test, 627
Drug(s). See also specific drugs
  hypothermia and, 315
  prescription of, legal issues concerning, 50
  renal effects of, 301t, 301–302
  street, prohibition by major sports organizations, 184t
Drug abuse, 133–146
  of alcohol, 141–142, 142t
  of anabolic-androgenic steroids, 133–136, 134t, 135t, 153
  of androstenedione, 144–146
  of bromantan, 144
  of cocaine, 140–141
  of creatine monohydrate, 144
  drugs and methods prohibited by IOC and, 133, 134t
  of erythropoietin, 138–139
  following injury and rehabilitation, 201
  of human growth hormone, 136–138
  of marijuana, 142–143
  of mesocarb, 143–144
  of smokeless tobacco, 143
  of sympathetic amines, 139t, 139–140
Drug testing, 151–174
  circumvention techniques for, 171–173
    prohibition by major sports organizations, 183t
  cost of, 173
  doctor-patient relationship and, 160
  of endurance events, 42
  false positive and false negative results with, 167–170
  intent of, 156
  legal issues in, 156–157, 173
  methodologies for, 160–167
    by drug group, 164–167
  origins of, 151–153, 154t–155t, 156

policy for
  chain of custody and, 158–159, 159t
  consequences of positive tests and, 159–160
  informed consent and, 157–158
  scheduling and, 158
  reliability of, 170–171
  in weightlifting, 611
Dwarf Athletic Association of America, 116

E
Eating disorders, 185–189
  definitions of, 185, 186t
  in female athletes, 104t, 104–106, 105t
  following injury and rehabilitation, 201–202
  identifying athletes with, 188, 188t
  long-term health effects of, 187–188
  prevalence among athletes, 185–186, 186f
  prevention in athletes, 189
  risk factors for, 186–187, 187t
  treatment of, 188–189
  weight loss recommendations and, 189
Echocardiography, with athlete's heart, 255–257
Ederle, Gertrude, 93
Education
  about injury and rehabilitation, 195–196
  about skiing, 559
Education Amendments Act (1972), Title IX of, 94
Education of All Handicapped Children Act (1975), 223
Effort-exertion headaches, 284
Elbow
  avulsion injuries about, 416
  biomechanics of, in tennis, 580
  Little League, 398–399
  of overhead thrower, 447
Elbow injuries. See also specific injuries
  dislocations, martial arts and, 528
  football and, 482
  golf and, 496
  rowing and, 539, 539f
  swimming and, 572
  volleyball and, 599
  weightlifting and, 619–621
Electrocardiogram (ECG)
  with athlete's heart, 253–255, 254f–256f
  exercise, in diabetes mellitus, 290
Elementary and Secondary Education Act, 1967 amendments to, 223
Elevation, in PRICE concept of injury management, 666–667
Emergencies. See also On-the-field emergencies
  associated with headaches, 281, 282t
Emergency medical services notification, of endurance events, 42
Emotional reactions, to injury, 193–194
Empowerment, by sports participation, for people with disabilities, 225–226
"Empty beer can test," 618
Endurance events
  medical coverage of, 33–45, 34t
    administrative responsibilities and, 38
    for bike races, 44
    drug testing and doping control and, 42

first aid and treatment stations for, 42–43, 43t
hospital and emergency services notification and, 42
medical director's objectives and goals and, 39
medical protocols for, 39, 40f, 41
for multiday races, 44
for Nordic skiing races, 44
for physically challenged athletes, 44–45
postrace operations and, 45
preparticipation medical questionnaire and examination and, 38
prerace contestant information and, 38
prerace operations and, 33–35
race day communication and surveillance for, 42
race day transportation for, 42
record keeping for, 41, 41t
risk assessment and risk reduction and, 35–38
staffing medical teams for, 41
for swim races, 43–44
for triathlons, 43
for ultraendurance events, 44
volunteer education for, 42
medical disqualification of athletes for, 37–38
Environment, rehabilitation, 647–648
Environmental conditions, endurance events and, 36–37
Enzyme immunoassay (EIA), for drug testing, 161, 162t
Enzyme-linked immunosorbent assay, for drug testing, 166t
Enzyme-multiplied immunoassay technique (EMIT), for drug testing, 161
l'Epée, Abbe de, 222
Epicondylar apophysitis, medial, 398–399
Epicondylar fractures, medial
  avulsion, 416
  weightlifting and, 620
Epicondylitis
  cycling and, 458, 458f
  lateral
    tennis and, 583–584
    volleyball and, 599
    weightlifting and, 620
  medial
    rowing and, 539, 539f
    tennis and, 584
    weightlifting and, 620
Epidermal cysts, testicular, 376f
Epididymitis, 375, 376f
Epidural hematomas, 335, 336f, 336–337
Epigastric hernia, 360
Epilepsy, 265–271
  definition of, 265
  prognosis of, 267–268
  seizure classification and, 265–266
  sports participation and, 268, 270
  sports-specific considerations for patients with, 268–270
    in contact and collision sports, 269–270
    in water sports, 268–269, 269t
  treatment of, 266–267
Epinephrine, for pulmonary emergencies, 27
Epiphysitis. See Traction apophysitis
Epistaxis, 31
Epitestosterone, to circumvent drug testing, 173
Epstein-Barr virus (EBV), 239–240. See also Infectious mononucleosis (IM)
Erectile dysfunction, cycling and, 466
Erythrasma, 233

Erythromycin, for erythrasma, 233
Erythropoietin (EPO), 138–139
  for blood boosting, 297
  prohibition by major sports organizations, 183t
  testing for, 165, 166t, 167, 169
Ethical issues, in medical practice, 8
Evaporation, heat exchange by, 312
Exercise, therapeutic value of, for people with disabilities, 226
Exercise-induced acute renal failure (EIARF), 306, 306f
Exercise-induced anaphylaxis (EIAna), 27, 261, 262–264
  diagnosis of, 263–264
  epidemiology of, 263
  food-dependent, 262–263
  pathophysiology of, 263
  prevention of, 264
  treatment of, 264
  variant-type, 261, 262
Exercise-induced asthma (EIA), 261, 273–277
  clinical presentation of, 274
  conditioning and, 277, 278f
  diagnosis of, 276–277
  pathophysiology of, 274
  treatment and prevention of, 274–275, 275f
    drugs used for, international competition and, 275, 276t
    nonpharmacologic measures for, 275–276
Exercise-induced bronchospasm (EIB), 27
  in rowers, 540
Exercise-induced hypoglycemia, 288, 289, 289t
Exercise-induced urticaria (EIU), 261–262
  diagnosis of, 263
  epidemiology of, 263
  pathophysiology of, 263
  prevention of, 264
  treatment of, 264
Exertional hemolysis, 295
  hematuria due to, 304
Exertion-related headaches, 284
Extensor carpi ulnaris tendinitis, golf and, 496
Extensor carpi ulnaris tendon sheath rupture, golf and, 496
Extensor carpi ulnaris tendon subluxation, weightlifting and, 623
Extensor pollicis longus tendon rupture, weightlifting and, 623
Extensor tenosynovitis, rowing and, 539
Extracorporeal cardiopulmonary bypass, for hypothermia, 316
Eye injuries
  lacrosse and, 517, 518
  soccer and, 564

F

Face mask removal, 24, 26f
Facet joint arthropathy, rowing and, 536
Facet syndrome, lateral, rowing and, 539
Facial injuries
  ice hockey and, 505
  lacrosse and, 517–518
  soccer and, 564
False negative drug test results, 167–168
False positive drug test results, 167–168
Famciclovir (Famvir), for herpes infections, 232t
  dermatologic, 231
Fatalities. See Deaths
Fatty hernia of the linea alba, 360

Fear, of reinjury, mental training for, 199
Fédération International de Lutte Amateur (FILA), 637
Fédération Internationale de Medecine Sportive (FIMS), 4
Feet
  cycling and, 465–466
  trauma to, preventing in diabetes mellitus, 290
Female athletes, 93–110
  adult, 94–97
    aerobic performance of, 95–96
    anaerobic performance of, 96–97
    body composition of, 94–95, 95–96
    menstrual cycle effects on performance and, 97
    skeletal differences in, 95
    strength of, 95
    thermoregulation in, 97
  athlete's heart in, 255
  cycling by
    bicycle-seat discomfort and, 467
    dyspareunia and, 467
    nipple friction and pain and, 467
    tampon use and, 467
    vulvar swelling and, 467
  female athlete triad and, 103–109
    amenorrhea and, 106–107
    disordered eating and, 104t, 104–106, 105t
    osteopenia and osteoporosis and, 107–108
  genital injuries in, 378–379
    perineal, 378–379, 379t
    vaginal, 379, 379t
  historical background of, 93–94
  iron-deficiency anemia in, 294–295
  iron deficiency in, 108
  musculoskeletal injuries in, 98–103
    arthritic disorders and, 103
    of lumbar spine, 102–103
    rates of, 98–99
    risk factors for, 99–101
  physiologic parameters and, 94, 94t
  prepubescent, 97–98, 98t
  stress urinary incontinence in, 108–109
Femoral anteversion, rowing and, 539
Femoral hernias, 360–361
Field hockey, 519–523
  catastrophic injuries in, 323
  conditioning and injury prevention in, 522
  head injuries in, 332, 332t, 333, 333t
  historical background of, 519–520
  injury demographics in, 520
  injury types in, 520f, 520–521
  mechanisms of injury in, 521–522
    of contact injuries, 521–522
    of noncontact injuries, 521
Fifth metatarsal, traction apophysitis at base of, 409f, 409–410
Filtration factor (FF), exercise and, 299–300
Fingers
  crushing injuries of, weightlifting and, 624
  dislocations of, volleyball and, 599
  sprains of, volleyball and, 599
Finkelstein test, 622
First aid stations, of endurance events, 42–43, 43t
Fixx, James, 541
Flail chest, 28
Flexor carpi radialis tendinitis
  golf and, 496
  weightlifting and, 623
Flexor carpi ulnaris tendinitis
  golf and, 496
  weightlifting and, 623

Flexor digitorum profundus, avulsion of, 415
  football and, 484
Flexor hallucis tendinitis, due to dance, 475
Fluconazole, for tinea corporis/cruris, 232
Fluid balance, exercise and, 301
Fluid replacement, for cardiovascular emergencies, 27
Fluid resuscitation, for hypothermia, 317
Fluorescence polarization immunoassay (FPIA), for drug testing, 161, 162t
Focal brain injury, 334, 335f–337f, 335–337
Folliculitis, 232t
  cycling and, 459
Football, 477–489, 478t. See also National Football League (NFL)
  catastrophic injuries in, 322t, 322–323, 327
  elbow injuries in, 482
  foot and ankle injuries in, 488–489
  forearm injuries in, 482
  head injuries in, 332, 332t, 333, 333t, 334, 484
  injury risk factors in, 478–480
  knee injuries in, 486–488
  leg injuries in, 488
  lumbar spine injuries in, 484
  pelvic and hip injuries in, 484–485
  shoulder injuries in, 480–482
  thigh injuries in, 485–486
  wrist and hand injuries in, 482–484
"Footballer's migraine," 283
Foot deformities, in athletes with cerebral palsy, 124
Foot injuries. See also specific injuries
  avulsion injuries, 423–425
  football and, 488–489
  soccer and, 565
  swimming, 574
  volleyball and, 593, 594, 595–596
  weightlifting and, 628
Footstrike hemolysis, 295
  hematuria due to, 304
Footwear
  for dance, 471
  football injuries and, 479
  musculoskeletal injuries in female athletes and, 102
  for snow skiing, 558
  frostbite and, 314, 314f
  traction apophysitis due to, 397
Footwork, for tennis, 588
Forefoot pain, chronic, running and, 550
Fractures. See also specific sites
  abdominal injuries with, 357
  avulsion. See Avulsion injuries
  compound, 30
  due to dance, 474, 474f
  occult, imaging of, 66, 66f
  physeal. See Physeal injuries
  rupture of, 595
  stress. See Stress fractures
Freestyle wrestling, 637
Freiberg's disease, running and, 550
Frostbite, 234, 311, 313–314, 314f
Functional evaluation, 646–647, 647f–649f
Functional feeding, 653
Furuncles, cycling and, 459

G

Galen, Claudius, 3–4, 23
Gamekeeper's injury, imaging of, 63–65, 64f, 65f
Ganglia, weightlifting and, 624
Ganglion cysts, weightlifting and, 623

Gas chromatography (GC), for drug testing, 161
Gas chromatography/high resolution mass spectrometry (GC/HRMS), for drug testing, 163, 163t
Gas chromatography/mass spectrometry (GC/MS), for drug testing, 162, 163t
Gastrocnemius strain, volleyball and, 597
Gastrointestinal emergencies, 28
Gender, 215–219. See also Female athletes
  circumspection of physical activity based on, 217–218
  definition of, 215–216
  exclusion from physical activity based on, 216
  skiing injuries and, 557
  soccer injuries and, 566
Gender typing, of physical activity and sport, 217
General Assembly of International Federation of Sports, 611
Generalized seizures, 266
Genital injuries, 373–379. See also specific injuries
  in females, 378–379
    cycling and, 467
    perineal, 378–379, 379t
    vaginal, 379, 379t
    vulvar, 467
  in males, 373–378
    penile, 375–376, 466
    perineal, 378, 378f
    prostatic, 378
    testicular and scrotal, 373–375, 374f, 376f
    urethral, 376–378, 377f, 466
  prostatic, 466
Genitofemoral nerve, irritation of, in bicyclists, 376
Genitourinary emergencies, 29
Genu valgum, rowing and, 539
Glasgow Coma Scale (GCS), 339, 340t
Glenohumeral instability, football and, 481–482
Glomerular filtration rate (GFR), exercise and, 299
Glycoprotein hormones
  prohibited by major sports organizations, 183t
  testing for, 165, 167, 169
Goal setting, for rehabilitation, 196
Golf, 493–497, 494t
  elbow injuries in, 496
  low back injuries in, 494–495
  mechanics of swing in, 493–494
  shoulder injuries in, 495
  wrist injuries in, 496–497
Goniometry, knee, 456
Goode, Ben, 5
Gracilis syndrome, 366
Grand mal seizures, 266
Greater trochanter avulsion, 403, 419–420
Greater trochanteric bursitis, weightlifting and, 625
Groin injuries. See also specific injuries
  contusions, football and, 484
  ice hockey and, 510
Groin pain
  running and, 550
  soccer and, 565
Growth arrest, after physeal injuries, 389, 390
  treatment of, 390–391
Growth hormone. See Human growth hormone (hGH)
Guttman, Ludwig, 115

Guyon's canal syndrome, weightlifting and, 623–624
Gymnastics
  catastrophic injuries in, 324, 328, 329
  head injuries in, 332t

H

Haglund's disease
  running and, 550
  weightlifting and, 629
Hamartomas, in female genital tract, 379
Hamate fractures, golf and, 497
Hamstrings
  injuries of, running and, 550
  tight, cycling and, 465
Hand, neuropathies of, weightlifting and, 623
Hand injuries, 517. *See also specific injuries*
  avulsion, 413–415
  field hockey and, 520, 520f
  football and, 482–484
  fractures, lacrosse and, 517
  lacrosse, 517
  soccer and, 564
  swimming and, 572
  volleyball and, 599–600
Hapkido, 525. *See also* Martial arts
Haüy, Valentin, 222
Hawkin's sign, 597
Headaches, 281–284
  emergencies associated with, 281, 282t
  exertion-related, 284
  migraine, 282t, 282–283
  nonorganic, 284
  posttraumatic, 283
  tension, 283–284
  tumor-related, 281–282
Head concussion, 338
Headgear, in martial arts, 527
Head injuries, 331–350
  baseball and, 332, 332t
  basketball and, 332, 332t
  bicycling and, 334
  boxing and, 348
  in children, 90
  classification systems for, 342–343, 344t–345t
  complications and sequelae of, 341–342, 342t
  definitions related to, 334
  epidemiology of, 331–334, 332t, 333t
  evaluation of athletes with, 339–341, 340f, 340t, 341f
  new methods for, 346–347
  field hockey and, 332, 332t, 333, 521
  focal, 335f–337f, 335–337
  football and, 332, 332t, 333, 334, 489
  gymnastics and, 332t
  ice hockey and, 332t, 332–333, 334, 505, 508
  lacrosse and, 332t, 333
  martial arts and, 526–528
  mechanisms and pathophysiology of, 338–339
  nonfocal, 337t, 337–338
  as on-the-field emergency, 23–24, 24f–26f, 26–27
  recurrent, 342, 527
  return-to-play guidelines for, 343, 345–346
  soccer and, 332, 332t, 333, 348–349, 349f, 564
  softball and, 332t
  volleyball and, 332, 332t, 600
  wrestling and, 332, 332t
Healing imagery, 197–198, 198f

Health, "gender-appropriate" sports and, 218
Health maintenance organizations (HMOs), 7
Heart. *See also* Athlete's heart
  cooling of, in hypothermia, 315
  volume of, in female athletes, 96
Heat balance, in cold conditions, 311
Heat exchange, 311–312
Heating blankets, for hypothermia, 316
Helmets
  for football, 480
  head injury reduction by, 334
  in lacrosse, 516–517
  for skiing, 558
Hematocele, 374
Hematocrit, of female athletes, prepubescent, 98, 98t
Hematological problems, 293–297
  anemia, 293–295
  bleeding and clotting disorders, 296–297
  blood boosting and, 297
  footstrike hemolysis, 295
  in infectious mononucleosis, 244
  sickle-cell trait, 295–296
Hematomas
  auricular, 30
  epidural, 335, 336f, 336–337
  of rectus sheath, 363–364
  subdural, 335, 335f, 336–337
Hematuria, 303t, 303–306
  "raver's," 306, 306f
  workup for, 305, 305f, 305t
Hemoglobin
  altitude training to increase concentration of, 297
  of female athletes, 96
    prepubescent, 98, 98t
Hemolysis, footstrike (exertional), 295
  hematuria due to, 304
Hemorrhage, cerebral, 336, 336f, 337f
Hepatitis B virus (HBV) infections
  prevalence of, 247
  prevention guidelines for, 249–250
  testing for, 249
  transmission of, 248
Hepatomegaly, in infectious mononucleosis, 356
Hernias, 359f, 359–362
  acquired, 360
  epigastric, 360
  femoral, 360–361
  incisional (ventral), 359, 359f
  inguinal, 360, 376f
  Littre, 361
  "sports," 361
    weightlifting and, 625
  treatment of, 361–362
  umbilical, 360
Herniography, 361–362
Herodicus, 3
Herpes infections
  dermatologic, 231, 232f
  herpes simplex, 232t
  herpes zoster, 232t
High-performance liquid chromatography (HPLC)
  for drug testing, 162–163, 163t
  with ultraviolet visible-particle beam mass spectrometry, for drug testing, 166t
Hip
  abnormalities of, in athletes with cerebral palsy, 124
  apophysitis of. *See* Traction apophysitis, of hip and pelvis
  biomechanics of, 463–464
  labrum of, imaging of, 72–74, 74f
  "turning out," in dance, 471–472, 472f, 473f

Hip injuries. *See also specific disorders*
  avulsion, 418–420
  dislocations, football and, 484–485
  football and, 484–485
  running and, 550
  weightlifting and, 624–626
Hippocrates, 3
Hippocratic Oath, 8
Hip pointers, football and, 484
Hip spica, taping procedure for, 661, 662f
Hitchcock, Edward, 4
Hockey. *See* Field hockey; Ice hockey
Hogshead, Nancy, 273
Hormones. *See also specific hormones*
  peptide
    prohibited by major sports organizations, 183t
    testing for, 165, 167, 169
  renal tubules and, 300, 300t
Hospital notification, of endurance events, 42
Hughston, Jack C., 5
Hughston Orthopaedic Clinic, 6
Human chorionic gonadotropin (hCG)
  to circumvent drug testing, 173
  prohibition by major sports organizations, 183t
  testing for, 165, 167, 169
Human growth hormone (hGH)
  abuse of, 136–138
  prohibition by major sports organizations, 183t
  renal effects of, 301, 301t
  testing for, 165, 166t, 167, 169
Human immunodeficiency virus (HIV) infections
  exercise and, 248–249
  prevalence of, 247
  prevention guidelines for, 249–250
  testing for, 249
  transmission of, 247–248
Humeral ligament, transverse, ruptured, test for, 617–618
Humerus, contusions of, football and, 481
Hydrocele, 376f
  benign, 375
Hydrocortisone, for pulmonary emergencies, 27
Hypercoagulability, 297
Hyperexia, hematuria due to, 304
Hyperhydration, seizures due to, 268
Hypermobile joints, in female athletes, 99
Hyperthermia
  seizures due to, 268
  in wheelchair athletes, 122
Hypertrophic cardiomyopathy, athlete's heart versus, 257
Hyperventilation, seizures due to, 268
Hyphema, 30
Hypoglycemia, exercise-induced, 288, 289, 289t
Hypothermia, 311, 314–317
  in wheelchair athletes, 122
Hypoxia
  hematuria due to, 304
  seizures due to, 268

I

Ice, in PRICE concept of injury management, 666
Ice hockey, 499–511
  abdominal injuries in, 510
  axillary nerve injury in, 510
  boot-top tendon lacerations in, 510
  catastrophic injuries in, 324, 325, 328
  face injuries in, 508

head injuries in, 332t, 332–333, 333t, 334, 508
incidence of injury in, 499–500, 500t, 501t, 502
injury severity in, 502, 502t
injury sites in, 503, 504t, 505
injury types in, 502–503, 503t
mechanism of injury in, 505, 506t
medical risks in, 509–510
musculoskeletal injury in, 499
period of play and injury in, 507, 507t
player position and injury in, 505, 507, 507t
rule changes in, injury incidence and, 510
spine injury in, 508f, 508–509
Idiopathic thrombocytopenic purpura (ITP), 296
Iliac apophysis, 403–404
Iliac crest, avulsion fractures of, 419
Iliac spine, anterior, avulsion fractures of, 418
Iliotibial band (ITB) syndrome
  cycling and, 464f, 464–465
  rowing and, 539
  running and, 545–546
  volleyball and, 597
Imagery, healing, 197–198, 198f
Imaging, 57–84. *See also specific modalities*
  of bone, 61–67, 62f–67f
  bone scintigraphy for, 59
  of cartilage, 67–74, 68f–74f
  computed tomography for, 57–58, 58f
  conventional tomography for, 57
  for head injury assessment, 336–337, 347
  of ligaments and tendons, 74f–80f, 75–76, 78f–80f
  magnetic resonance imaging for, 59–61, 60f, 61f
  of muscles, 80f–83f, 80–84
  plain film radiography for, 57
  ultrasound for, 58
Impingement syndromes
  dance and, 474f, 474–475, 475f
  test for, 618
  weightlifting and, 618
Impotence, cycling and, 466
Incisional hernia, 359, 359f
Infectious mononucleosis (IM), 239–245
  clinical course of, 242–243, 245
  complications of, 243–244, 244t
  diagnosis of, 241f, 241–242, 242f, 242t
  epidemiology of, 239–240
  pathophysiology of, 239
  return-to-play decisions and, 245, 245t
  signs and symptoms of, 240f, 240–241
  splenic rupture in, 356, 356f
  treatment of, 243, 243t
Inferior iliac spine, anterior, avulsion of, 402
Informed consent, 50–51
  for drug testing, 157–158
Inguinal hernias, 360, 376f
Injuries. *See also specific injuries*
  career-ending, 202
  catastrophic. *See* Catastrophic injuries
  direct, 321
  fatal, 202
  "gender-appropriate" sports and, 218
  health-related values, attitudes, and beliefs and. *See* Sport, health-related values, attitudes, and beliefs in
  indirect, 321

Injuries (contd.)
  psychological impact of. See Psychological impact of injury and rehabilitation
Insulin
  dosage of, exercise of, 289
  injection site for, exercise of, 290
Intergluteal area, lichenification of, 236, 236f
Internal rewarming, for hypothermia, 316–317
International Amateur Wrestling Federation (FILA), 637
International Association of Sports Medicine (AIMS), 4
International Federation of Bodybuilding, 611
International Federation of Sports Medicine (FIMS), 4
International Olympic Committee (IOC)
  drugs prohibited by, 133, 134t, 176t–184t
  drug testing by, cost of, 173
  drug testing policy of, 154t
    penalties for positive tests and, 159–160
    procedures and, 164, 165, 167
    specimen collection procedures and, 159, 159t
  Medical Committee of, 5, 152
  methods prohibited by, 133, 134t
International Powerlifting Federation, 611
International World Games Association, 611
Interphalangeal joints, injuries of
  football and, 483–484
  proximal, avulsion, 414
Intersection syndrome
  golf and, 496–497
  weightlifting and, 622–623
Intertrigo, 233
Intestinal injuries, 357f, 357–358
Iron-deficiency anemia, 294–295
  in female athletes, 108, 294–295
Ischemia, hematuria due to, 304
Ischial avulsion fractures, 418–419, 419f
Ischial bursitis, weightlifting and, 625–626
Ischial tuberosity
  avulsion of, 402–403
  pain in, cycling and, 459
Iselin's disease, 409f, 409–410
Itraconazole (Sporanox), for tinea corporis/cruris, 232

J
Jackson, R. W., 5–6
Javelin, catastrophic injuries in, 329
Jaw-thrusts, 24, 26f
Jensen, Kurt Enemar, 151–152
Jerk test, 627
Jersey finger, football and, 484
Jock itch, cycling and, 461
Jogger's nipples, 235, 236f
Joint laxity, in female athletes, 99
Joubert, Laurent, 4
Joyner-Kersee, Jackie, 273
Judo, 525. See also Martial arts
Jumper's knee
  running and, 545
  volleyball and, 596

K
Karate, 525. See also Martial arts
Kehr's sign, 353
Ketoconazole, for tinea versicolor, 233
Kidneys. See also Renal entries; specific injuries
  injuries of, 28, 29f
  solitary, 307

Knee, meniscus of, imaging of, 69–70, 70f–72f
Knee effusions, recurrent, running and, 549
Knee goniometry, 456
Knee injuries. See also specific injuries
  avulsion, 420–423
  cycling and, 461–465
  dislocations, 29
    martial arts and, 528
  football and, 486–488
  lacrosse and, 517
  rowing and, 539–540
  skiing and, 555, 555t
  soccer and, 565
  swimming and, 574
  volleyball and, 596–597
  weightlifting and, 612–614, 613t, 614t, 626–628
Knowledge bases, associated with sports medicine
  clinical, 8
  nonclinical, 9
Koch, Bill, 273
Kung fu, 525. See also Martial arts

L
Lachman test, 627
Lacrosse, 513–519
  catastrophic injuries in, 325, 326, 329
  conditioning and injury prevention in, 519
  historical background of, 513
  injury demographics in, 513–515
    in men's lacrosse, 513–514
    in women's lacrosse, 514f, 514–515
  injury types in, 515, 515f
  mechanisms of injury in, 307
    ball-to-body contact and, 518
    body-to-body contact and, 516f, 516–517
    body-to-playing surface contact and, 518f, 518–519
    noncontact injuries and, 515–516
    stick-to-body contact and, 517f, 517–518
LaFontaine, Pat, 192
Laparoscopic surgery, for hernia repair, 362
Late asthmatic response, 274
Legal issues, 47–56
  athlete's responsibility to protect own health, 52–53
  concerning drug testing, 156–157, 173
  court cases
    Chuy v. Philadelphia eagles Football Club, 51
    Dailey v. Winston, 50
    Gardner v. Holifield, 49–50, 54
    Gathers v. Loyola-Marymount University, 51–52
    Gillespie v. Southern Utah State College, 53
    Hendy v. Losse, 54
    Knapp v. Northwestern University, 55
    Krueger v. San Francisco Forty Niners, 51
    Lillard v. State of Oregon, 52
    Mendenhall v. Oakland Raiders, 50
    Mikkelson v. Haslam, 51, 53
    Montalvo v. Radcliffe, 55
    Murphy v. Blum, 49
    Pahulu v. University of Kansas, 55–56
    Penny v. Sands, 52
    Rosensweig v. State, 49
    School Board of Nassau County, Florida v. Arline, 55

    Sorey v. Kellett, 54
    Speed v. State, 49
    Vernonia (Oregon) School District 47J v. Acton, 156–157
    Welch v. Dunsmuir Joint Union High School District, 50
  diagnosis and treatment of athletes, 49–50
  enforceability of liability waivers, 53
  immunity from malpractice liability, 53–54
  informed consent and medical clearance, 50–52
  judicial resolution of athletic participation disputes, 54–56
  physician-athlete relationship and, 47–48
  physician's general legal duty of care, 48
  preparticipation and screening examinations, 48–49
  prescription of drugs, 50
Legislation, on disability and sport, 223
Leg-length discrepancy, 455–456
  correcting for, 456
  measuring and evaluating leg length and, 455–456, 456f
Leg muscle strains, tennis and, 585
Lesser trochanter, avulsion of, 403, 419
Liability waivers, legal enforceability of, 53
Lichenification, of intergluteal area, 236, 236f
Life-threatening injuries, volleyball and, 600
Ligaments, imaging of, 74f–80f, 75–76, 78–80
Limb amputations, athletes with, 125–126
Linburg's syndrome, weightlifting and, 623
Linear force, head injury due to, 349, 349f
Lippman's test, 617
Liquid chromatography, with ultraviolet absorbance detection, for drug testing, 166t
Little League elbow, 398–399
Little League shoulder, 391, 399–400, 400f
Littre hernias, 361
Liver, fatty, in infectious mononucleosis, 244
Liver injuries, 28, 356f, 356–357, 357t
Logroll technique, 24, 25f
Lombardo, John, 6
Loss of consciousness (LOC), with head injury, 334
Low back injuries
  field hockey and, 520–521
  golf and, 494–495
Low back pain
  cycling and, 459
  rowing and, 533–537, 534f, 535t, 536t
  tennis and, 584–585
  weightlifting and, 616–617
Lower extremity injuries. See also specific injuries
  cycling and, 461–465
  field hockey and, 520
  football and, 488
  martial arts and, 528
  soccer and, 565
  traction apophysitis, 404–410
    at base of fifth metatarsal, 409f, 409–410
    calcaneal apophysitis, 408f, 408–409, 409f
    medial malleolus apophysitis, 407–408

    Sinding-Larsen-Johansson syndrome, 406–407, 407f
    tibial tubercle apophysitis, 404f, 404–406, 405f
Ludington's test, 617
Lumbar spine injuries
  avulsion, 417–418
  football and, 484
  golf and, 495
  musculoskeletal, in female athletes, 102–103
Lunate dislocations, football and, 483

M
Magnetic resonance arthrography
  of cartilage, 70–71, 72f, 73f
  of shoulder, 70–71, 72f, 73f
Magnetic resonance imaging (MRI), 59–61, 60f, 61f
  of bone, 63, 64f–67f, 64–65, 66–67
  of cartilage, 67–70, 68f–72f, 72–74, 74, 74f
  of hip, 72–74, 74f
  of ligaments and tendons, 74f–80f, 75–76, 78–80
  of muscles, 80, 80f–83f, 81–83
  of muscle strains, 363
  of physeal injuries, 387–388, 388f
  of stress fractures, 433–434
Major League Baseball (MLB)
  drugs prohibited by, 176t–184t
  drug testing policy of, 155t
Malleolus
  lateral, avulsion fractures of, 423
  medial
    apophysitis of, 407–408
    avulsion fractures of, 423
Mallet finger, with avulsion fracture of distal phalanx, 414–415
Malpractice liability, immunity from, 53–54
Mannitol, for head injuries, 27
Marathons, 541
Marijuana
  abuse of, 142–143
  prohibition by major sports organizations, 183t
  testing for, 169–170, 170t
Martial arts, 525–530
  disqualifying athletes from, 530
  extremity injuries in, 528
  head injuries in, 526–528
  injury trends in, 525–526, 526t, 527t
  medical disorders commonly seen in participants of, 530
  physician's responsibility at competitions, 530
  trunk injuries in, 528–529, 529f
  types of, 525
Martin, Casey, 224
Masking agents, to circumvent drug testing, 172, 173
Mass spectrometry (MS), for drug testing, 162, 163t
Medial collateral ligament (MCL)
  injuries of, football and, 486
  instability of, football and, 482
Medial synovial plica syndrome, swimming and, 574
Medial tennis elbow
  tennis and, 584
  weightlifting and, 620
Medical clearance, 51–52
Medical collateral ligament (MCL) injuries, swimming and, 574
Medical team, for endurance events, 41
Meningeal irritation, nuchal rigidity and, 281
Meniscal cysts, imaging of, 70, 71f
Meniscal injuries
  football and, 487
  weightlifting and, 627

Meniscotibial ligament sprain, weightlifting and, 626–627
Menstrual cycle
  amenorrhea and, 106–107
  effect on performance, 97
Mentally retarded athletes, competition for, 116
Mental training, 197–199
  biofeedback in, 198
  continued performance enhancement, 197
  for fear of reinjury, 199
  healing imagery in, 197–198, 198t
  for pain management, 198–199, 199t
  rehabilitation rehearsal in, 197
Mercuriali, Geronimo, 4
Mesenchymal syndrome, weightlifting and, 620
Mesocarb, abuse of, 143–144
Metabolic demands, in tennis, 580–581
Metacarpals
  avulsion injuries of, 413
  fractures of, football and, 482
Metacarpophalangeal joint
  dislocation of, football and, 483
  of thumb, avulsion injuries of, 413–414, 414f
Metatarsals
  fifth, proximal, fractures of, 425
  fractures of
    stress, treatment algorithm for, 435, 436f
    volleyball and, 595
Microhematuria, 303
Migraine headaches, 282t, 282–283
Millard, Keith, 192
Miller, Johnny, 495
Mind-body-spirit integration, by recreational sport, for people with disabilities, 226
Miserable malalignment syndrome, 100, 100f
Molluscum contagiosum, 233–234, 234f
Morgan, William G., 591
Morton's neuroma
  volleyball and, 595–596
  weightlifting and, 631
Motor firing patterns, in tennis, 581
Mottin, Yves, 152
Multiday races, 35
  medical coverage of, 44
Multiplanar tomography, of physeal injuries, 387
Multiple sclerosis, athletes with, 124–125
  classification of, 124
  exercise physiology and, 124–125
Murphy, Robert, 222
Muscle(s)
  anomalous, weightlifting and, 623
  imaging of, 80f–83f, 80–84
  oxidative capacity of, of female athletes, 96
Muscle function, 649–650
Muscular strength, of overhead thrower, 448t, 448–449
Musculoskeletal base, evaluation of, for tennis, 581–582
Musculoskeletal injuries, 28. See also specific injuries
  emergencies, 29–30
  in female athletes, 98–103
    arthritis and, 103
    of lumbar spine, 102–103
    rates of, 98–99
    risk factors for, 99–101
  muscle contusions, 362–363
  muscle strains
    abdominal, 362, 363
    football and, 485–486

Myofascial pain syndrome, weightlifting and, 619

N
Nails, blackened, weightlifting and, 631
Narcotics
  prohibited by major sports organizations, 180t–181t
  testing for, 164, 169
Nasal injuries, 31
National Association of Intercollegiate Athletics (NAIA), 6
National Athletic Trainers Association (NATA), 3, 5
National Basketball Association (NBA)
  drugs prohibited by, 176t–184t
  drug testing policy of, 153, 154t
National Collegiate Athletic Association (NCAA), 6
  drugs prohibited by, 176t–184t
  drug testing policy of, 153, 155t, 156
  Injury Surveillance System (ISS) of, 332, 333, 638
National Football League (NFL), drug testing policy of, 153, 154t
National Junior College Athletic Association (NJCAA), 6
National Wheelchair Athletic Association (NWAA), 116
National Wheelchair Basketball Association, 115
Neck injuries. See also Cervical spine injuries
  cycling and, 457
  ice hockey, 505
  lacrosse, 518
  soccer and, 564
  volleyball and, 600
  wrestling and, 639, 639f
Neer test, 597, 618
Nerve entrapment syndromes. See also specific syndromes
  in wheelchair athletes, 121–122
Neurologic disorders. See also specific injuries
  in infectious mononucleosis, 244
Neuromuscular control, overhead throw and, 449f, 449–450
Neuropsychological testing, following head injury, 346–347
Nicklaus, Jack, 494–495
Nitrogen dioxide toxicity, in ice arenas, 509–510
Nonarticular osteochondritis. See Traction apophysitis
Nonorganic headaches, 284
Nonsteroidal anti-inflammatory drugs (NSAIDs), renal effects of, 301, 301t
Nordic skiing races, medical coverage for, 44
Nuchal rigidity, 281

O
Oath of Hippocrates, 8
Ober's test, 625
Obturator neuropathy, 366–367
Ocular injuries, 30
O'Donoghue, Don, 5
Olecranon
  apophysitis of, 399
  avulsion fractures of, 416
Olecranon bursitis, volleyball and, 599
Olecranon-triceps tendinitis, weightlifting and, 620
Olinger, Ford, 224
Olympiad, 3
Olympic Games. See also International Olympic Committee

(IOC); United States Olympic Committee (USOC)
  drug testing at, 152
  female participation in, 93, 94
  physical examination requirement of, 4
  rowing in, 531
  team physicians and, 6
  weightlifting in, 609
  wrestling in, 637
Olympic weightlifting, 609, 610, 610f, 611. See also Weightlifting
On-the-field emergencies, 23–30
  cardiovascular, 27
  eye, ear, nose, and throat, 30
  gastrointestinal, 28
  genitourinary, 29
  head injuries, 23–24, 24f–26f, 26–27
  kidney injuries, 28, 29f
  liver injuries, 28
  muscle injuries, 28
  musculoskeletal, 29–30
  pancreatic injuries, 28–29
  pulmonary, 27–28
  splenic, 28
Oral contraceptives, amenorrhea and, 107
Osgood-Schlatter's lesion (OSL), 404f, 404–406, 405f
  cycling and, 463
Osteitis, of clavicle, weightlifting and, 618
Osteitis pubis, 364–367, 365f, 366f
  football and, 485
  rehabilitation following, 368, 369t
Osteochondritis. See Traction apophysitis
Osteochondritis dissecans (OCD)
  imaging of, 69, 69f
  volleyball and, 597
Osteomyelitis, of pubic symphysis, football and, 485
Osteopathic Oath, 8
Osteopenia, in female athletes, 107–108
Osteoporosis, in female athletes, 107–108
Os trigonum fractures, volleyball and, 594
Otitis externa, swimming and, 574
Otolaryngologic disorders, in infectious mononucleosis, 244
Overhead throw, 441–442
  biomechanics of, 442f, 442–446, 443f
    of acceleration phase, 444–445
    of cocking phase, 443–444, 444t
    of deceleration/follow-through phase, 445–446
    of windup phase, 442–443, 443f
  elbow and, 447
  muscular strength and performance and, 448t, 448–449
  neuromuscular control and, 449f, 449–450
  rehabilitation following injuries and, 450, 450t
  shoulder and, 446f, 446–447
    laxity of, 447
Over-the-counter (OTC) medications, containing prohibited substances, 179t–180t
Overtraining, swimming and, 574–575

P
Pain. See also specific sites
  "gender-appropriate" sports and, 218
  health-related values, attitudes, and beliefs and. See Sport, health-related values, attitudes, and beliefs in
  injury-related, 192–193

social structures of sport and, 207–208
  sociology of sport and, 205–207
  tolerance of, 201
Pain management, mental training for, 198–199, 199t
Pancreatic injuries, 28–29, 358, 358f
Paralympics, 116, 221, 223
  weightlifting in, 611, 631–632
Paralympics for Persons with Mental Handicaps, 223
Parameniscal cysts, imaging of, 70, 72f
Paraplegia, 117. See also Wheelchair athletes
Paraumbilical hernia, 360
Parrot beak tears, of meniscus, imaging of, 70, 71f
Pars defects, of lumbar spine, in female athletes, 103
Partial seizures, 266
Participation disputes, judicial resolution of, 54–56
Passive rewarming, for hypothermia, 316
Patella
  avulsion fractures of, 422–423
  subluxation of, volleyball and, 596–597
Patellar tendinitis
  running and, 545
  volleyball and, 596
Patellar tendinosis, cycling and, 463, 463f
Patellofemoral injuries
  football and, 487–488
  rowing and, 539
  swimming and, 574
  volleyball and, 596
Patellofemoral ligament, inflammation of, cycling and, 464
Patellofemoral pain syndrome (PFPS), in female athletes, 101
Patellofemoral stress syndrome (PTSS), running and, 543, 544–545
Pectineus muscle, avulsion of, weightlifting and, 625
Pelvic injuries
  apophysitis. See Traction apophysitis, of hip and pelvis
  avulsion, 418–420
  football and, 484–485
  soccer and, 565
  weightlifting and, 624–626
Penile injuries, 375–376
Peptide hormones
  prohibited by major sports organizations, 183t
  testing for, 165, 167, 169
Perilunate dislocations, football and, 483
Perineal injuries, in females, 378–379, 379t
Perineal nodules, subcutaneous, in bicyclists, 378, 378f, 459
Peroneal tendon injuries, weightlifting and, 630
Pes anserine tendinitis, cycling and, 464, 464f
Petit mal seizures, 266
Phalen's sign, 623
Phelps, Winthrop, 5
Physeal injuries, 381–393
  anatomy and, 381–383, 382f
  biomechanics and, 383
  classification of, 383–386, 384f–385f
  embryology and, 381, 382f
  epidemiology of, 386–387
  evaluation of, 387–389, 388f
  microscopic analysis of, 386, 386f
  prognosis of, 390

Physeal injuries (contd.)
    treatment of
        of anterior cruciate ligament injury in skeletally immature athletes, 391–392
        of physeal arrest, 390–391
        principles of, 389–390
        referral to orthopedist for, 392–393
        of stress-related and apophyseal injuries, 391
Physical examination, preparticipation. See Preparticipation physical examination (PPE)
Physically challenged athletes, 35, 115–127. See also Wheelchair athletes
    with arthritis, 126
    athletes with
        classification of, 125
        prevention and treatment of injuries in, 125–126
    blind, 116, 125
        snow skiing for, 126
    with cerebral palsy, 116, 123–124
        classification of, 123
        exercise physiology and, 123–124
        prevention and treatment of injuries in, 124
    deaf, 116, 126
        World Games for the Deaf and, 115
    historical background of, 115–117
    with limb amputations, 125–126
        classification of, 125
        prevention and treatment of injuries in, 125–126
    medical coverage for, 44–45
    with multiple sclerosis, 124–125
        classification of, 124
        exercise physiology and, 124–125
    with polio/postpolio syndrome, 125
    preparticipation physical examination for, 117
    snow skiing for, 126
    sports organizations for, 127
    World T.E.A.M. sports for, 126–127
Physicians
    legal duty of care of, 48
    physician-athlete relationship and, 47–48
    drug testing and, 160
    team. See Team physicians
Piriformis injuries
    running and, 550
    weightlifting and, 626
Pitching. See Overhead throw
Pityriasis versicolor, 232f, 232t, 232–233, 233f
Pivot shift test, 627
Plain film radiography, 57
    of bone, 61–62, 63f
Planes of motion, 649, 650f, 650t
Plantar fascia, rupture of, weightlifting and, 630–631
Plantar fasciitis
    running and, 548–549
    tennis and, 586–587
    volleyball and, 595
    weightlifting and, 630–631
Plantar neuromas
    volleyball and, 595–596
    weightlifting and, 631
Plantar warts, 232t
Plasma volume, of female athletes, 96
Playing surfaces
    football injuries and, 478–479
    lacrosse injuries and, 518f, 518–519
Plica, cycling and, 464
Pneumothorax, 27
Pole vault, catastrophic injuries in, 328–329

Polio, athletes with, 125
"Popeye syndrome," weightlifting and, 621
Postconcussive syndrome, 341–342, 342t
Posterior cruciate ligament (PCL) injuries
    football and, 487
    tears, imaging of, 78, 78f, 79f
Posterior tennis elbow, weightlifting and, 620
Postexercise proteinuria (PEP), 302–303, 303f
Postpolio syndrome, athletes with, 125
Posttraumatic headaches, 283
Postural sway, for head injury assessment, 347
Powerlifting, 609, 610, 610f. See also Weightlifting
Prednisone, for infectious mononucleosis, 243
Prehabilitation, for tennis, 588
Preparticipation physical examination (PPE), 11–21
    for disabled athletes, 117
    for endurance events, 38
    frequency of, 12
    guidelines for participation and, 18t–20t
    history form for, 13, 14f–16f
    laboratory tests in, 13
    legal issues concerning, 48–49
    musculoskeletal, 17f, 21
    Olympic Games requirement for, 4
    for physically challenged athletes, 117
Prepatellar bursitis, cycling and, 464
Pressure sores, in wheelchair athletes, 121
PRICE concept of injury management, 665–667
Principle-centered rehabilitation. See Rehabilitation, principle-centered
Probenecid, to circumvent drug testing, 173
Problem solving approaches, 7–8
Professional Golf Association (PGA), Martin's participation in, 224
Pronation, 650–653
Pronator syndrome, weightlifting and, 621–622
Prostate injuries, 378
Prostatitis, cycling and, 466
Protection, in PRICE concept of injury management, 665
Protective equipment. See also Helmets
    for football, 480
Proteinuria, postexercise, 302–303, 303f
Pseudoanemia, athletic, 294
Pseudoephedrine, abuse of, 140
Psychological impact of injury and rehabilitation, 191–202
    assessment of, 194t, 194–195
    compliance and, 201
    eating disorders and, 201–202
    pain tolerance and, 201
    psychological antecedents to injury and, 200, 200f
    psychological response and, 192–194
        affective cycle of injury and, 193–194
        pain and, 192–193
        stresses of injury and, 192, 192t
    psychological treatment and, 195–199
        education as, 195–196
        goal setting for, 196
        mental training for, 197–199

social support for, 196–197
referral process and, 199–200, 200t
with severe injury, 202
substance abuse and, 201
Pudendal neuropathy
    in bicyclists, 376
    cycling and, 466
Puffer, Jim, 6
Pulmonary emergencies, 27–28
Punch-drunk syndrome, 527–528
Pupillary assessment, in head injury, 339–340

Q
Quadri, Jean-Louis, 152
Quadriceps contusions, football and, 485
Quadriceps tendinosis, cycling and, 463
Quadriceps tendon rupture, weightlifting and, 628
Quadriplegia, 117. See also Wheelchair athletes
Quigley, Thomas "Bart," 5

R
Races. See Endurance events; Marathons
Radial nerve, entrapment of, weightlifting and, 621
Radial stress injuries, distal, 391
Radiation, heat exchange by, 311–312
Radiography, plain film, 57
    of bone, 61–62, 63f
Radioimmunoassay (RIA), for drug testing, 161, 162t
Ramazzini, Bernardino, 4
"Raver's hematuria," 306, 306f
Rebagliati, Ross, 160
Record keeping, medical, for endurance events, 41, 41t
Recreational sport, for people with disabilities, 225–226
Rectus femoris muscle strain, weightlifting and, 626
Rectus sheath hematomas (RSHs), 363–364
Red blood cell mass, of female athletes, prepubescent, 98, 98t
Refractory period, in asthma, 274
Rehabilitation
    for abdominal injuries, 367–368, 368f, 369t, 370f, 370–371, 371f
    of overhead athlete, 450, 450t
    principle-centered, 645–652
        approach of, 645–646
        compensations and, 648–649, 649t
        environment for, 647–648
        functional evaluation in, 646–647, 647f–649f
        functional feeding and, 653
        muscle function and, 649–650
        planes of motion and, 649, 650f, 650t
        pronation and supination and, 650–653
        strategy for, 652–653
    psychological impact of. See Psychological impact of injury and rehabilitation
    for tennis injuries, principles of, 587
    for weightlifting injuries, 615–616
Rehabilitation Act (1973), 54, 223
Rehabilitation rehearsal, 197
Reinjury, fear of, mental training for, 199
Renal blood flow (RBF), exercise and, 299, 300t
Renal disorders
    acute renal failure, 306, 306f

hematuria, 303t, 303–306, 305f, 305t
postexercise proteinuria, 302–303, 303f
traumatic, 306–307
Renal function, 299–307
    drugs and, 301t, 301–302
    hydration and, 301
    physiology of, 299–300, 300t
    solitary kidney and, 307
Renal trauma, 306–307
    hematuria due to, 304
Renal tubule function, 300, 300t
Renin-angiotensin system (RAS), postexercise proteinuria and, 302
Resistive training, for tennis, 588
Rest, in PRICE concept of injury management, 665–666
Retinopathy, in diabetes mellitus, exercise and, 290–291
Return to play
    following head injury, 343, 344t–345t, 345–346
    following stress fractures, 437
    with infectious mononucleosis, 245, 245t
Rewarming
    for frostbite, 314
    for hypothermia, 316–317
Rib injuries
    lacrosse and, 517
    rowing and, 537f, 537–538, 538f
    weightlifting and, 617
Rice, Jerry, 192
Rotational force, head injury due to, 349, 349f
Rotator cuff injuries
    football and, 480–481
    golf and, 495
    volleyball and, 597–598
Rotator cuff tendinitis, tennis and, 583
Rowing, 531–540
    back injuries in, 533–537, 534f, 535t, 536t
    biomechanics of, 531–532, 532f–534f
    dermatologic disorders and, 540
    elbow and wrist injuries in, 539, 539f
    exercise-induced bronchospasm and, 540
    knee injuries in, 539–540
    rib and thorax injuries in, 537f, 537–538, 538f
    shoulder and upper extremity injuries in, 538–539
Running, 541–552. See also Endurance events; Marathons
    accessory navicular injuries and, 550–551
    Achilles tendon and calf injuries and, 547–548
    anatomic location and types of injuries in, 543–544
    calluses and, 235f
    etiology of injuries in, 542–543
    forefoot pain and, chronic, 550
    groin pain and, 550
    Haglund's deformity and, 550
    hip pain, posterior thigh pain, and sciatica and, 550
    iliotibial band syndrome and, 545–546
    jogger's nipples and, 235, 236f
    knee effusions and, recurrent, 549
    lichenification of intergluteal area and, 236, 236f
    medial arch pain and, 549–550
    medial tibial stress syndrome, shin pain, and tibial stress fracture and, 544, 546–547
    patellar tendinitis and, 545

patellofemoral stress syndrome and, 543, 544–545
plantar fasciitis and, 548–549
tarsal tunnel syndrome and, 551
training schedule for, 541–542
treatment of running injuries and, 551

S

Saddle sores, cycling and, 459–460
Safety equipment, for cyclists, 453–454
Sag test, 627
Saphenous nerve, entrapment of, weightlifting and, 628
Scaphoid fractures
 football and, 483
 weightlifting and, 621
Scapula, avulsion fractures of, 417, 417t
Scapula syndrome, cycling and, 457–458
Scheduling, of drug testing, 158
Sciatica, running and, 550
Scoliosis, adolescent, in female athletes, 103
Screening examinations, legal issues concerning, 48–49
Scrotal injuries
 evaluation of, 375, 376f
 of skin, 373–374
Seagasser's sign, 353
Seborrheic dermatitis, 232t
Second impact syndrome (SIS), 283, 342
Segond fractures, 420f, 420–421
 imaging of, 63–64, 64f
Seizures, 265–266. See also Epilepsy
 definition of, 265
 generalized, 266
 with head injury, 341
 partial, 266
 revised classification of, 266
 treatment of, 266–267
Selenium sulfite, for tinea versicolor, 233
Sesamoid fractures, football and, 488
Sesamoiditis
 volleyball and, 596
 weightlifting and, 631
Shin splints, 544, 546–547
 volleyball and, 597
Shivering, thermogenic, 315
Shoes. See Footwear
Shorter, Frank, 541
Shot put, catastrophic injuries in, 329
Shoulder
 biomechanics of, in tennis, 579–580
 labrum of, imaging of, 70–72, 72f, 73f
 laxity of
  in female athletes, 102
  in overhead throwers, 447
 Little League, 391, 399–400, 400f
 of overhead thrower, 446f, 446–447
 swimmer's, 571
Shoulder girdle injuries, lacrosse and, 516, 516f
Shoulder impingement syndrome, volleyball and, 597–598
Shoulder injuries. See also specific injuries
 avulsions, 416–417
 dislocations, 29–30
  volleyball and, 598
 football and, 480–482
 golf and, 495
 ice hockey and, 505
 lacrosse and, 517
 rowing and, 538–539
 soccer and, 564
 subluxation, volleyball and, 598
 swimming and, 571–572
 volleyball and, 597–599, 598f

weightlifting and, 617–619
 in wheelchair athletes, 121
Shoulder pain, in female athletes, 102
Shoulder spica, taping procedure for, 662–663, 663f
Sickle-cell trait (SCT), 295–296
Simpson, Tommy, 152
Sinding-Larsen-Johansson syndrome (SLJS), 406–407, 407f
Single photon emission computed tomography (SPECT), of physeal injuries, 388–389
Ski boots, 558
 frostbite and, 314, 314f
Skiing. See Snow skiing; Water-skiing
Skill level, skiing injuries and, 557
Skin. See Dermatologic problems; specific dermatologic problems
Ski poles, 558
Skull fractures, 341
 basilar, 340, 340f, 340t, 341f
Sliding inguinal hernia, 360
"Slipping rib syndrome," weightlifting and, 617
Smith, Edwin, 3
Smokeless tobacco, abuse of, 143
"Snapping scapula," weightlifting and, 618
Snow skiing, 553–559
 catastrophic injuries in, 324, 325
 incidence of injuries in, 553–554
 injury prevention in, 557–559
 injury trends in, 554t, 555, 555t
 mechanisms of injury in, 555–557, 556f
 Nordic skiing races and, medical coverage for, 44
 for physically challenged athletes, 126
 risk factors for injury and, 557
Soccer, 563–567
 catastrophic injuries in, 327, 329
 head injuries in, 332, 332t, 333, 333t, 348–349, 349f, 564
 injury trends in, 566
 leg, knee, ankle, and foot injuries in, 565
 neck injuries in, 564
 pelvic injuries in, 565
 prevention of injuries in, 566–567
 shoulder, arm, wrist, and hand injuries in, 564
 trunk and back injuries in, 564–565
Social structures of sport, pain and injury and, 207–208
Social support, 196–197
Sociology of sport, pain and injury in, 205–207
Sodium, urinary excretion of, exercise and, 300
Softball
 catastrophic injuries in, 325–326, 329
 head injuries in, 332t, 333t
Soft tissue injuries
 lacrosse and, 518
 in wheelchair athletes, 121
Solar plexus, blows to, martial arts and, 528
Somatropin, testing for, 167
Special Olympics International, 116, 223
Spectator medical care, 35
Speed training, for tennis, 588
Spermatocele, 376f
Spine injuries
 cervical
  swimming and, 573
  weightlifting and, 617
 ice hockey and, 508f, 508–509
 thoracic, swimming and, 573
Splenectomy, for infectious mononucleosis, 244

Splenic injuries, 28, 353–354, 354f–356f, 354t–356t, 356
 rupture, in infectious mononucleosis, 243–244
Splenomegaly, in infectious mononucleosis, 356, 356f
Spondylolisthesis, weightlifting and, 617
Spondylolysis
 football and, 484
 of lumbar spine, in female athletes, 102–103
 rowing and, 536
 volleyball and, 600
 weightlifting and, 616
Sport
 health-related values, attitudes, and beliefs in, 208–212
  interview and ethnographic research on, 210–211
  recommendations and, 212–213
  sport ethic and, 208–209
  studies of athletic trainers and, 211–212
  surveys of coaches, students, and student athletes and, 209–210
 social structures of, 207–208
 sociology of, 205–207
 therapeutic value of, for people with disabilities, 226
Sport ethic, 208–209
 "gender-appropriate" sports and, 217–218
Sports anemia, 294
"Sports hernias," 361, 625
Sports medicine, content of, 7
Sports organizations. See also specific organizations
 for physically challenged athletes, 127
Sprint/interval training, for tennis, 588
Stabilization exercises, following abdominal injuries, 370f
Steadman, J. Richard, 193
Stener lesions, imaging of, 63, 64, 65f
Stenosing tenosynovitis
 golf and, 496
 weightlifting and, 622
Sternoclavicular dislocations, football and, 481
Steroids. See Anabolic-androgenic steroids (AASs); Corticosteroids
Stevens, Mal, 5
Stimulants
 prohibited by major sports organizations, 176t–179t
 testing for, 164, 168–169
Stinton, Bill, 5
Stoke-Mandeville wheelchair games, 115
Stomach injuries, 357
Street drugs, prohibition by major sports organizations, 184t
Strength, of female athletes, 95
 prepubescent, 98, 98t
Strength training, in children, 90
Stress, of injury, 192, 192t
Stress fractures, 429–438
 in athletes with cerebral palsy, 124
 cause of, 430f, 430–432
 confirmatory studies for, 433t, 433–434
 diagnosis of, 432–433
 epidemiology of, 429–430, 430t
 in female athletes, 101–102
 football and, 489
 future research directions for, 438
 of hip, weightlifting and, 625
 historical background of, 429
 prevention of, 437–438
 return to sport following, 437

of ribs
  rowing and, 537f, 537–538, 538f
  weightlifting and, 617
 rupture of, 595
 tibial, running and, 547
 treatment of, 434–437, 435f–437f
 volleyball and, 597
Stress urinary incontinence, in female athletes, 108–109
Students, health-related values, attitudes, and beliefs of, 209–210
Subdural hematomas, 335, 335f, 336–337
Substance abuse. See Drug abuse; Drug testing
Subungual hematomas, weightlifting and, 631
Sudden death, preperformance physical examination and, 12–13
Sunburn, 234, 234f
Superior iliac spine, anterior, avulsion of, 402
Supination, 650–653
Suprascapular neuropathy, volleyball and, 598f, 598–599
Surfer's nodules, 235–236
Surveillance, of endurance events, 42
Swimmer's ear, 574
Swimmer's shoulder, 571
Swimming, 571–575
 ankle injuries in, 574
 back injuries in, 572–573
 catastrophic injuries in, 324, 325, 328, 329
 elbow injuries in, 572
 foot injuries in, 574
 hand injuries in, 572
 knee injuries in, 574
 medical coverage for races and, 43–44
 medical problems associated with, 574–575
 shoulder injuries in, 571–572
Sympathomimetic amines
 abuse of, 139t, 139–140
 prohibited by major sports organizations, 182t
 testing for, 164

T

Tackling techniques, football injuries and, 479–480
Tae kwon do, 525. See also Martial arts
Talon noir, 235
Talus, lateral process of, avulsion fractures of, 424–425
Tandem mass spectrometry (MS/MS), for drug testing, 163, 163t, 166t
Taping procedures, 653–663
 Achilles tendon, 659, 659f
 for arch
  longitudinal, 656f, 658
  modified "low-dye," 657f–658f, 658
 for hip spica, 661, 662f
 preventive, 654f–655f, 655, 657
 for shoulder spica, 662–663, 663f
 thumb, 658, 661, 661f
 turf toe, 658, 660f
 wrist, 661, 662f
Tarsal tunnel syndrome
 running and, 551
 weightlifting and, 631
Tarsometatarsal joint, strain or sprain of, weightlifting and, 631
Tarsonavicular fractures
 avulsion, 425
 treatment algorithm for, 435, 437f
Team physicians, 3–10
 ancient, 3–4
 issues confronting, 7–9
  associated clinical knowledge bases, 8

Team physicians (contd.)
  associated nonclinical knowledge bases, 9
  content of sports medicine, 7
  ethical, 8
  problem solving approach, 7–8
  modern, 6–7
  needs of, 9
  in recent past, 4–6
  roles of, 9–10
Teeth, fractures and avulsions of, 31
Temperature, endurance events and, 36
Tendinopathy, imaging in, 75f–77f, 75–76
Tendons, imaging of, 74f–80f, 75–76, 78–80
Tennis, 577–588
  biomechanics of, 579–580
  catastrophic injuries in, 326
  conditioning for, 587–588
  injury analysis in, 577–579, 578t, 579f
  injury evaluation in, 582–587
    for Achilles tendinitis, 585–586
    for ankle sprains, 586
    for lateral epicondylitis, 583–584
    for leg muscle strains, 585
    for low back and trunk pain, 584–585
    for medial epicondylitis, 584
    for plantar fasciitis, 586–587
    process of, 582f, 582–583
    for rotator cuff tendinitis, 583
  injury prevention strategies for, 586–587
  macrotrauma injuries in, 577, 579f
  microtrauma injuries in, 577–578, 579f
    model for causation of, 578–579, 580f
  pathology in, 578
  musculoskeletal base evaluation and, 581–582
  physiology and, 580–581
  rehabilitation principles for injuries in, 587
Tennis elbow
  tennis and, 583–584
  weightlifting and, 620
"Tennis leg," 585
Tennis toe, 235
Tension headaches, 283–284
Tension pneumothorax, 27
Terfenadine, for tinea corporis/cruris, 232
Testicles, "accessory," 378, 378f, 459
Testicular injuries, 29, 373, 374f, 374–375
  contusions, 374
  dislocation, 375
  highball syndrome, 375
  lacrosse and, 518
  rupture/lacerations, 374
  soccer and, 565
  torsion, 374f, 374–375
Testicular nip, 313
Testicular tumors, 376f
  carcinomas, 375
Thermogenic shivering, 315
Thermoregulation, 311, 312
  in female athletes, 97
  prepubescent, 98, 98t
  in wheelchair athletes, 122
Thigh injuries
  cycling and, 459
  football and, 485–486
  soccer and, 565
  weightlifting and, 624–625, 626
Thigh pain, posterior, running and, 550
Thin-layer chromatography (TLC), for drug testing, 161, 162t

Thoracic outlet syndrome, weightlifting and, 618–619
Thorndike, Angus, 5
Throat injuries, lacrosse and, 518
Thrombocytopenic purpura, idiopathic, 296
Throwing, overhead. See Overhead throw
Thumb
  metacarpophalangeal joint of, avulsion injuries of, 413–414, 414f
  taping procedure for, 658, 661, 661f
Tibia fractures, skiing and, 554t, 555
Tibialis anterior tendinosis, cycling and, 465
Tibial spine, avulsion fractures of, 421
Tibial stress fractures, running and, 547
Tibial stress syndrome, medial
  running and, 544, 546–547
  volleyball and, 597
Tibial tendinitis, posterior, weightlifting and, 630
Tibial torsion, external, rowing and, 539
Tibial tubercle
  apophysitis of, 404f, 404–406, 405f
  avulsion fractures of, 421f, 421–422, 422f
Tinea infections, 231–233, 232f, 233f
  tinea corporis, 232, 232t
  tinea cruris, 232
  tinea pedis, 231–232, 232t
  tinea versicolor, 232f, 232t, 232–233, 233f
Tinel's sign, 623
Tobacco, smokeless, abuse of, 143
Tonic-clonic convulsions, 265
Tonic convulsions, 265
Track, catastrophic injuries in, 326, 328–329
Track bite, in rowers, 540
Traction apophysitis, 397–410
  epidemiology of, 397
  of hip and pelvis, 400–404, 401f, 401t
    avulsion of anterior inferior iliac spine, 402
    avulsion of anterior superior iliac spine, 402
    avulsion of greater trochanter, 403
    avulsion of ischial tuberosity, 402–403
    avulsion of lesser trochanter, 403
    of iliac apophysis, 403–404
  of lower extremity, 404–410
    at base of fifth metatarsal, 409f, 409–410
    calcaneal apophysitis, 408f, 408–409, 409f
    medial malleolus apophysitis, 407–408
    Sinding-Larsen-Johansson syndrome, 406–407, 407f
    tibial tubercle apophysitis, 404f, 404–406, 405f
  predisposing factors for, 397–398, 398t
  of upper extremity, 398–400
    acromial apophysitis, 400
    Little League shoulder, 399–400, 400f
    medial epicondylar apophysitis, 398–399
    olecranon apophysitis, 399
Trainers, health-related values, attitudes, and beliefs of, 211–212
Training
  excessive, traction apophysitis due to, 397

following abdominal injuries, 368, 368f
mental. See Mental training
schedule for, of runners, 541–542
for tennis, 587–588
with weights, 610
Transportation, of endurance events, 42
Triathlons, 35
  medical coverage of, 43
Triceps rupture, weightlifting and, 620
Triceps tendinitis
  volleyball and, 599
  weightlifting and, 620
Triquetrum, avulsion injuries of, 415
Trunk, biomechanics of, in tennis, 580
Trunk injuries. See also specific injuries
  soccer and, 564–565
  tennis and, 584–585
Trusses, for hernias, 362
Tumor-related headaches, 281–282
Turf toe
  football and, 488
  taping procedure for, 658, 660f
Type 1 diabetes, 287–291, 288t
  exercise in
    benefits of, 287, 288t
    contraindications for, 290–291
    guidelines for, 287–290

U
Ulnar artery, thrombosis or aneurysm of, weightlifting and, 623
Ulnar carpal ligament (UCL), injury of, football and, 483
Ulnar collateral ligament, imaging of, 79–80, 80f
Ulnar fractures, weightlifting and, 621
Ulnar neuropathy
  cycling and, 458f, 458–459
  in wheelchair athletes, 122
Ulnar styloid, avulsion injuries of, 415
Ultramarathon races, 35
  medical coverage of, 44
Ultrasound
  of ligaments and tendons, 76
  of muscles, 80
  with splenic injuries, 354, 354t
Umbilical hernia, 360
U.S. Association for Blind Athletes, 116
United States Olympic Committee (USOC), drugs prohibited by, 176t–184t
Upper extremity injuries. See also specific injuries
  of forearm
    football and, 482
    fractures, lacrosse and, 517, 517f
    martial arts and, 528
    rowing and, 538
    soccer and, 564
  traction apophysitis, 398–400
    acromial apophysitis, 400
    Little League shoulder, 399–400, 400f
    medial epicondylar apophysitis, 398–399
    olecranon apophysitis, 399
Urethral injuries, 376–378
  anterior, 376–377, 377f
  mechanical urethritis, 377–378
  posterior, 377, 377f
Urinary catheterization, to circumvent drug testing, 171
Urinary problems
  cycling and, 466
  stress incontinence, in female athletes, 108–109

urinary stasis, in wheelchair athletes, 122–123
Urine
  dilution of, to circumvent drug testing, 172
  output of, exercise and, 300
  substitution of, to circumvent drug testing, 171
Urticaria, cholinergic, 261–262
  diagnosis of, 263
  epidemiology of, 263
  pathophysiology of, 263
  prevention of, 264
  treatment of, 264
USA Powerlifting, 611
USA Wrestling, 637

V
Vaginal infections, crotch dermatitis and, 461
Vaginal water injection injuries, 379, 379t
Valacyclovir (Valtrex), for herpes infections, 232t
  dermatologic, 231
Values, health-related. See Sport, health-related values, attitudes, and beliefs in
Van Dyken, Amy, 273
Vasopressin, renal function and, 300, 300t
Ventral hernia, 359, 359f
Viet Nam Challenge, 127
Volleyball, 591–600
  ankle and foot injuries in, 593–596
  back injuries in, 600
  basic skills for, 591, 592f
  catastrophic injuries in, 329
  elbow injuries in, 599
  hand and wrist injuries in, 599–600
  head injuries in, 332, 332t
  injury incidence in, 591–593, 593t
  knee and leg injuries in, 596–597
  life-threatening injuries in, 600
  shoulder injuries in, 597–599, 598f
  skin injuries in, 600
  "Volleyball shoulder," 598f, 598–599
Volunteer education, of endurance events, 42
von Willebrand's disease (VWD), 296
Voy, Bob, 6

W
Warm-up exercises, in asthma, 275–276
Warm water immersion, for hypothermia, 316
Warts, 233–234
  common, 232t
  plantar, 232t
"Water-loading," to circumvent drug testing, 172
Water polo, catastrophic injuries in, 323–324
Water-skiing, 603–607
  classification of injuries in, 605t, 605–607, 606f
  epidemiology of injuries in, 604, 604t
  factors contributing to injuries in, 604–605
  safety guidelines for, 607, 607t
  tournament skiing injuries in, 607
Water sports. See also specific sports
  with epilepsy, 268–269, 269t
Watkins, A. L., 5
Weight control, "gender-appropriate" sports and, 217–218
Weight gain, blood glucose control and, in diabetes mellitus, 290
Weightlifting, 609–632
  anabolic steroid use in, 614, 616
  chest and back injuries in, 616–617

elbow injuries in, 619–621
foot and ankle injuries in, 628–632
forearm, wrist, and hand injuries in, 621–624
knee injuries in, 612–614, 613t, 614t, 626–628
pelvis, hip, and thigh injuries in, 624–626
prevention of injuries in, 615
rehabilitation for injuries in, 615–616
shoulder injuries in, 617–619
types of, 609, 610f
Weight loss
　recommendations for, 189
　in wrestlers, 639–641

Weight training, 610
Wendell, Susan, 224, 225
Wheelchair athletes, 117–123
　classification of, 117–118, 118f, 119t
　competitions for, 115–116
　exercise physiology and, 118–120
　prevention and treatment of injuries in, 120–123
Wheelchair Sports USA, 116
Wills, Helen, 93
Winter sports. *See also specific sports*
　catastrophic injuries in, 324–325, 325t, 326t
Woodson, Rod, 192
Work/rest intervals, in tennis, 581

World Games for the Deaf, 115, 223
World T.E.A.M. sports, 126–127
"Wrestler's ear," 638f, 638–639
Wrestling, 637–641
　catastrophic injuries in, 324, 325, 325t, 328
　head injuries in, 332, 333t
　injuries in, 637–639, 638f, 639f
　types of, 637
　weight loss in wrestlers and, 639–641
"Wringing out," 571
Wrist
　biomechanics of, in tennis, 580
　taping procedure for, 661, 662f

Wrist injuries
　avulsion, 415
　football and, 482–484
　golf and, 496–497
　rowing and, 539
　soccer and, 564
　volleyball and, 599–600

X

Xerosis, 232t

Y

Yergason test, 617

Z

Zambonis, nitrogen dioxide emissions of, 509–510